VOLUME 2

Comprehensive Management of Head AND Neck TUMORS

EDITORS

Stanley E. Thawley, M.D.

William R. Panje, M.D.

ASSOCIATE EDITORS

John G. Batsakis, M.D.

Robert D. Lindberg, M.D.

1987

W. B. SAUNDERS COMPANY

Philadephia □ London □ Toronto □ Mexico City
Rio de Janeiro □ Sydney □ Tokyo □ Hong Kong

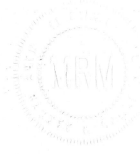

W. B. Saunders Company: West Washington Square
                          Philadelphia, PA   19105

Library of Congress Cataloging in Publication Data

Main entry under title:

Comprehensive management of head and neck tumors.

1. Head—Cancer.   2. Neck—Cancer.   I, II.
    Thawley, Stanley E., Panje, William R.   [DNLM: 1.
    Head and Neck Neoplasms—therapy.   WE 707 C737]

RC280.H4C66 1987   616.99′291   85–8352

ISBN 0–7216–8825–X

Editor: Staff
Designer: Terri Siegel
Production Manager: Bob Butler
Manuscript Editors: Carol Wolf/Lee Walters
Illustration Coordinator: Walt Verbitski
Page Layout Artist: Patti Maddaloni
Indexer: Ruth Low

Volume I ISBN   0–7216–8823–3
Volume II ISBN   0–7216–8824–1
Set ISBN   0–7216–8825–X

Comprehensive Management of Head and Neck Tumors

Last digit is the print number: 9   8   7   6   5   4   3   2   1

To my family, Betty, David, and Mark, for sharing and supporting me with this project and for keeping me oriented as to what life is all about.

To all of my teachers over the years; each one of them is a part of me.

To my residents and students, who challenge and force me to learn along with them.

To my parents, who laid the foundation.

S.T.

To my patients,
who have endured my desire to cure them.

W.P.

To the Department of Head and Neck Surgery,
University of Texas System Cancer Center,
M.D. Anderson Hospital, Houston.

J.B.

To Gilbert Fletcher, M.D.,
as a mentor of 20 years.

R.L.

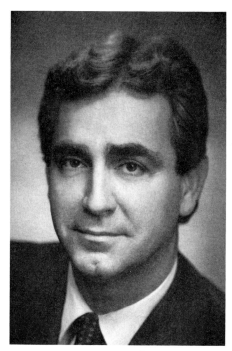

Stanley E. Thawley, M.D.

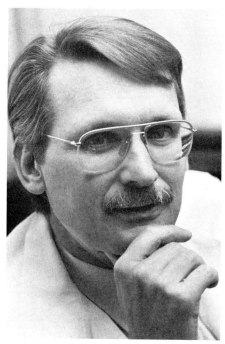

William R. Panje, M.D.

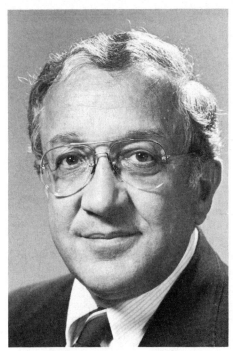

John G. Batsakis, M.D.

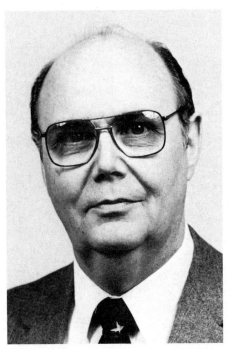

Robert D. Lindberg, M.D.

Contributors

LARRY H. ALLEN, M.D.

Fellow, Ocular Oncology and Orbital Clinic, University of British Columbia, Vancouver, Canada.

Clinical Evaluation and Pathology of Tumors of the Eye, Orbit, and Lacrimal Apparatus

PETER R. ALMOND, Ph.D.

Professor and Vice Chairman, Department of Radiation Oncology, University of Louisville, School of Medicine, Louisville, Kentucky.

Physics of Radiation Therapy of Head and Neck Tumors

RICHARD L. ANDERSON, M.D., F.A.C.S.

Professor of Ophthalmology, Director of Oculoplastic, Orbital and Oncology Services, University of Utah Medical Center, Salt Lake City. Staff, University of Utah Hospital, Holy Cross Hospital, and Primary Children's Hospital.

Treatment of Tumors of the Eye, Orbit, and Lacrimal Apparatus

EDGAR T. BALLARD, M.D.

Associate Professor of Pediatrics and Pathology, University of Cincinnati, Cincinnati, Ohio. Attending Staff, Children's Hospital; Associate Medical Staff, University Hospital, Cincinnati.

Tumors of the Head and Neck in Children

JANUSZ BARDACH, M.D.

Professor of Plastic Surgery, Department of Otolaryngology–Head and Neck Surgery, and Department of Surgery, University of Iowa, Iowa City.

Reconstruction of the External Ear: Surgical Reconstruction

JOHN G. BATSAKIS, M.D.

Ruth Legget Jones Professor of Pathology, University of Texas System Cancer Center, M.D. Anderson Hospital, Houston. Chairman, Division of Pathology, M.D. Anderson Hospital, Houston.

Pathology of Tumors of the Nasal Cavity and Paranasal Sinuses; Pathology of Tumors of the Oral Cavity

OLIVER H. BEAHRS, M.D.

Professor of Surgery, Emeritus, Mayo Medical School, Rochester, Minnesota.

Controversy in the Management of Tumors of the Thyroid and Parathyroid Glands

STEPHEN P. BECKER, M.D.

Assistant Professor, Northwestern University Medical School, Chicago, Illinois. Attending Staff, Northwestern Memorial Hospital and Children's Memorial Hospital, Chicago; Attending Staff, Skokie Valley Hospital, Skokie.

Controversy in the Management of Tumors of the Nasal Cavity and Paranasal Sinus

ROBERT E. BERKTOLD, M.D.

Instructor, Northwestern University Medical School, Chicago, Illinois. Associate Attending Physician, Northwestern Memorial Hospital; Attending Physician, Veterans Administration Lakeside Medical Center and Cook County Hospital, Chicago.

Controversy in the Management of Tumors of the Nasal Cavity and Paranasal Sinus

HUGH F. BILLER, M.D.

Professor and Chairman of Otolaryngology, The Mount Sinai School of Medicine, New York, New York.

Glottic and Subglottic Tumors

WILLIAM H. BLAHD, M.D.

Professor of Medicine, University of California School of Medicine, Los Angeles. Chief, Nuclear Medicine Ultrasound Service, Wadsworth Division, Veterans Administration Center, West Los Angeles, California.

Nuclear Medicine Therapy of Thyroid Cancer

MELVIN A. BLOCK, M.D., Ph.D.

Clinical Professor of Surgery, University of California, San Diego. Chairman, Department of Surgery, Green Hospital of Scripps Clinic and Research Foundation, La Jolla, California.

Surgical Therapy of Thyroid Tumors

WILLIAM G. BOWEN, M.D.

Assistant Professor of Clinical Medicine and Attending Cardiologist, Washington University, St. Louis, Missouri. Assistant Physician, Barnes Hospital and Jewish Hospital; Cardiology Consultant, John Cochran Veterans Administration Hospital, St. Louis.

Medical Management of Head and Neck Surgery Patients

NEIL A. BRESLAU, M.D.

Associate Professor of Clinical Medicine, University of Texas Health Science Center at Dallas, Southwestern Medical School,

Dallas. Assistant Director, General Clinical Research Center; Attending Physician, Parkland Memorial Hospital, Dallas.

Clinical Evaluation of Parathyroid Tumors

RANDY A. BROWN, M.D.

Clinical Instructor of Medicine, University of Texas Southwest, San Antonio. Staff Physician, Bexar County Hospital District; Staff Appointment, Southwest Texas Methodist Hospital and Humana Hospital of San Antonio.

Chemotherapy and Immunotherapy of Head and Neck Tumors

ROBERT M. BUMSTED, M.D.

Professor and Director, Division of Rhinology, Department of Otolaryngology–Head and Neck Surgery, University of Iowa, Iowa City. Staff, University of Iowa Hospital and Clinics and Veterans Hospital, Iowa City.

Surgical Therapy of Skin Tumors

NICHOLAS J. CASSISI, D.D.S., M.D.

Professor and Chief, Division of Otolaryngology, Department of Surgery, University of Florida, Gainesville, Florida. Assistant Chief of Staff and Attending Surgeon, Shands Teaching Hospital, Gainesville.

Clinical Evaluation of Pharyngeal Tumors

ROGER I. CEILLEY, M.D.

Assistant Clinical Professor, Department of Dermatology, University of Iowa College of Medicine, Iowa City, Iowa. Senior Staff, Iowa Methodist Medical Center, Des Moines.

Surgical Therapy of Skin Tumors

VAROUJAN A. CHALIAN, D.D.S., M.S.D.

Professor and Chairman, Department of Maxillofacial Prosthetics, Indiana University School of Dentistry, Professor, Department of Otorhinolaryngology, Indiana School of Medicine, Indianapolis. Staff, Indiana University Hospital, Veterans Administration Hospital, Methodist Hospital, and St. Vincent Hospital, Indianapolis.

Reconstruction of the External Ear: Prosthetic Reconstruction

SHARON L. COLLINS, M.D.

Assistant Professor, Department of Otolaryngology–Head and Neck Surgery, Loyola University Medical Center, Maywood, Illinois. Attending Physician, Foster G. McGraw Hospital, Maywood; Chief, Section of Head and Neck Surgery, Hines Veterans Administration Hospital, Chicago, Illinois.

Controversies in Management of Cancer of the Neck

JOHN CONLEY, M.D.

Professor Emeritus, Otolaryngology, Columbia University, New York, New York.

Controversies Regarding Therapy of Tumors of the Salivary Glands

ROBIN T. COTTON, M.D., F.A.C.S., F.R.C.S.(C)

Professor of Otolaryngology and Maxillofacial Surgery, University of Cincinnati College of Medicine, Cincinnati, Ohio. Director, Otolaryngology and Maxillofacial Surgery, Children's Hospital Medical Center, Cincinnati.

Tumors of the Head and Neck in Children

STANLEY W. COULTHARD, M.D.

Professor, Section of Otolaryngology, Department of Surgery, University of Arizona Health Sciences Center, Tucson. Attending Otolaryngologist, University of Arizona Health Sciences Center, Veterans Administration Medical Center, Kino Community Hospital, Tucson. Associate Staff, Tucson Medical Center, St. Joseph's Hospital, El Dorado Hospital, and Northwest Hospital, Tucson.

Clinical Evaluation of Tumors of the Salivary Glands

ROGER L. CRUMLEY, M.D.

Clinical Professor, Department of Otolaryngology–Head and Neck Surgery, University of California, San Francisco. Staff, University of California Medical Center, San Francisco.

Rehabilitation of the Patient with Tumors of the Salivary Glands

CHARLES W. CUMMINGS, M.D.

Professor and Chairman, Department of Otolaryngology, University of Washington. Staff, University Hospital, Seattle, Washington.

Controversy in the Management of Tumors of the Oral Cavity

LAWRENCE W. DAVIS, M.D.

Professor and Chairman, Department of Radiation Therapy, Albert Einstein College of Medicine, Bronx, New York. Chairman, Radiation Therapy, Montefiore Medical Center, North Central Bronx Hospital, and Jacobi Hospital, Bronx.

Controversy in the Management of Laryngeal Tumors: Radiation Therapy Perspective

WILLIAM E. DAVIS, M.D., M.S.P.H.

Professor of Surgery (Otolaryngology), University of Missouri, Health Sciences Center, Columbia, Missouri. Staff, University of Missouri, Health Sciences Center, Columbia.

Statistics of Head and Neck Cancer

LAWRENCE W. DE SANTO, M.D.

Professor of Otolaryngology–Head and Neck Surgery, Mayo Medical School, Rochester, Minnesota. Staff, Mayo Clinic, St. Mary's Hospital, Rochester Methodist Hospital, Rochester.

Treatment of Tumors of the Oropharynx: Surgical Therapy; Controversy in the Management of Laryngeal Tumors: Surgical Perspective

PAUL J. DONALD, M.D., F.R.C.S.(C)

Professor, Department of Otorhinolaryngology–Head and Neck Surgery, University of California, Davis. Attending Otolaryngologist/Head and Neck Surgeon, University of California, Davis Medical Center, Sacramento.

Intranasal and Paranasal Sinus Carcinoma; Diagnosis of Tumors of the Paranasal Sinuses and Nasal Cavity: Surgical Evaluation

STANLEY J. DUDRICK, M.D.

Clinical Professor of Surgery, The University of Texas Medical School, Houston. Director, Nutritional Support Services, St. Luke's Episcopal Hospital, Houston.

Nutritional Management of Head and Neck Tumor Patients

JONATHAN J. DUTTON, M.D., Ph.D.

Assistant Professor of Ophthalmology; Chief of Oculoplastic and Orbital Surgery and Ophthalmic Oncology Service, Duke

University Medical Center, Durham, North Carolina. Attending Faculty, Duke University Medical Center; Attending Faculty, Consultant, Durham Veterans Administration Medical Center, Durham.

Treatment of Tumors of the Eye, Orbit, and Lacrimal Apparatus

EDWARD ELLIS III, D.D.S., M.S.

Assistant Professor, Department of Oral and Maxillofacial Surgery, The University of Michigan, Ann Arbor.

Surgical Treatment of Non-odontogenic Tumors; Management of Odontogenic Cysts and Tumors

JOHN T. FAZEKAS, M.D.

Clinical Professor of Radiation Therapy, New York University, New York, New York. Director, Department of Radiation Therapy, Booth Memorial Medical Center, Flushing, New York.

Controversy in the Management of Laryngeal Tumors: Radiation Therapy Perspective

PETER J. FITZPATRICK, M.B., B.S., F.R.C.P.(C), F.R.C.R.

Professor of Radiology (Oncology) and Staff Physician, University of Toronto and Princess Margaret Hospital, Toronto, Canada.

Radiation Therapy of Tumors of the Skin of the Head and Neck

TERENCE J. FLEMING, D.D.S.

Assistant Clinical Professor, University of Texas Dental Branch; Associate Professor of Dental Oncology (Maxillofacial), M.D. Anderson Hospital, Houston, Texas. Associate Dental Oncologist, M.D. Anderson Hospital and Tumor Institute, Houston.

Rehabilitation of the Nasal and Paranasal Sinus Area: The Irradiated Patient

GILBERT H. FLETCHER, M.D.

Professor of Radiotherapy, University of Texas, M.D. Anderson Hospital and Tumor Institute, Houston.

Radiation Therapy of Tumors of the Neck

RAYMOND J. FONSECA, D.M.D.

Associate Professor and Chairman, Department Oral and Maxillofacial Surgery, University of Michigan, Ann Arbor.

Management of Odontogenic Cysts and Tumors

KAREN K. FU, M.D.

Professor, Department of Radiation Oncology, University of California, San Francisco.

Treatment of Tumors of the Nasopharynx: Radiation Therapy

DENNIS FULLER, Ph.D.

Assistant Professor at Washington University Medical School, St. Louis, Missouri. Staff, Barnes Hospital, St. Louis Children's Hospital, Irene Walter Johnson Rehabilitation Institute, St. Louis.

Speech Rehabilitation

MOKHTAR GADO, M.D.

Professor of Radiology, Washington School of Medicine, St. Louis, Missouri. Radiologist, Barnes Hospital and St. Louis Children's Hospital, St. Louis.

Diagnosis of Tumors of the Paranasal Sinuses and Nasal Cavity: Radiologic Evaluation

MICHAEL E. GLASSCOCK III, M.D., F.A.C.S.

Clinical Professor of Surgery (Otology/Neurotology), Vanderbilt University School of Medicine, Nashville, Tennessee; Clinical Professor of Otolaryngology, University of Tennessee College of Medicine, Memphis. Active Staff, Baptist Hospital and West Side Hospital, Nashville. Consulting Staff, Park View Hospital, Nashville General Hospital, St. Thomas Hospital, Vanderbilt University Hospital, and Veterans Administration Medical Center, Nashville.

Therapy of Glomus Tumors of the Ear and Base of Skull: Surgical Methods

JOEL A. GOEBEL, M.D.

Instructor, Department of Otolaryngology, Washington University School of Medicine, St. Louis, Missouri. Staff, Barnes Hospital, St. Louis Children's Hospital, Regional Hospital, St. Louis.

Clinical Evaluation of Glomus Tumors of the Ear and the Base of the Skull

JACQUELYN A. GOING, M.D.

Staff, Georgetown Memorial Hospital, Black River Road, Georgetown, South Carolina.

Tumors of the Head and Neck in Children

JEROME C. GOLDSTEIN, M.D.

Visiting Professor of Otolaryngology, Head and Neck Surgery, Johns Hopkins University School of Medicine, Baltimore, Maryland. Adjunct Professor of Surgery, Albany Medical College, Albany, New York. Consultant, Lochraven Veterans Administration Hospital, Baltimore; Walter Reed Army Medical Center, Washington, D.C.

Rehabilitation of Patients with Tumors of the Larynx

JOSEPH H. GRABOYES, M.D.

Attending Staff, Children's Hospital of Wisconsin and St. Michael's Hospital, Milwaukee, Wisconsin.

Lymphoreticular and Granulomatous Disorders of the Head and Neck

ROBERT O. GREER, Jr., D.D.S., Sc.D.

Professor and Chairman, Division of Oral Pathology and Oncology, University of Colorado School of Dentistry, Denver; Professor, Department of Pathology, University of Colorado School of Medicine. Pathology Staff, Rose Medical Center; Staff, University Hospital and Denver Children's Hospital, Denver.

Non-odontogenic Tumors: Clinical Evaluation and Pathology

HERMES C. GRILLO, M.D.

Professor of Surgery, Harvard Medical School, Boston, Massachusetts. Chief of General Thoracic Surgery, Massachusetts General Hospital, Boston.

Management of Tumors of the Trachea

CORDELL E. GROSS, M.D.

Associate Professor of Neurosurgery, University of Colorado Health Sciences Center, Denver. Staff, University Hospital,

Children's Hospital, Denver Veterans Administration Hospital, Denver General Hospital, and Rose Hospital, Denver.

Treatment of Tumors of the Nasopharynx: Surgical Therapy

D.F.N. HARRISON, M.D., F.R.C.S.

Chairman, Professorial Unit, Royal Nation Throat, Nose and Ear Hospital; Professor of Laryngology and Otology, University of London, England. Senior Surgeon, Royal National Throat, Nose and Ear Hospital, London.

Controversy in the Management of Tumors of the Pharynx; Surgical Therapy of the Larynx: Surgical Anatomy

FRED J. HODGES III, M.D.

Professor of Radiology, Washington School of Medicine, St. Louis, Missouri. Radiologist, Barnes Hospital and St. Louis Children's Hospital, St. Louis.

Diagnosis of Tumors of the Paranasal Sinuses and Nasal Cavity: Radiologic Evaluation

G. RICHARD HOLT, M.D.

Professor of Otorhinolaryngology and Oral and Maxillofacial Surgery; Assistant Dean for Student Affairs, The University of Texas Health Science Center at San Antonio. Attending Physician, Medical Center Hospital, Audie L. Murphy Memorial Veterans Hospital, and Santa Rosa Children's Hospital, San Antonio, Texas.

Surgical Therapy of Oral Cavity Tumors: Lip Tumors

NED B. HORNBACK, M.D.

Professor and Chairman of Radiation Oncology, Indiana University School of Medicine, Indianapolis. Radiation Oncologist, Indiana University Medical Center, Indianapolis.

Radiation Therapy of Tumors of the Salivary Glands

VINCENT J. HYAMS, M.D.

Distinguished Scientist, Armed Forces Institute of Pathology, Washington, D.C. Professor of Pathology, Uniformed Services University of Health Sciences, Bethesda, Maryland.

Pathology of Tumors of the Ear

RHONDA F.K. JACOB, D.D.S., M.S.

Assistant Professor of Clinical Dental Oncology, Department of Dental Oncology, University of Texas System Cancer Center, M.D. Anderson Hospital and Tumor Institute, Houston; Clinical Assistant Professor, Restorative Dentistry (Maxillofacial), University of Texas Health Science Center, Dental Branch, Houston. Assistant Dental Oncologist (Maxillofacial), Department of Dental Oncology, University of Texas System Cancer Center, M.D. Anderson Hospital and Tumor Institute, Houston.

Dental Complications of Head and Neck Surgery; Rehabilitation of the Nasal and Paranasal Sinus Area: Surgical Obturation of Palatal Defects

MICHAEL E. JOHNS, M.D.

Andelot Professor and Chairman, Johns Hopkins University School of Medicine, Baltimore, Maryland. Otolaryngologist-in-Chief, Johns Hopkins University School of Medicine, Baltimore.

Surgical Therapy of Tumors of the Salivary Glands

MICHAEL J. KAPLAN, M.D.

Assistant Professor of Otolaryngology–Head and Neck Surgery, University of California School of Medicine, San Francisco. Staff, University of California Medical Center, San Francisco. Chief, Otolaryngology, Veterans Administration Medical Center, San Francisco.

Surgical Therapy of Tumors of the Salivary Glands

GORDON E. KING, D.D.S.

Professor of Restorative Dentistry (Maxillofacial Prosthetics), University of Texas, Dental Branch, Houston. Dental Oncologist and Professor of Clinical Dental Oncology and Chairman, Department of Dental Oncology, University of Texas, M.D. Anderson Hospital, Houston. Consultant Staff, Methodist Hospital, Hermann Hospital, and Veterans Administration Medical Center, Houston.

Rehabilitation of the Nasal and Paranasal Sinus Area: The Foundation of Rehabilitation; Obturator-Restored Function and Limitations

SAM E. KINNEY, M.D.

Head, Section of Otology and Neurotology, Department of Otolaryngology and Communicative Disorders, Cleveland Clinic Foundation, Cleveland, Ohio.

Tumors of the External Auditory Canal, Middle Ear, Mastoid, and Temporal Bone

J. CAMERON KIRCHNER, M.D.

Assistant Professor of Surgery (Otolaryngology), Yale University School of Medicine, New Haven, Connecticut. Attending Physician, Yale–New Haven Hospital, New Haven. Consultant, Veterans Administration Medical Center, West Haven.

Reconstructive Surgery of the Sinuses

CHARLES F. KOOPMANN, Jr., M.D., F.A.C.S.

Associate Professor of Surgery, University of Arizona, Health Sciences Center, Tucson. Staff, University Medical Center, Veterans Administration Medical Center, Tucson Medical Center, Northwest Hospital, St. Joseph's Hospital, and Kino Community Hospital, Tucson.

Head and Neck Surgery in the Aged Patient

ALAN D. KORNBLUT, M.D., F.A.C.S.

Clinical Professor of Surgery (Otolaryngology), Uniformed University of Health Sciences, Bethesda, Maryland; Clinical Associate Professor of Surgery (Otolaryngology), Georgetown University School of Medicine, Washington, D.C. Consultant in Otolaryngology, National Institute of Allergy and Infectious Disease, Bethesda.

Clinical Evaluation of Tumors of the Oral Cavity

DONALD C. KRAMER, D.D.S., M.S.

Associate Professor of Dental Oncology, University of Texas, System Cancer Center, Houston. Associate Dental Oncologist, M.D. Anderson Hospital, Houston.

Rehabilitation of the Nasal and Paranasal Sinus Area: The Definitive Obturator

JOHN F. KVETON, M.D.

Attending Neurologist/Otologist, Lahey Clinic Medical Center, Burlington, Massachusetts.

Therapy of Glomus Tumors of the Ear and Base of Skull: Surgical Methods

MICHAEL KYRIAKOS, M.D.

Professor of Pathology and Surgical Pathology, Washington University School of Medicine, St. Louis, Missouri. Surgical Pathologist, Barnes Hospital; Consultant in Pathology, St. Louis Children's Hospital and Shriner's Hospital for Crippled Children, St. Louis.

Pathology of Selected Soft Tissue Tumors of the Head and Neck

WILLIAM E. LA VELLE, D.D.S., M.S., F.A.C.D., F.A.C.P.

Professor of Otolaryngology and Maxillofacial Surgery; and Professor of Removable Prosthodontics, University of Iowa Colleges of Medicine and Dentistry, Iowa City. Staff Prosthodontist, University Hospital; Consultant, Veterans Administration Hospitals, Knoxville and Iowa City.

Dental Management and Rehabilitation

WILLIAM LAWSON, M.D., D.D.S.

Professor of Otolaryngology, The Mount Sinai School of Medicine, New York.

Glottic and Subglottic Tumors

HOWARD LEVINE, M.D.

Senior Staff Physician, Department of Otolaryngology and Communicative Disorders, Cleveland Clinic Foundation, Cleveland, Ohio.

Auricular and Periauricular Cutaneous Carcinomas

ROBERT D. LINDBERG, M.D.

Professor and Chairman, Department of Radiation Oncology, University of Louisville School of Medicine, Louisville, Kentucky.

Radiation Therapy of Tumors of the Neck

RALEIGH E. LINGEMAN, M.D.

Morgan Professor and Chairman, Department of Otolaryngology–Head and Neck Surgery, Indiana University School of Medicine, Indianapolis, Active Staff, Indiana University Hospitals, Wishard Memorial Hospital, and Veterans Administration Hospital, Indianapolis. Consulting Staff, Methodist Hospital and St. Vincent Hospital, Indianapolis.

Surgical Management of Tumors of the Neck: Malignant Tumors

VIRGINIA A. LI VOLSI, M.D.

Professor of Pathology, Department of Pathology and Laboratory Medicine, University of Pennsylvania School of Medicine, Philadelphia. Director, Surgical Pathology Section, Department of Pathology and Laboratory Medicine, Hospital of the University of Pennsylvania, Philadelphia.

Pathology of Thyroid Tumors

FRANK E. LUCENTE, M.D.

Professor, Department of Otolaryngology, New York Medical College, Valhalla, New York. Chairman, Department of Otolaryngology, New York Eye and Ear Infirmary, New York, New York.

Psychological Problems of the Patient with Head and Neck Cancer

MARIO A. LUNA, M.D.

Professor of Pathology, and Staff, The University of Texas, M.D. Anderson Hospital and Tumor Institute, Houston.

Pathology of Tumors of the Salivary Glands

JAY MARION, M.D.

Assistant Professor of Clinical Medicine, Washington University School of Medicine, St. Louis, Missouri. Staff, Barnes Hospital, St. Louis.

Diagnosis and Treatment of Lymphomas; Chemotherapy and Immunotherapy of Head and Neck Tumors

JAMES E. MARKS, M.D.

Professor of Radiotherapy, Loyola University, Stritch School of Medicine, Chicago, Illinois. Chief of Radiotherapy, Foster G. McGraw Hospital, Maywood, and Edward Hines, Jr., Hospital, Hines, Illinois.

Treatment of Tumors of the Hypopharynx: Radiation Therapy; Radiation Therapy of Laryngeal Tumors: Planned Combined Radiotherapy and Surgery

JACK W. MARTIN, D.D.S., M.S.

Assistant Dental Oncologist (Maxillofacial) and Assistant Professor of Dental Oncology, University of Texas System Cancer Center, M.D. Anderson Hospital and Tumor Institute, Houston; Clinical Assistant Professor, Department of Prosthodontics, University of Texas Heath Science Center, Dental Branch, Houston. Chief, Maxillofacial Prosthodontics Section, Department of Dental Oncology, Division of Surgical Services, Houston.

Rehabilitation of the Nasal and Postnasal Sinus Area: Transition from Surgical to Interior Obturation

BRIAN F. MC CABE, M.D.

Professor and Chairman, Department of Otolaryngology–Head and Neck Surgery, The University of Iowa, Iowa City.

Controversy in the Management of Tumors of the Ear

KENNETH D. MC CLATCHEY, M.D., D.D.S.

Associate Professor of Pathology, Associate Professor of Dentistry; and Associate Chairman, Department of Pathology, University of Michigan, Ann Arbor.

Pathology of Lymphoreticular Disorders

FRED M. S. MC CONNEL, M.D.

Associate Professor of Surgery (Head and Neck), Section of Otolaryngology, Emory University School of Medicine, Atlanta, Georgia. Staff Physician, Emory University Hospital and Grady Memorial Hospital, Atlanta.

Rehabilitation of Patients with Tumors of the Pharynx

R. KEITH MC DANIEL, B.A., D.D.S., M.S.

Professor, Department of Pathology and Radiology, The University of Texas Health Science Center at Houston, Dental Branch, Houston, Texas.

Odontogenic Cysts and Tumors: Clinical Evaluation and Pathology

MARIA J. MERINO, M.D.

Associate Chief, Surgical Pathology and Postmortem Sections,

Laboratory of Pathology, National Cancer Institute, National Institutes of Health, Bethesda, Maryland.
Pathology of Thyroid Tumors

RODNEY R. MILLION, M.D.

Professor, Radiation Therapy Division, University of Florida College of Medicine, J. Hillis Miller Health Center, Gainesville, Florida. Medical Director, Radiation Therapy Division, Shands Teaching Hospital, J. Hillis Miller Health Center, Gainesville.
Radiation Therapy of Tumors of the Oral Cavity; Treatment of Tumors of the Oropharynx: Radiation Therapy

ELEANOR D. MONTAGUE, M.D.

Professor of Radiotherapy, University of Texas, M.D. Anderson Hospital and Tumor Institute, Houston.
Therapy of Glomus Tumors of the Ear and Base of Skull: Radiation Procedures

WILLIAM T. MOSS, M.D.

Professor and Chairman, Department of Radiation Therapy, Oregon Health Sciences University, Portland, Oregon.
Radiation Therapy for Tumors of the Nasal Cavity and Paranasal Sinuses

CHARLES M. MYER III, M.D.

Assistant Professor, Children's Hospital Medical Center, Department of Pediatric Otolaryngology; and University of Cincinnati College of Medicine, Department of Otolaryngology and Maxillofacial Surgery, Cincinnati, Ohio. Staff, Children's Hospital Medical Center, Veterans Hospital, University Hospital, and Shriner's Hospital for Crippled Children, Cincinnati.
Tumors of the Head and Neck in Children

RONALD H. NISHIYAMA, M.D.

Professor of Pathology, University of Vermont School of Medicine, Burlington, Vermont. Chief, Anatomic Pathology, Department of Laboratory Medicine, Maine Medical Center, Portland, Maine.
Pathology of Parathyroid Tumors

JOSEPH J. O'DONNELL, M.D.

General Surgery Resident, The University of Texas Medical School, Houston/Hermann Hospital, Houston.
Nutritional Management of Head and Neck Tumor Patients

ROBERT C. PACKMAN, M.D.

Professor of Clinical Medicine, Washington University, St. Louis, Missouri. Staff, Barnes Hospital, Jewish Hospital of St. Louis.
Medical Management of Head and Neck Surgery Patients

CHARLES Y. C. PAK, M.D.

Don Seldin Professor of Internal Medicine, University of Texas Health Service Center at Dallas, Southwestern Medical School, Dallas, Texas. Director, General Clinical Research Center; Attending Physician, Parkland Memorial Hospital, Dallas.
Clinical Evaluation of Parathyroid Tumors

WILLIAM R. PANJE, B.S., M.S., M.D., M.S. (Otol.), F.A.C.S.

Professor, The University of Chicago Pritzker School of Medicine, Chicago. Chairman, Division of Ear, Head, and Neck Surgery (Otolaryngology)–Head and Neck Center, Pritzker School of Medicine. Attending Physician, The Bernard Mitchell Hospital and Wyler's Children's Hospital, University of Chicago Medical Center, Chicago.
Immediate Reconstruction of the Oral Cavity; Treatment of Tumors of the Nasopharynx: Surgical Therapy

JAMES T. PARSONS, M.D.

Assistant Professor, Radiation Therapy Division, University of Florida College of Medicine, J. Hillis Miller Health Center, Gainesville, Florida. Radiation Therapist, Shands Teaching Hospital, J. Hillis Miller Health Center, Gainesville.
Radiation Therapy of Tumors of the Oral Cavity; Treatment of Tumors of the Oropharynx: Radiation Therapy

ROBERT L. PEAKE, M.D.

Clinical Professor of Internal Medicine, University of Texas Medical Branch, Galveston, Texas. Attending Physician, St. Mary's Hospital, Galveston.
Clinical Evaluation of Thyroid Tumors

BRUCE W. PEARSON, M.D., F.R.C.S.(C), F.A.C.S.

Associate Professor of Otolaryngology, Mayo Medical School, Rochester, Minnesota. Consultant in Otolaryngology and Head and Neck Surgery, Rochester; St. Mary's Hospital of the Sisters of Charity, Rochester.
Surgical Therapy of the Nasal Cavity and Paranasal Sinuses: Surgical Anatomy

LESTER J. PETERS, M.D.

Radiotherapist and Professor of Radiotherapy; Head, Division of Radiotherapy; and Chairman, Department of Clinical Radiotherapy, The University of Texas, M.D. Anderson Hospital and Tumor Institute, Houston.
Biology of Radiation Therapy

JAMES C. PHERO, D.M.D.

Associate Professor of Clinical Anesthesia; and Assistant Professor of Surgery, University of Cincinnati Medical Center, Cincinnati, Ohio. Assistant Director, Pain Control Center, University of Cincinnati. Staff Anesthesiologist, University Hospital, Holmes Hospital, Veterans Administration Medical Center, Children's Hospital, Cincinnati.
Pain Control in Cancer of the Head and Neck

JOHN C. PRICE, M.D.

Associate Professor, Department of Otolaryngology, Head and Neck Surgery, The Johns Hopkins University School of Medicine, Baltimore, Maryland. Chief of Otolaryngology, Head and Neck Surgery, Lochraven Veterans Administration Hospital, and The Johns Hopkins University Hospital, Baltimore.
Rehabilitation of Patients with Tumors of the Larynx

P. PRITHVI RAJ, M.D.

Professor of Anesthesiology, University of Cincinnati College of Medicine, Cincinnati, Ohio. Director, Pain Control Center, University Hospitals, Cincinnati.

Pain Control in Cancer of the Head and Neck

DALE H. RICE, M.D.

Professor and Chairman, Department of Otolaryngology–Head and Neck Surgery, University of Southern California, Los Angeles. Director, Department of Otolaryngology, Head and Neck Surgery, Los Angeles County–USC Medical Center. Head, Department of Otolaryngology, Head and Neck Surgery, Kenneth Norris Cancer Hospital. Attending Staff, Hollywood Presbyterian Hospital, Los Angeles.

Surgical Therapy of Nasal Cavity, Ethmoid Sinus, and Maxillary Sinus Tumors

MICHAEL D. ROHRER, D.D.S., M.S.

Associate Professor of Oral Pathology and Pathology, Colleges of Dentistry and Medicine, University of Oklahoma, Health Sciences Center, Oklahoma City. Staff, Oklahoma Memorial Hospital, Oklahoma Children's Memorial Hospital, and Veterans Administration Hospital, Oklahoma City.

Non-odontogenic Tumors: Clinical Evaluation and Pathology

JACK ROOTMAN, M.D., F.R.C.S.(C)

Professor of Ophthalmology and Pathology, University of British Columbia, Vancouver, Canada. Active Staff, Vancouver General Hospital and British Columbia's Children's Hospital. Chairman, Ocular and Orbital Oncology Group, British Columbia Cancer Institute, Vancouver.

Clinical Evaluation and Pathology of Tumors of the Eye, Orbit, and Lacrimal Apparatus

KLAUS SARTOR, M.D.

Associate Professor of Radiology, Washington University School of Medicine, St. Louis, Missouri; Radiologist, Barnes Hospital and St. Louis Children's Hospital, St. Louis.

Diagnosis of Tumors of the Paranasal Sinuses and Nasal Cavity: Radiologic Evaluation

CLARENCE T. SASAKI, M.D.

Professor of Surgery; and Chief, Section of Otolaryngology, Yale School of Medicine, New Haven, Connecticut. Attending Physician, Yale–New Haven Hospital, New Haven. Consultant, Veterans Administration Hospital, West Haven; St. Mary's Hospital and Waterbury Hospital, Waterbury; William W. Backus Hospital, Norwich; and Windham Community Memorial Hospital, Willimantic, Connecticut.

Reconstructive Surgery of the Sinuses

FRANKLIN L. SCAMMAN, M.D.

Associate Professor, Department of Anesthesia, University of Iowa College of Medicine and University of Iowa Hospitals, Iowa City.

Anesthesia for Surgery of Head and Neck Tumors

BERTRAM SCHNITZER, M.D.

Professor of Pathology, University of Michigan, Ann Arbor. Director, Hematopathology Laboratory, Ann Arbor.

Pathology of Lymphoreticular Disorders

VICTOR L. SCHRAMM, Jr., M.D., F.A.C.S.

Associate Professor, University of Pittsburgh School of Medicine, Pittsburgh, Pennsylvania. Chief, Veterans Administration Hospital, Pittsburgh. Staff, Eye and Ear Hospital and Children's Hospital, Pittsburgh.

Craniofacial Surgery for Sinus Tumors

DAVID E. SCHULLER, M.D.

Professor and Chairman, Department of Otolaryngology, The Ohio State University, Columbus. Director, Head and Neck Oncology Program, The Ohio State University Comprehensive Cancer Program, Columbus. Staff, The Ohio State University Hospitals and Columbus Children's Hospital, Columbus.

Clinical Evaluation of Tumors of the Neck

MITCHELL K. SCHWABER, M.D.

Clinical Assistant Professor, University of Florida and Medical College of Georgia. Active Staff, St. Vincent's Medical Center, Jacksonville, Florida.

Clinical Evaluation of Glomus Tumors of the Ear and the Base of the Skull

RICHARD F. SCOTT, D.D.S., M.S.

Assistant Professor, Department of Oral and Maxillofacial Surgery, The University of Michigan, Ann Arbor. Staff, University of Michigan Hospitals, Ann Arbor Veterans Administration Hospital, and Westland Medical Center, Ann Arbor.

Surgical Treatment of Non-odontogenic Tumors

DONALD G. SESSIONS, M.D.

Professor of Otolaryngology, Washington University School of Medicine, St. Louis, Missouri. Assistant Otolaryngologist, Barnes Hospital, St. Louis.

Surgical Therapy of Hypopharyngeal Tumors; Surgical Therapy of Supraglottic Tumors

JATIN P. SHAH, M.D., F.A.C.S.

Associate Professor of Surgery, Cornell University Medical College, New York, New York. Associate Attending Surgeon, Head and Neck Service, Memorial Sloan-Kettering Cancer Center, New York.

Surgical Therapy of Oral Cavity Tumors: Buccal Mucosa, Alveolus, Retromolar Trigone, Floor of Mouth, Hard Palate, and Tongue Tumors

ROBERT H. SHELLHAMER, Ph.D.

Professor of Anatomy, Indiana University School of Medicine, Indianapolis, Indiana.

Surgical Management of Tumors of the Neck: Malignant Tumors

LARRY J. SHEMEN, M.D., F.R.C.S.(C)

Program Director and Assistant Attending Surgeon, Manhattan Eye, Ear, and Throat Hospital, New York, New York. Attending Surgeon, St. Vincent's Hospital and Medical Center, New York.

Surgical Therapy of Oral Cavity Tumors: Buccal Mucosa, Alveolus, Retromolar Trigone, Floor of Mouth, Hard Palate, and Tongue Tumors

HOMAYOON SHIDNIA, M.D.

Associate Professor of Radiation Oncology, Indiana University School of Medicine, Indianapolis. Radiation Oncologist, Indiana University Medical Center, Indianapolis.

Radiation Therapy of Tumors of the Salivary Glands

BERNARD L. SHORE, M.D.

Instructor in Clinical Medicine, Washington University School of Medicine, St. Louis, Missouri. Assistant Physician, Barnes Hospital and Jewish Hospital, St. Louis.

Medical Management of Head and Neck Surgery Patients

GREGORIO A. SICARD, M.D.

Associate Professor of Surgery, Washington University School of Medicine, St. Louis, Missouri. Staff Surgeon, John Cochran Veterans Administration Hospitals; Assistant Surgeon, Barnes Hospital; Attending Surgeon, St. Louis County Hospital and St. Louis Children's Hospital; and Director, Vascular Service, Barnes Hospital.

Surgical Therapy of Parathyroid Tumors

BARBARA A. SIGLER, R.N., M.N.Ed.

Assistant Clinical Instructor, University of Pittsburgh School of Medicine, Pittsburgh, Pennsylvania. Adjunct Clinical Instructor, University of Pittsburgh, School of Nursing. Clinical Nurse Specialist, Head and Neck Oncology, Eye and Ear Hospital of Pittsburgh.

Nursing Care for Head and Neck Tumor Patients

CRAIG L. SILVERMAN, M.D.

Assistant Professor, Department of Radiotherapy, Stritch Medical School, Loyola University, Chicago, Illinois. Attending Radiotherapist, Foster G. McGraw Hospital, Loyola University, and Edward Hines Veterans Hospital, Chicago, Illinois.

Radiation Therapy of Laryngeal Tumors: Planned Combined Radiotherapy and Surgery

GEORGE A. SISSON, M.D.

Professor and Chairman, Northwestern University Medical School, Chicago, Illinois. Chairman, Otolaryngology–Head and Neck Surgery, Northwestern Memorial Hospital, Chicago. Staff, Cook County Hospital and Children's Memorial Hospital, Chicago. Consultant, Veteran's Administration Lakeside Medical Center, Chicago. Consultant, Delnor Hospital, St. Charles, Illinois.

Controversy in the Management of Tumors of the Nasal Cavity and Paranasal Sinus

J. LESLIE SMITH, Jr., M.D.

Professor of Pathology, M.D. Anderson Tumor Hospital, Houston, Texas.

Pathology of Skin Tumors of the Head and Neck

PETER G. SMITH, M.D., Ph.D.

Assistant Professor, Department of Otolaryngology, Washington University School of Medicine, St. Louis, Missouri. Staff, Barnes Hospital, St. Louis. Consultant, Jewish Hospital and John Cochran Veterans Administration Medical Center, St. Louis.

Clinical Evaluation of Glomus Tumors of the Ear and Base of the Skull

STEVEN M. SOBOL, M.D.

Associate Professor of Otolaryngology, Head and Neck Surgery, New York Eye and Ear Infirmary, New York Medical College, New York, New York. Attending Surgeon, New York Eye and Ear Hospital and Lenox Hill Hospital, New York.

Surgical Management of Tumors of the Neck: Benign Tumors

ROBERT B. STANLEY, Jr., M.D.

Assistant Professor and Vice Chairman, Department of Otolaryngology, Head and Neck Surgery, University of Southern California, Los Angeles. Assistant Director, Department of Otolaryngology–Head and Neck Surgery, Los Angeles County–USC Medical Center, Los Angeles. Assistant Head, Department of Otolaryngology–Head and Neck Surgery, Kenneth Norris Cancer Hospital, Los Angeles. Attending Staff, Hollywood Presbyterian Hospital, Los Angeles.

Surgical Therapy of Nasal Cavity, Ethmoid Sinus, and Maxillary Sinus Tumors

JAMES J. STRAIN, M.D.

Professor of Clinical Psychiatry, Mount Sinai School of Medicine, New York, New York. Director, Psychiatric Consultation and Liaison Service, Mount Sinai Medical Center, New York.

Psychological Problems of the Patient with Head and Neck Cancer

ELLIOT W. STRONG, M.D., F.A.C.S.

Professor of Surgery, Cornell University Medical College, New York, New York. Attending Surgeon and Chief, Head and Neck Service, Memorial Sloan-Kettering Cancer Center, New York.

Surgical Therapy of Oral Cavity Tumors: Buccal Mucosa, Alveolus, Retromolar Trigone, Floor of Mouth, Hard Palate, and Tongue Tumors

DANIEL TABAK, M.D.

Senior Fellow, Department of Hematology–Oncology, Washington University School of Medicine, St. Louis, Missouri. Staff, Barnes Hospital, St. Louis.

Chemotherapy and Immunotherapy of Head and Neck Tumors

THOMAS D. TAYLOR, D.D.S., M.S.D., F.A.C.P.

Associate Professor of Prosthodontics; and Director, Maxillofacial Prosthodontics, University of Washington School of Dentistry, Seattle. Consultant, Veterans Administration Hospital, Seattle.

Dental Management and Rehabilitation

JERRY TEMPLER, M.D.

Associate Professor of Surgery in Otolaryngology, University of Missouri, Columbia. Staff, University of Missouri Health Science Center and Harry S Truman Memorial Veterans Administration Hospital, Columbus.

Clinical Evaluation of the Larynx

STANLEY E. THAWLEY, M.D.

Associate Professor of Otolaryngology, Washington University School of Medicine, St. Louis, Missouri. Staff Otolaryngologist, Barnes Hospital; Chief, Otolaryngology–Head and Neck Surgery Service, Veterans Administration Hospitals, St. Louis.

Surgical Therapy of the Larynx: Surgical Anatomy; Surgical Therapy of Hypopharyngeal Tumors; Treatment of Tumors of the Oropharynx: Surgical Therapy; Surgical Therapy of Supraglottic Tumors

RICHARD B. TOWBIN, M.D., F.A.A.P.

Associate Professor of Radiology and Pediatrics and Medical Student Advisor, University of Cincinnati College of Medicine, Cincinnati, Ohio. Attending Radiologist, University Hospital, Cincinnati. Staff Radiologist, Division of Radiology; Head, Section of Neuroradiology; and Head, Section of Special and Interventional Procedures, all at Children's Hospital Medical Center, Cincinnati.

Tumors of the Head and Neck in Children

ARIYADASA UDAGAMA, D.D.S., M.S.D.

Associate Professor of Clinical Dental Oncology, University of Texas, Houston. Chief, Section of Facial Prosthetics, University of Texas, M.D. Anderson Hospital and Tumor Institute, Houston

Rehabilitation of the Nasal and Paranasal Sinus Area: Prosthetic Restoration of the Nose and Midface

A. W. PETER VAN NOSTRAND, M.D., F.R.C.P.(C)

Professor of Pathology and Otolaryngology, University of Toronto, Canada. Chief of Surgical Pathology, Toronto General Hospital, Toronto.

Pathology of Laryngeal Tumors

KATHERINE VERDOLINI, M.S.

Speech Therapist, Washington University School of Medicine, St. Louis, Missouri.

Swallowing Rehabilitation

C. C. WANG, M.D.

Professor of Radiation Therapy, Harvard Medical School, Boston, Massachusetts. Radiation Therapist and Head, Division of Clinical Services, Department of Radiation Medicine, Massachusetts General Hospital, Boston.

Radiation Therapy of Laryngeal Tumors: Curative Radiation Therapy

LOUIS H. WEILAND, M.D.

Professor of Pathology, Mayo Medical School, Rochester, Minnesota. Consultant, Surgical Pathology, Mayo Clinic, Rochester.

Pathology of Pharyngeal Tumors

SUSAN WEINMANN-WINKLER, R.D./L.D., M.S. & Hyg.

Assistant Director, Clinical Nutrition, Education and Nutritional Support Assessment, St. Luke's Episcopal Hospital, Texas Heart Institute and Texas Children's Hospital, Houston.

Nutritional Management of Head and Neck Tumor Patients

DUANE C. WHITAKER, M.D.

Assistant Professor, Director of Dermatologic Surgery, University of Iowa Hospitals and Clinics, Iowa City.

Clinical Evaluation of Tumors of the Skin

KWAN Y. WONG, M.B.B.S.

Associate Professor of Pediatrics, University of Cincinnati College of Medicine, Cincinnati, Ohio. Attending Pediatrician and Assistant Director, Division of Hematology/Oncology, Children's Hospital Medical Center, Cincinnati.

Tumors of the Head and Neck in Children

JOHN E. WOODS, M.D., Ph.D.

Professor of Plastic Surgery, Mayo Clinic and Mayo Medical School, Rochester, Minnesota.

Controversy in the Management of Tumors of the Skin

DAVID A. WYATT, Th.M.

Chaplain (retired), Barnes Hospital, St. Louis, Missouri.

Psychological Problems of the Patient with Head and Neck Cancer

STEPHEN KENT YOUNG, D.D.S., M.S.

Associate Professor of Oral Pathology and Pathology, Colleges of Dentistry and Medicine, University of Oklahoma, Health Sciences Center, Oklahoma City. Staff, Oklahoma Memorial Hospital, Oklahoma Children's Hospital, and Veterans' Administration Hospital, Oklahoma City.

Non-odontogenic Tumors: Clinical Evaluation and Pathology

MARY ANN ZAGGY, M.S.

Senior Speech Pathologist, Department of Otolaryngology, Barnes Hospital/Washington University Medical School, St. Louis, Missouri.

Swallowing Rehabilitation

Foreword

We live in language. Literally, every minute of our waking lives is concerned with our interaction as neurobiologic beings with the physical world around us, and this occurs in language. This involves our cultural heritage, our experience, our education and training, and our vision, and we integrate all of this in language. Curiously and intentionally, we observe and interpret and then attempt to impose order on the physical world and create meaning and value out of so doing. Related to this process is the willingness on the part of some not only to study and perform in the arena but also to lead and teach about the process.

Comprehensive Management of Head and Neck Tumors is a text created by practitioners who have devoted their lives to the study and treatment of patients with tumors occurring in the anatomic area of the head and neck. The avowed purpose of the book is to provide comprehensive information about tumors of the head and neck from experts in the multiple disciplines that deal in this field. The authors provide their considered opinions based on a professional lifetime of experience, and it is exciting that in describing specific tumors of the head and neck, the judgments, interpretations, and treatment recommendations are often seemingly different and sometimes diametrically opposed to each other. This results in a situation that may cause some discomfort to the reader. For although we would like for there to be a "sure" or "best" way to handle each case, this is seldom possible. Each chapter addresses individual and collective issues that arise in managing patients with difficult treatment problems and provides insight into the multiple valid management approaches available. The text, by adding clarity to a complex situation, enlarges our perspective about the specific problem discussed, demands an engagement with the material, and requires the reader to formulate the "best" recommendation for each patient on an individual basis.

A good part of the maturation of a physician involves the opening up of areas of inquiry that were previously thought to be already mastered. As time goes by, areas of medical knowledge we thought we knew well come into question. As physicians, we have a professional and societal thrownness to have answers to all medical questions, especially in areas of our announced expertise. When answers show up around these areas, it makes us "comfortable" again in our ability to handle patients with these medical problems. These answers, however, are a disaster in the domain of the inquiry—for once we have the answer, our natural inclination is to end the inquiry. The power of this book lies in the editors' unwillingness to simplify the approaches to the management of head and neck tumors. The language and scientific rigor of this text indicate the authenticity of the authors, with the result that there is little arrogance expressed in these chapters.

Patients with head and neck cancers have difficult problems with which to deal. Multiple factors, including medical, psychological, nutritional, societal, and economic, must be taken into account. The specific management to be recommended for individual patients often is not clear. Various forms of therapy available to treat these patients often result in severe functional and cosmetic sequelae. Each time a patient presents to us with a head and neck tumor, we enter into a relationship that ultimately results in our recommendation of some form of treatment. What we recommend is often determined by our prior education and training and, particularly, by our experience in the specific area. The power of this book lies in the multidimensional presentation of the issues in a measured and scientific manner. The sections on controversial issues are stimulating because of the many significant questions that are raised. This is important, because breakthroughs are created not from known answers, but from our interaction with the issues and the continual generation of more questions.

DONALD SESSIONS

Preface

The management of head and neck tumors has a long and interesting history characterized by various phases of development. At times, the therapeutic emphasis has been on surgical ablation; at others, radiation therapy has been the popular modality. While treatment advanced, our understanding of tumor pathology and behavior also matured. Restoration of function and maintenance of quality of life continue to improve as surgical reconstruction and prosthetics become more sophisticated. The management of patients with head and neck tumors has become so complex that no single clinician can be a master of all the required knowledge and also be proficient in all of the techniques. Practitioners of multiple specialties are commonly involved, and patients receive the expertise of a head and neck surgeon, a radiation therapist, a prosthodontist, social worker, and nursing staff. The time has come to amalgamate the information of this multispecialty approach into one source and to provide those involved in the management of patients with head and neck tumors a comprehensive reference.

The purpose of this publication is to present a wealth of information on head and neck tumors in one source. Both general and specific information is offered for anyone who desires a comprehensive understanding of the subject. *Comprehensive Management of Head and Neck Tumors* was designed to be as thorough as possible. The specialists involved in the care of patients with head and neck tumors who will find this book useful are head and neck surgeons, radiation therapists, pathologists, anesthesiologists, oral surgeons, medical oncologists, nurses, dentists, prosthodontists, radiologists, nutritionists, speech therapists, social workers, and psychiatrists.

I especially wanted to avoid creating a book that would be identified as a surgical- or radiation-oriented text; likewise, it does not represent the orientation of any particular university or any geographical area. Editors were selected from the specialities of head and neck surgery, radiation therapy, and pathology from different universities. Each had the responsibility of recruiting the leading experts in his field to present thorough and current coverage of the current knowledge. The reader is offered a wealth of facts, personal opinions and experience, philosophies, and techniques. Some information may overlap but, finally, the reader benefits from this multispeciality presentation. Responsibility rests on the clinician to read, interpret, understand, and make logical decisions for each patient.

The format of the book offers detailed discussions of tumors affecting each area of the head and neck: ear, nose and paranasal sinuses, oral cavity, pharynx, larynx, neck, salivary glands, and skin. Each section includes separate chapters on diagnosis and clinical presentation, pathology, radiation therapy, surgical therapy, and rehabilitation plus a chapter on controversies contributed by a specially chosen authority. There are additional chapters on dental, thyroid, tracheal, orbit, and pediatric tumors, and separate chapters on speech therapy, chemotherapy, nutrition, statistics of head and neck tumors, anesthesia, nursing, and dental management.

It is not our intent to recommend the "best" treatment for each tumor. Our purpose is to provide an extensive source of information about these lesions, to offer the reader the combined knowledge of multiple specialists, to encourage the clinician to be flexible and innovative, to stimulate the imagination, and to give physicians the background information to make the best, educated, responsible decisions for their individual patients.

Because each tumor site is discussed individually, there is no single chapter on general behavior of head and neck tumors; however, the interested reader is directed particularly to Chapter 56. Although this chapter concerns neck tumors, it provides stimulating and provocative discussion for our thinking concerning the general disease entity of head and neck tumors. Most of all, this chapter stimulates our imagination and challenges us to open our minds and think.

It is hoped that this book will allow a more intelligent understanding of head and neck tumors, resulting in skillful treatment to maximize the patient's chance of cure and to preserve the highest quality of life.

STAN THAWLEY

Acknowledgments

This project has been lifted out of the planning stages and carried to fruition by a great number of individuals who have worked with me over the past several years. I am truly grateful and appreciative of all of their contributions and wish to acknowledge them and offer my sincere thanks for allowing a dream to become a complete reality.

My editors, William Panje, M.D., John Batsakis, M.D, and Robert Lindberg, M.D., without whose help this project would have been impossible.

My colleagues, who accepted the challenge of writing and contributed the numerous excellent chapters.

The Department of Otolaryngology at Washington University School of Medicine in St. Louis for support of this project. This department has provided a stimulating atmosphere over the years, allowing me to learn and develop professionally. I am especially grateful to my former chairman, the late Dr. Joseph Ogura, and to his successor, Dr. John Fredrickson, for their great leadership and support.

My secretaries, Pat Kerbel, Sally Jones, Kathy Florence, and Jean Mayo, for typing, phone calls, and patience with me.

Tim Dyches, M.D., Jill Dyches, Sue Lyon, and Mark Thawley, for their artistic contributions.

Sue Witte, for her numerous illustrations, her willingness to revise, her pleasantness, and her interest to learn.

Don Davis, my photographer for many years, who contributed many of the photographs.

Dianne Pechmann, for her typing of manuscripts and the endless revisions.

Mike Grannon, Stan Kiger, and Mike Vannier, M.D., for the computer head and neck images that inspired the cover design. It was great fun being allowed to create these images on their computers.

A special thanks to Rhonda Krulik, my secretary, for her efficient management of my office, allowing me to direct a project of this size and to maintain an active head and neck practice. She does all of this with a pleasantness that makes my work truly enjoyable.

Numerous workers at W. B. Saunders—Suzanne Boyd, my editor, who had patience and who really sparked the initiation of the project; Bob Butler and Carol Wolf, for their detailed final manuscript production; and Terri Siegel, for her skill and patience in executing my cover design.

STAN THAWLEY

Acknowledgments

Janusz Bardach, M.D., for teaching me the concept of plastic and reconstructive surgery.

Brian F. McCabe, M.D., for allowing me the opportunity to develop in head and neck oncology.

John J. Conley, M.D., for instilling the ethics to treat head and neck cancer.

William Montgomery, M.D., for his friendship.

Helen, Nikki, and Megan, for their understanding, happiness, and support.

WILLIAM R. PANJE

Contents

PART II
Tumors of the Ear

PART III
Tumors of the Nasal Cavity and Paranasal Sinuses

PART IV
Tumors of the Oral Cavity

PART V
Tumors of the Pharynx

PART IX
Tumors of the Neck

PART X
Dental and Jaw Tumors

PART XI
Tumors of the Thyroid and Parathyroid Glands

PART XII
Tumors of the Trachea

PART XIII
Tumors of the Eye, Orbit, and Lacrimal Apparatus

PART XIV
Special Topics

Tumors of the Salivary Glands

CHAPTER 41

Clinical Evaluation of Tumors of the Salivary Glands

Stanley W. Coulthard, M.D.

The clinical evaluation of salivary gland tumors requires the physician to rely heavily on previous experience, a thorough knowledge of head and neck anatomy, and an understanding of the biologic behavior of the numerous histologically varied tumors that can occur in this system of glands. Historically, the salivary gland neoplasms were vaguely classified until Foote and Frazell presented their correlation of histopathologic and biologic behavior in 1953.[13] The early ambiguity in histologic classification and biologic characteristics for salivary gland tumors meant that therapy was poorly directed prior to the 1950s. McFarland in 1933 stated that surgical treatment of these neoplasms was unnecessary.[19] The integration of pathologic and clinical knowledge along with more sophisticated surgical and anesthetic methods during the last three decades has led to more appropriate and effective treatment.

The majority of masses in the major salivary glands represent neoplasms.[14] It is the physician's responsibility to determine the benign or malignant nature of these tumors and to counsel the patient appropriately. A thorough history and physical examination along with selected radiographic and pathologic tests allow for these therapeutic decisions. It is the selection of tests and the decisions that are made on the basis of these tests that are becoming more and more crucial as the cost-effectiveness of therapy is examined more closely and the physician is scrutinized more closely by a consumer-conscious public. The physician has been confronted with numerous new tests and pressure to supply the patient with more and more information concerning disease processes and possible complications and outcomes from therapeutic measures. Often when evaluating a patient for the first time it is difficult to immediately recommend an operative procedure that may be extensive and involve major complications of head and neck deformity. This is the dilemma of the salivary gland surgeon and specifically the parotid gland surgeon who deals with the facial nerve. It is at this point that the physician may feel pressured to order ancillary tests even though they may be superfluous to the actual decision-making process.

This chapter examines the process of clinical evaluation of salivary gland neoplasms. We will utilize the history and physical examination as the foundation for this evaluation and selectively recommend supplemental examinations with computed tomography (CT), sialography, nuclear imaging, and aspiration needle biopsy.

ETIOLOGY

The etiology of salivary gland neoplasms, like that of most neoplasms, has been elusive. Other than a few reports of radiation-induced neoplasms, the mechanisms of induction of abnormal growth in these complex glands is unknown.[23] The greatest insight into the understanding of these neoplasms and their cellular origins is gained by looking at the histogenesis of salivary gland neoplasms.[22]

Embryologically the salivary glands originate from the aerodigestive tract as small buds off the oral cavity. This occurs at the end of the second week of gestation. Full differentiation is probably not completed until 6 weeks after birth.[21]

In the fully developed salivary gland, the differentiated tissues have formed mucous and serous acini. The acini lead into the intercalated duct, which leads to the striated duct and then into the extralobular excretory duct. Around the acini and intercalated duct are the myoepithelial cells. The myoepithelial cell is a contractile cell that actively forces secretions from the acini and the intercalated ducts. Multiple myofilaments are found in the myoepithelial cells on electron microscopy (Fig. 41–1).[5]

The ductal component of the salivary gland unit consists first of a relatively undifferentiated intercalated duct and a well-differentiated striated duct. The striated duct cells show deep basal membrane invaginations and many intracellular mitochondria. The function of these cells is thought to be water and electrolyte transport.

The basal cell is found in the area of the intercalated duct and the excretory duct. These cells are thought to represent progenitor cells. Their capacity to differentiate into other salivary gland cells and tumor cells is an important aspect of the salivary gland histogenesis.[12]

Theoretically, there are two possible explanations for the histogenesis of salivary gland neoplasms. The first would require differentiated cells to dedifferentiate into the multiple cell types. The second theory utilizes the progenitor cell (basal cell) present in the intercalated duct and excretory duct to explain differentiation into the various histologically varied neoplasms. Regezi and Batsakis organized the latter theory into the cell differentiation shown in Table 41–1.[22]

The benign mixed cell tumor contains two types of cells—epithelial and myoepithelial. Each tumor is represented by a certain concentration of each cell type.

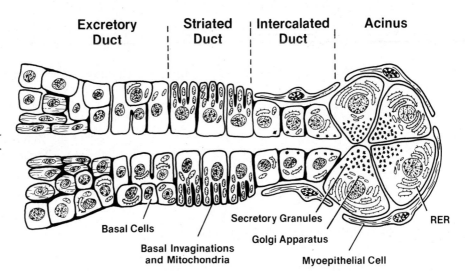

Figure 41–1. The cellular composition of the salivary duct structure.

The majority of neoplasms of this type contain an epithelial preponderance, although on rare occasion the monomorphic type appears which has mainly epithelial or myoepithelial elements.

The adenoid cystic carcinoma contains cells that resemble the intercalated duct cells. The major controversy has centered around the reports of two types of cell types in this neoplasm.

The squamous cell carcinoma or mucoepidermoid carcinoma theoretically can originate from any of the salivary gland cell types because of their epithelial anlage.

The oncocytic neoplasms contain the oncocyte, which is generally found along the entire salivary gland unit as an individual ages. The oncocytes contain hyperplastic and pleomorphic mitochondria. They are thought to represent a form of cellular degeneration.

Acinous cell carcinoma contains cells that have secretory granules. It is thought that the cell of origin is the intercalated duct reserve cell. It is also thought that the adenocarcinomas arise from the intercalated duct reserve cells.

INCIDENCE

The physician must keep in mind that palpable lesions in the major salivary glands are almost always neoplasms. Statistics show that 95 per cent of palpable parotid lesions will demonstrate neoplastic growth.[10] Parotid neoplasms are the most numerous and will account for approximately 80 per cent of salivary neoplasms. The submandibular gland makes up 10 per cent, and other glands make up the other 10 per cent.[17] The palate is the most common location for involvement of the minor salivary glands.

The most common parotid tumor is in the lower pole of the gland and is in the superficial lobe. Eighty per cent of tumors in the parotid are in this location. The remainder of tumors are in the upper pole and in the deep lobe, and only about 1 per cent or less account for the so-called "dumbbell" tumor.

Tumors of the salivary glands are indeed rare. They account for less than 3 per cent of all neoplasms in the head and neck region.[3] The overall incidence of salivary gland neoplasms as reported by Biorklund from the Karolinska Institut in Stockholm is 40 cases per million persons. The incidence of malignancy among these neoplasms is nine cases per million population.[3] The incidence of salivary gland tumors has been found to be similar around the world. Benign neoplasms far outweigh the malignant ones. In general, 80 per cent of parotid tumors will be benign, whereas two thirds of submandibular and one half of palatal salivary gland neoplasms will be benign.

Childhood salivary gland neoplasms are commonly separated into benign and malignant (Table 41–2). The benign tumors contain the vascular lesions such as the lymphangioma and hemangioma. Schuller and McCabe reported the lymphangioma as the most common vascular neoplasm and the benign mixed tumor as the most common nonvascular benign neoplasm of the salivary glands.[24] Figure 41–2 shows a lymphangioma of the left parotid gland and neck. The history revealed that the mass had been present since the child's birth, and physical examination revealed easy transillumination of the mass. The mucoepidermoid carcinoma is the most common malignant neoplasm in children. Their report made special note of a high incidence of malignant neoplasms in the salivary glands of this childhood group. When only the nonvascular neoplasms were considered, they found a 57.5 per cent incidence of malignancy in childhood salivary gland masses.

TABLE 41–1. Histogenic Scheme for Salivary Gland Neoplasms*

Normal Structure	Cell of Origin	Neoplasm
Excretory duct	Excretory duct reserve cell	Squamous cell carcinoma Mucoepidermoid carcinoma
Acinus	Intercalated duct reserve cell	Acinic cell carcinoma Mixed tumor Monomorphic adenoma Myoepithelioma
Intercalated duct		Adenoid cystic carcinoma
Myoepithelium		Adenocarcinoma
Striated duct		Oncocytic tumors

*From Regezi JA, Batsakis JG: Otolaryngol Clin North Am, *10*:300, 1977.

TABLE 41—2. Parotid Tumors in Children*

Benign	
Mixed	22
Hemangioma	16
Lymphangioma	5
Cystic Hygroma	1
Plexiform Neurofibroma	1
Lipomatosis	1
Schwannoma	1
Malignant	
Mucoepidermoid	13
Acinic Cell	4
Metastatic	4
TOTAL	66

*From Chong GC, Beahrs OH, Chen ML, Hayles AB: Mayo Clinic Proc., *50*:279, 1975.

There is no demonstrable sex difference among the salivary gland neoplasms in Caucasians, but in the nonwhite population in the United States and Africa the salivary gland neoplasms are most commonly found in females. The African Negro presents most often with mixed tumors of the minor or lesser salivary gland rather than the parotid or submandibular gland.[8]

Breast cancer and salivary gland cancer correlations have been reported in the literature. Even though this remains a controversial subject, the statistics presented appear to make strong evidence for this association.[2]

CLASSIFICATION

The salivary glands are said to give rise to more types of histologically varied neoplasms than any other system

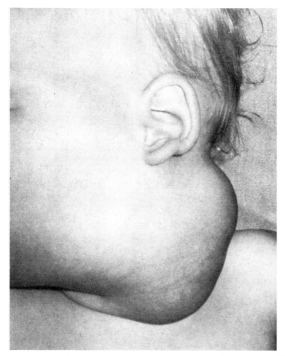

Figure 41—2. A child with lymphangioma involving the parotid and neck.

of the body. This fact is exemplified by the great difficulty which pathologists and clinicians have had in classifying these tumors. Batsakis has proposed the most extensive classification of salivary gland tumors based on histopathologic data (Table 41–3).[1] A listing of other classifications can be found in Tables 41–4 and 41–5. A comparison of Tables 41–1 and 41–3 demonstrates the extensive clinicopathologic entities that Batsakis has further divided. The difficulty and controversy in this area are related to the rarity of these neoplasms and the lack of large experience in any one medical center. Only the added experience of the future will help to solidify these concepts.

The TNM tumor *staging scheme* was first proposed by Denoix in 1946. It was an effort to correlate the state of a tumor prior to treatment with the biologic severity of

TABLE 41—3. Classification of Epithelial Salivary Gland Tumors*

Type of Lesion	Variations
Benign	Mixed tumor (pleomorphic adenoma)
	Papillary cystadenoma lymphomatosum (Warthin's tumor)
	Oncocytoma (oncocytosis)
	Monomorphic tumors
	Basal cell adenoma
	Glycogen rich adenoma (?)
	Clear cell adenoma
	Membranous adenoma
	Myoepithelioma
	Sebaceous tumors
	Adenoma
	Lymphadenoma
	Papillary ductal adenoma (papilloma)
	Benign lymphoepithelial lesion
	Unclassified
Malignant	Carcinoma ex pleomorphic adenoma (carcinoma arising in a mixed tumor)
	Malignant mixed tumor (biphasic malignancy)
	Mucoepidermoid carcinoma
	Low-grade
	Intermediate-grade
	High-grade
	Adenoid cystic carcinoma
	Acinous cell (acinic) carcinoma
	Adenocarcinoma
	Mucus-producing adenopapillary and nonpapillary carcinoma
	Salivary duct carcinoma (ductal carcinoma)
	Other adenocarcinomas
	Oncocytic carcinoma (malignant oncocytoma)
	Clear cell carcinoma (nonmucinous and glycogen-containing or nonglycogen-containing)
	Primary squamous cell carcinoma
	Hybrid basal cell adenoma/adenoid cystic carcinoma
	Undifferentiated carcinoma
	Epithelial-myoepithelial carcinoma of intercalated ducts
	Miscellaneous (includes sebaceous, Stensen's duct, melanoma and carcinoma ex lymphoepithelial lesion)
	Metastatic
	Unclassified

*From Batsakis JG: Tumors of the Head and Neck. 2nd ed. Baltimore, Williams & Wilkins Co., 1979, p. 9.

TABLE 41–4. W.H.O. Classification of Salivary Gland Tumors*

Epithelial tumors
  Adenomas, pleomorphic adenoma (mixed tumor)
Monomorphic adenomas
  Adenolymphoma
  Oxyphilic adenoma
  Other types
Mucoepidermoid tumor
Acinic cell tumor
Carcinomas
  Adenoid cystic
  Adenocarcinoma
  Epidermoid carcinoma
  Undifferentiated
  Carcinoma in pleomorphic adenoma (malignant mixed tumor)
Nonepithelial tumors
Unclassified tumors
Allied conditions
  Benign lymphoepithelial lesion
  Sialosis
  Oncocytosis

*From Thackray AC, Sobin LH: Histological Typing of Salivary Gland Tumors. Geneva, World Health Organization, 1972.

TABLE 41–5. Soft-Tissue Tumors of the Major Salivary Glands and Paraglandular Tissues*

Vascular
  Primary hemangioma of the parotid gland
  Lymphangioma
  Arteriovenous fistula (aneurysms)
  Angiosarcoma

Lymphoreticular
  Lymphoma (primary and secondary)
  Atypical lymphoreticular hyperplasia (pseudolymphoma)
  Histiocytosis
  Lymphoepithelial lesion (with or without Sjögren's syndrome)
  Benign, reactive hyperplasia

Neurogenous
  Neurofibroma
  Neurofibrosarcoma
  Neurilemoma
  Traumatic neuroma
  Neuroepithelial tumor (sarcoma)
  Granular cell tumor
  Meningioma

Skeletal muscle
  Rhabdomyosarcoma
  Rhabdomyoma
  Infantile rhabdomyoma
  Masseteric hypertrophy
  Smooth muscle
  Leiomyoma
  Leiomyosarcoma

Fibroblastic and histiocytic
  Fibrous scar or keloid
  Fibrosarcoma
  Fibromatosis
  Histiocytoma and variants

*Batsakis JG: Tumors of the Head and Neck. 2nd ed. From Baltimore, Williams & Williams Co., 1979, p. 9.

TABLE 41–6. Clinical Staging, Parotid Gland*

Stage T1	Stage T2	Stage T3
0–3 cm in diameter	3.1–6 cm in diameter	6 cm or more in diameter
Solitary	Solitary	Multiple nodules
Freely mobile	Freely mobile or skin fixation	Ulceration
		Deep fixation
Cranial nerve VII intact	Cranial nerve VII intact	Cranial nerve VII dysfunction

*Modified from Spiro RH et al: Am J Surg *130*:452, 1975.

the disease. Spiro first proposed a staging system for cancer of the parotid gland in 1975.[27] This scheme is presented in Table 41–6.

Levitt has more recently in 1981 presented a more involved system of staging (Table 41–7).[18] Unfortunately, the experience with these classification systems is limited, and it appears that use of the methods is slow to gain popularity.

PATIENT EVALUATION

The patient presenting with a salivary gland mass may have a variety of signs and symptoms because of the vast number of possible locations between the major and minor salivary glands. Certainly, for practical pur-

TABLE 41–7. Proposed TNM Classification of Levitt

T0	No clinical evidence of primary tumor
T1	Tumor 0.1 to 2 cm in diameter without significant local extension
T2	Tumor 2.1 to 4 cm in diameter without significant local extension
T3	Tumor 4.1 to 6.0 cm in diameter without significant local extension
T4a	Tumor >6 cm in diameter without significant local extension
T4b	Tumor of any size with significant local extension
N0	No evidence of regional lymph node involvement (including palpable but not suspicious regional lymph nodes)
N1	Evidence of regional lymph node involvement (including palpable and suspicious regional lymph nodes)
Nx	Regional lymph nodes not assessed
M0	No distant metastases
M1	Distant metastases, such as to bone or lung

Stage		
I	T1, N0, M0	
	T2, N0, M0	
II	T3, N0, M0	
III	T1, N1, M0	
	T2, N1, M0	
	T4a, N0, M0	
	T4b, N0, M0	
IV	T3, N1, M0	
	T4a, N1, M0	
	T4b, N1, M0	
	Any T, Any N and M 1	

poses the parotid and submandibular glands can be stressed in this discussion. The minor salivary gland tumors may cause signs and symptoms from the oral pharynx into the laryngopharyngeal region and tend to have less consistency in presentation.

The most common presentation of the parotid or submandibular gland neoplasm is a lump noted incidentally while washing the face or shaving. The history of duration is usually indefinite and not too meaningful. The location of the glands in relatively inconspicuous areas of the head and neck leads to this inaccuracy in time of onset and duration. The most common site for parotid neoplasms is the lower pole, or tail, of parotid area. Figure 41–3 shows a moderate-sized tail of parotid neoplasm presenting in the tail of the parotid gland. The mass in Figure 41–4 is more subtle than the mass in Figure 41–3 and represents a mixed cell tumor. Figure 41–5 illustrates a left parotid mass that was metastatic carcinoma from a nasopharyngeal primary. This location frequently remains unobserved by patients and may even be missed by physicians. Also, changes in the deep portions of the gland may go unnoticed for long periods of time. If the patient or family gives a history of definite rapid enlargement or change in growth pattern, the physician must pay particular attention to the possibility of malignancy or infection. It must always be remembered that the major salivary glands may be the location for metastases from other areas of the body. The majority of metastases are from squamous cell carcinoma of the skin or melanoma.[7] Figure 41–6 demonstrates a parotid mass that is a lymph node involved with squamous cell carcinoma metastatic from the ear.

The benign neoplasm located in the superficial lobe of the parotid will have no other signs or symptoms.

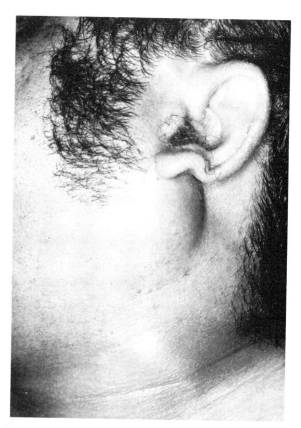

Figure 41–4. Left tail of parotid mass that was a mixed cell tumor.

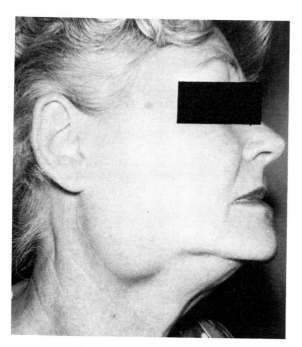

Figure 41–3. A right tail of parotid mass that represented a Warthin's tumor.

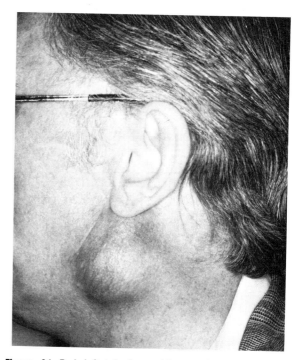

Figure 41–5. A left tail of parotid mass that was metastatic squamous cell carcinoma from a nasopharyngeal primary tumor.

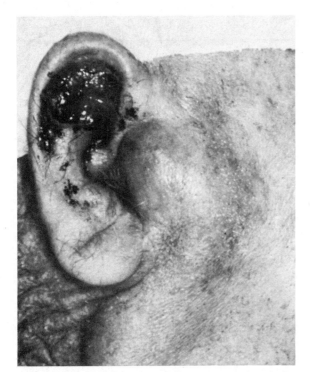

Figure 41–6. The parotid mass is a metastatic lymph node from the squamous cell carcinoma of the ear.

The physical examination will demonstrate a mobile nontender mass. The mass will usually be firm and solitary. The presence of multiple masses would be indicative of primary malignancy or metastatic disease. An exception would be the recurrent benign mixed tumor, which may have many foci of seeding.

A parotid region mass may indeed represent other anatomic structures in the area. The diagram in Figure 41–7 demonstrates the location of possible areas of confusion. The mandibular coronoid process and condyle may be prominent in the cheek and preauricular area, respectively. The masseter may be markedly hypertrophied (Fig. 41–8) and may cause confusion. The angle of the mandible may be prominent, and the transverse process of the second cervical bone will frequently present in the retromandibular region as a mass.

The lesion that involves the deep lobe of the parotid gland may be extending into the parapharyngeal space. These lesions can be examined intraorally by performing a thorough head and neck examination. The parapharyngeal space is bounded cephalad and laterally by the base of skull and mandible, respectively.[20] These boundaries make medial and caudal growth the path of least resistance (Fig. 41–9). In general, the patient notes minimal changes in voice or deglutition until the mass is large. As a mass in the parapharyngeal space enlarges, the nasopharynx, eustachian tube, and lateral oropharynx may be affected, as is demonstrated in the computerized tomographic (CT) scan in Figure 41–10, in which a parapharyngeal paraganglioma is displacing the pharynx and parotid. The most common history is probably the incidental finding of the lesion on medical or dental examination (Fig. 41–11).

On occasion, the history may include that of previous biopsy. The examiner may notice scarring and fibrosis of the palate. This practice means by definition that the constrictor and palatal musculature has been violated if the neoplasm has been entered and a successful biopsy has been obtained. Such a method of preoperative clinical evaluation is to be discouraged. It not only makes surgical removal more difficult in the palatal and pharyngeal area but also is commonly unsuccessful because of the depth of the neoplasm.

If the tumor is isolated to the parapharyngeal space, no palpable mass in the lateral face or neck will be observable or palpable. If the lesion is the true "dumbbell" tumor described by Thackray, it will pass through

Figure 41–7. Parotid region anatomic sites of confusion in physical examination. (1) Coronoid process; (2) angle of mandible; (3) condyle of mandible; (4) masseter muscle; and (5) transverse process.

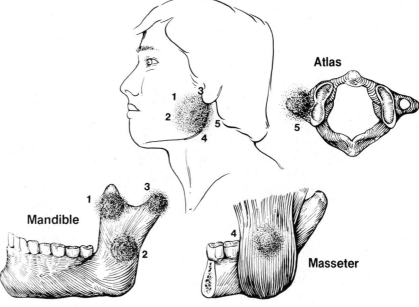

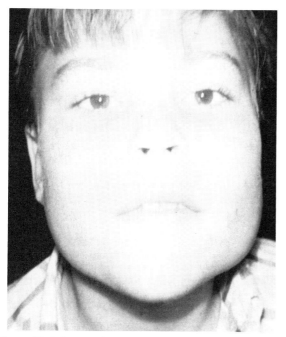

Figure 41–8. A parotid region prominence caused by masseter hypertrophy.

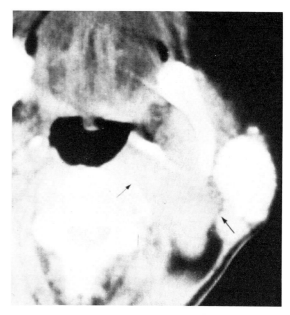

Figure 41–10. Computerized tomographic sialogram showing displacement of parotid laterally by parapharyngeal paraganglioma.

the stylomandibular tunnel into the retromandibular area.[4] The great vessels of the neck and the ninth, tenth, eleventh, and twelfth cranial nerves are located in this space. It is extremely rare to have nerve involvement by a tumor unless it is of neurogenous origin or is malignant. These tumors are now most clearly defined by using CT studies of the base of skull and neck.[6] Computerized radiographic imaging of the body tissues has helped the salivary gland surgeon mainly with the deep lobe tumors in preoperative planning and patient counseling. The CT scan in Figure 41–12 shows the combined use of sialography and CT to demonstrate a deep lobe mass.

Facial nerve paralysis or weakness associated with a salivary gland neoplasm is accepted as an extremely ominous sign. Conley and Haymaker report an incidence of facial paralysis in malignant neoplasms of the salivary gland as 12 per cent.[6] Eneroth reported an incidence of 14 per cent and a mortality rate of 100 per cent.[9] Adenoid cystic carcinoma is commonly associated with perineural invasion of the nerves. This is thought

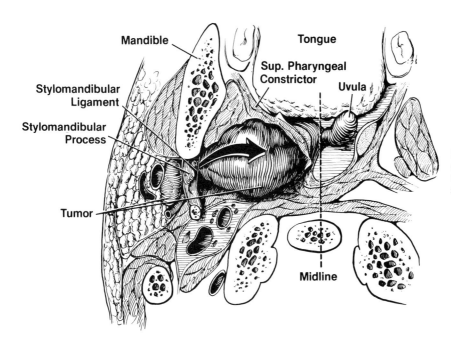

Figure 41–9. Diagram showing a dumbbell tumor and the anatomic relationships in the parapharyngeal space.

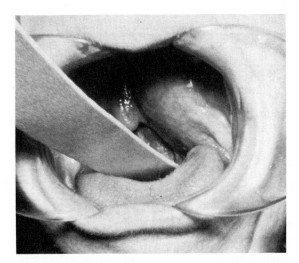

Figure 41–11. The patient demonstrates a palatal presentation of a parapharyngeal tumor.

to be the major route of spread and to lead to its poor long-term prognosis.

Metastatic lymph node involvement in primary salivary gland neoplasms in general occurs late in the course of the disease. Conley records an incidence of 60 per cent for metastasis in patients having facial paralysis.[6] A recent development of examining the neck with CT scanning for occult nodes may supplement the physical examination of the neck. Figure 41–13 shows a CT examination of the neck showing nodes that were not palpable on physical examination.

Eneroth examined pain as a possible indicator of malignancy and found 5.1 per cent of benign neoplasms presented with pain and 6.5 per cent of malignant neoplasms presented with pain.[9] Spiro and associates found that those malignant neoplasms presenting with pain carry a poorer prognosis.[27] He reported that the group presenting with pain had a 35 per cent 5-year survival rate compared with the nonpain group survival rate of 68 per cent.

The physical examination of the patient with a salivary gland mass requires that the physician note specifically several areas of the head and neck examination. It is particularly helpful to discern whether the primary mass is extraglandular or intraglandular. If an extraglandular mass is identified, a thorough examination of the head and neck for possible skin neoplasms should be performed. Squamous cell carcinoma and malignant melanoma are the most common malignancies metastatic to the parotid region. These malignancies may arise from relatively hidden areas of the hair-bearing scalp and eye. A complete examination of these areas along with the mucous membrane surfaces of the aerodigestive tract may uncover a primary lesion. Figure 41–14 demonstrates the large number and distribution of extraglandular lymph nodes in the parotid and submandibular region. In general, superficial or extraglandular nodes are mobile, and in the instance of the submandibular region the nodes may be rolled over the edge of the mandible. This is not possible if the mass is intraglandular because of the fascial attachments from the gland to the mandible. Careful scalp and eye examinations may reveal inconspicuous primary lesions metastatic to the salivary gland regions. The area of the retromandibular parotid gland extension is a difficult

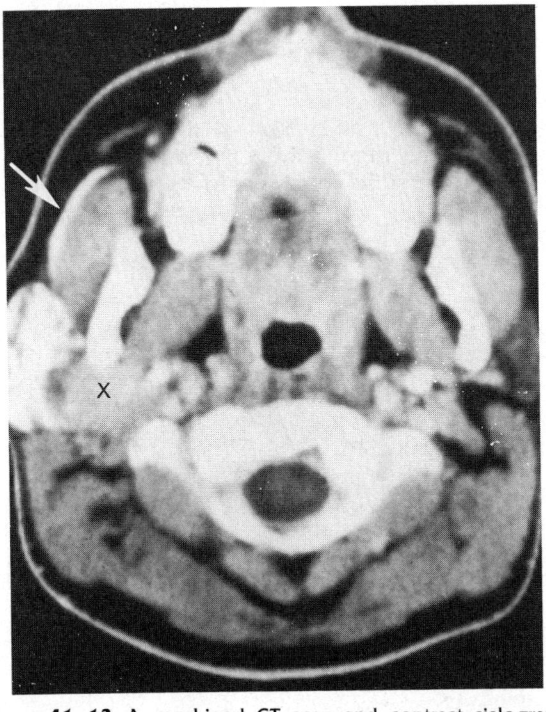

Figure 41–12. A combined CT scan and contrast sialogram demonstrating a deep lobe mass. The arrow demonstrates the parotid duct, and X shows the deep lobe mass.

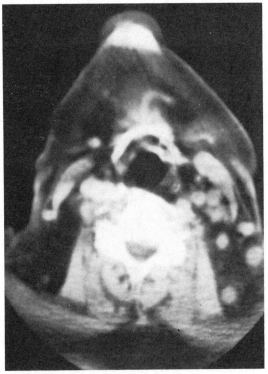

Figure 41–13. A CT scan showing nodes in the neck not palpable on physical examination.

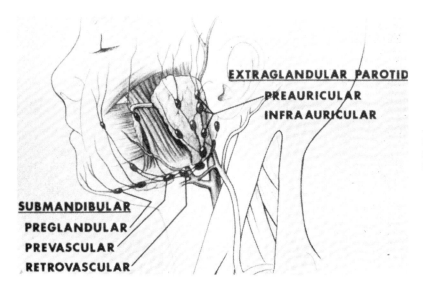

Figure 41–14. This diagram demonstrates the large number of extraglandular lymph nodes in the parotid and submandibular region.

area to evaluate and should be noted specifically in these patients (Fig. 41–15). The pharyngeal examination should note the presence of a parapharyngeal mass. Cranial nerve examination should be systematically performed and recorded in the record. Finally, the cervical lymph node chain should be palpated and suspicous nodes noted.

RADIOLOGY

The advances in radiographic imaging of body tissues have been phenomenal in the last decade. The sophisticated techniques of computed tomography have added much to the evaluation of many head and neck prob-

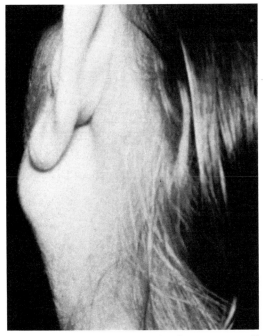

Figure 41–15. A posterior view of a large retromandibular parotid mass.

lems. Even though the salivary gland surgeon has seen these significant additions made to his armamentarium of diagnostic tests, there are only a few occasions when any procedures beyond the complete head and neck history and physical examination are warranted in evaluating salivary gland neoplasms.

It is imperative that the physician put the various diagnostic tests in perspective and be selective in ordering them. This is important from a cost-effective standpoint and also from that of the patient, who needs to understand that in the majority of salivary gland masses only an adequate microscopic examination of tissue will allow the physician the important information for decision-making regarding therapy. The ordering of multiple tests must not be done to delay the decision of salivary gland surgery. The decision to perform surgery can usually be made after the first examination of a salivary gland mass. It may be prudent to have an initial interview with the patient and schedule a follow-up appointment to further discuss surgery and allow the patient to adjust to the surgical recommendation.

In general, supplemental diagnostic tests should be reserved for the 10 per cent or fewer salivary gland masses that are located in the retromandibular and parapharyngeal region of the parotid or are in debilitated patients unable to tolerate surgery.

Plain Radiography

The plain radiograph is used in salivary gland evaluation when calculi are suspected. The majority of calculi are radiopaque concretions that can be seen on plain radiographs. The radiopaque submandibular calculi are easily visualized on plain radiographs (Figs. 41–16 and 41–17). There is no indication for a plain radiograph in routine evaluation of salivary gland masses. If base of skull involvement or mandibular erosion is suspected, much more information can be obtained from a computed tomography study.

Sialography

Contrast sialography is indicated in inflammatory diseases of the salivary glands in an effort to delineate

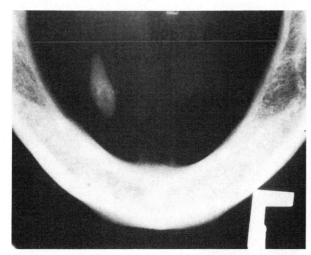

Figure 41–16. Plain film showing submandibular duct calculus.

their etiology. Salivary gland sialectasis, calculi, or strictures are the main problems to be identified by this method. It is seldom indicated and can be contraindicated in salivary gland neoplasms. The potential problem with performing contrast sialography in an obstructive situation is the possibility of inciting an inflammatory or infectious episode by injecting foreign material under pressure into the duct system. The exception may be the combined use of contrast sialography and computed tomography in studying deep lobe and parapharyngeal space masses (Fig. 41–18).

The technique utilizes a catheter placed in the parotid or submandibular gland duct for contrast introduction into the gland. The contrast is injected until the patient feels considerable pressure or slight pain. Many radiologists will allow the patient to perform the injection. A set of films are taken when filling is complete. These are followed by giving the patient a sialogogue to empty the ductal system. A normal gland will empty in less than 5 minutes. Follow-up films in 30 minutes may be helpful to observe delayed function of the gland.

Normally the ductal system will fill to the intercalated ducts. In strictures usually multiple areas of ductal narrowing can be identified. Calculi, if radiolucent, will be seen as a bubble in the duct (Fig. 41–19). Radiopaque calculi will be seen on a plain film taken prior to contrast injection. Sialectasis is diagnosed by observing areas of punctate, globular, or cavitary widening at the end of the duct (Fig. 41–20). Salivary gland neoplasms will distort the ductal architecture and leave areas of the gland devoid of contrast material.[15]

Radiosialography

Radiosialography is based on the concentrating ability of the salivary gland striated ductal epithelium.[26] The cells of this portion of the salivary gland unit have the ability to extract ^{99m}Tc (pertechnetate) from the capillary network of the salivary glands. Gamma emissions from the radioactive material secreted by the ducts can then be identified during scanning of the gland.

Radiosialography has been most useful in the presence of salivary gland masses in the elderly or debilitated. The scan will identify a mass lesion and delineate the location, size, and activity. The presence of a "hot" mass is usually indicative of a Warthin's tumor or oncocytoma (Fig. 41–21). However, several reports have indicated that "hot" masses can also represent malig-

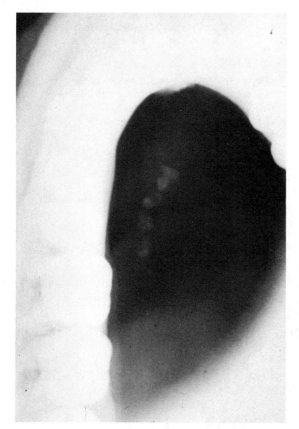

Figure 41–17. Submaxillary duct stones demonstrated on a plain radiograph.

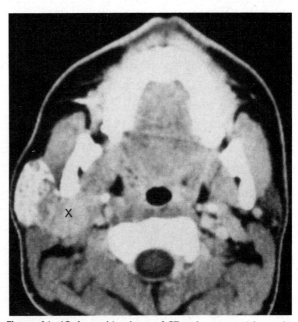

Figure 41–18. A combined use of CT and contrast sialography; X identifies a deep lobe tumor.

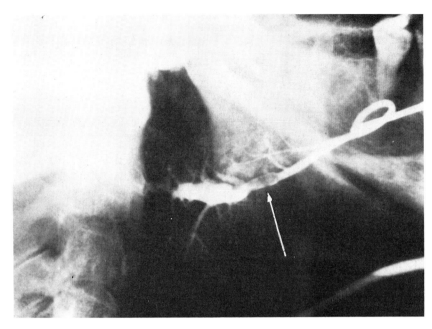

Figure 41–19. A sialogram outlining a calculus in the parotid duct.

nancy. A malignant neoplasm usually appears as a "cold" nodule (Fig. 41–22). Neoplasms such as a benign mixed tumor may on occasion appear cold. I have found the ^{99m}Tc scan to be helpful in counseling the elderly and high-risk surgical patient who presents with a salivary gland mass.

Computed Tomography

The advances in the field of computed tomography have revolutionized diagnostic medicine. This is certainly true of the head and neck region. These techniques allow the head and neck physician to investigate in a noninvasive manner the base of the skull and the retromandibular and parapharyngeal spaces. The study of a deep lobe mass extending into the parapharyngeal

space is an elegant application of this method of evaluation.

Several reports in the literature have advised the combination of contrast sialography and computed tomography for further delineation of the glandular tissue and neoplastic growth[11] (Fig. 41–23). It is probable that as the sophisticated new generations of equipment for computed tomography and nuclear magnetic resonance become available, this will be unnecessary.

Angiography

The use of conventional intra-arterial angiography or digital subtraction venous angiography (DSVA) for the evaluation of salivary gland neoplasms has limited application. Vascular studies of the deep lobe and para-

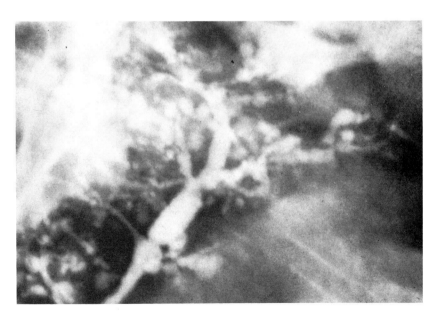

Figure 41–20. A sialogram demonstrating multiple punctate areas and widening of the ducts.

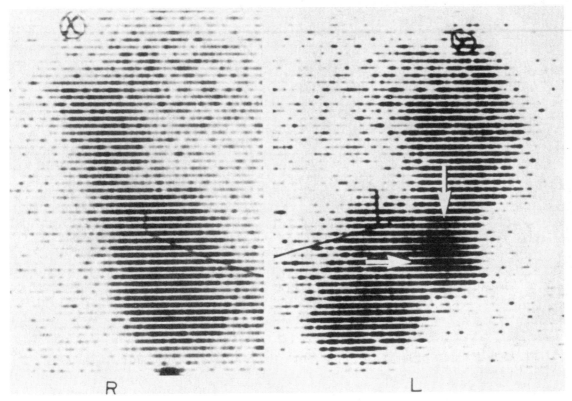

Figure 41–21. A radiosialogram demonstrating a Warthin's tumor as a "hot" spot on the scan.

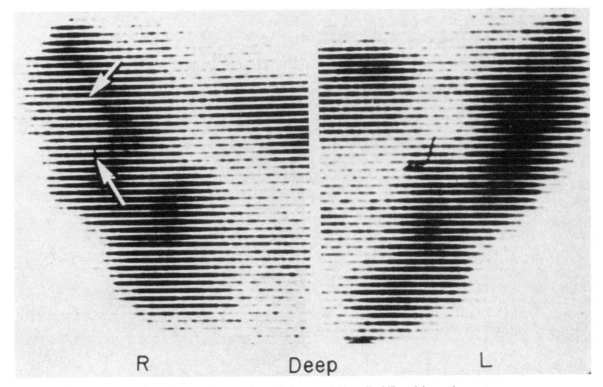

Figure 41–22. A radiosialogram demonstrating a "cold" nodule on the scan.

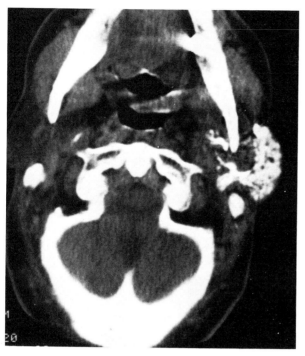

Figure 41–23. This patient had a combined study using sialography and CT scanning.

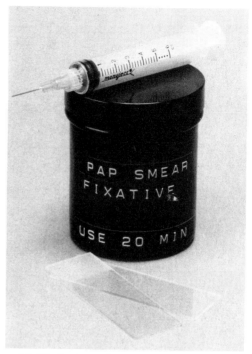

Figure 41–24. Basic equipment needed for a fine needle operation.

pharyngeal space tumors are useful in diagnostic and preoperative planning efforts. If a mass is suspected to be of vascular origin, a screening DSVA study is helpful. This study is performed on an outpatient basis and requires only a venous injection. If a vascular neoplasm or involvement is identified, further study utilizing conventional angiography may be necessary to selectively study the vascular supply to the area.

DIAGNOSTIC TECHNIQUES

Other diagnostic techniques short of excisional biopsy include core-needle biopsy and fine-needle aspiration biopsy. Techniques such as sialometry, scintigraphy, and radiosialometry are function tests that give no useful information in a diagnostic evaluation of salivary gland neoplasms.

Fine-Needle Aspiration Biopsy

The fine-needle aspiration biopsy was developed in the Scandinavian countries during the 1950s.[25] It has been advocated as a direct and inexpensive method of salivary gland neoplasm diagnosis. The method as described by Zajicek involves introducing a 22-gauge needle into the mass in question and obtaining an aspirate of tissue by applying negative pressure. The pressure is then allowed to equalize before removing the needle. The aspirate is then applied to a glass slide and is fixed in 95 per cent ethyl alcohol and Papanicolaou solution (Fig. 41–24). It must be stressed that this is a cytologic examination and requires a pathologist well versed in salivary gland pathologic appearance and cytologic methods. Sismanis and associates report an 82.2 per cent concurrence between cytologic diagnosis and subsequent histologic diagnosis.[25]

Complications from this method are minimal when the operator and pathologist are adept at the procedure. Suggestions that seeding along the tract of the needle may occur have not been substantiated by review of numerous cases.

Core-Needle Biopsy

In contrast to the fine-needle aspiration biopsy, which utilizes cytologic methods of evaluation, the core-needle biopsy actually uses a core of tissue for histologic examination. This should be viewed as an incisional biopsy and utilized when definitive surgery is not possible because of tumor size or patient disability. The large reticulum cell sarcoma (Fig. 41–25) is an example of a parotid mass successfully biopsied with a core biopsy.

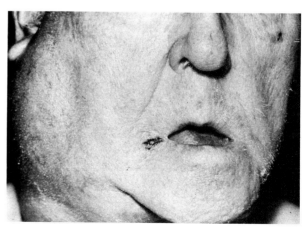

Figure 41–25. A large right parotid mass in a debilitated patient which was biopsied utilizing a core biopsy.

In contrast to the fine-needle aspiration biopsy, reports of seeding the tract of the needle path have appeared in the literature. These reports have occurred with the Vim-Silverman needle. It is now more common to use the disposable Medi-Cut needle, which brings about a smoother operation.

After all tests and examinations are performed, the excisional biopsy provides the physician and patient the most useful information. In the majority of patients, the biopsy is both diagnostic and therapeutic.

REFERENCES

1. Batsakis JG: Tumors of the Head and Neck. 2nd ed. Baltimore, Williams & Wilkins Co., 1979, p 9.
2. Berg JW et al: The unique association between salivary gland and breast cancer. JAMA 204:771, 1968.
3. Biorklund A, Eneroth CM: Management of parotid gland neoplasms. Am J Otolaryngol 1:155, 1980.
4. Carter BL, Karmody CS, Blickman JR, Panders AK: Computed tomography and sialography. 1. Normal anatomy. J Comput Assist Tomogr 5:42, 1981.
5. Chisholm DM, Waterhouse JP, Kraucunas E, Sciubba JJ: A quantitative ultrastructural study of the pleomorphic adenoma (mixed tumor) of human minor salivary glands. Cancer 34:1631, 1974.
6. Conley J, Haymaker RC: Prognosis of malignant tumors of the parotid gland with facial paralysis. Arch Otolaryngol 101:39, 1975.
7. Coulthard SW: Metastatic disease of the parotid gland. Otolaryngol Clin North Am 10:437, 1977.
8. Edington GM, Sheiham A: Salivary gland tumours and tumours of the oral cavity in Western Nigeria. Br J Cancer 20:20, 1966.
9. Eneroth CM: Facial nerve paralysis: A criterion of malignancy in parotid tumors. Arch Otolaryngol 95:300, 1972.
10. Eneroth CM: Salivary gland tumors in the parotid gland, submandibular gland and the palate region. Cancer 27:1415, 1971.
11. Eneroth CM, Franzen S, Zajicek J: Cytologic diagnosis on aspirates from 1000 salivary gland tumors. Acta Otolaryngol (Suppl) 244:167, 1967.
12. Eversole LR: Histogenic classification of salivary tumors. Arch Pathol 92:433, 1971.
13. Foote FW Jr, Frazell EL: Tumors of the major salivary glands. Cancer 6:1065, 1953.
14. Gallia LJ, et al: The incidence of neoplastic versus inflammatory disease in major salivary gland masses diagnosed by surgery. Laryngoscope 91:512, 1981.
15. Gates GA: Sialography and scanning of the salivary glands. Otolaryngol Clin North Am 10:379, 1977.
16. Gates GA: Radiosialographic aspects of salivary gland disorders. Laryngoscope 82:115, 1972.
17. Leegaard T, Lindeman H: Salivary gland tumors: Clinical picture and treatment. Acta Otolaryngol 263:155, 1970.
18. Levitt SH, et al: Clinical staging system for cancer of the salivary gland: A retrospective study. Cancer 47:2712, 1981.
19. McFarland J: Tumors of the parotid region. Surg Gynecol Obstet 57:104, 1933.
20. Patey DH, Thackray AC: The pathological anatomy and treatment of parotid tumors with retropharyngeal extension (dumbbell tumors). J Surg 44:352, 1956.
21. Redman RS, Sreabny LM: The prenatal phase of the morphosis of the rat parotid gland. Anat Rec 168:127, 1971.
22. Regezi JA, Batsakis JG: Histogenesis of salivary gland neoplasms. Otolaryngol Clin North Am 10:300, 1977.
23. Schneider AB, Favus MJ, Stachura ME, et al: Salivary gland neoplasms as a late consequence of head and neck irradiation. Ann Intern Med 87:160, 1977.
24. Schuller DE, McCabe BF: Salivary gland neoplasms in children. Otolaryngol Clin North Am 10:399, 1977.
25. Sismanis A, Strong MS, Merriam J: Fine needle aspiration biopsy diagnosis of neck masses. Otolaryngol Clin North Am 13:421, 1980.
26. Sour PM, Biller HF: The combined computerized tomography—sialogram. A technique to differentiate deep lobe parotid tumors. Ann Otol Rhinol Laryngol 88:590, 1979.
27. Spiro RH, Huvos AG, Strong EW: Cancer of the parotid gland. A clinicopathologic study of 288 primary cases. Am J Surg 130:452, 1975.

CHAPTER 42

Pathology of Tumors of the Salivary Glands

Mario A. Luna, M.D.

Although salivary gland tumors are relatively seldom observed, they have occasioned much interest and debate because of the variability in their structure and behavior. The difficulty of histologic diagnosis of some tumors of these glands is a matter of fairly general agreement among pathologists. As the result of several excellent clinical investigations, publications of numerous long-term follow-up studies, and the widespread participation of pathologists in seminars and workshops, many of the problems have been at least partially solved over the past decade. Still, some biologically proved cancers that lack the familiar histologic features of malignancy remain, as well as an apparently increasing number of benign lesions whose morphologic resemblance to cancer leads the alert pathologist to suspect carcinoma where none exists.

In addition to the rarity of salivary gland tumors and therefore the comparatively little experience of the pathologists with them, there are other reasons for the difficulties in histologic diagnosis. One is the overlying of histologic features found in different salivary gland tumors; for example, mixed tumors and adenoid cystic carcinomas may exhibit a similar growth pattern in localized areas. Another is that the histologic pattern in any given tumor may vary from field to field; thus, most malignant mixed tumors will contain both areas of completely benign mixed tumor and areas of overt carcinoma. In this event, a small biopsy specimen of such a lesion may lead to an incorrect diagnosis. Again, several different classifications of salivary gland tumors may be found in the literature,[9, 33, 37, 94] leading to the confusion of the pathologists and the clinicians.

DISTRIBUTION

In our experience, from 80 to 90 per cent of salivary gland tumors arise in the major glands, approximately 70 to 85 per cent of these being in the parotid gland and the remainder in the submaxillary glands.[3, 8, 32, 84] Tumors originate only rarely in the sublingual glands. Not only does the overall incidence of tumors differ strikingly, but the ratio between benign and malignant tumors depends largely upon the gland of origin. Benign tumors constitute from 65 to 80 per cent of the parotid neoplasms, 45 to 60 per cent of the submaxillary gland tumors, and 50 to 60 per cent of neoplasms in the minor accessory glands. The majority of tumors of the sublingual glands are malignant.[79]

The cause of the pronounced difference that exists in the relative incidence of the types of tumors in the major, lesser major, and accessory glands is unknown. Warthin's tumors, sebaceous tumors, and acinic cell carcinomas are virtually confined to the parotid gland, and adenoid cystic carcinomas account for most of the submaxillary tumors.[17, 25, 85]

GROSS EXAMINATION

To be most effective, the gross examination of specimens of the salivary glands should involve some foreknowledge of the reason for the surgical procedure. For parotid tumors, the specimen generally consists of the superficial lobe of the gland, sometimes of the entire gland, and occasionally of the contents of the neck and associated structures. In the presence of a submaxillary tumor, the gland and the contents of the submaxillary triangle constitute the surgical specimen.

When the specimen is received in the laboratory, the pathologist should orient it carefully in its normal anatomic position, then clean and dry it with gauze. As with any other neoplasm, three maneuvers are important in the gross examination: (1) measurement of the tumor, (2) delineation of the surgical margins, and (3) a description of the gross characteristics of the lesion, including circumscription, encapsulation, multilobulation, and apparent satellite nodules. All surfaces of the specimen representing the surgical margins should be painted with India ink and allowed to dry for 5 minutes. The pathologist next prepares blocks and sections for histologic study to demonstrate (1) the proximity of the lesion to the surgical margins and (2) the relationship of normal glandular tissue to the tumor.[77] Samples should also be taken of the lymph nodes and any other anatomic structure removed.

BIOPSY

The biopsy is the foundation upon which the diagnosis and treatment plan of any neoplasm is based. Therefore, biopsy becomes the sine qua non of oncologic surgery. The frozen section technique, the preoperative needle aspiration cytologic examination, the needle biopsy, and the incisional and excisional biopsy are discussed.

Frozen Section. The diagnosis of salivary gland tumors from *frozen sections* presents no more problems than it does of those elsewhere in the body.[77] Generally, one should have no trouble in identifying the types of tumors usually encountered. Most problems arise in studies of histologically exceptional mixed tumors, in some monomorphic adenomas, and in lymphomas.[47, 64] Unless a precise diagnosis modifies the surgical procedure, the indication for frozen section is to evaluate the margins of excision.[77] The plan for surgical treatment for tumors of the parotid and submaxillary glands is based primarily upon their size and clinical stage, rather than upon their histologic type.[51, 89] These variables cannot be assessed accurately until the tumor is surgically exposed.

Needle Biopsy. Needle biopsy is helpful in differentiating neoplastic from non-neoplastic diseases, and in diagnosing metastatic and inoperable cancers. In other circumstances, needle biopsy is not reliable; two of the most prevalent neoplasms, mixed tumors and adenoid cystic carcinomas, are at times indistinguishable by this method.[3]

Preoperative Needle Aspiration. For the cytologic diagnosis of salivary gland tumors, this technique has become popular during the past 20 years.[56] This procedure requires a highly qualified cytologist and a well-trained procurer of the specimen in order to ensure a correct interpretation. As documented in the medical literature, the diagnostic accuracy of the fine needle technique for tumors of the salivary glands is quite high, although the clinical value of the technique remains to be substantiated.[3, 56]

Excisional Biopsy. For tumors in the lateral lobe of the parotid gland, the minimal biopsy procedure is superficial or lateral parotidectomy, whereas for lesions located in the deep lobe it is almost total parotidectomy.[85] The latter procedure allows the surgeon to remove the tumor in question in its entirety, to identify the facial nerve and its branches, and to remove the parotid lymph nodes. In addition, it provides the pathologist with the best possible diagnostic material. The same considerations apply to tumors in the submaxillary glands, although the glands should be removed completely and in such a way as to include the connective tissue and the regional lymph nodes. This technique allows the surgeon to determine clearly the relation between the gland, the tumor, and the lingual, hypoglossal, and mylohyoid nerves.[17]

Incisional Biopsy. Except perhaps for tumors in the sublingual glands, incisional biopsy should not be encouraged.

HISTOCHEMISTRY

Hematoxylin and eosin have long been the standard tissue stains for examination by pathologists; in the large majority of cases, this alone permits an accurate diagnosis. Histochemistry, immunocytohistochemistry, enzyme histochemistry, and electron microscopy are ancillary, rather than diagnostic, methods.[3, 9]

No specific histochemical battery, however, is unique for the demonstration of disease of the salivary glands.[3, 12] The histochemistry of mucins and enzymes in tumors of these glands has been extensively studied, though its value as a diagnostic measure has not been particularly impressive.[3] The same thing may be said of immunocystohistochemistry.

Mucin stains (mucicarmine, and alcian blue, pH 2.5) and PAS (periodic acid–Schiff) with and without diastase digestion are the most useful special stains for establishing a diagnosis. Mucoepidermoid carcinomas are differentiated from squamous carcinoma by the presence of goblet or signet ring cells with large mucicarmine- and alcian blue–positive droplets in their cytoplasm.[1, 14, 86] The cytoplasm of at least some of the cells in acinic cell carcinomas contains PAS-positive, diastase-resistant secretory granules.[77] Clear cell carcinomas of salivary gland origin and metastatic renal cell carcinomas do not exhibit PAS-positive, diastase-resistant granules in the cytoplasm, and they may or may not contain glycogen.[26, 77] In addition, these tumors do not have mucicarmine- or alcian blue–positive secretions.[11, 43]

ELECTRON MICROSCOPY

The extent to which electron microscopy can aid in identifying neoplasms of the salivary glands varies. It may provide a specific diagnosis not otherwise obtainable, or it may offer information that is as easily available on routine light microscopy.[69, 72, 83] Despite its variable contribution, it is especially reliable in the identification of atypical acinic cell carcinomas, in questionable oncocytic tumors, and in distinguishing undifferentiated carcinomas from lymphomas.[3] It is pointed out, however, that electron microscopy does not distinguish benign from malignant tumors.

EMBRYOGENESIS AND HISTOLOGY OF MAJOR SALIVARY GLANDS

Embryogenesis

All the major salivary glands are ectodermally derived, and they arise in fundamentally the same manner by the growth of oral epithelium into the underlying mesenchyme.[9, 34] The epithelial buds that form the parotid and submaxillary glands appear in the sixth week of embryonic life, and those of the sublingual glands appear during the seventh to eighth weeks.

At the future site of the exit of the excretory ducts of the salivary glands, the oral epithelium thickens and forms a solid bud of epithelial cells that grow into the underlying mesenchyme. Cell proliferations and cleavages between terminal cell groups eventually result in the development of a multiple-branched structure of epithelial strands. Each of these strands is completely surrounded by a richly vascularized mesenchymal tissue. Terminal clusters of epithelial cells are found at the tips of the most distal branches. A tubuloalveolar pattern is formed when terminal cell clusters differentiate into round or oblate alveoli.[3] After this tubuloalveolar character is established, the individual cells undergo further cytodifferentiation of ductal and secretory end pieces in preparation for their various functions.[3] The secretory end pieces are connected to the developing ductal system by the terminal tubule complex.[2] It is generally accepted that the reserve cells of the excretory duct and the intercalated duct act as stem cells for the most differentiated cells of the salivary gland unit. Excretory duct stem cells give rise to the columnar and squamous cells of that duct, and intercalated duct stem cells give rise to the acinar cells, other intercalated duct cells, striated duct cells, and probably to the myoepithelial cells.[2, 34] The first gland to appear is the parotid, followed by the submaxillary and sublingual, when the embryo is about 10, 18, and 22 mm, respectively, in crown-to-rump length.

Histologic Appearance

Salivary glands in histologic sections appear as a number of lobules, separated from each other by connective tissue septa. The entire structure of each gland is surrounded by a connective tissue capsule, which may be substantial in some glands and rather insignificant in others.

The ducts of the salivary glands form a tree-like pattern. The finest branches are the intercalated ducts; the larger branches and the stem form the excretory ducts. Striated ducts usually are present between the intercalated and excretory ducts. The acini are terminally located at the tips of the intercalated ducts. Excretory and striated ducts are located in the connective tissue septa, and smaller striated ducts, intercalated ducts, and acini make up the bulk of the lobules (Fig. 42–1).

The acini consist of a number of pyramidal cells arranged around a central lumen, myoepithelial cells being interposed between them and the basement membrane. The acinar cells may be serous, mucinous, and seromucinous. Serous cells are found predominantly in the parotid gland and in variable amounts in the submaxillary gland. Mucinous cells are found in sublingual and submaxillary glands, in many accessory glands, and in small amounts in the parotid glands of young individuals.[9] Seromucinous cells are found in the sublingual

and many minor salivary glands. The intercalated ducts are formed by a single layer of cuboidal cells; myoepithelial cells may appear between these cells and the basal lamina (Fig. 42–1). The striated ducts are lined by a single layer of tall to low columnar eosinophilic cells, and fine striations are present at the basal portion of the cytoplasm. The excretory ducts are located entirely within connective tissue septa; they are lined by multiple (usually two) layers of epithelial cells, which may vary in shape from cuboidal to squamous (Fig. 42–1).

The most active part of the salivary gland duct unit is at the junction of the intercalated ducts and the acini. Intercalated ducts probably are the source of reserve cells. Under certain influences the reserve cells may proliferate and differentiate into a number of cellular types, such as acinar cells, intercalated duct cells, and myoepithelial cells. It is also from this cellular zone of the salivary duct unit that most tumors of the salivary glands arise.[2, 34]

HISTOGENESIS AND CLASSIFICATION

Three types of tumors must be distinguished in the region of the salivary glands:

1. *Sialadenoma*, or *sialoma*, a tumor of the salivary gland parenchyma.

2. *Synsialadenoma*, or *synsialoma*, a tumor that arises within the salivary gland capsule from the supporting connective tissues, such as blood vessels and nerves.

3. *Parasialadenoma*, or *parasialoma*, a neoplasm of the surrounding tissues that may simulate a salivary gland.

Tumors of the salivary parenchyma, or sialomas, are the most common and by far the most important of all neoplasms involving these structures.

Current classifications of tumors of the salivary gland parenchyma are based upon their morphologic, cytologic, and biologic features.[9, 33, 37, 94] Because observers do not universally agree as to their cell of origin, for the present, histogenic classifications are premature.[34] Most classifications of salivary gland tumors are based

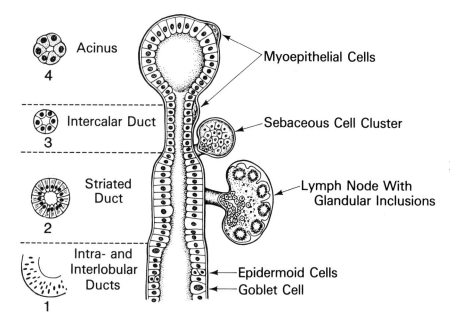

Figure 42–1. Schematic diagram of the microanatomy of the salivary unit.

upon the scheme devised by Foote and Frazell[37]; with some modification, it is one that offers flexibility and usefulness. The main modification of this classification relates to the accepted view of the clinical behavior of mucoepidermoid and acinic cell carcinomas. This author strongly feels that mucoepidermoid and acinic cell carcinomas must be classified as cancers, but with variable histologic grades and corresponding behavioral patterns. The classification used in this chapter, presented in Table 42–1, deals only with epithelial tumors of either neoplastic or presumed neoplastic origin.

Eversole[34] and Batsakis[2] postulate that the reserve or stem cell of the salivary duct system is the cell responsible for neoplasia. Two ductal reserve cells are important: the intercalated and the excretory. Application of the oncogenic-carcinogenic stimulus upon the process of morpho- and cytodifferentiation results in the formation of different neoplastic types according to the stage of development at which the stimulus acts. Whether the result of this epigenetic neoplastic event is benign or malignant will depend upon the overall extent of some differentiation within reserve cell components. Anaplastic carcinomas arise from undifferentiated cells, analogous to the embryonic primordium before the first regulatory event in cytodifferentiation.[2] Under this hypothesis, the intercalated duct reserve cells are the epithelial source for adenoid cystic carcinoma, acinic cell carcinoma, mixed tumor, and monomorphic adenoma.[2, 34] Stimulated excretory duct reserve cells are the source for mucoepidermoid carcinoma, papillary mucinous adenoma, squamous carcinoma, and intraductal papilloma.[2, 34]

The myoepithelial cells play an important role in the composition and growth of several salivary gland tumors. With the exception of the myoepithelioma, it is doubtful that the myoepithelial cell is the primary cell of origin for any salivary gland tumor; however, its participation in mixed tumor, in adenoid cystic carci-

noma, in salivary duct carcinoma, and in intercalated duct carcinoma cannot be denied.[7]

GROSS PATHOLOGIC FEATURES

The gross configuration of the tumor, the appearance of its cut surface, and the relationship between neoplasm and normal tissue often provide strong clues to the diagnosis.[77] A tumor bulging out of the cut surface is usually benign (mixed tumor, monomorphic adenoma, or Warthin's tumor) (Fig. 42–2). Malignant mixed tumor without capsular invasion may have a similar appearance. According to LiVolsi and Perzin,[60] this type of malignant mixed tumor does not metastasize; hence, the most important question before the pathologist is the adequacy of the surgical margins of the tumor.

Most of the benign tumors of the salivary glands consists of a single mass of tissue with well-circumscribed margins. In contrast, malignant tumors are often composed of multiple separate nests of cells of variable size and configuration. These nests usually lie in a dense fibrous stroma that lacks the myxoid or cartilaginous appearance of mixed tumors. If the tumor has ill-defined margins and appears to infiltrate normal tissue, it is usually malignant. Oncocytoma, Warthin's tumor, and neurofibroma are three of the benign tumors that may have this appearance. Adenoid cystic carcinoma, high-grade mucoepidermoid carcinoma, poorly differentiated adenocarcinoma, and invasive malignant mixed tumor characteristically have indistinct, highly invasive borders (Fig. 42–3). A tumor with pushing margins and a cystic or partially cystic cut surface may turn out, on microscopic examination, to be a low-grade mucoepidermoid carcinoma, acinic cell carcinoma, monomorphic adenoma, Warthin's tumor, or branchial cleft cyst (Fig. 42–4).

Solid tumors with pushing margins and brown, ho-

TABLE 42–1. Classification of Epithelial Salivary Gland Tumors

Benign
    Mixed tumor
    Warthin's tumor
    Monomorphic adenoma
        Basal cell adenoma, dermal analogue tumor
        Salivary duct adenoma
        Oncocytoma
        Myoepithelioma
        Sebaceous lymphadenoma
    Lymphoepithelial lesion
Malignant
    Mucoepidermoid carcinoma
    Adenoid cystic carcinoma
    Acinic cell carcinoma
    Malignant mixed tumor
    Adenocarcinoma; NOS
    Salivary duct carcinoma
    Intercalated duct carcinoma
    Terminal duct carcinoma
    Squamous cell carcinoma
    Miscellaneous (sebaceous, oncocytic, lymphoepithelial)
    Undifferentiated carcinoma
    Metastatic
    Unclassified

NOS = Not otherwise specified.

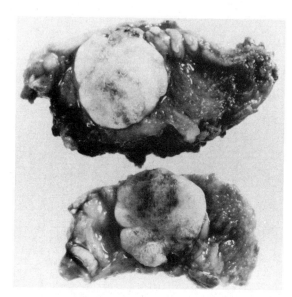

Figure 42–2. A tumor that bulges out of the cut surfaces is usually benign. Mixed tumor, Warthin's tumor, monomorphic adenoma, and preinvasive malignant mixed tumor may have this gross appearance.

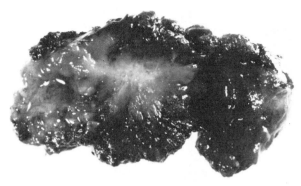

Figure 42–3. A tumor with indistinct and highly infiltrative borders is almost always malignant. Adenoid cystic carcinoma, high-grade mucoepidermoid carcinoma, undifferentiated carcinoma, and malignant mixed tumor have highly invasive borders.

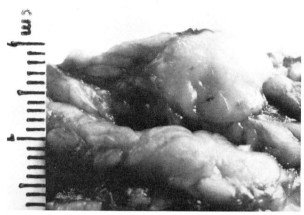

Figure 42–5. Solid tumors with pushing margins and brown homogeneous cut surfaces usually are Warthin's tumor, oncocytomas, enlarged lymph nodes, or acinic cell carcinomas.

mogeneous cut surfaces usually are oncocytomas, Warthin's tumors, or acinic cell carcinomas (Fig. 42–5). The majority of the solid tumors with lobulated margins and a firm, gray surface are of the mixed type. All these lesions can be readily differentiated on microscopic examination. Recurrent mixed tumors and some monomorphic adenomas (skin analogue tumors) often consist of multiple nodules of tissue (Fig. 42–6). The pathologist should study carefully the relationship of the tumor to the adjacent normal tissue. Monomorphic adenomas and recurrent mixed tumors, regardless of the pattern, should have circumscribed margins with pushing borders and should not invade adjacent tissue.[4, 11, 77]

A well-circumscribed parotid mass consisting of fish-flesh gray tissue may be an enlarged intraparotid lymph node. These lymph nodes may become enlarged because of nonspecific reactive hyperplasia, toxoplasmosis, granulomatous diseases, metastatic carcinoma, or malignant lymphoma. Warthin's tumor is the neoplasm that more often arises in ectopic ductal epithelium within parotid lymph nodes. Rarely, mixed tumor,

monomorphic adenoma, and acinic cell carcinoma may develop within ectopic salivary gland tissues.[4, 5, 13, 75, 78]

BENIGN EPITHELIAL TUMORS

Mixed tumor (pleomorphic adenoma) and Warthin's tumor are the most common benign salivary gland tumors.[33, 94] Warthin's tumor and sebaceous lymphadenoma are observed almost exclusively in the parotid gland, whereas the other benign tumors may be found in any major gland (Table 42–2). Warthin's tumor, oxyphilic cell adenoma, and benign lymphoepithelial lesions may be bilateral and multiple.[96] Mixed tumor, basal cell adenoma, and sebaceous adenoma rarely are bilateral. The benign lymphoepithelial lesion probably represents a type of autoimmune process, rather than a neoplastic disease.[9, 67]

Mixed Tumors

Mixed tumors (*pleomorphic adenomas*) represent 60 or 70 per cent of all neoplasms of the major glands.[32, 33, 37, 94] Although the distribution of these tumors varies widely, a superficial lobe of the parotid gland is the usual site; approximately 84 per cent are located in the parotid glands, 8 per cent in the submaxillary glands, 6.5 per cent in the accessory glands of the upper aerodigestive tract, and 0.5 per cent in the sublingual glands.[11, 33] Bilateral tumors are extremely rare.[96]

Grossly, mixed tumors are often irregular, lobulated, and bosselated. The cut surface is gray or blue, depending upon the amount of chondroid tissue present. The tumors are enclosed within an uneven connective tissue capsule, which is well developed and thick in some areas, and thin and incomplete in others (Fig. 42–7). Regardless of the completeness of the capsule or its absence, the tumor is clearly demarcated.[37] Multiple nodules often protrude from the main mass, but all are connected to the main tumor by slender strands of neoplastic tissue. Only 0.5 per cent of the mixed tumors are multicentric.[96] Recurrent mixed tumors have a strong tendency to be multinodular.

Microscopically, it is characteristic of mixed tumors

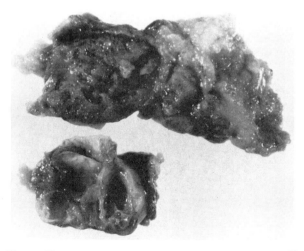

Figure 42–4. A tumor with pushing margins and cystic or partially cystic cut surfaces may be Warthin's tumor, branchial cleft cyst, monomorphic adenoma, low-grade mucoepidermoid carcinoma, or acinic cell carcinoma.

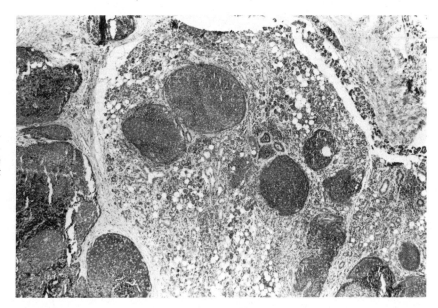

Figure 42–6. Multiple, well-circumscribed nodules are often seen in recurrent mixed tumor, dermal analogue monomorphic adenoma, and recurrent low-grade carcinomas.

that their histologic appearance also varies, not only in different tumors, but in different parts of the same tumor as well. A mixture of ductal, myoepithelial, and mesenchymal cells may be observed (Fig. 42–8). The ductal cells are of many types and are arranged in numerous patterns; they form glands, tubules, solid nests, ribbons, or files. Frequently, metaplastic changes (squamous, oncocytic, or sebaceous) are present in the ductal cells. The stroma of the mixed tumor is also pleomorphic and consists of admixtures of mucoid, myxoid, chondroid, and hyaline tissues and, on rare occasions, of bone or fat. The myoepithelial cells are of two types: spindle and plasmacytoid. The spindle cells are often grouped in a palisade arrangement, thus simulating a benign neoplasm of smooth muscle, and the plasmacytoid cells are usually arranged in solid nests or cords.

Related to, if not directly responsible for, the structural complexity and pleomorphism of the mixed group of neoplasms is the role of the myoepithelial cells. A number of authors have suggested that these cells are responsible for the production of the myxoid, chondroid, and osseous matrix, and that they may differentiate into myxoid, clear, myoid, and hyaline cells.[7, 27] Electron microscopic studies of mixed tumors have demonstrated cells of ductal and myoepithelial character, with precursor cells and transitional forms.[27, 61] The

proportion between ductal, myoepithelial, and mesenchymal elements, as well as the degree of stromal and epithelial metaplasia, are responsible for the structural variation and diversity of the histologic appearance of one lesion from another and in different parts of the same tumor.

Occasionally, one may find it difficult to distinguish between benign and malignant mixed tumors. The malignant mixed tumor is a destructive, infiltrating lesion, in stark contrast to the benign tumor with its expanding, encapsulated margins. No single criterion qualifies the malignancy of these tumors. Some useful diagnostic features of borderline tumors are as follows:

1. Micronecrosis.
2. Dystrophic calcification.
3. Atypical mitosis.
4. Extensive hyalinization of the residual mixed tumor.
5. Solid areas resembling lobular carcinoma of the breast.[11, 60]

When all these features are observed in a mixed tumor, it is qualified as malignant.

In a few cases, a mixed tumor might be confused with an adenoid cystic carcinoma. The most helpful feature in distinguishing between the two is the presence of myxoid or chondroid stroma in the mixed tumor, as opposed to the poorly cellular collagenous stroma of the adenoid cystic carcinoma. The mucoid change, however, which is so typical of the mixed tumor, sometimes is found in an adenoid cystic carcinoma. Here, the distinguishable feature is the clear demarcation between epithelial cells and mucoid intercellular material in adenoid cystic carcinoma, whereas ·the cells in mixed tumors often appear to blend with the mucin. Other features that confirm a diagnosis of adenoid cystic carcinoma are its highly invasive growth pattern and its tendency to involve nerves. Diagnostic problems usually can be resolved if a sufficient amount of tissue from the tumor is examined.

The clinical course of a mixed tumor depends on the type of initial treatment, rather than on the microscopic appearance of the tumor.[11, 31, 33, 68] Foote and Frazell[37]

TABLE 42–2. Benign Salivary Gland Tumors, Distribution by Site*

Site	Parotid (n = 208)	Submaxillary (n = 22)
Mixed	75%	56%
Warthin's tumor	16%	—
Adenoma	4%	4%
Hemangioma	3%	9%
Lymphangioma	1%	9%
Miscellaneous	1%	22%

*Data extracted from Skolnik EM, et al: Tumors of the major salivary glands. Laryngoscope 87:834, 1977.

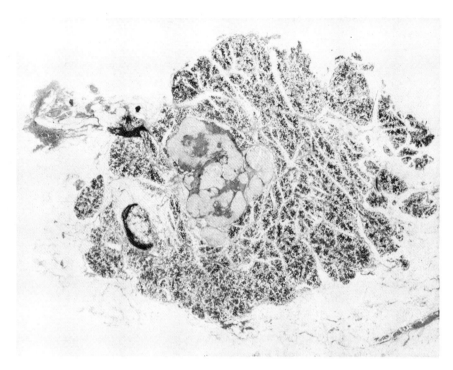

Figure 42–7. Whole organ section of a mixed tumor with varying thickness of capsule.

classified mixed tumors into these categories: (1) principally myxoid, (2) equally myxoid and cellular, (3) predominantly cellular, and (4) extremely cellular. They reported that the cellular and extremely cellular variants tend to have the highest recurrence rate. This observation has not been reported by others; in fact, in two recent investigations, most recurrent mixed tumors were found to be hypocellular, with abundant chondromyxoid stroma.[57] The rate of recurrence of parotid mixed tumors following lateral lobectomy or total parotidectomy, as indicated by the position of the tumor, varies from zero to 2 per cent, in contrast to a much higher recurrence rate for enucleation of the tumor.[11, 85]

Recurrent Mixed Tumor

A recurrent mixed tumor is grossly characterized by the presence of multiple, round, well-circumscribed

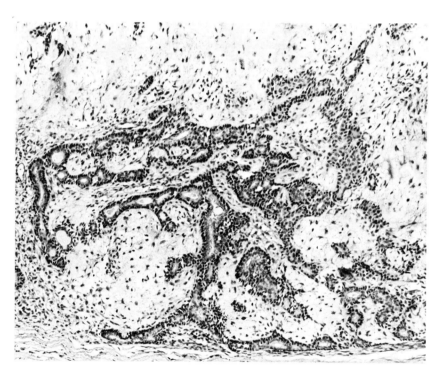

Figure 42–8. This mixed tumor contains the characteristic mixture of epithelial and mesenchymal components.

nodules growing in the salivary gland tissue, in the adipose tissue adjacent to the gland, or in scar tissue from a previous surgical procedure. Histologically, recurrent mixed tumors exhibit the same growth pattern observed in other benign mixed tumors, and the tumor cells have benign cytologic features (Fig. 42–9).

Carcinoma may arise in recurrent mixed tumors; therefore, when a resection has been performed for the recurrence, each nodule should be examined microscopically because carcinoma may be found in any one of the nodules.[77]

Warthin's Tumor (Papillary Cystadenoma Lymphomatosum)

Warthin's tumor accounts for 2 to 6 per cent of all parotid tumors and is the second most common benign neoplasm of the salivary glands. It almost always involves only the parotid gland, although it may arise in lymph nodes superficial or medial to this gland.[9, 13] A significant number of patients have bilateral or multiple growths, or both. In the review by Dietert,[28] 21 tumors were bilateral and four of these were bilateral simultaneously.

Warthin's tumor may develop in patients of any age, although it is usually observed in those over 40. The incidence is eight times higher in men than in women.

Grossly, Warthin's tumor is well circumscribed, soft and cystic. The lumen contains a creamy substance resembling pus or caseous material. Microscopically, the tumor is composed of papillary elements lining cystic spaces in a lymphoid stroma (Fig. 42–10). The epithelium typically is arranged in two layers, the inner layer consisting of tall, cylindric, oncocytic cells, and the outer layer consisting of cuboidal cells abutting the basement membrane. Other types of epithelial cells, such as goblet, sebaceous, and squamous cells, may also be found. The associated lymphoid tissue is benign, yet it may manifest varying degrees of reactivity. The lymphoid stroma is composed predominantly of E rosette-forming T lymphocytes, and a smaller number of

surface immunoglobulin-positive B lymphocytes. The relative distribution of the T and B lymphocytes is similar to that found in normal and reactive lymph nodes.[48, 95]

According to the most widely accepted theory concerning its histogenesis, Warthin's tumor originates in a heterotopic salivary gland duct in the lymph nodes of the parotid gland, both inside and outside the parenchyma. Functional immunologic studies, in conjunction with morphologic observations, support the concept that the lymphoid component of Warthin's tumor is derived from a pre-existing lymph node.[48, 95]

Convincing documentation of malignant transformation of Warthin's tumor has been reported in only six cases in the American literature.[63] Spontaneous malignant propensity is of such a low order as to be nonexistent.

Monomorphic Adenomas

Monomorphic adenomas are benign growths in which the epithelium forms a regular pattern, usually glandular, and in which there is no evidence of the mesenchyma-like tissue so characteristic of mixed tumor. Table 42–3 depicts the histogenic and histologic classification of monomorphic adenomas, as proposed by Batsakis, Brannon, and Sciubba.[5]

BASAL CELL ADENOMA

Basal cell adenoma accounts for approximately 54 per cent of all monomorphic adenomas and represents 1 to 3 per cent of the tumors of the major salivary gland.[5, 69] Although it is most often observed in females over 60 years of age, the broad range of age distribution (32 to 87 years) indicates that basal cell adenoma should be considered in the differential diagnosis of salivary gland tumors, even in persons in the eighth and ninth decades of life.[5, 33] The parotid gland and the minor salivary glands of the upper lip are the usual sites of this type

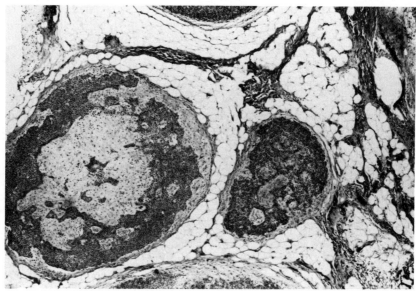

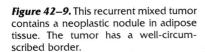
Figure 42–9. This recurrent mixed tumor contains a neoplastic nodule in adipose tissue. The tumor has a well-circumscribed border.

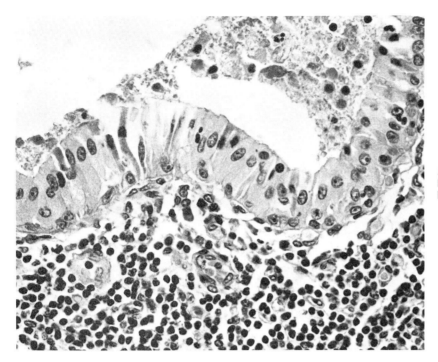

Figure 42–10. Warthin's tumor, exhibiting a double row of epithelial cells in lymphoid tissue.

of tumor. Basal cell adenoma of a submaxillary gland is more rare.

Grossly, basal cell adenomas are round or oval in shape and are encapsulated by fine fibrous connective tissues. The cut surface is grayish-white. In many cases, cystic formations containing mucinous fluids are present in the center of the tumor. In general, the adenomas tend to be smaller than mixed tumors, their greatest diameter being less than 2 cm.

Three basic histologic patterns are found in basal cell adenomas: (1) trabecular-tubular, (2) solid, and (3) canalicular.[5, 33, 69] The trabecular-tubular and solid types are often combined, and this finding serves to demonstrate that there is no dividing line between these histologic subtypes. Microscopically, the tumors are composed of

TABLE 42–3. Histogenetic Classification of
Monomorphic Adenoma*

A. **Terminal duct origin**
   1. Basal cell adenomas
      a. Solid
      b. Trabecular
      c. Canalicular
   2. Dermal analogue tumor
   3. Salivary duct adenoma
   4. Clear cell adenoma (?)
B. **Terminal or striated duct origin**
   1. Sebaceous adenoma
   2. Sebaceous lymphadenoma
C. **Striated duct origin**
   1. Oncocytoma
   2. Cystadenolymphoma
D. **Proximal duct origin**
   1. Mucinous adenoma
   2. Epidermoid papillary adenoma

*From Batsakis JG, Brannon RB, Sciubba JJ: Clin Otolaryngol 6:129, 1981. Permission granted by Blackwell Scientific Publications Ltd., Oxford.

dark, round to oval nuclei set in a scant basophilic cytoplasm. The cells are arranged in solid nests, buds, and cords with palisading peripheral rows (Fig. 42–11); in the minor glands, the tumor cells are usually arranged in tubules, rather than in solid nests. The parenchyma and stroma are well demarcated by a prominent basement membrane.

The monomorphic appearance and the absence of chondroid tissue and myxoid stroma differentiate basal cell adenoma from mixed tumor. The basal cell adenoma has sometimes been mistaken for adenoid cystic carcinoma. The two features that help to distinguish these lesions are (1) the circumscription of the basal cell adenoma, in contrast to the invasive pattern of adenoid cystic carcinoma, and (2) the lack of vascularity in the microcystic areas of adenoid cystic carcinoma, which contrasts with the numerous endothelial cells lining channels in basal cell adenoma. The vascular pattern should be interpreted with caution, however, especially in limited biopsy material. This author has observed focal areas in adenoid cystic carcinoma of the same vascular pattern as is encountered in basal cell adenoma. Similarly, the vascular pattern of the basal cell adenoma can be obscured in the presence of fibrosis. In the experience of the author and others, special stains are of no value in distinguishing between these tumors.[5, 70]

The recurrence rate of basal cell adenoma is quite low. Unequivocal acceptance of malignant transformation of the tumor cannot be made in light of the fact that, in reported cases, identification of a still recognizable residual benign tumor is not possible.[5]

Batsakis and Brannon[4] have used the term *dermal analogue tumors* to describe *membranous monomorphic adenomas*. The biologic behavior of these monomorphic adenomas appears to be somewhat different from that of other monomorphic adenomas; in three of the eight cases they observed, evidence of recurrence was apparent.[4]

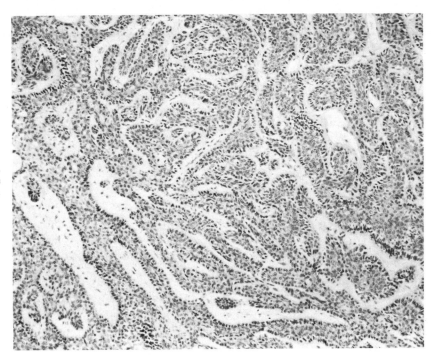

Figure 42–11. Basal cell adenoma, showing nests of cytologically benign basaloid cells with peripheral palisading.

Dermal analogue tumors are often multicentric and multilobular. Usually they are not encapsulated (Fig. 42–6); as a consequence, an invasive quality is imparted to this group, with lobular and cellular extensions separated by stroma. Microscopically, these adenomas are characterized by excessive production of an eosinophilic basal laminar material presenting the following features:

1. Hyaline cuffs around blood vessels within the tumor.

2. Small droplets surrounded by epithelial cells.

3. Large coalescent masses entrapping pyknotic cells (Fig. 42–12).

The parenchymal cells are similar to those found in solid basal cell adenomas and, like many of them, manifest epidermoidal changes, keratinization, and, less often, sebaceous differentiation.

Although the majority of these adenomas are located in the parotid gland, they have been observed in the submaxillary gland and arising within peri- or intraparotid lymph nodes.[4] Synchronous or metachronous ad-

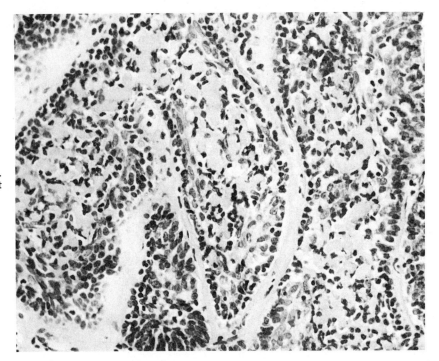

Figure 42–12. Dermal analogue tumor. Note abundant interepithelial basement membrane material.

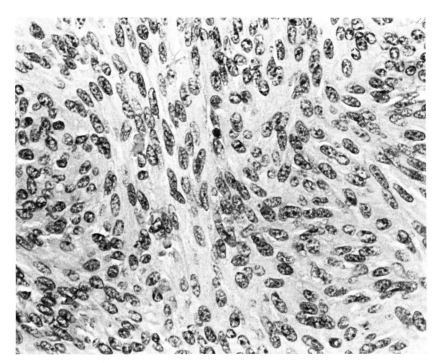

Figure 42–13. Spindle-cell myoepithelioma.

nexal cutaneous tumors, including dermal cylindromas, trichoepitheliomas, and eccrine spiradenomas, have been reported in patients with salivary dermal analogue adenomas.[45] No other monomorphic adenoma exhibits such combinations.

MYOEPITHELIOMA

Myoepithelioma is a rare type of monomorphic adenoma, accounting for less than 1 per cent of all salivary gland tumors.[83] Its distribution, clinical behavior, and gross appearance upon clinical presentation is similar to that of the mixed tumor. Most of the patients with this tumor are in their sixth decade of life.

Microscopically, myoepitheliomas exhibit three cellular types: spindle, plasmacytoid, and mixed cell. The spindle cells have centrally located nuclei; tend to be bipolar, with eosinophilic, granular to fibrillar cytoplasm; and are often arranged in fascicles, resembling tumors of smooth muscle (Fig. 42–13). The cytoplasm of the plasmacytoid cells contains distinctive eosinophilic hyaline material, and their nuclei are crowded to one pole (Fig. 42–14). The mixed cell type of myoepithelioma is composed of an admixture of spindle and plasmacytoid cells. The pattern of growth ranges from predominantly solid lesions with minimal myxoid stroma to those with a significant amount of background. This adenoma is often mistaken for neurilemoma, smooth muscle tumor, fibroma, and sarcomas of different types. A malignant variant is extremely

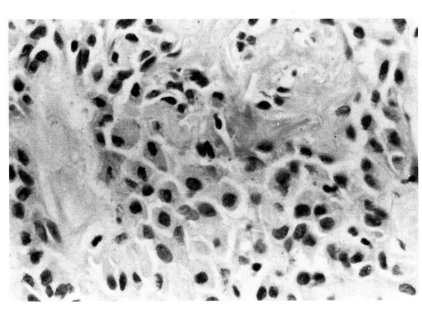

Figure 42–14. Plasmacytoid hyaline cells in a myoepithelioma.

unusual.[5, 11, 83] In the author's experience, this variant is a frequently observed component of malignant mixed tumor.

ONCOCYTOMA

Oncocytoma, or *oxyphilic adenoma*, arises in the parotid gland, the submaxillary glands, and the minor salivary glands. It accounts for less than 1 per cent of all salivary gland tumors. Patients with this tumor usually are in the older group, the average age being 72 years.[9, 52]

When found in the major salivary glands, oncocytoma is well circumscribed and usually has a solid, yellow-tan cut surface. Microscopically, it is composed of large polyhedral cells of varying sizes and shapes, with abundant eosinophilic granular cytoplasm (Fig. 42–15). The nuclei usually are single and pyknotic. The cells are arranged in columns, solid cords, or in a few tumors, in tubular or acinar formations. Occasionally, multiple small foci aggregates of oncocytes are found in glands that may also harbor adenomatous nodules and may be appropriately regarded as nodular oncocytic hyperplasia or oncocytosis.[9]

The hallmark of oncocytomas is the presence of true oncocytes that contain large numbers of mitochondria (Fig. 42–16); in the absence of these mitochondria, the oncocyte cannot be conclusively identified. The demonstration of the oncocyte in controversial lesions ultimately requires ultrastructural examination,[9, 52] because histochemical reactions, such as phosphotungstic acid hematoxylin, Bensley's aniline–acid fuchsin, and periodic acid–Schiff stains, are not reliable.[9] Cells with oncocytic features may be identified focally in acinic cell carcinomas, mixed tumors, malignant mixed tumors, and mucoepidermoid carcinomas. The diagnosis of oncocytoma should be made only when the entire lesion contains oncocytic cells. Solid oncocytic nodules should be considered neoplastic.

Pure oncocytomas are rarely malignant. Johns and associates[52] accepted only 11 cases reported as of 1977. The diagnosis of oncocytic carcinoma can be made only when unequivocal evidence of destructive invasion is apparent. Features such as local recurrence, cellular pleomorphism, and hyperchromatism, while implying local aggressiveness, do not necessarily imply malignancy.[9, 52]

SEBACEOUS CELLS

Sebaceous cells are commonly present within normal salivary gland tissue, yet neoplasms consisting partially or entirely of such cells within salivary glands are seldom observed. Sebaceous cell neoplasms of salivary glands exhibit two forms: sebaceous lymphadenoma and sebaceous adenoma.[42]

SEBACEOUS LYMPHADENOMA

Sebaceous lymphadenoma is a distinct, benign tumor of the parotid gland.[42] As the name implies, the growth is composed of sebaceous glands and ducts in a lymphoid tissue background (Fig. 42–17). It has a tendency to arise in middle-aged or older women. In nature and origin, the sebaceous lymphadenoma is comparable to Warthin's tumor. Both types of tumors arise from salivary gland ducts enclosed within lymph nodes; the sebaceous lymphadenoma probably arises from the small intralobular salivary ducts, while Warthin's tumor originates in striated ducts.[9]

SEBACEOUS ADENOMA

Sebaceous adenoma consists of numerous sebaceous glands and large cystic cavities lined by epithelium and supported by a fibrous tissue stroma (Fig. 42–18). Only

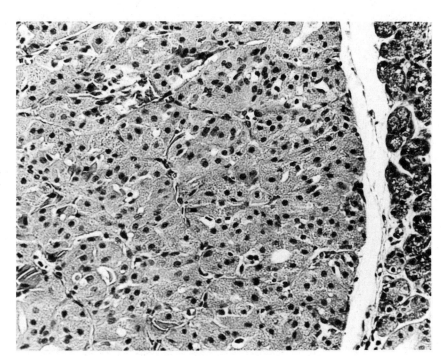

Figure 42–15. Oncocytoma containing oxyphilic granular cells with centrally located nuclei.

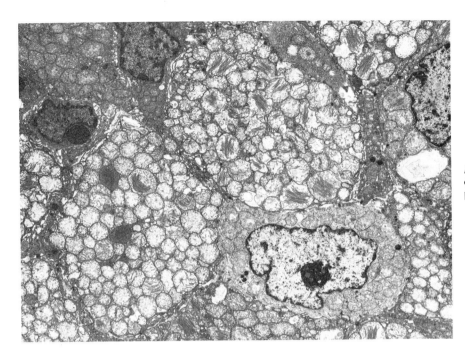

Figure 42–16. Oncocytoma. This electron micrograph shows multiple mitochondria in cytoplasm.

six cases in which the tumor arose outside the parotid gland have been described.[42] Because of the rarity of sebaceous adenoma, Batsakis and associates[11] regard it as a poorly established entity.

ADDITIONAL MONOMORPHIC ADENOMAS

Other monomorphic adenomas of the major glands, such as the *salivary duct adenomas, mucinous adenomas,* and *epidermoid papillary adenomas,*[5] have been described in the literature; these adenomas are unusual. The clear

cell tumors, glycogen-rich or glycogen-negative, which are considered benign by some authors, should always be regarded as at least low-grade carcinomas.[8, 26] They will be discussed with the malignant tumors.

Benign Lymphoepithelial Lesions

Incidence figures for benign lymphoepithelial lesions (BLEL) are not routinely reported in the literature. Duplessis[30] found three BLEL in 200 patients with parotid masses. Evans and Cruickshank[33] suggested a

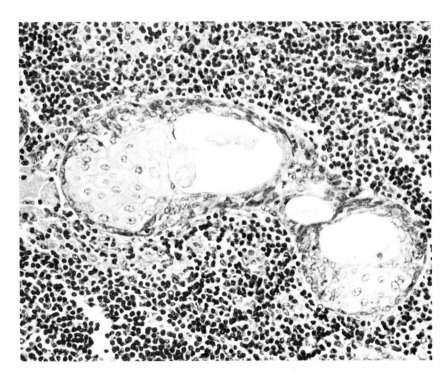

Figure 42–17. Sebaceous lymphadenoma. Nests of sebaceous epithelium are seen in a lymphoid stroma.

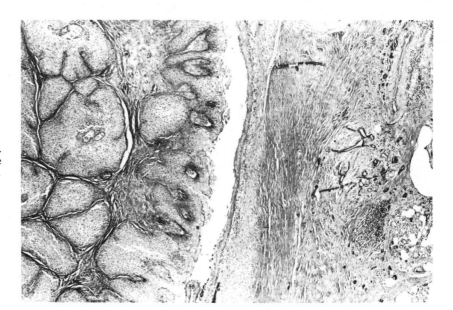

Figure 42–18. Sebaceous adenoma. Nests of sebaceous epithelium are separated by connective tissue bands.

much higher incidence in patients with concurrent Sjögren's syndrome and reported that 10 per cent of a large rheumatoid clinic population with polyarthritis had BLEL. These lesions are most often observed in women, particularly those with Sjögren's syndrome. Morgan and Castleman[66] reported 18 cases, including 15 in females. Eight patients had multiple lesions and four had the sicca syndrome. The ages of the patients at the onset of symptoms ranged from 15 to 70 years, the majority being in the fifth and sixth decades of life. Bernier and Bhaskar[13] described 55 cases, including 30 in males and 25 in females. All except six patients had solitary lesions and none had the sicca syndrome. Their ages at onset of symptoms ranged from 2 to 74 years. The small number of cases involving multiple glands and the unusual male predominance in this series may be explained by the fact that the cases were drawn from the files of the Armed Forces Institute of Pathology.

The BLEL may be diffuse or focal.[13] Focal lesions may be encapsulated or nonencapsulated. Diffusely involved glands retain their lobular pattern surrounded by fibrous septa, and the individual lobules may be enlarged. The cut surface exhibits a rubbery, smooth, glistening parenchyma, either pink or tan in color. The capsule of the salivary gland remains intact.

The BLEL is a disease process characterized histologically by replacement of the salivary parenchyma with lymphoid tissue containing epithelial islands that are often referred to as "epimyoepithelial" (Fig. 42–19). The early histologic manifestation of the BLEL is a focal, periductal infiltration of lymphocytes and plasma cells. Initially, the lymphoid infiltrate involves only the interlobular ducts; subsequently, it progresses until the parenchyma is entirely replaced by lymphoid cells and only remnants of ducts remain. The lymphoid component of the lesion often appears as diffuse infiltration (often

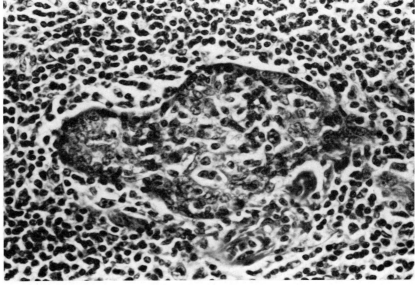

Figure 42–19. Epimyoepithelial islands in lymphoid stroma from a benign lymphoepithelial lesion.

with germinal centers) and consists of plasma cells, mature lymphocytes, and immunoblasts. The epithelial islands are of two distinct cellular types: a round cell with a small nucleus, and a cuboidal cell with a large, dark-staining nucleus.

The preceding histopathologic description contrasts sharply with the complex clinical diseases and syndromes with which BLEL is associated. Many authors have expressed the view that the BLEL is one of the manifestations of Mikulicz's disease and Sjögren's syndrome.[36] The latter disease complex is characterized by keratoconjunctivitis, xerostomia, polyarthritis, hyperglobulinemia, and enlargement of the salivary glands. Mikulicz's disease is believed to be a minor variety of Sjögren's syndrome, in which the salivary glands are involved in the absence of any systemic disorder. It is important to emphasize, however, that the BLEL is not diagnostic of Sjögren's syndrome; it may be found in patients who have localized, limited (unilateral or unifocal) disease of a salivary gland.

Moutsopoulos[67] separates Sjögren's syndrome into primary and secondary forms, depending upon the presence or absence of a coexisting autoimmune disease. The primary form is an exocrinopathy resulting from a lymphocyte-mediated destruction of exocrine glands (major and minor salivary glands, sometimes lungs and gastrointestinal tract), leading to decrease or absence of glandular secretions and consequent mucosal dryness. The secondary form of the syndrome is defined as exocrinopathy preceded or followed by another autoimmune systemic disease. The reader is referred to a selected bibliography for the clinical manifestations and immunologic alterations of this syndrome.[36, 67]

Data presented by Moutsopoulos indicates a relative risk of lymphoma in women with Sjögren's syndrome of more than 40 times that of control subjects. Thus far, the majority of malignant lymphomas complicating the course of Sjögren's syndrome have been extrasalivary and have been classified as large cell lymphomas, probably of the immunoblastic type.[82] There is, however, increasing evidence of the origin of lymphoma in the salivary glands.[82] Histopathologic changes in the salivary glands in patients with Sjögren's syndrome may be monitored by performing biopsies of the minor salivary glands in the lip, palate, and nasal mucosa.[67]

The differential diagnosis between BLEL and primary malignant lymphomas of the salivary glands may be at times extremely difficult. Differential features include:

1. Loss of normal salivary gland lobular architecture in lymphomas.
2. Cytologic atypia of lymphoid cells in lymphomas, especially in large cell and in undifferentiated types.
3. Invasion of the salivary gland capsule and surrounding structures by malignant lymphoid cells.
4. Lymphomatous involvement of adjacent lymph nodes and distant sites, including bone marrow.

According to Schmid and associates,[82] the early evidence of primary lymphoma in a BLEL is the presence of confluent proliferation of immunoblasts and lymphoplasmacytoid cells, which exhibit a monotypic immunoglobulin pattern with the immunoperoxidase technique (PAP).

Unlike the lymphoma arising in relation to a preexisting BLEL, the development of carcinomas from the metaplastic epithelial islands has not been associated with clinical evidence of a systemic autoimmune disorder.[80] Carcinomatous transformation is extremely unusual; in several series of cases reported in this country, it manifested a definite racial disposition, being most prevalent in Eskimos and American Indians.[3] Metastatic carcinoma from the upper respiratory tract should always be excluded.

MALIGNANT EPITHELIAL TUMORS

Malignant salivary gland tumors constitute a group of lesions about which accurate statistical data are lacking. In most reports it is estimated that the incidence of primary salivary gland carcinomas is 10 to 15 per cent of all salivary tumors.[32, 37, 85] The ratio of malignant tumors of the three major salivary glands—parotid, submaxillary, and sublingual—is 40:10:1, respectively.[32, 85] The majority of tumors of the sublingual salivary glands are malignant.[79]

The incidence of the different types of tumor varies. The most common malignant tumor of the parotid gland is mucoepidermoid carcinoma, followed by malignant mixed tumor and acinic cell carcinoma. Among the submaxillary and sublingual gland neoplasms, adenoid cystic carcinoma predominates (Table 42–4).

Mucoepidermoid Carcinoma

Mucoepidermoid carcinomas are observed in most of the major glands, especially in the parotid gland, which is the primary site of 89 per cent of all the mucoepidermoid carcinomas of the salivary glands.[108] The neoplasms probably originate in the epithelial cells of the interlobar or intralobular salivary ducts.[1, 2, 34] As the name implies, they contain mucin-producing and epithelial cells of the epidermoid type. Electron microscopic studies indicate that both of these varieties of cells may differentiate from intermediate cells of undeterminate type, and these cells are also a feature of the tumors.[73] Myoepithelial cells are not found.

The prevalence of mucoepidermoid carcinoma is highest among persons in the fifth decade of life, though it is the most common malignant salivary gland tumor in children.[22, 58] In the majority of reported series, its predominance in females is striking, ranging from two to four times the incidence in males.[46, 86] Approximately 60 to 70 per cent of the tumors are located in the parotid gland, 15 to 20 per cent in the oral cavity, and 6 to 10

TABLE 42–4. Malignant Epithelial Salivary Gland Tumors, Distribution by Site*

Type	Parotid (n = 288)	Submaxillary (n = 54)	Sublingual (n = 15)
Mucoepidermoid	50%	31%	40%
Malignant mixed	18%	7%	—
Acinic cell	12%	—	13.3%
Adenocarcinoma	10%	16%	—
Adenoid cystic	7%	31%	40%
Squamous cells	3%	7%	—
Undifferentiated	—	8%	6.7%

*Data extracted from Conley J, et al, Ann Otolaryngol 18:323, 1972;[25] Rankow RM, Mignogna F, Am J Surg 118:790, 1969;[79] and Spiro RH, et al, Am J Surg 130:452, 1975.[89]

per cent in the submaxillary glands. Occasionally, this tumor is observed centrally located in the mandible, where clinically it resembles ameloblastoma.[6]

Since the introduction of the term "mucoepidermoid" by Stewart and associates,[92] the biologic behavior of these lesions has been the subject of controversy. In particular, it has been questioned whether there is a benign variety of mucoepidermoid carcinoma. Some authors believe that benign and malignant forms can be separated on the basis of morphology and history,[14] whereas others maintain that they are all carcinomas.[1, 46, 86] The fact is, the subtle blending of one form into another would preclude the possibility of absolute separation of these neoplasms into benign and malignant forms. Today, most authorities recognize that even the best differentiated tumors do at times metastasize. The author believes that all mucoepidermoid tumors should be classified as malignant, yet a histologic difference should be noted between the locally aggressive, rarely metastasizing, well-differentiated tumor and the high-grade carcinoma with a pronounced tendency to metastasize. The designation of "tumor" should be dropped except as used in a generic sense.[1, 6]

Traditionally, on the basis of their histologic appearance and degree of anaplasia, mucoepidermoid carcinomas have been classified as well differentiated (low grade), or as poorly differentiated (high grade), although careful study will show that many of the lesions have histologic features intermediate between these two extremes.[46, 86] The degree of differentiation correlates with the extent of local invasion, with the incidence of lymph node metastasis, and with the overall survival.[86]

Tumors of low-grade malignancy manifest themselves clinically in a manner similar to that of benign mixed tumor and generally undergo a prolonged period of painless enlargement. Highly malignant tumors grow rapidly and are often accompanied by pain and ulceration. The mean time interval between the initial swelling and histologic verification of low-grade tumors is quite long, being an average of 6.8 years, while that of high-grade lesions is approximately 1.5 years.[6]

Grossly, tumors of low-grade malignancy resemble the mixed variety. They are usually well circumscribed, and the cut surfaces often show dilated cystic structures containing mucous material. Although low-grade tumors vary in size, they rarely measure more than 3 cm. Intermediate and high-grade carcinomas are poorly circumscribed, and infiltration of adjacent tissues is a prominent feature. The cut surfaces lack the cystic formation usually observed in the low-grade tumors.

Microscopically, the majority of low-grade mucoepidermoid carcinomas consist of multiple well-developed granular or microcystic structures lined by mucin-producing, intermediate, or epidermoid cells (Fig. 42–20). Keratinization is seldom found. Microcystic formations coalescing into larger cysts are often prominent. If the mucinous material present in the cysts escapes into the stroma, an intense inflammatory reaction may obscure the true neoplastic character of the lesion. Low-grade carcinomas generally grow in a relatively broad advancing front (Fig. 42–21) and are not highly invasive.

As mucoepidermoid carcinomas become less differentiated, the nests of the tumor cells become larger, more irregular, and more solid, and fewer cystic spaces containing mucous secretions are apparent. In intermediate carcinomas, the nests are composed of epidermoid or even squamous cells, or intermediate basaloid elements; if the latter cells predominate, fewer goblet cells are present (Fig. 42–22).

As these carcinomas become poorly differentiated (high grade), they exhibit more extensive local invasion and are likely to have infiltrated beyond a point visible to the naked eye. Microscopically, the high-grade carcinomas tend to form solid nests or cords composed of intermediate and epidermoid cells, with a few mucin-producing cells. The degrees of anaplasia, atypical mitosis, nuclear pleomorphism and invasion of normal structures are obvious (Fig. 42–23). Perineural invasion and lymph node metastases are frequently associated. In the metastases, all these cell types are present, though not necessarily in the same proportion as in the primary tumor.[1]

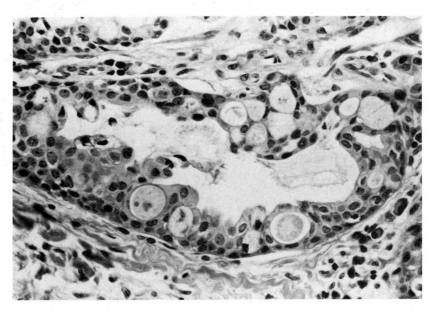

Figure 42–20. Low-grade mucoepidermoid carcinoma. Cystic spaces are lined with mucin and epidermoid cells. The nuclei exhibit only minimal pleomorphism.

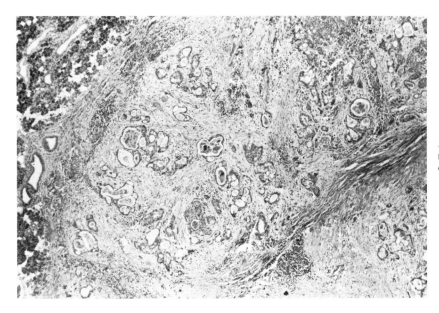

Figure 42–21. Low-grade mucoepidermoid carcinoma. Note pushing margins of the tumor.

Many benign mixed tumors contain prominent areas of squamous metaplasia, and thus may create a diagnostic problem. Mucoepidermoid carcinomas of any grade of malignancy, however, exhibit no evidence of myoepithelial cells or of chondroid or myxochondroid stroma, all of which are so characteristic of mixed tumor.

High-grade mucoepidermoid carcinoma is differentiated from squamous carcinoma by the presence of intracellular mucin. If mucin-producing cells are entirely lacking, the lesion is classified as squamous carcinoma. The confinement of cytologically benign squamous epithelium to the pre-existing lobular pattern of the salivary gland distinguishes lobular regeneration from mucoepidermoid carcinoma.[10]

Recurrence rates for mucoepidermoid carcinoma are rather high in most series. Stevenson and Hazard[91] reported a 75 per cent rate, whereas a 30 per cent recurrence rate was reported by Batsakis[1, 6] and Healey.[58]

The 15-year "cure" rate varies according to the grade of the tumor. In the series of Spiro and associates,[86] the 15-year "cure" rate was 48 per cent for patients with low-grade carcinomas, as compared to 25 per cent for patients with intermediate and high-grade carcinomas.

Acinic Cell Carcinoma

These tumors affect chiefly middle-aged and elderly patients, although they may be encountered in patients of any age. They are more prevalent in women than in men, and frequently arise in the salivary glands of children. A few cases have been reported to arise in ectopic salivary gland tissue in the middle and low cervical lymph nodes.[75] The tumors are believed to be derived from the reserve cells of the terminal ducts or intercalated ducts. Less often, they develop in more mature acinar cells.[1, 2] In 99 per cent of the cases, the

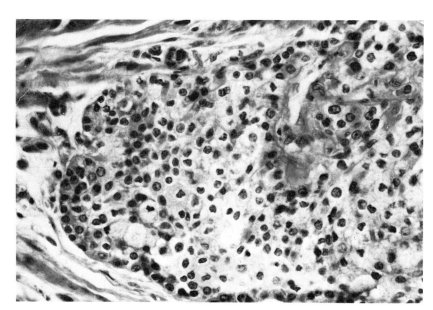

Figure 42–22. Moderately differentiated mucoepidermoid carcinoma. Solid nests of intermediate cells are seen with occasional mucinous cells.

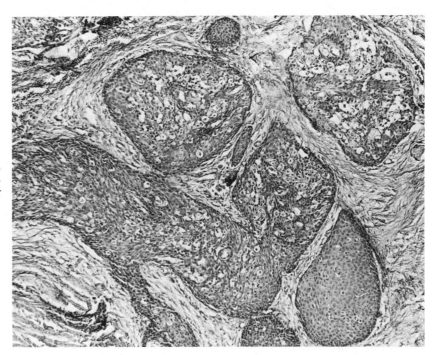

Figure 42–23. High-grade mucoepidermoid carcinoma. Solid nests of epidermoid cells are seen, with a few clear cells containing stainable mucin.

parotid gland is the primary site[1]; rarely, they originate in the submaxillary gland and the oral cavity.

Acinic cell carcinomas account for between 2 and 4 per cent of all parotid gland tumors and between 12 and 17 per cent of all cancers of this gland. They rank second only to Warthin's tumor in bilaterality, the incidence of bilaterality in the parotid glands being approximately 3 per cent.[1, 76, 87, 96]

Upon gross examination, acinic cell carcinomas are frequently fairly well circumscribed by a large layer of dense fibrous tissue. They are of much the same consistency and color as the normal salivary gland. Upon low-power examination, many can be seen growing in large, fairly well circumscribed nests composed of cells with a basophilic cytoplasm (Fig. 42–24). The tumor cells are arranged in different patterns, including acini, tubules, follicles, solid nests, or cystic papillary structures.[1] The stroma is sparse and consists of fibrovascular septa. Lymphoid infiltrate may be prominent; it is sometimes arranged in germinal centers (Fig. 42–25). The margins of the tumors are usually of the pushing type, though the more aggressive tumors may have

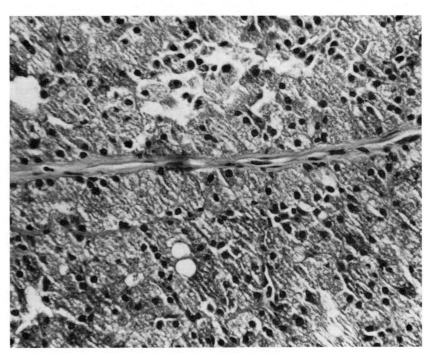

Figure 42–24. Acinic cell carcinoma with basophilic granular cells.

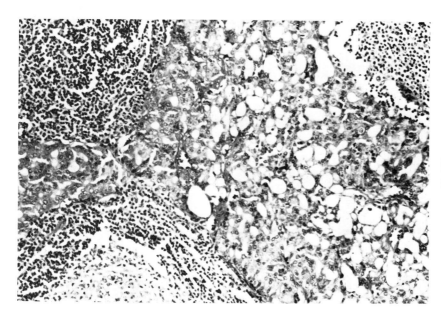

Figure 42–25. Acinic cell carcinoma arising in a lymph node. The tumor is composed of small cystic structures.

destructive infiltrating margins with vascular or lymphatic invasion.[87]

The cytoplasm of at least some of the cells in acinic cell carcinoma contains PAS-positive diastase-resistant secretory granules. The number of granules varies from field to field and from tumor to tumor. Electron microscopic examination reveals three types of cells:

1. Ductular cells with few cytoplasmic organelles and microvilli oriented toward irregular lumina.

2. Serous cells with abundant cytoplasmic organelles in the form of rough endoplasmic reticulum, and large secretory granules having a variable electron-dense content.

3. Undifferentiated cells with sparse cytoplasm and without secretory granules. These epithelial cells are situated between the ductular and the serous cells.[6]

Acinic cell carcinomas must be differentiated from the clear cell variant of mucoepidermoid carcinoma, metastatic renal cell carcinoma, and intercalated duct carcinoma. In the vast majority of acinic cell carcinomas, the histologic pattern, the cytoplasmic granularity with basophilia, and the post-diastase PAS-positive reaction are the most distinguishing features.[77] Mucoepidermoid carcinoma, renal cell carcinoma, and intercalated duct carcinoma are recognized by the fact that they contain cells rich in glycogen. Electron microscopic examination is valuable in the differential diagnosis of atypical acinic cell carcinomas.[6]

As a group, acinic cell carcinomas behave as low-grade malignant tumors in that they have a strong tendency to recur locally yet they seldom metastasize. Thus, patients with this tumor should be followed for long periods of time. In Spiro's series,[87] the "determinate cure" rates were 76, 63, and 55 per cent at 5, 10, and 15 years, respectively. Perzin and LiVolsi[76] reported the determinate 5-, 10-, and 15-year survival rates at 76, 63, and 44 per cent, respectively.

Adenoid Cystic Carcinoma

Adenoid cystic carcinomas (*cylindromatous carcinomas*) are the most common malignant tumors arising in the submaxillary, sublingual, and accessory salivary glands. They account for 14 per cent of cancers of the parotid gland and 31 per cent of those of the submaxillary glands.[74, 88] The majority of the patients are between the ages of 40 and 60 years. Tumors in the submaxillary glands are generally observed in females, whereas those arising in the accessory glands exhibit no predilection for either sex. The primary site of these tumors is believed to be the reserve epithelial cells in the intercalated ducts, which can differentiate into epithelial and myoepithelial cell forms.[2, 10]

In the usual histologic pattern of adenoid cystic carcinoma, the majority of the cells are small and darkly stained and have a scant cytoplasm. The cells are arranged in nests that are fenestrated by round or oval spaces, creating the characteristic "cribriform" pattern (Fig. 42–26). Occasionally, the tumors present a predominantly solid cellular pattern, having an anaplastic appearance with few fenestrations (Fig. 42–27). Tubular structures with minimal stratification of the lining epithelium are often mixed with the classic cribriform and solid areas (Fig. 42–28).

If the surgical specimen is large, the diagnosis of adenoid cystic carcinoma can be made without difficulty. In small biopsy specimens, however, the distinction from mixed tumor, basal cell adenoma and poorly differentiated mucoepidermoid carcinoma may be a problem. Mucoepidermoid carcinoma can be determined by the presence of glandular structures composed of mucinous, transitional and squamous cells. The histologic differences between adenoid cystic carcinoma, basal cell adenoma, and benign mixed tumor have already been discussed.

In a recent study of adenoid cystic carcinomas by Perzin and associates,[74] the important factor influencing prognosis was found to be the presence or absence of tumor at the margins of resection. The same authors classified adenoid cystic carcinomas according to their predominant histologic pattern—tubular, cribriform, or solid. Tumors containing many tubular structures carried the most favorable prognosis, and those consisting predominantly of solid nests had the worst. These

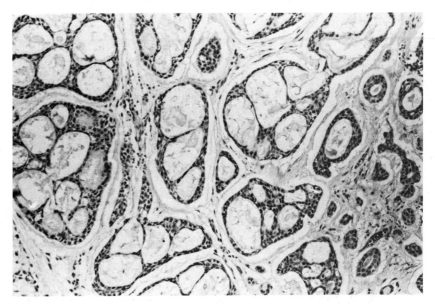

Figure 42–26. Adenoid cystic carcinoma, cribriform pattern.

observations have also been made in other studies and more recently have been corroborated by Chilla and associates[21] and by Szanto and associates.[93]

As a rule, adenoid cystic carcinomas grow slowly and spread relentlessly into adjacent tissues. Hematogenous metastases to the lungs and bones are observed late in the course of the disease. Metastasis to the lymph nodes takes place in a few cases.[10, 16] Grahne and associates[44] found that metastasis to the lungs was three times more prevalent than metastasis to the lymph nodes.

These tumors also have a strong tendency to invade perineural spaces and extend for long distances by this route. In Perzin's series, 59 per cent of all tumors of this type exhibited perineural invasion.[74] An extremely long period of observation is required if the prognosis is to be judged with any degree of reliability; the "determinate" cure rate at 5, 10, 15, and 20 years is 31, 18, 10, and 7 per cent, respectively.[88]

Malignant Mixed Tumor

Approximately 75 per cent of malignant mixed tumors arise in the parotid gland, the primary site of the remainder being the submaxillary and accessory salivary glands.[60, 90] Patients with malignant mixed tumors are approximately 10 to 20 years older than those with benign mixed tumors.

Malignant mixed tumors account for between 3 and 12 per cent of all cancers of the salivary glands and 2 per cent of all tumors in these locations.[90] The number of malignant mixed tumors detected depends upon the diligence with which the pathologist searches the cancerous material for areas of residual benign mixed tumor. The malignant component of a mixed tumor may so greatly overgrow the areas of origin that it becomes extremely difficult to prove the presence of a residual benign mixed tumor. This point is well illustrated by

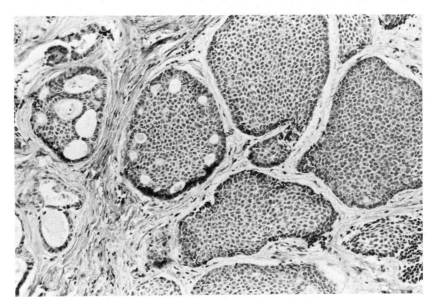

Figure 42–27. Adenoid cystic carcinoma. This tumor consists of solid nests of cells as well as cribriform structures.

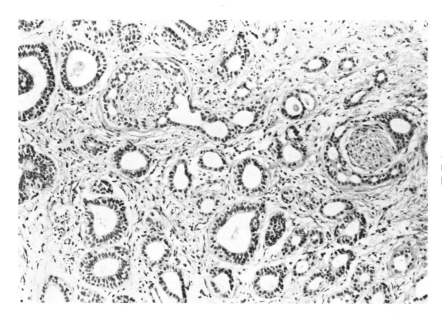

Figure 42–28. Adenoid cystic carcinoma, tubular variant. Note intra- and perineural invasion.

the report of Beahrs and coworkers,[12] who, in reviewing the surgical specimens from 178 cases of parotid carcinomas, type not specified, discovered 29 in which benign mixed tumor was associated with carcinoma in the same lesion.

There are four variants of malignant mixed tumor:

1. Carcinoma in mixed tumor or carcinoma ex-pleomorphic adenoma is by far the most common form. The malignant component is usually a poorly differentiated adenocarcinoma (Fig 42–29), and the metastases contain only carcinoma.[11, 65, 90] An origin of adenoid cystic carcinoma, mucoepidermoid carcinoma, or acinic cell carcinoma in benign mixed tumor seldom can be demonstrated.

2. The next variant is the true or primary malignant mixed tumor, or carcinosarcoma, in which the malignant components are carcinoma and sarcoma (Fig. 42–30) and the metastases contain both elements.[11, 41]

3. Metastasizing mixed tumor, in which both the original tumor and the metastases consist of structures typical of benign mixed tumor, is the most rare variant of malignant mixed tumor; only a few authentic cases having been reported.[20]

4. In situ, or noninvasive carcinoma, in a mixed tumor, is a term that was introduced by LiVolsi and Perzin.[60] It applies to those tumors without evidence of invasion of the capsule or adjacent tissue, and therefore is a malignant neoplasm of no clinical or biologic significance. If no invasion outside the main mass is identified, the carcinoma should not metastasize.

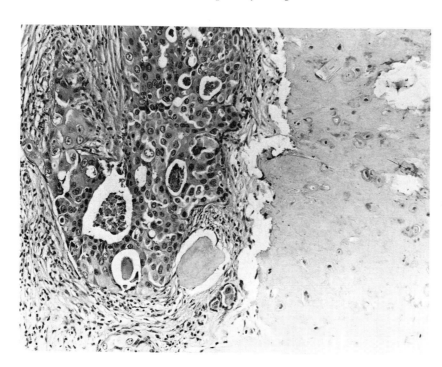

Figure 42–29. Carcinoma in mixed tumor. The adenocarcinoma is invading surrounding tissues.

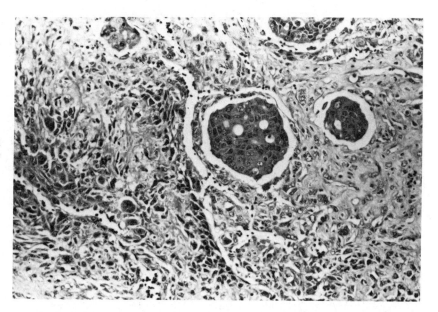

Figure 42–30. Primary malignant mixed tumor. Malignant glandular and spindle cells are present.

The lesion most frequently confused by the pathologist with malignant mixed tumor is adenoid cystic carcinoma.[60] The carcinoma in malignant mixed tumor is usually composed of large irregular nests or solid cords in a myxoid or chondroid stroma. In contrast, adenoid cystic carcinoma contains regular cords, tubules with lumina, and often cribriform areas in a fibrotic background. As pointed out by Evans and Cruickshank,[33] adenoid cystic carcinoma seldom, if ever, has a chondroid or myxoid stroma.

The pathologist must also differentiate recurrent benign mixed tumor from malignant mixed tumor. In the former, all the histologic features of a benign mixed tumor are identified. It must be remembered that recurrent mixed tumor is frequently composed of multiple, well-circumscribed nodules in the salivary gland, in adipose tissue, or in the scar of the previous excision. These nodules do not exhibit the features of cell anaplasia and invasiveness that characterize malignant mixed tumors.[77] Points of difference between benign mixed tumor, adenoid cystic carcinoma, and malignant mixed tumor have already been discussed in sections on benign neoplasms.

Invasive carcinomas in mixed tumors and true or primary malignant mixed tumors are highly aggressive. The recurrence rate over a 5-year period or longer is between 40 and 70 per cent and the rate of metastasis to regional lymph nodes is 25 per cent and to distant organs, 33 per cent.[12, 65] In the series of Spiro and associates,[90] the "determinate" cure rates 5, 10, and 15 years after treatment were 40, 24, and 17 per cent, respectively.

Adenocarcinoma

A proportion of salivary gland tumors are adenocarcinomas of various types, such as mucin-producing, clear cell, ductal, intercalated, neuroendocrine, papillary, solid, anaplastic, cylindric, and others.[10, 37] The true incidence of those originating in the major salivary glands is difficult to define, though they probably do not constitute more than 4 per cent of all tumors of these glands. Although they may arise from any portion of the salivary duct system, the majority originate from the larger intralobular duct or excretory ducts.[2, 10]

This is a heterogeneous group of neoplasms, which, although capable of being separated into specific histologic categories, are nonetheless of such low incidence when separated by categories that a detailed statistical analysis is extremely difficult. There is much need of clinical studies, however, in order to promote a clear understanding of the clinical behavior and natural history of these tumors.

Mucinous Adenocarcinoma. Blanck,[15] in studying a series of 1678 parotid tumors, found that 2.8 per cent were *mucinous adenocarcinomas*. These usually originate in the parotid gland. Microscopically, they are characterized by papillary structures composed of mucinous cylindric cells and by solid sheets of polymorphic cells (Fig. 42–31). Blanck separated these tumors into invasive and noninvasive. By this criterion, 20 per cent of patients with invasive tumors lived 20 years, as compared with 41 per cent of those with noninvasive tumors.

Salivary Duct Carcinoma. Kleinsasser and associates[55] described a group of malignant neoplasms composed of mixed epithelial and myoepithelial elements that morphologically resembled ductal carcinoma of the breast, that is, intraductal papillary proliferation, comedocarcinoma variant, cribriform pattern, and occasional areas like sclerosing adenosis (Fig. 42–32). He called this group *salivary duct carcinoma*.

These tumors appear predominantly in the parotid gland of elderly people, affecting males three times more often than females. A ductal origin is supported by the presence of dysplasia and carcinoma *in situ* within otherwise normal ducts. Intraductal spread of the tumor into acini is at times demonstrable. Although some carcinomas of the salivary gland duct grow slowly and metastasize late,[10, 40, 55] the majority are rapidly progressive, metastasizing early to the regional lymph nodes and lungs.

Intercalated Duct Carcinoma. A rather distinctive

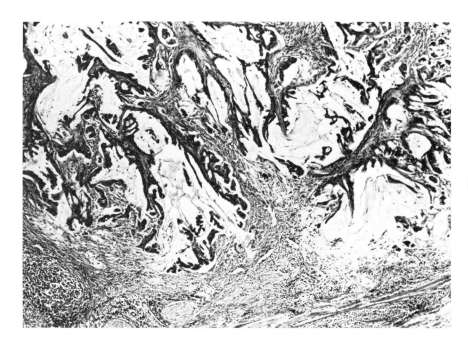

Figure 42–31. Adenocarcinoma with papillary structures.

form of adenocarcinoma has been designated by Donath and coworkers[29] as "epithelial myoepithelial carcinoma of intercalated duct origin" or *"intercalated duct carcinoma."* This term embraces those tumors previously described as glycogen-rich carcinoma or adenoma, clear cell adenoma or carcinoma, tubular carcinoma, and adenomyoepithelioma.[11] In the series reported by Corio and associates,[26] the neoplasms arose chiefly in women in the seventh and eighth decades of life. Most of the tumors originated in the parotid gland.

Microscopically, intercalated duct carcinomas are composed of small ducts lined by cuboidal epithelial cells surrounded by clear cells resting on a basement membrane (Fig. 42–33). In our experience, they constitute 0.7 per cent of all salivary gland tumors and behave like a low-grade carcinoma; the survival rate at 10 years is 92 per cent, and the recurrence rate is 60 per cent.[43] Similar observations have been reported in other series.[26, 29]

Undifferentiated Carcinoma

Undifferentiated carcinomas of the salivary glands are malignant epithelial neoplasms that do not fulfill histologic criteria that permit them to be placed in other categories. Areas of undifferentiated carcinoma may be associated with benign mixed tumor, mucoepidermoid carcinoma, adenoid cystic carcinoma, or acinic cell carcinoma. Thus, when the pathologist studies an undifferentiated carcinoma in a salivary gland, the entire tumor should be sectioned and searched for a better differentiated area in which the carcinoma might have

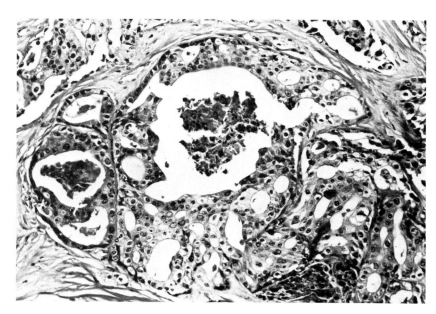

Figure 42–32. Salivary duct carcinoma. Note the similarity to breast carcinoma.

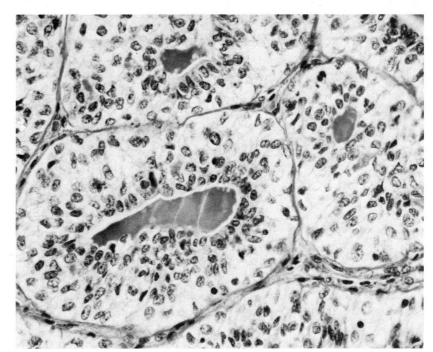

Figure 42–33. Intercalated duct carcinoma. The duct is surrounded by clear cells resting in a well-developed basement membrane.

arisen.[12, 77] If such an area is not identified, the lesion may be classified as an undifferentiated carcinoma.

These tumors account for no more than 3 per cent of all neoplasms of the parotid gland.[70] Most of the patients are in their sixth or seventh decade of life. The 5-year survival rate is 20 to 30 per cent.[70]

Microscopically, undifferentiated carcinomas are arranged in solid or trabecular patterns of small hyperchromatic cells with scant cytoplasm, resembling oat cell carcinoma of the lung (Fig. 42–34). Histologically, they are divided into large and small cell types.

Squamous Cell Carcinoma

The submaxillary glands are more often the sites of origin of squamous cell carcinomas than is the parotid gland. Approximately 3.5 per cent of all of these tumors in the submaxillary glands are squamous cell carcinomas, but in the parotid gland only 0.3 to 0.8 per cent are of this type.[6, 8, 25] The difference in incidence exhibited by the two major salivary glands is attributed to the much higher percentage of obstructive duct disease in the submaxillary glands.[3, 6, 8] The majority of patients

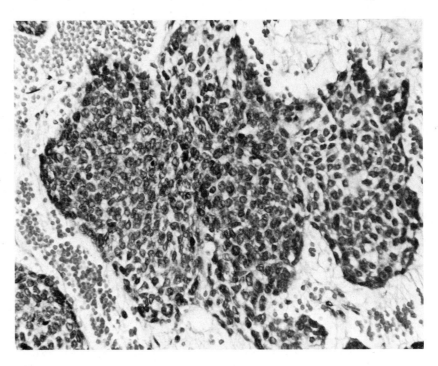

Figure 42–34. Undifferentiated carcinoma.

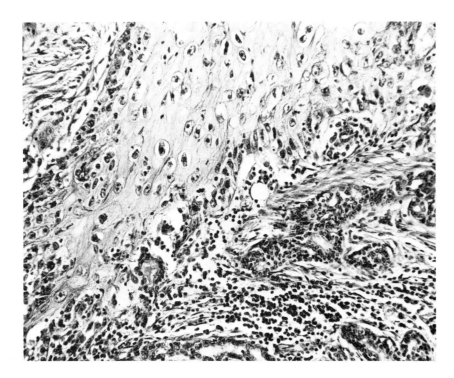

Figure 42–35. Primary squamous carcinoma of parotid gland.

with primary squamous cell carcinoma of the salivary glands are over the age of 60 years.

The microscopic appearance of squamous cell carcinoma originating in a salivary gland is identical to that of squamous carcinoma in other tissues. Intracellular keratinization, intercellular bridges, and keratin pearl formation are often observed (Fig. 42–35). No mucin is present. Before ascribing squamous carcinoma to a major salivary gland as the primary site, one must exclude mucoepidermoid carcinoma and metastasis or extension to the gland from an extrasalivary glandular source.[6, 8, 86]

The usual course of the disease following treatment for the primary tumor is local recurrence and metastasis to the regional lymph nodes.

Other Salivary Carcinomas

Sebaceous carcinoma, malignant oncocytic neoplasms, lymphoepithelial carcinomas, and myoepithelial carcinomas of the major salivary glands have been reported in the literature,[33, 42, 52] although they are seldom encountered. The majority of these tumors follow an aggressive clinical course.

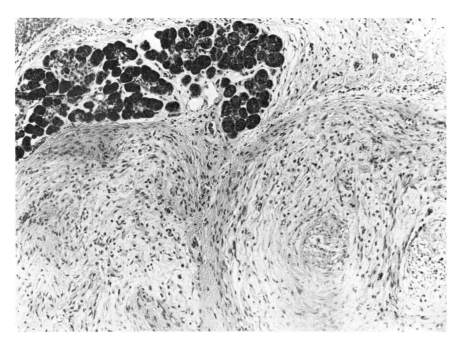

Figure 42–36. Plexiform neurofibroma of parotid gland. (Courtesy of Stanley Weitzner, M.D.)

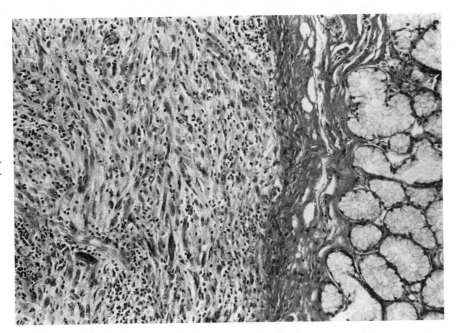

Figure 42–37. Malignant fibrous histiocytoma of soft tissue invading submaxillary gland.

NONEPITHELIAL TUMORS

Nonepithelial tumors, both benign and malignant, constitute less than 5 per cent of all neoplasms in the salivary glands of adults.[85] Collectively, they are termed synsialomas or synsialadenomas. They arise in the supporting tissues of the salivary glands, such as blood and lymphatic vessels, nerves, nerve sheets, and surrounding connective tissue. Angiomas, lipomas, neurofibromas, neuromas, and hemangiopericytomas are the most frequently observed benign synsialomas.[62, 85, 98] With the exception of neurofibromas, these tumors have been reported only in the parotid gland[98] (Fig. 42–36). Benign mesodermal tumors comparatively often arise in the parotid glands of children; the majority of these are hemangiomas, which are discussed subsequently in the section on "Tumors in Children."

Grossly, many mesenchymal tumors are poorly demarcated, the infiltrating margins suggesting malignancy. The microscopic patterns and histologic criteria are identical to those of tumors in other tissues. Lipoma and neurofibroma may penetrate deeply into the intraglandular septa and may recur.

Sarcomas arising primarily in the major salivary glands, or growing into them, make up an interesting group of neoplasms. They affect all age groups, although they are more prevalent in patients under 40 years of age. They cover almost the entire gamut of mesenchymal tumors: rhabdomyosarcomas, fibrohistiocytomas, fibrosarcomas, neurosarcomas, and synovial sarcomas (Fig. 42–37). Although they are unusual, these are the most often reported types of sarcomas involving the major salivary glands.[35, 84]

Primary malignant lymphomas of the salivary glands are rarely encountered; Batsakis and Regezi[8] found two among 589 tumors of the parotid gland. Freeman and associates,[38] reviewing 1467 cases of extranodal lymphomas, discovered 69 in the major salivary glands. The parotid glands are involved much more often than the submaxillary glands, the ratio being 5 to 1. The sublin-gual glands are seldom affected by lymphomas; as of 1980, only two cases had been reported.[23] Most patients with salivary gland lymphomas are in the sixth or seventh decade of life.[23, 38, 49]

Lymphomas in the salivary glands require the same type of staging as those in the cervical lymph nodes. Colby and Dorfman,[23] in a study of 59 patients with lymphomas involving the salivary glands, discovered that 37 had evidence of lymphoma distant from the head and neck region. Hyman and Wolff[49] established the following criteria to qualify a lymphoma as of salivary gland origin:

1. Enlargement of a salivary gland must be the first clinical manifestation of the disease.

2. Histologic proof that the lymphoma involves salivary gland parenchyma, rather than being confined to soft tissues or a lymph node in the area.

3. Architectural and cytologic confirmation of the malignant nature of the lymphoid infiltrate (Fig. 42–38).

The majority of lymphomas of the salivary glands are of the nodular type; of these, poorly differentiated lymphocytic tumors have the highest incidence, followed closely by that of diffuse large cell lymphomas. Noteworthy is the fact that all subtypes of lymphoma are encountered in the salivary glands, though Hodgkin's lymphoma appears to be extremely unusual.[23, 38, 49]

A malignant lymphoma must be distinguished from nonspecific chronic sialadenitis, benign lymphoepithelial lesions, and undifferentiated carcinoma. Of these, nonspecific chronic sialadenitis undoubtedly is more often observed. In this disease, the infiltrate consists of mature cells and an admixture of lymphocytes and plasma cells appearing in paraductal locations and later involving the interstitium of the gland. The histologic differences between lymphoma and benign lymphoepithelial lesions have already been discussed.

Undifferentiated carcinoma may at times mimic lymphoma. Special stains, including mucin and PAS, may help in making the distinction. The cytoplasm of the epithelial cells may contain mucopolysaccharide. It must

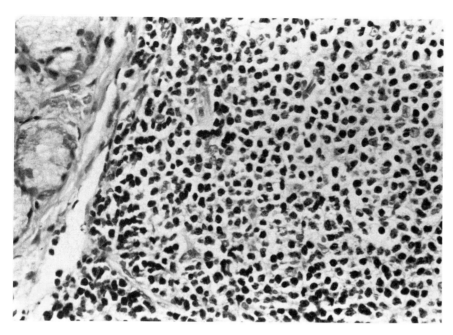

Figure 42–38. Malignant lymphoma.

be admitted, however, that some of these tumors may be difficult to recognize, even with the electron microscope.[77]

The end result of therapy of patients with lymphoma of the salivary glands is discouraging. Regardless of the histologic type of tumor, approximately 30 per cent are free of disease after a 5-year follow-up period.[23, 38, 49]

METASTASIS TO SALIVARY GLANDS

Metastasis to the major salivary glands may take place by (1) lymphatic spread, (2) hematogenous dissemination, or (3) contiguous extension. The last is especially likely of sarcomas arising from facial bones or soft tissues as well as cancers of the skin.[50] The majority of lymphatic and hematogenous metastases to the major vary glands are found in the parotid glands. The submaxillary glands are seldom invaded. The absence of intraglandular lymph node is the apparent reason for the rarity of lymphatic metastatic lesions.[3] Hematogenous disseminations of carcinoma of a lung or breast to the submaxillary glands occasionally has been reported.[3]

Secondary neoplastic involvement of the parotid gland is probably less rare than the literature would lead one to believe. Yarington,[100] in a series of 250 consecutive parotidectomies performed for clinically primary parotid tumors, found 10 (4 per cent) metastatic neoplasms from an unsuspected primary source. Similar experiences have been described by Rees and associates[81] and by Nichols and associates.[71]

As noted by Conley and Arena,[24] the parotid gland contains as many as 20 to 30 lymph nodes and a rich network of intercommunicating lymph vessels. Paraparotid lymph nodes are present around the external surface of the gland, being particularly numerous in the pretragal and supratragal areas. Intraglandular and par-

aglandular lymph nodes communicate freely with each other and drain into the cervical chains.

Since the lymphatic drainage of the scalp, face, external ear, eyelids, and nose is to both intraglandular and periglandular parotid lymph nodes, it is not surprising that cutaneous squamous cell carcinoma and melanoma arising in these areas are the metastatic malignant tumors most often found in the parotid lymph nodes (Fig. 42–39). In a review of 81 cases of secondary parotid lesions, Conley and Arena[24] found that 40 per cent were squamous cell carcinomas and 42 per cent were melanomas. Other authors have observed the propensity of cutaneous tumors of the head and neck to metastasize to the parotid lymph nodes. Occasionally, the palate, tonsil, and nasopharynx are sites of origin of metastases to the intra- or paraparotid lymph nodes.[24, 71]

Blood-borne metastatic carcinomas from infraclavicular organs to the parotid gland region arise, first, from a primary tumor in a lung and, less often, from one in a breast or kidney or the gastrointestinal tract.[100] When it becomes difficult to assign a given salivary gland neoplasm to a particular category, the pathologist must remember that it may possibly be a secondary tumor (Fig. 42–40).

Malignant secondary neoplasms of the parotid gland carry a grave prognosis: the overall 5-year survival rate is estimated at 12.5 per cent.[3, 24, 71] Survival is influenced by the cell type, regional spread of the disease, site of origin of metastases, and prevention of local recurrence. Jackson and Ballantyne[50] and Rees and associates[81] have reported a 67 per cent survival rate of 5 years for cutaneous metastatic squamous carcinoma. The 5-year survival rate for metastatic melanoma to the parotid lymph nodes varies from 10 to 30 per cent. Metastatic parotid tumors that arise from noncutaneous sites also have a poor prognosis: the 5-year survival rate is less than 5 per cent, indicating the systemic metastatic

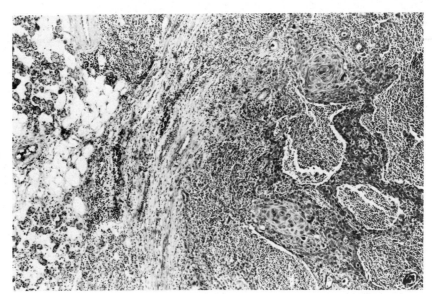

Figure 42–39. Metastatic squamous carcinoma.

nature of carcinomas of the lungs, breasts, kidneys, and tonsillar and nasopharyngeal regions.[3, 81]

TUMORS OF THE MAJOR SALIVARY GLANDS IN CHILDREN

Neoplasms of the major salivary glands seldom arise in children; they make up less than 5 per cent of all tumors of the salivary glands in all age groups.[85] Beahrs and Chong[22] found that among 1600 patients of all ages treated for parotid tumors at the Mayo Clinic, only 3 per cent were less than 16 years old at the time of diagnosis. Castro and associates[19] reported 38, or 1.7 per cent, in children in a series of 2135 patients who were treated at Memorial Sloan-Kettering Cancer Center for tumors of the major salivary glands. In a review of

their cases at the Armed Forces Institute of Pathology (AFIP), Krolls and coworkers[58] discovered 168 tumors of the major salivary glands in children, representing 4.3 per cent of the total number of tumors of the salivary glands observed in that institution. In all reported series, neoplasms of the parotid gland predominate over those of the submaxillary glands in a ratio of 7 to 1. Mixed tumors, hemangiomas, and mucoepidermoid carcinomas are the types usually observed (Table 42–5). If mesenchymal tumors are excluded, a disproportionately large number (50 per cent) of salivary gland tumors in children are malignant.[19, 22, 58]

In general, hemangiomas and lymphangiomas are present at birth; because surgical treatment is usually delayed until later, the average age at operation is 4.8 years.[62] Patients with epithelial neoplasms, such as benign mixed tumor, mucoepidermoid carcinoma, and acinic cell carcinoma, are older.[19, 22, 58]

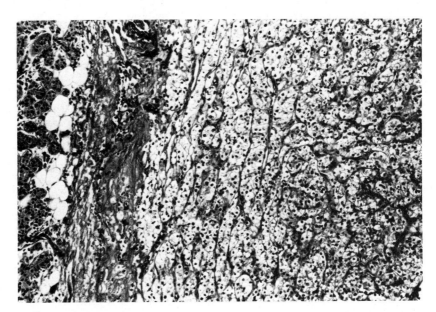

Figure 42–40. Metastatic renal cell carcinoma.

TABLE 42–5. Salivary Gland Tumors in Children

Histologic Type	Chong et al[22]	Castro et al[19]	Kroll et al[58]	Kaufman and Stout[54]	Byers et al[18]	Total
Mixed tumor	22	18	55	6	7	108
Monomorphic adenoma			1			1
Warthin's tumor			2			1
Lymphoepithelial lesion		1				1
Papillary cyst adenoma			2			2
Mucoepidermoid carcinoma	13	15	20	5	15	68
Acinic cell carcinoma	4	2	12	3	2	23
Adenocarcinoma		1	3		5	9
Adenoid cystic carcinoma				1	2	3
Undifferentiated carcinoma				4	2	6
Malignant mixed tumor		1				1
Metastatic	4		2			6
Hemangiomas	16		35	11	3	65
Lymphangiomas	5					9
Cystic hygroma	1					1
Neurofibroma	2		7			9
Lipoma	1					1
Sarcoma			6			6
Lymphoma			6	1		7
Unclassified			5	1		6
Totals	68	38	160	32	36	334

Benign Tumors

Mixed Tumors. The mixed tumors are by far the most often observed benign epithelial neoplasms of the salivary glands in children (Table 42–5), despite the fact that they are rare in this age group. Of a total of 3875 mixed tumors accessioned at the AFIP, 55 (1.4 per cent) were in the pediatric population. Only 1 per cent of 712 tumors reviewed by Kaufman and Stout[54] at the Columbia Presbyterian Medical Center affected children. Castro and associates[19] found 18 mixed tumors at the Sloan-Kettering Institute and counted 19 reported in the literature. The peak incidence of these tumors is at 10 years of age.

The biologic behavior and the morphologic appearance of mixed tumors in children do not differ from those in adults. In the series of Chong and associates,[22] collected from the Mayo Clinic, three of 22 children with mixed tumors had recurrences over periods varying from 1 to 50 years. Following parotidectomies for the recurrences, all three patients were still apparently free of their disease at 9, 12, and 50 years later.

Hemangiomas. The incidence of hemangiomas is the next highest. Krolls and associates[58] encountered 55 mixed tumors and 39 vascular proliferations in 117 cases of benign salivary gland tumors in children. The parotid gland is by far the favorite site of vascular tumors; only a few in the other salivary glands have been described.[62, 68]

Of the mesenchymal neoplasms of these glands in infants and children, hemangiomas predominate, yet they constitute less than 10 per cent of all causes of parotid swelling.[53] They generally affect Caucasian females. Massarelli and associates[62] state that 54 of 61 reported lesions were observed during the first year of life, the fourth through the sixth month being the period of maximum growth.

Hemangiomas are located at the angle of the mandible. They may be well defined, although they are more often diffuse, their margins extending below the ramus of the mandibile and into the neck itself. The masses seem to increase in size with crying or straining. A concomitant hemangioma or telangiectasia in the overlying skin is fairly common. Another important clinical observation is the bluish discoloration of the overlying skin transmitted from the cavernous component of the hemangioma. Also, while a small number of the tumors are firm in consistency, the majority are soft, doughy, and compressible. These findings should leave little doubt about the diagnosis of a vascular tumor of the parotid gland that appears during the first year of life.[73] Arteriography and sialography are of diagnostic value in complicated cases.[73]

Although hemangiomas of the parotid gland may be considered a single clinical entity, Welch[99] has recognized three groups of tumors, representing their variable natural history:

1. The slowly growing spongy and cavernous tumors.
2. The more rapidly growing firm and cellular types.
3. Those that function as arteriovenous fistulas and have a very rapid growth phase.

The controversy over whether these lesions are true neoplasms or vascular malformations has not been resolved. The cavernous form, observed in older children, is best considered a malformation.

Grossly, the involved gland is hypertrophied, apparently incident to an increase in the size of individual lobules; the latter are purple-red, spongy, and distinctly congested. Microscopically, numerous capillary blood vessels ramify in the parenchyma of the gland (Fig. 42–41). Occasionally, endothelial cells with mitoses are present in the capillary lumina. Nuclear pleomorphism and atypism are lacking.

Approximately 50 per cent of hemangiomas will undergo spontaneous involution, particularly during the second and third years of life.[73] After excision of the tumors, recurrence is unusual, although it is more likely if the patient is less than 4 months old.[62, 73, 99]

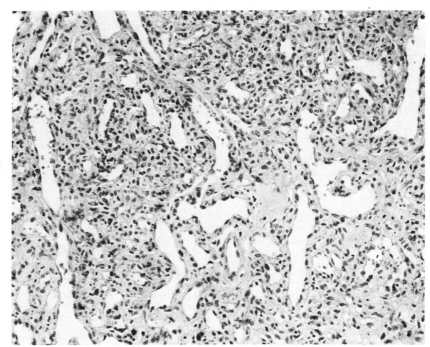

Figure 42–41. Hemangioma of parotid gland. This lesion is composed of proliferating capillaries.

Warthin's Tumor. Warthin's tumor and benign lymphoepithelial lesions have also been reported in children.[19, 22, 58] Both these tumors are similar biologically and morphologically to those encountered in adults.

Malignant Salivary Gland Tumors In Children

Three characteristics of malignant neoplasms of the major salivary glands in children deserve emphasis:

1. The biologic activity of malignant epithelial tumors in children does not differ from that of their counterparts in adults.[19, 58]

2. The tumors may be of epithelial or mesenchymal origin.

3. Well-differentiated mucoepidermoid carcinoma is the malignant neoplasm usually observed.

Mucoepidermoid carcinoma and acinic cell carcinoma together account for almost 60 per cent of the malignant salivary gland tumors in children. The incidence of acinic cell carcinoma, adenocarcinoma, undifferentiated carcinoma, and rhabdomyosarcoma is lower (Table 42–5).

MUCOEPIDERMOID CARCINOMA

Mucoepidermoid carcinomas are the most common malignant epithelial tumors of the salivary glands that affect children; 20 of 35 malignant tumors reviewed by Krolls and associates[58] at the AFIP and 13 of 17 malignant parotid epithelial tumors found at the Mayo Clinic by Chong and associates[22] were mucoepidermoid carcinomas. The majority arise in the parotid gland. The AFIP series included 14 primary tumors in the parotid gland, four in the submaxillary glands, and two in the accessory salivary glands.[58]

The histologic appearance and clinical behavior of mucoepidermoid carcinomas in children are similar to those of these same tumors in adults. The majority are of the low-grade type and are seldom fatal. Of 15 mucoepidermoid carcinomas reported by Byers and associates[18] from The M. D. Anderson Hospital, 13 were of low-grade malignancy; all the 13 patients survived from 2 to 24 years. In contrast, the high-grade carcinomas carried a comparatively unfavorable prognosis; patients with this type had a 5-year survival rate of 50 per cent. Of 27 mucoepidermoid carcinomas in children reviewed by Kaufman and Stout,[54] only one child died of widespread metastases. Five others had metastases in lymph nodes, though none of these was known to have died. Seven others had local recurrences.

ACINIC CELL CARCINOMA

The second most frequently observed malignant epithelial tumor is *acinic cell carcinoma*. Twelve of 35 malignant epithelial tumors at AFIP and four of 17 reported by Chong and associates[22, 58] at the Mayo Clinic were in this category. The majority of children with acinic cell carcinoma are girls, their chief complaint being a mass of several years' duration in the parotid gland. Even in this age group, acinic cell carcinoma retains its usual characteristics of slow growth, local invasion, and late metastases.

Of the 10 tumors of the parotid gland in the AFIP series, only one recurred. In the Mayo Clinic series, all four children with acinic cell carcinoma were free of disease at 8 to 16 years after treatment.

ADENOID CYSTIC CARCINOMA, ADENOCARCINOMA, AND UNDIFFERENTIATED CARCINOMA

Of these malignant epithelial neoplasms of the salivary glands that have been reported in children, Kaufman and Stout[54] considered the undifferentiated carcinoma the most malignant. Six of nine patients in the cases reviewed by these authors had metastases, five of whom were known to have died of the tumor.

Two cases of *embryomas*, an extremely rare form of congenital epithelial tumors of the parotid gland, have been described by Vawter and Tefft.[97] They were recognized in newborns, having developed during fetal life, and recurred after removal of the original tumor.

MALIGNANT LYMPHOMA AND SARCOMA

Malignant lymphomas and sarcomas, such as rhabdomyosarcoma and fibrosarcoma are seldom observed in children, although they should be considered in the differential diagnosis of an enlargement of any of the major salivary glands. Rhabdomyosarcoma accounted for five of the six sarcomas at the AFIP.[58] Karlan and Snyder reported three sarcomas of the parotid gland, one an undifferentiated sarcoma, one a neurosarcoma, and one a rhabdomyosarcoma.[53]

Although the incidence of *non-Hodgkin's lymphoma* varies during childhood and adolescence, involvement of the salivary glands appears to be a rarity in these age groups. Of 59 patients with lymphomas in the salivary glands reported by Colby and Dorfman,[23] only four were under 16. All these patients had *lymphoblastic lymphoma*, three in the parotid gland and one in an accessory gland. Krolls and associates[58] found only six cases of non-Hodgkin's lymphoma in 158 salivary gland tumors in children.

ANATOMIC AND PATHOLOGIC FEATURES INFLUENCING PROGNOSES

The anatomic and pathologic features that appear to influence the clinical course of malignant salivary gland tumors include the following:

1. Histologic type.
2. Size of the tumor and structures involved.
3. Site of origin.
4. Presence or absence of tumor at the margin of resection.
5. Histologic grade.

Table 42–6 depicts the influence of these prognostic factors upon survival of patients with malignant salivary gland tumors most often observed.

Histologic Type

The histologic type of a tumor of a salivary gland is one of the factors of most significance in the outcome; it correlates not only with the clinical stage of the lesion but also with the length of survival of the patient.[39–51] For example, the 10-year survival rate for a patient with a parotid tumor 2 cm or less in size, that is solitary, freely movable, and not associated with evidence of dysfunction of the facial nerve (Stage I) is 97 per cent for low-grade mucoepidermoid carcinoma, 68 per cent for acinic cell carcinoma, 47 per cent for adenoid cystic carcinoma, and 36 per cent for malignant mixed tumor (Table 42–6). Spiro and associates,[89] correlating the clinical stage with the histomorphologic appearance, found that low-grade mucoepidermoid carcinoma, low-grade adenocarcinoma, and acinic cell carcinoma were least likely to metastasize to cervical lymph nodes or distant sites, and that more than 70 per cent of patients with these tumors had Stage I disease. In contrast, about 50 per cent of the adenoid cystic carcinomas, malignant mixed tumors, and high-grade mucoepidermoid carcinomas were more aggressive, being in Stage III category when the patient was first observed.

Size of Tumor

The size of the tumor and the structures involved are prominent considerations in predicting behavior. Spiro and associates[89] correlated the size of the tumor with the incidence of lymph node and distant metastasis. They reported 5-year survival rates of 85 per cent for tumors less than 2 cm in diameter (T1), 67 per cent for cancers between 2 and 4 cm (T2), and 14 per cent for lesions between 4 and 6 cm (T3). In their series of adenoid cystic carcinomas, 47 per cent of the patients with tumors of 2 cm or less in diameter were alive and well at 10 years. The same authors were also able to correlate recurrence rates with the size of the tumors. T1 lesions recurred in only 7 per cent of the cases,

TABLE 42–6. Anatomic and Pathologic Factors Influencing Survival*

Factors	Mucoepidermoid	Adenoid Cystic	Acinic Cell	Malignant Mixed
Less than 2 cm	97	47	68	36
2.1 to 4 cm	83	11	68	—
4.1 cm or more	28	21	0	13
Positive LNS	20	22	44	10
Negative LNS	80	32	99	30
Bone positive	46	7	—	—
Bone negative	82	32	—	—
Positive margins	43	8	37	77
Negative margins	97	34	86	100
Low grade	66	70	71	—
Intermediate grade	—	51	—	—
High grade	36	12	33	—
Parotid gland	64	77	61	26
Submaxillary gland	45	29	—	20

*Numbers indicate percentage of patients alive and well 10 years after treatment. Data extracted from Healey WV et al,[46] LiVolsi VA et al,[60] Perzin KH et al,[74, 76] Spiro RH et al,[86–88, 90] and Szanto PA et al.[93]
LNS = Lymph nodes.

whereas T3 lesions had 58 per cent recurrence rate. The presence of metastases to the lymph nodes is another important factor. In the study by Spiro and associates,[89] 2 per cent of patients with tumors less than 4 cm in diameter, and with negative cervical lymph nodes (Stage I), had an incidence of distant metastases, in contrast to 39 per cent of patients with metastases from tumors of the same size but with positive cervical lymph nodes (Stage III). For example, patients with metastatic acinic cell carcinoma in lymph nodes had a survival rate of 20 per cent at 10 years, as compared with a survival rate of 60 per cent of patients with negative nodes.

Invasion of bone is an ominous sign; in our series of adenoid cystic carcinoma, only one of 24 patients with bone involvement was free of the disease at 15 years.[93] A similar experience has been reported by Spiro and associates.[88]

The previously mentioned factors—size and structures involved—are likewise significant in *staging* cancers of the parotid gland. Fu and coworkers[39] and Levitt and associates,[59] using the same staging system as Spiro and associates,[89] found a 10-year survival rate of 83 per cent for patients with Stage I cancers of the parotid gland, 76 per cent for those with Stage II, and 32 per cent for those with Stage III cancers.

Site of Origin

The location of the tumor is also a consideration in the prognosis. Tumors in the submaxillary glands are usually more aggressive than identical parotid tumors.[32] Szanto and associates[93] found that patients with adenoid cystic carcinomas in the parotid gland had better prognoses (the cumulative survival rates at 15 years being 38 per cent) than patients with submaxillary gland tumors, who had a cumulative survival rate of 10 per cent for the same period of time (Fig. 42–42). The incidence of cervical lymph node metastases in mucoepidermoid carcinoma and adenoid cystic carcinoma is also higher for submaxillary gland tumors (28 per cent) than for parotid tumors (52 per cent).[16, 56] The prognosis

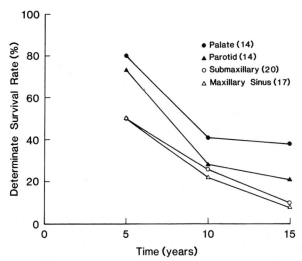

Figure 42–42. Determinate survival rates of patients with adenoid cystic carcinoma, according to the site of origin of the primary tumor.

of patients with acinic cell carcinoma in the deep lobe of the parotid gland is less favorable than it is if the lateral lobe of the gland is the primary site. The 10-year survival rates reported by Spiro and associates[87] was 14 per cent for patients with tumors of the deep lobe, as compared to 61 per cent for those with tumors in the lateral lobe.

Presence or Absence of Tumor at Surgical Margin

In our series of adenoid cystic carcinomas, only two of 24 patients (8.3 per cent) whose surgical margins were positive were alive without evidence of disease at 15 years after operation.[93] In the series reported by Perzin and associates,[74] two of 46 patients (4 per cent) with positive margins were alive and without evidence of recurrent tumor between 5 and 21 years postoperatively. LiVolsi and Perzin,[60] studying malignant mixed tumors, found that demonstrable tumor in the margin of excision correlated with an increased local recurrence rate as well as increased mortality rate. Of 26 patients with tumor at the surgical margin, 14 (54 per cent) had a local recurrence, eight (31 per cent) exhibited metastasis, and six (23 per cent) had died of the disease. In contrast, of 14 subjects with negative margins, two (14 per cent) had a local recurrence and 7 per cent had regional lymph node metastases, but none had died of their tumor from 5 to 13 years after treatment. Similar results have been described by Healey and Perzin[46] for patients with mucoepidermoid carcinomas and by Perzin and LiVolsi[76] for those with acinic cell carcinomas.

Histologic Grade

Over the years, the grading of histologic malignancy into low-, intermediate-, and high-grade types, based upon differentiation, has been applied to several tumors of the salivary glands, including mucoepidermoid carcinoma, adenoid cystic carcinoma, acinic cell carcinoma, and adenocarcinoma. A good clinicopathologic correlation has been reported for mucoepidermoid carcinoma[46] and, more recently, for adenoid cystic carcinoma.[74] Even on the latter, the size, anatomic location, and status of the surgical margin play a prominent role.

Healey and Perzin[46] and Spiro and associates[86] classified mucoepidermoid carcinomas into low, intermediate, and high grades. These authors discovered a definite correlation between histologic appearance, lymph node metastases, recurrence, and overall survival. Stage I lesions were usually of low histologic grade and were effectively controlled by conservative surgical procedures. In contrast, most of the patients with Stage III lesions had high-grade carcinomas and seldom were cured of the tumor. Healey and Perzin[46] reported a recurrence rate of 6 per cent for low-grade, 20 per cent for intermediate-grade, and 78 per cent for grade III lesions. In the series of Spiro and associates,[87] 66 per cent of patients with low-grade carcinoma were alive and without evidence of recurrence 10 years after treatment, as compared with 36 per cent of the patients with lesions of intermediate and high grades. The incidence of metastasis to regional lymph nodes in patients with low-grade mucoepidermoid carcinoma was zero, in contrast to 44 per cent of those with high-grade carcinomas.

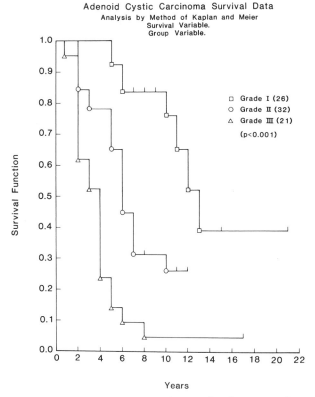

Figure 42–43. Cumulative survival rates of patients according to histologic grade of differentiation of adenoid cystic carcinoma.

The histologic grading of *adenoid cystic carcinoma* into high and low grades had produced inconsistent findings[88] until Perzin and associates[74] graded these carcinomas according to their predominant histologic pattern, whether tubular, cribriform, or solid. Tumors with a predominantly solid pattern were larger, had an aggressive clinical behavior, recurred frequently, and usually proved to be fatal within 4 years after treatment of the patient. Tumors composed predominantly of tubular structures tended to be smaller, were generally amenable to complete surgical excision, and had a protracted clinical course. The predominantly cribriform lesions appeared to follow a clinical and pathologic course between the other two forms. These observations also have been made in other studies[21, 93] (Fig. 42–43).

REFERENCES

1. Batsakis JG: Mucoepidermoid and acinous cell carcinomas of salivary tissues. Ann Otolaryngol 89:91, 1980.
2. Batsakis JG: Salivary gland neoplasia: An outcome of modified morphogenesis and cytodifferentiation. Oral Surg 49:229, 1980.
3. Batsakis, JG: Tumors of the Head and Neck. 2nd ed. Baltimore, Williams & Wilkins Co., 1981.
4. Batsakis JG, Brannon RB: Dermal analogue tumors of major salivary glands. J Laryngol Otol 95:155, 1981.
5. Batsakis JG, Brannon RB, Sciubba JJ: Monomorphic adenomas of salivary glands: A histologic study of 96 tumors. Clin Otolaryngol 6:129, 1981.
6. Batsakis JG, Chinn E, Repola DA: The pathology of head and neck tumors: Salivary glands, Part 2. Head Neck Surg 1:167, 1978.
7. Batsakis, JG, Kraemer B, Sciubba JJ: The pathology of the head and neck tumors: The myoepithelial cell and its participation in salivary gland neoplasia, Part 17. Head Neck Surg 5:222, 1983.
8. Batsakis JG, Regezi JA: Selected controversial lesions of salivary tissues. Otolaryngol Clin North Am 10:309, 1977.
9. Batsakis JG, Regezi JA: The pathology of head and neck tumors: Salivary glands. Part 1. Head Neck Surg 1:59, 1978.
10. Ibid., Part 4. Head Neck Surg 1:340, 1979.
11. Batsakis JG, Regezi JA, Block D: The pathology of head and neck tumors: Salivary glands, Part 3. Head Neck Surg 1:260, 1979.
12. Beahrs OH, Woolner LB, Kirklin JW, Devine KD: Carcinomatous transformation of mixed tumors of the parotid gland. Arch Surg 75:605, 1957.
13. Bernier JL, Bhaskar SN: Lymphoepithelial lesions of salivary glands. Histogenesis and classification based on 186 cases. Cancer 11:1156, 1958.
14. Bhaskar SN, Bernier JL: Mucoepidermoid tumors of major and minor salivary glands. Cancer 15:801, 1962.
15. Blanck JG: Mucus-producing adenopapillary (nonepidermoid) carcinoma of the parotid gland. Cancer 28:676, 1971.
16. Bosch A, Brandenburg JH, Gilchrist KW: Lymph node metastases in adenoid cystic carcinoma of the submaxillary gland. Cancer 45:2872, 1980.
17. Byers RM, Jesse RH, Guillamondegui OM, Luna MA: Malignant tumors of the submaxillary gland. Am J Surg 126:458, 1973.
18. Byers RM, Piorkowski R, Luna MA: Malignant parotid tumors in children. Arch Otolaryngol 110:232, 1984.
19. Castro EB, Huvos AG, Strong EW, et al: Tumors of major salivary glands in children. Cancer 29:312, 1972.
20. Chen KTK: Metastasizing pleomorphic adenoma of the salivary gland. Cancer 42:2407, 1978.
21. Chilla R, Schorth R, Eysholdt V, Droese M: Adenoid cystic carcinoma of the head and neck. J Otorhinolaryngol Relat Spec 42:346, 1980.
22. Chong GC, Beahrs OH, Chen ML, Hayles AB: Management of parotid gland tumors in infants and children. Mayo Clin Proc 50:279, 1975.
23. Colby TV, Dorfman RF: Malignant lymphomas involving the salivary gland. Pathol Annu 14:307, 1979.
24. Conley J, Arena S: Parotid gland as a focus of metastasis. Arch Surg 87:757, 1963.
25. Conley J, Meyers E, Cole R: Analysis of 115 patients with tumors of the submandibular gland. Ann Otolaryngol 18:323, 1972.
26. Corio RL, Sciubba JJ, Brannon RB, Batsakis JG: Epithelial myoepithelial carcinoma of intercalated duct origin. Oral Surg 53:280, 1982.
27. Dardick I, Van Nostrand AWP, Phillips MJ: Histogenesis of salivary gland pleomorphic adenoma with an evaluation of the role of the myoepithelial cell. Hum Pathol 13:62, 1982.
28. Dietert SE: Papillary cystadenoma lymphomatosum (Warthin's tumor) in patients in a general hospital over a 24-hour period. Am J Clin Pathol 63:866, 1975.
29. Donath K, Seifert G, Schmitz R: Zur Diagnose und Untrastruktur des tubularen Speichelgangcarcinoms. Epithelial-myoepitheliales Schaltstuckcarcinom. Virchows Arch (Pathol Anat) 356:16, 1972.
30. Duplessis DJ: The problem of Mikulicz's disease. S Afr Med J 32:265, 1958.
31. Eneroth CM: Mixed tumors of major salivary glands: Prognostic role of capsular structure. Ann Otol Rhinol Laryngol 74:944, 1965.
32. Eneroth CM: Salivary gland tumors in the parotid gland, submandibular gland and the palate region. Cancer 27:1415, 1971.
33. Evans RW, Cruickshank AH: Epithelial Tumors of the Salivary Glands. Philadelphia, W. B. Saunders Co., 1970.
34. Eversole LR: Histogenic classification of salivary tumors. Arch Pathol 92:433, 1971.
35. Fayemi AO, Ali M: Fibrous histiocytoma of the parotid gland. Mount Sinai J Med 47:290, 1980.
36. Ferlito A, Cattai N: The so-called "benign lymphoepithelial lesion" (Part 1—explanation of the term and of its synonymous and related terms). J Laryngol Otol 94:1189, 1980.
37. Foote FW Jr, Frazell EL: Tumors of the major salivary glands. Cancer 6:1065, 1953.
38. Freeman C, Berg JW, Culter SJ: Occurrence and prognosis of extranodal lymphomas. Cancer 29:252, 1972.
39. Fu KK, Leibel SA, Levine ML, et al: Carcinoma of the major and minor salivary glands. Cancer 40:2882, 1977.
40. Garland TA, Innes DJ, Fechner RE: Salivary duct carcinoma. Lab Invest 48:28A, 1983.
41. Gerughty RM, Scofield HH, Brown RM, et al: Malignant mixed tumors of salivary gland origin. Cancer 24:471, 1969.
42. Gnepp DR: Sebaceous neoplasms of salivary gland origin. Pathol Annu 18:71, 1983.

43. Gomez L, Luna MA: Clear cell tumors of the parotid gland. Am J Clin Pathol 77:245, 1982.

44. Grahne B, Lavren C, Holsti LR: Clinical and histological malignancy of adenoid cystic carcinoma. J Laryngol Otol 91:743, 1977.

45. Headington JT, Batsakis JG, Beals TF, et al: Membranous basal cell adenoma of parotid gland, dermal cylindromas and trichoepitheliomas. Cancer 39:2460, 1977.

46. Healey WV, Perzin KH: Mucoepidermoid carcinoma of salivary gland origin. Cancer 26:368, 1970.

47. Hillel AD, Fee WE: Evaluation of frozen section in parotid gland surgery. Arch Otolaryngol 109:230, 1983.

48. Howard DR, Bagley C, Batsakis JG: Warthin's tumor. A functional immunologic study of the lymphoid cell component. Am J Otolaryngol 3:15, 1982.

49. Hyman GA, Wolff M: Lymphomas of the salivary glands. Am J Clin Pathol 65:421, 1976.

50. Jackson GL, Ballantyne AJ: Role of parotidectomy for skin cancer of the head and neck. Am J Surg 142:464, 1981.

51. Johns ME: Parotid cancer: A rational basis of treatment. Head Neck Surg 3:132, 1980.

52. Johns ME, Regize JA, Batsakis JG: Oncocytic neoplasms of salivary glands: An ultrastructural study. Laryngoscope 87:862, 1977.

53. Karlan MS, Snyder WH: Salivary gland tumors and sialadenitis in children. Calif Med 108:423, 1968.

54. Kaufman SC, Stout AP: Tumors of the major salivary glands in children. Cancer 16:1317, 1963.

55. Kleinsasser O, Hubner G, Klein HJ: Talgzellcarcinoma der Parotis. Arch Klin Exp Ohren Nasen Kehlkopfheikd 197:59, 1970.

56. Kline TS, Merrian JM, Shapshay SM: Aspiration biopsy cytology of the salivary gland. Am J Clin Pathol 76:263, 1981.

57. Krolls SO, Boyers RC: Mixed tumors of salivary glands: Long-term follow-up. Cancer 30:276, 1972.

58. Krolls SO, Trodahl JN, Boyers RC: Salivary gland lesions in children. A survey of 430 cases. Cancer 30:459, 1972.

59. Levitt S, McHugh RB, Gomez-Marin O, et al: Clinical staging system for cancer of the salivary gland. Cancer 47:2712, 1981.

60. LiVolsi C, Perzin KH: Malignant mixed tumor arising in salivary glands. Cancer 39:2209, 1977.

61. Lomax-Smith JD, Azzopardi JJ: The hyaline cell: A distinctive feature of mixed salivary tumors. Histopathology 2:77, 1978.

62. Massarelli G, Tanda F, Fois V, Oppia L: Hemangiopericytoma of the parotid gland. Report of a case and review of the literature. Virchows Arch (Pathol Anat) 368:81, 1980.

63. McClatchey KD, Appelblatt NH, Langin JL: Carcinoma in papillary cystadenoma lymphomatosum. Laryngoscope 98:98, 1982.

64. Miller RH, Calcaterra TC, Paglia DE: Accuracy of frozen section diagnosis of parotid lesions. Ann Otol Rhinol Laryngol 88:573, 1979.

65. Moberger JG, Eneroth CM: Malignant mixed tumors of the major salivary glands; special reference to the histologic structure in metastasis. Cancer 21:1198, 1968.

66. Morgan WS, Castleman B: A clinicopathologic study of "Mikulicz's disease." Am J Pathol 29:471, 1953.

67. Moutsopoulos HM: Sjögren's syndrome (sicca syndrome): Current issues. Ann Intern Med 92:212, 1980.

68. Naeim R, Forsberg MI, Waisman J, et al: Mixed tumor of the salivary gland. Growth pattern and recurrence. Arch Pathol Lab Med 100:271, 1976.

69. Nagao K, Matsuzaki T, Saiga H, et al: Histopathologic studies of basal cell adenoma of the parotid gland. Cancer 50:736, 1982.

70. Nagao K, Matsuzaki T, Saiga H, et al: Histopathologic studies of undifferentiated carcinoma of the parotid gland. Cancer 50:1572, 1982.

71. Nichols RD, Pinnock LA, Szymanowski RT: Metastasis to parotid nodes. Larynogoscope 90:1324, 1980.

72. Nicolatou O, Harwick RD, Putong P, Leifer C: Ultrastructural characterization of intermediate cells of mucoepidermoid carcinoma of the parotid. Oral Surg 48:324, 1979.

73. Nussbaum M, Tan S, Som ML: Hemangiomas of the salivary glands. Laryngoscope 86:1015, 1976.

74. Perzin KH, Gullane P, Clairmont AC: Adenoid cystic carcinomas arising in salivary glands. Cancer 42:265, 1978.

75. Perzin KH, LiVolsi VA: Acinic cell carcinoma arising in ectopic salivary gland tissue. Cancer 45:967, 1980.

76. Perzin KH, LiVolsi VA: Acinic cell carcinomas arising in salivary glands. A clinicopathologic study. Cancer 44:1434, 1979.

77. Perzin KH: Systematic approach to the pathologic diagnosis of salivary gland tumors. Progr Surg Pathol 4:137, 1982.

78. Pesavento G, Ferlito A: Benign mixed tumor of heterotopic salivary gland tissue in upper neck. J Laryngol Otol 90:577, 1976.

79. Rankow RM, Mignogna F: Cancer of the sublingual salivary gland. Am J Surg 118:790, 1969.

80. Redondo C, Garcia A, Vazquez F: Malignant lymphoepithelial lesion of the parotid gland. Cancer 48:289, 1981.

81. Rees R, Maples M, Lynch JB, Rosenfeld L: Malignant secondary parotid tumors. South Med J 74:1050, 1981.

82. Schmid U, Helbron D, Lennert K: Development of malignant lymphoma in myoepithelial sialadenitis (Sjögren's syndrome). Virchows Arch (Pathol Anat) 395:11, 1982.

83. Sciubba JJ, Brannon RB: Myoepithelioma of salivary glands. Cancer 49:562, 1982.

84. Shmooker BM, Enzinger FM, Brannon RB: Orofacial synovial sarcoma. A clinicopathologic study of 11 new cases and review of the literature. Cancer 50:292, 1982.

85. Skolnik EM, Friedman M, Becker S, et al: Tumors of the major salivary glands. Laryngoscope 87:834, 1977.

86. Spiro RH, Huvos AG, Berk R, et al: Mucoepidermoid carcinoma of salivary gland origin. A clinicopathologic study of 367 cases. Am J Surg 136:301, 1978.

87. Spiro RH, Huvos AG, Strong EW: Acinic cell carcinoma of salivary origin. A clinicopathologic study of 67 cases. Cancer 41:924, 1978.

88. Spiro RH, Huvos AG, Strong EW: Adenoid cystic carcinoma of salivary origin. A clinicopathologic study of 242 cases. Am J Surg 128:512, 1974.

89. Spiro RH, Huvos AG, Strong EW: Cancer of the parotid gland. Am J Surg 130:452, 1975.

90. Spiro RH, Huvos AG, Strong EW: Malignant mixed tumor of salivary gland origin. A clinicopathologic study of 146 cases. Cancer 39:388, 1977.

91. Stevenson GF, Hazard JB: Mucoepidermoid carcinoma of salivary gland origin. Cleve Clin Q 20:445, 1953.

92. Stewart FW, Foote FW, Becker WF: Mucoepidermoid tumors of salivary glands. Ann Surg 122:820, 1945.

93. Szanto PA, Luna MA, Tortoledo ME, White RA: Histologic grading of adenoid cystic carcinoma. Cancer 54:1062, 1984.

94. Thackray AC, Lucas RB: Tumors of the Major Salivary Glands. Atlas of Tumor Pathology. Series 2. Fasc 10. Washington, D.C., Armed Forces Institute of Pathology, 1975.

95. Tubbs RR, Sheibani KS, Weiss RA, et al: Immunohistochemistry of Warthin's tumor. Am J Clin Pathol 74:795, 1980.

96. Turnbull AD, Frazell EL: Multiple tumors of the major salivary glands. Am J Surg 118:787, 1969.

97. Vawter FG, Tefft M: Congenital tumors of the parotid gland. Arch Pathol 82:242, 1966.

98. Weitzner S: Plexiform neurofibroma of the major salivary glands in children. Oral Surg 50:53, 1980.

99. Welch K: Presalivary glands. In Mustard WT, Ravitch MM, Synder WH Jr, et al: Pediatric Surgery. 2nd ed. Chicago, Year Book Medical Publishers, 1969.

100. Yarington CT: Metastatic malignant disease to the parotid gland. Larynogoscope 91:517, 1981.

CHAPTER 43

Radiation Therapy of Tumors of the Salivary Glands

Homayoon Shidnia, M.D. • **Ned B. Hornback, M.D.**

Salivary gland tumors constitute 3 to 4 per cent of all head and neck neoplasms.[10, 24] The parotid glands are involved in 70 to 80 per cent of all tumors of the salivary glands, the submaxillary gland in 10 to 20 per cent, the minor salivary glands in 7 to 10 per cent, and the sublingual glands in 1 per cent.[4, 6, 8, 10]

In patients who present with salivary gland tumors, the percentage of those tumors having malignant components will vary, depending upon which gland is involved. The percentage of malignant involvement in salivary gland tumors is lowest in the parotid gland (20 to 30 per cent),[7] with increased involvement in the submaxillary gland (40 to 60 per cent),[1, 29, 51] accessory minor salivary gland (50 to 60 per cent)[9, 57] and highest in the sublingual gland (80 to 90 per cent).[1]

The behavior of salivary tumors has been best described by Ackerman and del Regato:[2] "The usual salivary tumor is a tumor in which the benign variant is less benign than the usual benign tumor and the malignant variant is less malignant than the usual malignant tumor."

Surgery alone has been the sole treatment for benign tumors of the salivary gland. When only radical surgery is used for the treatment of malignant tumors of the salivary glands, two major distressing sequelae have been noted: facial paralysis (86 per cent) and recurrence of the tumor in the surgical field (27 to 64 per cent).[53–58] The role of radiation therapy in treatment of both benign and malignant tumors in the past has been unclear. Prior to the 1950s, radiation had occasionally been used in the treatment of infectious conditions of the salivary gland[60] with varied results or, in some instances, as the only modality of treatment for malignant mixed tumors.[3, 4]

It is difficult to evaluate the results of treatment by radiation alone in these tumors, and the few good responses are usually anecdotal in nature. The opinion of many surgeons and radiation oncologists that salivary gland tumors are radioresistant may be changed as better results are seen as a result of improved treatment field design and delivery of optimal doses of radiation. When proper radiation therapy is given in combination with surgery, facial nerve function can be salvaged and local recurrence rates can be reduced with only minimal risk of increased complications.[20, 27, 30, 37, 38]

HISTORICAL CONSIDERATIONS

According to Ahlbom,[3] the surgical approach to parotid tumors started in the late 18th and early 19th centuries, and Warren[44] is credited for the first reported total parotidectomy. The superficial parotidectomy with conservation of the facial nerve was suggested by Taylor and Garcelon in 1948;[56] however, a radical parotidectomy had been recommended by Ahlbom as early as 1935[3] and Kirklin in 1944.[34]

As far as radiation therapy is concerned, Kirmission in 1904 and 1905 suggested the use of radiation therapy for the treatment of parotid mixed tumors.[35] In 1912, Villard, with radiation alone, observed a good tumor response in the treatment of recurrent carcinoma of the parotid.[44] The superficial application and/or an interstitial implant of radioactive sources was recommended by Wickham and Degrais as well as Abbe in 1911.[44] In 1922, Burrows also reported good results in 19 cases that were treated with radiation therapy.[46] The combination of x-rays and radium was also attempted by Harmer and Russell and later by Merritt in 1922.[45] In 1915, Kuttner recommended the use of postoperative radiation therapy.[45]

In 1935, Ahlbom reported a large series of 254 cases treated (radiosurgically) between 1909 and 1932 at Radiumhemmet with preoperative and postoperative radiation therapy[3] and also a group of patients treated with radiation therapy alone.[3] He concluded that "all cases of mucous and salivary tumors should be treated with radiation except on those with distant metastasis" and recommended that "treatment should be given as early as possible, and should be initiated with fractional external radiation." He adds that "radio-resistant tumors should be treated with surgery" and advises that operable or inoperable (malignant tumors) should be given a large dose of external radiation: "It is wiser to use radiosurgery for most parts of this type of tumors." In closing, he suggested that a lymph node dissection should not be performed unless lymph nodes were suggestive of tumor, in which case radiation should be applied to the surgical scar as well as the lymph node metastasis.

In 1937, Kaplan recommended a moderate dose of radiation therapy (by today's standard) for the treatment of this malignancy.[33] Lederman in 1942 suggested the routine use of postoperative radiation therapy.[37] Blocker and Desaive in 1960 suggested the routine use of tele-radium and telecobalt for postoperative radiation.[19, 23]

ANATOMIC AND PHYSIOLOGIC CONSIDERATIONS

Because the salivary glands are incidentally within the treatment volume of most portals of the oral cavity, nasopharynx, and oropharynx, the review of anatomy and physiology of this area is very important when radiation therapy is contemplated.

Parotid Gland. The parotid gland is ensheathed by cervical fascia, which is dense superficially but is very thin in the deep portions adjacent to the parapharyngeal space. Neoplastic involvement of the deep part of the gland may present as a primary pharyngeal mass. The parotid overlies the masseter muscle anteriorly, extends superiorly to the zygomatic arch, is grooved inferiorly by the posterior belly of the digastric muscle, and extends posteriorly to the mastoid process.

The branches of the facial nerve divide the parotid gland into two lobes joined by parotid tissue called the *isthmus*. The deep lobe relates deeply to the styloid process and transverse process of C2. Of the two lobes of the parotid gland, the superficial lobe is larger and is the most common site of neoplastic involvement. The incidence of tumors arising from the deep lobe is 11 to 12 per cent (Figs. 43–1 and 43–2).[31, 39]

Normally, the parotid gland does not extend anteriorly along the Stensen's duct (which is approximately at the level of the second upper molar), but occasionally there is an accessory lobe in this location.

The superficial lymphatic drainage of the parotid is to the preauricular nodes anterior to the tragus. This can also be the site of metastases from the scalp and lip rather than from the parotid gland. Deep lymphatic drainage of the parotid gland is to the subdigastric nodes. The intra- and periparotid lymph node may also become involved.

Submaxillary Gland. The submaxillary gland is encased by the superficial layer of deep cervical fascia.

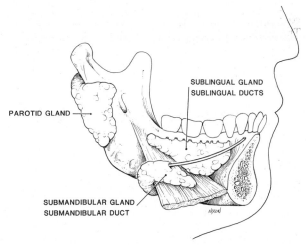

Figure 43–2. Medial view of salivary glands of left side.

Part of it lies on the external surface of the mylohyoid muscle. The deep portion of the gland extends around the mylohyoid muscle, and lies on the lateral aspect of the hyoglossal muscle. The submaxillary gland drains via Wharton's duct to papillae adjacent to the frenulum of the tongue.

The lymphatic drainage of the submaxillary gland is to the submaxillary nodes and the upper jugular nodes are second-echelon nodes.

Sublingual Gland. Located immediately beneath the mucosa of the floor of the mouth and mylohoid muscle, the sublingual gland drains by 5 to 15 ducts in to the floor of the mouth in the sublingual region (Rivinus's ducts). This gland is rarely the site of a primary tumor; however, any neoplastic process in this area should be considered malignant unless proven otherwise.

The primary lymphatic drainage of this gland is to the submental and submaxillary regions.

Minor Salivary Glands. The minor salivary glands will be discussed in the section on tumors of the oral cavity and other sites of origin.

PHYSIOLOGY

According to Schneyer and Levin, 47 per cent of all saliva is secreted by the main salivary glands.[48] Approximately two thirds, or 70 per cent, of the saliva is from the submaxillary gland, 25 per cent is from the parotid gland, and 5 per cent is from the sublingual gland. Between meals, saliva is secreted at the rate of 0.25 ml/min, or 15 ml/hr, and 600 to 1500 ml/24 hr.

Mixed saliva is slightly acidic and hypotonic, with a pH of 6.8, composed of 99.5 per cent water, and a specific gravity of 1.002 to 1.012. During sleep, saliva is secreted at the rate of 0.03 to 0.05 ml/hr. The lowest amount of saliva is secreted in the morning, with the peak being at 4:00 to 6:00 P.M. Males secrete more saliva than do females, and persons between the ages of 6 and 14 have more saliva.[59]

Mechanical stimulation, low pH, and mucosal irritation are physiologic stimuli. The parotid gland contains serous glands, which are responsible for stimulated saliva. Submaxillary glands are mixed serous and mu-

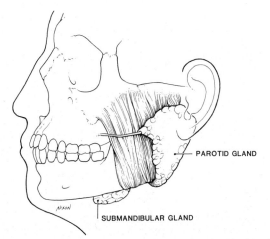

Figure 43–1. Lateral view of parotid and submaxillary gland.

cous, mainly responsible for saliva secreted during rest. The sublingual glands are mixed glands. Serous glands are more sensitive to radiation therapy, and damage to these glands is greater than that to mucous glands. After a course of radiation therapy, saliva is reduced and becomes more acidic and thicker.

EFFECTS OF RADIATION ON SALIVARY GLANDS

Even with the high number of salivary glands being incidentally in the field of radiation, our knowledge of the early or late effects of radiation is limited and based on only a few studies. Many questions remain to be answered, such as recovery of the salivary glands from radiation damage, change in composition of the saliva after treatment, temporary or permanent changes in taste, and the relationship between saliva and dental caries.

Most experimental work is based on a single dose of 1000 to 2000 centigray (cGy) which has no practical clinical value for daily practice of fractionated radiation therapy. Six to 12 hours after a dose of 180 to 200 cGy, a few patients will develop pain and swelling of the parotid or submaxillary glands if the gland was in the treatment field. This is normally a self-limited process, and moderate doses of aspirin or cold compresses will relieve the symptoms. The process lasts 2 to 3 days; normally there is no need for interruption of treatment, and additional treatment will not worsen the condition.

After radiation, according to Rubin and Cassaret,[47] histologically there is a predominance of lymphoid cells, plasma cells, and polymorphonuclear cells in the treated area. The interlobular capsule may also show some edema. The earlier changes would be seen in the serous glands rather than in the mucous glands. As treatment progresses, dryness becomes a problem factor. By the end of the first week of treatment, or at approximately 1000 cGy, the flow of saliva is reduced to 50 per cent. At the beginning of the second week, taste acuity is decreased. At the end of the third week, or at approximately 3000 cGy, salivary flow is reduced to 25 per cent and the sweet and salty taste sensations are reduced. By the fifth week, or at 5000 cGy, all four taste sensations (sweet, salt, acid, and bitter) will be suppressed. A mucosal reaction in the buccal mucosa will appear, and the salivary flow will be approximately 10 per cent. If the dose is limited to 5000 cGy, there is a full recovery of the salivary glands.

PATHOPHYSIOLOGY

Benign Tumors of the Salivary Glands

Benign tumors make up 60 per cent of all tumors of the salivary glands and about 85 per cent of parotid tumors.

Benign Mixed Tumors. Benign mixed tumors constitute 65 per cent of all neoplasms of the parotid glands. These usually are located in the tail of the parotid. The age group most commonly affected is between 20 and 40 years.[11] A recurrence rate of 30 per cent is associated with simple enucleation. According to Rafla-Demetrious,[45] recurrence rate can be reduced to 2.7 per cent

by giving 3500 to 5000 cGy in 3 to 5 weeks. Postoperative radiation therapy for unresectable tumors or incompletely resectable tumors is highly recommended.

Papillary Cystadenoma Lymphomatosum (Warthin's Tumor). This tumor constitutes approximately 9 per cent of all benign tumors of the salivary glands.[28] These tumors are usually unilateral and are normally completely excised by surgery. No radiation therapy is recommended.

Benign Lymphoepithelial Lesions (Godwin's Tumor). Some authors have included Mikulicz's disease and adenolymphoma in this group of tumors. This tumor represents approximately 5 per cent of all benign tumors of the salivary glands.[1] As long as these lesions are unilateral, they are successfully treated with surgery alone. In bilateral cases, or if there is the risk of facial nerve damage, this type of tumor can be successfully treated with radiation therapy to a dose of 3000 cGy in 3 weeks.

Oncocytoma. This rare tumor accounts for approximately 1 per cent of all benign tumors of the salivary glands, and surgery is the treatment of choice.

Basal Cell Adenoma. This type of tumor is rare, and the treatment of choice is surgery.

Malignant Tumors of the Salivary Glands

Since the pattern of failure and spread of disease as well as the clinical presentation of each histopathologic type of tumor is different, we will consider each separately. A summary of the various types of tumors is presented in Table 43–1.

Acinic Cell Tumors. Acinic cell tumors account for 2.5 to 4 per cent of all tumors of the salivary gland and represent 13 per cent of all malignant tumors of the parotid gland.[14] These tumors are very slow-growing and more commonly occur in females in the fifth decade of life. They rarely metastasize to the lymph nodes, and the incidence of facial nerve involvement is 3 per cent. If the entire tumor has been removed, no additional therapy is needed. Late local recurrence can be a problem and sometimes may be multifocal.

Adenoid Cystic Carcinoma (Cylindroma). Cylindroma accounts for 2 to 5 per cent of all tumors of the salivary glands. The most malignant tumor of the minor salivary glands and submaxillary gland is equally common in males and females.[12] The incidence of facial nerve involvement is 26 per cent. In half of the patients, microscopic evidence of perineural involvement is seen. The incidence of cervical node metastasis at presentation is about 15 per cent.[55] In the treatment planning of patients with this type of tumor, the entire path of the nerve, including the base of the skull, should be within the treatment field. Because "skip areas" of involvement may occur, one cannot be comfortable with negative neural margins on frozen sections. Long-term survivals of 10 to 20 years, even with the presence of lung metastasis, have been reported, but most patients with pulmonary metastasis succumb in 3 to 5 years.

Low-Grade Mucoepidermoid Carcinoma. This tumor accounts for 10 to 12 per cent of all tumors of the salivary glands[25, 51, 54] and can be successfully treated by adequate surgery.[13] Low-grade tumors account for 65 per cent of all mucoepidermoid tumors. They usually do not involve the facial nerve, and the recurrence rate

TABLE 43–1. Summary of Clinical Histologic Presentations in Malignant Tumors of the Salivary Gland

Histology	Incidence (%)	Age Predilection (Decade)	Sex Predilection	Favored Site	Node Metastasis (%)	7th Nerve Involvement (%)	Recurrence (%)	Distant Metastasis (%)	Specific
Acinic cell carcinoma	4	5th	F>M	Parotid	10	3	10–22	Rare	Multifocal, sometimes bilateral
Adenoid cystic carcinoma	2–5	5th–6th	F = M	Minor salivary glands and submaxillary glands	15	26	High*	28	Pain is presenting symptom; long-term survival with distant metastasis not unusual
Mucoepidermoid carcinoma									
Low grade	17–20	1st–2nd 4th–5th	M>F	No	60	8	17	33	More patients have low-grade type; half of histology of children in this type
High grade		6th				High*	75		
Malignant mixed tumor	4	7th	M>F	Parotid and submaxillary glands	33	14	30–40	31	Tumor slow-growing; starts sometimes in pre-existing pleomorphic adenoma
Squamous cell carcinoma	0.1–3	None	None	Parotids and salivary duct	High*	High*	70	High*	Rapid-growing; nerve palsy a frequent presentation
Adenocarcinoma	2.8	5th–6th	None	Parotid	50	9	67	19	Painless mass usual presentation
Undifferentiated carcinoma	3	7th–8th	F>M	None	50	23	High*	30	May start within pre-existing pathology such as mixed, cylindroma, or adenocarcinoma

*A high incidence in few cases.

is approximately 15 per cent. If a tumor is close to the surgical margins, postoperative radiation therapy with electron beam radiation is recommended,[30, 31] although adequate surgical excision of residual disease is also an alternative.

High-Grade Mucoepidermoid Carcinoma. This is a very aggressive tumor that often presents with lymph node metastasis and sometimes distant metastasis. The majority of mucoepidermoid carcinomas are low grade (65 per cent); approximately 35 per cent are high grade.[25, 51] The recurrence rate after surgery also is 60 to 75 per cent,[29] and the incidence of facial nerve involvement is high. This tumor should be treated with postoperative radiation therapy. Sixty-six per cent of the patients will have metastases to the neck nodes and 33 per cent will have cutaneous, pulmonary, cerebral, and/or bone metastases.

Malignant Mixed Tumors. This type of tumor accounts for 4 per cent of all tumors of the salivary glands and is very aggressive. Approximately 14 per cent of all patients with this type of tumor develop facial nerve paralysis. One third of the patients will have lymph node metastasis and should be treated with postoperative radiation therapy. Without radiation therapy, the recurrence rate is approximately 30 to 40 per cent.

Squamous Cell Carcinoma. Tumors with squamous cell histology account for 0.1 to 3 per cent of all tumors of the salivary gland and should be differentiated from squamous cell carcinoma of the skin with metastasis to the parotid gland, which usually occurs in older patients.[29] Tumors arising from the parotid are very aggressive, and nerve paralysis is a usual presentation. Cervical lymph node metastasis is a prominent feature, and the local recurrence rate is very high. These patients should always receive postoperative radiation therapy.

Adenocarcinoma. These tumors account for 5 to 8 per cent of all tumors of the salivary gland and are very

aggressive. More than 50 per cent of patients with adenocarcinoma develop lymph node metastasis.[18] Nerve paralysis can be a clinical presentation, and these tumors should be treated with postoperative radiation therapy.

Undifferentiated Carcinomas. These tumors comprise 3 per cent of all tumors of the salivary glands and 4 to 5 per cent of all malignant neoplasms of the parotid gland. The incidence of facial nerve paralysis is 23 per cent. The incidence of cervical node metastasis is high, approximately 50 per cent.[15] These tumors are very aggressive and should be treated with postoperative radiation therapy.

Extranodal Malignant Lymphoma. In our series of 64 patients with non-Hodgkin's lymphomas of the head and neck area, six had tumors located in the salivary gland. The majority of these tumors were of the large cell (or histiocytic) type. Five of the six patients experienced a relapse, and in three of these five patients the failure was in an adjacent lymph node.[49]

In the treatment planning of this type of tumor, elective irradiation of non-involved areas in the neck should be considered. The primary tumor responds very well to radiation therapy.

TREATMENT

Pretreatment Work-up

The work-up required for patients who are to undergo radiation therapy for malignant tumors of the parotid gland should include a history and general physical examination; routine blood studies; biopsy; examination of the skin (especially looking for skin malignancies in the head and neck area); careful evaluation of the cranial nerves; extensive ear, nose, and throat examination; computed tomography (CT) scanning through the in-

TABLE 43–2. TMN Staging of Salivary Tumors

Primary Tumor (T)	Nodal Involvement (N)
1. TX: Minimum requirements to assess the tumor unable to be met	1. NX: Nodes cannot be assessed
2. T0: No evidence of primary tumor	2. N0: No clinically positive nodes
3. T1: Tumor 2 cm or less in diameter, solitary, freely mobile, facial nerve intact*	3. N1: Single clinically positive homolateral node 3 cm or less in diameter
4. T2: Tumor more than 2 cm but not more than 4 cm in diameter, solitary, freely mobile or reduced mobility or skin fixation, and facial nerve intact*	4. N2: Single clinically positive homolateral node more than 3 cm but not more than 6 cm in diameter or multiple clinically positive homolateral nodes, none more than 6 cm in diameter
5. T3: Tumor more than 4 cm but not more than 6 cm in diameter, or multiple nodes, skin ulceration, deep fixation, or facial nerve dysfunction*	5. N2a: Single clinically positive homolateral node more than 3 cm but not more than 6 cm in diameter
6. T4: Tumor more than 6 cm in diameter and/or involving mandible and adjacent bones	6. N2b: Multiple clinically positive homolateral node, none more than 6 cm in diameter
	7. N3: Massive homolateral node(s), bilateral nodes or contralateral node(s)
	8. N3a: Clinically positive homolateral node(s) more than 6 cm in diameter
	9. N3b: Bilateral clinically positive nodes (in this situation, each side of the neck should be staged separately, that is, N3b: right, N2a; left, N1)
	10. N3c: Contralateral positive node(s) only
	Distant Metastasis (M)
	1. MX: Not assessed
	2. M0: No (known) distant metastasis
	3. M1: Distant metastasis present; specify _____

*Applicable to parotid tumors only.

volved gland; chest x-ray examination, bone scan, and dental evaluation.

Taste Test

A *taste test* can be performed by using four standard solutions:

1. Sweet—simple syrup, one sixth (⅙) strength.
2. Salt—sodium chloride solution 0.9 per cent.
3. Acid—acetic acid solution 0.31 per cent.
4. Bitter—quinine sulfate solution 0.0125 per cent.

Evaluation of the salivary flow with mechanical stimuli can be determined by having the patient chew a dry sponge or wax for 2 to 5 minutes. The difference in the weight of the sponge represents the total amount of saliva produced during that time period.

Staging

The American Joint Committee TMN system of classification for salivary tumors is given in Table 43–2.

Irradiation Technique

The major role of radiation therapy in the treatment of salivary gland tumors is adjunctive to surgery in the form of postoperative irradiation; however, *preoperative irradiation* as well as *radiation therapy alone* has been considered by some oncologists.[2–5, 24, 26, 27, 37, 44–46, 50]

Parotid Gland

The minimal treatment volume would cover the entire parotid compartment, including the drainage of lymph nodes in the preauricular and upper neck areas. In tumors of high-grade histology, the entire neck on the same side should be included within the treatment field. There does not appear to be a dose-response curve based on different histologies. A dose of 6000 cGy in 6 to 7 weeks postoperatively is well tolerated by the majority of patients. However, with close margins a dose of 6500 cGy is required. When there is gross residual disease, a dose of 7000 cGy with a reducing field technique is recommended. With evidence of peri-

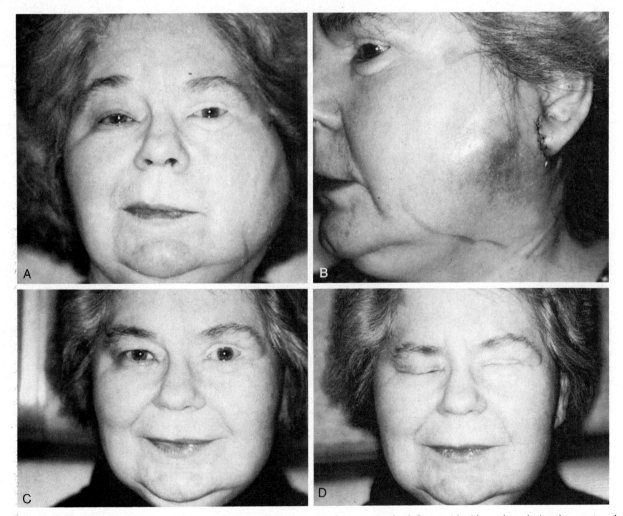

Figure 43–3. Treatment of 63-year-old white female with a history of a mass in the left parotid with neck node involvement and left-sided facial paralysis. (*A*) Anterior view before treatment. (*B*) Lateral view before treatment. (*C* and *D*) Frontal view 4 months after completion of 5000 cGy in 5 weeks, via a 19-MeV electron beam and twice weekly 433 MHz microwave therapy for 30 minutes.

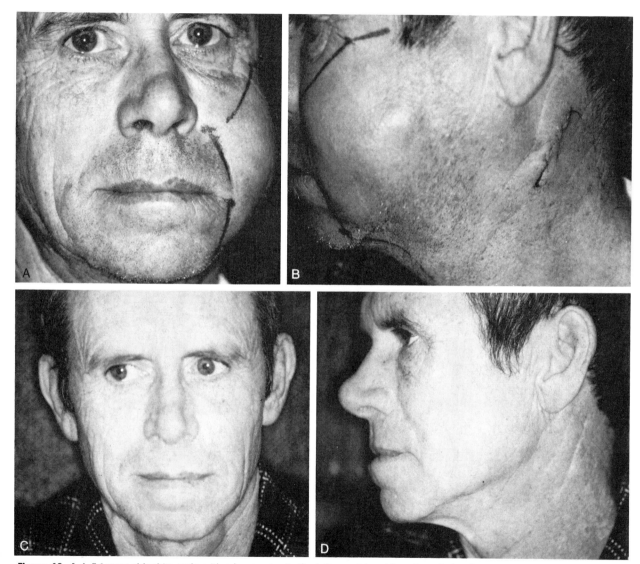

Figure 43–4. A 56-year-old white male with a large mass in the left parotid and lymph node involvement. A biopsy proved poorly differentiated squamous cell carcinoma. (*A*) Anterior view before treatment. (*B*) Lateral view. (*C*) Anterior view 8 months after completion of 5000 cGy in 5 weeks via a 19-Mev electron beam and twice weekly 433 MHz microwave therapy. (*D*) Lateral view.

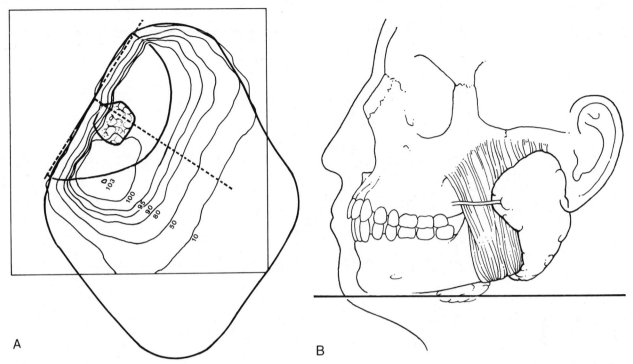

Figure 43–5. Isodose curves. (*A*) Single lateral beam 16-Mev electrons. (*B*) Isodose curve at the level of the submaxillary gland.

neural involvement, especially in adenoid cystic carcinoma, the field of therapy should extend to the base of the skull to include the nerve pathway.

Indications for Radiation Therapy. Radiation is recommended for:

1. All high-grade tumors, including adenoid cystic carcinoma.

2. Tumors that are transected during surgery or specimens that have close surgical margins.

3. Tumors involving the facial nerve.

4. Recurrent disease.

5. Documented lymph node metastasis.

6. Bone or connective tissue involvement.

In all of the above cases, postoperative radiation therapy should be used. Occasionally an exceptionally good response to a moderate dose of radiation therapy alone can be achieved (Figs. 43–3 and 43–4) where surgery cannot be performed. When considering all histologies, postoperative radiation therapy is expected to reduce the recurrence rate from 29.6 to 9.1 per cent.[31]

In general, patients who are accepted for postoperative radiation therapy will begin treatment 3 to 4 weeks following surgery or as soon as the surgical incision has healed. Facial nerve grafts, when required, have *not* been deleteriously affected by radiation (in our experience), and radiation therapy has not delayed the recovery of the nerve graft.[41] The treatment volume for the primary tumor site is similar in preoperative, postoperative, and radiation therapy alone. The recommended method of therapy is a high-energy photon beam, a high-energy electron beam, or a combination of the two.

Technique. Place the patient in a supine position with a shaped field. Choose a single lateral electron beam

oppositional to contour (Fig. 43–5) or a pair of back-to-back 45-degree wedged fields tilted 50 to 60 degrees according to the isodose curve, with only photon or electron beams (Fig. 43–6) or the best combination 2:1 in favor of the electron beam (Fig. 43–7). Angle the field posteriorly to avoid radiation to the eye and other salivary glands and to include the surgical scar. Extend the treatment field superiorly to the ridge of the zygoma, inferiorly below the angle of the mandible, posteriorly to include the external auditory canal and tip of the mastoid process, and anteriorly to the border of the masseter, including the opening of the parotid duct (Figs. 43–8 and 43–9).

In patients with a high-grade histology or lymph node metastasis, also include the homolateral lower neck within the field of therapy. This is done by continuing the field from the inferior border of the primary tumor field, which should include the medial two thirds of the clavicle and a 2-cm margin beyond the surgical scar. The total given dose to the neck nodes should be 6000 cGy in 6 to 7 weeks. This field can also be treated through a single anterior field with high-energy photons or through a lateral field with electron beams. Use bolus build-up in the surgical scar when necessary.

In the case of perineural involvement or adenoid cystic disease, the base of the skull should be included in the field of therapy. A combination of high-energy electron and high-energy photon beams should be used for uniformity of the radiation dose and for lowering the dose to the temporomandibular joint.

In any case, the depth of coverage should include the lateral wall of the pharyngeal wall on the same side of the primary tumor.

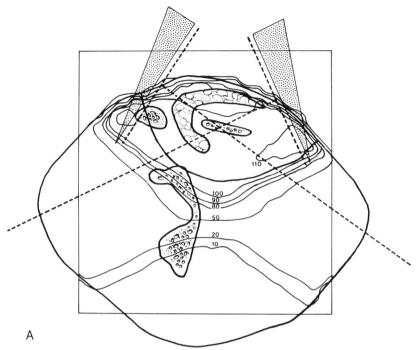

A

Figure 43–6. (*A*) Isodose curves. Cobalt 60 with a pair of 45-degree wedge filters. (*B*) Isodose curve at the level of the parotid gland.

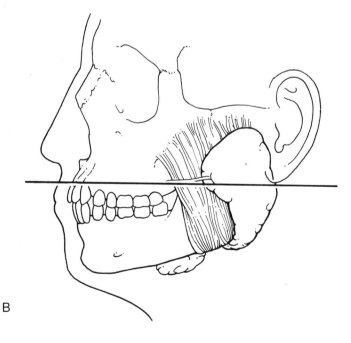

B

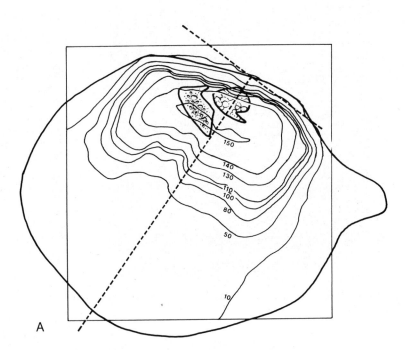

A

Figure 43–7. Isodose curves. (*A*) Combined 25-Mev photon and 16-Mev electron beams with 2:1 loading for electrons. (*B*) Isodose curve at the superior margin of the parotid gland.

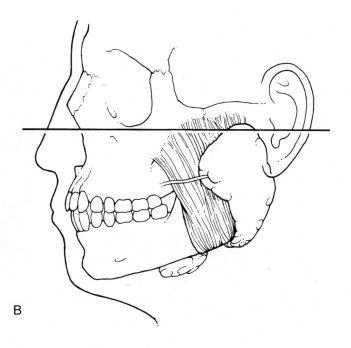

B

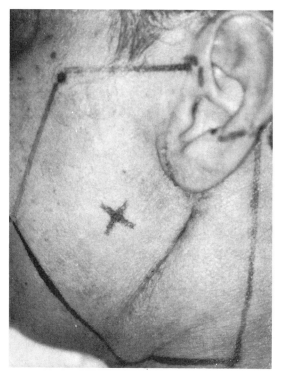

Figure 43–8. Postoperative portal with no neck node involvement.

Dose. Give a daily dose of 180 to 200 cGy to a total of 4500 to 5000 cGy with the use of the high-energy electron beam. Continue via a 20- to 25-Mev photon beam for an additional 2000 to 2500 cGy for a total of 6500 to 7000 cGy in 7 to 8 weeks.

Shielding. Because of the curvature of the neck, the dose should be calculated to the spinal cord and should not exceed 4500 cGy. The opposite salivary glands and opposite eye should be carefully excluded from the field of therapy.

Submaxillary Gland Tumors

Indications. Indications are the same as for tumors of the parotid gland.

Technique. Place the patient in the supine position with a cork and tongue depressor in the mouth. The superior border is 1 cm above the border of the tongue as seen in a lateral x-ray. The inferior border line is parallel to the hyoid bone. The posterior border includes the base of tongue and jugulodigastric region. The anterior border includes the entire oral cavity, excluding 1 cm from the soft tissue of the chin to prevent an excessive reaction of the lower lip and chin. The posterior aspect of the symphysis of the mandible should be within the field of therapy.

Method. Use an electron beam or a combination of a high-energy photon beams with a pair of 45-degree wedged filters tilted 40 to 60 degrees according to the isodose curve. The coverage should include the midline of the tongue, and if inclusion of the lower neck is desired, use the same technique as for treatment of parotid gland tumors.

Dose. Give a daily dose of 180 to 200 cGy to a total of 4500 to 5000 cGy with the use of an electron beam. Continue via a reducing field with electron or photon beams for an additional 2000 to 2500 cGy for a total of 6500 to 7000 cGy in 7 to 8 weeks.

Sublingual Gland Tumors

Indications. Indications and methods are the same as for tumors of the parotid gland.

Technique. The technique is identical to that used in the treatment of carcinoma of the submaxillary gland.

Dose. Use cobalt-60 teletherapy or high-energy photon beams through parallel opposing fields to a total tumor dose of 5000 cGy in 5 weeks. Additional therapy may be given with the use of a submental field with electron beams for an additional 1500 to 2000 cGy. Treatment can be either by hyperextension of the neck through a submental field or by placing the patient in a lateral position with neck extended using an angled table and directing the submental field to the vertex from the symphysis of the mandible to the level of the hyoid bone. A shrinking field can also be used via a high-energy photon beam. The time-dose fractionation is similar to that used for tumors of the submaxillary gland. If treatment of the lower neck is indicated, bilateral neck irradiation is recommended to a total dose of 5000 cGy in 5 weeks.

Results of Treatment

Historically, malignant tumors of the salivary gland treated with radiation or surgery as a single modality have had a high risk of recurrence (27 to 64 per cent).[53] As early as 1909, combinations of radiation therapy and

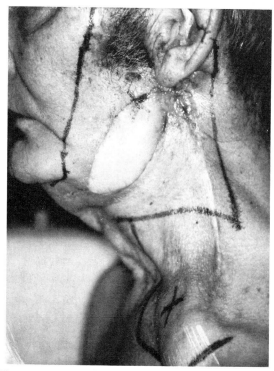

Figure 43–9. Two-field portal with neck node involvement.

TABLE 43–3. Incidence of Local Failures in Malignant Tumors of the Parotid—Surgery Alone or Surgery and Irradiation*

	Surgery Alone 1945–December 1965 Analysis, 1973	Surgery + Irradiation 1948–July 1973 Analysis, June 1976
Squamous cell carcinoma	—	0/3
Adenocarcinoma	4/10	0/4
Malignant mixed tumor	5/24	1/7
Adenocystic carcinoma	4/8	1/7
Mucoepidermoid carcinoma	3/12	1/12
Total	16/54 (29.6%)	3/33 (9.1%)

*From Guillamondegui OM, Byers RM, Luna MA, et al: AJR *123*:49, 1975.[31]

surgery had been suggested by several physicians. In 1935, Ahlbom in an excellent review of 254 patients treated with preoperative radiation, postoperative radiation, and radiation and surgery alone reported that the recurrent rate for 91 patients with benign tumors was 2½ per cent; in addition, 33 patients with semimalignant tumors had a recurrence rate of 17 per cent. In a total of 124 patients with malignant tumors, half received radiation alone, and the other half were treated with combined radiation and surgery. The 2-year survival rate in both groups was 45 per cent, 5-year survival rate 31 per cent, and 11-year survival 20 per cent.

Benign Tumors. The treatment of benign salivary gland tumors is adequate surgical excision. This usually means superficial lobectomy for parotid tumor (unless deep lobe is involved). In benign mixed tumors, however, a recurrence rate of 20 per cent in 10 to 15 years has been reported.[39] In my experience, postoperative radiation therapy decreases the recurrence rate to 2.7 per cent. In patients with bilateral lymphoepithelial tumors, a moderate dose of radiation therapy of 3000 cGy in 3 weeks to a small field can produce good tumor regression with an excellent cosmetic result.

Malignant Tumors. In high-grade malignant tumors, postoperative radiation therapy may reduce the recurrence by one third. In the experience of M. D. Anderson Hospital, a course of postoperative radiation therapy can reduce the recurrence rate from 29.6 to 9.1 per cent (Table 43–3).[31]

TABLE 43–4. Site of Failure in 94 Patients with Salivary Tumors: Minimum of 2-Year Survival*

| Histopathology | Site | | | |
	Parotid	Submaxilla	Sublingual	Total
Acinic cell carcinoma	6/8	1/1	0/0	7/9
Adenocarcinoma	8/15	2/5	1/2	11/22
Adenoid cystic carcinoma	3/5	4/4	1/1	8/10
Epidermoid carcinoma	4/12	1/3	0/0	5/15
Malignant mixed tumors	1/4	1/2	0/0	2/6
Mucoepidermoid tumors	12/16	0/2	1/1	13/19
Undifferentiated carcinoma	2/8	0/1	0/0	2/9
Other	1/3	0/0	0/1	1/4
Totals	37/71	9/18	3/5	49/94

*Seven patients died of other causes.

TABLE 43–5. Type of Failure in 94 Patients with Salivary Tumors

Histology	Persistent	Recurrent	Metastatic
Acinic cell carcinoma	2	0	0
Adenocarcinoma	5	4	1
Adenoid cystic carcinoma	0	0	2
Epidermoid carcinoma	8	2	0
Malignant mixed	3	0	0
Mucoepidermoid	4	2	0
Undifferentiated	3	3	1
Other	2	1	0
Total	27	12	4

Two patients were lost to follow-up.
*From Shidnia H, Hornback NB, Hamaker R, et al: Carcinoma of Major Salivary Glands. Cancer *45*:693, 1980.[50]

In our series of 74 patients with T$_1$ and T$_2$ lesions, in aggressive histologies treated with a combination of surgery and local and regional radiotherapy, the control rate was 100 per cent, whereas the with surgery alone the control rate was 75 per cent. Patients with T$_3$ and T$_4$ lesions treated with combined modalities had a 66 per cent 5-year survival; with surgery alone the rate was 28.5 per cent survival.[54] Many facial nerves can be saved with a combination of radiation therapy and surgery. As in the experience of other centers,[41] we have not experienced any compromise of nerve grafts after postoperative radiation therapy. Tables 43–4 through 43–7 summarize the experience at Indiana University Medical Center and M. D. Anderson Hospital concerning the treatment results and patient failures.

Complications of Treatment

Dryness of the mouth is one of the major complications, but it can be avoided by the well-planned use of combined electron beams and photon beams and the sparing of other salivary glands. Also, commercially available synthetic saliva such as Moi-Stir, VA-OraLube, or Salivart may be used to alleviate this condition.

Trismus has not been a major complication as long as the dose to the temporomandibular joint and masseter muscle is kept at the level of 5000 cGy. This can be done by reducing the treatment field to include only the primary tumor bed.

The possible occurrence of *otitis media* should be discussed with the patient. Normally this complication is handled by conservative treatment. *Hair loss* and *skin changes* do occur, but have not been of major significance.

Dental complications, such as decreased sensitivity of teeth and development of dental caries, can occur but can be prevented by good dental hygiene. To a great extent, these complications can be avoided by the prophylactic treatment of teeth.

Information regarding *radiation-induced salivary gland tumors* is based on retrospective studies of patients who received radiation therapy for benign conditions, survivors of atomic bomb explosion at Hiroshima and Nagasaki, and in a few instances, the period following curative therapy for malignant tumors of the head and neck region. Unfortunately, there is insufficient information available regarding the quality of the radiation

TABLE 43–6. Minimum 2-Year Absolute Survival According to Histology and
Staging in 94 Patients with Salivary Tumors

Histology	Stage				Total	Per Cent
	I	II	III	IV		
Acinic cell carcinoma	4/5	0/0	2/3	1/1	7/9	78%
Adenoid cystic carcinoma	1/1	0/1	4/5	3/3	8/10	80
Adenocarcinoma	3/3	3/3	4/6	1/10	11/22	50
Epidermoid carcinoma	2/2	0/1	3/4	0/8	5/15	33
Malignant mixed tumors	1/1	1/1	0/2	0/2	2/6	33
Mucoepidermoid carcinoma	7/7	4/5	2/3	0/4	13/19	68
Undifferentiated carcinoma	1/1	1/2	0/1	0/5	2/9	22
Others	1/1	0/1	0/2	0/0	1/4	25
Total	20/21 (95.2%)	9/14 (64%)	15/26 (57.7%)	5/33 (15.2%)	49/94 (52.2%)	52.2%

*Minimum 2 years absolute survival.

beam, total dosage received, or dose distribution to determine risk of radiation in patients with these tumors. There is, however, an *increasing incidence of tumors in children* who received low-dose radiation therapy for benign conditions such as thymic enlargement or tinea capitis. The latent period averages approximately 13.3 years. Lawson and Som,[36] in a survey of 97 radiation-induced salivary gland tumors, reported 80 per cent to be located in the parotid gland. The incidence of malignant to benign tumors was 47:53. The most common type of malignant tumor was mucoepidermoid, followed by adenocarcinoma. The most common benign tumor was the mixed type. The calculated dose in most cases ranged from 350 to 400 cGy but as high as 2000 cGy was used. In an epidemiologic study of survivors of the atomic bomb reported by Belsky and colleagues in 1972,[17] the incidence of salivary neoplasia was reported to be five times greater than that expected in the "normal" population.

TABLE 43–7. Absolute 5-Year Survival in 120 Patients with Parotid Gland Cancer Treated at M.D. Anderson Hospital (1944–1965)

Histopathology	Number of Patients	Percentage of Patients
Acinic cell carcinoma	12	92
Mucoepidermoid (low grade)	28	76
Adenocarcinoma	12	56
Malignant mixed	27	50
Adenoid cystic	10	50
Squamous cell	6	50
Mucoepidermoid (high grade)	13	46
Undifferentiated	12	33

From Guillamondegui OM, Byers RM, Luna MA, et al: AJR 123:49, 1975.

REFERENCES

1. Ackerman LV, del Regato JA: Cancer Diagnosis, Treatment and Prognosis, 4th ed. St. Louis, C. V. Mosby, 1970, p. 535.
2. Ibid., p. 537.
3. Ahlbom HE: Mucous and salivary gland tumours. Acta Radiol Supp 23, 1935.
4. Alaniz F, Fletcher GH: Place and technics of radiation therapy in the management of malignant tumours of the major salivary glands. Radiol 84:412, 1965.
5. Bardwil JM, Juna MA, Healey JE Jr: Salivary glands. In Maccomb WS, Fletcher GH (eds). Cancer of the Head and Neck. Baltimore, Williams and Wilkins, 1967, p. 62.
6. Ibid., p. 358.
7. Ibid., p. 370.
8. Ibid., p. 379.
9. Ibid., p. 382.
10. Batsakis JG: Tumors of the Head and Neck, 2nd ed. Baltimore, Williams and Wilkins, 1979, pp. 15–16.
11. Ibid., p. 22.
12. Ibid., p. 31.
13. Ibid., p. 35.
14. Ibid., p. 40.
15. Ibid., p. 46.
16. Ibid., p. 57.
17. Belsky JL, Takechi N, Yamamoto T, et al: Salivary gland neoplasms following atomic radiation: Additional cases and reanalysis of combined data in a fixed population 1957–1970. Cancer 35:555, 1975.
18. Blanck C, Eneroth CM, Jokobsen PA: Mucus-producing adenopapillary (nonepidermoid) carcinoma of the parotid gland. Cancer 28:676, 1971.
19. Blocker TG Jr: Treatment of parotid tumours. Am J Surg 100:805, 1960.
20. Conley JJ: Surgical management of tumours of the parotid gland. Trans Am Acad Ophthalmol Otolaryngol 61:499, 1957.
21. Conley J, Arena S: Parotid gland as a focus of metastasis. Arch Surg 87:757, 1963.
22. Conley J, Hamaker RC: Prognosis of malignant tumors of the parotid gland with facial paralysis. Arch Otolaryngol 101:39, 1975.
23. Desaive P: The tumours of salivary glands. Rev Belg Sci Med 8:170, 1936.
24. DeVita VT Jr, Hellman S, Rosenberg SA: Cancer Principles and Practice of Oncology. Philadelphia, Lippincott, 1982, p. 382.
25. Eversole LR: Mucoepidermoid carcinoma. Preview of 815 reported cases. J. Oral Surg. 28:490, 1970.
26. Fletcher GH: Textbook of Radiotherapy, 3rd ed. Philadelphia, Lea and Febiger, 1980, p. 427.
27. Ibid., p. 434.
28. Foote FW Jr, Frazell EL: Tumors of the major salivary glands. Cancer 6:1065, 1953.
29. Frazell EL: Clinical aspect of tumours of the major salivary glands. Cancer 7:637, 1954.

30. Fu KK, Leibel SA, Levine ML, et al: Carcinoma of the major and minor salivary glands: Analysis of treatment results and sites and causes of failures. Cancer 40:2882, 1977.

31. Guillamondegui OM, Byers RM, Luna MA, et al: Aggressive surgery in treatment for parotid cancer: The role of adjunctive postoperative radiotherapy. AJR 123:49, 1975.

32. Hanna DC, Gaisford JC, Richardson GS, Bindra RN: Tumors of the deep lobe of the parotid gland. Am J Surg 116:524, 1968.

33. Kaplan I: Radiation Therapy. New York, Oxford Medical Publications, 1937, p. 164.

34. Kirklin J, McDonald JR, Harrington SW, New GB: Parotid tumours: Histopathology, clinical behaviour and end results. Surg Gynecol Obstet 92:721, 1951.

35. Kirmisson E: Precis de Chirurgie Infantile. Paris, Masson, 1906, p. 1.

36. Lawson W, Som ML: Second primary cancer after irradiation of laryngeal cancer. Ann Otol Rhinol Laryngol 84:771, 1975.

37. Lederman M: Mucous and salivary gland tumours: A report on a series of 57 cases with special reference to radium treatment. Br J Radiol 14:329, 1941.

38. Lott JS: Clinical experience with radiation therapy in the management of parotid tumors. J Can Assoc Radiol 14:70, 1963.

39. McFarland J: The histopathologic prognosis of salivary gland mixed tumors. Am J Med Sci 203:502, 1942.

40. McFarland J: Tumors of the parotid region. Surg Gynecol Obstet 57:104, 1933.

41. McGuirt WF: Effect of radiation therapy on facial cable autografts. Trans Am Acad Ophthalmol Otolaryngol 82:487, 1976.

42. Nigro MF, Spiro RH: Deep lobe parotid tumors. Am J Surg 134:523, 1977.

43. Rafla-Demetrious S: Mucous and Salivary Gland Tumours. Springfield, Ill., Charles C Thomas, 1970, p. 11.

44. Ibid., p. 12.

45. Ibid., p. 13.

46. Ibid., p. 107

47. Rubin P, Cassaret GW: Clinical Radiation Pathology, vol. 1. Philadelphia, W. B. Saunders Co., 1968, p. 255.

48. Schneyer LH, Levin LK: Rate of secretion by exogenously stimulated salivary gland pairs of man. J Appl Physiol 7:609, 1955.

49. Shidnia H, Hornback NB, Barlow P: Extranodal lymphoma of the head and neck area. American Journal of Clinical Oncology: Cancer Clinical Trials. Proc of the American Radium Society, 65th Annual Meeting, p. 143, Savannah, Ga., April 5–9, 1983.

50. Shidnia H, Hornback NB, Hamaker R, et al: Carcinoma of major salivary glands. Cancer 45:693, 1980.

51. Siefert G, Rich H, Donath K: Classification of the tumors of the minor salivary glands: Pathohistologic analysis of 160 cases (Germ). Laryngol Rhinol Otol 59/7:379, 1980.

52. Simons JN, Beahrs OH, Woolner LB: Tumours of the submaxillary gland. Am J Surg 108:485, 1964.

53. Singleton AO: Tumours of the salivary glands, benign and locally malignant. Surg Gynecol Obstet 74:569, 1942.

54. Spiro RH, Koss LG, Hajdu SI, Stang EW: Tumors of minor salivary gland origin: A clinicopathologic study of 492 cases. Cancer 31:117, 1973.

55. Spiro RH, Huvos AG, Stang EW: Adenoid cystic carcinoma of salivary origin: A clinicopathologic study of 242 cases. Am J Surg 128:512, 1974.

56. Taylor GW, Garcelon GG: Tumors of salivary gland origin. N Eng J Med 238:766, 1948.

57. Vellios F, Shafer WG: Tumors of the intra-oral accessory salivary glands. Surg Gynecol Obstet 108:450, 1959.

58. Ward GE, Hendrick JW: Diagnosis and Treatment of Tumours of the Head and Neck. Baltimore, Williams and Wilkins, 1950, p. 396.

59. Yoel J: Pathology and Surgery of the Salivary Glands. Springfield, Ill., Charles C Thomas, 1975, p. 14.

60. Ibid., p. 1390.

CHAPTER 44

Surgical Therapy of Tumors of the Salivary Glands

Michael E. Johns, M.D. · Michael J. Kaplan, M.D.

The management of salivary gland tumors has long been a challenge for the head and neck surgeon. Cancers of the salivary glands occur with relative infrequency. The American Cancer Society estimates their incidence to be between one and one and a half per 100,000 population.[1] It is further estimated that fewer than 750 deaths occur each year as a result of cancers of the salivary glands. It is apparent, then, that most surgeons have had limited experience with these tumors. The management of salivary gland cancer is further complicated by its intricate interaction with the complex anatomy of the head and neck. A further challenge lies in the numerous histopathologic possibilities associated with the salivary gland mass (both neoplastic and nonneoplastic) and the limited amount of pretreatment information available at the time of surgery.

Furthermore, salivary gland cancers have a variable biologic course and do not follow the familiar survival pattern of squamous cell carcinomas of the head and neck. Three- and 5-year follow-up periods are inadequate for reviewing survival rates among patients with parotid cancer. In fact, many of these lesions are so slow in their growth that a 20-year survival with active disease is possible.

The salivary glands can be divided into two groups: (1) the *major* salivary glands, composed of the parotid, submandibular, and sublingual glands; and (2) the *minor* salivary glands, which represent some 600 to 1000 small glands distributed in the oral cavity, pharynx, and sinuses. The *parotid* gland is the most common site for salivary gland neoplasm, accounting for approximately 80 to 85 per cent of these tumors. The *submandibular gland* is the next most frequent, with the *sublingual* and *minor salivary glands* accounting for 5 per cent or fewer of these neoplasms. Approximately 80 per cent of parotid gland tumors are benign, 50 to 60 per cent of submandibular gland tumors are benign, and 45 to 55 per cent of minor salivary gland tumors are benign (Tables 44–1 and 44–2).

The fundamental goal in the management of salivary gland neoplasms is no different than the management of neoplasms anywhere else in the body: Eliminate all the tumor with a minimum of deformity, and reconstruct any residual defect when reasonable.

HISTORY

Head and neck oncologists who are particularly interested in the historical aspects of salivary gland anatomy and surgery should refer to the first chapter in *Diseases of the Salivary Glands*, which extensively reviews the historical aspects of salivary gland anatomy and surgery.[40a] The earliest surgical procedures directed at the salivary glands involved the excision of ranula and removal of calculi via the oral route. It was not until 1802 that Bertrandi[22] outlined the first surgical approach to parotidectomy for the treatment of a tumor. Velpeau[59] described a method for submandibular gland excision that served as a model for current techniques. Today's modern techniques of surgery are the result of the accumulative wisdom of many surgeons in history. In the review by Micheli-Pellegrini and Polayes,[40a] it is apparent that the surgical approaches in the 1800s were well thought out and probably limited only by the difficulties with anesthesia and postoperative care.

ANATOMY

The physician who wishes to treat diseases of the salivary glands will find that an understanding of their anatomy is essential to success. It is not the glands themselves that make this knowledge critical but rather the complex interweaving of major vessels, cranial nerves, and muscles with these glands that complicates the treatment of salivary gland diseases.

Embryology. The major salivary glands are considered to be ectodermal in origin. There is some controversy over the germ cell origin of the parotid gland. Some embryologists believe it arises from the endodermal side of the stomadeal plate. A frequent finding of sebaceous gland elements in the parotid gland supports the ectodermal theory of origin.

Both the major and minor salivary glands arise in the same histologic fashion, that is, by the proliferation and ingrowth of a solid anlage of cells into the underlying mesenchymal tissues. As these ingrowths develop, they hollow out and arborize, forming tubules composed of a double layer of cells. These will go on to differentiate

TABLE 44–1. Parotid Gland Tumors: Histologic Diagnosis in Reported Series

Classification	Foote/Frazell[24] (N=766)	Bardwill[3] (N=153)	Eneroth[18] (N=763)	Lambert[37] (N=83)	Hugo et al[33] (N=194)
Mixed Tumor	447 (57.6%)	36 (23.5%)	569 (70.9%)	44 (53.3%)	93 (47.2%)
Benign (pleomorphic adenoma)	46 (5.9%)	34 (22.2%)		1	8 (4.1%)
Malignant (biphasic malignancy)	50 (6.4%)	5 (3.3%)	41 (5.1%)	16 (19.3%)	35 (17.8%)
Papillary cystadenoma lymphomatosum (Warthin's tumor)					18 (9.1%)
Mycoepidermoid carcinoma					
Low-grade	45 (5.8%)	32 (20.9%)	34 (4.2%)	5 (6.0%)	
High-grade	45 (5.8%)				
Adenoid cystic carcinoma	16 (2.1%)	13 (8.5%)	19 (22.4%)	2 (2.4%)	12 (6.1%)
Acinous cell (acinic) carcinoma	21 (2.7%)	8 (5.2%)	36 (4.5%)	3 (3.6%)	2 (1.0%)
Adenocarcinoma (miscellaneous)	32 (4.1%)	16 (10.4%)	17 (2.1%)		6 (3.0%)
Oncocytic cell tumor	1 (0.1%)	1 (0.7%)	4 (4.8%)	1 (1.2%)	2 (1.0%)
Squamous cell carcinoma	26 (3.4%)	8 (5.3%)	1 (0.1%)	4 (4.8%)	2 (0.5%)
Miscellaneous					
Benign	3 (0.4%)				14 (17.1%)
Malignant			15	5 (6.0%)	3 (1.5%)
Unclassified					
Unclassified					
Benign	4 (0.5%)				
Malignant	30 (3.9%)			2 (2.4%)	

into the ductal system, the acini, and other component cells of the salivary gland unit. The proximal portion of the original primordium becomes the main duct of the gland. The surrounding mesenchyme divides the gland into lobules and envelops it to form a capsule.

This process begins at the fourth to sixth week of development (Fig. 44–1). The parotid anlage is the first to appear, but is the last to become encapsulated. This allows lymph nodes to become entrapped within the substance of the parotid gland. Occasionally, a normal cervical lymph node containing salivary gland elements may be found.

Developmental anomalies of the salivary gland parenchyma are unusual and include hypoplasia and aplasia of the glands. The parotid gland can be part of first branchial cleft anomalies.

Histology. The salivary gland secretory unit is composed of acini, intercalated ducts, striated ducts, and the excretory duct. Other cells, such as myoepithelial cells, oncocytes, and sebaceous cells, may be found.

The acinar cells may be serous or mucous cells. The acinar cells of the parotid gland are serous and secrete a thin, watery saliva (Fig. 44–2). The mucous cells, which predominate in the sublingual and oral minor salivary glands, secrete a viscous, sticky solution (Fig. 44–3). The submandibular gland is a mixed gland containing both mucous and serous cells (Fig. 44–4).

Electron microscopy of these acinar cells demonstrates numerous secretory granules (Fig. 44–5). The Golgi vesicles and rough endoplasmic reticulum (Fig. 44–6) are the factories producing the cellular secretions of the acinar cells. Electron microscopy can play a helpful role in classifying undifferentiated tumors. The demonstration of such secretory granules can be most helpful in differentiating a primary salivary gland tumor from a metastatic squamous cell carcinoma.

The myoepithelial cells are contractile supporting cells surrounding the acini and intercalated ducts. They have been shown to contain contractile filaments and are said to aid in moving secretions along in the ductal system.

The oncocyte is found in the aging salivary gland, particularly the parotid gland, and along with sebaceous cells has no known function in the salivary glands.

TABLE 44–2. Incidence of Submandibular Gland Tumors

Author	Total Cases (% Benign/ % Malignant)	Adenoid Cystic Carcinoma (%)	Adenocarcinoma (%)	Mucoepidermoid Carcinoma (%)
Conley et al.[14]	115(53/47)	31	15	31
Spiro et al.[51]	217(44/56)	35	12	19
Eneroth et al.[22]	157(61/39)	40	0	10

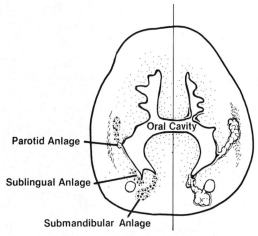

Figure 44–1. Embryologic development of the major salivary glands. Composite drawing of 8 weeks' development on left and later stage right. (From Johns ME: The salivary glands: Anatomy and embryology. Otolaryngol Clin North Am 10:262, 1977, with permission from W. B. Saunders Co.)

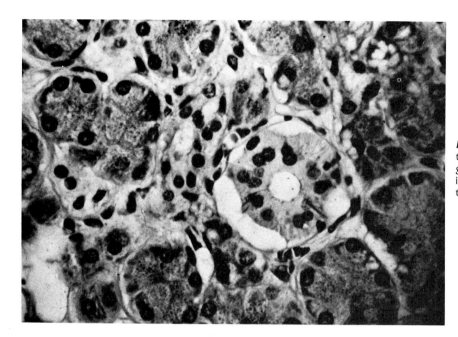

Figure 44–2. Microphotograph of the acinar structure of the parotid gland. The acinar cells are all serous in nature. Note the striated duct in the center of the figure.

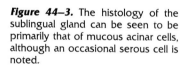

Figure 44–3. The histology of the sublingual gland can be seen to be primarily that of mucous acinar cells, although an occasional serous cell is noted.

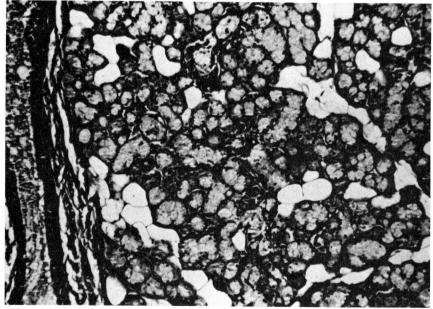

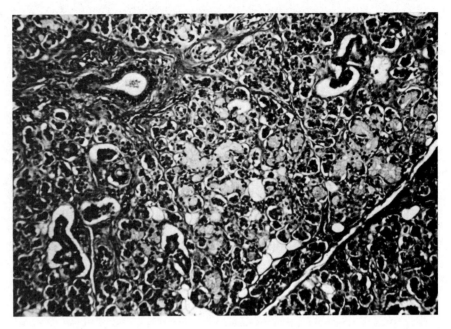

Figure 44—4. The normal submandibular gland is a mixed gland containing both mucous and serous acinar cells.

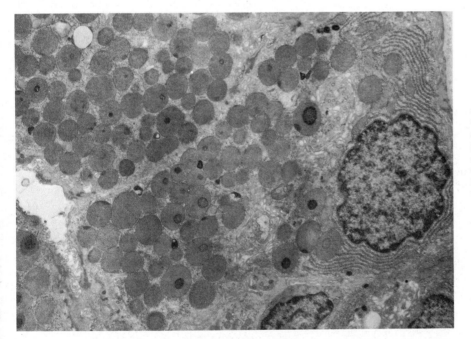

Figure 44—5. Electron micrograph of acinar cells containing numerous secretory granules of varying density. Note acinar lumen (left) and golgi vacuoles and rough endoplasmic reticulum lamellae surrounding nucleus (right). (Courtesy of Joseph Regezi, D.D.S., University of Michigan.)

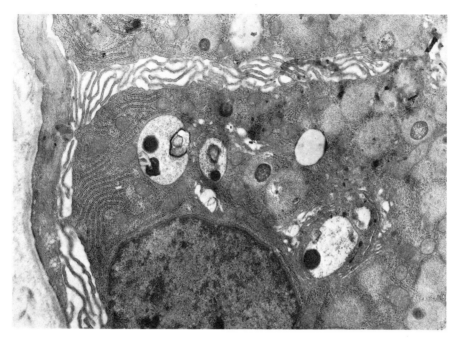

Figure 44–6. Electron micrograph of two adjacent acinar cells containing numerous secretory granules of varying density. Golgi vesicles and rough endoplasmic reticulum lamellae are located near nucleus. The cytoplasm of a myoepithelial cell lies along the basal portion of the acinar cells on the left. (Uranyl acetate and lead citrate, × 11,000.) (Courtesy of Joseph Regezi, D.D.S., University of Michigan.)

The anatomy of the major salivary glands will be presented with an emphasis on the *parotid gland*, which has the most complex anatomic interrelationships. However, a knowledge of the detailed anatomy of all of these glands is essential for the physician who performs surgical procedures on them.

Parotid Gland

Parotid Compartment

The parotid compartment is a space located in front of the ear containing the parotid gland, the facial nerve

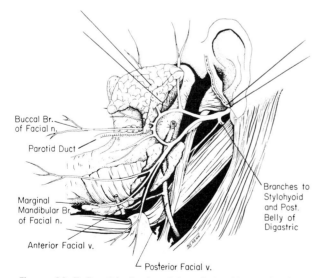

Figure 44–7. Parotid gland and its relationship to the facial nerve and surrounding anatomic structures. Note the relationships of the facial nerve and branches to the tragal pointer, parotid duct, and posterior facial vein. (From Johns MD: The salivary glands: Anatomy and embryology. Otolaryngol Clin North Am *10:*262, 1977, with permission from W. B. Saunders Co.)

and other nerves, and blood and lymphatic vessels (Fig. 44–7 and Table 44–3). This three-dimensional structure is somewhat triangular in shape and has height, width, and depth. When considering the anatomic relationships of this compartment, one must keep in mind these three-dimensional relationships.

The *anterior border* of the compartment is diagonal and extends from the anterior end of the superior and inferior boundaries of the compartment overlying the masseter muscle. From superficial to deep the anterior boundaries are the masseter muscle, the ramus of the mandible, and internal pyterygoid muscle. *Superiorly,* the compartment is bounded by the zygomatic arch. The *posterior border* is composed of the external auditory canal (bony and cartilaginous), the mastoid process, and the base of the styloid process. The *inferior borders* are the sternocleidomastoid muscle and the posterior belly of the digastric muscle.

The deep portion is in close proximity to the lateral pharyngeal space and rests on a floor composed of the

TABLE 44–3. Contents of the Parotid Compartment

Nerve Compartment (Superficial Portion)
1. Great auricular nerve
2. Auriculotemporal nerve
3. Facial nerve

Venous Compartment (Middle Portion)
4. Superficial temporal vein, uniting with
5. Internal maxillary vein, to form
6. Posterior facial vein, which divides into
7. Anterior branch of posterior facial vein and
8. Posterior branch of posterior facial vein, which joins
9. Posterior auricular vein to form
10. External jugular vein

Arterial Compartment (Deep Portion)
11. External carotid artery
12. Internal maxillary artery
13. Superficial temporal artery

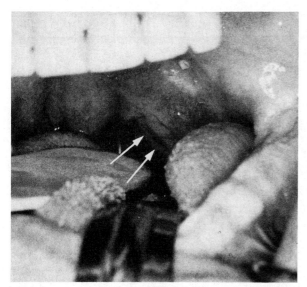

Figure 44–8. A common presenting finding of a parapharyngeal space tumor is a shift of the tonsil and palate toward the midline. In this example, the left tonsil is being pushed medially (arrows).

styloid process and its muscles, the stylomandibular ligament and membrane, and the carotid sheath. The transverse process of the atlas can frequently be felt through the skin and sometimes is mistaken for a tumor in the tail of the parotid gland. It is the close relationship to the lateral pharyngeal space that allows neoplasms to occasionally present intraorally in the lateral pharyngeal space (Fig. 44–8). These have been described as "dumbbell" or round tumors. The dumbbell tumor penetrates between the mandible and the stylomandibular ligament to present in the lateral pharyngeal space. It has a waist-like constriction at the area of the stylo-

mandibular ligament, thus assuming a dumbbell shape (Fig. 44–9). The round tumor passes posterior to the stylomandibular ligament into the lateral pharyngeal space; it does not have a waist-like constriction (Figs. 44–10 and 44–11).

The parotid gland is covered by skin and subcutaneous fatty tissue and has an irregular wedge shape. Although the topic has been debated in the past, there are no true lobes of the parotid gland. It is a unilobular gland. There is a small waist-like constriction of the gland between the ramus of the mandible and the posterior belly of the digastric muscle. This constriction has been designated as the *isthmus* of the gland. The facial nerve splits into its major branches around this isthmus and separates the gland into two portions—a *lateral portion* above the facial nerve and a portion deep to the nerve, which is frequently called the *deep lobe*. We re-emphasize that *there are no anatomic lobes* and that this is a product of surgical dissection.

There are three superficial processes of the parotid parenchymal tissue that have been described but are not always found in each gland:

1. The *condylar process*, found in the condylar area of the temporomandibular joint.

2. The *meatal process*, found in the medial area of the incisura of the external auditory canal.

3. The *posterior process*, projecting between the mastoid and the sternocleidomastoid muscle.

There are also two deep processes:

1. The *glenoid* process, resting on the vaginal process of the tympanic portion of the temporal bone.

2. The *stylomandibular* process, projecting anteromedially above the stylomandibular ligament (Fig. 44–12).

It is these small processes that makes it extremely difficult to perform a total parotidectomy without leaving some portion of parotid tissue.

The parotid (Stensen's) duct lies topographically on a

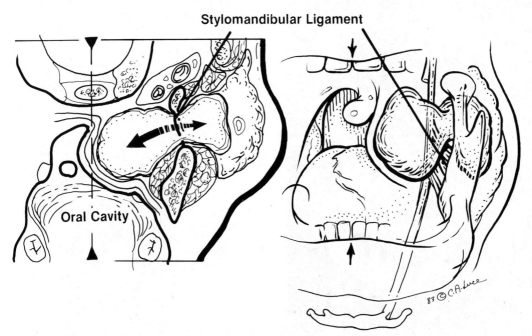

Figure 44–9. Relationship of "dumbbell" tumor to stylomandibular ligament (axial and coronal diagrams). The dumbbell tumor penetrates between the mandible and the stylomandibular ligament to present in the parapharyngeal space.

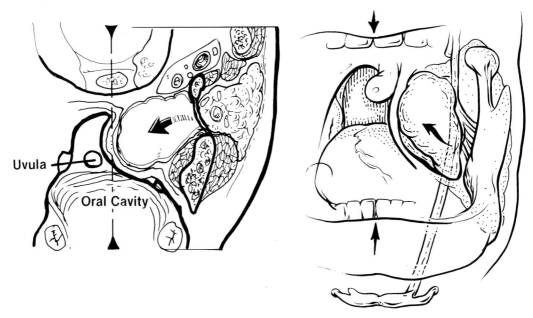

Figure 44–10. The round tumor passes posterior to the stylomandibular ligament, presenting as a mass in the parapharyngeal space (axial and coronal diagrams).

line drawn from the floor of the external auditory meatus to just above the commissure of the lips. It courses from the anterior border of the gland below the zygoma, crosses the masseter muscle and the buccal fat pad, and turns deep to penetrate the buccinator muscle, finally opening intraorally opposite the second upper molar tooth. The duct varies in length from 4.0 to 7.0 cm. An accessory parotid gland is occasionally found to accompany the parotid duct. This accessory gland may vary in size.

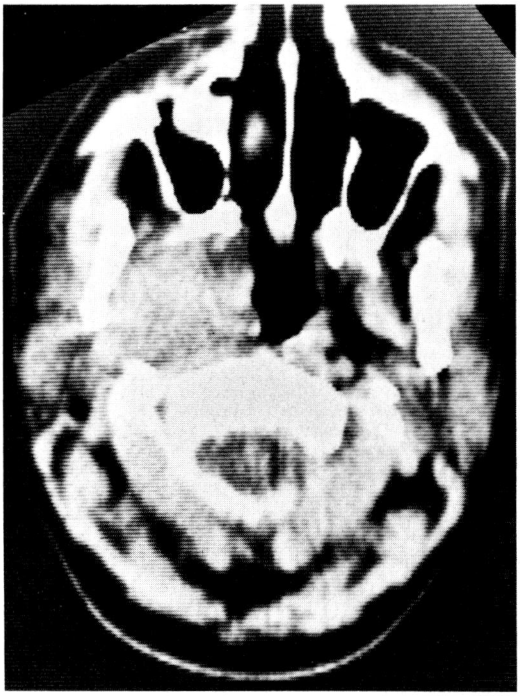

Facial Nerve

The facial nerve is intimately associated with the parotid gland. As it courses through the gland itself, it divides into its main terminal branches. After traversing the temporal bone, the facial nerve exits at the base of the skull through the stylomastoid foramen. This foramen is immediately posterior to the base of the styloid process and anterior to the attachment of the digastric muscle to the mastoid tip. As a rule, the main trunk of the facial nerve is constantly found between the base of the styloid process and the mastoid process (see Figure 44–26). In difficult cases, the facial nerve can be found here by knocking off the mastoid tip with a chisel and finding the facial nerve in the descending portion of the

Figure 44–11. CT scan of a round tumor (an adenoid cystic carcinoma in this example) in the parapharyngeal space.

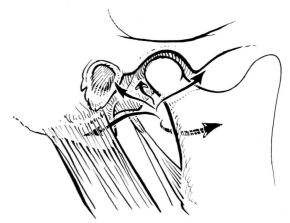

Figure 44–12. Processes of the parotid gland (see text).

facial canal as it exists through the stylomastoid foramen (see Figure 44–28). The facial nerve from this point courses anteriorly and laterally to enter the substance of the parotid gland. Before entering the gland, the nerve has three branches: (1) to the posterior auricular muscle, (2) to the posterior belly of the digastric muscle, and (3) to the stylohyoid muscle. As the nerve enters the gland, it is superficial to the external carotid artery and posterior facial vein. The nerve then branches into two divisions: (1) the upper temporal-facial division and (2) a lower cervical-facial division. This point of branching is known as the pes anserinus (see Figure 44–32). From this point in the gland, the nerve divides into at least five branches that will exit the gland and supply innervation to the muscles of facial expression. It is common to find multiple interconnecting branches between the five main nerve trunks. Figure 44–13 shows some of the more common branching patterns of the facial nerve described by Davis and associates.[15] The different approaches to finding the facial nerve in surgery are discussed later in this chapter.

The blood supply of the parotid gland is derived from the external carotid artery. The venous return is from the gland to the retromandibular vein. The lymph drainage of the gland occurs via intraglandular and extraglandular lymph nodes and then to the jugulodigastric nodes of the deep cervical chain (Fig. 44–14).

Submandibular Gland

The submandibular glands are paired salivary glands that lie below and in front of the angle of the mandible (Figs. 44–15 and 44–16). They contain both serous- and mucous-secreting glandular elements and constitute the second largest of the salivary glands, weighing 10 to 15 gm apiece.

The gland is somewhat irregular in shape, having a deep and superficial portion; the deep portion lies below the mylohyoid muscle, and the superficial portion lies above the mylohyoid muscle (Fig. 44–16). It extends anteriorly, sometimes as far as the anterior belly of the digastric and posteriorly to the stylomandibular ligament, which keeps the submandibular gland separate from the parotid gland. The upper part of the superficial lobe lies against the body of the mandible and partially on the medial pterygoid muscle. The lateral portion of the superficial process is covered by the skin, superficial fascia, platysma muscle, and the superficial layer of deep cervical fascia. It is crossed by the anterior facial vein and often by the marginal mandibular and cervical branches of the facial nerve. Its deep lobe lies between the mylohyoid muscle and the hyoglossal muscle. The facial artery grooves the deep portion of the gland as it courses inferior to superior and must be ligated twice when excising the gland.

The submandibular (Wharton's) duct is about 5 cm long. It runs between the mylohyoid and hyoglossal muscles anteriorly onto the genioglossal muscle and opens into the oral cavity at the side of the lingual frenum. The important relationships of the duct, as it takes it course, are the *hypoglossal nerve*, which lies below, and the *lingual nerve*, which lies above the duct.

The arterial supply to the gland is from the lingual and facial arteries, and the venous drainage is through

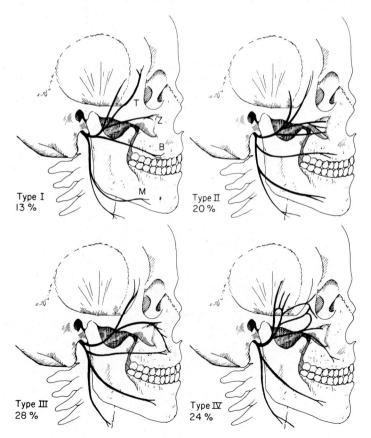

Figure 44–13. Common variations of the facial nerve branching. (Adapted from Davis, R. A., et al.: Surg Gynecol Obstet *102*:385, 1956.)

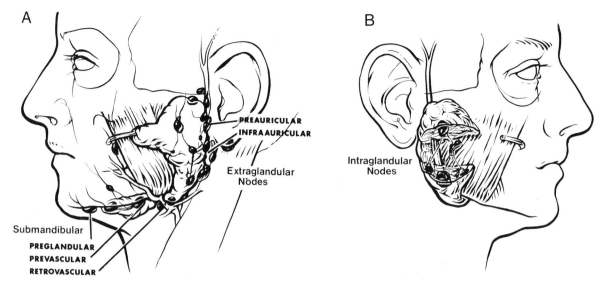

Figure 44–14. The parotid lymph nodes are divided into (*A*) extraglandular and (*B*) intraglandular groups. The submandibular nodes (*A*) are separated into prevascular, retrovascular, and preglandular groups.

the anterior facial vein. The lymphatic drainage is into the submaxillary node and then to the jugular chain.

Sublingual Gland

The sublingual gland is the smallest of the salivary glands, weighing about 2 gm. It lies in the sublingual depression on the inner surface of the mandible near the symphysis of the mandible under the mucosa of the floor of the mouth (Fig. 44-16). It is located above the mylohyoid line of the mandible and rests on the mylohyoid muscle. There is not as discrete a capsule around the sublingual gland as surrounds the other major salivary glands. There are between 8 to 20 ducts emanating from the superior surface of the gland, which opens separately along the sublingual fold of the floor

of the mouth. The sublingual gland receives its blood supply from the sublingual branch of the lingual artery and the submental branch of the facial artery. The lymph drainage is to the submental and submandibular lymph node groups. The mucous cell type predominates in the sublingual gland.

Minor Salivary Glands

The minor salivary glands have been estimated to number between 600 to 1000. They are small, independent, predominantly mucous glands that are found in almost every part of the oral cavity, the superior poles of the tonsils (Weber's glands), and tonsillar pillars. These glands are particularly abundant in the buccal, labial, palatal, and lingual areas. Each gland has its own

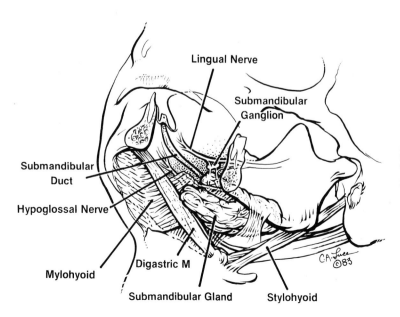

Figure 44–15. Relationships of the submandibular gland to the adjacent muscles and nerves. Take note of the close relationship of the hypoglossal and lingual nerves to Wharton's duct.

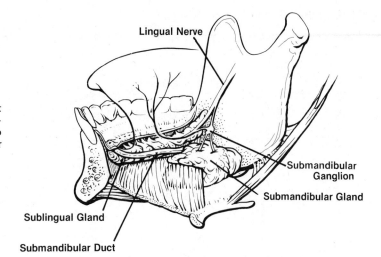

Figure 44–16. Anatomic view from the medial aspect of the mandible. Note the relationship of the superficial and deep lobes of the submandibular gland to the mylohyoid muscle, which forms the muscular floor of the mouth.

small separate duct that opens into the oral cavity directly. Tumors of the minor salivary glands are most commonly in the palate, upper lip, and cheek.

NEURAL CONTROL OF SALIVATION

Salivation is controlled and regulated by the autonomic nervous system. The efferent pathway is via the parasympathetic and sympathetic components of the autonomic nervous system. The afferent portion of the reflex contributing to the salivary secretion may be triggered by a number of physical, psychic, and pharmacologic factors.

The *parotid gland* receives its parasympathetic supply in a complicated and interesting pathway. Preganglionic parasympathetic fibers originating in the inferior salivatory nucleus join with the glossopharyngeal nerve and, after passing through the jugular foramen, give off a tympanic branch. The tympanic branch of the glossopharyngeal nerve, known as *Jacobson's nerve*, enters the middle ear through a canaliculus between the internal jugular vein and the internal carotid artery. The nerve passes to the promontory of the middle ear. Here the nerve anastomoses with the caroticotympanic branch containing sympathetic fibers from the superior cervical ganglia which form the sympathetic plexus on the external carotid artery. This anastomosis is known as the *tympanic plexus*.

The *lesser superficial petrosal nerve* is then formed from this plexus and travels vertically to reach a small canal below the tensor tympani muscle and courses through the temporal bone receiving branches from the geniculate ganglion and greater petrosal nerve. It leaves the temporal bone from its anterior surface through a small opening just lateral to the hiatus for the greater petrosal nerve. The lesser superficial petrosal nerve then leaves the middle cranial fossa through the foramen ovale, where it joins the otic ganglion near the base of the skull just medial to the mandibular division of the trigeminal nerve. The parasympathetic fibers synapse here, and postganglionic fibers along with the sympathetic fibers pass with the *auriculotemporal nerve* to supply the parotid gland (Fig. 44–17).

Disruption of this network by tympanic neurectomy has been advocated as treatment for chronic parotitis, excessive salivation, and glossopharyngeal otalgia.

The *submandibular and sublingual glands* receive their parasympathetic innervation by fibers originating in the superior salivatory nucleus, which leave the brain stem as the nervus intermedius portion of the seventh cranial nerve. These parasympathetic fibers follow the course of the *chorda tympani nerve* through the tympanic cavity to join the lingual branch of the mandibular division of the fifth cranial nerve. The preganglionic fibers synapse in the submandibular ganglion and are distributed to the submandibular and sublingual glands. The sympathetic innervation to these glands, as well as to the parotid gland, arises from the superior cervical ganglion and is distributed to the glands along blood vessels from the carotid system (Fig. 44–18).

PHYSIOLOGY

In a 24-hour day the glands produce 1000 to 1200 ml. of salivary fluid; 45 per cent is derived from the parotid glands, 45 per cent from the submandibular glands, and 5 per cent from the sublingual glands. The remaining 5 per cent is derived from the minor salivary glands. The salivary flow rate is markedly reduced when there is no stimulation from an external source, but will increase tenfold when there is external stimulation. It is obvious, therefore, that the greater salivary flow occurs during eating. In addition, there seems to be a diurnal rhythm associated with salivary flow. However, because the flow rate of the major salivary glands is less than 0.05 ml. per minute when there is no external stimulation, this diurnal variation probably has very little effect on the total production of saliva.

Three types of cells are associated with the production and composition of saliva: (1) *serous acinar cells*, (2) *mucous acinar cells*, and (3) *lining cells* of the ducts. Mucous and serous acinar cells differ qualitatively and quantitatively in the type of saliva produced. The parotid gland, which is primarily composed of serous acinar cells, secretes a saliva that is relatively low in

Parasympathetic to Parotid Gland

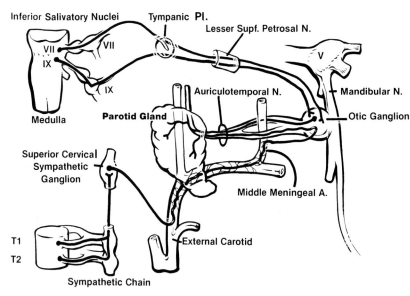

Figure 44–17. Sympathetic and parasympathetic innervation of the parotid gland.

calcium compared with the secretion of the submandibular gland, composed of both mucous and serous acinar cells. It is interesting to speculate that perhaps this low concentration of calcium in the parotid secretions may be the reason for fewer stones being found in the parotid gland than the submandibular gland, although there is no evidence to suggest that the level of calcium in the salivary secretions is associated with calculus formation.

The initial production of saliva occurs in the terminal acini of the salivary glands. Here an isotonic solution is secreted resulting in a high-sodium, low-potassium se-

cretion. As the fluid passes through the intercalated and striated ducts, it is modified. The striated duct cells have similar histology to the cells of the convoluted tubules of the kidney and function in a similar fashion. They are capable of secreting or reabsorbing water, which affects the calcium, chloride, bicarbonate, sodium, and potassium levels of these fluids passing by the cell surfaces. As previously mentioned, these processes are controlled and altered by the autonomic nervous system. The electrolyte concentrations of parotid fluids, stimulated and unstimulated, are presented in

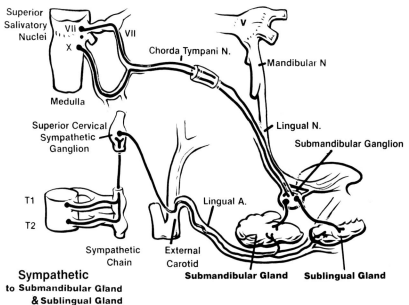

Figure 44–18. Sympathetic and parasympathetic innervation of the submandibular and sublingual glands.

Table 44–4. It is apparent that by the time the saliva reaches the end of the parotid duct, the high-sodium, low-potassium ratio has changed and a fluid with a different electrolyte composition than that originating in the acini has evolved. It is no longer isotonic and is markedly different from the plasma levels also shown in Table 44–4.

Components of Saliva

Saliva is composed of electrolytes, enzymes, other protein, and various vitamins and hormones; as shown in Table 44–4, the components of saliva are quite varied. In general, the concentration of these components in the parotid is somewhat higher than that of the submandibular gland. The major exception to this is the level of calcium, which is twice as concentrated in submandibular saliva as in parotid saliva. The electrolyte concentration of saliva is unaffected by the plasma concentrations.

Many factors affect the composition of the saliva, e.g., whether it is whole saliva or specific saliva obtained from one gland, whether the saliva is stimulated or unstimulated, the age of the patient, drugs the patient may be taking, diet, various hormonal imbalances, and systemic or local diseases (Table 44–5).

Whole saliva is a mixture of submandibular, sublingual, and minor salivary gland secretions mixed with food debris, bacteria, cells, and other particulate matter found in the oral cavity. *Specific saliva* is obtained by either cannulating a duct of one of the specific glands or using some other device to gather saliva that is uncontaminated by saliva produced at other sites or by other contaminants in the oral cavity. It is quite obvious that whole saliva will be considerably different from specific saliva.

The flow rate has a considerable effect on the concentrations of the electrolytes found in saliva. As flow rates increase, certain electrolytes will increase and others will decrease.

Age also plays a role in the composition of the saliva. This is due to change in the flow rate as one ages and atrophic changes that occur in the salivary glands with aging.

Many drugs can affect the flow and composition of saliva, including digitalis and atropine-like substances such as pro-Banthine. A list of other factors is presented in Table 44–5.

TABLE 44–4. Parotid Saliva Composition in Normal Adults

Eq/liter	Stimulated*	Unstimulated†	Plasma
Sodium	23.0	2.6	140.00
Potassium	20.0	36.7	4.00
Chloride	23.0	24.8	104.00
Bicarbonate	20.0	1.0	0.27
Magnesium	0.2	0.3	2.00
Calcium	2.0	3.0	5.00
Phosphate	6.0	15.3	2.50

*Adapted from Mandel ID: Saliva. *In* Grant D, et al (eds): Periodontics: A Concept—Theory and Practice, 4th ed. St. Louis, C. V. Mosby, 1972.
†Adapted from Shannon IL: A Formula for Parotid Fluid Collected without Exogenous Stimulation. U.S. Air Force, Aerospace Medical Division, Report No. SAM-TDR-66-52, 1966.

TABLE 44–5. Factors Affecting Salivary Flow

Drugs
  Cocaine
  Reserpine
  Scopolamine
  Antihistamines
  Antiparkinsonian

Endocrine Diseases
  Aldosteronism
  Cushing's disease
  Addison's disease

Metabolic Diseases
  Alcoholism
  Diabetes mellitus
  Cystic fibrosis

Glandular Atrophy
  Irradiation
  Chronic inflammation

Others
  Bell's palsy
  Ductal stones
  Smoking
  Dehydration

Levels of aldosterone and corticosteroids have a definite influence on the concentration of sodium in saliva.

Functions of Saliva

Saliva performs many important functions in the oral cavity, including lubrication of mucous membranes and cleansing of food, cellular debris, and bacteria from the gingiva and other areas of the oral cavity. It plays an important role in the protection of teeth, providing minerals, calcium, and phosphate and forming a film over the teeth to reduce wear caused by nutrition and abrasion. In addition, saliva has an antibacterial activity and contains secretory immunoglobulin A, which is effective against a number of viruses and bacteria. In addition, saliva contains lysozyme, which is capable of breaking up the cell walls of many bacteria.

CLASSIFICATION OF PAROTID TUMORS

In the past, one of the major obstacles in establishing principles of treatment for parotid neoplasms had been the lack of a universally accepted classification system. As recently as 1976, Kagan and associates[35] lumped all parotid cancers into two groups—squamous cell carcinoma and adenocarcinoma—in an effort "to avoid making the complexities of pathology incomprehensible." Unfortunately, as we shall see, such attempts only serve to make the reporting of data on parotid cancer incomprehensible.

An accurate histopathologic diagnosis must be the keystone of any treatment plan. At present, the splitting of parotid neoplasms into different categories based on their histologic appearance seems necessary because the biologic course appears to be different for each histologic type. In fact, some histopathologic varieties of parotid cancer are so rare that the biologic course of these tumors is not clear, and, as such, they should be kept separate until it can be determined from their behavior whether they should be placed within a more general histologic category. In a series of four articles on salivary gland neoplasms, Batsakis and co-workers described the reasons for their classification system,[4-8] and their categories of epithelial salivary gland tumors are shown in Table 44–6.

DIAGNOSTIC AIDS

Sialograms, radionuclide images, computed tomography (CT), ultrasonograms, and combinations thereof have all been advocated as aids in the diagnosis of salivary gland tumors. In most instances, however, the results of these tests do not differentiate between benign or malignant neoplasms and they rarely alter the therapeutic approaches. As such, their routine use is not cost-effective or recommended.

Sialography, CT Scans. The use of sialography, CT scanning, or combinations has its greatest, and perhaps only, value for those salivary gland masses in which there is a question as to disease extent or involvement of vital structures that would suggest inoperability. For the majority of parotid neoplasms that occur in the superficial lobe, particularly the tail of the parotid, no

TABLE 44–6. Classification of Epithelial Salivary Gland Tumors*

I. Benign lesions
   A. Mixed tumor (pleomorphic adenoma)
   B. Papillary cystadenolymphoma (Warthin's tumor)
   C. Oncocytosis, oncocytoma
   D. Monomorphic adenoma
     1. Basal cell adenoma
     2. Glycogen-rich adenoma and clear cell adenoma
     3. Others
   E. Sebaceous adenoma
   F. Sebaceous lymphadenoma
   G. Benign lymphoepithelial lesion
II. Malignant lesions
   A. Carcinoma ex pleomorphic adenoma (carcinoma arising in or from a mixed tumor)
   B. Mucoepidermoid carcinoma
     1. Low grade
     2. Intermediate grade
     3. High grade
   C. Hybrid basal cell adenoma, adenoid cystic carcinoma
   D. Adenoid cystic carcinoma
   E. Acinous cell carcinoma (acinic carcinoma)
   F. Adenocarcinoma
     1. Mucus-producing adenopapillary and nonpapillary carcinoma
     2. Salivary duct carcinoma (ductal carcinoma)
   G. Oncocytic carcinoma (malignant oncocytoma)
   H. Clear cell carcinoma
   I. Epithelial or myoepithelial carcinoma of intercalated ducts
   J. Squamous cell carcinoma
   K. Undifferentiated carcinoma
   L. Miscellaneous (including sebaceous, Stensen's duct, melanomas, and carcinoma ex lymphoepithelial lesion)
   M. Metastatic carcinoma

*This system is based on findings by Batsakis (J Laryngol Otol 93:325, 1979; Head Neck Surg 1:59, 1978; 1:167, 1978; 1:260, 1979; 1:340, 1979.[4-8]

useful pretreatment information is gained from these evaluations.

Radionuclide Scans. In the past, radionuclide imaging of salivary gland neoplasms was felt to be useful when there was a high suspicion of the benign Warthin's tumor or oncocytoma (which scan "hot") in a patient who is a high surgical risk. However, these tumors are very easily diagnosed by needle aspiration biopsy and, as such, we presently see no indication for using radionuclide scans in the diagnosis of parotid tumors.

Fine-Needle Aspiration Biopsy. In many centers, this technique has become a valuable pretreatment diagnostic test. It requires a pathologist skilled in its use and familiar with the cytologic appearance of the varied parotid neoplasms. The surgeon must have an understanding of what the pathologist is saying when he tenders a diagnosis. The pathologist must err to the side of "not able to make a diagnosis" if there is any question in his mind. As such, this takes close cooperation of surgeon and pathologist in the use of this diagnostic technique. Today a growing number of medical centers employ pathologists who are skilled in this technique. Aspiration biopsy of the parotid mass has been approximately 75 per cent accurate in providing the correct diagnosis.[25, 48, 50] The incidence of "tumor seeding" in the head and neck area with the fine-needle aspiration biopsy must be exceedingly low, since there have been no reported cases in the literature and we have *not* seen a single case in more than 800 aspiration biopsies at our institution. Nevertheless, it is a theoretical possibility.

Frozen Section. The use of frozen sections is potentially risky and controversial. For tumors that clinically appear to be malignant and in which the needle aspiration biopsy has not provided a tissue diagnosis, we use this technique. If a firm diagnosis of malignancy is returned from the pathologist, we proceed with the surgical approach appropriate for the malignancy. In most instances, however, we perform a parotidectomy and wait for a permanent section diagnosis.

The use of frozen sections should be done only in institutions where the pathologist has had experience with salivary gland tumors. This is available in a selected few places. If this is available to you, we suggest that the specimen be taken to the pathologist and the frozen sections reviewed with him directly so that clinical correlation can be made and problems in communication avoided. If this approach is not available, do not use a frozen section on which to base aggressive surgery. It would be regrettable if the permanent section diagnosis were changed from malignant to benign. It would be better to wait for the permanent section diagnosis and then, if malignant, to return to the operating room in the next day or two to complete the surgery.

Open Biopsy. Open biopsy is rarely used, being employed only when there is an obvious malignancy, the patient is not a surgical candidate, and the needle aspiration has not provided a diagnosis. In these cases, open incisional biopsy is used to make a diagnosis and provide histopathologic guidance for the use of palliative radiation or chemotherapy.

Classic Biopsy. The classic biopsy approach to parotid tumors has been the superficial parotidectomy with preservation of the facial nerve. For 80 to 90 per cent of parotid neoplasms, this procedure is both diagnostic and therapeutic if one considers that excision of the tumor with a cuff of normal tissue is adequate surgical therapy for 85 per cent of parotid tumors.

Incisional Intraoral Biopsy. *Incisional intraoral biopsy of a parapharyngeal tumor should be avoided.* Such a biopsy contaminates the oral mucosa, necessitating its excision during the definitive procedure. It will frequently result in considerable inflammation, edema, and possible infection, causing delay of the surgical procedure. Because of the location of the tumor, en bloc resection is not feasible and the need for a tissue diagnosis is not critical, since it will not, in most cases, alter the surgical approach. We routinely obtain a CT scan (see Fig. 44–11), with and without contrast and injected intravenously, to rule out a vascular tumor and to determine the location of the carotid artery. Needle aspiration biopsy can be done using a 22-gauge needle via an extraoral or intraoral route.

FACTORS INFLUENCING SURVIVAL

In order to develop a treatment plan for tumors at any site, one must be aware in advance of the factors that affect survival. We have identified the following factors:

1. Histopathologic diagnosis.
2. Incidence of lymph node metastasis.
3. Pain.
4. Facial nerve paralysis.
5. Skin involvement.
6. Stage.
7. Location.
8. Incidence of recurrence.
9. Distant metastasis.
10. Radiation sensitivity.
11. Chemotherapeutic sensitivity.

The head and neck surgeon who understands the roles played by these risk factors will be better prepared to develop a rational therapeutic approach. Although the primary treatment for salivary gland tumors has been and still is surgical, a role for adjuvant radiation therapy and possibly the future role of chemotherapy must be kept in mind.

Submandibular and minor salivary gland tumors occur considerably less frequently than parotid tumors; thus there is less known regarding the clinical behavior and biologic course of salivary gland neoplasms at these sites. In general, it can be said, however, that the submandibular gland malignancies seem to have a somewhat more aggressive behavior than parotid malignancies. Minor salivary gland malignancies, in which adenoid cystic carcinoma predominates, appear to behave yet even more aggressively.

Because of the limited amount of information available in the literature regarding these risk factors for the submandibular and minor salivary gland tumors, the following review of data is directed at parotid malignancies. Where appropriate, comments regarding submandibular and minor salivary gland tumors will be mentioned.

Salivary gland neoplasms in children are uncommon. However, the presence of such a tumor in a child requires careful diagnostic evaluation in view of the higher frequency of malignancies in children than in adults. In a review of 428 salivary gland neoplasms in children (both epithelial and nonepithelial) by Schuller and McCabe,[48] malignant neoplasms were responsible for 35 per cent (149 of 428) of the salivary gland tumors (Table 44–7). The most common benign tumor was the hemangioma; the most common malignant tumor, the mucoepidermoid carcinoma. Of the benign epithelial tumors, the mixed tumor was the most common. It should be noted that although malignant tumors occur more frequently in children than in adults, the benign mixed tumor is still the most frequently seen nonvascular tumor in the pediatric age group.

In order to expand the data on parotid tumors beyond the limited experience that any one surgeon may accrue in a lifetime, we have reviewed the current literature along with the experience at the University of Virginia (Table 44–8). Only data from series in which the tumors were classified according to the system proposed by Batsakis are included. We have made no attempt to draw conclusions regarding the miscellaneous group of rare cancers because data are insufficient for analysis.

Histopathology

The prerequisite for adequate treatment of parotid tumors is an accurate histopathologic diagnosis, since the biologic aggressiveness of these tumors correlates with their histology. The correlation of histopathology with biologic behavior has allowed these tumors to be divided into two groups:

1. *Low-grade* cancers include acinous cell carcinoma and low-grade mucoepidermoid carcinoma.

2. *High-grade* cancers include adenoid cystic carcinoma, high-grade mucoepidermoid carcinoma, carcinoma ex mixed tumor, squamous cell carcinoma, and adenocarcinoma.

Five-year survival statistics for these tumors are shown in Table 44–8. As seen in Table 44–9, the survival rates continue to fall at 10 years, with only the mucoepidermoid and acinous cell carcinomas having 10-year survival rates comparable with the 5-year survival rates. Ten-year or greater survivals have been reported by only a few authors.[12, 21, 26, 54] Their data also demonstrate

TABLE 44–7. Salivary Gland Neoplasms in Children (Total: 428)*†

Benign		Malignant	
Hemangioma	111	Mucoepidermoid carcinoma	73
Mixed tumor	94	Acinous cell carcinoma	18
"Vascular proliferative"	40	Undifferentiated carcinoma	14
Lymphangioma	18	Undifferentiated sarcoma	9
Lymphoepithelial tumor	3	Carcinoma ex mixed tumor	11
Cystadenoma	3	Adenocarcinoma	11
Warthin tumor	3	Adenoid cystic carcinoma	6
Plexiform neurofibroma	2	Squamous cell carcinoma	3
Xanthoma	2	Mesenchymal sarcoma	2
Neurilemmoma	1	Rhabdomyosarcoma	2
Adenoma	1	Malignant epithelial tumor	1
Lipoma	1	Ganglioneuroblastoma	1
Total	279	Total	149

*Adapted from Schuller DE, McCabe BF: Otolaryngol Clin North Am 10:399, 1977.[48]

†From the literature, 392; from the University of Iowa, 36.

TABLE 44–8. Five-Year Survival Rates Among Patients with Parotid Carcinoma

Histologic Type of Carcinoma	Eneroth[21] (%)	Spiro[54] (%)	Hollander[32] (%)	Fu[26] (%)	University of Michigan[34] (%)	Conley[12] (%)	University of Virginia (%)
Mucoepidermoid			75	96	83		63
Low-grade	97	86				94	
High-grade	56	22				35	
Acinous cell	90	66	90	80	47	86	90
Adenoid cystic	75	45	42	65	82	82	55
Adenocarcinoma	75	75	25	72	16	49	55
Arising from mixed tumor	50	63	36	—	62	77	5
Squamous cell	—	30	25	57	47	42	36
Undifferentiated	30	—	—	44	—	30	100

that survival rates continue to decrease even after 5 years. In fact, Eneroth and Hamberger[21] reported 20-year determinate survival rates and found that the only tumor types in which the 5-year survival predicted long-term survival were the low-grade mucoepidermoid and squamous cell carcinomas. Even the survival rate associated with acinous cell carcinoma, a low-grade tumor, decreased from 80 per cent at 5 years to a 60 per cent determinate survival rate at 20 years.

Until recently, the mucoepidermoid carcinoma was the only malignant parotid tumor that could be histologically classified as low or high grade. More recently, there have been attempts to correlate histologic features with survival in adenoid cystic carcinoma and acinous cell carcinoma.

Eby and associates[16] in 1972 divided adenoid cystic carcinoma into two histologic types: a cribriform and a solid pattern. They felt that the solid tumor behaved more aggressively than the cribriform tumor. Spiro and colleagues[53] attempted to correlate survival with the histologic classification of Eby's for patients with adenoid cystic carcinoma, but were not able to do so. Perzin and co-workers[43] divided their cases of adenoid cystic carcinoma into three histologic groups: (1) a "tubular" pattern, (2) a "cribriform" pattern, and (3) a "solid" pattern. They found recurrence rates of 59 per cent for patients with tubular adenoid cystic carcinoma, of 89 per cent for patients with cribriform lesions, and of 100 per cent for patients with solid neoplasms. Patients with the tubular pattern had the longest survival intervals, averaging 9 years before death; the average survival interval for the cribriform pattern was 8 years and for solid tumors, 5 years. Despite these findings, there still seems to be considerable controversy among patholo-

gists regarding the histologic subclassification of adenoid cystic carcinoma. It is not unusual for a single adenoid cystic carcinoma to have all three patterns present. It seems, then, that histologic variants should not be used to establish management principles at this time.

An attempt to classify acinous cell carcinoma histologically was carried out by Batsakis and associates.[5] In a retrospective review, they classified 35 acinous cell carcinomas according to high- and low-grade histologic patterns. Their findings showed a high degree of correlation between survival and histologic pattern; 58 per cent of patients with high-grade tumors died of the neoplasm, but only 5 per cent of patients with low-grade neoplasm died of the disease.

Spiro and co-workers[55] classified acinous cell carcinoma into three groups: *Group 1* included tumors that were completely encapsulated; *group 2*, those in which encapsulation was incomplete and in which there was evidence of blood vessel or capsule invasion; and *group 3*, tumors that showed a papillary-cystic histologic pattern. They found the 10-year survival rates to be 71 per cent in group 1, 33 per cent in group 2, and 0 per cent in group 3.

Although retrospective classification of carcinomas as high- and low-grade lesions based on histologic patterns may correlate with the ultimate biologic outcome, it is unlikely that such classifications will be helpful during the intraoperative procedure through the analysis of frozen sections. Nevertheless, these factors should be kept in mind, and the use of adjuvant radiation therapy or chemotherapy may be indicated when permanent section analysis demonstrates high-grade histologic patterns.

TABLE 44–9. Five- and Ten-Year Survival Rates among Patients with Parotid Carcinoma

Histologic Type of Carcinoma	Eneroth[18] 5-Year	Eneroth[18] 10-Year	Spiro[54] 5-Year	Spiro[54] 10-Year	Fu[26] 5-Year	Fu[26] 10-Year	Conley[12] 5-Year	Conley[12] 10-Year
Mucoepidermoid					96%	95%		
Low-grade	97%	97%	92%	90%	—	—	94%	94%
High-grade	56%	54%	49%	42%	—	—	35%	28%
Acinous cell	90%	80%	—	—	80%	80%	86%	—
Adenoid cystic	75%	60%	45%	28%	65%	29%	82%	77%
Adenocarcinoma	75%	60%	—	—	72%	62%	49%	41%
Arising from mixed tumor	50%	30%	63%	39%	—	—	77%	—
Squamous cell	—	—	—	—	57%	57%	42%	—
Undifferentiated	30%	25%	—	—	44%	22%	30%	—

Lymph Node Metastasis

Radical neck dissection has frequently been proposed as a concomitant part of the management of parotid cancer whether or not lymph node metastases are present (Fig. 44–12). Today it is well accepted that if a patient has a clinically positive node, the prognosis is altered and surgical management is indicated. However, indications for a prophylactic neck dissection are quite controversial. Many head and neck surgeons might agree that if there is a 25 per cent or greater likelihood of occult metastases, a neck dissection would be indicated. Others might argue, however, that there is no evidence showing clearly that waiting for the occult metastasis to become clinically manifest adversely affects the ultimate outcome of the disease process.

In an effort to determine which of the histologic classes of tumors have a propensity for lymphatic metastasis, the pooled data available in the literature[12, 32, 46, 54] and the experience at the University of Virginia were studied to determine the incidence of cervical metastases that develop at any time in the course of the disease (i.e., those present on initial exam, occult metastases discovered at neck dissection, or metastases occurring later). As shown in Table 44–10, only the high-grade mucoepidermoid and squamous cell carcinomas have a greater than 25 per cent propensity for neck metastasis. The incidence of cervical node metastasis present at the time of initial presentation in all parotid cancers is said to be 13 per cent.[54] Spiro and co-workers[54] found the incidence of occult cervical nodes to be 16 per cent or less for all parotid cancers except for squamous cell carcinoma, where they found a 40 per cent incidence of occult metastasis (Table 44–11). In their series, only ten (16 per cent) of 64 high-grade mucoepidermoid carcinomas had occult metastasis. Using a modification of the current American Joint Committee (AJC) staging system (Fig. 44–19) for cancer of the parotid gland, Spiro[54] found that stage I tumors of the parotid had a 1 per cent incidence of neck metastasis, stage II tumors a 14 per cent incidence, and stage III tumors a 67 per cent incidence. Fu and coworkers[26] found that stage I tumors had a 13 per cent incidence of neck metastasis, stage II tumors a 13 per cent incidence, and stage III tumors a 33 per cent incidence.

In a review of the experience with adenoid cystic carcinoma of the parotid and submandibular glands seen at the University of Virginia, Marsh and Allen[40] reported that regional spread occurs by contiguous growth and rarely, if ever, by lymphatic extension. The incidence of neck metastasis in acinous cell carcinoma

TABLE 44–11. Rates of Occult Lymph Node Metastasis among Patients with Parotid Carcinoma

Histologic Type of Carcinoma	No with Metastasis/ Total (%)
Mucoepidermoid (high-grade)	10/64 (16%)
Malignant mixed	0/48 (0%)
Acinous cell	2/31 (6%)
Adenocarcinoma	2/23 (9%)
Adenoid cystic	0/19 (0%)
Squamous cell	4/10 (40%)

is almost equally as rare. In 1974, Eneroth and Hamberger[21] recommended neck dissection as routine treatment for acinous cell carcinoma, but in a more recent review,[10] Eneroth no longer recommended neck dissection for this tumor.

Treatment planning can be modified when, during parotidectomy, the first-echelon lymph nodes are exposed. These parotid and subdigastric nodes are where metastases would most likely occur first. Any suspicious node can be biopsied at dissection. If postoperative irradiation is to be employed as an adjunct to surgery, this in itself may control any occult metastasis.

The evidence suggests that in untreated parotid cancers the incidence of cervical metastasis is quite low. More important, occult metastasis is rare in all but squamous cell carcinoma. T3 parotid cancers and cancers associated with facial nerve paralysis, however, do have a high association with regional lymph node metastasis. Eneroth[19] reported a 77 per cent incidence, and Conley and Hamaker[13] a 66 per cent incidence of lymph node metastasis in patients who presented with facial nerve paralysis.

There is, however, no information to suggest that the clinically negative neck is best treated by a prophylactic radical neck dissection. We include the neck in the radiation port in the postoperative irradiation of these advanced tumors.

Considering these facts, we have evolved the following philosophy for treatment of the clinically negative neck. Since parotidectomy is the biopsy procedure used, the upper jugular nodes and posterior submandibular triangle nodes are inspected, and suspicious nodes are either biopsied or included in the parotid dissection. Whether further surgery will be carried out and whether postoperative radiation therapy will be used will then be based on the pathology report.

Pain

The significance of pain as a presenting complaint is not entirely clear. In reviewing 802 parotid tumors, Eneroth[18] found pain to be an initial symptom in 34 (5.1 per cent) of 665 patients with benign tumors and in 9 (6.5 per cent) of 137 patients with malignant tumors. He concluded that pain could not be used as a criterion of malignancy. When Spiro's group[54] studied the significance of pain in patients with malignant parotid tumors, they found that patients complaining of pain had a 5-year survival rate of 35 per cent, whereas asymptomatic patients had a 5-year survival rate of 68 per cent. Mustard and Anderson[41] reported a similar 5-year sur-

TABLE 44–10. Rates of Lymph Node Metastasis among Patients with Parotid Carcinoma

Histologic Type of Carcinoma	No. with Metastasis/ Total (%)
Mucoepidermoid (high-grade)	62/140 (44%)
Acinous cell	8/60 (13%)
Adenoid cystic	3/58 (5%)
Adenocarcinoma	37/144 (26%)
Arising from mixed tumor	24/177 (21%)
Squamous cell	24/65 (37%)
Undifferentiated	15/64 (23%)

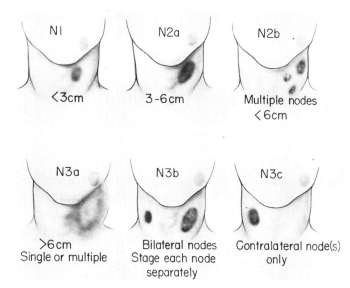

Figure 44–19. 1980 American Joint Commission Staging System for nodal metastasis in head and neck cancer. (From Johns ME: Head Neck Surg 3:131, 1980.)

vival rate of 33 per cent for those presenting with pain.

It appears, then, that pain is not a criterion of malignancy, but when it does occur in a patient with malignant tumor, it is associated with a poor prognosis and most likely is a sign of nerve invasion by the tumor.

Facial Nerve Paralysis

Facial nerve paralysis associated with a parotid mass indicates malignancy, carries an adverse prognosis, and occurs with varying frequency, depending on the histologic type (Table 44–12). Eneroth[19] found no cases of facial nerve paralysis in a series of 1790 benign parotid tumors, but did find 46 cases in 378 malignant parotid tumors. In the latter group, the mortality rate was 100 per cent at 5 years and the average survival interval after onset of paralysis was 2.7 years. In a multi-institutional study published later, Eneroth and coworkers[20] reviewed 1029 cases of malignant parotid tumors and found an incidence of facial nerve paralysis of 14 per cent and a 5-year survival rate of 9 per cent for these patients. Reviewing 279 malignant parotid tumors, Conley and Hamaker[13] did not find that facial nerve paralysis was quite as hopeless a prognostic indicator: nine of 34 patients were free of disease at 5 years, and four of 26 patients who were available for 10-year follow-up were free of disease at 10 years. Spiro and co-workers[54] found a 5-year survival rate of 14 per cent in 43 patients with facial nerve paralysis. Thus, facial nerve paralysis occurring in the presence of a

parotid mass apparently indicates both malignancy and a poor prognosis (Table 44–13).

Skin Involvement

No reports are available on the significance of skin involvement by parotid tumors. An unusual occurrence today, it does indicate advanced malignancy and decreased survival. When seen, it is usually in a massive tumor and requires wide resection including the facial skin (Fig. 44–20).

Stage

In the *Manual for Staging of Cancer*,[2] the size of the mass is a prominent factor in staging parotid gland cancer (Table 44–14). Size is the major distinguishing feature among various lesions: T1 (0 to 2 cm), T2 (2 to 4 cm), T3 (4 to 6 cm), and T4 (6 cm). Although the staging system has not been fully evaluated, Spiro,[52, 54, 55] did a considerable amount of work correlating stage of disease with prognosis, incidence of lymph node metastasis, and distant metastasis. Spiro's staging system is somewhat different from the AJC system in that he used diameters of 0 to 3 cm for T1 lesions, 3 to 6 cm for T2, and 6 cm for T3. He reported 5-year survival rates of 85 per cent for T1 cancers, 67 per cent for T2, and 14 per cent for T3.[54] Using the same staging system, Fu and co-workers[26] found a 5-year survival rate of 88 per cent and a 10-year determinate survival rate of 83

TABLE 44–12. Frequencies of Facial Nerve Paralysis among Patients with Malignant Parotid Carcinoma

Histologic Type of Carcinoma	Eneroth[19]	Conley[13]	Eneroth[19] and Conley[13]
Mucoepidermoid	8%	11%	16/171 (9%)
Acinous cell	2%	0%	1/83 (1%)
Adenoid cystic	22%	11%	15/86 (17%)
Adenocarcinoma	8%	15%	10/92 (11%)
Arising from mixed tumor	9%	5%	5/70 (7%)
Squamous cell	—	19%	4/21 (19%)
Undifferentiated	24%	23%	27/114 (24%)
Total			78/637 (12%)

TABLE 44–13. Malignancy and Prognosis among Patients with Parotid Carcinoma and Facial Nerve Paralysis

	Percentage with Neck Metastasis	Ten-Year Survival Rate
Eneroth[19]	77%	0%
Conley[13]	84%	14%

TABLE 44–14. Proposed Staging System for Major Salivary Gland Cancer*

T0	No clinical evidence of primary tumor
T1	Tumor 0.1–2 cm in diameter without significant local extension
T2	Tumor 2.1–4 cm in diameter without significant local extension
T3	Tumor 4.1–6.0 cm in diameter without significant local extension
T4a	Tumor >6 cm in diameter without significant local extension
T4b	Tumor of any size with significant local extension
N0	No evidence of regional lymph node involvement (including palpable but not suspicious regional lymph nodes)
N1	Evidence of regional lymph node involvement (including palpable and suspicious regional lymph nodes)
NX	Regional lymph nodes not assessed
M0	No distant metastases
M1	Distant metastases (e.g., bone, lung, etc.)
	Stage I T1N0M0
	T2N0M0
	Stage II T3N0M0
	Stage III T1N1M0
	T2N1M0
	T4aN0M0
	T4bN0M0
	Stage IV T3N1M0
	T4aN1M0
	T4bN1M0
	Any T Any N and M1

*From the American Joint Committee for Cancer Staging and End-Results Reporting. Manual for Staging of Cancer. Chicago, 1980.[2]

per cent for stage I cancers, a 5-year survival rate of 76 per cent and a 10-year survival rate of 76 per cent for stage II cancers, and a 5-year survival rate of 49 per cent and a 10-year survival rate of 32 per cent for stage III cancers.

The correlation of stage with distant metastases is quite notable in Spiro's studies;[52–55] stage I lesions had a 2 per cent incidence of distant metastasis, whereas stage III cancers, 39 per cent. Furthermore, recurrence rates were correlated with the stage of disease: T1 lesions recurred in only 7 per cent of cases, T3 lesions, in 58 per cent. In their study of mucoepidermoid carcinoma,[52] they found that lymph node mestastasis, distant metastasis, recurrence, and overall survival correlated well with the stage of disease.

In 1981, a multi-institutional study of the staging system for cancer of the salivary glands was published and formed the basis for the 1980 AJC staging for major salivary gland cancers.[38] The results of this retrospective study of 861 patients led to the proposal of a new TNM classification system for these tumors. This system involves the use of five clinical variables: (1) size of tumor, (2) local extension, (3) palpable regional lymph nodes, (4) suspicion of involvement by tumor of palpable regional lymph nodes, and (5) presence of distant metastases. In this system, it should be noted that the T classification is based solely on the size and that T4 is divided into two subheadings, a and b, based on whether or not significant local extension exists.

Because the initial evidence suggests that prognosis appears to be dependent more on size and stage than on histology, the staging of salivary gland cancers should play a fundamental role, perhaps the most significant role, in treatment planning.

Location

The parotid gland is not truly divided anatomically into two lobes, but the facial nerve divides the gland into two portions, the superficial and the deep portions. The deep portion is less accessible surgically, and one might conclude that a malignant tumor of the deep lobe would have a less favorable prognosis than one in the superficial lobe. Nigro and Spiro[42] studied 36 patients with malignancies of the deep lobe and found no difference in survival for those patients in comparison to all patients with carcinoma of the parotid. The 5-, 10-, and 15-year survival rates for deep-lobe tumors were 61, 52, and 48 per cent, respectively. These figures

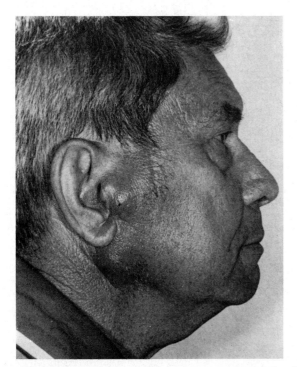

Figure 44–20. Advanced malignant parotid tumor with facial skin involvement.

compare favorably with survival rates for malignancies in all sites of the parotid. However, a decreased survival rate occurred when the mass presented in the oral cavity along the parapharyngeal space.

In planning therapy it might be kept in mind that after Warthin's tumor, the acinous cell carcinoma is the next most frequent to occur bilaterally and multicentrically. Clong and colleagues[11] suggest the need for total parotidectomy because of the potential for multicentricity; they report improved rates of local control for total parotidectomy compared with partial parotidectomy in this histologic group of tumors.

Recurrence

Recurrence rates in parotid carcinoma are quite high. Spiro and coworkers[54] found that 27 per cent of parotid cancers in their series recurred. Woods and colleagues[60] reported a 36 per cent incidence of recurrence in 226 parotid cancers and found recurrence to be particularly frequent in the highly malignant tumors (Table 44–15). Hodgkinson and Woods[31] reported a 38 per cent local recurrence in 5 years. It is particularly significant that in 64 per cent of the patients the facial nerve was sacrificed. This finding suggests that recurrences are frequent for parotid cancer, even with aggressive surgical maneuvers, and further supports the need for adjunctive treatments such as irradiation.

Kagan and co-workers[35] found a total of 109 recurrences in 56 patients with parotid gland cancer—an average of two recurrences per patient. The average survival interval from the first recurrence was 3.7 years. Hanna and coworkers[29] reviewed the survival rates for recurrent malignant parotid tumors and found a 5-year disease-free rate of 37 per cent. In several studies reviewing survival in recurrent parotid carcinomas, the rates varied from a low of 17 per cent to a high of 49 per cent.[35, 40] Compared with 5-year survival rates of 67 per cent for nonrecurrent cancers, it is clear that recurrence in parotid cancer is a poor prognostic sign, indicating the need for aggressive management.

Distant Metastasis

Distant metastasis obviously indicates a poor prognosis. The incidence of distant metastasis in parotid cancer is 20 per cent overall (Table 44–16) and is as high as 50 per cent in adenoid cystic carcinomas.[26, 44, 65] The most frequent site of metastasis is the lung, and the next most frequent site is bone. The aggressive behavior

TABLE 44–15. Incidence of Local Recurrence in Patients with Malignant Parotid Carcinoma

Histologic Type of Carcinoma	No. with Recurrence/ Total
Mucoepidermoid	3/62
Acinous cell	5/34
Adenoid cystic	17/28
Adenocarcinoma	25/54
Arising from mixed tumor	9/15
Squamous cell	14/22
Undifferentiated	7/11

TABLE 44–16. Incidence of Distant Metastasis among Patients with Parotid Carcinoma

Histologic Type of Carcinoma	No. with Metastasis/ Total (%)
Mucoepidermoid	14/183 (8%)
Acinous cell	2/14 (14%)
Adenoid cystic	22/53 (42%)
Arising from mixed tumor	3/14 (21%)
Squamous cell	2/13 (15%)
Adenocarcinoma	25/91 (27%)
Undifferentiated	10/28 (36%)
Total	78/396 (20%)

of parotid cancers as manifested by this high incidence of distant metastasis (higher than that seen in squamous cell cancer of the head and neck) suggests the need for adjuvant chemotherapy programs to decrease the chance of failure at the distant site. At present, little experience is available in this area.

Radiation Sensitivity

There is a need for treatment adjunct to surgery. The use of irradiation in salivary gland cancers has been controversial. In the past, these tumors have been reported as being radiation-resistant.[23] There is mounting evidence, however, that radiation therapy is effective in the treatment of salivary gland carcinoma in certain clinical situations.

King and Fletcher[36] in 1971 reported local control in 81 per cent of their patients with recurrent or inoperable parotid cancers, although the follow-up time varied from 2 to 20 years. Rossman[47] reported similar findings in 11 patients treated with irradiation as the only modality. Five of the 11 patients received a nominal standard dose (NSD) of greater than 1800 rets, and local control was achieved in all five patients at 2 to 6 years.* Six of the 11 patients received doses of less than 1800 rets, and local control was achieved in only one of them.

Elkon and co-workers[17] irradiated 19 patients, most of them for advanced disease (base of skull or cervical node involvement). Control was achieved in only two of the 19 patients, one with adenoid cystic carcinoma and the other with squamous cell carcinoma.

Data such as these suggest that irradiation can affect some salivary gland cancers and may be more effective when there is only minimal disease. Combining this experience with that seen in squamous cell cancer, one might hypothesize that irradiation may be effective in the treatment of patients who have minimal residual disease or a high likelihood of recurrence.

Rossman[47] found that recurrence in patients treated with a combination of surgery and irradiation was only 17 per cent, whereas patients treated with surgery alone had a 65 per cent recurrence rate. Elkon and others[17] found a local recurrence rate of 6 per cent in 17 patients treated with irradiation for microscopic residual dis-

---

*The NSD (rets) is calculated according to the formula $D/(N^{0.24} \times T^{0.11})$, where D = dose in rad, N = number of fractions, and T = time elapsed.

eases. Tapley,[57] in a review of the experience at the M.D. Anderson Hospital in Houston, reported a 30 per cent local failure rate in 54 patients treated with surgery alone and a 9 per cent incidence in 33 patients treated with surgery and irradiation. Shidnia and co-workers[49] noted a 50 per cent rate of treatment success with surgery alone and a 70 per cent rate of freedom from disease when combination treatment was employed. Fu and co-workers[26] reported that in 35 patients known to have microscopic tumor at or close to the surgical margin, local control was achieved with postoperative irradiation in 86 per cent of the cases, whereas in 13 patients with similar margins treated with surgery alone, control was achieved in only 46 per cent of the cases. An interesting retrospective study by Tu and colleagues[58] from the People's Republic of China demonstrated the superiority of combined therapy, i.e., surgery and postoperative irradiation in the management of parotid cancer. In the study, 59 patients were treated by surgery and an equal number received surgery and postoperative radiation therapy. In their study, postoperative radiation therapy increased local control in comparison to surgery alone (1) if there was evidence of locally advanced disease, (2) if the tumor belonged to one of the high-grade categories, (3) if the tumor was recurrent, or (4) if the facial nerve was involved by the tumor. In all of these series, however, the follow-up period was variable and rarely exceeded 5 years, which is a short follow-up interval for this group of cancers. Nevertheless, compared with recurrence rates at 5 years in other series of patients receiving only surgical treatment, these results are more than just encouraging.

Such data, although not final, dispel the long-held assertions that salivary gland cancer is radiation-resistant and that there is no role for radiation therapy in this group of malignancies. Combining radiation therapy with surgery will reduce the incidence of local and regional tumor recurrence in selected instances. We agree with and use the seven indications of Guillamondegue et al[28] for postoperative irradiation:

1. High-grade cancers.
2. Recurrent cancers.
3. Deep-lobe cancers.
4. Gross or microscopic residual disease.
5. Tumor adjacent to the facial nerve.
6. Regional node metastasis.
7. Invasion of muscle, bone, skin, nerves, or any extra parotid extension.
8. Any T3 parotid cancer.

All of these parameters are indicators of a poor prognosis, and surgical management alone in these situations has not provided adequate local and regional control. Furthermore, we have added to this list an eighth indication—any T3 lesion—to indicate that even low-grade T3 lesions indicate a poor survival and should be treated aggressively.

Chemotherapeutic Sensitivity

We are in an evolving process in the treatment of parotid cancers. Only 30 years ago, Foote and Frazell introduced an acceptable classification system that has allowed study of these malignancies.[24] More recent studies of their pathology have added further knowledge to their histology.[3, 7, 18, 33, 37, 48] We have learned the

limitations of surgery and have begun to use radiation therapy as an adjunct to improve local control. We are now aware of the frequency of distant metastasis in this group of cancers and the potential value of adjunctive chemotherapy. To make further progress in the understanding of this group of infrequent malignancies, multi-institutional cooperative studies will be needed to accumulate adequate numbers of cases for studying the value of adjunctive therapy in this deadly group of cancers over long follow-up intervals.

Suen and Johns[56] have published a multi-institutional survey of the results of chemotherapy in salivary gland cancers in an attempt to come to some conclusion as to what might be useful drug regimens for specific histologic types of salivary gland cancers. A total of 85 cases of salivary gland cancers were available for review. There seems to be little question that salivary gland cancers will respond to chemotherapy (Table 44–17). All of the patients in the study represented treatment for palliation. There is still too little information available to draw definite conclusions; however, we noted trends that provide some guidelines.

The salivary gland cancers reviewed in the study represented major and minor types. There appeared to be no obvious difference as to the site of origin, but histologic type did seem to be important with regard to which drugs were effective. Although each histologic type is different, there seemed to be two groups: (1) the adenocarcinoma-like cancers (adenoid cystic, adenocarcinoma, carcinoma ex mixed tumor, and acinous cell), which respond best to Adriamycin, cis-platinum, and 5-fluorouracil; and (2) the squamous-like cancers (squamous cell carcinoma and mucoepidermoid), which respond best to methotrexate and cis-platinum.

It is not known whether combination regimens have an advantage over single drugs. In a future study, it would seem most sensible to begin with single drugs if it were known that the drugs selected had proved effective. After identification of the effective single drugs, combinations of these effective drugs could then be tried to improve the response rates.

TREATMENT

Treatment Principles for Parotid Tumors

Based on the distillation of available data from the literature and the experience at the University of Virginia, a treatment plan composed of four categories has

TABLE 44—17. Histologic Type of Carcinoma and Response Rate

Type	No.	Complete Response	Partial Response	No Response
Adenoid cystic carcinoma	53	4	17	32
Mucoepidermoid carcinoma	9	2	3	4
Adenocarcinoma	10	2	3	5
Carcinoma or mixed tumor	9	1	2	6
Acinous cell carcinoma	3	0	2	1
Squamous cell carcinoma	1	0	0	1
Total	85	9 (10%)	27 (32%)	49 (58%)

*Data from Suen JY, Johns ME: Laryngoscope 92:235, 1982.[56]

been formulated based on the factors that influence survival (Table 44–18). Treatment becomes progressively more aggressive from group I to group IV.

Group I includes the T1 and T2N0 low-grade malignancies. Removal of the tumor with a cuff of normal tissue (usually total parotidectomy) is adequate treatment. The digastric triangle lymph nodes should be evaluated at the time of surgery. Although some data suggest that T1 high-grade mucoepidermoid carcinomas and perhaps other T1 cancers may respond to this same treatment, we are currently placing these high-grade tumors in group II.

Group II includes T1 and T2N0 high-grade malignant tumors. Treatment includes total parotidectomy with regional resection of digastric nodes and preservation of the facial nerve (except those branches involved by the tumor grossly). If the nerve is involved, it is resected back to clear margins (frozen section) and immediate nerve grafting is performed. If the nerve is not grossly involved by the tumor, it is preserved, since all patients in this group receive radiation therapy to a wide field, including the upper-echelon nodes. The vital function of the facial nerve can be preserved in such situations without sacrificing the chance for cure.

Group III includes T3N0 or any N+ high-grade cancers and recurrent cancers. A radical parotidectomy (sacrifice of facial nerve) and modified neck dissection for N0 or radical neck dissection for N+ neck metastasis is carried out. If there is evidence of facial nerve involvement into the mastoid, the surgeon should be prepared to follow the nerve into the mastoid until negative margins are achieved. Primary facial nerve grafting is carried out at the time of surgery. All patients receive postoperative irradiation to a wide field that includes the primary

lesion on the same side of the neck from the skull base to the clavicle, including the mastoid bone.

Group IV includes tumors greater than 6 cm or with extraparotid extension. Aggressive radical surgery to achieve adequate margins is indicated. In addition to radical parotidectomy and neck dissection, surgery in this group *may* include resection of the masseter muscle, buccal fat pad, skin, mandible, ear canal, mastoid, or other involved structures as indicated. Postoperative irradiation is used routinely. The facial nerve is reconstructed by grafting techniques; however, in this situation, with a potentially avascular bed for the nerve graft, additive procedures (such as dynamic muscle transfers using the masseter or temporalis muscle performed at the time of primary surgery) may provide important functional and cosmetic reconstruction. The chances for long-term survival are low, and the treatment results in considerable morbidity.

Treatment Principles for Submandibular Tumors

A treatment plan using similar factors for submandibular gland tumors is outlined in Table 44–18. For *group I*, which includes tumors smaller than 4 cm of the low-grade histology, we recommend wide excision of the submandibular triangle. All nerves are preserved unless there is evidence of involvement. No radiation therapy is used.

In *group II*, which includes the T1 and T2 high-grade tumors, wide excision of the submandibular triangle with preservation of all nerves is done unless there is evidence of nerve invasion. In this group, however, postoperative radiation therapy is given.

In *group III*, with or without positive nodes, a radical

TABLE 44–18. Principles of Treatment for Parotid Carcinoma

	I	II	III	IV
		Treatment Group		
Tumor type	T1 and T2 low-grade	T1 and T2 high-grade		T4
	Mucoepidermoid low-grade	Adenocarcinoma	T3, N0 or N+	
		Malignant mixed		
	Acinous cell	Undifferentiated	Any recurrent tumors not in Group IV	
		Squamous cell		
Treatment				
Parotid gland	Superificial or total parotidectomy	Total parotidectomy with resection of first-echelon lymph nodes	Radical parotidectomy (sacrifice of seventh nerve with immediate reconstruction)	Radical parotidectomy with resection of skin, mandible, muscles, mastoid tip, as indicated
	Preservation of seventh nerve		Neck dissection for N+ neck only	Sacrifice of seventh nerve with immediate reconstruction
			Postoperative irradiation	Neck dissection Postoperative irradiation
Submandibular[14, 51]	Submandibular triangle resection	Wide excision of submandibular triangle	Radical neck dissection to include 12th nerve and lingual nerve	Surgery to fit disease extent
		Preserve nerves unless involved		
		Postoperative radiation therapy	Postoperative radiation therapy	

neck dissection includes the 12th nerve and the lingual nerve. Postoperative radiation therapy is also administered. If the tumor does not involve the 11th nerve, this nerve might be preserved.

For *group IV* tumors, the surgery must be designed to fit disease extent. This may well include resection of the mandible, floor of mouth, tongue, and marginal mandibular nerve along with a radical neck dissection specimen.

As in all malignancies, treatment cannot be based on tumor factors alone. Age, emotional condition, medical condition, and various sociologic factors often require that surgeons modify their treatment routines and tailor them to specific patient needs.

Surgical Techniques

Having discussed principles of treatment and treatment planning, we now present the surgical techniques themselves. Minor salivary gland tumors will not be addressed as far as the technical aspects of treatment are concerned, since they must be treated in relationship to the anatomic region in which they are found. Reference to chapters on the oral cavity and on the nose and paranasal sinuses will be made and surgical techniques described in those chapters used. Our primary emphasis is directed toward the submandibular and parotid glands and, in particular, the various approaches to the parotid and parapharyngeal spaces.

Positioning, "Prepping," and Draping

To perform a *parotidectomy*, the patient is positioned on the operating table with the head turned facing away from the surgeon and with a pad beneath the shoulder on the same side needed for the surgery. A solution of fresh 1:100,000 epinephrine is injected subcutaneously along the planned incision line. No local anesthetic is used, since this may result in temporary paralysis to the facial nerve. The epinephrine-induced vasoconstriction decreases bothersome arteriolar bleeding at the time of the incision. The solution is prepared by diluting $\frac{1}{10}$ ml of 1:1000 epinephrine with 10 ml of sterile water for injection.

Some surgeons have recommended the installation of methylene blue into the ductal system, the principle being that the ducts and acinar system will take on a blue hue and the facial nerve will be white and thus stand out from the underlying salivary tissue. It seems to us, however, that overinjection of methylene blue could possibly lead to rupture into the soft tissues, thus complicating the surgical dissection. Transection of the salivary gland could also lead to leakage of the methylene blue into the operative field. Most important, however, is the fact that a surgeon who is skilled in parotid surgery does not require color contrast or color coding to identify and preserve the facial nerve.

Routine draping is carried out; however, a clear plastic drape, instead of towel draping, is placed over the face to include the eye and mouth anterior to the proposed incision site and thus provides a window to observe facial muscle function on the operative side. In order to do this effectively, no towel draping is placed across the eye or mouth on the operative side. The plastic drape is positioned away from the incision site but over the rest of the face.

Incision

A properly designed incision to allow exposure and the most cosmetic end result should be used. We prefer an incision that begins anterior to the attachment of the anterior helix at the zygomatic area and descends to the tragus. At this point, the incision is hidden behind the inner free margin of the tragus and then directed behind the lobule of the pinna in a soft curve and continues anteriorly onto the neck (Fig. 44–21). The incision is carried down to the parotid fascia. This fascia has a silvery sheen that is easily identifiable. The skin is then elevated from the parotid gland anteriorly until this anterior skin flap is 1 cm beyond (anterior to) the gland. If greater exposure is needed, the incision can be carried up into the temporal hairline and then a horizontal extension brought anteriorly. Inferiorly the incision can be extended to the hyoid bone. With these extensions, a facial flap can be elevated almost to the midline. Once the skin flap is elevated, it may be sutured anteriorly in place to eliminate the need for retraction.

Resection

The next step is to incise the fascia extending from the sternocleidomastoid muscle onto the parotid. This allows the tail of the parotid to be separated from the sternocleidomastoid muscle (Fig. 44–22). This generally requires sectioning the great auricular nerve; however, on occasion it may be mobilized and reflected posteriorly (Fig. 44–23). In most cases when superficial parotidectomy is being performed, the posterior facial vein can be preserved because the dissection will be superficial to it. Once the tail of the parotid is mobilized, the sternocleidomastoid can be retracted and the digastric muscle identified (Fig. 44–24). Later identification of the facial nerve may be aided if the digastric muscle is

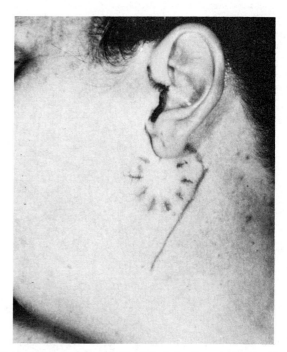

Figure 44–21. The skin is marked for the surgical incision employed for parotidectomy.

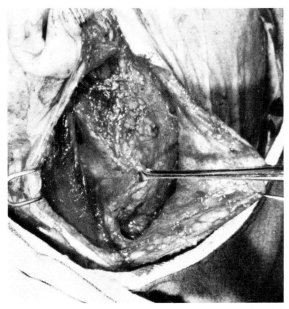

Figure 44–22. The anterior skin flap has been elevated, and the tail of the parotid gland is freed from its facial attachments to the sternocleidomastoid muscle.

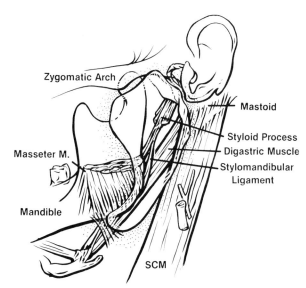

Figure 44–24. The anatomy of the parotid bed is diagrammed. The relationship of the digastric muscle, styloid process, and anterior border of the sternocleidomastoid muscle should be noted.

followed superiorly toward the mastoid tip and digastric groove where the muscle inserts.

Next, the parotid gland is bluntly dissected from its attachments to the cartilage of the external auditory canal. As one does this, the so-called tragal pointer is identified (Fig. 44–25). The facial nerve will lie approximately 1 cm deep and slightly inferior and anterior to the tragal pointer. The tympanomastoid suture line can also be palpated at this point of dissection. The facial nerve will exit the skull base approximately 6 to 8 mm deep to the inferior end of the tympanomastoid suture line. This is a nearly constant relationship. With the preceding mobilization now complete, the index finger can palpate the styloid process and the attachment of

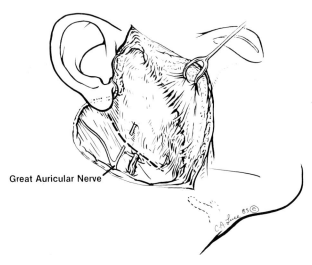

Figure 44–23. Separation of the tail of the parotid from the sternocleidomastoid usually requires sectioning the greater auricular nerve.

the digastric muscle to the digastric ridge. The facial nerve lies between these two structures (Fig. 44–26). Careful dissection of this small area with a narrow hemostat in the direction of the facial nerve will separate the soft tissues until the facial nerve is identified. For the majority of parotid tumors, this approach will lead to the easy identification of the facial nerve as it exits the stylomastoid canal (Fig. 44–26).

Occasionally, however, the tumor mass may be sitting over the main trunk of the facial nerve or previous surgery or recurrent tumor may obscure the anatomy. Alternative approaches to the facial nerve should then be employed. Perhaps the most commonly used optional approach to identifying the facial nerve is to follow carefully the posterior facial vein superiorly as it enters the parotid gland (Fig. 44–27). As this is done, one can see the marginal mandibular nerve crossing superficial to posterior facial vein. This is nearly a constant anatomic finding. Once the marginal mandibular nerve is seen crossing superficial to the posterior facial vein, it can be followed posteriorly to the main trunk.

Another technique that is very useful for patients who have had previous surgery or heavy scarring or recurrent tumor in the area of the main trunk involves removing the mastoid tip and identifying the facial nerve as it exits to the styloid mastoid canal. This can be done using a mallet and gouge or, in a more controlled fashion, an otologic drill (Figs. 44–28 and 44–29). If recurrent tumor sits in the region of the stylomastoid canal, we recommend starting with this approach because it allows one to identify the facial nerve in a nonoperated area. In these cases, the facial nerve is frequently indistinguishable from the scar tissue, thus making the intratemporal approach most valuable.

In addition to the two principal alternate methods for identifying the facial nerve, another method involves identifying the buccal branch as it courses parallel to the parotid duct. This requires identification of the

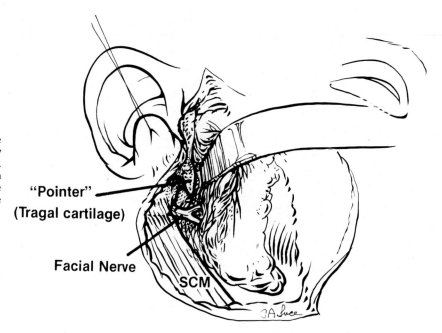

Figure 44–25. Blunt dissection of the parotid gland from the external auditory canal cartilage reveals the tragal pointer. The facial nerve lies approximately 1 cm deep and slightly anteroinferior to the pointer, or 6 to 8 mm deep to the tympanomastoid suture line.

"Pointer"
(Tragal cartilage)

Facial Nerve

SCM

parotid duct anteriorly as it crosses the masseter muscle (Fig. 44–27).

Once the main trunk of the facial nerve is identified, a tunnel is created just above the facial nerve and the parotid tissue in that area is incised, splitting the gland up to the pes anserinus (Fig. 44–30A). At this point the facial nerve branches are identified. The surgeon can then start with the branch most distal from the tumor

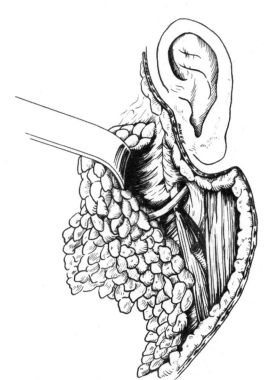

Figure 44–26. The facial nerve exits the stylomastoid foramen to run anteriorly between the styloid process and attachment of the digastric muscle to the digastric ridge.

and follow it out to the periphery of the gland. As a tunnel is created between the nerve and the gland, use a No. 12 blade to cut the overlying parotid tissue (Fig. 44–30B). Once the first branch is completely followed out to its point of exit from the gland, the surgeon returns to find the next lower branch. By creating a second tunnel, the surgeon sharply connects this tunnel to the previously dissected parotid space, observing the facial nerve branch that was previously dissected. This pattern is successively followed inferiorly. The gland is reflected downward in the plane of the facial nerve by serial identification of each nerve branch until the entire superficial portion of the gland is reflected inferiorly and freed from the most inferior branch of the facial nerve. This gives an intact superficial portion of the gland that includes the tumor (Fig. 44–31A, B). Thus, the superficial parotidectomy progressively mobilizes the gland from the underlying facial nerve branches, from superior to inferior.

Deep Lobe Tumors

The majority of tumors of the parotid gland arise in the superficial portion of the gland. About 10 to 12 per cent of tumors of the parotid lie in the deep portion of the gland medial to the facial nerve. Tumors involving the deep lobe can generally be removed by the standard external approach, preserving the facial nerve branches. These tumors are, however, more difficult to remove with a margin of normal salivary gland tissue while still preserving the facial nerve. The superficial gland is first removed as described above (Fig. 44–32). The exposed branches of the facial nerve are then dissected from the deep lobe, and rubber "spaghetti" bands are placed under the branches to allow general retraction of the facial nerve during dissection. The deep-lobe tissue, along with the tumor, is then dissected from the mandible and stylomandibular membrane by patient and diligent mobilization of the gland from all four sides and its deep attachments (Fig. 44–33).

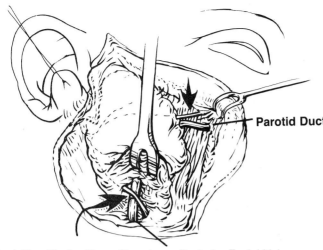

Marginal Mandibular Nerve Branch   Posterior Facial Vein

Parotid Duct

Figure 44–27. The marginal mandibular nerve can be reliably found by tracing the posterior facial vein superiorly. The marginal division almost always crosses superficial to the vein. Also diagrammed is the relationship of the buccal division to the parotid duct.

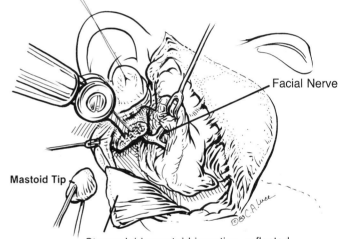

Facial Nerve

Mastoid Tip

Sternocleidomastoid insertion, reflected

Figure 44–28. Finding the main trunk of the facial nerve within the mastoid bone by removing the mastoid tip is particularly helpful when doing surgery in a previously operated field.

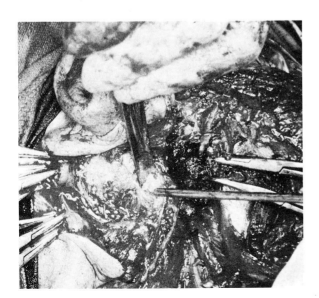

Figure 44–29. In this case, a radical parotidectomy was done for cancer. The mastoid tip is being removed from the mastoid bone to obtain adequate margin and a proximal site for nerve grafting.

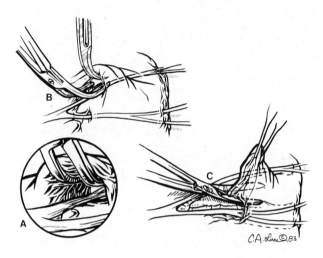

Figure 44–30. The technique of following each branch of the facial nerve is demonstrated. (*A*) A tunnel is created in the plane of the nerve. (*B*) The overlying parotid tissue is cut with a No. 12 blade. (*C*) Each successive tunnel is then connected to the prior tunnel.

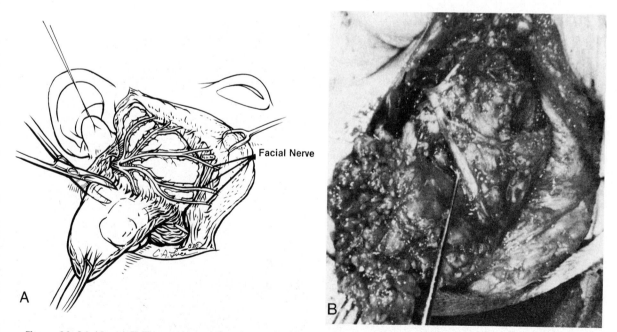

Facial Nerve

Figure 44–31. (*A* and *B*) The nearly completed process with the tumor within the intact superficial parotidectomy specimen.

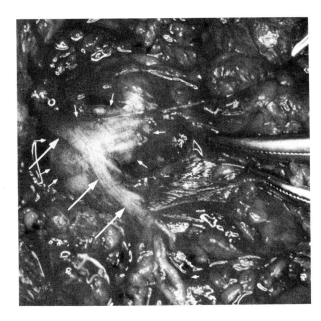

Figure 44–32. Following superficial parotidectomy, a deep lobe mixed tumor is seen sitting under the pes anserinus.

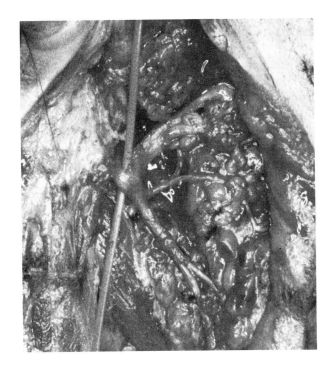

Figure 44–33. Following removal of a deep lobe tumor, the facial nerve is intact.

Parapharyngeal Space Tumors

Tumors that involve the parapharyngeal space or retromandibular area can be approached in two ways:

1. *Submandibular approach*—simpler and applicable in most cases.

2. *Osteotomy* of the mandibular ramus, with reflection of the mandible superiorly to expose the parapharyngeal space.

SUBMANDIBULAR APPROACH

The first step in obtaining exposure is excision of the submandibular gland. Because removal of the gland and lymph nodes of the submandibular space is an integral part of a radical neck dissection, the surgical technique is discussed in detail in the chapter on neck dissection. We review it only briefly here.

The skin incision is made in the natural skin crease 3 to 4 cm inferior to the mandible and extends from the greater cornu of the hyoid bone posterolaterally toward the level of the angle of the mandible. This incision is an easy extension of the inferior part of a parotidectomy incision (Fig. 44–34). The incision is extended through the subcutaneous tissue and platysma to the superficial layer of the deep cervical fascia. Anteriorly the anterior belly of the digastric muscle and posteriorly the anterior border of the sternocleidomastoid are identified. The anterior facial vein, running just superficial to the deep cervical fascia, is then ligated and divided. The marginal mandibular nerve generally runs just superficial to the anterior facial vein. Therefore, it is commonly taught that retraction of the superior ligature on the anterior facial vein will protect the nerve as the fascia is reflected superiorly. Although this is true, we nevertheless recommend its positive identification as the best method to ensure its preservation.

Elevation of the fascia exposes the gland. The gland is dissected superiorly where the external maxillary artery (facial artery) is ligated and divided (Fig. 44–35). Retraction of the mylohyoid muscle anteriorly and the gland itself posteroinferiorly exposes the lingual nerve

and Wharton's duct (Fig. 44–36). The submandibular ganglion with its venous plexus is ligated and divided as is the duct itself. Division of the ganglion allows the lingual nerve to retract superiorly out of harm's way.

The hypoglossal nerve lies between the mylohyoid and hyoglossal muscles. Inferior retraction of the anterior belly and tendon of the digastric muscle exposes this nerve, which is easily preserved as the inferior border of the submandibular gland is dissected free and the facial artery ligated and divided (Fig. 44–37). If not already done, Wharton's duct is ligated and divided, and the gland is removed.

Following the submandibular gland excision, a superficial parotidectomy is completed to identify and preserve the facial nerve. If the tumor involves the tail of the parotid, the superficial portion of the parotid gland can be reflected from superior to inferior. This will allow for identification and protection of the facial nerve and leaves the attachment of the tumor to its parapharyngeal extension. The stylomandibular ligament is then sharply incised and detached from the mandible (Fig. 44–38). This allows for anterior dislocation of the mandible to improve access to the parapharyngeal space (Fig. 44–39). This approach provides sufficient exposure so that most tumors can then be bluntly dissected with the index finger (Figs. 44–40 through 44–42).

MANDIBULAR OSTEOTOMY

Larger tumors or those encircling the neurovascular bundle of the carotid sheath require an approach to the parapharyngeal space using a mandibular osteotomy. The facial nerve is identified, and the lateral portion of the parotid is removed by the superficial parotidectomy technique. An incision is then made along the inferior body and angle of the mandibular ramus. The marginal mandibular nerve is carefully preserved. Using a periosteal elevator, the surgeon elevates the masseter muscle from the angle of the mandible. Holes for rewiring the mandible are drilled into the bone prior to creating the osteotomy. Once this is accomplished, a step or V-

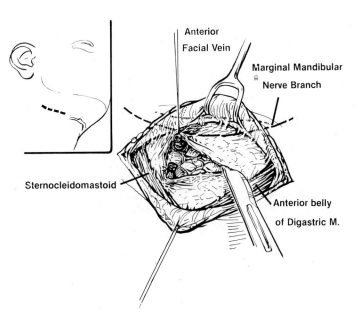

Figure 44–34. Submandibular gland incision. The incision is made in a natural skin crease 3 to 4 cm inferior to the mandible. The marginal mandibular nerve generally runs just superficial to the anterior facial vein.

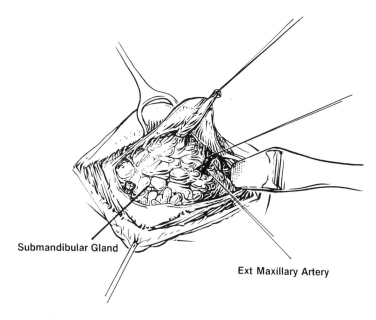

Submandibular Gland

Ext Maxillary Artery

Figure 44–35. Submandibular gland excision. The external maxillary artery is identified.

Figure 44–36. Submandibular gland excision. The mylohyoid is retracted anteriorly and the gland posteriorly, exposing the lingual nerve, submandibular ganglion, and Wharton's duct.

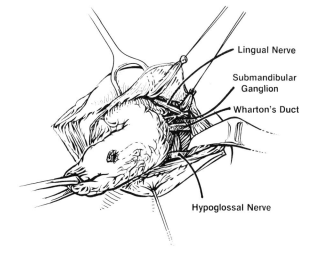

Lingual Nerve

Submandibular Ganglion

Wharton's Duct

Hypoglossal Nerve

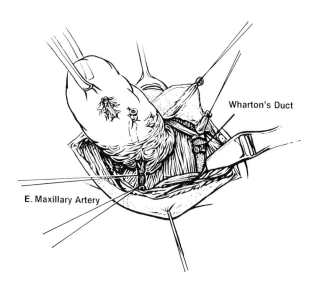

Wharton's Duct

E. Maxillary Artery

Figure 44–37. Submandibular gland excision. The hypoglossal nerve runs between the hypoglossus and the mylohyoid muscle. The external maxillary artery will be again divided.

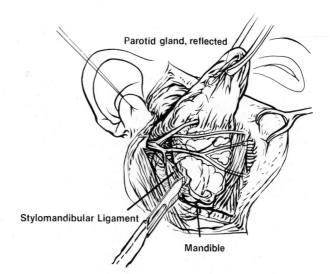

Figure 44–38. Resection of parapharyngeal space tumor. Following completion of the superficial parotidectomy and submandibular gland excision, access to the parapharyngeal space is obtained by first incising the stylomandibular ligament.

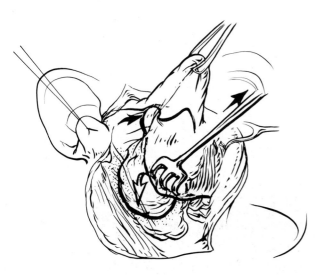

Figure 44–39. Resection of parapharyngeal space tumor. The mandible can be retracted or dislocated anteriorly.

Figure 44–40. Resection of parapharyngeal space tumor. Access to the parapharyngeal space has been obtained by first a superficial parotidectomy and submandibular gland excision. Incising the stylomandibular ligament has allowed anterior dislocation of the mandible. The tumor can be seen just posterior to the angle of the mandible and just superior to the posterior belly of the digastric tendon.

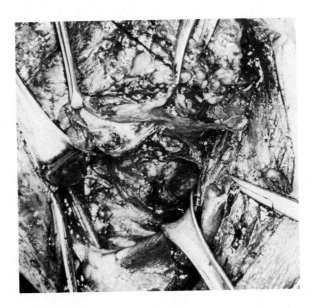

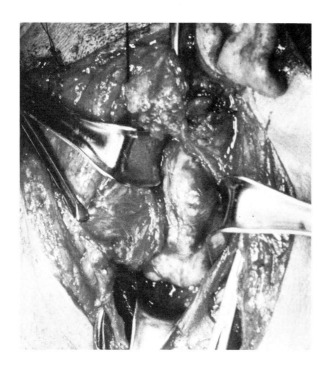

Figure 44–41. Resection of parapharyngeal space tumor. The tumor has been partially dissected and is now clearly visible.

Figure 44–42. Resection of parapharyngeal space tumor. The tumor has been completely mobilized with blunt finger dissection.

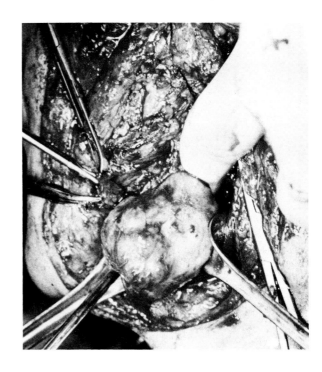

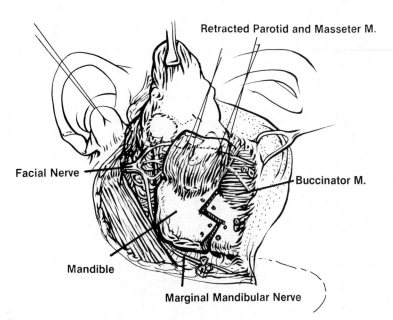

Figure 44–43. Resection of parapharyngeal space tumor. Larger parapharyngeal tumors or those encircling the carotid sheath require the wider exposure obtained via a mandibular osteotomy. A parotidectomy and submandibular gland excision having been completed and the masseter and internal pterygoid muscles separated from the mandible. Holes to rewire the step-osteotomy have been drilled and the osteotomy cut to take advantage of all possible favorable mandibular fracture configurations.

type osteotomy is made at the angle of the mandible (Fig. 44–43). The internal pterygoid muscle can then be detached and the bony segment swung superiorly. This allows exposure of the parapharyngeal and pterygoid areas for direct removal of the tumor (Fig. 44–44). Once the tumor is completely removed, the mandible is reapproximated with a "figure-8" wire placed in the previously created drill holes. If the mandible is reapproximated carefully, significant inferior alveolar nerve regeneration will occur within 6 months to a year.

After tumor resection, the wound is irrigated with saline and a drain is placed for suction. We prefer the Jackson-Pratt drains when radical neck dissection is not used. If the parotid surgery is in conjunction with a radical neck dissection, large suction drains are preferred. The wound is closed in layers, and the drain is generally left in place from 24 to 48 hours, depending upon the amount of drainage.

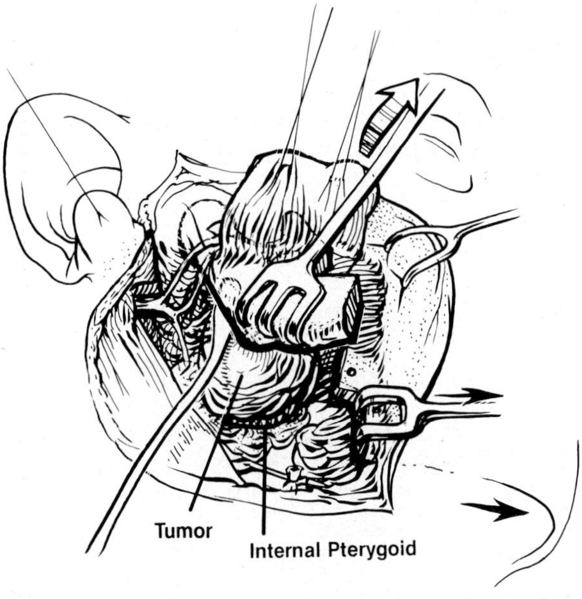

All of the approaches described work well for benign tumors that are confined to those described portions of the gland. When the tumor crosses these various planes, or is malignant, however, the surgeon must use a combination of methods, keeping in mind that removal of the tumor with a margin of normal tissue is paramount. The resection of malignant tumors may require resection of the facial nerve, masseter muscle, or mandible or may even a mastoidectomy. The extent of surgery is determined by the extent of the tumor; there is no "standard" approach.

The approach to the facial nerve for parotid tumors must be direct. For benign tumors, the facial nerve may be dissected away from the tumor mass. The facial nerve must be sacrificed in the rare benign case of the repeatedly recurrent mixed tumor, which surrounds and encases this nerve. This may well be the only possible approach that will cure the patient of the tumor.[61]

When the facial nerve is resected, a frozen section of the proximal and distal stumps is obtained to rule out perineural spread. The nerve is resected back to clear margins. Facial nerve reconstruction is carried out at the time of primary resection.

COMPLICATIONS

The complications of parotid surgery include facial nerve injury, hematoma, infection, gustatory sweating, and salivary fistulae.

Facial Nerve Injury. See Chapter 45.

Hematoma. Postoperative hematomas occur infrequently and are generally related to inadequate hemostasis being obtained at the time of the procedure. Treatment involves, quite simply, evacuation of the hematoma and control of the bleeding points.

Figure 44–44. Resection of parapharyngeal space tumor. Separating the internal pterygoid muscle from the mandible thus allows the mandible to swing anteriorly and laterally, providing access to the parapharyngeal space.

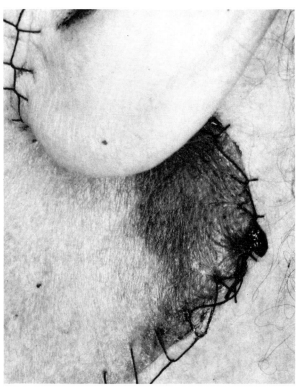

Figure 44–45. Necrosis of distal tip of skin flap.

Infection. Infection is exceedingly rare postoperatively in parotid surgery. Prophylactic antibiotics are generally not indicated unless surgery is being carried in a chronically infected gland or if entry into the oral cavity is a part of the procedure. Occasionally, a small distal tip of the skin flap will be lost (Fig. 44–45).

Gustatory Sweating. *Frey's syndrome*, or auriculotemporal syndrome, is a complex of symptoms that include localized facial sweating and flushing during mastication of food. This is said to occur in 35 to 60 per cent of patients who have undergone parotidectomy with facial dissection.[27, 30] It may be a result of aberrant regeneration of nerve fibers from the postganglionic secretomotor parasympathetic innervation to the parotid gland occur-

ring through the severed axon sheaths of the postganglionic sympathetic fibers that supply the sweat glands of the skin (Fig. 44–46). It is important to note that this syndrome may also occur in the distribution of the great auricular nerve or the branches of the cervical plexus. The syndrome will usually present itself several months after surgery. Once it does present, it will be persistent in varying degrees of severity and more or less socially handicapping.

The area of gustatory sweating can be objectively documented by performing the Minor's starch-iodine test. This involves painting the skin of the infected area on the face with a solution of 3 gm of iodine, 20 gm of castor oil, and approximately 200 ml of absolute alcohol. Once this solution dries, the painted area is dusted with starch powder. The patient is then asked to chew a sialagogue, such as a lemon wedge, for 2 minutes to produce a salivary response. The area affected by Frey's syndrome will be demonstrated by sweat, which dissolves the starch powder and reacts with the iodine to produce dark blue-black spots (Fig. 44–47).

The treatment of this syndrome is supportive in most cases. The majority of patients are not significantly affected to cause them to seek therapy. Numerous treatments have been proposed, including tympanic neurectomy, the subdermal insertion of fascia lata grafts, or the rotation of sternocleidomastoid muscle flaps over the parotidectomy bed. Perhaps the most promising approach to therapy was pioneered by Hayes and colleagues,[30] which evaluated the use of glycopyrrolate prepared as a 1 per cent roll-on lotion. They reported on 14 of 16 patients using a concentration up to 2 per cent roll-on lotion. The side effects of this therapy using 1 per cent solution were very low, but included the anticholinergic symptoms of blurred vision or dry mouth.

Guidelines for treatment for gustatory sweating include the following:

1. Confirm the location of the gustatory sweating using the Minor starch-iodine test.

2. Avoid installation of glycopyrrolate into the nose, mouth, or eyes.

3. Do not apply to a cut or infected skin.

4. Topically applied anticholinergic agents are contraindicated in patients with glaucoma.

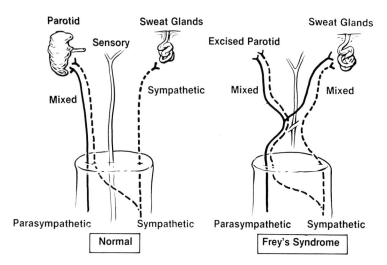

Figure 44–46. Proposed mechanism of gustatory sweating (Frey's syndrome).

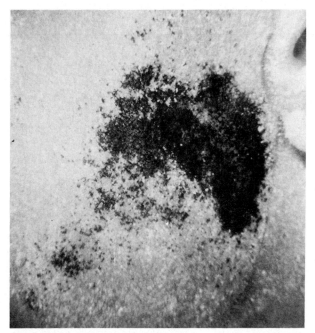

Figure 44–47. Minor's starch-iodine test in a patient with moderately severe Frey's syndrome.

5. Twice-a-day application increases effectiveness.

6. Wash hands well afterwards, and avoid contact with eyes or eyelids following application.

7. Treat significant side effects; blurred vision or dry mouth should be treated by temporarily discontinuing the use of the drug.

It is likely that most patients would prefer to try glycopyrrolate before fascia lata transfers or tympanic neurectomies. It should be noted, however, that at the present time this drug is under development and is not yet approved for general use by the Food and Drug Administration.

Salivary Fistulae. Rarely will a salivary fistula develop postoperatively. It generally presents as an opening in the suture line just below the lobule of the pinna. Clear drainage will obviously be saliva. Occasionally the wound heals and salivary accumulation occurs under the flap. This will most frequently occur following ligation of the duct after superficial parotidectomy. The remaining parotid tissue lying deep in the facial nerve will then exude saliva into the wound. In most instances this is a self-limited problem that will respond to pressure dressing.

REFERENCES

1. American Cancer Society: Cancer Facts and Figures. New York, 1983.
2. American Joint Committee for Cancer Staging and End-results Reporting: Manual for Staging of Cancer. American Joint Committee, Chicago, 1980.
3. Bardwill JM: Tumors of the parotid gland. Am J Surg 114:498, 1967.
4. Batsakis JG, Chinn E, Regezi JA, Repola DA: The pathology of head and neck tumors: Salivary glands, part 2. Head Neck Surg 1:167, 1978.
5. Batsakis JG, Chinn EK, Weimert TA: Acinic cell carcinoma: A clinicopathologic study of thirty-five cases. J Laryngol Otol 93:325, 1979.
6. Batsakis JG, Regezi JA: The pathology of head and neck tumors: Salivary glands, part 1. Head Neck Surg 1:59, 1978.
7. Ibid., Part 4. Head Neck Surg 1:340, 1979.
8. Batsakis JG, Regezi JA, Bloch D: The pathology of head and neck tumors: Salivary glands, part 3. Head Neck Surg 1:260, 1979.
9. Bertrandi A: Trattato Delle Operazioni di Chirurgia. Tomo 1. Torino, Botta, prato e Paravia, 1802.
10. Bjorkland A, Eneroth CM: Management of parotid gland neoplasms. Am J Otolaryngol 1:55. 1980.
11. Chong CG, Beahrs OH, Woolner LB: Surgical management of acinic cell carcinoma of the parotid gland. Surg Gynecol Obstet 138:65, 1974.
12. Conley J: Salivary glands and the facial nerve. New York, Grune & Stratton, 1975.
13. Conley J, Hamaker RC: Prognosis of malignant tumors of the parotid gland with facial paralysis. Arch Otolaryngol 101:39, 1975.
14. Conley J, Meyers E, Cole R: Analysis of 115 patients with tumors of the submandibular gland. Ann Otol Rhinol Laryngol 81:323, 1972.
15. Davis RA, Anson BJ, Budinger JM, Kurth LE: Surgical anatomy of the facial nerve and parotid gland based upon a study of 350 cervicofacial halves. Surg Gynecol Obstet 102:385, 1956.
16. Eby LS, Johnson DS, Baker HW: Adenoid cystic carcinoma of the head and neck. Cancer 29:1160, 1972.
17. Elkon D, Colman M, Hendrickson FR: Radiation therapy in the treatment of malignant salivary gland tumors. Cancer 41:502, 1978.
18. Eneroth CM: Histological and clinical aspects of parotid tumors. Acta Otolaryngol (Suppl) 191:1, 1964.
19. Eneroth CM: Facial nerve paralysis: A criterion of malignancy in parotid tumors. Arch Otolaryngol, 95:300, 1972.
20. Eneroth CM, Andreasson L, Beran M, et al: Preoperative facial paralysis in malignant parotid tumors. ORL 39:272, 1977.
21. Eneroth CM, Hamberger CA: Principles of treatment of different types of parotid tumors. Laryngoscope 84:1732, 1974.
22. Eneroth CM, Hjertman L, Moberger G: Malignant tumors of the submandibular gland. Acta Otolaryngol 64:514, 1967.
23. Evans JC: Radiation therapy of salivary gland tumors. Radiol Clin Biol (Basel) 35:153, 1966.
24. Foote FW Jr, Frazell EL: Tumors of the major salivary glands. Cancer 6:1065, 1953.
25. Frable WJ, Frable MA: Thin needle aspiration biopsy: The diagnosis of head and neck tumors revisited. Cancer 43:1451, 1979.
26. Fu KK, Leibel SA, Levine ML: Carcinoma of the major and minor salivary glands. Cancer 40:2882, 1977.
27. Gordon AB, Fiddian RV: Frey's syndrome after parotid surgery. Am J Surg, 132:54, 1976.
28. Guillamondegue OM, Byers RM, Luna MA, et al: Aggressive surgery in treatment for parotid cancer: The role of adjunctive postoperative radiotherapy. Am J Roentgenol 123:49, 1975.
29. Hanna DC, Dickason WL, Richardson GS, Gaisford JC: Management of recurrent salivary gland tumors. Am J Surg 132:453, 1976.
30. Hays LL, Novack AJ, Worsham JC: The Frey syndrome: A simple, effective treatment. Otolaryngol Head Neck Surg 90:419, 1982.
31. Hodgkinson DJ, Woods JE: The influence of facial nerve sacrifice in surgery of malignant parotid tumors. J Surg Oncol 8:425, 1976.
32. Hollander L, Cunningham MP: Management of cancer of the parotid gland. Surg Clin North Am 53:113, 1973.
33. Hugo NE, McKinney P, Griffith BH: Management of tumors of the parotid gland. Surg Clin North Am 53:105, 1973.
34. Johns ME, Coulthard SW: Survival and follow-up in malignant tumors of the salivary glands. Otolaryngol Clin North Am 10:455, 1977.
35. Kagan AR, Nussbaum H, Handler S, Shapiro R: Recurrences from malignant parotid salivary gland tumors. Cancer 37:2600, 1976.
36. King J, Fletcher G: Malignant tumors of the major salivary glands. Radiology 100:381, 1971.
37. Lambert JA: Parotid gland tumors. Milit Med 136:484, 1971.
38. Levitt SH, McHugh RB, Gomez-Marin O, et al: Clinical staging system for cancer of the salivary gland: A retrospective study. Cancer 47:2712, 1981. Parotid tumors. Acta Otolaryngol Suppl (Stockh) 191:1, 1963.
39. Lingberg LG, Ackerman M: Aspiration cytology of salivary gland tumors: Diagnostic experience from six years of routine laboratory work. Laryngoscope 86:584, 1976.
40. Marsh WL, Allen MS: Adenoid cystic carcinoma: Biologic behavior in 38 patients. Cancer 43:1463, 1979.
40a. Micheli-Pelligrini VC, Polayes IM: Historical background. In Rankow RM, Polayes IM (eds): Diseases of the Salivary Glands. Philadelphia, W. B. Saunders Co., 1976, pp. 1–16.
41. Mustard RA, Anderson W: Malignant tumors of the parotid. Ann Surg 159:291, 1964.

42. Nigro MF Jr, Spiro RH: Deep lobe parotid tumors. Am J Surg *134*:523, 1977.
43. Perzin KH, Gullane P, Clairmont AC: Adenoid cystic carcinoma arising in salivary glands: A correlation of histologic features and clinical course. Cancer *42*:265, 1978.
44. Rafla S: Malignant parotid tumors natural history and treatment. Cancer *40*:136, 1977.
45. Rafla-Demetrious SR: Mucous and Salivary Gland Tumors. Springfield, Ill, Charles C Thomas, 1970.
46. Rosenfeld L, Sessions DG, McSwain B, Graves H: Malignant tumors of salivary gland origin. Ann Surg *163*:726, 1966.
47. Rossman KJ: The role of radiation therapy in the treatment of parotid carcinomas. Am J Roentgenol *123*:492, 1975.
48. Schuller DE, McCabe BF: Salivary gland neoplasms in children. Otolaryngol Clin North Am *10*:399, 1977.
49. Shidnia H, Hornback NB, Hamaker R, Lingeman R: Carcinoma of major salivary glands. Cancer *45*:693, 1980.
50. Sismanis A, Merriam JM, Kline TS, et al: Diagnosis of salivary gland tumors by fine needle aspiration biopsy. Head Neck Surg *3*:482, 1981.
51. Spiro RH, Hajdn SI, Strong EQ: Tumors of the submaxillary gland. Ann J Surg *132*:463, 1976.
52. Spiro RH, Huvos AG, Birk R, Strong EW: Mucoepidermoid carcinoma of salivary gland origin: A clinicopathologic study of 367 cases. Am J Surg *136*:461, 1978.
53. Spiro RH, Huvos AG, Strong EW: Adenoid cystic carcinoma of the salivary origin: A clinicopathologic study of 242 cases. Am J Surg *128*:512, 1974.
54. Spiro RH, Huvos AG, Strong EQ: Cancer of the parotid gland. Am J Surg *130*:452, 1975.
55. Spiro RH, Huvos AG, Strong EW: Acinic cell carcinoma of salivary origin: A clinicopathologic study of 67 cases. Cancer *41*:924, 1978.
56. Suen JY, Johns ME: Chemotherapy for salivary gland cancer. Laryngoscope *92*:235, 1982.
57. Tapley ND: Irradiation treatment of malignant tumors of the salivary glands. Ear Nose Throat J *56*:110, 1977.
58. Tu G, Hu Y, Jiang P, Qin D: The superiority of combined therapy (surgery and postoperative irradiation) in parotid cancer. Arch Otolaryngol *108*:710, 1982.
59. Velpeau ALM: Nuovi Elementi de Medicina Operatora. Prima versione italiana del Dottore Antonio Rignacca con aggiunte di Guiseppe Spairani. Milano, Truffi e Co., 1933.
60. Woods JE, Chong GC, Beahrs OH: Experience with 1360 primary parotid tumors. Am J Surg *130*:460, 1975.
61. Work WP, Batsakis JG, Bailey DH: Recurrent benign mixed tumor in the facial nerve. Arch Otolaryngol *102*:15, 1976.

CHAPTER 45

Rehabilitation of the Patient with Tumors of the Salivary Glands

Roger L. Crumley, M.D.

Rehabilitation following salivary gland surgery concerns itself with facial nerve reconstruction. The intimate relationship of the parotid gland and facial nerve dictates that facial nerve continuity be sacrificed occasionally for certain neoplastic lesions. This devastating insult to emotional expression is never entirely overcome after the facial nerve is transected.

Although patients are told that facial paralysis will follow such operations, it is difficult to communicate to them the full impact of facial paralysis. Movies or videotapes are probably the most effective means of preparing them, and still photographs may help somewhat. Naturally, cancer ablation takes precedence over saving nerve branches; hence, the patient should not be told preoperatively that a certain branch will be preserved while others will be sacrificed, as intraoperative findings may dictate total nerve resection. These preoperative discussions are a key factor in the patient's understanding and acceptance of surgical treatment, which in many cases is the only form of treatment with curative potential.

Salivary side effects of such surgery must also be reviewed preoperatively. Patients undergoing irradiation will experience a drastic diminution in salivary flow from the remaining glands. In addition, many cancer patients have decreased saliva production due to advanced age. Removal of one parotid or submaxillary gland further decreases saliva production; hence, one of the most common complaints following head and neck cancer treatment is that of dry mouth, and it is best to have discussed this thoroughly in the planning phases of treatment.

Following wide-field parotid and submaxillary resections, a varying degree of cosmetic deformity results. When salivary gland resection is combined with mandibulectomy or temporal bone resection, a further cosmetic defect is incurred. The effects of surgical scarring and radiation make these concave defects difficult to reconstruct. The surgeon must generally encourage the patient to accept them, rather than promote false hope for rehabilitation.

This chapter deals with the paralytic, cosmetic, and functional problems of patients undergoing salivary gland cancer surgery. The major emphasis will be on facial nerve rehabilitation, and Frey's syndrome and other disabilities will also be discussed.

GENERAL CONSIDERATIONS

Motor and Sensory Nerves Other Than the Facial Nerve

Certainly the most devastating aspect of salivary gland tumor surgery is facial nerve sacrifice. However, other nerves are often transected in radical ablations of parotid, submandibular, or other salivary glands. The facial nerve is routinely reconstructed and or grafted following transection; however, other nerve injuries and their effects should be described when transection is inevitable. Such problems include hypoglossal and lingual nerve injury for high-grade cancers of the submandibular gland; the anesthesia of the ear following greater auricular nerve transection; and auriculotemporal nerve paresthesias, hypoesthesia, and anesthesia.

Facial Cosmesis

Submandibular gland removal, or submaxillary triangle exenteration, has negligible impact on facial cosmesis. If the marginal mandibular branch of the facial nerve is transected, lower lip asymmetry will result. This will be discussed further later in this chapter. However, the anatomic defect resulting from submaxillary gland surgery is rarely problematic.

Parotid gland removal, on the other hand, may result in a deep concavity in the preauricular region. Depending on the amount of parotid tissue, periglandular fat, and intraglandular lymph nodes, this resulting hollowed-out defect can be substantial (Fig. 45–1). The cutaneous scar resulting from parotidectomy is seldom a cosmetic problem.

Irradiation

The use of gamma irradiation for salivary gland neoplasms has its own list of sequelae. Dry mouth, skin atrophy, radiation caries, and radiation-induced neoplasia are all considerations. An experienced radiation therapist and a dentist should discuss these problems with the patient in the pretreatment period.

The Facial Nerve

Although the preceding considerations are important, the most crucial aspect of rehabilitation is that of facial

1139

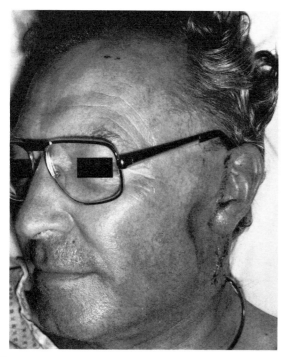

Figure 45–1. Typical superficial parotidectomy defect, 48 hours after surgery. Superior aspect of superficial lobe remains and appears to accentuate the defect.

nerve reconstruction. Many factors determine which form of reanimation should be used, and the surgeon must review each case with these factors in mind (Table 45–1).

Although facial nerve reconstruction is indicated following virtually any procedure that results in facial paralysis, it is known that facial muscle reinnervation may occur spontaneously. This is thought to arise via facial nerve or trigeminal nerve pathways, although the exact source and route of reinnervation are not clear. Interestingly, in the first report of this phenomenon by Hayes Martin, it was noted that a re-excision of the parotid fossa and facial nerve for recurrent tumor did not abolish the reinnervated movement. This confirmed that another pathway (hypothesized by Martin to be via the trigeminal nerve) was responsible.[22] This, of course, is not offered as support of omitting facial nerve reconstruction as part of a parotid resection requiring nerve sacrifice, but it is of historical and physiologic significance.

One must consider first the patient's *needs* in relation

TABLE 45–1. Factors Influencing Type and Timing of Facial Reanimation Procedure

Objective factors
    Nerve and muscle status
    Tumor status
    Radiation
Relative factors
    Age
    Life-style and vocation
    Nutritional and metabolic status

to surgical planning for facial paralysis. *No* surgical procedure can produce normal function on the paralyzed side. Muscle transfers generally result in less normal facial function than do cable grafts and cranial nerves XII and VII crossovers, which result in innervation of the muscles of facial expression.

However, there are situations in which the patient requires immediate rehabilitation of one component of the facial paralysis, as in the case of the sagging oral commissure of a terminally ill patient who is unable to eat without drooling or a paralytic ectropion with exposure keratitis. In such situations it would be inappropriate to perform nerve grafting or transfer alone, because a fascial sling, muscle transfer, or tarsorraphy could rehabilitate the patient immediately.

The "donor" consequences of nerve or muscle transfer should be considered. If the masseter and temporalis are weak on the nonparalyzed side, transfer of these muscles on the side of the facial paralysis might leave the patient incapable of chewing properly. Similarly, contralateral hypoglossal nerve injury or tongue deformity might be grossly exaggerated by a hypoglossal-facial anastomosis on the side of the facial paralysis.

Anatomic factors are perhaps the most important. Nerve grafting or transfer procedures are designed to allow axon regeneration to the facial muscles distally. Hence, a healthy proximal nerve capable of mounting a regenerative effort is a prerequisite to axon growth through a nerve graft.

It is known that the facial nerve contains approximately 7000 motor nerve fibers (axons).[12] Although it is not essential that each and every one of these fibers regenerate to the periphery, it is important that the regenerating nerve be given its best opportunity for regeneration; that is, the nerve selected for grafting should have a relatively large number of endoneurial tubules and should be harvested atraumatically, sutured without tension, unirradiated, and unquestionably free of tumor.

Proximal Nerve

Many parotid cancers are fixed to the pes anserinus. When resecting the proximal facial nerve, it is sometimes tempting to cut the nerve somewhat close to the tumor in order to leave a cuff of proximal nerve to which to suture the nerve graft. This, of course, is oncologically unsound. In these situations, it is preferable to amputate the tip of the mastoid process or more proximal portions of the temporal bone when appropriate. This results in transection of the facial nerve in its more distal portion toward the pes anserinus. Such procedures require an additional 1 to 1½ hours of surgical time, but they result in increased local control and a healthier proximal nerve stump for grafting.

The cell body (soma, perikaryon) and proximal nerve stump determine the regenerative potential in nerve grafting repair and procedures. A history of prior mastoid or middle ear surgery, Bell's palsy, or temporal bone injuries should be elicited because any of these processes may weaken the regenerative potential of the proximal nerve. In any event, should the (parotid) surgeon be unfamiliar with intratemporal facial nerve techniques (mastoidectomy, microneural instruments, nerve rerouting), it would be advisable to employ the services of an otologic consultant, because transection and grafting to the mastoid portion of the nerve may allow one additional plane between the surgical margin and parotid tumor.

Distal Nerve

The nerve graft must be sutured to a distal facial nerve or nerve branches that are in continuity with the motor end plates of their respective facial muscles. At the time of parotid resection, when facial nerve sacrifice is planned, the facial nerve branches should be identified and isolated well distal to the neoplasm. This allows for attachment of branches, or the main distal portion, of the nerve graft.

When nerve grafting is done at some time *after* parotidectomy and nerve sacrifice, the nerve stimulator cannot be used for identification of the distal branches. In these situations the distal branches may be quite difficult to find. As a result the surgeon may be forced to route a nerve graft directly to the most important facial muscles (orbicularis oculi, zygomaticus major and minor, orbicularis oris) *or* to perform masseter or temporalis muscle transfer. Hence, the integrity, viability, identification, and "tagging" of distal nerve branches is most important at time of tumor resection.

Facial Muscles

Unless there has been longstanding facial paralysis, the facial muscles will usually be viable and capable of reinnervation. This is a most important determination, because nerve grafting or transfer is futile when the facial muscles have degenerated or are otherwise absent. This might occur following extended parotidectomy or other facial tumor surgery when important muscles (such as zygomaticus major and minor, and levator labii superioris) have been resected. In longstanding facial paralysis (as in a patient who had parotidectomy, facial nerve sacrifice, and no facial nerve rehabilitation procedure) following periods of 2 or more years, the facial muscles will undergo denervation atrophy. Facial nerve grafting would yield no facial movement in these cases.

The viability of the facial muscles can be determined by electromyography (EMG). The surgeon should be present and should actively assist the electromyographer at the time of EMG. The muscles needing reinnervation should be evaluated selectively so that the capability for reinnervation is known prior to nerve grafting or transfer. If fibrillation ("denervation") potentials are seen in the target muscles, a nerve transfer or facial nerve cable graft can be expected to reinnervate the muscle. If voluntary potentials are seen when the patient tries to contract the muscle, there is facial nerve continuity with the muscle. In some instances this may be "subclinical"; that is, there is no detectable muscle movement. These muscles are also capable of being reinnervated, provided that the "subclinical innervation" (existing facial nerve) is transected. If a thorough search of the facial muscle region is completed with the EMG electrode and no potentials are found, this "electrical silence" may mean denervation atrophy has occurred. (In these situations muscle transfer or static suspension would be preferred to nerve grafting or neural transfer.[9])

Status of Hypoglossal Nerve

In the event that the proximal facial nerve is absent or of questionable viability, the hypoglossal nerve is the next most appropriate neural source for facial reanimation. The above-mentioned considerations (status of facial muscles, integrity of distal facial nerve) also apply in planning hypoglossal-facial anastomosis. The hypoglossal nerve must be intact and capable of regenerating nerve fibers through a nerve anastomosis. An operative note may explain whether the hypoglossal nerve was transected during prior surgery.

Physical examination for tongue protrusion can assess the viability of the twelfth cranial nerve. The examiner should also place the index finger against the ipsilateral hemitongue and ask the patient to protrude the tongue forcefully. Comparison of the two sides will allow detection of hypoglossal nerve weakness when protrusion is symmetric. Patients with hypoglossal paresis or paralysis should not undergo hypoglossal-facial anastomosis.

Trigeminal Nerve Integrity

Whenever masseter or temporalis muscle transfer is contemplated, the trigeminal nerve motor branches to these muscles must be evaluated. Again, prior operative notes may describe sacrifice of portions of the masseter muscle or nerve during radical parotid surgery. This, of course, would preclude masseter transfer for facial reanimation. Other neurologic lesions, such as petrous apicitis, epidural abscess, or congenital cholesteatoma, which may cause facial nerve weakness, may produce trigeminal nerve deficits as well. Masseter and temporalis muscle function may be tested by palpation of each muscle during forceful closure of the jaws. The masseter is palpated immediately above the mandibular angle, and the temporalis is palpated in its midportion, 1½ in. above the middle third of the zygomatic arch.

Length of Time Since Nerve Transection

Long-standing, complete paralysis produces several obstacles to facial reanimation. The most important of these factors is *atrophy* of the facial muscles. Denervation atrophy, which may occur after 18 months of complete denervation, is sometimes difficult to determine.[15] Electromyography is currently the most accurate method for determining the status of the muscles.

A complete description of the technique of electromyography is beyond the scope of this chapter. However, Table 45–2 summarizes the common electromyographic potentials and their meaning for the patient with facial paralysis. *Voluntary action potentials* recorded during attempted facial movements mean that motor axons of the facial nerve are "in continuity" from brain stem to motor end plates. There may or may not be visible facial movement with this finding. Reanimation surgery that requires facial nerve transection (such as hypoglossal-facial anastomosis) should not be attempted in this setting unless there has been no improvement in facial movement in over 18 months. If voluntary potentials are present after this time period, and there is no apparent facial movement, *"subclinical" innervation* is present. This means that the facial nerve innervates

TABLE 45–2. Electromyography (EMG) Correlations

EMG Potential	Meaning	Surgical Implications
Voluntary	Facial nerve continuity	Do not attempt reanimation*
"Nascent" or polyphasic	Muscle reinnervation	Facial reanimation surgery contraindicated until end result apparent
Fibrillation	Muscle denervation	Facial muscles viable, but denervated; optimal for "cable graft" or graft of cranial nerves XII and VII
Electrical silence	Absent muscles	Muscle transfer indicated

*In some instances, *subclinical* innervation may warrant nerve transection and reinnervation surgery.

certain facial muscles, but without sufficient axon population to trigger visible or meaningful movement. In this situation, nerve transection and reinnervation surgery may be warranted.[9]

Both *"nascent"* and *polyphasic* potentials may be seen during the active phases of reinnervation. They mean that neural regeneration is occurring within the facial nerve. Facial reanimation surgery is contraindicated until the end result is apparent. These potentials may become normal voluntary potentials, or so-called giant motor potentials.

Fibrillation or denervation potentials mean that the EMG electrode tip is located in denervated muscle. This means that the facial muscle in question is viable but has no nerve supply. This is an optimal situation for cable grafting, if the proximal facial nerve is present and otherwise normal, or for cranial nerves XII and VII anastomosis if it is not.

Electrical silence is the absence of all electrical EMG potentials. If it is a persistent finding on repeated EMG examinations, it usually means that the muscles of facial expression have undergone denervation atrophy. Obviously, nerve grafting or transfer would be futile in this instance. Muscle transfers are indicated.

Neural Scarring

Prior reports have indicated that endoneural scarring may occur following long time lapses. Whether this represents an obstacle to reinnervation is not known at this time. It is known, however, that the neuron's ability to regenerate declines with time. This may be a consequence of peripheral scarring or diminishing regenerative vitality of the cell body in the brain stem. Hence, it is always preferable to perform facial reanimation surgery as soon as possible following the onset of paralysis, provided that the surgical procedure does not interfere with ongoing regeneration in the facial nerve.

Age

It is well known that young, vigorous subjects repair injured organ systems more rapidly than do their older counterparts. This is also true with regard to nerves.[10] Accordingly, a 75-year-old patient will not have as complete, nor as active, facial reanimation as would a 20-year-old individual. This factor should be considered when dealing with facial paralysis in the older patient. Hypoglossal facial anastomosis will require 8 to 12 months before satisfactory facial tone is seen, and the clinical situation (needs of the patient) may mandate masseter or temporalis muscle transfer for immediate rehabilitation, particularly in the elderly.

Radiation Therapy

Several studies have offered conflicting data regarding the effects of radiotherapy on nerve regeneration. Although these studies were concerned with facial nerve grafts, their data can be extrapolated to hypoglossal-facial anastomosis as well. McGuirt and McCabe showed that irradiation did not preclude facial nerve reinnervation following grafting.[24] Pillsbury and Fisch demonstrated that irradiation produced a delay and a decreased reinnervation but confirmed that grafting could successfully reinnervate facial muscles in such patients.[29] Miehlke's work concurred.[26]

Radiation may affect the neovascularization of the nerve graft as well as the proximal and distal segment of the facial nerve. However, the most important impact of irradiation on nerve regeneration is the dose received by the cell body in the brain stem. Fortunately, most patients with salivary gland tumors do not receive high midline doses, and hence, the facial nerve nucleus is usually spared.

Diabetes

Whether it be due to impaired metabolism at the cellular level, or on the basis of microangiopathy, diabetics are relatively poor regenerators of injured nerves. This factor would not, taken alone, preclude nerve grafting or transfer, but in combination with radiation, advancing age, or similar factors, it might warrant consideration of muscle transfer or facial suspension rather than a nerve anastomotic procedure.

SURGICAL CONSIDERATIONS

Generally, the sacrifice of facial nerve branches is determined intraoperatively by location, degree of malignancy, and nature of the neoplastic process. The particular type of rehabilitation procedure can, and should, be planned preoperatively whenever possible.

When the entire facial nerve trunk or pes anserinus must be resected, a nerve cable graft should be performed. The patient should be advised of the necessity of an incision on the opposite side for harvesting of a greater auricular nerve graft or of a lower leg incision for a sural nerve graft.

When smaller neoplasms are located anteriorly, superiorly, or inferiorly in the parotid, the possibility of selective branch resection and reconstruction occurs. These opportunities are not common, but they should be anticipated, as they present the best chances for nearly normal function following nerve resection. Certainly, branch resection alone should not be done if the surgeon feels the entire nerve trunk should be resected, but whenever possible, it provides excellent facial movement with a minimum of synkinesis.

Other authors, notably Fisch,[13] have described branch-to-branch transposition (cervical to marginal mandibular, or buccal branch) for lesions requiring single-branch resection, but this requires that the uninvolved branch can be transposed, will reach the distal end of the transected branch, and is "less important" (minimal donor deficit) in terms of overall facial function. This author has not had satisfactory results in the few cases in which this has been possible, and hence, the technique cannot be strongly endorsed.

Radical Parotidectomy with Facial Nerve Sacrifice (Acute)

It is standard practice to employ "cable" nerve grafting when parotid tumors require facial nerve resection. This should generally be performed at the time of tumor ablation. The two most commonly used donor nerves are the greater auricular and the sural nerve(s).

The *ipsilateral* greater auricular nerve should not be used because it may be involved with tumor. The opposite neck should be prepared and draped for harvesting the contralateral greater auricular nerve. The surgical landmarks are well defined: a line is drawn from the mastoid tip to the angle of the mandible. This line is then bisected by a perpendicular line that crosses the sternocleidomastoid muscle from inferoposterior to anterosuperior and courses toward the parotid gland. The greater auricular nerve is directly beneath this latter line. By dissecting the nerve superiorly, a multibranch graft can be harvested for grafting from the facial nerve trunk to its peripheral branches.

We prefer the sural nerve because of its greater neural connective tissue ratio and large diameter.[37] It is also ideal when long grafts are needed, as up to 35 cm of nerve can be obtained.

Proximally, the sural nerve is formed by the junction of the medial sural cutaneous nerve and the peroneal nerve between the two heads of the gastrocnemius muscle. The nerve lies immediately deep to and behind the lesser saphenous vein. A pneumatic tourniquet is applied to the thigh, and a transverse incision is then made immediately behind the lateral malleolus. Multiple "stair-step" horizontal incisions can be used, or a vertical incision coursing over the length of the nerve allows for excellent exposure. The surgeon should avoid tugging on the sural nerve while harvesting.

Many techniques have been described for anastomosis of nerves (acrylic glue, perineural suture, tissue glue), but epineurial repair with 9–0 or 10–0 monfilament nylon suture on a 75-micron cutting needle is generally preferred. The needle must pass through epineurium only. This technique appears to induce less neural injury than those using larger suture or using other suture techniques. The proximal end of the facial nerve should be transected cleanly, using a sterile razor blade, and the proximal end of the nerve graft is managed similarly. Four epineurial sutures are usually necessary to seal the epineurium around the anastomosis and prevent axonal escape. The nerve graft and its branches must be long enough to allow 1 cm of excess length at each anastomosis. Suture at the distal end of the nerve graft is performed similarly, except that when peripheral branches are involved, only two or three epineurial

sutures are necessary, owing to the much smaller diameter. Suction drains must be kept away from the neural anastomosis sites and the nerve graft for obvious reasons. Pressure dressings are to be avoided.

The patient should be advised that return of function can be expected in 6 to 9 months. Axon penetration of the nerve graft begins in the first month, and subsequently, the axon sprouts advance approximately 1 mm per day until the motor end-plate region of the muscle is reached. Neuromuscular activity is not seen for another 6 to 12 weeks, during which time the nucleus converts its enzymatic production to acetylcholinesterase and other neural excitatory metabolites.[10]

When the proximal stump at the stylomastoid foramen is of inadequate length, suturing the proximal anastomosis should be done in the mastoid. This, of course, requires mastoidectomy and preparation of the nerve at that site. When dealing with adenoid cystic carcinoma, the proximal stump should be biopsied and submitted for frozen section so that the proximal nerve resection is known not to contain tumor. A surgical "no man's land" exists from 1 cm above to 1 cm below the stylomastoid foramen. Here the nerve is tightly bound by epineurium and periosteum and is extremely difficult to dissect free for anastomosis. Accordingly, it is best to identify the nerve with the operating microscope in the *midmastoid* portion. The extra length required by this procedure may necessitate use of the longer sural nerve, rather than the greater auricular nerve, as a cable graft.

Cable Grafting (Delayed)

When more than 3 days have elapsed following nerve transection, the technique of cable grafting differs from the preceding procedure because the distal nerve segment(s) may not be easily found. (The nerve stimulator cannot be used to find the distal branches after 72 hours have elapsed.) Accordingly, the surgeon wishing to cable graft in such delayed cases must have a preconceived "map" to find these distal branches. In these situations, the prior operative report describing facial nerve anatomy is essential. The anatomy from the operative report must then be correlated with a topographic facial nerve "map." The map used by the author is shown in Figure 45–2. The pes anserinus of the facial nerve is deep (approximately 2 cm) to a point 1 cm anterior and 2 cm inferior to the tragus. The superior division of the facial nerve follows a slightly curvilinear course, convex posterosuperiorly from that point to the lateral end of the eyebrow, its zygomatic branch passing to the orbicularis oculi, slightly lateral to the lateral canthus.

The buccal branch, or its most significant contribution, passes from the pes anserinus anteriorly, paralleling, and 1 cm below, the inferior border of the zygomatic arch.

The inferior division (marginal mandibular and cervical branch) passes between the pes anserinus' point and a 2 cm circle, the center of which is over the angle of the mandible. This division then courses anteriorly, remaining 1 to 2 cm below the inferior border of the mandible until it reaches the facial artery, where it passes superiorly over the inferior border to innervate the depressor labii inferioris and depressor anguli oris (Fig. 45–2).

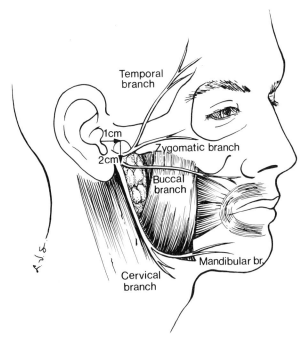

Figure 45–2. Topographic map of facial nerve and branches. Pes anserinus is 1 cm anterior and 2 cm inferior to tragus. Superior division curves toward lateral aspect of eyebrow, with convexity above. Buccal branch parallels inferior border of zygomatic arch, and 1 cm below it. Inferior division passes toward mandibular angle.

Utilization of this map will generally allow the surgeon to find at least the buccal and marginal mandibular branches, and hence will allow cable grafting despite the electrical nonexcitability of the distal facial nerve (Fig. 45–3).

The proximal site for cable grafting may be any portion from the brain stem distally, depending on the site and nature of the facial nerve injury. When oncologic factors dictate partial or complete temporal bone resection, it is possible to graft from the mastoid, tympanic, labyrinthine, or cerebellopontine portions of the facial nerve. One can route the nerve graft anteriorly from the internal auditory canal directly to the face via a bone window near the posterior root of the zygomatic arch, or from the posterior fossa, a long sural graft can be routed to the face through a small dural window near the sigmoid sinus.

Conley and Baker have described excellent results with over 170 cases treated with these techniques.[4, 6] Millesi has described fascicular or interfascicular nerve repair, indicating that individual fascicles or fascicle groups might be selectively repaired, thereby eliminating synkinesis or mass movement.[27] Such fascicular repairs, a distinct technologic advance in other motor nerves, appear to have limited utilization for the facial nerve, however. This is because the intraneural topography of the facial nerve remains in question.

This author, May, and Miehlke have reported that discrete, spatially oriented nerve fascicles are present in the area near the stylomastoid foramen; others, notably Sunderland and Thomander, report data showing that the various portions of the face are represented *randomly* in the proximal facial nerve.[7, 23, 25, 38, 39] In addition, the

varying fascicular patterns in the parotid portion versus the mastoid and tympanic portions (which often contain monofascicular nerve) make fascicular matching difficult.[8]

Cross-Face Nerve Graft (Faciofacial Anastomosis)

The cross-face nerve graft procedure, introduced by Scaramella in 1970, offered great hope for patients with facial paralysis in the 1970s. Other authors have added their modifications and reported varying results. This technique is ingenious in design, by "borrowing" appropriate facial nerve fibers from the normal side and routing them to the paralyzed side of the face.

As reviewed by Baker and Conley, the technique must be classified at this time as of marginal value.[5, 6] Samii reported only one of 10 cases with "good" facial movement; Anderl described 15 cases in which five had "good" symmetry, and five had "fair" symmetry with some degree of movement.[32] The technique appears to suffer from a lack of sufficient axonal population and neural excitatory "fire-power." It should *not* be performed by occasional facial nerve surgeons, as other techniques offer a better chance for facial reanimation.

Nerve Transposition

Ordinarily the surgical removal of malignant parotid tumors results in a proximal stump of facial nerve in the parotid or temporal bone. Because cable nerve grafting is preferred to nerve substitution or transposition, such procedures should be reserved for unique cases in which cable grafting is not appropriate.

However, for certain patients in whom temporal bone surgery (for preparation of a proximal nerve stump) is not feasible, transposition should be considered. Other than the cross-face nerve transposition procedure, the hypoglossal, spinal accessory, and phrenic nerves have all been utilized for anastomosis to the facial nerve trunk. Each of these nerves has the capability of bringing new axons to the distal facial nerve for reactivation of the facial musculature.

The hypoglossal-facial anastomosis appears to be the most successful of these procedures. Hypoglossal nerve transection results in far less disability than sacrifice of either the spinal accessory or the phrenic nerve. In addition, the hypoglossal is an excellent size match for the facial. Stennart described the physiologic similarities between the facial nerve and the hypoglossal nerve.[36] Similarly, each nerve has an afferent reflex relationship with the trigeminal nerve. Owing to these and other similarities, the hypoglossal nerve is as ideal a substitutional neural source as is available.

For purposes of salivary and temporal bone tumors, hypoglossal-facial nerve anastomosis would most commonly be used for failed attempts at cable grafting. One should rule out tumor recurrence as a cause of failure prior to embarking upon hypoglossal-facial anastomosis. In Conley's series, 122 cases (95 per cent of the patients) regained satisfactory tone in repose, with some mass facial movement.[3] Fifteen per cent of his cases developed hypertonia and excessive mass movement in the middle part of the face. However, none of the patients upon questioning stated that they would prefer paralysis to the excessive movement. Excessive move-

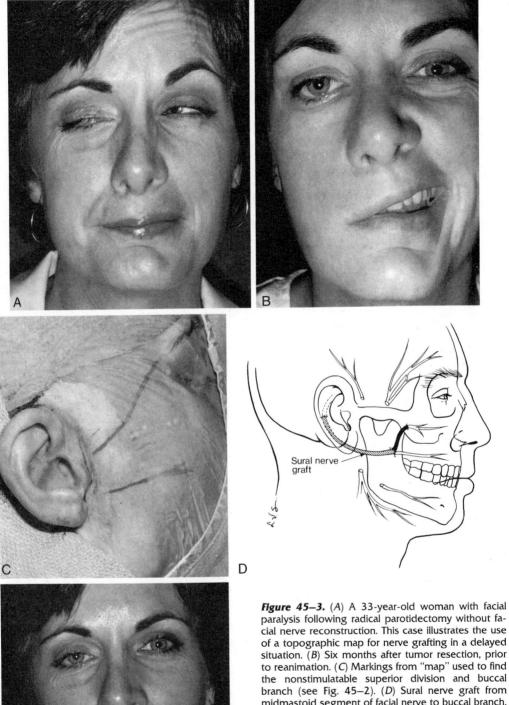

Figure 45–3. (*A*) A 33-year-old woman with facial paralysis following radical parotidectomy without facial nerve reconstruction. This case illustrates the use of a topographic map for nerve grafting in a delayed situation. (*B*) Six months after tumor resection, prior to reanimation. (*C*) Markings from "map" used to find the nonstimulatable superior division and buccal branch (see Fig. 45–2). (*D*) Sural nerve graft from midmastoid segment of facial nerve to buccal branch. Note "jump graft" from sural-buccal anastomotic site to zygomatic branch. No attempt was made to reanimate temporal or marginal mandibular branches. (*E*) Eight months after reanimation. Note mimetic movement in buccal branch distribution and tone in orbicularis oculi. Hair styling camouflages paralyzed frontals.

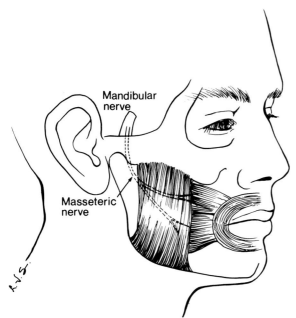

Figure 45–4. Masseter anatomy pertinent to transfer procedures. If muscle is split longitudinally, nerve supply will be divided.

ment was found to decrease gradually over 10 to 20 years. Conley's data implied that minimal intraoral crippling resulted from ipsilateral hypoglossal nerve sacrifice. Seventy-eight per cent of the patients had moderate or severe tongue atrophy, and 22 per cent showed minimal atrophy. This large series and several smaller ones confirm that hypoglossal-facial anastomosis is a mainstay in the armamentarium for treating facial paralysis.

Muscle Transfer

Like hypoglossal-facial anastomosis, muscle transfers are infrequently necessary in patients with parotid or ear malignancies because cable grafting is the preferred technique. However, when the proximal facial nerve is not available, and particularly when the hypoglossal nerve has been sacrificed, no neural source may be available for reinnervation of the paralyzed facial muscles. In addition, patients who have gone 2 or more years following facial nerve transection may have no facial muscles available for reinnervation. In such situations, consideration must be given to transfer of the masseter, temporalis, or other muscles into the face for reanimation.

Baker and Conley have reviewed muscle transposition for relief of facial paralysis.[1, 2] Lexer is generally given credit for the first muscle transposition (masseter) in 1908.[21] Subsequently, many authors have modified muscle transposition techniques.

Masseter muscle transposition is generally performed for the elevation and rehabilitation of the paralyzed oral commissure and buccal branch muscles. It can be accomplished externally via a parotidectomy incision, or intraorally using a mucosal incision immediately lateral to the ascending ramus of the mandible. Avoidance of the masseteric nerve supply is achieved by staying deep to the muscle belly and transposing the entire antero-posterior diameter of the muscle (Figs. 45–4, 45–5, and 45–6).

The external incisions are made just medial to the nasolabial fold, at the lateral oral commissure, and at the vermilion-cutaneous junction of the lower lip. These incisions are then connected to the tunnel in the cheek to allow transfer of the masseter muscle (Fig. 45–5).

The distal muscle is sutured to the dermis or (as proposed by May[23]) to the mucocutaneous line behind the orbicularis muscle. Gross overcorrection is essential to obtain satisfactory long-term results.

Combining the masseter transfer with facial nerve grafting allows for creative possibilities culminating in segmental facial reanimation. This has been discussed and refined in recent communications.[31, 36] Additional combinations include use of the masseter muscle for the oral commissure and transposition of the temporalis

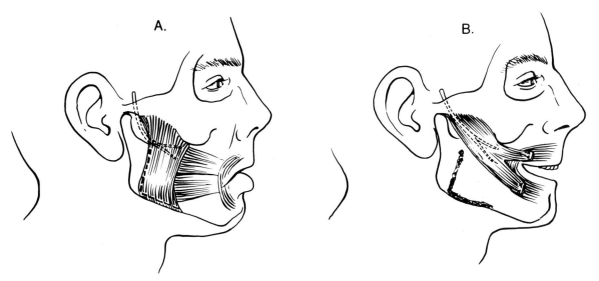

Figure 45–5. Masseter transposition. All, or nearly all, of the muscle is transferred. Interrupted sutures of 4–0 clear nylon attach the muscle to the lower and upper halves of the orbicularis oris muscle. Overcorrection is essential.

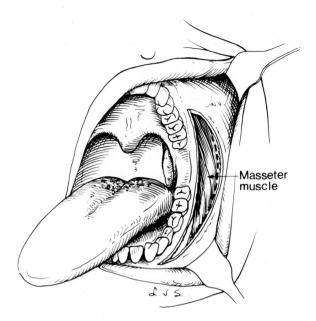

Figure 45–6. Intraoral approach to masseter transfer procedure. Blunt dissection lateral to the muscle allows transfer of entire muscle. Tunneling of the muscle through the soft tissues of the cheek is similar to that used in the external approach.

muscle for the orbicularis oculi and periorbital region (see following discussion).

Temporalis Muscle Transposition

Sir Harold Gillies is frequently given credit for introducing the temporalis transposition for facial paralysis.[14] However, in the United States much credit must be given Rubin for refining the goals of the operation and the surgical technique.[30]

The deep origin of the temporalis muscle is from the periosteum of the entire temporal fossa. The muscle belly passes deep to the zygomatic arch and inserts on the entire coronoid process and a portion of the ascending ramus of the mandible. The muscle is exposed through an incision that passes above the ear and then courses somewhat anteriorly to expose the entire upper portion of the muscle (Fig. 45–7). Rubin's technique consists of dissecting the muscle free from the periosteum, and then attaching muscle or fascial strips to the temporalis muscle as it is turned downward over the zygomatic arch. The fascial strips are necessary, as the muscle's length is not sufficient to reach the lateral oral commissure. Conley and Baker report a modification of the technique in which the epicranium deep to the muscle is turned inferiorly and used for suture to the oral commissure, rather than attaching muscle or fascial

Figure 45–7. Temporalis transfer. The entire muscle is transferred after vertical splitting (B) divides the muscle into two eyelid and two oral commissure strips. Tunnel superficial to zygomatic arch must be at least 1½ in. wide to minimize bulging. Fascial strips are sutured to muscle (D) to achieve adequate length.

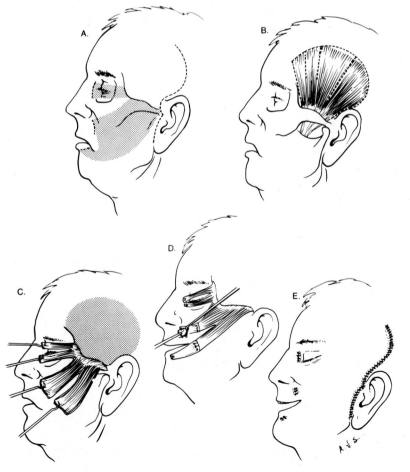

strips.[6] A tunnel at least 1½ in. wide over the zygomatic arch is necessary to allow the muscle to turn inferiorly and not produce an unsightly bulge. The muscle is attached to the dermis just medial to the nasolabial fold so that this natural crease is reproduced by the muscle pull. As with the masseteric operation described previously, a marked overcorrection is necessary on the operating table to allow satisfactory results several months later.

Two objections to the temporalis operation have been voiced: (1) The bulge of temporalis muscle over the zygomatic arch is quite conspicuous. The tunnel used for this procedure will allow the muscle to be "spread out" over the arch. This renders the bulge less unsightly. (2) The concave defect in the temporal fossa is sometimes conspicuous. Rubin suggests a soft silicone block to fill in this depression.[30]

Closure of the eye can also be accomplished with the temporalis procedure. Muscle strips, fascial strips, or epicranium are reinforced to the upper end of the muscle as it is turned forward. These strips are then passed through the upper and lower eyelid and sutured at the medial canthus.

With both masseter and temporalis transfer, the impulse for the facial movement originates from the trigeminal nerve, which is activated by chewing or biting. Some patients may learn how to incorporate these induced movements to imitate an emotional reaction. Generally, however, patients should be told that these procedures will not allow any emotional reanimation but rather to expect, at best, symmetry and tone at rest with some induced and learned movement activated by closing the jaw.

Other Techniques

The Neural Muscular Pedicle

Tucker has devised an ingenious operative procedure consisting of transfer of branches of the ansa hypoglossi nerve and small muscle blocks at the end of the transposed branches.[41] This procedure, initially described for reinnervation of the paralyzed vocal cords, has now been adapted for use in selected patients with facial paralysis.

The basic concept of the procedure is to transfer innervated motor end plates to the denervated facial muscles without a delay period, which is seen with free nerve grafts and nerve transfers.

This operation, first reported for facial paralysis in 1976, has not achieved universal acceptance owing to its limited applicability (it is used only for the perioral muscles, depressor anguli oris, and the zygomaticus muscle).[41] In addition, other investigators have serious doubts whether the procedure achieves a functioning transfer of new innervation.

Free Muscle Grafts

Hakelius and Thompson have independently reported use of free autogenous muscle grafts in the treatment of facial paralysis.[16, 40] Thompson's technique consists of transfer of the palmaris longus muscle, the tendon of which is attached to the zygomatic arch on the paralyzed side. The muscle belly is then sutured to the oral commissure and orbicularis oris muscle. Reinnervation of this graft occurs from the orbicularis oris muscle fibers on the nonparalyzed side. For eye closure, muscle grafts of the extensor digitorum brevis are approximated to the orbicularis oculi muscle of the normal side, and tendons are passed in a tunnel behind the nasal bones. These tendons are then attached to the lateral canthal ligament on the paralyzed side and are said to induce eye closure, which is triggered by the normal side.

Harii has described free muscle grafts of gracilis, latissimus dorsi, or extensor digitorum brevis muscles transferred with the microvascular anastomosis. He has shown electromyographic evidence of reinnervation with the technique.[17] Hakelius has described 107 free muscle transplants in 89 patients, reporting that 88 per cent of patients were improved.[16]

This procedure has achieved neither unanimous support nor everyday usage in the United States. Perhaps these authors, and others in future years, will demonstrate a useful role for this technique in facial paralysis treatment.

Z-Plasty

When immediate rehabilitation of the oral sphincter is necessitated by troublesome drooling, the nasolabial Z-plasty described by Pickrell and associates should be considered.[28] This technique utilizes transfer of the entire lateral oral commissure upward by transposing a triangular nasolabial flap in classic Z-plasty fashion. It should be recognized that this does not produce a dynamic or reanimated perioral region and should not be performed in preference to nerve or muscle transfers. It does, however, achieve an immediate improvement in appearance and function, and it may be helpful in certain clinical situations in which prompt rehabilitation is mandatory.

PROTECTION OF THE EYE

Many of the preceding techniques are effective *long-term* treatments for paralysis of the orbicularis oculi muscle. However, the surgeon should be thinking specifically of eye protection whenever the facial nerve must be sacrificed. The consequences of exposure keratitis may range from short-term extreme discomfort to long-term visual loss. During the immediate postoperative period, the paralyzed eyelids should be taped during sleep. Frequent instillation(s) of wetting solutions such as LacriLube, physiologic saline, or other occlusive techniques (Saran Wrap) must be used to prevent drying. Frequently, a temporary tarsorrhaphy or lid adhesion is helpful during the postoperative period while one awaits the return of facial nerve function via a nerve graft or transposed nerve. It is outside the scope of this chapter to attempt to describe all treatments of paralysis of the orbicularis oculi muscle; however, many treatments have been proposed.

In addition to the preceding techniques, the following may be useful: scleral shells, soft contact lenses, Silastic tubing encirclement, palpebral wire springs, upper lid weights, and small surgical magnets.[20]

FREY'S SYNDROME (GUSTATORY SWEATING)

Sweating of the ipsilateral face following parotidectomy has been known since 1757.[11] It is extremely common following operations on the parotid gland. Generally the symptoms are not troublesome enough to warrant treatment. The syndrome consists of flushing and cutaneous discomfort, as well as sweating, in the distribution of the auriculotemporal nerve.

Pathophysiology of the syndrome is the misdirected regeneration of parasympathetic and sympathetic fibers (both cholinergic) to the cholinergic receptors of the skin's sweat glands. In afflicted patients, noticeable sweat flow may be seen during chewing, deglutition, or even when thinking of food. Chewing of bland substances such as paraffin does not produce the phenomenon.

Treatment is directed toward blocking the abnormal neural pathway. The parasympathetic fibers leave the brain via the glossopharyngeal nerve and enter the middle ear as Jacobson's nerve. Here they may be sectioned via tympanic neurectomy. They exit the middle ear as the lesser petrosal nerve. Here they could be severed via a middle cranial fossa approach. They then enter the infratemporal fossa via the "unnamed canal of Vesalius." The pathway is not then easily approachable until the auriculotemporal nerve sends the aberrant branches toward the skin.

Suggested treatments have included the following:

1. Topical application of scopolamine hydrobromide cream (3 per cent). (This may cause atropinic symptoms such as blurred vision or dry mouth.[19])

2. Division or avulsion of the auriculotemporal nerve.

3. Intracranial sectioning of the glossopharyngeal nerve.

4. Alcohol injection of the ganglion.

5. Excision of the affected skin with grafting of the defect.

6. Systemic atropine.

7. Tympanic neurectomy.

Unfortunately, all of these methods have been associated with a high recurrence rate.

Hemenway stated that 90.9 per cent of cases treated by tympanic neurectomy had a "satisfactory postoperative result."[18] He considered Jacobson's neurectomy the procedure of choice for symptomatic gustatory sweating.

Because these and prior authors had occasionally found chorda tympani neurectomy to be necessary in addition to tympanic neurectomy, Sessions and associates sought a more direct method of denervating the offending sweat glands.[34, 35] They described attachment of fascia lata under the abnormally sweating skin as being successful in four cases. They noted that careful mapping of the involved skin with starch-iodine was mandatory. After tattooing the boundaries of this area with a needle dipped in methylene blue, the periparotid skin is elevated. A large piece of fascia lata is then fashioned to the approximate size and shape, and sutured to the subcutaneous scar bed from the prior surgery. This procedure produced excellent results in four patients.[34] An additional advantage of this technique is the partial reconstruction of the parotidectomy concavity.

In patients with moderate symptoms and an aversion

to surgery, "heavy duty" antiperspirants have decreased sweat flow in several cases.[33]

REHABILITATION OF PAROTIDECTOMY DEFECTS

Most patients are willing to accept a cutaneous concavity in the parotid fossa as a sequela of parotidectomy and other tumor ablations of this region (Fig. 45–8). However, in certain individuals the defect is less acceptable, and the highly motivated patient may request surgical rehabilitation.

Several variables account for the wide range in severity of these defects. These will be mentioned briefly, in order that the possibilities for reconstruction can be put in the proper perspective.

Superficial lobectomy alone leaves a definite concavity (see Fig. 45–1) but as it is usually performed for benign disease, most commonly it is not followed with radiation therapy. As a result, the surrounding skin and hair are normal and are more easily able to disguise the existing defect.

Radiation therapy is a major obstacle to tissue transfer for postparotidectomy defects. Decreased vascularity due to radiation vasculitis and scarring preclude the use of free grafts such as fat or muscle in these situations.

As mentioned earlier, patient motivation is one of the most important aspects of planning for reconstruction. The patient who is willing to undergo two or more operations to achieve improved facial and cheek symmetry is a good candidate as far as motivation is concerned.

Availability of arteries and veins for microvascular anastomosis is an important variable in selected cases. Prior operative notes, prior radiation therapy and phys-

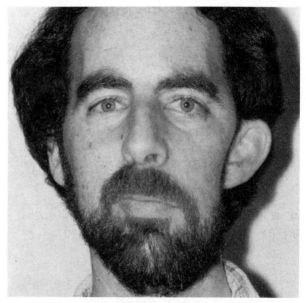

Figure 45–8. Typical deformity after radical parotidectomy, partial mandibulectomy, facial nerve resection and reconstruction, and partial temporal bone resection. Reconstruction of the concave defect is difficult owing to the heavy irradiation, which precludes use of free grafts.

ical findings are helpful in evaluating the patient for this mode of reconstruction.

As indicated, the highly motivated patient with a superficial parotidectomy defect, a benign tumor, no irradiation, and (if a free flap technique is contemplated) a palpable superficial temporal pulse represents the ideal candidate for reconstruction of the fossa defect. Prior authors have proposed free fat or muscle grafts. Walter proposed a free dermal-fat graft at the time of initial parotidectomy for reconstruction of the concavity and reported that the technique also eliminated Frey's syndrome.[42]

Baker and associates described six cases in which radical parotidectomy defects were successfully rehabilitated with free groin flaps transferred via microvascular anastomosis. One of these anastomoses was to the distal (superior) stump of the superficial temporal artery,[2] indicating that the technique can be used despite prior ligation of the superficial temporal artery.

REFERENCES

1. Baker DC, Conley J: Regional muscle transposition for rehabilitation of the paralyzed face. Clin Plast Surg 6:317, July 1979.
2. Baker D, Shaw W, Conley J: Reconstruction of radical parotidectomy defects. Am J Surg 138:550, 1979.
3. Conley J: Hypoglossal crossover—122 cases. Trans Am Acad Ophthalmol Otolaryngol 84:763, 1977.
4. Conley J: Facial rehabilitation: New potentials. Clin Plast Surg 6:421, July 1979.
5. Conley J: Myths and misconceptions in the rehabilitation of facial paralysis. Plast Reconstruct Surg 71:538, 1983.
6. Conley J, Baker DC: The surgical treatment of extratemporal facial paralysis. Head Neck Surg 1:12, 1978.
7. Crumley R: Spatial anatomy of facial nerve fibers: A preliminary report. Laryngoscope 90:274, 1980.
8. Crumley RL: Interfascicular nerve repair. Arch Otolaryngol 160:313, 1980.
9. Crumley R: Pathophysiology of facial nerve injury. In Gibbs A, Smith M (eds): Otolaryngology I. London, Butterworth Scientific, 1982.
10. Ducker T, Kauffman F: Clinical Neurosurgery, Vol. 24. The Congress of Neurological Surgeons. Baltimore, The Williams and Wilkins Company, 1977, pp 406–408.
11. Duphenix (1757) cited in Spiro R, Martin H: Gustatory sweating following parotid surgery and radical neck dissection. Ann Surg 165:118, 1967.
12. Esslen E: The Acute Facial Palsies. Heidelberg, Springer-Verlag, 1977, pp 7–8.
13. Fisch U: Facial nerve grafting. Otolaryngol Clin North Am 7:517, 1974.
14. Gilles HD: Facial paralysis. Proc R Soc Med 27:1372, 1934.
15. Gutman E, Young J: The reinnervation of muscle after various periods of atrophy. J Anat 78:15, 1944.
16. Hakelius L: Free muscle grafting. Clin Plast Surg 6:301, 19 .
17. Harii K: Microneurovascular free muscle transplantation for reanimation of facial paralysis. Clin Plast Surg 6:361, 1979.
18. Hemenway WG: Gustatory sweating and flushing. Laryngoscope 70:84, 1960.
19. Laage-Hillman JE: Treatment of gustatory sweating and flushing. Acta Otolaryngol (Stockholm) 49:132, 1953.
20. Levine H: Management of the eye in facial paralysis. Otolaryngol Clin North Am 7:531, 1974.
21. Lexer E, Eden R: Uber die chirurgische Behandlung der peripheren Facialislahmung. Beitr Klin Chir 73:116, 1911.
22. Martin H: Spontaneous return of function following excision of the seventh nerve. Ann Surg 146:715, 1957.
23. May M: Anatomy of the facial nerve. Laryngoscope 83:1311, 1973.
24. McGuirt WF, McCabe BF: Effect of radiation therapy on facial nerve cable autografts. Laryngoscope 87:415, 1977.
25. Miehlke A: Topography of the course of fibers in the facialis stem. Arch Klin Exp Ohren Nasen Kehlkopfkunde (Berlin) 56:171, 1958.
26. Miehlke A: Factors influencing results in extratemporal facial nerve repair. In Fisch U (ed): Facial Nerve Surgery. Birmingham, Aesculapius Publishing Co., 1977, pp 216–226.
27. Millesi H: Nerve suture and grafting to restore the extratemporal facial nerve. Clin Plast Surg 6:333, 1979.
28. Pickrell K, Puckett C, Peters C: Transposition of the lips for the correction of facial paralysis. Plast Reconstruct Surg 57:427, 1976.
29. Pillsbury HC, Fisch U: Extratemporal facial nerve grafting and radiotherapy. Arch Otolaryngol 105:441, 1979.
30. Rubin LR: Entire temporalis muscle transposition. In Rubin LR (ed): Reanimation of the Paralyzed Face: New Approaches. St. Louis, C. V. Mosby Co., 1977, pp 294–315.
31. Sachs M, Conley J: Dual simultaneous systems for facial reanimation. Arch Otolaryngol 109:137, 1983.
32. Samii M: Nerves of the head and neck. In Omer GE, Spinner M (eds): Management of Peripheral Nerve Problems. Philadelphia, W. B. Saunders Co., 1979.
33. Schindler D: Personal communication, 1983.
34. Sessions R, Roark O, Alford B: Frey's Syndrome. A technical remedy. Ann Otol 85:734, 1976.
35. Smith R, Hemenway W, Stevens K et al: Jacobson's neurectomy for Frey's syndrome. Am J Surg 120:478, 1970.
36. Stennert E: Hypoglossal facial anastomosis: Its significance for modern facial surgery. Clin Plast Surg 6:471, 1979.
37. Sunderland S: Factors influencing the course of regeneration and the quality of recovery after nerve suture. Brain 75:19, 1952.
38. Sunderland S: Mass movements after facial nerve injury. In Fisch U (ed): Facial Nerve Surgery. Birmingham, Aesculapius Publishing Co., 1977, pp 285–289.
39. Thomander L, Aldshogius H, Grant G: Motor fiber organization of the facial nerve in the rat. In House GM (ed): Disorders of the Facial Nerve. New York, Raven Press, 1980, pp 75–82.
40. Thompson N: Autogenous free grafts of skeletal muscle. Plast Reconstruct Surg 48:11, 1971.
41. Tucker HM: Human laryngeal reinnervation: Long-term experience with the nerve-muscle pedicle technique. Laryngoscope 88:598, 1978.
42. Walter C: The free dermis fat transplantation as adjunct in the surgery of the parotid gland (author's transl). Laryngol Rhinol Otol (Stuttgart) 54:435, 1975.

CHAPTER 46

Controversies Regarding Therapy of Tumors of the Salivary Glands

John Conley, M.D.

Controversies in the treatment of salivary gland tumors are to be expected, and, hopefully, will ultimately prove productive. Controversies may be a manifestation of the highest type of analytical thought, or be merely an expression of opposing views or a derivative of confusion. They can lead to brilliant precepts and acceptable consensus or nonproductive quarreling. I will attempt to analyze some features of their genesis in salivary gland tumors, the significance of these differences, and their possible evolution.

All rational treatment programs should be preceded by an investigative and diagnostic analysis that establishes the reason and the style of management. There is certainly no fixed dictum regarding only one type of treatment. One would therefore expect nuances in management, depending on the therapist's analysis, professional background, and emotional attitudes regarding the disease and its treatment. This type of individual freedom in any therapeutic program introduces variations that will, hopefully, eventually lead to the truth.

Controversies in therapy are the direct derivative of our reaction to the problems associated with neoplasia in salivary glands. The anatomy, the diagnosis, the biologic behavior, new surgical techniques, new concepts of management, irradiation, and chemotherapy generate discrepancies in results and the reporting of these results so that a variety of opinions may emerge. These differences naturally lead to controversies which are debated and ultimately settled by empiricism. Controversies are usually relative, contemporary, and personal, and most are ultimately relegated to oblivion.

BIOPSY

There are some controversies in the method of diagnosis of these tumors. No one disputes the essentiality of the history and physical examination, but the question of biopsy has evolved through open incisional biopsy to needle aspiration biopsy to lateral lobectomy with frozen section diagnosis, which in some instances is an excisional biopsy. One would naturally expect some difference of opinion in such a broad approach. It is obvious that no single diagnostic procedure is applicable every time, nor is it expected to be eternally infallible.

Open incisional biopsy is rarely performed today and is reserved for certain problem cases that defy routine methods of diagnosis. A possibly malignant tumor of the deep lobe in a teen-age girl who has questionable early facial paresis, and when the family group insists on a definitive pretherapeutic diagnosis, may necessitate an open biopsy if needle aspiration biopsy has proved to be inconclusive.

Aspiration biopsy has the advantage of penetrating the tumor without incision and, hopefully, harvesting sufficient germane tissue to justify an accurate histologic diagnosis. The difficulties with this technique are associated with the not infrequent pleomorphic structure of the tumor, the possibility that a representative portion of tumor may not be retrieved, and that the pathologist may not be able to establish the correct diagnosis or may request additional tissue for study purposes. If the pathologist's interpretation is incorrect and the patient receives treatment complying with this inaccuracy, there will certainly be controversy. In spite of these potential hazards, aspiration biopsy may be very helpful. It has the capability of differentiating benign from malignant tumors and identifying inflammatory disease under ideal circumstances. The responsibility for error or misjudgment with this technique rests with those who use it and who are sensitive to its strengths and weaknesses. It will obviously not solve all problems, but it can solve some.

The technique of lateral lobectomy has become a standard operation in the management of parotid tumors. It is particularly useful in tumors located in the lateral lobe, and it is indeed both diagnostic and curative for all benign tumors and many low-grade malignant tumors localized in this portion of the gland. It has the advantage of exposure and protection of the facial nerve and of removing the major portion of the parotid gland while preserving the nerve. It establishes technical and biologic security, and supplies the pathologist with sufficient tissue for immediate frozen section examination. There is, of course, always the possibility that a frozen section diagnosis may be ambiguous. If it is, the surgeon has the option of waiting for the final definitive diagnosis and then advising the patient as to what should be done, or proceeding with conservative surgery immediately, without mutilation, to gain the maximum effectiveness during the primary operation.[3]

One word should be said regarding microscopic diagnosis of salivary gland tumors. It is a product of the training, interest, and experience of a pathologist or a group of pathologists. If the microscopic sections are examined by only one pathologist in a hospital that has a small volume of salivary gland tumors, there will be little controversy but perhaps an increased chance for misinterpretation. In large medical centers, there may be a consensus after a conference and discussion. In some instances, the responsible surgeon or patient may wish a second opinion. Both must be aware that a change of diagnosis or opinion can occur in over 10 per cent of the complicated cases and that this is not a fault, but a fact.[4, 9]

TREATMENT

Today there is general agreement that salivary gland tumors require treatment.[2, 11, 14] For decades, however, it was not uncommon for the physician to advise the patient "not to operate a salivary gland tumor until it bothered him." This naïve concept of management has been replaced by treatment of all of these tumors, in light of the fact that approximately 25 per cent in the parotid gland, 50 per cent in the submandibular gland, and 65 per cent in the minor salivary glands are malignant. There is rarely ulceration of the skin or mucous membrane. These threatening data leave little choice beyond an attempt to accurately diagnose and then institute a therapeutic program. Sialography, technetium scanning, and response to conservative treatment, combined with clinical evaluation, inevitably lead to the proposition of a histologic diagnosis when tumor is suspected. Because of the difficulties encountered in certain histopathologic types of tumors in salivary glands, a variety of concepts of management have developed. These concepts include observation, conservative surgery, radical surgery, rehabilitative surgery, surgery in combination with irradiation, irradiation alone, chemotherapy, and combinations of these modalities.

Differences of opinion are normative for such a complex set of situations occurring in the salivary glands. These controversies are reduced in scope by a general consensus that the majority of benign tumors are treated surgically,[13] that the majority of malignant tumors of epithelial origin are also treated surgically, that all lymphomas and Hodgkin's neoplasms are treated by irradiation and chemotherapy, and that the majority of the pernicious, recurrent, and high-grade cancers are treated by a combination of surgery and irradiation. There are obvious exceptions and overlapping in all therapeutic trials. In general, the controversies do not dominate management and hopefully point the way to a more effective program.

The basic surgical approach is by lateral lobectomy operation or removal of the submandibular or minor salivary gland combined with the advantage of frozen section information. The lateral lobectomy operation has proved effective in all benign tumors of the lateral lobe and isthmus and as a surgical preparation for benign tumors of the deep lobe and in some low-grade malignant tumors in the lateral lobe. This facilitates the management of approximately 85 per cent of all primary tumors of the parotid gland. Excisional biopsy in all other salivary glands is usually curative for benign tumors, but always requires reoperation if the tumor proves to be malignant. It is in this latter circumstance that some physicians and some patients hope that the biopsy excision has cured the malignant tumor and prefer to "wait and see" what happens or to have

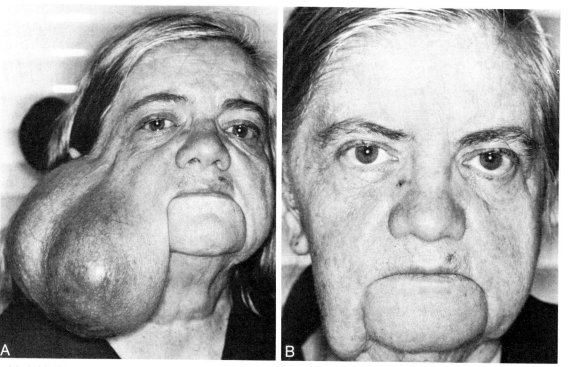

Figure 46–1. (A) This patient delayed treatment of a benign mixed tumor for 30 years. (B) After total conservative treatment. There should be no controversy about removing these tumors when they are first diagnosed.

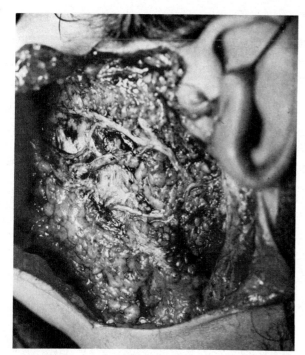

Figure 46–2. Subtotal parotidectomy (lateral lobectomy) for benign tumors of the lateral lobe and isthmus. There is controversy in applying this technique for carcinoma.

irradiation. This decision, which is primarily based on wishful thinking, often proves disastrous. The alternative to this is to have discussed the possibility of malignancy in advance with the patient and to be prepared to carry out a radical ablation on the basis of a frozen section diagnosis or to reoperate after clarification with the patient.

Some surgeons have expressed insecurity about accepting a frozen section diagnosis. There is always, of course, a possibility for error, and this responsibility must be measured by the surgeon in realistic terms that relate to the pathologist's experience and firmness upon open interrogation concerning the reliability of the diagnosis. If there is any doubt whatsoever on the part of the surgeon or the pathologist, the surgeon should not proceed with a mutilating operation without the patient's knowledge and consent.

There is little difference of opinion regarding the treatment of benign tumors of the salivary glands.[5] In the vast majority of cases, the benign tumor is removed along with the gland in which it arises. Some surgeons do not perform a lateral lobectomy in the parotid gland, but prefer enucleation. When this is performed outside the capsule, when the tumor is spheroid and compact without significant lobulations, and when it is removed without spillage, there is an equal chance of a low recurrence rate comparable to that associated with the lateral lobectomy technique. If these criteria, however, cannot be met, the incidence of recurrence will markedly increase. Under ideal circumstances, the rate of recurrence will be approximately 1 per cent.

There is mild controversy and a slight misunderstanding regarding the management of recurrent benign mixed tumors in the parotid gland.[6, 16] The vast majority of these conditions are due to spillage and seeding during the primary operation. The incidence of local recurrence with the uncomplicated benign mixed tumor undergoing lateral lobectomy is in the neighborhood of 1 per cent. Before reoperating on anyone with a recurrent tumor, one should confirm the microscopic diagnosis of benignity and review the original operative report, if that is available. An assessment of the recurrent tumor will provide the information for the most rational reoperation. If there is a single focus of recurrence and the facial nerve is intact, every effort should be made to conservatively remove the isolated tumor and preserve the nerve. If the more likely situation of multiple recurrences presents at the operative site, a conservative resection should again be considered, but the situation is obviously more complex. Recurrence rates for recurrent benign mixed tumor go up to 25 per cent after multiple failures at conservative attempts. When recurrent tumors have enmeshed the facial nerve and there are confluent masses of tumor about the area of the primary operation, the surgeon has few alternatives to an operation that would encompass the nerve. Under these circumstances, the facial nerve should be rehabilitated immediately by autogenous facial nerve grafting. Even with these aggressive efforts, the patient must be cautioned regarding the possibility of local recurrence. Some patients will not accept this type of operation and prefer either to remain under observation or to receive irradiation. Keeping a benign tumor under observation may please the patient for an indefinite period of time, but over a period of decades it always presents the slight possibility of the development of cancer and also of expanding to an inoperable status. Irradiation will retard the growth of the vast majority

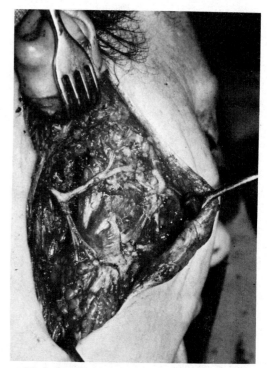

Figure 46–3. "Total" parotidectomy applicable to benign tumors, chronic recurring parotitis, and certain low-grade cancers of the lateral lobe. There is little controversy here.

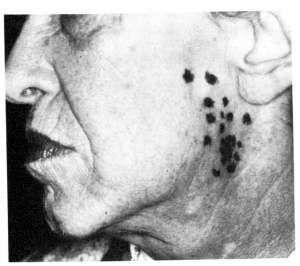

Figure 46—4. This patient was operated on in 1962 for benign mixed tumor. The recurrence was recognized in 1976. This patient has elected to keep the tumor under observation. There is the risk of inoperability and cancer in the future, and this causes controversy.

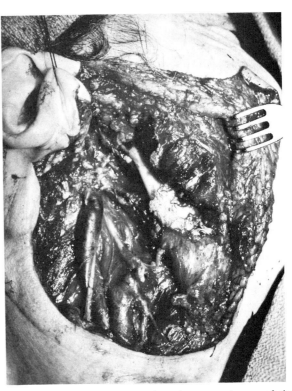

Figure 46—6. Basic operation for primary carcinoma of the parotid with sacrifice of the facial nerve. This may be reduced or extended according to the pathologic process. The facial nerve is immediately rehabilitated. There is some controversy regarding the extent of radicality.

of these tumors, but carries the biologic risks associated with its use in the treatment of benign tumors.

There is a substantial difference of opinion regarding certain specific aspects of the treatment of malignant tumors in the salivary glands.[7, 8] This difference is generated by the variations in the histologic and biologic behavior of individual tumors, the teaching background of the surgeon or radiotherapist involved, and the emotional reactions of the patient to the problem. Most surgeons agree that all high-grade malignant tumors, all malignant tumors with preoperative facial paralysis or gross metastases, all large malignant tumors of the deep lobe or those that have invaded adjacent structures, and most recurrent malignant tumors require an aggressive ablative resection, usually including the total parotid, facial nerve, paraglandular structures, possibly the mandible, and some type of neck dissection. Neck dissection is, of course, more applicable in these types of tumors in the parotid gland and submandibular gland than in minor salivary glands. In cancers of the parotid gland, one may be forced to include the ear, a portion of the mastoid or temporal bone, the mandible, and infratemporal space contents. In such cancers arising in the submandibular gland, one may be obligated to carry out not only a neck dissection, but often resection of associated skin, a portion of the parotid, floor of the mouth, and a portion of the tongue. In such large resections, some type of regional flap is usually necessary to rehabilitate the wound. In such salivary gland cancers arising in the sinuses, palate, or oral cavity, large areas of not only the specific site of origin but also the adjacent tissue must often be sacrificed simultaneously. Most surgeons would also agree that the majority of these cases would be candidates for postoperative radiotherapy. The variability and aggressiveness of the different types of malignant tumors, their approximation to important aesthetic and functional structures,

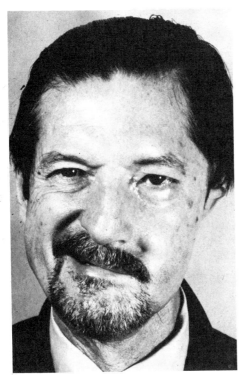

Figure 46—5. There is no controversy as to radical surgery and postoperative irradiation in preoperative facial paralysis, as manifested by this patient.

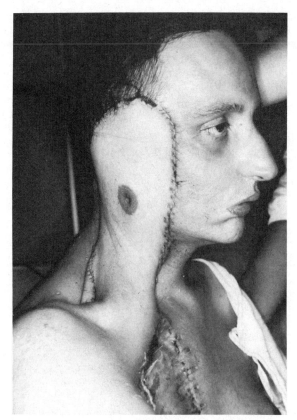

Figure 46–7. This patient had recurrent mucoepidermoid carcinoma for 30 years. It was treated by conservative surgery and irradiation upon multiple occasions. The tumor became undifferentiated and required massive palliative resection. Controversy might raise the question of delayed adequate treatment.

and the promise of therapeutic enhancement from postoperative irradiation have created a mixture of biologic insecurity and emotional hopefulness that has made the assessments of therapeutic options more difficult. The patient's involvement in the decision-making process is often influenced by the instinctual desire to maintain the integrity of the body and the "quality of life." These forces could understandably lead to controversy in a management program containing these variables. A consultation is always helpful.

In low-grade malignant tumors of the salivary glands, there is a realistic possibility for some degree of conservatism. Low-grade mucoepidermoid and low-grade acinic cell cancers are candidates for some of these modifications. Small tumors that are readily accessible surgically and have not approached or invaded adjacent structures, and tumors for which there has been a specific request to preserve the facial nerve or mandible or adjacent soft tissues and for which there is a planned intent to use postoperative irradiation as complementary treatment, also qualify for some type of conservation modification.

There is no question that preserving all or some part of the facial nerve in malignant tumors of the parotid gland has gained considerable popularity.[1, 10, 12, 15] Many of these advocates propose "peeling" the cancer off the nerve sheath and preserving the integrity of the nerve regardless of the proximity, size, or biologic aggressiveness of the cancer. At times they may be willing to sacrifice a secondary or tertiary branch. These attitudes and judgments contain an increased risk, and this is compensated for by the use of postoperative irradiation. It is generally agreed today that the complementary use of irradiation in a combined program has great merit and will improve prognosis in certain cases. Saving the

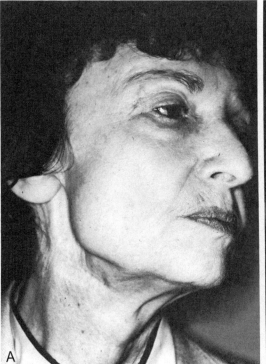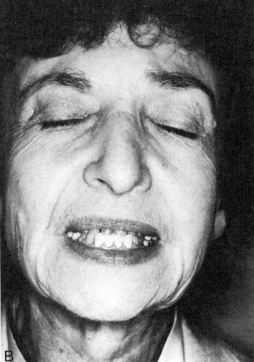

Figure 46–8. (*A*) A small undifferentiated carcinoma of the parotid gland. It was treated by total parotidectomy with preservation of the facial nerve and postoperative irradiation. (*B*) Normal movement of the face 8 years after surgery. Patient participated in the decision to preserve the facial nerve.

TABLE 46–1. Analysis of Surgical Results in Patients with Malignant Tumors of the Parotid Gland

	Patients (%)	Type of Surgery
Extent of surgery	68%	Radical ablation
	32%	Some variety of conservation
Results	26%	Facial nerve graft
	32%	All or part of nerve intact
	42%	Not grafted, but other types of reconstruction (e.g., masseter muscle, 12th cranial nerve, temporal muscle, use of alloplastic substance)

facial nerve in specific and hazardous circumstances may, indeed, be justified in a combined program. The decision for this type of management understandably contains the risks of spillage and gross subtotal resection of the cancer and the biologic possibility that any microscopic residual cancer may not respond to irradiation. The concept of conservation is emotionally very appealing and is being strongly advocated, but its ultimate role in therapy must await additional trials and data.

An analysis of my experience with these variations in malignant tumors of the parotid gland indicated that 68 per cent of the patients had radical ablative surgery and 32 per cent had some type of conservation surgery. Approximately 32 per cent had preservation of some of the branches of the facial nerve, 26 per cent had facial nerve grafts, and 42 per cent had other types of reconstructive procedures. These results are summarized in Table 46–1.

There are obvious exceptions to the preceding philosophical concepts. Some patients will not accept mutilating procedures. Some radiotherapists are willing to treat a large variety of malignant tumors, and even some benign tumors, with irradiation as the primary method of management. Other radiotherapists approve of a reduction in the scope of the operation, with the hope that postoperative irradiation will eradicate any possible residual cancer. Some radiotherapists are reluctant to use irradiation in children because of the severe sequelae in arrested development, gross deformity, and

biologic hazards. Some surgeons have not accepted radicality with any degree of enthusiasm and attempt to organize effective palliation in advanced cases. Many of these differences are reflections of philosophical and emotional reactions to the complexity intrinsic in the management of some of these life-threatening and potentially deforming neoplasms. In dealing with a system of malignant tumors for which the cure rate varies from 20 to 95 per cent, it is realistic to have differences of opinion and controversy. There should never be a rigid protocol of therapy until the treatment advances to the stage at which a fixed protocol is justified.

REFERENCES

1. Alaniz F, Fletcher GR: Place and technics of radiation therapy in the management of malignant tumors of the major salivary glands. Radiology 84:412, 1965.
2. Beahrs OH, Woolner LB, Carveth SW, Devine ED: Surgical management of parotid lesions. AMA Arch Surg 80:890, 1960.
3. Conley J: Salivary Glands and the Facial Nerve. Stuttgart, Georg Thieme, 1975.
4. Conley J: Pathology enigmas for the surgeon. In Salivary Glands and the Facial Nerve. Stuttgart, George Thieme, 1975, pp. 77-79.
5. Conley J: Concepts in Head and Neck Surgery. New York, Grune & Stratton, 1970.
6. Conley J: Recurrent mixed tumors of the parotid. Laryngoscope 90:880, 1980.
7. Conley J, Hamaker RC: Prognosis of malignant tumors of the parotid gland with facial paralysis. Arch Otolaryngol 101: 39, 1975.
8. Eneroth CM: Facial nerve paralysis: A criterion of malignancy in parotid tumors. Arch Otolaryngol 95:300, 1972.
9. Evans RW, Cruikshank A: Epithelial tumors of the salivary glands. In Major Problems in Pathology. Philadelphia, W.B. Saunders Co., 1970.
10. Fletcher GH, Tapley N du V, Patricio MB: Irradiation: Radiotherapist's concept. In Conley J (ed): Concepts in Head and Neck Surgery. New York, Grune & Stratton, 1970.
11. Frazell EL: Clinical aspects of tumors of the major salivary glands. Cancer 7:637, 1954.
12. King JJ, Fletcher GH: Malignant tumors of the major salivary glands. Radiology 100:381, 1971.
13. Lathrop FD: Benign tumors of the parotid gland: A 25-year review. Laryngoscope 72:992, 1962.
14. Lescher TC, Hollingshead WH, Remine WH: Surgical management of benign parotid disease. Am J Surg 113:743, 1967.
15. Tapley N du V, et al: In Fletcher GH (ed): Textbook of Radiotherapy, 2nd ed. Philadelphia, Lea & Febiger, 1973, pp 348–365.
16. Work WP, Batsakis JG, Bailey DG: Recurrent benign mixed tumor and the facial nerve. Arch Otolaryngol 102:15, 1976.

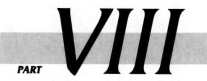

PART **VIII**

Tumors of the Skin

CHAPTER 47

Clinical Evaluation of Tumors of the Skin

Duane C. Whitaker, M.D.

The skin of the head and neck amounts to less than 10 per cent of the body surface area, yet a large majority of all cutaneous tumors occur in this area. The increased incidence of epithelial cell tumors in this area is undoubtedly due to the increased exposure to ultraviolet light (UVL) and to other environmental insults.[18, 36, 56] However, whether this exposure accounts for tumors of other tissues such as those of vascular, neural, or muscular origin remains to be determined. Furthermore, metastatic skin cancer from any organ in the body can be expressed in the skin, and the head and neck region is often the site of these metastatic lesions. From the pathologist's point of view, the first decision is to determine whether the tumor is benign or malignant and the second is to determine if it arose from the skin or if it is metastatic from another site. Benign growths of the skin are much more common than malignancies; however, the diagnosis of some benign lesions such as seborrheic keratoses, compound nevi, sebaceous hyperplasia, pyogenic granuloma, trichoepithelioma, and even viral-induced verrucae can be confusing at times. The purpose of this chapter is to aid clinicians in the recognition and diagnosis of some of the more common tumors arising from the skin of the head and neck, as well as providing some guidelines on the probable degree of tumor extension.

Head and neck skin tumors frequently are so readily visible that it may be unavoidable for inspection to precede history taking. However, it goes without saying that the proper approach always includes an assessment of the patient's general health by history and physical examination. For instance, it is important to specifically ask about previous radiation therapy, which predisposes to skin cancer. In evaluating a case of recurrent basal cell carcinoma after radiation therapy, one can usually anticipate that the tumor will be deeply infiltrative and may require extensive treatment.

Attention, then, must be directed toward the lesion in question. Good lighting is essential, and frequently the light source must be redirected to different angles in order to examine the lesion with the best advantage. Some of the fine points that are important to note are as follows: Recognition of the pearly, translucent rim of basal cell carcinoma, as well as clinical estimation of the margin extent, is best accomplished with tangential lighting from various angles. It is essential to be able to note irregularities of pigmentation and loss of a distinct margin. In the examination of a melanotic lesion, both signs may suggest malignant degeneration. Loss of normal skin lines or obliteration of follicular orifices adjacent to a tumor is usually indicative of further subclinical extension beyond the obvious limit.

Sometimes a clinical impression can be altered by distinguishing between "scale" and "crust." Scale is defined as the accumulation of products of the keratinization process due to both excessive production and decreased shedding. In contrast, crusts are made up of the products of exudation and therefore indicate that injury has extended at least through the epidermis to the level of the most superficial dermal vessels. These fine points may be of extreme importance in evaluating several types of neoplasms, such as sebaceous carcinoma of the eyelid, apocrine carcinoma, or Paget's disease of the external auditory canal. These carcinomas are frequently treated for years as blepharitis or otitis externa without biopsy. However, these two latter dermatitic conditions should not normally be expected to produce chronic accumulation of crust and eschar once appropriate therapy has been instituted. A history of persistence of crusting after adequate therapy is a clear indication for biopsy.

Finally, the feel of the tumor, its base, and adjacent tissues is important, as well as palpation of regional lymph nodes. Sometimes tumors are friable or secondarily infected, making direct palpation difficult.

After a history is obtained, the lesion is examined both visually and by touch of the lesion. Biopsy is usually indicated. Depending on the suspected tumor type, duration, and location, the method of biopsy may vary. However, skin tumors are readily accessible to this definitive diagnostic procedure, and the rule states: when in doubt, always biopsy. (This applies to lesional biopsy, not lymph node aspiration or biopsy.) Special diagnostic studies are indicated in certain situations to further define tumor extent and to plan therapy. These points are discussed at length in this chapter.

ETIOLOGY

Skin tumors can occur anywhere on the body, but it is well documented that a disproportionate number occur on the head and neck. In fact, the head and neck account for 90 per cent of all skin cancers in white males and 85 per cent among white females.* Not all types of tumors are found with such high incidence in this region. For instance, tumors that arise from appendageal structures such as the sweat gland and sebaceous carcinoma do not show a preference for sun-exposed areas. They occur more frequently where there is higher concentration of the parent cell types. Thus, most sebaceous carcinomas arise in the eyelids, and apocrine tumors arise from the axillas, inguinal area, or external auditory canal. However, cancers that arise from keratinocytes and melanocytes of the epidermis, such as basal cell carcinomas, squamous cell carcinomas, and melanomas, do show a tendency to occur more frequently on exposed skin. The predominance of melanoma is not as great; still, the head and neck area is overrepresented in the incidence of melanoma in relation to its surface area. It is interesting to note that the area of highest concentration of melanocytes in the human body is the malar area. Lentigo maligna, a precursor of melanoma found in older individuals, occurs almost exclusively in the malar/temporal area.

Fair-skinned individuals with greater ultraviolet light exposure via occupation, leisure activities, or geographic location are at greater risk for basal cell carcinoma or squamous cell carcinoma.[36, 56] Thus, the genetic background, as well as environmental exposure, seems to play a role. In addition, these types of tumors are seen more frequently with increasing age of the patient and are more common and more aggressive in immunosuppressed patients. Basal cell and squamous cell carcinomas occur more frequently in sites of irradiated skin; furthermore, both types of tumors can be seen in patients with a history of chronic inorganic arsenic ingestion as well as in those exposed to chemical carcinogens. Known carcinogens include polycyclic hydrocarbons, pitch, and tar compounds.

The etiology of melanoma is a more complex subject. Clearly the genetic background, ultraviolet light, and the presence of congenital nevi are etiologic agents in the genesis of melanoma. Patterns of familial melanoma have been described, and it is important to recognize that irregular nevi may be a clue to the recognition of the dysplastic nevus familial melanoma syndrome. It seems clear that ultraviolet light exposure plays a role in genesis of melanoma; however, that role is less well understood than in the case of basal cell or squamous cell carcinoma.

INCIDENCE AND EPIDEMIOLOGY

The yearly incidence of melanoma in the United States is 9000, and the incidence of all other skin cancers is conservatively estimated at 300,000. The incidence of all types of cancer other than skin cancer is about 600,000 per year.[36, 56] Thus, skin cancer accounts for a major portion of the newly diagnosed cancer lesions each year. The numbers may be even greater, since true figures of skin cancer are probably greatly underreported. In a 3-year study, the U.S. National Cancer Institute found skin cancer to be so grossly underre-

ported that the true incidence might be twice the reported figures.[56] A 22-year study ending in 1966 showed that half of all individuals with a first diagnosis of skin cancer were over the age of 65 years at the time.[36] Also, there was a median delay of 3 years from the first symptom to diagnosis of skin cancer. These figures do not reflect the considerable increase in the past 10 years in basal cell carcinomas seen in the younger population. These often are individuals who, by choice or necessity, may have nearly year-round sun exposure. It is no longer rare to find basal cell carcinoma on the faces of individuals in their late twenties or thirties. The study cited, however, does illustrate that there is frequently excessive delay before seeking treatment for skin cancer. One fourth of individuals with skin cancer have more than one lesion at the time of first diagnosis. Basal cell carcinomas account for 60 to 70 per cent; squamous cell 20 to 30 per cent; and other types approximately 10 per cent of all types of skin cancers.[28, 36] Rates of incidence in skin cancer may vary considerably with geography and climate as well as the skin color of the predominant population. The incidence is highest in those living closer to the Equator. Furthermore, the fairer the skin of the population, the more susceptible they are to skin cancer. Even within the United States, the incidence of skin cancer in some Southern cities is twice that of some Northern cities. The association of outdoor occupations such as farming and sailing to skin cancer has long been appreciated.[18] Basal cell and squamous cell carcinomas are diseases in which early treatment could all but eliminate fatalities and drastically reduce the rate of morbidity.

Twenty per cent of all melanomas are seen in the head and neck.[21] Superficial spreading melanoma accounts for 70 per cent of melanomas, and nodular melanoma, which has the worst prognosis, accounts for 15 to 20 per cent of melanomas.[2] The peak incidence of melanoma is as much as 10 to 20 years earlier than that of basal cell and squamous cell carcinomas. Although the incidence of all types of skin cancer appears to be on the rise, the incidence of melanoma, in particular, has doubled in the past 20 years based on data gathered from within the United States and other countries.[56] The Connecticut Tumor Registry has shown an increased incidence in melanoma of more than 500 per cent in the past four decades.[52] Melanoma accounts for about 1 per cent of all cancer deaths, and although overall 5-year survival has improved, the long-term survival of stage II and stage III disease has been essentially unaffected by medical treatment.[52] Thus, the need for increased patient education and awareness, as well as better training in recognition and treatment of skin cancer, has never been greater.

CLASSIFICATION AND STAGING

Basal Cell Carcinoma

Basal cell carcinoma is not a homogenous entity. Several methods have been used to correlate histopathologic classification with biologic behavior. From the clinical standpoint, the most useful clinical pathologic classification is (1) nodular or noduloulcerative; (2) morphea or sclerosing; and (3) superficial multicentric. Fur-

---

*Blacks very seldom develop sun-induced skin cancer, and these figures do not apply to them.

ther differentiation and subtyping can be done, but this adds little to planning the correct therapeutic regimen. Sixty to 80 per cent of all basal cell carcinomas are nodular in type and may be solid or show cystic or adenoid differentiation under the microscope.[32] Clinically, these lesions may be either nodular and exophytic or friable and ulcerative. Basal cell carcinomas that clinically show extensive ulceration usually are more ominous and infiltrative, even though they may show no distinctive histopathologic changes. The pathology report that reads "metatypical basal cell" or basal cell with "squamous differentiation" may reflect a more aggressive variant or may indicate an inability on the part of the pathologist to give a definitive interpretation based on the specimen presented. The morpheaform basal cell carcinoma often is clinically unimpressive and may actually look like a depressed scar. The morpheaform basal cell carcinoma, however, is more aggressive biologically and shows deep invasion, as well as wider peripheral spread.[33, 44, 49] It tends to invade with finger-like projections or tentacles that do not always show contiguous growth. This must be taken into consideration when planning therapy. Superficial multicentric basal cell carcinomas occur predominantly on the trunk and will be mentioned only briefly in this discussion. These lesions usually present as an eczematous patch that tends to advance peripherally with minimal deep invasion.

As a rule, basal cell carcinomas do not metastasize so that the TNM concept of staging is not often used in reference to this type of carcinoma. Only 78 cases of proven metastatic basal cell carcinomas were found in an extensive review published in 1977. Half of the reported metastatic lesions involved the lymph nodes, and the other half involved the lung, bone, liver, and other viscera. Considering the fact that there are probably at least 300,000 new basal cell carcinomas in the United States each year, the incidence of metastatic disease is obviously slight.[32] When distant metastases do occur, however, the cancer is as severe as any other metastatic lesions, with death due to the cancer in about 10 months being the rule. Some authors have suggested that the adenocystic subtype is more likely to metastasize as well as show local recurrence. However, based on our present knowledge, the anatomic location, the long duration of the tumor, and multiple treatment failures (especially tumors recurrent after radiation therapy) are factors that are at least as important as the histologic subtype in predicting which basal cell carcinoma will show more invasive behavior. Thus, when dealing with a multiply recurrent or very large tumor, it is important to be sure that one is dealing with localized disease, as is the usual case.

Squamous Cell Carcinoma

This chapter confines discussion of squamous cell carcinoma to those arising from cutaneous epithelium of the head and neck, thus excluding squamous cell carcinoma of the vermilion, lip, and oral cavity. The clinical staging system similar to that used in melanoma (Table 47–1) is applicable to squamous cell carcinomas. Fortunately, most squamous cell carcinomas arising from keratinizing epithelium of the skin present as stage I lesions. A few patients will show palpable regional

TABLE 47–1. Clinical and Histopathologic Stages of Melanoma

Stage	Clinical Findings	Histologic Description
I	Localized disease (no clinically palpable lymph nodes)	Absence of histologic evidence of tumor in regional lymph nodes
II	Palpable regional lymph nodes	Histologic evidence of melanoma in regional lymph nodes
III	Presence of distant metastases	Histologic documentation of distant metastases

lymph nodes (stage II), and rarely, distant metastases are seen (stage III). Even though regional lymph node spread is not common, the lymph nodes should be palpated routinely, even with quite small lesions. Further breakdown of staging usually is not required or useful. However, when further classification is needed, the TNM system can be used. Once again, as in the case of basal cell carcinoma, the next essential step is to combine information obtained clinically and histopathologically to assess the extent of the lesion and determine appropriate therapy. Solar or actinic keratoses are UVL-induced precancerous lesions, which occur almost exclusively on sun-exposed areas. If untreated, approximately 10 to 20 per cent of actinic keratoses may progress to squamous cell carcinomas.[28] In general, squamous cell carcinomas arising from actinically damaged skin are considered to be less aggressive than those arising in other sites. However, this general rule should not be applied blindly, as quite poorly differentiated and aggressive squamous cell carcinomas can arise on sun-exposed skin. Squamous cell cancers may also arise de novo or from a previously injured area, such as a burn scar or radiation site. These tumors may be more aggressive.

Histopathologically, squamous cell carcinoma may be classified as typical squamous cell carcinoma or variants that show adenocarcinoma or spindle cell elements. Additionally, squamous cell carcinoma is graded by degree of differentiation, atypicality, and depth of invasion.[32] If microscopic examination shows well-differentiated squamous cell carcinoma with minimal invasion of the dermis and solar elastosis, this forms the histologic picture of a less invasive lesion.

Keratoacanthoma may represent a variant of squamous cell carcinoma and can usually be differentiated on the basis of a history of rapid growth, clinical appearance, and histopathologic form. The patient usually will describe that the lesion developed over a period of 6 to 8 weeks or less. The rapid growth will be quite striking to the patient. Keratoacanthoma usually occurs on sun-exposed areas. Generally, these present as dome-shaped nodules with a keratinous central plug. When this is the suspected diagnosis, either an excisional biopsy or incisional biopsy, as discussed below, should be done to establish diagnosis.

Melanoma

Melanoma is classified as lentigo maligna melanoma (LMM), which has the best prognosis; superficial spreading melanoma (SSM); or nodular melanoma

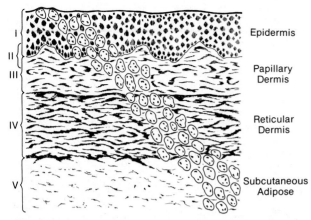

Figure 47–1. The Clark levels of melanoma are shown diagramatically. *Level I:* Melanoma confined to epidermis. *Level II:* Any invasion of melanoma cells into the papillary dermis. (Thus, the integrity of the basement membrane separating dermis and epidermis has been disrupted by the melanoma). *Level III:* Melanoma cells invade and fill the papillary dermis. *Level IV:* Invasion into the reticular dermis. *Level V:* Invasion into the subcutaneous adipose.

(NM), which has the worst prognosis. These classifications have identifying clinical and histopathologic characteristics, which will be discussed later. Melanoma can be staged as shown in Table 47–1.[2, 21]

Unfortunately, medical and surgical therapy has not improved the chance of survival of patients with stage II and stage III melanoma, for nearly all these patients eventually die of the disease. Fortunately, particularly with early diagnosis, most melanomas are stage I.[52] Here, further classification based on the depth of the lesion can be accomplished, and this subdividing is of prognostic importance. Clark and his coworkers originally proposed level criteria of melanoma based on depth of the lesion with respect to anatomic levels of the skin[8a] (Fig. 47–1). Level I lesions are confined to the epidermis, and their diagnosis as a melanoma is even doubted by some. Level II lesions invade into the papillary dermis, with level III lesions filling the papillary dermis and extending to the reticular dermis. Level IV lesions involve the reticular dermis, and the deepest, level V, shows invasion into the subcutaneous fat.

More recently, Breslow has refined the depth classification by precisely measuring the thickness of melanoma using a micrometer.[6] The measurements are made from the top of the epidermis to the deepest melanoma cells in the dermis. He and subsequent workers found break points in measurements that seem to correlate well with likelihood of metastases and predicted 5-year survival. Patients with stage I melanoma whose tumor measures less than 0.85 mm in depth have approximately a 98 per cent 5-year survival rate and very low incidence of metastases. Intermediate levels of 0.85 to 1.69 mm and 1.70 to 3.64 mm present relatively greater risk, with those tumors greater than 3.65 mm in thickness being most likely to metastasize and cause the patient's death. For patients with clinical stage I disease, tumor thickness is useful in prognosis. Another risk factor is the location of the lesion. This is particularly important with regard to what is called the BANS regions (back, posterolateral arms, posterolateral neck, and posterior scalp).[52] These areas present greater risk in terms of survival.

Figures that document an improvement in the 5-year survival rate for all melanomas probably reflect an increased recognition and excision of early stage I melanomas. Within the category of clinical stage I disease, further categorization regarding prognosis and therapy can be made by combining the clinical and histopathologic information with the depth of tumor measurement. Thus, within clinical stage I, a thicker lesion and an anatomic location in the BANS region both indicate poor prognosis.[52]

CLINICAL EVALUATION

Basal Cell Carcinoma

Basal cell carcinoma is the single most common neoplasm in the skin, and a recent review shows that over 90 per cent of all basal cell carcinomas occur on sun-exposed areas of the head and neck. Although they may occur anywhere, particular sites of predilection are the nose and paranasal area, auricle, periauricular region, canthi, lid margins, cheek, and temple. The primary nodular or ulcerative basal cell carcinoma is readily visible to inspection and usually causes the patient no pain. The only symptom may be recurrent bleeding or ulceration of a site. If the patient extensively manipulates the lesion or has poor hygiene, it may become infected and purulent. Nodular basal cell carcinomas begin as small, smooth-surfaced, translucent or "pearly" papules or nodules with tiny telangiectatic vessels (Fig. 47–2). They may be smooth or ulcerated centrally with a rolled border. Although they are firm to palpation, they may bleed easily with mild trauma. Occasionally, small benign nevi or areas of sebaceous gland hyperplasia will look like basal cell carcinoma. These benign lesions, however, do not ulcerate or bleed spontaneously. Basal cell carcinomas tend to grow very slowly,

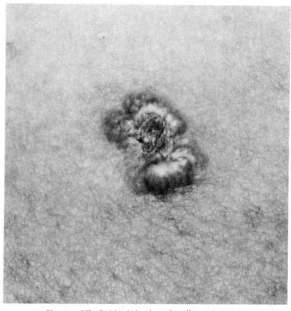

Figure 47–2. Nodular basal cell carcinoma.

and patients will sometimes claim to have noticed no increase in size for a year or longer.

Often patients are quite inaccurate in their estimation of how long the lesion has been present. In the case of larger tumors, they generally underestimate because they may understand the question to be, "How long has it been this bad?" or they may be hesitant to admit that they avoided treatment for so long. Thus, when one is really interested in the growth rate of a particular tumor, it is helpful to ask the question in several different ways at different times.

As lesions become larger, a central dimple appears and then ulceration occurs with frequent crusting and eschar. There may be central healing while the tumor continues to enlarge peripherally and deeply. The recurrent ulceration and partial healing cycle may result in a very ragged appearance to the ulcer, thus giving it the unaesthetic historical name of "rodent ulcer" (Fig. 47–3). Because of the unsightly clinical appearance, patients may try various home remedies to cover the lesion. However, in the natural state, the description "translucent telangiectatic nodule with ulceration" has come to be virtually synonymous with basal cell carcinoma in the language of dermatologists.

Morpheaform basal cell carcinoma accounts for about 10 to 20 per cent of all basal cell carcinomas.[32] This subtype, however, can be quite deceptive, and it is important to be aware of its existence. Morpheaform lesions tend to show greater subclinical extension and therefore are likely to result in a disproportionate number of recurrent tumors. Because of their extension, the morpheaform subtype is correlated with a greater risk to the patient and more aggressive behavior.[22, 33, 50] Morpheaform basal cell carcinomas usually are single, slightly depressed, white or yellow plaques without sharp margination. Loss of the follicular dimpling and the vellus hairs of normal skin around these tumors may indicate further dermal spread (Fig. 47–4). Typically, there is no ulceration or exophytic growth and no history of recurrent

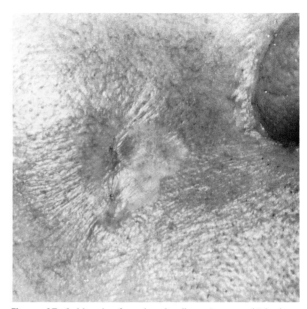

Figure 47–4. Morpheaform basal cell carcinoma, which shows scar-like appearance and lack of ulceration.

bleeding. Therefore, morpheaform basal cell carcinomas are less bothersome, and except for those patients who are quite appearance-conscious, the patient may seek care only after considerable delay. These lesions generally occur on sun-exposed areas of the head and neck. Hauben found the morpheaform lesions to be more common in younger age groups.[22] This type of lesion is also more difficult for the physician to recognize. Punch or excisional biopsy is required for diagnosis. The definition of this lesion by the pathologist is of extreme importance because morpheaform lesions often have deep and peripheral extension requiring a wider surgical margin. Morpheaform basal cell carcinoma of the nasolabial fold, nasal tip, and auricle are particularly difficult to assess clinically. A reliable method of excision with an examination of multiple frozen sections of the lateral and deep margins is required.

So far, we have discussed primary basal cell carcinoma. Evaluation of these tumors is relatively straightforward compared with that of recurrent basal cell carcinomas. Because the majority of basal cell carcinomas do not metastasize, in some instances these lesions are treated with an offhand approach, which may reflect the outlook that if the lesion is not eradicated in the first go around, another attempt can be made with little disadvantage to the patient. This outlook, coupled with the misconception that all basal cell carcinomas are the same, can result in gross underestimation of the aggressive behavior of some of these tumors. Some patients have undergone multiple, unsuccessful treatments at tremendous cost in dollars, not to mention patient illness, time lost from work, and psychological stress. Thus, by the time the patient is seen by the specialist, he or she is likely to have the impression that it is an incurable tumor. This is inexcusable both in terms of patient education and the surgical management of the tumor, which if treated properly, should have close to a 99 per cent cure rate. The assessment of a recurrent lesion is much more difficult. Obviously, the history of prior treatment is important, particularly since

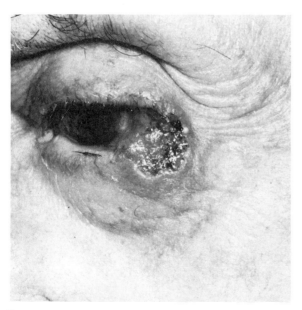

Figure 47–3. Ulcerated basal cell carcinoma of the lateral canthus.

remnants of previous graft or flap may be covering the tumor. This has been proved time and again by demonstrating the extent of tumor with microscopically controlled excisional technique.[12] Multiple biopsies are often indicated in order to assess the extent of recurrent lesions, as well as to confirm the diagnosis (Fig. 47–5). Regional node examination, as well as special studies such as radiographic or computed tomography (CT), nuclear magnetic resonance (NMR), or sonography may be indicated if it is suspected that the tumor has penetrated deep structures beyond the subcutaneous adipose tissue. For tumors of longstanding duration or multiple recurrent tumors, radiographs of the underlying structures are recommended in order to anticipate possible extent.

There are other special circumstances that should be considered. For instance, periorbital tumors tend not to spread down onto the cheek or into the eyebrow. Instead, they tend to advance fairly rapidly and deeply toward the globe and frequently into the deep soft tissue of the orbit. This is particularly true in tumors that arise from the medial canthus. Therefore, computerized tomography (CT) is helpful in evaluating these extensive periorbital tumors when there is suspicion that it may have penetrated into the orbit and displaced the globe. Ultrasound may also be helpful in evaluating the integrity of the globe.

Another factor of importance is clinical knowledge of adjacent anatomy. For example, basal cell carcinomas of the nasolabial fold and auricular sulci are notoriously difficult to eradicate. This appears to be due to merging of embryonic fusion planes resulting in tissues that offer variable resistance to tumor growth.[43, 44] Thus, quite eccentric tumor extension and deep invasion along certain planes may be seen. As many as 10 per cent of all basal cells may show neurophilic behavior, and the tumor may track along a nerve sheath for great distances.[12] Thus, if the patient develops pain at the site of a previously excised basal cell carcinoma, particularly if

located over nerve foramina, this may be indicative of residual neurophilic tumor. It is also useful to know that primary basal cell carcinomas uncommonly invade directly into the perichondrium or periosteum, unless the integrity of these tissues has been disrupted by previous surgery or irradiation. Cartilage invasion is also uncommon; rather, the usual mode of extension is lateral spread along these planes without direct invasion in the bone or cartilage. However, in recurrent or previously radiated basal cell carcinoma all bets are off, and direct invasion into deep structures can occur.[17, 25, 28, 33, 57] Clearly, tumors that invade periosteum or perichondrium have revealed themselves as aggressive regardless of the cell type. Furthermore, tumors that are proved to be unresponsive to multiple therapies are likely to be more aggressive, as are those lesions which are seen in immunologically suppressed patients.[59] Thus, there is no single test or specific histologic finding that identifies the more difficult basal cell carcinoma. Rather, all factors relating to the tumor and its host, as discussed previously, must be taken into consideration when evaluating basal cell carcinoma.

Squamous Cell Carcinoma

Squamous cell carcinoma accounts for 20 to 30 per cent of all cutaneous tumors, and like basal cell carcinoma, the sites of predilection are sun-exposed areas.[31] However, there are clearly other inciting factors. Nearly all fair-skinned individuals who have outdoor occupations or who spend considerable time in outdoor leisure activities will develop some evidence of solar damage by the time they are in their mid-50s or younger. These actinic changes are particularly common on the helix, anthelix, nose, malar area, temples, bald scalp, and dorsum of the hands and arms. Examination of the skin will reveal a multiplicity of clinical signs including hyper- or hypopigmentation, loss of elasticity, mild atrophy, telangiectasia, chronic erythema, and persistent scaling in the absence of any irritant. Against this background, actinic keratoses, which are precursors of squamous cell carcinomas, are frequently seen (Fig. 47–6). They show persistent and often adherent scale. They may be erythematous to gray or tan in color and often have surface telangiectasia. In addition to persistent scale, there may be crusting from periodic leakage of serum through the epidermis. Actinic keratoses generally are not symptomatic unless the patient becomes preoccupied with the lesion, and then because of secondary irritation it may become tender, inflamed, or pruritic. It is often easier to feel actinic keratoses, which are scaly or feel like sandpaper. Unless inflamed, actinic keratoses do not have a feel of thickness or induration. If there is induration, the diagnosis of squamous cell carcinoma should be considered. The majority of experienced physicians do not find it necessary to biopsy all lesions suspected as actinic keratoses. As a matter of fact, this would be nearly a physical impossibility in some instances, and with experience, clinical recognition can be quite accurate. Because 10 to 20 per cent of actinic keratoses will progress into squamous cell carcinoma, physicians treat actinic keratoses by various destructive or surgical techniques.[28] When in doubt about the diagnosis, either a tangential shave or an excisional punch biopsy can be done.

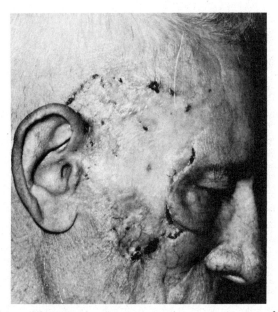

Figure 47–5. Basal cell carcinoma that was recurrent after multiple treatments.

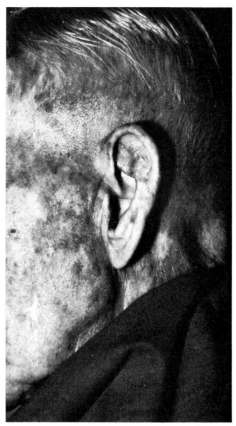

Figure 47–6. Patient with extensive actinic keratoses and chronic solar damage.

Not all squamous cell carcinomas arise from actinic keratoses. Even in areas of sun-damaged skin, a squamous cell carcinoma can still arise de novo, and failure to recognize it can result in incorrect assessment and therapy. This is particularly important because at least 8 per cent of all de novo squamous cell carcinomas of the skin will develop regional and distant metastases. Squamous cell carcinomas arising from the sites of inflammatory degenerative processes such as nonhealing ulcers or sinuses, burn scars, and radiation sites show even higher metastatic rates of 20 to 30 per cent or greater. Those patients who do have evidence of regional or distant metastases will ultimately die from that disease in 75 per cent of cases.[32] The vermilion of the lip is sun-exposed, and any squamous cell carcinoma at a mucocutaneous junction is well known to be at more risk for metastatic disease, as well as local recurrence (see Chapter 25). Thus, all squamous cell carcinomas deserve special attention, therapy, and follow-up. It is important to consider whether the tumor has arisen from an area of actinic degeneration or previous injury, as well as the condition of surrounding tissues, anatomic location, histopathologic appearance, and the status of the regional lymph nodes. In instances in which there is no actinic damage or other locally predisposing factors, and if pathologic examination shows poor differentiation, then it is incumbent upon the clinician to determine if the lesion might be metastatic from another primary site.

Squamous cell carcinomas arising from the skin are markedly variable in their rate of growth. Some show very slow doubling time, comparable to the least aggressive of basal cell carcinomas. However, others may multiply quite rapidly and invade deeply. The appearance of the lesion itself is important in predicting biologic behavior. Squamous cell carcinomas arising from actinic keratoses tend to be somewhat hyperkeratotic with minimal or no ulceration. Some induration will usually be present at the base of the lesion. The surrounding skin will show evidence of actinic damage. The biopsy specimen should show well-differentiated superficially invasive squamous cells with evidence of elastotic degeneration. However, the presentation of a nodule with significant induration and ulceration, particularly 2 cm or greater in diameter, is not the usual presentation of a squamous cell carcinoma arising from sun-damaged skin (Fig. 47–7). This should alert the clinician to the possibility of a more aggressive lesion. Squamous cell carcinoma arising in areas of chronic inflammation or other sites in nonhealing tissue can be the most deceiving of all clinically. They may be very hyperkeratotic and may show thickening of the dermis or atrophy with a chronically nonhealing ulcer. Squamous cell carcinoma in situ is known as *Bowen's disease* and histologically is defined as epidermal atypicality without dermal invasion. This occurs on either sun-exposed or covered areas and may be confused with a recalcitrant patch of dermatitis. The diagnosis of squamous cell carcinoma in these situations requires a strong clinical suspicion and willingness to biopsy any nonhealing area of greater than 1 year's duration.

Clinical differentiation of squamous cell carcinoma from basal cell carcinoma is not always possible. Therefore, biopsy is indicated to substantiate or rule out the clinical diagnosis. For small lesions, an excisional biopsy may be the most practical. For exophytic or large nodular lesions, a wedge of tissue obtained by incision or a punch biopsy will usually be required to establish a

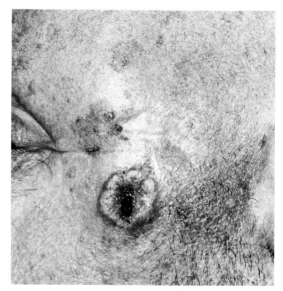

Figure 47–7. Squamous cell carcinoma with ulceration and a nodular margin.

diagnosis. Sometimes a deep shave biopsy will be adequate. However, if a lesion is suspicious for a *keratoacanthoma*, this type of technique usually will not give the pathologist adequate tissue to establish diagnosis. If one has a high degree of suspicion of a low-grade superficial squamous cell carcinoma arising from actinically damaged skin, full excisional biopsy and linear closure is often preferable.

Keratoacanthoma is somewhat of a peculiarity in that often it cannot be differentiated from squamous cell carcinoma on microscopic examination. Usually, a keratoacanthoma presents with a history of rapid growth over 1 to 2 months and grossly has a "heaped-up" crater configuration with a central keratin plug. It is preferable to fully excise keratoacanthoma so that when it is examined histologically, the configuration distinctive for keratoacanthoma is seen. In true keratoacanthoma, dermal invasion will not be found as in squamous cell carcinoma. Additionally, the literature indicates that these tumors do resolve spontaneously. However, involution, when it occurs, is slow, extending over a period of 6 months or longer.[32] Not all lesions involute, and there have been a few reports of metastatic disease. When it is not practical to fully excise a lesion or when the clinical diagnosis is not clear, a wedge-shaped incision extending through the margin with some normal adjacent tissue usually is required for the pathologist to differentiate the lesion from squamous cell carcinoma. An incisional biopsy from the center of the lesion may not demonstrate the overall configuration necessary for accurate microscopic diagnosis. Keratoacanthoma should be treated as low-grade squamous cell carcinoma.

Melanoma

Head and neck melanomas account for 20 per cent of all melanomas, and nearly 80 per cent of these arise from the skin. The remainder are of ocular or mucosal origin.[21] Considering the entire surface area of the body, the number of tumors arising from the head and neck skin make up a disproportionate percentage. As discussed previously, environmental exposure (UVL, heat, wind) are presumed to play a role in the pathogenesis of these lesions. However, the relationship is not as direct as in a basal cell carcinoma and squamous cell carcinoma because the majority of nodular melanomas do occur on covered areas.

The cheek is the single most common site of melanoma of the head and neck, followed by the scalp, ear, and neck.[21] Some of the melanoma, located on the malar area are *lentigo maligna*, the least aggressive form of melanoma. In contrast, melanomas that occur on the posterior scalp, the back and sides of the neck, and the postauricular skin probably present the greatest risk statistically of head and neck melanomas. Sober and associates have shown that certain areas (the BANS regions) are associated with a much poorer prognosis.[52]

Other lesions may on occasion be difficult to differentiate from melanoma. Differential diagnosis of any pigmented lesion of the face should include pigmented nevi, seborrheic keratoses, solar lentigines, pigmented basal cell carcinomas, and benign tumors, which may become infarcted or hemorrhagic giving a melanotic appearance. In the case of nevi, a history of long duration and unchanged appearance with features of sharp margination and regular color throughout are suggestive of that diagnosis. Histopathologically, nests of nevus cells are seen in the dermis or epidermis. The history is important because congenital pigmented nevi do present risk of malignant degeneration, as discussed below. *Seborrheic keratoses* appear in older patients and vary in color from black to light tan. These entirely benign epidermal growths can range in size from 3 mm to 2 cm; they are rarely larger. An irritated seborrheic keratosis can be confused with melanoma by those who are unfamiliar with these lesions. Seborrheic keratoses have a "stuck-on" appearance. The feel of the surface is rough and "warty" and slightly greasy. These lesions are easily shaved off tangentially with the skin, and normal appearing dermis is seen below. *Solar* or *senile lentigines* are flat, uniformly pigmented, brown or tan macules on sun-exposed areas. They are commonly referred to as "liver spots," or "age spots," by patients. They darken on sun exposure and usually are in the same age population as seborrheic keratoses. Solar lentigenes usually can be differentiated from lentigo maligna because they are generally multiple, entirely flat, and quite homogeneous in color. When in doubt, a biopsy should be obtained. When a *pigmented basal cell carcinoma* has the other characteristic features, including a rolled, pearly, telangiectatic margin, a few flecks of pigment in the lesion usually will not confuse the clinician (Fig. 47–8). However, if the lesion has diffuse dark brown or black pigment throughout the surface, it may look somewhat like a malignant melanoma. Occasionally, other benign growths such as skin tags, nevi, or vascular lesions are subjected to local irritation and trauma and acquire a darkened surface, which may be confused with a melanoma. A biopsy examination will be decisive in such cases.

Clinical inspection of melanoma is useful in categorizing the subtype as well as in providing some prognostic information. *Lentigo maligna* is a biologically benign, but

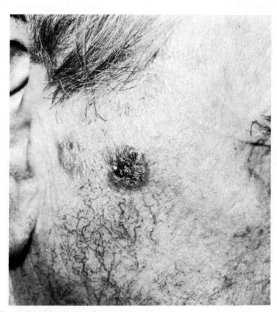

Figure 47–8. This basal cell carcinoma has considerable pigmentation centrally.

morphologically malignant, lesion.[32] Lentigo maligna is quite slow-growing and is found almost exclusively on the faces of elderly individuals. The mean age for patients with these lesions is 65 years. Lentigo maligna usually has been present for a number of years before the patient seeks care.[3, 5, 10] The lesions are macular and erythematous to tan-brown in color. Generally, their border is indistinct, which may help to differentiate them from benign senile lentigo. Lentigo maligna is usually singular and varies in size from 1 to 4 cm, although occasionally larger lesions may be seen (Fig. 47–9). Color may not be homogeneous throughout and may show darker areas of pigment accumulation or areas of spontaneous regression. Within the lesion, there may be small papules, which become darker in color. This usually signals the evolution of lentigo maligna to lentigo maligna melanoma and occurs very slowly, sometimes requiring 10 to 15 years or longer.[5, 10] Biopsy of lentigo maligna melanoma will show increased numbers of atypical melanocytes at the junction and invasion of melanoma cells into the dermis. Thus, lentigo maligna as a premalignant lesion shows radial or horizontal growth. When the transition into vertical or invasive growth starts, then the lesion is classified as a lentigo maligna melanoma. This invasive stage may have the physical characteristics of a nodular melanoma, but growth is slow and prognosis generally remains better. Clearly, the goal should be to establish an early diagnosis so that the in situ lesions of lentigo maligna can be treated prior to development of the invasive stage.

Superficial spreading melanoma accounts for about 70 per cent of all melanomas. These lesions favor the sun-exposed regions, although they also occur in non–sun-exposed areas.[12] Superficial spreading melanomas have the second-best prognosis to lentigo maligna melanoma; they are palpable, vary from slightly to definitely elevated, and show slow growth. They are usually irregular

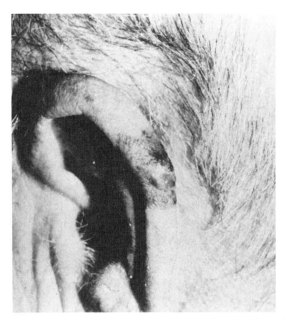

Figure 47–10. This superficial spreading melanoma shows irregular pigmentation with a central papule.

in configuration and pigmentation, are more wide than tall, and show spread of pigment onto the normal adjacent skin. Close inspection reveals small indentations ("notching") or protrusions of the margins. Color varies from brown or black to pink, rose, gray, or white (areas of depigmentation)[12] (Fig. 47–10).

Nodular melanomas are darkly pigmented nodules that are as tall as they are wide. They may be smooth or lobulated and may show ulceration (Fig. 47–11). Local satellite lesions are sometimes present, and there may be a remarkable play of color showing red, blue, black, or regression of pigment with an amelanotic appearance. Nodular melanomas usually show no anatomic site of preference in contrast to superficial spreading

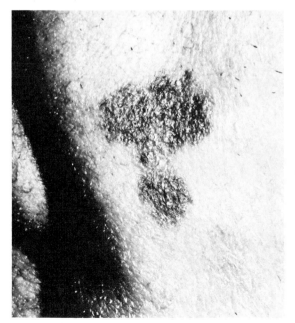

Figure 47–9. Lentigo malignas usually occur on the temple or cheek as pictured here.

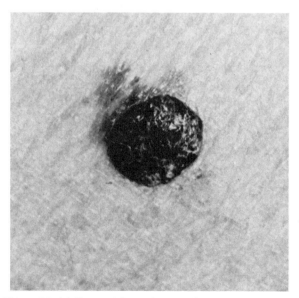

Figure 47–11. This nodular melanoma shows pigment spread onto the surrounding skin surface.

melanomas. They have a very short radial or horizontal growth phase. Unfortunately, they tend to invade early, often demonstrating both deep invasion as well as regional nodes at the time of diagnosis.

Day and associates found that in nodular melanoma, nodule size and ulceration were important in prognosis.[12] Those two features are found to be more important than size of the entire lesion or plaque. Their conclusions indicate that melanomas with either significant nodularity (larger size or greater number) or extensive ulceration may have the greater risk of metastases. This seems to be independent of depth or stage.

A fourth variant that has been recognized is *acrolentiginous melanoma*. These lesions usually occur on the palms and soles and may be seen in darker-skinned individuals. Biologically, they behave similar to nodular melanomas.

Whenever melanoma is suspected, if possible, it is preferable to do a complete excisional biopsy after field block anesthesia. However, both the size of a lesion and uncertainty as to clinical diagnosis may make it appropriate to do an incisional biopsy, especially since there is no convincing evidence that this increases the risk of metastases.[16, 45] When incisional biopsies are done, an adequate specimen with a generous amount of subcutaneous tissue should be taken, particularly because tumor depth seems to be the most useful prognosticator. Careful removal and handling of a good biopsy specimen is crucial to preserve the tissue relationships, which are critical to depth measurement.

Special diagnostic studies are indicated for patients suspected to have malignant melanomas. All patients, including those with the most superficial melanomas, require a minimum of thorough history and physical examination, total skin examination, hemogram, blood chemistries, and chest radiograph. The most significant clinical examination is determination of possible lymph node involvement. If there is obvious stage II disease, the clinician must rule out by further special studies the presence of blood-borne metastases. It is nearly impossible to predict the pattern of metastases based on a given primary site.[14] Beyond regional lymph nodes, the most common sites of organ metastases are lung and liver, although brain, bone, and other organs may be sites of metastases. Liver and bone scans have often been considered the next most important studies to perform. Poiron concluded that ultrasonography and CT were superior to radionuclide scanning in examination of the liver.[14] However, NMR studies may ultimately prove to be even more useful.

GENERAL PATIENT EVALUATIONS

Several syndromes are characterized by the development of skin cancers.

Nevoid Basal Cell Carcinoma Syndrome

The nevoid basal cell carcinoma syndrome (NBCC) represents a clinically important constellation of findings that require early recognition and diagnosis as well as appropriate therapy and regular follow-up care.[23, 32, 38] This syndrome is an autosomal dominant genodermatosis. Technically, the term "nevus" is misleading be-

cause the lesions are basal cell carcinomas, which are capable of invasive and destructive behavior. Initially, lesions develop during childhood as small nodules. These "nevoid collections of basal cells" are not physiologically invasive prior to puberty, but they cannot be differentiated histologically from basal cell carcinoma at any stage. There may be literally hundreds of lesions, which are nearly always on the face and neck, although they may appear on other exposed and non–sun-exposed skin surfaces. They seem to be especially common on the eyelids, central face, and scalp. During adulthood, these lesions enter a neoplastic stage and become invasive basal cell carcinoma. The rate of growth and destructive capability of the tumors vary greatly from one patient to the next (Fig. 47–12). The NBCC syndrome in its fullest expression consists of five major components:

1. Basal cell carcinomas.
2. Jaw cysts.
3. Congenital skeletal anomalies; spina bifida; and clavicle, long-bone, and metacarpal irregularities.
4. Ectopic lamellar calcification of the falx cerebri.
5. Pits of the palms and soles. Palmar pits 1 to 3 mm in diameter usually develop during the second decade of life and are found in about half of all NBCC patients (Fig. 47–13). This finding is said to be pathognomonic of NBCC, although palmar pits can also occur in patients with arsenical keratoses. In the latter instance, the pits are usually larger and more hyperkeratotic.

With close follow-up and regular therapy, some patients are able to lead fairly normal lives. In other cases,

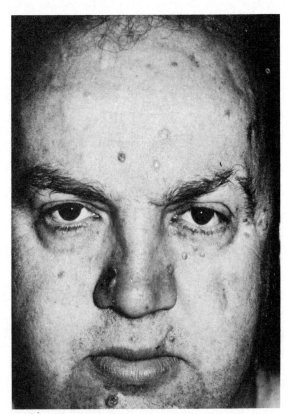

Figure 47–12. Over a dozen tumors are seen on the face of this man with nevoid basal cell carcinoma syndrome.

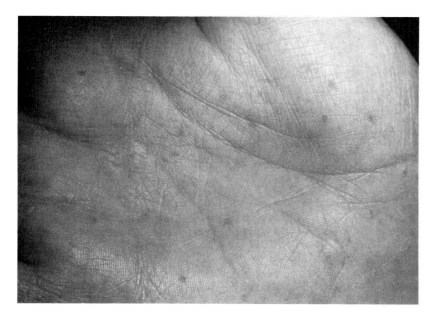

Figure 47–13. Palmar pits of nevoid basal cell carcinoma.

the lesions may be particularly destructive and mutilating in appearance, owing to both lesions and the associated therapy, greatly diminishing the patient's quality of life (Fig. 47–14). Furthermore, metastases to the lung, as well as direct extension into the orbit and brain, have been seen.[24, 38] Because of these complications, it is absolutely essential that the syndrome be identified early and rapport be developed with the patient so that

planned removal of all active lesions can be accomplished on a regular basis. Every attempt should be made to design therapy so that the initial excision is curative because recurrences are especially destructive and difficult to manage in NBCC patients. These patients need education regarding sun protection, and genetic counseling should be provided.

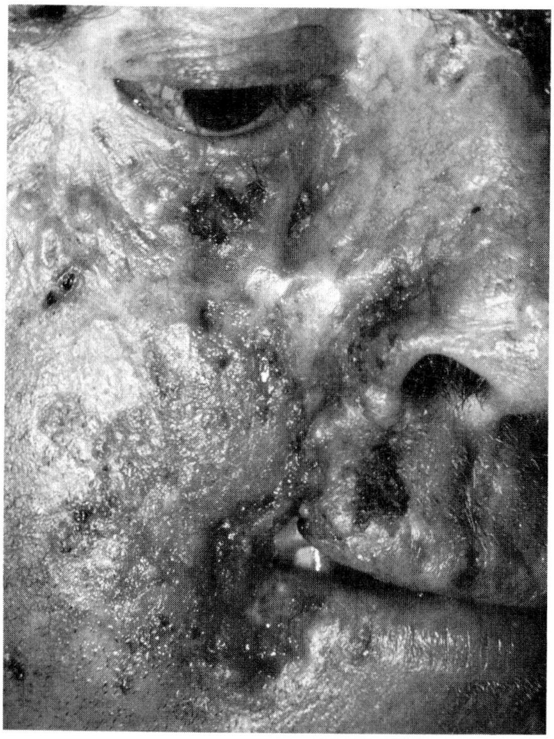

Trichoepithelioma

Trichoepitheliomas are benign hamartomas of hair follicle origin and can be mistaken for basal cell carcinoma.[32, 38] Multiple trichoepitheliomas occur as an autosomally dominant genodermatosis, which does not require treatment except for cosmetic reasons. Trichoepitheliomas may also appear as solitary lesions without a genetic pattern of inheritance. The lesions appear in childhood and increase in number, showing numerous round, skin-colored, firm papules and nodules usually 1 to 8 mm in diameter. They are commonly located in the nasolabial fold, but also occur on the nose, forehead, and upper lip[32] (Fig. 47–15).

Multiple trichoepitheliomas may be confused with basal cell nevi, although trichoepitheliomas usually do not ulcerate. In addition to NBCC, the differential diagnosis includes the angiofibromas of tuberous sclerosis (also known as adenoma sebaceum). Adenoma sebaceum may be differentiated clinically by the presence of other stigmata of tuberous sclerosis and also by the distinctive histopathologic appearance. Occasionally, multiple syringomas can be confused with the trichoepitheliomas. Syringomas are benign, nonulcerative papillomatous lesions 1 to 2 mm in size; they are soft in texture and usually occur on the eyelids. They frequently appear at puberty or later and are most frequently seen in females.

Dysplastic Nevus Syndrome

Described by Clark and associates in 1978, the dysplastic nevus syndrome establishes a familial basis for

Figure 47–14. This middle-aged man with severe expression of nevoid basal cell carcinoma had deeply destructive tumors over much of the face and scalp.

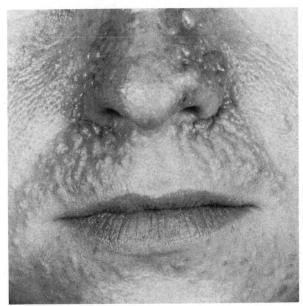

Figure 47–15. Multiple trichoepitheliomas heavily grouped on the lip and lateral side of the nose.

certain melanomas.[46] Familial malignant melanoma was found to be associated with dysplastic nevi, and many of the relatives of the melanoma patients had similar dysplastic nevi. Patients with the dysplastic nevus syndrome characteristically have nevi that are irregular in pigmentation and configuration. These nevi are frequently located on exposed skin and continue to form throughout adult life, as opposed to benign nevi. These dysplastic nevi are often somewhat larger, measuring 5 to 15 mm in diameter. They have a small central papular component in an otherwise flat lesion. Shades of brown, black, pink, and red may also be seen. A biopsy should be done for any new lesion with these characteristics.

Congenital Pigmented Nevus

Occurring in 1 per cent of the population, congenital pigmented nevi can be located anywhere on the body. The diagnosis is made on the basis of history of the lesion being present at birth, as well as examination. The lesions are tan to brown in color with a somewhat pebbly surface and often show hair growth. Margins are distinct and pigmentation is regular. Because the natural history of these lesions is darkening of the color into puberty, proper monitoring of the lesion by parents or physician may be difficult.

The management of these lesions is a complex problem. The decision to either surgically excise, observe and excise at a later time, or do nothing must be individualized. It is known that congenital pigmented nevi show a higher incidence of malignant degeneration than acquired nevi or normal skin. This rate of degeneration is reported to range from 2 to 30 per cent in the literature. In general, the larger the lesion, particularly when greater than 10 cm, the greater the risk. Therefore, if congenital pigmented nevi can be removed without severe disfigurement, excision is often preferable. However, the management is often far from satisfactory because the highest risk lesions are those in which

removal is the most disfiguring. Also, normal excisional techniques cannot guarantee a cure, for some of the potentially malignant melanocytes may be located in the subcutaneous adipose tissue, as well as in deeper structures, such as adipose and fascia. There is a case report in which a melanoma arose from subcutaneous tissue after complete removal of congenital nevus.[20, 52] Furthermore, giant nevi of the head and neck probably should be evaluated by CT scans because they can be associated with leptomeningeal melanocytosis and central nervous system symptoms or seizure disorder. If, for various reasons, a congenital nevus is not removed, the patient and the family should be instructed to monitor the lesion for noticeable changes in size, color, and configuration. If any of these occurs, a prompt biopsy is recommended.

Sebaceous Nevus

Another lesion, which is also congenital but often is not noticed until the patient reaches puberty, is sebaceous nevus. These lesions are usually tan, verrucous, and non–hair-bearing, proliferative growths that occur most commonly on the neck, face, and scalp (Fig. 47–16). They do not actually contain nevus cells, but prophylactic removal is recommended because basal cell carcinomas arise from the lesions.[32]

Xeroderma Pigmentosum

Xeroderma pigmentosum is a rare, autosomal-recessive disorder that shows excessive solar damage at a very early age. Usually actinic changes are noted as early as 1 to 2 years of age. This begins with diffuse erythema and freckling and then progresses over several years to telangiectasia with mottled pigmentation, solar keratoses, and finally frank carcinomas. Basal cell carcinomas, squamous cell carcinomas, and malignant melanomas all may occur. The epidermal changes noted

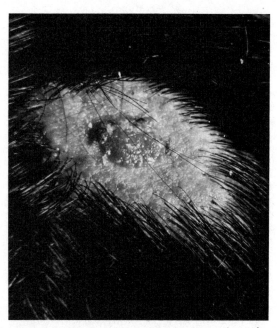

Figure 47–16. Sebaceous nevi usually occur on the scalp and are tan and yellowish in color with warty texture.

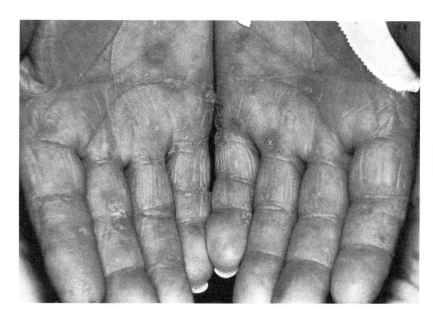

Figure 47–17. Multiple keratoses are seen on the palms and volar fingers in a patient with chronic arsenic ingestion.

previously occur most dramatically on heavily sun-exposed areas, though minimal exposure in other sites can result in similar changes. Photophobia and excessive lacrimation are seen early, and there may be a series of eye complications including keratitis, corneal ulcers, lid margin tumors, and ectropion. These patients frequently look as if they have chronic radiodermatitis.

Although the prognosis varies, depending on the severity of the condition, many patients may not survive past age 20.[32, 38] Metastatic melanoma frequently is the cause of death. Complete sun avoidance is essential, and radiotherapy should be avoided. Treatment of the skin cancers, when they develop, is otherwise similar to that of ordinary skin cancers.

Keratoses

Inorganic arsenic has an affinity for keratinizing epithelium, and after a latency period of 10 years or greater, individuals with a history of arsenic ingestion will begin to develop multiple punctate keratoses[18, 32] of the palms and soles. Keratoses seen on the palms and soles in these patients are usually quite hyperkeratotic and 2 to 5 mm in diameter (Fig. 47–17). More important, such patients may begin to develop basal cell and squamous cell carcinomas with a higher incidence rate than that found in the normal population. Arsenic was a major component of a number of herbicides and pesticides and historically was a component of some patent medications (Fowler's solution was probably the most common). In addition to the increased numbers of basal cell carcinomas and squamous cell carcinomas, these patients may have increased incidence of internal malignancy, although this point is controversial in the literature.

Other Syndromes

A series of rare *adnexal tumors* may be found on the skin. Those that arise from sweat glands (eccrine or apocrine) do not have a distinctive clinical appearance.

The apocrine tumors generally arise from the external auditory canal, eyelid, axillary, or inguinal region. Tumors that show hair follicle differentiation usually occur on the scalp, but they may arise also from any other site, except palms and soles.

In addition, the dermal tissues may be the source of malignant lesions. *Malignant angioendotheliomas* arising from vascular tissue have an affinity for the scalp and face of older individuals.[28] Rarely, malignant degeneration may occur in the lesions of von Recklinghausen's neurofibromatosis. *Liposarcomas* and *fibrosarcomas* are uncommon; when they occur in the skin, they usually present as subcutaneous nodules or masses.

Benign pilar or *epidermal cysts* are perhaps the most

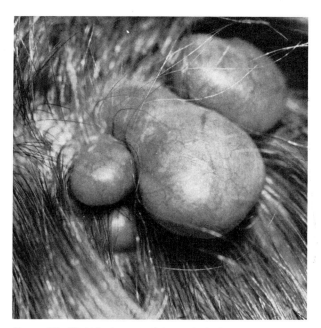

Figure 47–18. Cylindromas of the scalp become smooth with telangiectasia and may become quite large.

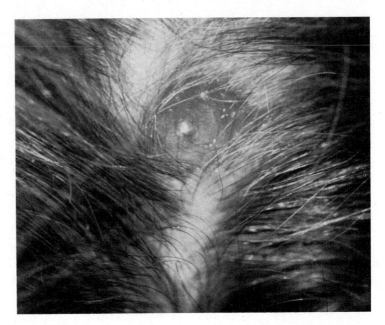

Figure 47–19. Renal cell carcinoma metastatic to the scalp.

common lesions of the scalp. However, two other tumors deserve special mention.

Cylindroma may be single or multiple and occurs as smooth nodules of the scalp. Cylindromas generally are only a few centimeters in diameter, but may be quite large and numerous (Fig. 47–18). When multiple, they frequently occur in association with multiple trichoepitheliomas of the face and show a dominant inheritance pattern. Cylindroma probably arises from apocrine structures and is generally a benign tumor, although occasional malignant degeneration has been reported.

Benign blue nevi occur as gray or bluish nodules anywhere on the skin or mucosa and usually are a centimeter or less in diameter. Malignant blue nevus is a rare tumor that may differ clinically from the benign form by presence of ulceration or by continued enlargement.[32] Malignant blue nevi may show either metastases limited to regional lymph nodes or quite aggressive spread with widespread metastases. Biopsy is required to establish diagnosis.

CUTANEOUS METASTASES OF THE SKIN

Cutaneous metastases are uncommon, occurring in less than 3 per cent of patients who have internal malignancies.[32] In women, breast carcinomas account for the greatest number of cutaneous metastases; in men, lung carcinomas are the most common cause of cutaneous metastases. Carcinoma of the large intestine is the second most common cause of cutaneous metastases in both sexes. Hematogenous dissemination is the usual mode of spread to the skin, although carcinomas of the breast or oral cavity may invade the skin directly through lymphatic channels. Cutaneous metastases may occur at any site, but the scalp is one of the most common sites of involvement. The outstanding characteristic is the extreme firmness of the metastatic nodules. Alopecia is common in scalp metastases (Fig. 47–19).

It is important to realize that cutaneous metastases from the hematogenous dissemination of an internal carcinoma may be apparent before the primary tumor is recognized. This is particularly true of carcinomas of the lung and kidney. In instances in which metastases occur early, usually only one or a few cutaneous nodules are encountered. However, in patients who develop late cutaneous metastases, the lesions are often multiple, and in these cases survival is only about 3 months, as a rule.[32]

REFERENCES

1. Albert RE: Skin carcinogenesis. *In* Andrade R (ed): Cancer of the Skin, vol. II. Philadelphia, W. B. Saunders Co., 1976.
2. Ariel IM: Malignant Melanoma. New York, Appleton-Century-Crofts, 1981.
3. Bagley FH, et al: Changes in clinical presentation and management of malignant melanoma. Cancer 47:2126, 1981.
4. Baker SR, Krause CJ: Cancer of the lip. *In* Suen JY, Myers EN (eds): Cancer of the Head and Neck. New York, Churchill Livingstone, 1981.
5. Becker FF: Lentigo maligna and lentigo maligna melanoma. Arch Otolaryngol 104:352, 1978.
6. Breslow A, Geelhoed GW: Tumor thickness as a guide to treatment in cutaneous melanoma. *In* Ariel IM (ed): Malignant Melanoma. New York, Appleton-Century-Crofts, 1981.
7. Burg G, et al: Histographic surgery: Accuracy of visual assessment of margins of basal cell epithelioma. J Dermatol Surg Oncol 1:21, 1975.
8. Casson P: Basal cell carcinoma. Clin Plast Surg 7:301, 1980.
8a. Clark WH Jr, from Bernadino L: The histogenesis and biologic behavior of primary human and malignant melanomas of the skin. Cancer Res 29:705, 1969.
9. Cohen C: Multiple cutaneous carcinomas and lymphomas of the skin. Arch Dermatol 116:687, 1980.
10. Colman WP III, et al: Treatment of lentigo maligna and lentigo maligna melanoma. J Dermatol Surg Oncol 6:476, 1980.
11. Crombie IK: Distribution of malignant melanoma on the body surface. Br J Cancer 43:842, 1981.
12. Day CL Jr, et al: Skin lesions suspected to be melanoma should be photographed. J Am Acad Dermatol 248:1077, 1982.
13. Dellon AL: Host-tumor relationships in basal cell and squamous cell carcinoma of the skin. Plast Reconstr Surg 62:37, 1978.

14. Doiron MJ: A comparison of noninvasive imaging modalities in the melanoma patient. Cancer 47:2581, 1981.
15. Epstein E: How accurate is a visual assessment of basal cell carcinoma margins? Br J Dermatol 89:37, 1973.
16. Epstein E, et al: Biopsy and prognosis of malignant melanoma. JAMA 208:1369, 1969.
17. Farmer ER, Helwig EB: Metastatic basal cell carcinoma: A clinicopathologic study of seventeen cases. Cancer 46:748, 1980.
18. Freeman RG: Carcinogenesis of skin neoplasms. In Anderson Hospital (ed): Neoplasms of the Skin and Malignant Melanoma. Chicago, Year Book Medical Publishers, 1976.
19. Freeman RG, Duncan WC: Recurrent skin cancer. Arch Dermatol 107:395, 1973.
20. Graham JH: Selected precancerous and mucocutaneous lesions. In Anderson Hospital (ed): Neoplasms of the Skin and Malignant Melanoma. Chicago, Year Book Medical Publishers, 1976.
21. Hamaker RC, Conley J: Melanoma of the head and neck. In Ariel IM (ed): Malignant Melanoma. New York, Appleton-Century-Crofts, 1981.
22. Hauben DJ, et al: The biologic behavior of basal cell carcinoma, parts 1 and 2. Plast Reconstr Surg 69:103, 110, 1982.
23. Howell JB: The roots of the nevoid basal cell carcinoma syndrome. Clin Exp Dermatol 5:339, 1980.
24. Howell JB, Anderson DE: Commentary: The nevoid basal cell carcinoma syndrome. Arch Dermatol 118:824, 1982.
25. Jackson R: Why do basal cell carcinomas recur (or not recur) following treatment? J Surg Oncol 6:245, 1974.
26. Jackson RJ: Pigmented tumors of the skin. J Surg Oncol 22:136, 1983.
27. Jackson R, Rowan HA: Horrifying basal cell carcinoma. J Surg Oncol 5:431, 1973.
28. Jansen GT, Westbrook KC: Cancer of the skin. In Suen JY, Myers EN (eds): Cancer of the Head and Neck. New York, Churchill Livingstone, 1981.
29. Khalil MK, et al: Sebaceous gland carcinoma of the lid. Can J Ophthalmol 15:117, 1980.
30. Kopf A, et al: Atlas of Tumors of the Skin. Philadelphia, W. B. Saunders Co., 1978.
31. Koplin I, Zarem MA: Recurrent basal cell carcinoma. Plast Reconstr Surg 65:656, 1980.
32. Lever WF, Shaumburg-Lever G: Histopathology of the Skin, 6th ed. Philadelphia, J. B. Lippincott Co., 1983.
33. Levine HL, Bailin PL: Basal cell carcinoma of the head and neck: Identification of the high risk patient. Laryngoscope 90:955, 1980.
34. Lillis PJ, Ceilley RI: Multiple tumors arising in nevus sebaceous. Cutis 23:3112, 1979.
35. Lynch PJ: Dermatology for the House Officer. Baltimore, Williams & Wilkins Co., 1982.
36. MacDonald EJ: Epidemiology of skin cancer. In Anderson Hospital (ed): Neoplasms of the Skin and Malignant Melanoma. Chicago, Year Book Medical Publishers, 1976.
37. MacKie RM: Clinical Dermatology: An Illustrated Textbook. New York, Oxford University Press, 1981.
38. McEvoy BF: Genodermatoses associated with malignancies. In Helm F (ed): Cancer Dermatology. Philadelphia, Lea & Febiger, 1979.
39. Menn H, Robins P, Kopf AW, et al: The recurrent basal cell epithelioma. Arch Dermatol 103:628, 1971.
40. Mohs FE: Chemosurgery: Microscopically Controlled Surgery for Skin Cancer. Springfield, Ill., Charles C Thomas, 1978.
41. Mora RG, Robins P: Basal cell carcinomas in the center of the face: Special diagnostic, prognostic, and therapeutic consideration. J Dermatol Surg Oncol 4:315, 1978.
42. Paletta FX: Squamous cell carcinoma of the skin. Clin Plast Surg 7:313, 1980.
43. Panje WR, Bumsted RM, Ceilley RI: Secondary intention healing as an adjunct to the reconstruction of mid facial defects. Laryngoscope 90:1148, 1980.
44. Panje WR, Ceilley RI: The influence of embryology of the mid face and the spread of epithelial malignancies. Laryngoscope 89:1914, 1979.
45. Rampen FHJ, et al: Incisional procedures and prognosis in malignant melanoma. Clin Exp Dermatol 5:313, 1980.
46. Reimer RR, Clark WH Jr, Greene MH, et al: Precursor lesions and familial melanoma: A new genetic preneoplastic syndrome. JAMA 239:744, 1978.
47. Rhodes AR, Lelski JW: Small congenital nevocellular nevi and the risk of cutaneous melanoma. J Pediatr 100:219, 1982.
48. Robins P: A dermatologist's approach to the management of skin cancer. Clin Plast Surg 7:421, 1980.
49. Robins P: Chemosurgery: My fifteen years' experience. J Dermatol Surg Oncol 7:779, 1981.
50. Robins P, Albon MJ: Recurrent basal cell carcinomas in young women. J Dermatol Surg Oncol 1:1, 1975.
51. Russell WG, et al: Sebaceous carcinoma of meibomian gland origin. Am J Pathol 73:504, 1980.
52. Sober AJ, et al: Primary melanoma of the skin. In Fitzpatrick TB, et al (eds): Dermatology in General Medicine: Update One. New York, McGraw-Hill Book Co., 1983.
53. Strauss M, Cohen C: Perineural invasion of the facial nerve: A case report with extension from cutaneous squamous cell carcinoma. Otolaryngol Head Neck Surg 89:831, 1981.
54. Taylor GA, Barisoni D: Ten years' experience in the surgical treatment of basal cell carcinoma. Br J Surg 60:522, 1973.
55. Thiers BH, Dobson RL (eds): The Yearbook of Dermatology. Chicago, Year Book Medical Publishers, 1982.
56. Vana J: Epidemiology. In Helm F (ed): Cancer Dermatology. Philadelphia, Lea & Febiger, 1979.
57. Waller G, Weindenbecher M: Recurrent basal cell carcinoma of the facial region—A clinico-pathological challenge. Arch Otorhinolaryngol 215:61, 1979.
58. Weimar VM, Ceilley RI: Basal cell carcinoma of the medial canthus with invasion of supraorbital and supratrochlear nerves: Report of a case treated by Mohs' technique. J Dermatol Surg Oncol 5:279, 1979.
59. Weimar VM, Ceilley RI, Goeken JA: Cell-mediated immunity in patients with basal and squamous cell carcinoma. Am Acad Dermatol 2:143, 1980.
60. Weimar VM, Ceilley RI: Aggressive biologic behavior of basal and squamous cell cancers in patients with chronic lymphocytic leukemia or chronic lymphocytic lymphoma. J Dermatol Surg Oncol 5:609, 1980.

CHAPTER 48

Pathology of Skin Tumors of the Head and Neck

J. Leslie Smith, Jr., M.D.

Tumors of the skin of the head and neck are more common than would be expected when the surface area of the head and neck is compared with that of the body as a whole. This is due primarily to the continuous exposure of this area to the environment, particularly solar irradiation. In addition, however, a wide variety of other tumors, unrelated to sun exposure, occur in this area; some are true neoplasms and others are developmental or hamartomatous in nature. A comprehensive discussion of the pathology of skin tumors of the head and neck would include the majority of all skin tumors. This presentation summarizes the clinicopathologic features of the important epithelial and melanocytic tumors occurring in this area.

EPIDERMAL LESIONS

Premalignant Epidermal Lesions

The most common premalignant epidermal lesion of the skin of the head and neck is *actinic keratosis*. Most of the other true premalignant lesions, the classical Bowen's disease and erythroplasia of Queyrat, occur in other areas of the body and have a different etiology. The epidermal changes in patients with xeroderma pigmentosum are similar, if not identical, to those of actinic keratosis, and the histologic features described for actinic keratosis apply to it as well.

The cumulative effect of sun exposure on the skin results in malignant transformation of epidermal epithelial cells. When the transformed cells are confined to the epidermis, the term "actinic" or "solar" keratosis is employed. At one time the term "senile" keratosis was used, but it was recognized that not all patients with such lesions are elderly and that its occurrence depended more on individual predisposition, with light-complexioned individuals being more predisposed than those with dark complexions.

The cytologic and histologic features of actinic keratosis are variable, both in degree and type.[25, 49] The basic change is that of dyskeratosis, or abnormal progression of maturation of the epidermal cells, generally beginning in the basal layer. The dyskeratosis varies from mild to moderate to severe, the latter being a fully developed carcinoma in situ (Fig. 48–1). The latter lesions are often qualified as "bowenoid type." Actinic keratoses, histologically as well as clinically, are usually not discrete solitary lesions, but multifocal. Other histologic features include hyperkeratosis, often alternating with parakeratosis. The intraepidermal eccrine pore is not involved in the process, and the keratin overlying a pore is of different character than that overlying the lesion. An underlying dermal chronic inflammatory response is common, the infiltrate frequently consisting largely of plasma cells. Actinic degenerative changes of dermal collagen and elastic tissue usually accompany the epidermal changes.

Within the histologic spectrum of actinic keratosis and carcinoma in situ there are several histologic subtypes:[67]

1. The *hypertrophic type* shows pronounced hyperkeratosis with moderate to marked acanthosis and occasionally papillomatosis. The hyperkeratosis, when marked, can result in the formation of a cutaneous horn.

2. The epidermis of the *atrophic type* is thinned and flattened and may show only slight hyperkeratosis.

3. The *acantholytic type* is characterized by areas of suprabasal acantholysis (Fig. 48–2). This type is common in the pre- and postauricular regions and is the precursor of the adenoid squamous carcinoma pattern.[64]

4. In the bowenoid type, the dyskeratosis is present through the full thickness of the epidermis, simulating the histologic pattern of classical Bowen's disease, which usually occurs on nonexposed areas.

Other variants of actinic keratosis, not included in the preceding classification, but which in my experience have distinctive cytologic features, include the clear cell type, spindle cell type, and the occasional lesion with markedly anaplastic and pleomorphic cells, all of which have corresponding invasive carcinoma counterparts.

Malignant Epidermal Tumors

The two most common malignant epidermal tumors are basal cell carcinoma and squamous cell carcinoma. The rare Merkel cell carcinoma is being included under this heading, since Merkel cells are normally present in the epidermis. However, it is recognized that not all Merkel cell carcinomas have shown a relationship to the epidermis.

Basal Cell Carcinoma

Basal cell carcinoma (basal cell epithelioma) is the most common of the malignant epidermal tumors of the head and neck. As indicated previously, basal cell

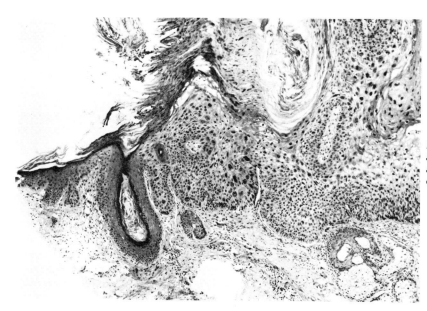

Figure 48–1. Actinic keratosis showing acanthosis with marked dyskeratosis and parakeratosis. Actinic degenerative changes are present in the dermis.

carcinomas do not form a homogeneous clinicopathologic entity. The classification considered most useful includes the (1) nodular or noduloulcerative, (2) the morphea or sclerosing, and (3) superficial multicentric types. Further histologic subclassification does not appear of value in selecting the best therapeutic regimen, but for completeness the other less common forms will also be described.

Nodular or Noduloulcerative Type. This is the most common histologic, as well as clinical, type. The tumor is composed of a solid nodule, or nodules, of uniform, basal type cells (Fig. 48–3). The cells at the periphery of the nests tend to be taller and more columnar with a palisading arrangement. Multiple sections may be required to demonstrate continuity with the epidermis or hair follicle. Not all the nests or nodules are solid, however, some exhibiting central cystic degeneration

for which reason the designation of cystic basal carcinoma is applied. Such lesions may be truly cystic with only a rim of viable tumor remaining. The nodules of other tumors may have an adenoid or adenoid cystic patterns in which there are gland-like spaces separated by interconnecting cords of basal cells, one or two cells in thickness. Keratinization may be present in some lesions, qualifying it for the keratotic type. Combinations of these patterns may be seen in the same tumor.

Morphea-like or Sclerosing Type. This histologic variant is characterized by irregular cords or strands of infiltrating basal cells in a dense sclerotic fibrous stroma. The compressed strands are occasionally only one or two cells in thickness. The thicker clusters of cells usually have an irregular outline with attenuated processes or branches. Unlike the nodular basal cell variant, the margins of the lesions and the extent of infiltration

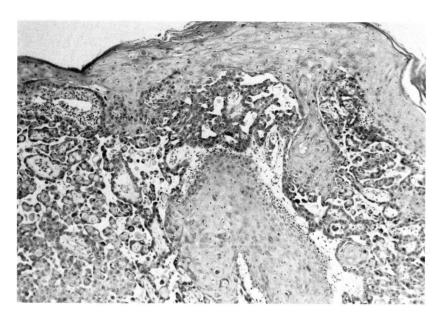

Figure 48–2. Adenoid squamous carcinoma showing acantholysis and pseudoglandular formations.

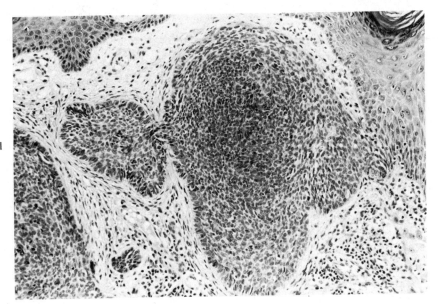

Figure 48–3. Solid nest of basal cell carcinoma with peripheral palisading.

may be ill defined. Thus, the adequacy of excision may be difficult to determine both clinically and histologically, accounting for the frequent recurrences of these tumors.

Superficial Multicentric Type. This variant is characterized by superficial multicentric proliferations of basal cells of the epidermis (Fig. 48–4). The proliferations are usually small, irregular, and only superficially invasive. They are solid with a well-defined border. The peripheral cells usually have a palisade arrangement. Varying degrees of dermal fibrosis are present around and between the proliferations.

Fibroepithelial Type (Fibroepithelioma of Pinkus). This variant, described by Pinkus in 1953, was not considered initially to be a basal cell carcinoma, but is now so considered.[48] The lesions often have a polypoid configuration. Histologically, they are characterized by thin cords or strands of basal cells that have multiple points of contact with the epidermis, forming an anastomosing network embedded in a prominent fibrous stroma, which is an integral part of the lesion (Fig. 48–5).

Pigmented Basal Cell Carcinoma. Basal cell carcinomas exhibit varying degrees of melanin pigmentation, ranging from virtually no pigment to those very heavily pigmented. The pigment is present in tumor cells and dendritic melanocytes. It may also be present in melanophages in the dermis. The significance of the pigmented tumors is that they may be confused clinically with malignant melanoma.

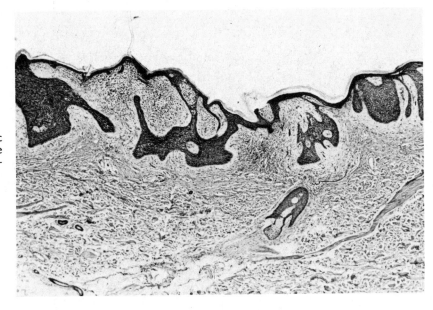

Figure 48–4. Superficial multicentric basal cell carcinoma showing multiple irregular superficial basal cell proliferations in continuity with the epidermis.

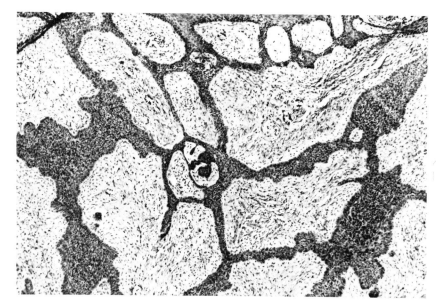

Figure 48–5. Fibroepithelial type of basal cell carcinoma showing anastomosing cords of basal cells imbedded in a prominent fibrous stroma.

Basosquamous Carcinoma (Metatypical Basal Cell Carcinoma). Occasional carcinomas exhibit histologic features of both basal cell and squamous carcinoma. The histogenesis of such tumors and their biologic behavior is still not entirely clear. The possibility of their representing a "collision tumor" is unlikely because transition between the two patterns can be observed in the same tumor. The evidence seems to favor their representing a histologic intermediate between the two carcinomas.[44] It has been suggested that its biologic behavior is somewhat more aggressive than the usual basal cell carcinoma, but convincing proof is lacking.

Basal Cell Carcinoma with Sebaceous Differentiation (Sebaceous Epithelioma). It is not uncommon for basal cell carcinoma to show some degree of differentiation. Their clinical features and biologic behavior are similar to those of typical basal cell carcinoma.[54]

Basal Cell Nevus Syndrome. Basal cell carcinomas observed in the basal cell nevus syndrome are indistin-guishable histologically from the usual varieties of basal cell carcinomas.[40]

Squamous Cell Carcinoma

"Squamous carcinoma" is a term for malignant epithelial tumors that exhibit cellular differentiation of the type seen in normal squamous epithelial tissues, such as the epidermis and squamous mucosal surfaces. It is a descriptive term that has little significance without knowledge of the site of origin. For example, squamous carcinomas arising from squamous mucosa of the lip are much more aggressive than those with similar degree of differentiation arising across the vermilion border on the skin side of the lip. It is also important to determine, if possible, its etiology for carcinomas with the same degree of differentiation, but different causes also can differ in biologic behavior. As an example, squamous carcinomas secondary to x-ray exposure may

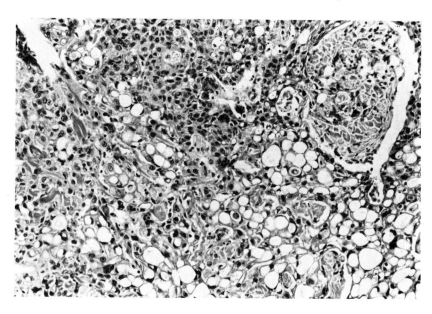

Figure 48–6. Clear cell squamous carcinoma pattern.

be highly aggressive, even though the pattern is well differentiated. Conversely, the majority of squamous carcinomas of skin in the head and neck region arising on the basis of actinic keratosis exhibit a nonaggressive biologic behavior and rarely metastasize. Other etiologic factors causing squamous carcinomas include thermal burns, chemicals, and chronic inflammation.[8] Squamous carcinomas arising from these causes are in general more aggressive than solar-induced tumors. Some squamous carcinomas appear to arise de novo, and these also are usually more aggressive than those arising on the basis of actinic keratosis.

In our experience the best indicator of biologic behavior of solar-induced squamous carcinomas is the size and depth of a lesion. If the biologic behavior of poorly differentiated squamous carcinomas and well-differentiated squamous carcinomas, of the same size and depth of invasion and arising on the basis of solar keratosis, are compared, our experience has been that the biologic behavior of the tumors are similar.

There are a variety of squamous cell carcinoma patterns, as well as degrees of differentiation, among which are the adenoid squamous carcinomas,[32, 64] the clear cell carcinomas, and the spindle cell carcinomas.[22] The adenoid squamous carcinomas are most common, though not exclusively, on or around the ear region. The preinvasive counterpart is acantholytic actinic keratosis. The adenoid squamous carcinoma pattern is characterized by cords or nests of invading carcinoma in which there is acantholysis, at times resulting in the formation of glandular or ductal patterns (Fig. 48–2). The clear cell (Fig. 48–6) and spindle cell squamous carcinomas are those in which those specific cell types predominate. It does not appear that the cell types have any particular significance with regard to the biologic behavior of the carcinoma.

Merkel Cell Carcinoma

Merkel cell carcinoma is an undifferentiated, malignant, small round cell neoplasm, commonly occurring in the skin of the head and neck (Fig. 48–7).[57] It was identified as a tumor of Merkel cells in 1978; before this time the tumors were often diagnosed as metastatic undifferentiated bronchogenic carcinoma or carcinomas of other origin. Ultrastructurally, the tumor cells show neuroendocrine granules, and for this reason the designation of neuroendocrine carcinoma has also been employed.[58] The lesions are usually solitary, although occasionally they are multiple. Their biologic behavior is aggressive, and death results from widespread metastases in a significant percentage of cases.

Benign Epidermal Tumors

The two important benign epidermal tumors of the head and neck are *seborrheic keratosis* and *keratoacanthoma*. Seborrheic keratosis, though usually not a diagnostic problem histologically, is important because of its frequency, and because clinically it can occasionally be confused with malignant melanoma. Keratoacanthoma is important because it must be distinguished from squamous cell carcinoma.

Seborrheic Keratosis

Histologically, as well as clinically, seborrheic keratoses are sharply demarcated, keratotic, and usually pigmented lesions, elevated above the level of the adjacent epidermis. They are characterized by acanthosis, hyperkeratosis, and papillomatosis and present a variety of histologic patterns. The most common type is the acanthotic type in which the epidermis shows

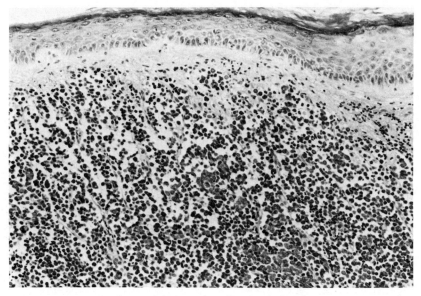

Figure 48–7. Merkel cell carcinoma consisting of undifferentiated malignant small cells.

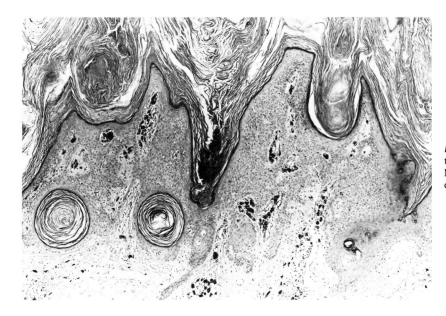

Figure 48–8. Seborrheic keratosis, acanthotic type, containing keratin tunnels. Numerous melanophages are present in dermis.

marked acanthosis, composed of compact cells, usually of basaloid type (Fig. 48–8). In some lesions the cells are more squamoid, or there may be combinations of the two cell types. Melanin pigmentation may range from slight to extremely heavy, for which reason the heavily pigmented lesions can be confused clinically with melanoma. Keratin cysts or tunnels are usually present within the acanthotic component. In the adenoid type thin anastomosing cords of cells, often two cells in thickness, are separated by dermal stroma (Fig. 48–9). Keratin cysts may or may not be present. In the "irritated" seborrheic keratosis varying numbers of "squamous eddies," small whorls of squamoid cells, are present. Hyperkeratosis may be the most prominent feature, for which reason it is designated hyperkeratotic type. Malignant transformation in a seborrheic keratosis has been reported, but it is exceedingly rare.

Keratoacanthoma

The diagnosis of keratoacanthoma is clinicopathologic.[1, 34, 35] A characteristic lesion develops over a 4- to 12-week period, during which time it assumes an elevated dome-shaped configuration with a central keratin plug. A typical lesion is characterized histologically by marked epidermal acanthosis, which assumes a cup-shaped configuration. The periphery of the cup is composed of irregular sheets and islands of squamous cells. On the surface, at the edge of the keratin plug, the squamous epithelial proliferation is in direct continuity with the epidermis.

The cytologic and histologic features vary according to the stage of evolution. Distinction from squamous cell carcinoma can be difficult in the early, rapidly proliferating phase, particularly if the specimen is sub-

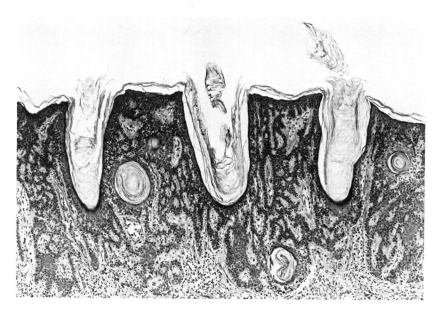

Figure 48–9. Seborrheic keratosis, adenoid type, showing thin anastomosing cords of basal cells and keratin tunnels.

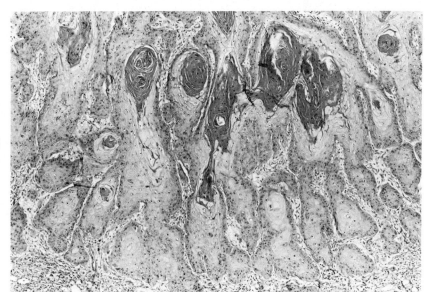

Figure 48–10. Base of keratoacanthoma showing irregular sheets and islands of squamous cells with central keratinization.

mitted piecemeal and is not representative. At this stage, mitotic figures may be frequent and the cells may appear immature. The cords or islands of cells around the base of the cup at this stage may appear irregular and ill-defined (Fig. 48–10). As the lesion "matures," however, the rate of cellular proliferation subsides, the cells composing the nests become better differentiated, and the nests are better defined with distinct borders. The progression of maturation of the squamous cells is toward the center of the cup, where a well-defined, irregular keratin plug is formed. As a lesion regresses, the epithelial mass becomes smaller and less cellular and the islands fewer in number. The epithelium at the base of the lesion ultimately flattens out, simulating normal epidermis, although it is depressed and hyperkeratotic. Following complete regression, there is a residual depressed scar at the site of the lesion. Regression may occur over several months. Distinction from squamous cell carcinoma is occasionally difficult under the best of circumstances. Without clinical information and representative or adequate tissue specimens, distinction from squamous cell carcinoma may not be possible.

ADNEXAL TUMORS

Tumors of the skin adnexa are very common in the head and neck region. Some are true neoplasms; others are hamartomas. For practical purposes, the clinician usually needs to know only whether such a lesion is benign or malignant. However, it is important to recognize that some benign tumors may simulate malignant tumors histologically, particularly if the specimen is submitted in pieces and is not representative.[28] It is very important that the clinician provide the pathologist with adequate clinical information as well as an adequate and representative specimen. The features of the more common adnexal tumors occurring in the head and neck region are summarized in the following paragraphs.

Hair Follicle Tumors

Pilar Cyst (Trichilemmal Cyst). Pilar cysts usually occur in the scalp region. They have no distinctive clinical features and are indistinguishable from epidermal inclusion cysts. Histologically, the cysts are lined by epithelial cells without intercellular bridges and the lining cells particularly near the surface are plump with abundant cytoplasm (Fig. 48–11). No granular cell layer is present as seen in epidermal inclusion cysts, and the cyst is filled with amorphous eosinophilic material rather than recognizable keratin material.

Proliferating Pilar Cyst. An occasional pilar cyst exhibits marked hyperplasia or proliferation of the pilar epithelial cells (proliferating epidermoid cyst, pilar tumor, giant hair matrix tumor, proliferating trichilemmal cyst). Such lesions may suggest malignancy both clinically and histologically, but their biologic behavior appears benign, yet recurrences may occur with incomplete excision.[7, 16, 74] The lesions are most commonly seen on the scalp, and the majority of patients have been elderly women. Lesions may be quite large, measuring several centimeters in diameter. Histologically, the proliferation forms well-defined, marginated lobules of squamous cells, often exhibiting some degree of dyskeratosis (Fig. 48–12). The center of the lobules may contain amorphous eosinophilic material of the type seen in simple pilar cysts. The tumor is usually dermarcated from the surrounding stroma, without suggestion of active invasion.

Trichoepithelioma. Patients with trichoepithelioma may have multiple lesions, or they may present with a solitary lesion.[27] The term "epithelioma adenoides cysticum" has been used for patients with multiple lesions. The patients present with multiple small tumors of the face, particularly in the paranasal region, which appear in childhood or around puberty. The scalp, neck, and back may also be involved. The lesions are asymptomatic, small skin-colored papules or nodules, ranging from a millimeter to a centimeter in size. Approximately two thirds of the patients with multiple lesions have a family history of the disease, which is transmitted as an

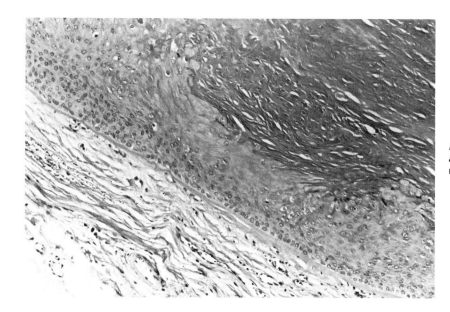

Figure 48–11. Pilar cyst containing amorphous material and lined by squamoid cells without a granular cell layer.

autosomal dominant trait. Solitary trichoepithelioma is not diagnostic clinically and may mimic a variety of other benign lesions.

The histologic features of the lesions which present as multiple lesions are identical with those that are solitary. They are hamartomatous in nature and are characterized by varying combinations of keratin cysts, occasionally immature hair follicles, islands of basoloid cells with peripheral palisading, epithelial tracts, and prominent stroma (Fig. 48–13). The islands of basaloid cells may be solid, but they often exhibit a lace-like arrangement that is intimately related to the surrounding stroma. Foreign-body granulomatous reaction is frequently encountered secondary to ruptured keratin cysts. Occasionally areas of calcification are present. Trichoepithelioma must be differentiated histologically from basal cell carcinoma, which it may closely resemble, particularly if a specimen is received in fragments

and is not representative. If a section of an intact lesion is available, differentiation is possible.

Trichofolliculoma. Trichofolliculoma usually occurs as a solitary lesion on the face, although less commonly it appears on the scalp or neck.[26, 50] They are small, dome-shaped nodules, averaging 4 mm in diameter, which are elevated slightly above the adjacent skin surface and have a central umbilicated opening. Some lesions may have a tuft of hair protruding through the opening, a feature which is virtually diagnostic clinically. Histologically, the lesion is characterized by a central dilated hair follicle that opens on to the skin surface. The dilated follicular space contains keratinous material in which small hairs may be seen. Occasional lesions may exhibit more than one dilated follicular space, each converging and opening onto the surface through the central opening. Multiple secondary hair follicle structures showing varying degrees of differen-

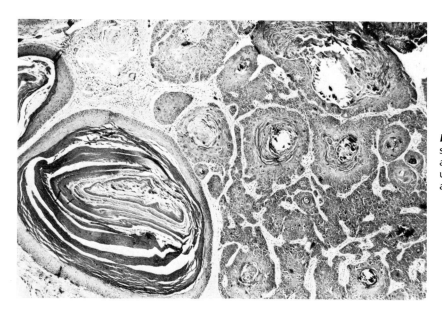

Figure 48–12. Proliferating pilar cyst showing a small, more typical pilar cyst and irregular proliferating nests or lobules with atypia. Focal foreign body reaction is present.

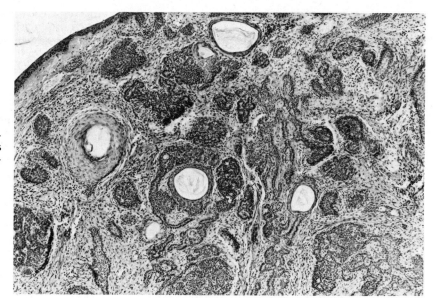

Figure 48–13. Trichoepithelioma containing keratin cysts and irregular islands and cords of basaloid cells in a prominent stroma.

tiation radiate perpendicularly from the epithelial lining (Fig. 48–14). Some are well-differentiated, miniature hair follicles forming small hairs, and others are composed of immature basaloid cells, which may not be readily recognizable as immature hair follicles. Some of the branching columns occasionally contain small keratinous cysts. The connective tissue intimately surrounding the lesion is well demarcated from the adjacent dermal stroma. When microscopic sections of a lesion are cut off-center, or when the specimen is received in fragments, the features of the lesion may not be recognizable and it is often diagnosed as basal cell carcinoma.

Pilomatrixoma. Known also as calcifying epithelioma of Malherbe, pilomatrixoma is a benign solitary hair follicle tumor common in young adults and children.[23] A high percentage of these lesions occur in the head and neck region. They present as firm, deep-seated cutaneous nodules ranging from a few millimeters to

several centimeters. The overlying skin is usually of normal color, and the lesions are asymptomatic.

Histologically, pilomatrixoma is characterized by a circumscribed tumor in the deep dermis, at times pushing into the subcutaneous tissue. It is composed of bands and sheets of epithelial cells with a convoluted configuration separated by connective tissue septa. The sheets are composed of two cell types, basophilic cells and shadow cells. The basophilic cells are considered to represent hair matrix cells. They are compact, of uniform cell type, and are present usually along the periphery of the convoluted sheets. The basophilic cells merge, usually gradually, into the shadow cells. Calcification is usually present, being observed at the periphery or end of a band of basophilic cells. Ossification may occasionally be seen. Some degree of squamous differentiation may be present. Foreign-body granulomatous reaction to the shadow cells is common. Specimens submitted

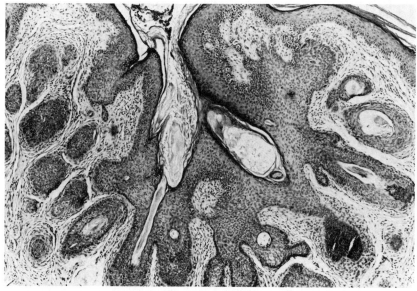

Figure 48–14. Trichofolliculoma showing a dilated follicle from which secondary immature hair follicles radiate.

to pathologists as fragments of tumor have on occasion been misdiagnosed as carcinoma.

Trichilemmoma. Trichilemmomas are small hair follicle tumors usually presenting as a solitary papule on the face.[9, 29] They are clinically not distinctive and may be misinterpreted as a basal cell carcinoma or verruca. Histologically, they are superficial lesions characterized by a lobule or lobules of cells extending from the epidermis into the dermis. The lobules are composed of variable numbers of clear cells containing abundant glycogen. Palisading of cells is present about the periphery of the lobules. The lobules are solid, except when there is a central identifiable hair follicle. Multiple trichilemmomas have been described as a part of Cowden's disease.

Sebaceous Gland Tumors

Senile Sebaceous Hyperplasia. Senile sebaceous hyperplasia occurs as one or several lesions in the head and neck region, particularly on the forehead and cheeks. The patients are usually of late middle age. The lesions appear as small, yellowish papules. Histologically, they are composed of mature, enlarged sebaceous lobules around a dilated, central keratin-containing duct or follicle. Clinically, they may be suspected of being basal cell carcinoma.

Nevus Sebaceus. Nevus sebaceus (nevus sebaceus of Jadassohn) is a pilosebaceous hamartoma, which is present at birth, usually on the scalp or in skin immediately around it.[10, 75] These lesions are irregular, slightly elevated plaques, devoid of hair, having a yellowish granular or verrucous surface. Histologically, they are characterized by poorly developed pilosebaceous structures that are situated at a higher level in the dermis than normal and that do not form normal hair (Fig. 48–15). The epidermis usually shows some degree of papillomatosis and acanthosis. The lesions may occur in conjunction with syringocystadenoma papilliferum. It has been reported that basal cell carcinoma develops in 6 to 10 per cent of the lesions.[19, 75]

Sebaceous Adenoma. True sebaceous adenomas are rare. They are clinically not distinctive, presenting as smooth, elevated nodules. Most lesions are solitary, although multiple sebaceous adenomas have been reported in association with visceral carcinomas, particularly carcinoma of the colon (Torre's syndrome).[53] Histologically, sebaceous adenomas are characterized by sharply demarcated irregular lobules of sebaceous type cells.[54] The cells composing the lobules are of two types: (1) the *germinative cells* of the type seen at the periphery of normal sebaceous glands and (2) the *differentiated sebaceous cells.* Transition between the two may be evident. Distribution of the two cell types within the lobules is variable, as are their proportions. Degeneration of sebaceous cells may result in cystic spaces. The term "sebaceous epithelioma" has been used for tumors that clinically present the features of basal cell carcinoma but histologically show some degree of sebaceous differentiation.

Sebaceous Carcinoma. The most common site of origin of sebaceous carcinoma is the meibomian gland of the eyelid.[4] It may occur in other skin sites, however. Although the clinical features are not distinctive, they are generally nodular and often ulcerated. The sebaceous carcinomas of the eyelid are solid and deep-seated and may or may not be ulcerated. They are aggressive and potentially metastatic, whereas on other skin sites they appear to have a low metastatic potential.[54] Cytologically and histologically they are similar to extraocular sebaceous gland carcinoma, although unlike those tumors, they often show pagetoid involvement of the conjunctival epithelium or overlying skin, or both.[55]

Eccrine Sweat Gland Tumors

Tumors of eccrine sweat glands are relatively uncommon. It is unnecessary for clinicians to be fully conversant with the complex classification of these tumors, not only because of the many types but also because of the multitude of terms, even for the same tumor. The diagnosis of benign or malignant eccrine sweat gland

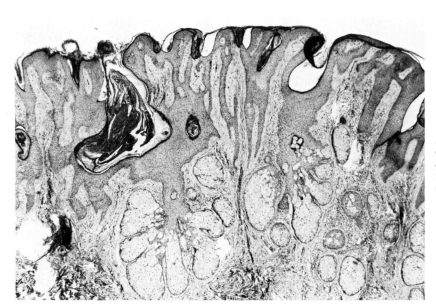

Figure 48–15. Nevus sebaceus of Jadassohn showing an irregular acanthotic and hyperkeratotic epidermis and abnormally developed and superficially located sebaceous glands.

tumor for practical purposes should be sufficient. Certain of the eccrine tumors, however, occur in the head and neck region more often than in other areas, and these will be summarized briefly.

Eccrine Hidrocystoma. Eccrine hidrocystoma is not a true tumor, it is a cystic dilatation of an eccrine sweat duct.[60] Though usually solitary, these lesions may be multiple. They are most frequently seen on the face, appearing as small translucent cystic nodules with a bluish hue, and range from 1 to 3 mm in diameter. Histologically, they are characterized by a small cystic structure lined by the two cell types that line normal eccrine ducts. If greatly distended, the cells may be flattened. Serial sections may demonstrate a normal eccrine duct in direct continuity with a cyst, and the coiled portion of the eccrine gland is frequently present beneath the cyst.

Syringoma. Syringomas present clinically as multiple small papules, often yellowish in color, in the skin of the lower eyelids and cheeks. They occur less frequently in other areas, such as the vulva, axilla, and groin. They usually become manifest around the time of puberty and are more common in females than males. Medical attention is usually sought for cosmetic reasons. Histologically, the lesions are characterized by multiple, small dilated eccrine sweat ducts in a fibrous stroma of the upper and middle dermis (Fig. 48–16). The cells lining the dilatations are usually flattened. Amorphous material is usually present in the lumen of the ducts. Epithelial strands often trail off from the ducts resulting in a common-like configuration. The strands may be seen in the stroma independent of cystic dilatations.

Dermal Eccrine Cylindroma. Cylindroma is probably the sweat gland tumor that clinicians most often associate with the head and neck area, probably because of the "turban tumors" often illustrated in textbooks. It is not uncommon, however, for the lesions to be solitary, and although the majority do occur in the head and neck region, they may occur in other body areas as well.[15] The tumor nodules range from a few millimeters to several centimeters. The skin overlying the nodules is smooth, often pinkish or reddish, occasionally with telangiectasia. Though the nodules may be numerous in the scalp area, forming the so-called "turban tumor," they more often occur singly or scattered. The lesions generally appear during adolescence or early adulthood, gradually increasing in size. Cylindroma of the multiple type is often dominantly inherited. Patients with multiple lesions may also have multiple trichoepitheliomas. Histologically, cylindroma is characterized by numerous islands or nests of basaloid epithelial cells forming nodules in the dermal stroma (Fig. 48–17). Characteristically, the nodules are irregular, of varying size, and form a compact, mosaic pattern. Each of the islands is surrounded by a layer of eosinophilic hyalin material, which though variable in thickness, in a given lesion is remarkably uniform. The hyalin material may be seen also as round deposits within the nests. The cells composing the nests are of two types, analogous to the cell types forming normal sweat ducts. One of the cells is small with a dark nucleus. These cells are usually at the periphery of the nests, where they may form a palisading pattern. The cells in the center of the nests tend to be larger with more vesicular nuclei. In some nests the two cell types may form a ductal structure with a lumen. The hyalin material stains positively with the periodic acid–Schiff (PAS) stain and is diastase-negative. It is important to recognize that the nests of cells may occur also as individual nests in the dermis apart from the tumor nodule. Of the various sweat gland tumor types, cylindroma is the one that tends to recur locally following excision (Fig. 48–17). This is explained by the presence of unrecognized nests that are left behind in the dermis at the time of excision. Malignant change may occur in cylindromas, but it is exceedingly rare. I have seen only one well-documented case. The case presented cytologic features of malignancy as well as aggressive local invasion.

Cylindroma of the skin should not be confused with adenoid cystic carcinoma of salivary gland origin, which in the past has also been referred to as "cylindroma and cylindromatous carcinoma." Other eccrine sweat gland

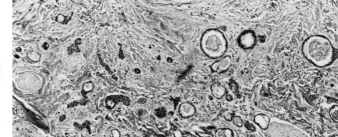

Figure 48–16. Syringoma illustrating multiple small cystic dilatations of eccrine sweat ducts.

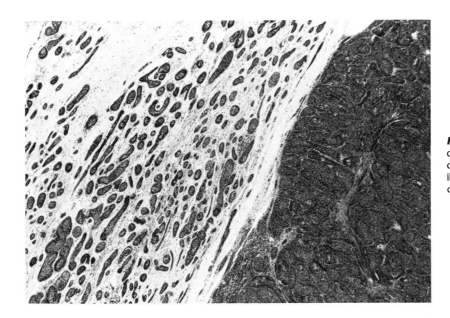

Figure 48–17. Dermal eccrine cylindroma consisting of islands of basaloid cells forming a mosaic pattern and similar islands lying separately in the adjacent dermis.

tumor types include eccrine poroma, eccrine acrospiroma, eccrine spiradenoma, and chondroid syringoma. Although these tumors may occur in the head and neck region, there is no particular predilection for them to do so and they will not be described in this presentation.

Apocrine Gland Tumors

Apocrine gland tumors, though rare, are most frequently encountered in the head and neck region. Apocrine tumors include apocrine hidrocystoma (apocrine cystadenoma), apocrine adenoma (including apocrine adenoma of ceruminous type, ceruminoma), and apocrine adenocarcinoma.

Apocrine Hidrocystoma. Apocrine hidrocystomas usually occur as solitary lesions on the face, ears, and scalp.[61] They may occur, however, in association with nevus sebaceus lesions and syringocystadenoma papilliferum. They have been described as often having a bluish color. If large, they present a cystic consistency. Their size may range from a millimeter to several centimeters. The cystic spaces are lined by two layers of cells, an inner layer of columnar cells with eosinophilic cytoplasm and basally situated nuclei, showing decapitation-type secretion.

Apocrine Adenoma of Ceruminous Type (Ceruminoma). Ceruminous glands present the cytologic, histologic, and ultrastructural characteristics of apocrine glands, and are therefore considered modified apocrine glands. Well-differentiated, benign localized proliferations of ceruminous glands form a variant of apocrine adenoma, referred to as *ceruminoma*.[18, 72] The histologic features are similar to apocrine adenomas in other body areas.

Syringadenoma (Syringocystadenoma) Papilliferum. Syringadenoma papilliferum is a hamartoma that appears to be as closely related to apocrine glands as any other adnexal structure. It occurs most commonly in the head and neck region and is usually noticeable at birth, although it may become more apparent at puberty.[28, 31] The lesions are not characterized by a tumor mass, but present as a slightly elevated, hairless plaque, at times papillomatous and crusty. Microscopically, the papillomatous appearance is due to irregular epidermal acanthosis with varying degrees of hyperkeratosis and the scattered cystic invaginations. In the depth of the cystic invaginations are micropapillations extending into the lumina of the cysts. The cysts and the papillae are lined by two layers of cells—an inner layer of cuboidal cells and an outer layer of columnar cells—occasionally showing decapitation secretion of apocrine gland type. The stromal core of the papillae is usually infiltrated by inflammatory cells, primarily plasma cells. Dilated apocrine glands are commonly present beneath the lesions. Basal cell carcinomas are reported to be associated with the lesions in about 10 per cent of the patients, and about one third of the cases are associated with nevus sebaceus of Jadassohn.

MELANOCYTIC TUMORS

The head and neck region is a common site for melanocytic lesions, both benign and malignant. These include hyperplasias, malformations or hamartomas (nevi), and true neoplasms. The majority of the lesions are the common variant of nevi and do not present major problems in diagnosis or treatment. However, a few of the benign melanocytic lesions can present problems in either histologic diagnosis or treatment. A brief review of the benign melanocytic lesions is presented in the following section, with emphasis given to those that can present these problems.

Benign Melanocytic Lesions

Ephelis. An ephelis, the common freckle, is a small, flat macular area of skin pigmentation occurring on the exposed skin surfaces, commonly of the head and neck. The macules are variable in size, most measuring 1 to 3 mm in diameter. They become clinically manifest during early childhood. Histologically, the ephelis is characterized by a localized increase in melanin pigment in an otherwise normal-appearing epidermis.

Lentigo. "Lentigo" is a nonspecific term for a flat, macular, hyperpigmented skin lesion. Unless qualified, such as in "lentigo maligna," the term refers to a benign lesion. There are two recognized forms: lentigo simplex and lentigo senilis (senile lentigo). Both are characterized by finger-like extensions or elongations of epidermis in which there is an increased amount of melanin pigment. In the head and neck area, lentigo senilis is the more important of the two. It is related to sun exposure and, in contrast to the ephelides and lentigo simplex, occurs in the later decades of life. It is more common in individuals with light complexions than in those with dark complexions. It is common to find the changes of actinic keratosis in the same specimen.

Melanocytic Nevi. A "nevus" is defined as a circumscribed new growth of skin of congenital origin. As such, it is a general term without specific reference to the tissue involved and implies a benign lesion unless specifically qualified, as in the rare "malignant blue nevus." "Melanocytic nevus" is employed for melanocytic lesions of this type. There are three general types of melanocytic nevi: the junction nevus, the intradermal nevus, and the compound nevus. The typical junction nevus is a flat, macular pigmented lesion, devoid of hair, which histologically is characterized by a well-demarcated nest of melanocytes (junction nevus cells) at the epidermal-dermal junction. In intradermal nevi, the melanocytic nevus cells are confined entirely to the dermis, and in compound nevi both junctional and intradermal nevus cells are present. Although these present a range of cytologic and histologic features, they are usually easily diagnosed histologically.[66]

The following variants of melanocytic nevi can present diagnostic and treatment problems.

HALO NEVUS (LEUKODERMA ACQUISITUM CENTRIFUGUM). A "halo nevus" is a descriptive clinical term for skin lesions characterized by a round peripheral zone of pigmentation about a centrally situated nevus.[24, 70] The head and neck area is a common site for the lesions, second only to the trunk, particularly the back. The majority of halo nevi occur during the first two decades. Males and females are affected with equal incidence. The halo nevus has a visible life cycle. Depigmentation, appearing at first around the periphery, in some instances progresses until the nevus disappears completely, leaving a round zone of vitiligo.[56] Histologically, the lesions in their early stage of evolution are characterized by the presence of a junction or compound nevus and a dermal chronic inflammation cell infiltration "hugging" and extending into the epidermis. The infiltration of inflammatory cells often obscures the dermal-epidermal junction and is associated with incontinence of pigment. Occasional lesions have been misinterpreted as malignant melanoma because of the inflammatory infiltrate and suggestion of dermal invasion. The nevus cells, however, are mature, of uniform type, and are similar to those in the junction nevus nests above or intradermal nevus cells in the dermis. As the active phase subsides, the inflammatory infiltrate becomes less intense. When a nevus disappears completely, it leaves a round area of depigmented epidermis.

SPINDLE AND EPITHELIOID CELL NEVUS (JUVENILE MELANOMA). The term "juvenile melanoma" was introduced in 1948 by Spitz to designate a melanocytic lesion in children, which, though disturbing cytologically and histologically, exhibited a benign biologic behavior.[65] The existence of such a lesion was confirmed, but the appropriateness of the term "juvenile melanoma" was questioned because the term "melanoma" carries a malignant connotation and such lesions are not confined to the juvenile period.[65] The term "spindle and epithelioid cell nevus" has been generally accepted by pathologists, although the designation of "Spitz nevus" is also used, particularly by clinicians.[21, 30, 46, 71] The spindle and epithelioid cell nevus is usually a solitary lesion, most often occurring in the head and neck region. Occasional patients have multiple lesions. The majority of lesions are observed in children and adolescents, but they also occur in adults. The lesions generally measure less than 1 cm in diameter, and clinically they are smooth, slightly elevated, hairless, and more often pink than brown, particularly in children. In children, the lesions are usually not recognized clinically as a nevus but more often are diagnosed as a hemangioma or pyogenic granuloma. Rarely, a patient may have multiple lesions. It is because of the atypical cytologic feature and the potential for misdiagnosis as malignant melanoma that the lesion is being emphasized. There is no one single histologic or cytologic feature that is diagnostic of these lesions, but the combination of features, of which the pathologist must be aware, and the clinical setting usually make correct diagnosis possible. Under the best of circumstances, such lesions can still present a diagnostic problem histologically.

CONGENITAL MELANOCYTIC NEVI. Congenital melanocytic nevi are melanocytic malformations present from birth.[51] The designation of "congenital giant hairy pigmented nevus" has been used for such lesions, but it is not entirely appropriate because not all such lesions are of "giant" size. Similarly, not all lesions are hairy. In the head and neck area, large lesions frequently involve the back of the neck, the "nuchal" variant. The concern of the patient and family is generally of a cosmetic nature. Another problem that has received increasing attention is the occurrence of malignant change in such a nevus.[33, 37, 45, 47] The true incidence of malignant change is not known because an accurate census of patients with giant congenital nevi is not available. Some have reported an incidence of 12 to 20 per cent, and for this reason excision of the entire lesion is often recommended. Complete excision often requires a deep and massive procedure, and the cosmetic results in our experience have been disappointing. It is the author's feeling that the incidence of malignant change is probably lower than reflected in the literature, but malignant change can occur. If it is not feasible to excise a lesion, the patient should be alerted to bring any change within the lesion to attention of the physician. Histologically, the bulk of the congenital nevus cells are of intradermal type. The nevus cells may produce marked thickening of the dermis and occasionally the subcutaneous tissue as well. Because of this, if surgical excision is performed for the purpose of eradicating the lesion, the subcutaneous tissue would have to be removed as well. The benign lesions, though often highly cellular, usually do not present diagnostic problems, cytologically or histologically. When malignant change does occur, it most often arises in the intradermal component. The diagnosis of malignancy is based on cytologically malignant cells, which often form a nodular, expansile growth within the lesion. Of importance also is the fact that patients with congenital melanocytic nevi, particularly the "nuchal" type, have a high incidence of meningeal melanocytosis, from which primary meningeal melanomas may arise.[59, 73]

BLUE NEVUS AND CELLULAR BLUE NEVUS. Blue nevus of the Jadassohn-Tieche type are most often observed on the dorsal surface of distal extremities, but they also occur commonly in the head and neck region. They are generally flat or only slightly elevated, blue-black, and hairless. It is unusual for a blue nevus to measure much more than a centimeter. The melanocytes composing the blue nevus are located in the dermis. They are bipolar and fusiform with tapering processes or stellate in configuration (Fig. 48–18). The melanocytes usually contain a large amount of melanin, although in some tumors the amount is minimal. The cells are often compressed and obscured by hypertrophic collagen bundles. At the margins of the lesion, the melanocytes usually fade into the adjacent connective tissue stroma. In the blue nevus category, it is the "cellular blue nevus" that may present a diagnostic problem histologically, not only because of its cellularity but also because of apparent extension in the subcutaneous tissue.[52] The cellular blue nevus is most often encountered on the sacral and buttock region and the dorsum of the foot and ankle, but it also occurs in the head and neck region. The majority of lesions are present at birth or appear during early childhood and thus are probably another form of congenital nevus. They are flat or slightly elevated, covered by smooth skin, and their color ranges from blue-black to gray-black. Most measure between 0.5 and 1.5 cm and unless subjected to trauma are asymptomatic. Patients usually seek medical attention because of the presence of a palpable mass and of pigmentation. Histologically, the cellular pattern

of the lesion is "biphasic," being composed of intertwining and intercommunicating well-defined fascicles and bundles of nevus cells, separated by stroma containing nevus cells of the more usual blue nevus type, though more cellular (Fig. 48–19).

DERMAL MELANOCYTOSIS (DERMAL MELANOCYTE HAMARTOMA). The "nevus of Ota" and the "nevus of Ito" are examples of dermal melanocytosis in the head and neck region.[11, 36, 42] These are malformations characterized by elongated, fusiform, or dendritic melanocytes, containing a variable amount of melanin pigment, interspersed between collagen bundles, usually in the middle and upper dermis. Cytologically, the melanocytes are similar, if not identical, to those seen in the blue nevus, though in blue nevi they are more numerous and localized.[20] In dermal melanocytosis the melanocytes are fewer in number and are distributed over a larger area. The "nevus of Ota" is a flat, macular, pigmented lesion, usually unilateral, involving the skin of the face, particularly the periorbital, temple, and malar regions, corresponding to the distribution of the first and second branches of the trigeminal nerve. The "nevus of Ito" differs from the "nevus of Ota" only by its location, which is usually the supraclavicular, scapular, or deltoid regions. The lesions are usually present at birth or appear shortly thereafter. The color of the lesions is variable, ranging from bluish gray to bluish black. The pigmentation is usually blotchy and irregular in outline. Though flat, the lesions may have slightly elevated areas within them. Dermal melanocytosis is not confined to the head and neck area, occurring on other body sites as well.

Premalignant Melanocytic Lesions

Lentigo Maligna. Lentigo maligna, or *melanotic freckle of Hutchinson*, is characterized clinically by a flat, slow-growing, irregular pigmented lesion that usually occurs

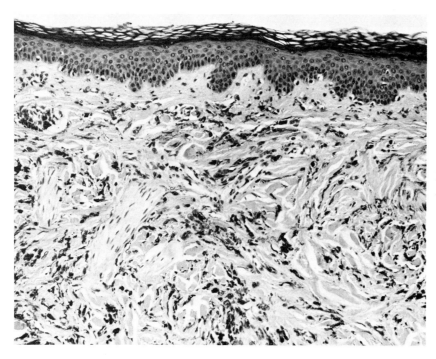

Figure 48–18. Blue nevus composed of pigmented fusiform melanocytic cells compressed between collagen bundles.

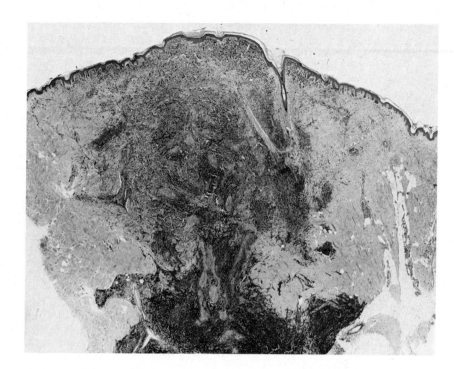

Figure 48–19. Cellular blue nevus extending from superficial dermis into subcutaneous tissue, illustrating biphasic pattern.

on the exposed skin of elderly individuals, particularly in the head and neck region.[13, 17, 41, 69] It is generally accepted as a premalignant melanocytic lesion. Initially it may be a relatively small macular lesion with a light tan color. Over a period of many years it may undergo progressive, irregular, peripheral spread. As it enlarges, the pigmentation becomes less uniform and more variegated, ranging from tan to light brown to dark brown. It is not common for the lesions to show areas of regression, manifested grossly by areas of depigmentation that at first may appear blue-gray but later becoming partially or completely depigmented. With continued growth, a lesion may reach several centimeters in size and the surface may become less regular. When

the pattern of pigmentation or rate of growth suddenly changes or nodularity develops in the lesion, the development of invasive melanoma is to be suspected. Lesions are present, on an average, 14 years before invasive melanoma develops. The histologic features of the early lesion are distinctive, characterized by an increase in the number of melanocytes in the basal layer of the epidermis, distributed over a relatively broad area in a single or double row (Fig. 48–20). The proliferation may extend down along hair follicles. The melanocytes in the early lesion are larger than normal melanocytes and have a clear or vacuolated cytoplasm and a hyperchromatic nucleus. As the melanocytic proliferation continues, the cells pile up, forming clusters, or *theques*, of

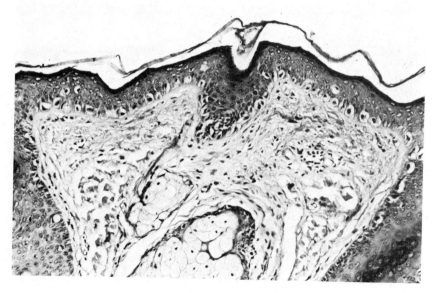

Figure 48–20. Lentigo maligna (melanotic freckle of Hutchinson), early lesion, showing atypical melanocytes distributed evenly in the basal layer of the epidermis.

cells. At this point it may be difficult to distinguish lentigo maligna from an in situ superficial spreading type of melanoma. The epidermal changes are almost invariably associated with actinic degenerative changes in the dermis. Once the lesion becomes invasive, it becomes a lentigo maligna melanoma.

Melanoma in Situ. The other type of flat melanoma, the superficial spreading melanoma, has a preinvasive or in situ phase also. Similarly, it is characterized by an intraepidermal proliferation of atypical or cytologically malignant melanocytes (Fig. 48–21). This form of melanoma is characterized by more rapid growth and an apparent tendency for earlier invasion than the lentigo maligna melanoma lesions. The term "melanoma in situ" has not become uniformly employed, however, for it is often difficult to define the dividing line between an atypical melanocyte and one that is frankly malignant. For this reason, some authors, including myself, often employ a descriptive designation of "atypical intraepidermal melanocytic proliferation," recognizing that some lesions could be, or are, in situ lesions. This terminology alerts the clinician to the atypical nature of the lesion but avoids giving the patient a melanoma diagnosis with all its connotations. Complete excision of lesions of this type is curative.

Malignant Melanoma

The diagnosis of malignant melanoma, unless otherwise qualified, such as malignant blue nevus or melanoma arising in a congenital nevus, refers to malignant neoplasms arising from the melanocytes of the epidermis. Clinically, malignant melanomas are generally flat or nodular. In 1969 Clark recommended the designations of "lentigo maligna melanoma" and "superficial spreading melanoma" for the flat varieties and "nodular melanoma" for the nodular variant.[12] "Acral lentiginous melanoma" has since been added to the flat melanoma

category, but this type does not occur in the skin of the head and neck.[14] These terms are now widely employed as clinicomorphologic types of melanoma. In recent years, questions have been raised, however, as to whether sharp lines of distinction exist between the melanoma categories,[2, 62] and in my experience there have been many lesions that have not readily fit into any of the specific categories. Yet, such a classification is generally considered useful.

The definitive diagnosis of melanoma, regardless of clinicomorphologic type, is based on the presence of unequivocal dermal invasion by cytologically malignant melanocytes from the epidermis.

In the flat lesions, the intraepidermal proliferation of atypical melanocytes does not exhibit an early tendency to invade, tending to "spread" peripherally before becoming invasive. The cells of the flat melanomas, once they become invasive, often exhibit loss of cohesion, and invasion usually occurs from multiple points of the epidermis (Fig. 48–22). Other cytologic and histologic features are looked for and noted in making a melanoma diagnosis, but these are used in support of the diagnosis, rather than as diagnostic features. These features include progression of the atypical melanocytes upward through the epidermis, the presence of mitotic figures, the presence of an inflammatory component, and the cytologic features of the invading cells.

In pure nodular melanomas, the melanocytic proliferation is more explosive, with a minimal intraepidermal component, suggesting origin de novo (Fig. 48–23). The rapid proliferation results in the formation of a nodule pushing into the dermis. Some flat lesions, at a point in time, may develop a superimposed nodule or nodules, a development having considerable prognostic significance.[62]

With regard to the prognostic significance of the clinicomorphologic melanoma types, there is a general impression that lesions diagnosed as lentigo maligna

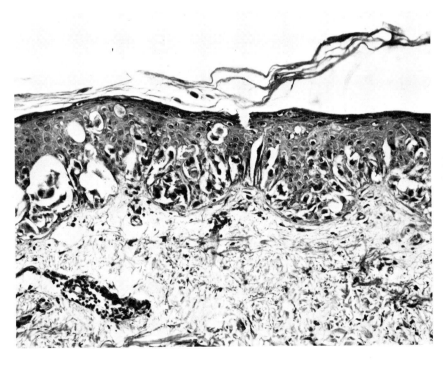

Figure 48–21. Melanoma in situ, superficial spreading type, characterized by an atypical intraepidermal melanocytic proliferation without invasion.

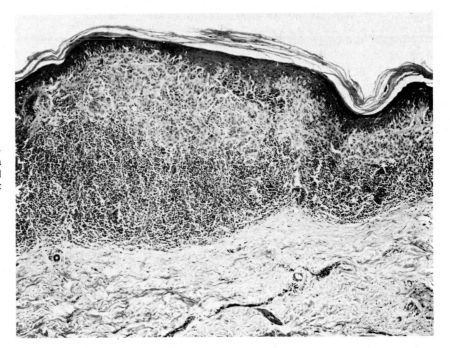

Figure 48–22. Low-power appearance of a flat malignant melanoma illustrating multiple points of epidermal melanocytic origin and a prominent inflammatory response.

melanoma are less aggressive than the other melanoma types. This has yet to be conclusively proved.[43] However, the superficial spreading melanomas are less aggressive than the nodular melanomas.[12, 62] The behavior of superficial spreading melanomas that develop superimposed nodularity is more aggressive than the pure flat lesion and more like that of nodular melanomas.[62]

Also, attempts have been made to determine a correlation between histologic features with behavior. In addition to the clinicomorphologic types just described, Clark recommended the use of "levels" of invasion for

documentation.[12] He defined a "level I" lesion as corresponding to melanoma in situ, a "level II" lesion as one in which invasion was confined to the papillary dermis, a "level III" lesion as one in which invasion extended to the junction of the papillary and reticular dermis, a "level IV" lesion as one in which there was invasion of the reticular dermis, and a "level V" lesion as one invading the subcutaneous tissue. A general correlation between the level of invasion and behavior was demonstrated, and the method was readily accepted and widely employed.[38, 68] A short time later,

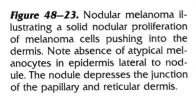

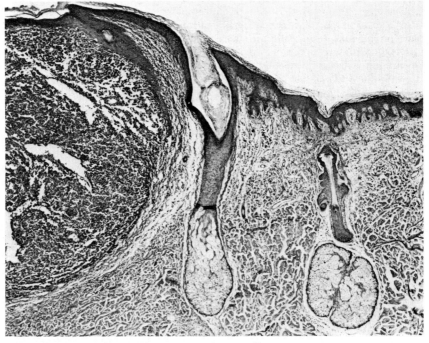

Figure 48–23. Nodular melanoma illustrating a solid nodular proliferation of melanoma cells pushing into the dermis. Note absence of atypical melanocytes in epidermis lateral to nodule. The nodule depresses the junction of the papillary and reticular dermis.

Breslow suggested that the measured thickness of a melanoma could also be correlated with behavior.[5, 6] Recognizing that there were problems in employing the levels system and that evidence supported a closer correlation between measured thickness and survival, many have accepted this method of documentation and at this time it is the documentation most often used.[3] In Breslow's original group of cases, no lesion smaller than 0.76 mm in thickness metastasized. In our institution, a routine melanoma report contains (1) diagnosis of malignant melanoma, (2) documentation as to whether it presents a primary or metastatic configuration, (3) the level of invasion, (4) the measured thickness, and (5) a statement regarding the adequacy of excision.

Cytologically, malignant melanoma is a great mimicker, capable of simulating a wide variety of other tumors. There is no one melanoma cell type, there being a very wide range, within the same lesion, as well as between different lesions. In my experience, it has been difficult to correlate specific melanoma cell types with behavior. Certain melanoma cell types are sufficiently distinctive, however, to have been given a descriptive cellular designation, such as desmoplastic melanoma and balloon cell melanoma.

The presence of inflammation in a melanoma appears to reflect the host's immunologic response to the lesion. It cannot serve as a specific diagnostic criterion because inflammation may be absent, or only slight, particularly in nodular melanomas, and may be present in benign melanocytic lesions, as in halo nevi. We also know that primary malignant melanomas undergo varying degrees of regression, at times complete, and that in the process of undergoing regression, it is the inflammatory infiltrate that is the most prominent feature.[63] Though the degree of inflammation cannot be used as a specific prognostic indicator, in general, patients with a moderate or marked inflammatory response exhibit longer survival than those with minimal or no inflammation.[62] Unfortunately, melanomas of some patients regress after having already metastasized, an immunologic paradox. Patients with metastatic malignant melanoma, but with no obvious primary lesion, may well have had unrecognized regression of a primary lesion and should be carefully examined for evidence of such regression.

Sex and age of patients can be correlated in a general way with behavior of melanomas, as can the location of the lesion.[39]

It is recognized that not all factors responsible for the biologic behavior of a malignant melanoma are reflected by the cytologic or histologic features observed by routine microscopy. Immunologic and other investigations may prove to be of value in this regard, but until these factors are identified and prove of value, light microscopy will remain the principal diagnostic modality, particularly of the primary lesion.

REFERENCES

1. Ackerman AB: Histopathology of keratoacanthoma. Andrade R, et al (eds): *In* Cancer of the Skin. Philadelphia, W. B. Saunders Co., 1976, p 781.
2. Ackerman AB: Malignant melanoma: A unifying concept. Hum Pathol 11:592, 1980.
3. Balch CM, et al: Tumor thickness as a guide to surgical management of clinical stage I melanoma patients. Cancer 43:883, 1979.
4. Boniuk M, Zimmerman LE: Sebaceous carcinoma of the eyelid, eyebrow, caruncle and orbit. Trans Am Acad Ophthalmol Otolaryngol 72:619, 1968.
5. Breslow A: Thickness, cross-sectional areas and depth of invasion in the prognosis of cutaneous melanoma. Ann Surg 172:902, 1970.
6. Breslow A: Prognostic factors in the treatment of cutaneous melanoma. J Cutan Pathol 6:208, 1979.
7. Brownstein MH, Arluk DJ: Proliferating trichilemmal cyst. Cancer 48:1207, 1981.
8. Brownstein MH, Rabinowitz AD: The precursors of cutaneous squamous cell carcinoma. Int J Dermatol 18:1, 1979.
9. Brownstein MH, Shapiro L: Trichilemmoma. Arch Dermatol 107:866, 1973.
10. Brownstein MH, Shapiro L: The pilosebaceous tumors. Int J Dermatol 16:340, 1977.
11. Burkhart CG, Gohara A: Dermal melanocyte hamartoma. Arch Dermatol 117:102, 1981.
12. Clark WH Jr, et al: Histogenesis and biologic behavior of primary human malignant melanoma of the skin. Cancer Res 29:705, 1969.
13. Clark WH Jr, Mihm MD: Lentigo maligna and lentigo-maligna melanoma. Am J Pathol 55:39, 1969.
14. Coleman WP, et al: Acral lentiginous melanoma. Arch Dermatol 116:773, 1980.
15. Crain RC, Helwig EB: Dermal cylindroma (dermal eccrine cylindroma). Am J Clin Pathol 35:504, 1961.
16. Dabska M: Giant hair matrix tumor. Cancer 28:701, 1971.
17. Davis J, et al: Melanotic freckle of Hutchinson. Am J Surg 113:457, 1967.
18. Dehner LP, Chen KTK: Primary tumors of the external and middle ear. Arch Otolaryngol 106:13, 1980.
19. Domingo J, Helwig EB: Malignant neoplasms associated with nevus sebaceus of Jadassohn. J Am Acad Dermatol 1:545, 1979.
20. Dorsey CS, Montgomery H: Blue nevus and its distinction from Mongolian spot and nevus of Ota. J Invest Dermatol 22:224, 1954.
21. Echevarria R, Ackerman LV: Spindle and epithelioid cell nevi in the adult. Cancer 20:175, 1973.
22. Evans HL, Smith JL: Spindle squamous carcinoma and sarcoma-like tumors of the skin. Cancer 45:2687, 1980.
23. Forbis R Jr, Helwig EB: Pilomatrixoma (calcifying epithelioma). Arch Dermatol 83:606, 1961.
24. Frank SB, Cohen HJ: The halo nevus. Arch Dermatol 89:367, 1964.
25. Graham JH, Helwig EB: Premalignant cutaneous and mucocutaneous disease. *In* Graham J et al (eds): Dermal Pathology. New York, Harper & Row, 1972, p 561.
26. Gray HR, Helwig EB: Trichofolliculoma. Arch Dermatol 86:619, 1962.
27. Gray HR, Helwig EB: Epithelioma adenoides cysticum and solitary trichoepithelioma. Arch Dermatol 87:1102, 1963.
28. Hashimoto K, Lever WF: Appendage Tumors of the Skin. Springfield, Ill., Charles C Thomas, 1968, p 46.
29. Headington JT, French AJ: Primary neoplasms of the hair follicle. Arch Dermatol 86:430, 1962.
30. Helwig EB: Seminar on the Skin Neoplasms and Dermatosis (Proceedings, 20th Seminar). American Society of Clinical Pathologists, 1955, p 63.
31. Helwig EB, Hackney VC: Syrinadenoma papilliferum. Arch Dermatol 71:361, 1955.
32. Johnson WC, Helwig EB: Adenoid squamous cell carcinoma (adenoacanthoma): A clinico-pathologic study of 155 patients. Cancer 19:1639, 1966.
33. Kaplan EN: The risk of malignancy in large congenital nevi. Plast Reconstr Surg 53:421, 1974.
34. Kern WH, McGray JK: The histopathologic differentiation of keratoacanthoma and squamous cell carcinoma of the skin. J Cutan Pathol 7:318, 1980.
35. Kopf AW: Keratoacanthoma—clinical aspects. Andrade R, et al (eds): *In* Cancer of the Skin. Philadelphia, W. B. Saunders Co., 1976, p 755.
36. Kopf AW, Weidman AI: Nevus of Ota. Arch Dermatol 85:195, 1962.
37. Kopf AW, et al: Congenital nevocytic nevi and malignant melanomas. J Am Acad Dermatol 1:123, 1974.
38. Lopansri S, Mihm MD Jr: Clinical and pathological correlation of malignant melanoma. J Cutan Pathol 6:180, 1974.
39. Marsden SB, et al: Malignant melanoma of the skin: The association of tumor depth and type, and patient sex, age and site with survival. Cancer 52:1330, 1983.
40. Mason JK, et al: Pathology of the nevoid basal cell carcinoma syndrome. Arch Pathol 79:401, 1965.
41. McGovern VJ, et al: Is malignant melanoma arising in Hutchinson's melanotic freckle a separate disease entity? Histopathology 4:235, 1980.

42. Mevorah B, et al: Dermal melanocytosis. Dermatologica 154:107, 1977.
43. Michalik EE, et al: Rapid progression of lentigo maligna to deeply invasive lentigo maligna melanoma. Arch Dermatol 119:831, 1983.
44. Okun MR, Edelstin LM: Gross and Microscopic Pathology of the Skin, vol. II. Dermatopathology Foundation Press, 1976, p 660.
45. Pack GT, Davis J: Nevus giganticus pigmentosus with malignant transformation. Surgery 49:347, 1961.
46. Paniago-Pereira C, et al: Nevus of large spindle and/or epithelioid cells (Spitz's nevus). Arch Dermatol 114:1811, 1978.
47. Penman HG, String HCW: Malignant transformation in giant congenital pigmented nevus. Arch Dermatol 103:428, 1971.
48. Pinkus H: Premalignant fibroepithelial tumors of the skin. Arch Dermatol Syph 67:598, 1953.
49. Pinkus H: Actinic keratosis—actinic skin. In Andrade R et al (eds): Cancer of the Skin. Philadelphia, W. B. Saunders Co., 1976, p 207.
50. Pinkus H, Sutton RLJ: Trichofolliculoma. Arch Dermatol 91:46, 1965.
51. Reed WB, et al: Congenital pigmented nevi, melanoma, and leptomeningeal melanocytosis. Arch Dermatol 91:100, 1965.
52. Rodriguez HA, Ackerman LV: Cellular blue nevus. Cancer 21:393, 1968.
53. Rulon DB, Helwig EB: Multiple sebaceous neoplasms of the skin: An association with multiple visceral carcinomas, especially of the colon. Am J Clin Pathol 60:745, 1973.
54. Rulon DB, Helwig EB: Cutaneous sebaceous neoplasms. Cancer 33:82, 1974.
55. Russell WG, et al: Sebaceous carcinoma of Meibomian gland origin: The diagnostic importance of Pagetoid spread of neoplastic cells. Am J Clin Pathol 73:504, 1980.
56. Shapiro L, Kopf AA: Leukoderma acquisitum centrifigum. Arch Dermatol 92:64, 1965.
57. Sidhu GS, et al: Merkel cell neoplasms. Am J Dermatopathol 2:101, 1980.
58. Silva E, Mackay B: Neuroendocrine (Merkel cell) carcinoma of the skin: An ultrastructural study of nine cases. Ultrastruct Pathol 2:1, 1981.
59. Slaughter JC, Hardman JM, Kempe LG, et al: Neurocutaneous melanosis and leptomeningeal melanomatosis in children. Arch Pathol 88:298, 1969.
60. Smith JD, Chernosky ME: Hidrocystomas. Arch Dermatol 108:676, 1973.
61. Ibid., Apocrine hidrocystoma (cystadenoma). Arch Dermatol 109:700, 1974.
62. Smith JL Jr: Histopathology and biologic behavior of malignant melanoma. In Neoplasms of the Skin and Malignant Melanoma. Year Chicago, Book Medical Publishers, 1976, p 293.
63. Smith JL Jr, Stehlin JS Jr: Spontaneous regression of primary malignant melanoma with regional lymph node metastases. Cancer 18:1399, 1965.
64. Smith JL, Tanaka T: Adenoacanthoma of the skin. In Tumors of the Skin. Chicago, Year Book Publishers, 1964, p 195.
65. Spitz S: Melanomas of childhood. Am J Pathol 24:591, 1948.
66. Stegmaier OC: Natural regression of the melanocytic nevus. J Invest Dermatol 32:413, 1959.
67. Strayer DS, Santa Cruz DJ: Carcinoma-in-situ of the skin: A review of histopathology. J Cutan Pathol 7:244, 1980.
68. Wanebo HJ, et al: Malignant melanoma of the extremities: A clinicopathology study using levels of invasion (microstage). Cancer 35:666, 1975.
69. Wayte DM, Helwig EB: Melanotic freckle of Hutchinson. Cancer 21:893, 1968.
70. Ibid.; Halo nevi. Cancer 22:69, 1968.
71. Weedon D, Little JH: Spindle and epithelioid cell nevi in children and adults: A review of 211 cases of the Spitz nevus. Cancer 40:217, 1977.
72. Wetli CV, et al: Tumors of ceruminous glands. Cancer 29:1169, 1972.
73. Williams HI: Primary malignant meningeal melanoma associated with benign hairy nevi. J Pathol 99:171, 1969.
74. Wilson-Jones E: Proliferating epidermoid cysts. Arch Dermatol 94:11, 1966.
75. Wilson-Jones E, Heyl T: Naevus sebaceus. Br J Dermatol 82:99, 1970.

CHAPTER 49

Surgical Therapy of Skin Tumors

Robert M. Bumsted, M.D. • Roger I. Ceilley, M.D.

Skin cancers involving the head and neck constitute the largest group of malignancies in this area. Malignancies in this location are readily visualized and are usually easily diagnosed, and with appropriate treatment a cure rate of over 95 per cent in early lesions can be achieved. Unfortunately, far-advanced tumors may extend deeply into the complex underlying anatomic structures of this region, requiring radical surgery, and these tumors carry a less favorable prognosis. Tumors involving certain anatomic locations such as the ears, nose, eyelids, and lip tend to have higher recurrence rates with greater morbidity and mortality than malignant neoplasms of the skin in general.

Prompt diagnosis and adequate treatment of skin cancers are extremely important. The fact that most skin cancers are curable tends to give many physicians a false sense of security when dealing with these lesions. All too often, biopsy confirmation of the pathologic diagnosis is not obtained prior to treatment because the lesion appears small, sharply circumscribed, and easily cured. Treatments based on these false premises may be inadequate. In addition, this attitude may lead to inadequate follow-up by the physician and neglect by the patient. The recurrent tumor (often lacking the typical appearance of a malignancy) may be dismissed as hypertropic scarring. Excessive concern with cosmesis in this region may also lead to inadequate extirpation.

The modern treatment of skin cancer encompasses surgical excision, electrosurgery, cryosurgery, Mohs' chemosurgery, chemotherapy, and, most recently, laser surgery. A thorough understanding of the indications for and limitations of these various therapeutic modalities is necessary in order to provide patients with optimal oncologic care. Proper selection of the method(s) of therapy depends on numerous factors, including:

1. Tumor type (primary or recurrent and cell type).
2. Size and depth of invasion.
3. Anatomic location.
4. Prior therapy (if any) and duration of tumor growth.
5. Skin type and degree of solar damage.
6. Age and general health of the patient.
7. Presence of solitary or multiple lesions.

In the most difficult cases a team approach including an oncologic and reconstructive surgeon, dermatologist, pathologist, medical oncologist, and rehabilitation specialist may be needed.

HISTORY

The search for an ideal approach to the management of cutaneous malignancies has led to many remarkable advances in medical knowledge and therapeutic techniques. In 1897, Gottheil stated that only early and superficial cases of skin cancer could be cured by operative or other methods of therapy.[13] At that time, treatment had consisted of excision, curettement, or destruction with cautery or various caustic agents. Advances in the 20th century have included radiation therapy; chemosurgery (1936); more recently, cryosurgery and medical oncology; and reconstructive surgery (in large part as a result of military surgical experience in the two great wars). A milestone in the progress of cutaneous oncology was the establishment of the New York Skin and Cancer Hospital in 1892. This was one of the first multispecialty hospitals in the world devoted to the study, prevention, and treatment of cancer. Now all major teaching hospitals in this country have such multidisciplinary oncologic activity. The first known causes of cancer (arsenic, tobacco, tars, radiation, thermal burns, sun damage, viruses, and injections) were discovered in part because they produced visible lesions of the skin or mucous membranes. Subsequent to these observations, the first experimentally produced malignancies were developed on the skin of laboratory animals by exposure to various chemical, physical, and infective carcinogens. This opened the avenue to modern research into carcinogenesis and oncologic therapy. Observations of the response of such experimental skin tumors have led to many of the modern therapeutic methods such as radiotherapy, chemosurgery, cryosurgery, immunotherapy, and chemotherapy.

ANATOMY

The anatomy of the head and neck, when compared with the rest of the body, appears to be unique in several ways in relation to cutaneous malignancies. These unique factors include cosmesis, vital function of certain structures, and the propensity for the spread of cutaneous facial malignancies along embryonic fusion planes.

The role of facial appearance in both the patients' feelings regarding themselves and the reaction of other individuals to this appearance is well known. Although minor degrees of cosmetic deformity may have minimal psychological and social effects, greater degrees of deformity can produce severe problems in these areas. The face is usually considered to be one's identity, as it is the focus of expression, perception, and outward countenance. In addition, it is a highly visible area that is difficult to cover with hair or clothes. Although the complete extirpation of cutaneous malignancies is always vital, the treating physician must always be cognizant of the effect of therapy on facial cosmesis so that psychologic and social problems can be recognized early and managed to minimize these effects during the post-therapeutic period.

Numerous structures on the face play a vital role in normal physiologic function in addition to cosmesis. The eyelids are necessary to maintain adequate hydration of the cornea to prevent desiccation and subsequent infection, ulceration, and possible visual loss. The lips are required for speech production and the maintenance of oral competency, which allows the patient to attain an adequate intake of liquids and food. The structure of the internal nose provides filtration, humidification, and warming of inspired air and also "recaptures" much of the heat and moisture given up to the inspired air during expiration. If the external nasal structure is destroyed, these functions may suffer a marked decrease in efficiency. The auricle appears to provide a minor contribution to directing sound waves into the external auditory canal. Although the effect of loss of the auricle in a young individual may be negligible, in an elderly patient with marginal hearing the loss of the auricle may result in an unsatisfactory social level of hearing.

In addition to these functional roles, the structure of the lower nose, auricle, and eyelids is also unique anatomically. Each has two closely approximated epithelial layers separated by a thin layer of cartilage. When invaded by a cutaneous malignancy, these structures often require complete excision of the involved area at a much earlier date than elsewhere in the body.

Cutaneous malignancies of the face also have a marked propensity to spread in a manner so that they remain between embryonic plane boundaries while they invade deeply at the site of embryonic fusion planes.[22, 24] This factor appears to be most significant in the nasal area (midportion of the nose, columella, mid upper lip, and nasolabial areas), intercanthal region, and auricle. When excising cutaneous malignancies in these areas of the face, the possibility of deep invasion along the embryonic fusion planes must always be considered, and attempts should be made to determine whether this is present.

DIAGNOSIS

Early diagnosis is one of the vital ingredients necessary to obtain optimal results in the treatment of cutaneous malignancies. In addition to early diagnosis, other vital factors include providing adequate treatment of the lesion itself and appropriate and prolonged postoperative care and follow-up.

Skin tumors of the head and neck are usually readily recognized and are easily detected by visual inspection (Fig. 49–1). Although advanced and large elevated lesions are easy to diagnose, the physician must be aware that even the most innocuous-appearing lesion can be malignant, and this possibility must be considered to obtain an early diagnosis. Any cutaneous lesion that increases in size, itches, bleeds, ulcerates, or changes in color has a higher risk of malignancy. A detailed history is also important and should include the general health of the patient as well as past exposure to carcinogens such as tobacco, radiation, arsenic, and ultraviolet light.

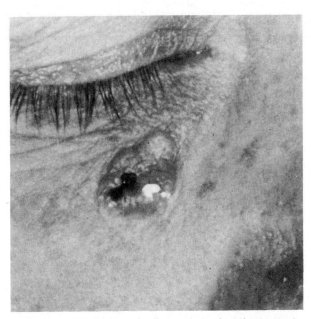

Figure 49–1. Nodular basal cell carcinoma, skin of right cheek.

Visual inspection of the lesion in question should be performed with an adequate light source that can be directed in several angles. The pearly translucent appearance of a basal cell carcinoma with its attendant telangiectasia is often best seen with tangential lighting. The pearly appearance can be best appreciated by gently stretching the skin while examining the lesion. The loss of a distinct margin, follicular dimpling, and fine vellus hairs of the adjacent skin may indicate dermal spread. Inflammatory lesions that do not respond to appropriate therapy should always raise the suspicion of malignancy and must undergo biopsy. This is especially true of the sebaceous carcinoma of the eyelid, apocrine carcinoma, and Paget's disease of the external auditory canal. These lesions are often treated for years as blepharitis or otitis externa before the correct diagnosis is made. Verrucous carcinoma of the nares and squamous cell carcinoma of the lip are also often misdiagnosed as benign inflammatory lesions. It is important to note irregularities of pigmentation or loss of a distinct tumor margin because these may be signs of a malignant melanoma. The tumor (and surrounding tissue) should be palpated with its base and margins carefully outlined. Palpation of regional lymph nodes is also an important part of the examination. The patient should be asked if any other lesions have been noted, and special attention should be given to those lesions and to areas of sun-exposed skin when the rest of the skin surface is examined. In our experience, approximately 25 per cent of patients will have a second primary skin tumor present.

If the history and examination suggest the possibility of malignancy, biopsies should always be performed even though dermatologists can often recognize most skin cancers by careful examination. Adequate and representative biopsies should be obtained to provide determination of tumor cell type and histologic aggressiveness, with estimation of the nature and depth of invasion (dermal or perineural spread). This allows adequate preoperative planning so that the best procedure may be undertaken to provide both complete extirpation (cure) and optimal cosmetic results. Care should be taken so that a shave or saucerization biopsy will provide adequate tissue for complete evaluation and that a punch or excisional biopsy is placed so that performing the definitive procedure (which may be necessary from the biopsy result) is not made more difficult.[3]

Close cooperation with the pathologist is important. (One with an oncologic orientation is best if available.) Adequate history and description of the lesion should be provided to the pathologist, who should be asked to comment on the degree of sclerosis and dermal spread. Ideally, the slides should be reviewed together; with difficult cases, consultation should be obtained with other pathologists. At no time should a potentially disfiguring procedure be performed without tissue confirmation of malignancy. If an excisional biopsy is performed, proper orientation, labeling, and mapping are essential. The specimen should be submitted with a map of the anatomic area showing reference landmarks with the specimen marked with sutures, dye, or a special map specimen container. A small board may be used, on which the excised tissue is attached with pins and appropriate labels. Tumor-free margins, both deep and lateral, are needed prior to closure, especially if undermining for primary or flap closure is performed. Reports of a "close margin" should be further excised and the margins re-examined prior to any reconstruction. Observation of the excision site for local recurrence rather than re-excision will often result in the development of more extensive recurrent lesions. In our opinion, positive margins should always be re-excised. Biopsy with frozen sections is sufficient for basal and squamous cell carcinomas. Frozen sections are not reliable for malignant melanoma and most fibrous tumors.

TREATMENT METHODS

Selection of Therapy

Since a number of methods of therapy are available for the management of malignant skin neoplasms, it is often difficult to choose the optimal method of treatment in the individual patient.[1] Accepted methods of therapy are listed in Table 49–1. Of these various therapeutic modalities, the *Mohs technique* has been repeatedly demonstrated to provide the highest cure rate for malignant neoplasms of the skin.[18-21, 31] Conventional surgery, though more commonly used, seems to be the second most effective method.

Although Mohs' technique is most useful, it is fre-

quently unavailable in the local community. This technique requires specialized training on the part of the surgeon, additional equipment and personnel, as well as increased time to perform the excision (compared with conventional surgery without frozen section control).

Selecting the method of treatment most suited to the individual patient should include several important factors. These are summarized in Table 49–2 and include:

1. Lesion location and size.
2. Histologic pattern (stromal invasion as in morphea-form basal cell carcinoma or anaplastic squamous cell carcinoma).
3. The patient's complexion, age, occupation, general health, medical status, personality, and personal wishes.

The latter two factors are important in psychologic consequences of scarring and possible secondary deformity, the patient's fear of cancer, and the reliability of follow-up, all of which need to be considered in selecting the method of therapy. The primary concern of the surgeon must be complete eradication of the tumor; cosmetic results are only an important secondary consideration. Complicated recurrent and aggressive neoplasms are best managed by a team approach consisting of the pathologist, head and neck surgeon, Mohs chemosurgeon, radiotherapist, and other specialists as needed.

Conventional Surgical Excision

An initial biopsy is always obtained unless an excisional biopsy is utilized as the therapeutic procedure (only in small lesions). Prior to excision, clinical margins of the tumor should be determined as close as possible by careful inspection with sufficient lighting and digital palpation as previously described. The margins determined are then marked with ink or dye. It is best to excise the lesion en bloc, obtaining adequate peripheral and deep margins. The primary consideration must always be complete tumor excision and not wound closure and cosmesis. Although these factors are important, they should be considered only secondarily after obtaining adequate excision margins. Width of these margins should be based on histologic type, whether the tumor is primary or recurrent, and location (dangerous areas such as the nasolabial fold) of the tumor. One must assume that the tumor extends with

TABLE 49–1. Methods of Therapy of Cutaneous Malignancies

Conventional surgical excision
Radiation therapy
Cryosurgery
Electrodesiccation and curettage
Topical chemotherapy
Chemosurgery (Mohs' technique)
Laser excision
Other modalities (immunotherapy, chemotherapy, laser incision)

TABLE 49–2. Factors in Selection of Method of Therapy for Skin Cancer of the Head and Neck

Lesion
Location
Size
Tumor
Primary or recurrent
Histologic type
Patient
Complexion
Age
Occupation
General health and medical status
Personality
Desires

small finger-like irregular projections into the surrounding clinically normal tissue.

No general "rule of thumb" can be given for determining the size of excision margins because the growth characteristics and behavior of tumors vary greatly with histologic type and anatomic location. Certain anatomic locations, such as the eyelid, may place severe limitations on the size of surgical margins, and lesions of the nasolabial fold are often deeply invasive. The typical small nodular basal cell carcinoma (less than 10 mm in diameter) usually requires excision margins of 5 to 7 mm. Smaller squamous cell carcinomas should ideally be excised with a 1-cm margin; however, larger lesions (greater than 10 mm in diameter) require wider and deeper margins with at least a 1-cm or greater margin. In addition, deep excision to the underlying fascia will result in fewer local recurrences. Recurrent tumors and those of longer duration should be more widely excised or are best treated similarly to lesions that are larger than 20 mm in diameter or that have indistinct clinical margins by microscopic controlled excision with frozen sections, such as Mohs' surgery. Complete frozen section control of all margins should be obtained when excising tumors in high risk locations such as the eyelids, lips, ears, nasal tip, ala, mid face triangle, and periauricular and periorbital areas.[6]

The margins for malignant melanoma are based on the depth of tumor invasion or Clark's classification. These margins are much more extensive than those previously described.

In general, the indications for conventional surgical excision may include:

1. Anatomic regions where the skin is mobile (cheeks, forehead, neck) and primary closure can be achieved after adequate margins are obtained.

2. Rapid healing and minimal postoperative morbidity important.

3. Intraoperative microscopic margins obtained.

4. Cosmetic factors.

5. Poorly differentiated squamous cell carcinoma or sclerosing basal cell carcinoma with deep invasion where cryosurgery, electrosurgery, and chemotherapy are difficult and less useful.

Advantages of conventional surgical excision include:

1. Rapid healing time.

2. A large resection tissue specimen available for complete microscopic evaluation of margins.

3. A good cosmetic result in most cases.

Disadvantages include:

1. Poor tolerance by older patients of the operative procedure and time required for frozen section evaluation of the excision margins.

2. Excessive bleeding in anticoagulated patients.

3. The potential tendency for surgeons to minimize margins in areas such as the nose, eyelids, and ears to allow primary closure.

4. Difficult primary closure in patients with multiple lesions such as basal cell nevus syndrome.

It is best not to do a primary reconstruction at the time of the excisional surgery with grafts, flaps, or wide undermining with primary closure if the excision margins are not certain. If reconstruction of this type is needed, complete frozen section control is essential prior to reconstruction. With the Mohs technique and adequate control of the excision margins, immediate reconstruction can be more safely utilized.[10]

Radiation Therapy

Radiation therapy can be a useful alternative to excision for certain selected skin cancers.[12] The inherent disadvantage of this technique is the absence of a histologic specimen for examination of the margins. It is especially useful for cancers on the eyelids, ears, nose, and lips. Unfortunately, radiochondritis may develop on the nose and ear; however, this can be minimized by proper dose fractionation. In sun-exposed skin of the head and neck, radiation produces increased aging of the skin, resulting in a scar with a poorer cosmetic appearance. The potential for future carcinogenesis limits its use in our practice to patients over 50 years of age.[23, 27] Although radiation therapy does eliminate the morbidity of a surgical procedure, it requires a prolonged period of time for completion of therapy. In addition, there is a higher rate of recurrence following this method of therapy as compared with conventional surgical excision or chemosurgery (Mohs' technique). Most chemosurgeons agree that recurrent tumors occurring after radiation therapy are often more difficult to treat and are frequently highly aggressive. The relative avascularity of the adjacent tissue also makes reconstructive procedures difficult. Radiation therapy may offer excellent palliative therapy for larger skin cancers in older patients. For a comprehensive review of the use of radiation therapy for skin cancer, refer to the review article by Goldschmidt and Sherwin[12] and to textbooks on radiotherapy.

Cryosurgery

Cryosurgery is an effective and versatile method for treating skin cancers. A high rate of cure can be achieved if proper degree, depth, and width of freeze are obtained. As with radiotherapy, however, it is a "field treatment" that does not provide a specimen for histologic examination of the margins and its use should be restricted to lesions in which the deep and lateral margins can be determined with a reasonable degree of certainty. A thorough treatise on the subject has been written by Zacarian.[32]

Some of the advantages of and indications for cryosurgery include:

1. Tumors located in areas with minimal movable underlying tissue, such as the nose, temple, ears, and eyelids.

2. Tumors located where tissue contraction is desirable, such as the eyelids, in selected cases.

3. Patients on anticoagulants or with a morbid fear of surgery.

4. Healing usually produces a soft and pliable scar that improves with time.

Disadvantages include:

1. Prolonged postoperative healing with necrosis and drainage followed by granulation and secondary intention healing that may take several weeks or even months.

2. Postoperative edema may be severe, especially on loose skin such as the eyelids.

3. Scar contracture may cause distortion of adjacent movable structures such as the eyelids or the lip.

4. Healed scars are usually hypopigmented with poor cosmesis in dark-complexioned individuals.

Contraindications for the use of cryosurgery include the following:

1. Carcinoma with poorly defined margins.
2. Most recurrent carcinomas.
3. Sclerosing basal cell carcinoma and poorly differentiated squamous cell carcinoma.
4. Location on eyebrows, scalp, and vermilion border of lips.
5. The presence of cryoglobulins, cryofibrogens, or cold agglutinins.[29]

Electrosurgery

Curettage and electrodesiccation have traditionally been the modality most frequently used by dermatologists for the treatment of skin cancer. This technique is being used less often, as dermatologists are now most commonly using conventional surgical excision and Mohs' chemosurgery. The most important aspect of this technique is the use of curettage. The experienced physician can remove the soft, mushy tumor with the curette, leaving behind the normal firm adjacent tissue. This method is also useful for debulking tumors prior to cryosurgery or Mohs' chemosurgery and to help determine margins prior to conventional excision surgery. It is quick and easily tolerated by the patient. For selected tumors, electrosurgery can provide a very high cure rate.[11, 15, 26]

The primary advantage of this technique is that it is a simple, cost-effective outpatient procedure. *Indications* for electrodesiccation and curettage include:
1. Small, primary nonsclerosing tumors less than 10 mm in diameter with clearly defined margins.
2. Multiple small tumors such as nevoid basal cell carcinoma or arsenical keratoses and tumors.
3. Nodular basal cell carcinoma, superficial multicentric carcinoma, and well-differentiated squamous cell carcinoma.

Disadvantages include:
1. The possibility of a hypertrophic or hypopigmented scar.
2. The absence of a histologic specimen being available for margin examination.
3. Prolonged healing (usually shorter than that after cryosurgery—3 to 6 weeks) requiring wound care with rare wound infection and postoperative bleeding.
4. Ineffectiveness in lesions greater than 10 mm in diameter, deep dermal spread or subcutaneous extension, or fibrotic (sclerosing basal cell carcinomas) or recurrent tumors.

Electrosurgery is *contraindicated* in patients with cardiac pacemakers and in areas with high recurrence rates or risk of contraction such as the eyelid, nasolabial fold, canthal areas, triangular area of the midface, margin of the vermilion of the lip, and the periauricular scalp regions.

Chemosurgery (Mohs' Technique)

Microscopic controlled excision with the Mohs technique gives the highest cure rate available for skin cancer.[1, 18–22, 31] This technique combines the modality of surgical excision with immediate pathologic examination of the margins. It was first developed by Frederick E. Mohs in 1936[18] and was named "chemosurgery" to describe the in situ fixation with zinc chloride fixative, which was followed by excision and complete microscopic control of tumor removal at the margins. Over the past half century, this technique has evolved, and since Tromovitch's report in 1974[30] on the "fresh tissue technique," nearly all tumors are removed with this approach. At the present time, Mohs' surgery more aptly refers to microscopically oriented histographic surgery or micrographic surgery.

The technique is performed in the following manner (Fig. 49–2): The surgical area is prepared and draped in the usual fashion, and the clinically apparent margins of the tumor are marked with gentian violet or other suitable marking dye. Local anesthesia is obtained by infiltrating 1 per cent lidocaine (Xylocaine) with epinephrine in a 1 to 100,000 ratio. After the entire obvious tumor mass, including a margin of normal tissue, is excised, a thin horizontal section of tissue approximately 2 mm in thickness is excised from the entire base and edges of the wound. This specimen is then divided into convenient portions that will fit an 8-mm slide, and the edges are marked with different colored dyes. Frozen sections are then obtained from the undersurface of each specimen. The location of residual tumor is marked on the map, and only the areas containing residual tumor are subsequently excised. With this system of mapping, the exact location of residual tumor is known. Thus, uninvolved tissue is spared. Surgical resection is continued until there is a microscopically proven tumor-free plane. Following the initial tumor excision, four more layers can usually be excised in the same day. Most tumors are removed in 1 day in contrast to the old fixed tissue technique, which often required several days. For large complicated cases, several days may be necessary with the fresh tissue technique. When perineural spread (Figs. 49–3 and 49–4) or bone or cartilage invasion (Fig. 49–5) is detected, more extensive ablative surgery is required. After completion of the tumor excision, the wound will be left open to heal by secondary intention, or if indicated, the defect is reconstructed with free grafts, flaps, or primary closure.

Advantages of the fresh tissue technique over the fixed tissue technique include:
1. Less time required.
2. Reduced morbidity of surrounding tissues (e.g., chondritis).
3. The possibility of immediate surgical reconstruction.
4. Reduced pain.

Both techniques allow planning of reconstructive procedures with unbiased resection of the tumor and maximum assurance of complete extirpation of the malignancy. The reconstructive surgeon can concentrate only on the repair and cosmesis, with less time wasted in the operating room waiting for frozen sections. This team approach can benefit the patient by having each specialist doing what he or she knows best.

Although Mohs' technique is an excellent modality for the treatment of all skin cancers, it is a time-consuming specialized technique and is not needed for the therapy of all cutaneous malignancies. Mohs' surgery should be strongly considered for the following lesions:
1. Recurrent cancers that have failed to respond to aggressive treatment with surgery, cryosurgery, or irradiation.
2. Large primary tumors of long duration.

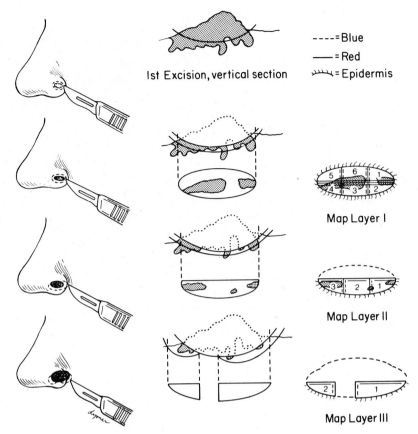

1st Excision, vertical section

- - - - = Blue
——— = Red
〜〜〜 = Epidermis

Map Layer I

Map Layer II

Map Layer III

Figure 49–2. Schematic diagram of the Mohs fresh-tissue technique.

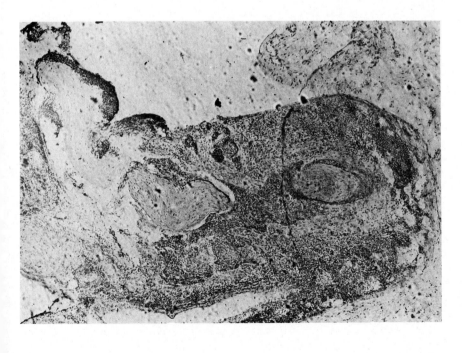

Figure 49–3. Photomicrograph showing strands of squamous cell carcinoma spreading along peripheral nerves.

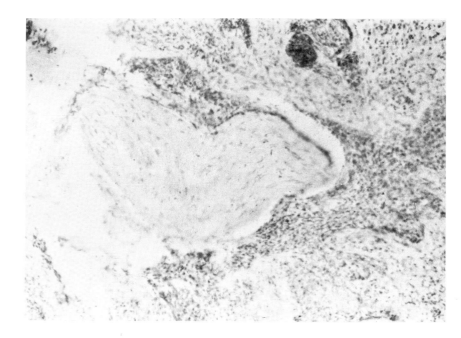

Figure 49–4. High-power view of Figure 49–3 showing tumor spread in perineural spaces.

Figure 49–5. Photomicrograph showing basal cell carcinoma with perichondrial spread and invasion.

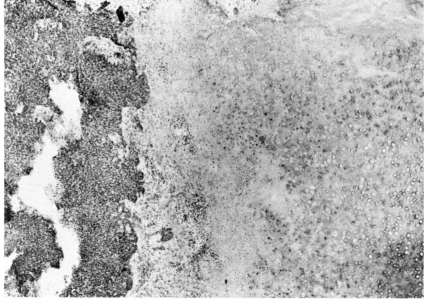

3. Poorly differentiated squamous cell carcinoma.

4. Sclerosing (morpheaform) basal cell carcinoma.

5. Tumors with poorly defined margins.

6. Tumors in difficult locations where the likelihood of deep invasion along the embryonic fusion planes or dermal spread is highly probable (nasolabial fold, nasal ala, ears, medial canthi and eyelid margins, periauricular area, and anywhere the skin is close to underlying bone or cartilage).

7. Areas where maximal preservation of normal tissue is essential for restoration of function or for surgical reconstruction.

The main *advantages* of microscopic controlled excision include:

1. The highest cure rate (especially for large and recurrent lesions).

2. Maximal sparing of normal tissue.

3. Minimal operative procedure (low morbidity and mortality rates, use of local anesthesia, usually performed on outpatient basis).

4. Its value as the only method of definitive treatment for certain patients (such as those with large lesions or radiation failures).

In addition, when used in conjunction with reconstructive surgery, the technique provides an objective method of tumor excision free of bias inherent in the desire to facilitate reconstruction. It allows the surgeon to plan the reconstruction and saves the patient operating room time. It also allows the surgeon to reconstruct with free grafts or local flaps with greater assurance that they are not covering up cancer, and it permits sparing of normal tissue in locations such as the nasal ala and eyelid where maximal tissue preservation is vital for optimal reconstruction.

Disadvantages of this technique include:

1. Its being a time-consuming and tedious procedure.

2. The requirement of training in both surgery and histopathology.

3. The necessity of an additional laboratory, cryostat, and technician to process the pathologic sections.

Mohs' technique is unnecessary in lesions that are well defined, less aggressive histologically, and not located in an area where recurrence would be a major concern or difficult to eradicate. In these situations, conventional surgical excision, curettage, and electrodesiccation and other modalities are appropriate methods of treatment. However, if the lesion is large, histologically aggressive, recurrent, or in a troublesome location, microscopic controlled excision is the treatment of choice. When combined with immediate or delayed reconstruction, this results in the highest cure rate for these difficult malignancies with optimal cosmesis. The most important feature of this technique is the microscopic control afforded by the systematic use of frozen sections to provide maximal probability of complete tumor excision, greatest preservation of non-involved tissue, and to allow planned surgical reconstruction with the highest assurance of tumor-free margins.

Other Modalities

A detailed discussion of other therapeutic modalities such as immunotherapy, chemotherapy, and laser excision are beyond the scope of this chapter. These modalities are either still in the investigative stages or are infrequently used.

Topical chemotherapy with 5-fluorouracil (5-FU) is very useful in the management of widespread actinic keratoses; however, its use for overt skin cancer is not recommended. The results are unpredictable, and the failure of the drug to penetrate the entire depth of the tumor may result in removal of only the superficial component. This in effect "drives the tumor deeper" giving a high recurrence rate with tumor that is deeply infiltrative and difficult to eradicate at the time the recurrence is evident clinically.

Therapy According to Tumor Type and Size

The factors that influence the choice of the therapeutic modality have been listed in Table 49–2.

When considering the tumor size and type, *electrosurgery* is adequate for small to medium-sized (less than 10 mm) superficial or nodular type basal cell carcinomas and for small to medium-sized well-differentiated squamous cell carcinomas.[16]

Conventional *surgical excision* is appropriate for nearly all tumors and has the advantage of available tissue for margin checks. In large lesions, sclerosing basal cell carcinoma, and recurrent tumors where grafts, flaps, or wide undermining were previously used for reconstruction, complete microscopic control is necessary as provided by the Mohs technique.

Radiation therapy is satisfactory for small to moderate-sized nodular basal cell carcinomas and well-differentiated squamous cell carcinomas. This technique should be avoided in sclerosing and superficial multicentric basal cell carcinomas, fibrous tumors, and malignant melanomas.

Cryosurgery is adequate for most small to moderate-sized nodular or superficial basal cell carcinomas and small, well-differentiated squamous cell carcinomas. It should be avoided in sclerosing basal cell carcinoma and poorly differentiated squamous cell carcinoma.

Mohs' surgery is excellent for tumors of all sizes and types. Its use for malignant melanoma is controversial. It is the treatment of choice for recurrent, sclerosing basal cell carcinomas and squamous cell carcinomas of all types.

Tumors with poorly defined margins should be treated with Mohs' surgery or, at the very least, with wide conventional excisional surgery with complete microscopic examination of all margins. The use of the curette may help to define these lateral margins prior to excision.

Tumors that invade deeply into the dermis or subcutaneous tissue should be treated with Mohs' surgery or with wide, deep surgical excision; again with complete examination of all margins.

Tumors in difficult locations (described previously) should be treated with Mohs' surgery. Tumors of very large size and long duration should be treated with wide surgical excision or with Mohs' surgery. A widespread or aggressive field of malignancy may be palliated by cryosurgery or radiation therapy.

Electrosurgery, *cryosurgery*, and *radiation therapy* are useful in elderly patients. However, many elderly patients can easily tolerate *conventional excision* and *Mohs' surgery* if procedures are not prolonged and anesthetics with epinephrine are minimized. *Cryosurgery* is helpful in patients on anticoagulants, with allergies to local anesthetics, and with cardiac pacemakers. *Radiation ther-*

apy should be avoided in patients less than 50 years of age because of the possibility of late induction of additional malignancies.

Recurrent tumors should usually be treated with wide *conventional excision* or *Mohs' technique*. *Radiation therapy* and *cryosurgery* should be avoided in these lesions except for palliation or with the initial recurrence of recent inadequately treated primary tumors.

The skilled surgeon should be able to excise "high-risk lesions" with wider margins and generally obtain an improved cure rate. One should not attempt techniques without prior training and experience but refer to or cooperate with other physicians skilled in these therapeutic modalities.

In *small lesions, electrosurgery* often produces a cosmetically pleasing scar that improves with time. *Cryosurgery* frequently results in hypopigmented scars that are undesirable, especially in dark-complexioned patients. *Radiation* scars tend to worsen with time, most commonly in areas of sun-exposed skin frequently found in the head and neck area. *Conventional excision* for medium-sized to large skin cancers usually gives an excellent cosmetic result. The cosmetic results of *Mohs'* surgery depend upon the method of reconstruction. The result of healing by secondary intention is comparable to that of electrosurgical scars in small lesions.

In some *medium-sized lesions*, especially in certain anatomic areas such as the medial canthus, *healing by secondary intention* may be preferable to free skin grafts or local flaps. Primary or flap closure after Mohs' surgery often gives superior cosmetic results because maximal conservation of normal tissue is possible with this technique and these methods minimize skin scarring and utilize the best cosmetically available tissue for reconstruction.

Excision followed by *primary closure* heals the fastest and requires the least postoperative care. Other modalities often prolong healing, and wound care may be needed for some time following the completion of the procedure to allow granulation and the completion of healing by secondary intention.

Radiation therapy requires multiple visits, which are inconvenient for all patients and may be especially difficult for elderly, weak, or disabled patients. *Cryosurgery* and *electrosurgery* are the least expensive for the initial therapy of cutaneous malignancies. However, when the cost of treatment of recurrence is considered, *Mohs' surgery* may be the most economical of all the techniques.

In difficult cases it is often helpful to have a "tumor board" to discuss the case and make recommendations for the therapeutic approach. This board can include a dermatologist, surgeon, head and neck reconstructive surgeon, radiotherapist, pathologist, medical oncologist, and rehabilitation specialist. Consideration of the disability and deformity to be incurred, as well as the techniques and timing of methods of management, should be discussed by the board and with the patient and the family. Special emphasis on the diagnosis, prognosis, and overall treatment plan must be provided in all cases. The nature of the problem should never be minimized by saying "it is just a skin cancer," and the patient must be informed of the risk of recurrence and the need for prolonged and regular follow-up.

Again, we emphasize that extirpation of the lesion should be the primary concern, with reconstruction and cosmesis considered secondarily. The best time to effect a cure is at the initial procedure.

Patient Follow-up

After the tumor is removed and rehabilitation is completed, the patient should be carefully followed for the remainder of his or her life, if possible. Although some authors feel that the duration of follow-up needs to be only 5 years, we feel that this is the minimum period of time required because recurrences may be missed with shorter times. Because many cutaneous malignancies are extremely slow-growing, they may recur clinically after this 5-year period. In addition, the likelihood of the patient's developing additional skin malignancies is greater than 25 per cent. In our practice, routine follow-up after the wound is healed is at 6 weeks, 3 months, 6 months, and then yearly. In patients at high risk for recurrence, the follow-up intervals are often shorter. In addition, the patient should be thoroughly educated as to the danger signs of skin cancer, premalignant lesions, and the use of sun protection in the future.

Therapy of Specific Anatomic Locations
The Ear

Malignant neoplasms of the external ear (Fig. 49–6) often begin as infiltrating growths spreading within the dermis and along perichondrium or embryonic fusion planes rather than the usual discrete exophytic lesions seen elsewhere in the body. This characteristic makes complete removal of cutaneous malignancies of the auricle difficult, even in small primary lesions. These malignancies tend to extend well beyond the clinically

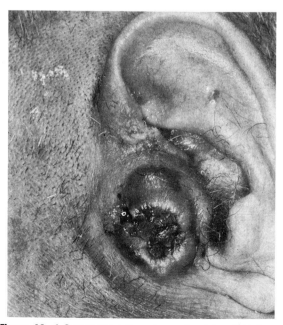

Figure 49–6. Squamous cell carcinoma involving the left ear.

apparent margins. Lesions located in the anterior and posterior auricular sulci may have invaded the parotid gland, causing the facial nerve to be jeopardized during surgical removal. Most authors feel that the prognosis for auricular cutaneous malignancies is worse than that for other areas of the body.[28]

In addition to the infiltrating nature of auricular malignancies, the anatomic structure of the auricle itself also poses a therapeutic problem. Much of the ear is composed of two layers of thin skin separated by auricular cartilage. Consequently, extensive or deep excision results in a severe cosmetic deformity. The use of conventional surgical excision for auricular malignancies is associated with both a high risk of inadequate excision and the excision of an excessive amount of normal tissue.[7] Our previously reported study indicated that high-risk lesions of the auricle included any tumor larger than 1 cm in diameter, all morpheaform basal cell carcinoma, and recurrent lesions of any size. *Radiation therapy* has a high incidence of recurrence when used for auricular malignancies. *Cryosurgery* has a greater risk for the development of chrondritis with subsequent deformity of the auricle. The therapeutic method of choice for all auricular neoplasms other than primary lesions less than 1 cm in size appears to be *Mohs'* *technique*. This therapeutic measure provides the highest cure rate and maximizes the retention of normal or noninvolved auricular tissue, resulting in less subsequent auricular deformity.

The Eyelid and Periorbital Area

Malignancies of the eyelid and periorbital area (Fig. 49–7) present a difficult therapeutic problem when compared with most other cutaneous malignancies. This is due to the close proximity of the tumor to vital structures, the functional requirements of the lids in preserving vision, and the difficulty in cosmetic reconstruction.

Again, these tumors frequently begin as infiltrating growths spreading into the dermis and along the tarsal plates rather than as the usual discrete exophytic lesion. This is especially true in recurrent malignancies. In addition to the characteristics of these tumors, there is a natural reluctance on the part of the surgeon to perform wide and radical excisions for fear of damaging the lacrimal or optic system.[2]

Although the majority (90 per cent) of cutaneous malignancies of this area are basal cell carcinomas,[4, 14, 17] the mortality rate from these malignancies has been reported to be between 2 and 11 per cent, with an even higher significant morbidity rate due to visual loss.[4, 5, 25] Because of this it would appear that the majority of lesions of this area are best treated by the use of the *Mohs technique*. This method of therapy maximizes the potential for complete excision of the tumor and also minimizes the amount of normal tissue excised during the therapeutic procedure.

Nasal and Midface Tumors

The nose is one of the most common sites of cutaneous malignancies on the face (Fig. 49–8). This is probably related to its unique position—exposing it to environmental damage from sunlight, weather, and smoke. The vast majority of these tumors are basal cell carcinomas.[24]

High-risk areas on the nose include the supratip area, the columella, the area of the nasolabial crease, and the upper nose near the medial canthal area. Tumors located in these areas, with the exception of very small superficial exophytic primary lesions, are best treated by the use of *Mohs' technique*. Other anatomic locations of nasal tumors may be successfully treated with *radiotherapy* and *conventional surgical excision*. However, the recur-

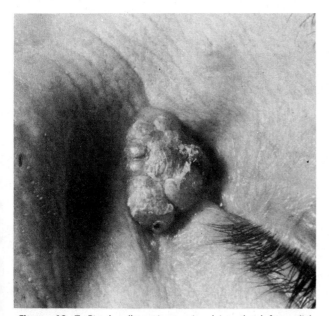

Figure 49–7. Basal cell carcinoma involving the left medial canthus.

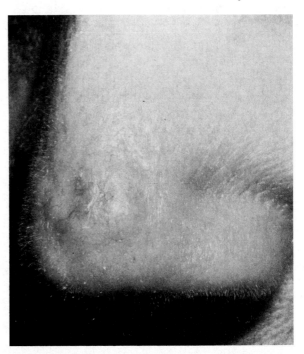

Figure 49–8. Infiltrative basal cell carcinoma involving nasal tip.

rence rate following radiotherapy is significantly higher than that following conventional surgical excision. Although the recurrence of nasal cutaneous malignancies infrequently causes death, these tumors have a long and protracted course with significant destruction of the midface. Because of this, complete excision should be obtained as early as possible.

RECONSTRUCTION

Numerous techniques are available for the reconstruction of defects created by the surgical excision of cutaneous malignancies. As shown in Table 49–3, these methods include:

1. Healing by granulation or secondary intention.
2. Primary closure.
3. Free grafts of skin or skin and underlying supporting structures (composite).
4. Flaps, which may be local, regional, or distant in origin. Tables 49–4 through 49–7 present detailed descriptions of these reconstructive techniques.

In the appropriate clinical setting, all of the methods may provide excellent cosmetic and functional results. Defects can frequently be satisfactorily reconstructed by several of these techniques, allowing the choice of several different methods of reconstruction.

Several factors are involved in the *selection of technique.* The primary factors are the tumor and defect, but the patient and surgeon also play a significant role. Important considerations in relation to the cutaneous malignancy include (1) whether tumor is primary or recurrent, (2) the histologic type, and (3) the probability of complete surgical excision. The size, location, and depth of the resulting defect also play a vital role. In addition, the patient's desires, condition of tissue adjacent to the defect, and the surgeon's prior training, experience, and personal preference are also important considerations.

In selected cases, the use of a prosthesis may be advisable until a period of time has passed to diminish the possibility of recurrence before performing surgical reconstruction.

Granulation (Secondary Intention)

Granulation, or secondary intention healing, will often provide excellent results in selected cases (Table 49–4). *Advantages* of this technique include (1) avoiding an additional surgical procedure and scar formation and (2) with proper patient selection the obtaining of excellent cosmesis (Fig. 49–9). *Disadvantages* include (1) the prolonged period required for complete healing; (2) use

TABLE 49–3. Methods of Reconstruction for Skin Cancers of the Head and Neck

Healing by granulation (secondary intention)
Primary closure
Free grafts
Skin
Composite
Flaps
Local
Regional or distant

TABLE 49–4. Granulation Healing Used in Reconstructive Surgery for Skin Tumors of the Head and Neck

Indications
Tumor, any type
Defect
Size—small and superficial best
Location—over firm underlying structure
Advantages
Additional procedures avoided
No additional scarring
Disadvantages
Prolonged healing
Cosmetic result—often poorer than in other methods
Limited by defect location, size, and depth

being limited by the defect location, size, and depth; and (3) an occasionally poor cosmetic result.

In general, the use of this technique is indicated in (1) defects that are small and superficial, (2) larger defects with a firm underlying structure that usually minimizes contracture produced secondary to granulation healing, and (3) locations that are immobile and do not perform a vital function. This method is frequently considered for highly aggressive primary or recurrent tumors.

The patient is instructed to clean the wound with hydrogen peroxide twice daily. Following this, an antibiotic ointment is applied to prevent excessive crusting. The duration required for complete healing depends on the size and depth of the defect and is usually 3 to 6 weeks.

Primary Closure

Reconstruction by primary closure is summarized in Table 49–5. This method provides rapid reconstruction and healing without creating any additional visible skin scars. It also frequently produces excellent cosmetic results.

The main *disadvantages* are that its use is often limited by defect size and location and there may be limited availability of adjacent tissue. In addition, extensive undermining is frequently required, producing additional adjacent subcutaneous scar tissue, which must be totally excised if the malignancy recurs, and this results in a very large defect. This is necessary, as recurrent malignancies often have noncontiguous nests of tumor cells interspersed throughout this scar tissue. Consequently, all adjacent scar tissue produced from previous methods of therapy must be excised in order to obtain complete removal of the recurrent malignancy.[6]

This technique is indicated when there is a high probability of complete tumor excision and adjacent tissue is available. The best cosmetic results are obtained by a layered closure using fine (6–0) sutures to approximate the skin margins.

The patient must be instructed to clean the suture line twice a day with hydrogen peroxide, followed by the application of an antibiotic ointment to prevent crust formation over the sutures. If a large crust does develop, the skin margins frequently will be disrupted when the sutures are removed, producing a poorer cosmetic result.

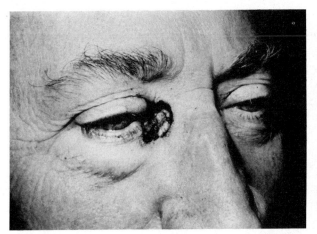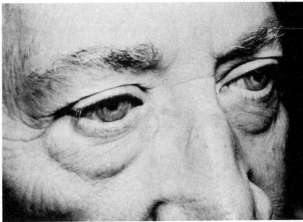

Figure 49–9. Defect and final result of granulation healing.

Free Grafts

Skin Grafts

Information regarding the use of free grafts is presented in Table 49–6.

Advantages include (1) the ability to reconstruct large defects; (2) the fact that no additional scar tissue adjacent to the defect is created; and (3) rapid healing and improved cosmesis compared with these results in granulation healing. *Disadvantages* include (1) the morbidity associated with obtaining the skin graft (donor site) and (2) the inability to use in defects that are full-thickness (through and through) or located where there is a large degree of motion or a vital function is necessary. In addition, the final cosmetic result is less satisfactory and healing duration is longer when compared with the use of local flaps or primary closure.

Free grafts are usually indicated in (1) aggressive primary tumors (usually morpheaform basal cell carcinoma); (2) moderate-sized or large recurrent tumors; and (3) those cases in which there is a higher probability of inadequate surgical excision. The best results are obtained when the defect is located over a firm underlying structure, as this decreases contracture during healing.

Skin grafts may be full- or split-thickness grafts. *Full-thickness* skin grafts consist of the entire epidermis and underlying dermis. Their survival depends on obtaining a vascular supply, the majority of which must be ob-

tained from the graft margins. The presence of fat on the undersurface of the graft markedly decreases the ingrowth of vessels from the underlying recipient bed. Consequently, the width of a full-thickness skin graft is limited, with best results usually obtained in defects 2 cm or less in width. Although the survival rate for full-thickness skin grafts is lower than that for split-thickness

TABLE 49–5. Primary Closure Used in Reconstructive Surgery for Skin Tumors of the Head and Neck

Indications
Tumor—high probability of complete excision
Defect
  Size—usually limited
  Location—availability of adjacent tissue
Advantages
Excellent cosmetic result
Rapid reconstruction
No additional skin scar
Disadvantages
Limited by defect size and location
Produces additional adjacent subcutaneous scar tissue

TABLE 49–6. Free Grafts Used in Reconstructive Surgery for Skin Tumors of the Head and Neck

Skin Graft
1. Indications
  a. Tumor—aggressive, higher probability of recurrence
  b. Defect
    (1) Size—any
    (2) Location—best over firm underlying structure
2. Advantages
  a. Reconstruction of large defects
  b. Avoids creation of additional adjacent scar
  c. Improved cosmetic result and healing duration over granulation
3. Disadvantages
  a. Donor site morbidity
  b. Limited by defect
    (1) Depth (full-thickness)
    (2) Location (motion or function, no firm underlying structure)
    (3) Poor cosmetic result and longer healing time than primary closure or local flap
4. Types
  a. Full-thickness
    (1) Greater tissue bulk, less contracture
    (2) Size limitation
  b. Split-thickness
    (1) No size limitation, higher survival
    (2) Increased contracture, donor site morbidity
5. Timing
  a. Immediate
  b. Delayed—after 21 or more days of granulation
    (1) Additional tissue bulk and improved cosmetic result
    (2) Correct technique vital
Composite Graft
1. Reconstruction of full-thickness defect without additional adjacent scar
2. Limited by
  a. Defect size (primarily)
  b. Donor availability

grafts, they do provide additional tissue bulk to the defect and frequently have less contracture during healing.

Split-thickness skin grafts consist of the entire epidermis and a portion of the dermis. Thus, both their margins and entire undersurface are available for ingrowth of vessels from the recipient bed. This allows an unlimited size of the split-thickness graft. Split-thickness skin grafts have a greater degree of contracture during healing than full-thickness grafts. In general, the thicker the split-thickness skin graft, the less the contracture.

Full-thickness skin grafts are usually obtained from the postauricular or supraclavicular area, with the donor site closed primarily. These areas are selected because the skin color is the most similar to that of the face. *Split-thickness* grafts are obtained with a battery-operated or mechanical dermatome. In general, thick grafts (18 to 21 thousandths of an inch) provide the best results. Improved color match is obtained by using sun-exposed skin, usually from the upper arm. However, when extremely large grafts are required, it may be necessary to use the thigh as a donor site.

Prior to obtaining the graft, a template of the defect is outlined on the donor site with gentian violet solution. When the graft has been obtained, it is then trimmed to the size of the previously marked defect. Split-thickness donor sites are either saturated with gentian violet solution and left open or are covered with a semipermeable polyurethane membrane (Op-Site). The graft is then sutured into the defect with multiple interrupted or running 5–0 absorbable sutures. Several small incisions are placed through the graft to allow drainage of any underlying fluid that may collect between the graft and the recipient site. The graft is then covered with a nonadherent bandage (Adaptic) followed by several layers of cotton gauze saturated with antibiotic ointment. This is used to create a bolster that is fixed in position with several 4–0 nylon sutures, which are placed well beyond the margins of the graft in order to avoid graft disruption when the bolster is removed. The absorbable sutures maintaining the graft position are not removed.

All patients are placed on a 5- to 7-day course of oral antibiotic therapy, which is usually initiated prior to the grafting procedure. Analgesics are used as necessary. The bolster is removed 7 to 10 days following the procedure. At this time, the graft is cleaned with hydrogen peroxide and a thick layer of a topical antibiotic ointment is applied. The patient is instructed not to do anything to the graft and to return 1 week later. The graft is again cleaned with hydrogen peroxide, antibiotic ointment is applied, and the patient is instructed to perform this procedure on a daily basis until healing is completed. When excessive contracture of the graft occurs, the initial therapy is a 5-minute digital massage of the graft performed by the patient twice daily, starting 6 to 8 weeks following the procedure. If the contracture persists, steroids (triamcinolone, 5 to 10 mg per ml) are injected beneath the graft site at 4- to 6-week intervals until the contracture resolves.

Most skin grafts are placed immediately or within a few days following the surgical excision. This provides more rapid healing than granulation and is best used in superficial defects. The initial defect and result obtained by the use of an immediate skin graft are shown in Figure 49–10. When the blood supply of the recipient bed is marginal or the defect is deep, improved results may be obtained by the use of delayed skin grafting.[8, 9] In this technique, a period of granulation healing is utilized prior to placing a thick split-thickness skin graft. We have found that a minimum of 21 days is the optimal duration of granulation healing. This provides significantly increased tissue bulk in deep defects and results in improved cosmesis. The technique of performing the delayed graft is vital for satisfactory results. Proper preparation of the recipient bed prior to placing the graft must be performed in all cases by excising a 1- to 2-mm strip of granulation tissue and regenerated epithelium from the entire circumference of the wound margin (Fig. 49–11). Following this, the central mass of granulation tissue is debrided in a manner to remove any superficial layer of overlying fibrin or necrotic material. Multiple deep incisions are then made through the remaining central mass of granulation tissue to completely "cross-hatch" this tissue. If this is not performed, significant contracture will result during the healing period and an unsatisfactory cosmetic result will

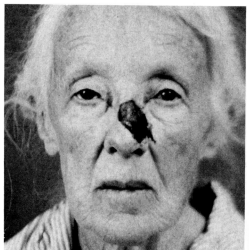
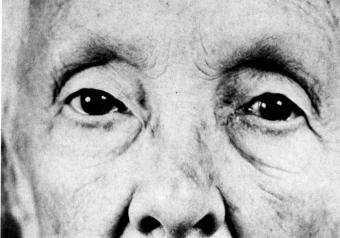

Figure 49–10. Defect and final result of an immediate split-thickness skin graft.

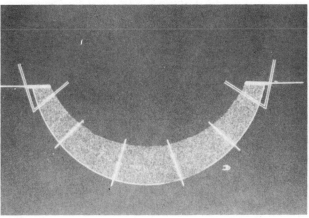
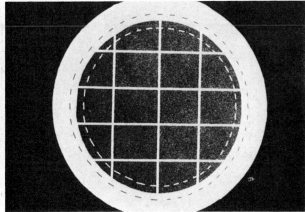

Figure 49–11. Cross-hatching of central mass of granulation tissue and excision of entire margin of regenerating epithelium and granulation tissue.

be obtained. The thick split-thickness skin graft is then placed in a manner similar to that previously described. The defect and result obtained by the use of delayed skin grafting are demonstrated in Figure 49–12.

Composite Grafts

Composite grafts are free grafts consisting of one or two layers of skin with the underlying supporting tissue, which is usually cartilage. They may be used to reconstruct full-thickness defects of the auricle or nose without creating any additional adjacent scar tissue. Free grafts of skin and cartilage may also be useful in eyelid reconstruction. These grafts must obtain their vascular supply from the margins of the defect and are limited in size. The best results are obtained when the center of the composite graft is 1 to 1.5 cm or less from the defect margins. However, longer grafts which are 1 cm or less in width may also survive.

Flaps

Local Flaps

Local flaps (Table 49–7 and Figure 49–13) usually produce an excellent cosmetic result by the skin color match, provide a large volume of vascularized tissue for immediate reconstruction, and have a high rate of success, since the tissue used for reconstruction does not need to obtain its vascular supply from the recipient site to survive.

Disadvantages include (1) the additional skin scar produced in obtaining the flap and the greatly increased subcutaneous scarring that is produced by the dissection necessary to close both the surgical defect and donor site; (2) the necessity of greater surgical expertise for satisfactory results; and (3) the fact that the availability of adjacent tissue may be limited, which would prevent the use of this method.

Local flap reconstruction should be used only when there is a high probability of complete tumor excision because recurrence will necessitate removal of all adjacent scar tissue, producing an extremely large defect following therapy of the recurrent lesion. Most defects may be reconstructed by local flaps, regardless of location or depth. However, extremely large defects may be limited by their size because of tissue availability adjacent to the defect. When local flaps are designed, care must be taken to avoid distortion of adjacent anatomic structures during closure of either the defect or the flap donor site.

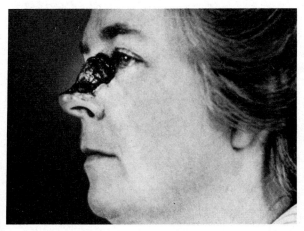
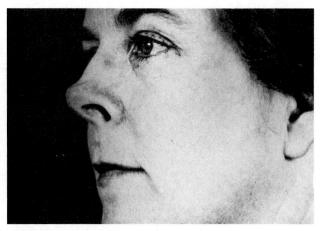

Figure 49–12. Defect and final result of a delayed split-thickness skin graft.

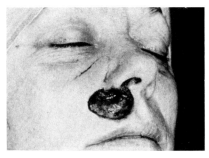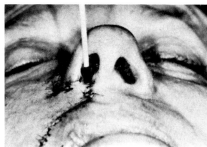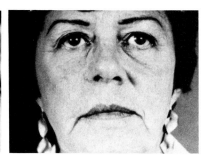

Figure 49–13. Local flap reconstruction showing the original defect and outlined flap, the transposed flap, and the final result.

Regional and Distant Flaps

Regional and distant flaps may be used for the reconstruction of massive facial defects without creating any additional scar adjacent to the defect. Their primary *disadvantages* are a poorer skin color match than that obtained from adjacent tissue and the multiple surgical procedures frequently required for reconstruction with this method. They are best used in extensive defects with a high probability of complete tumor excision. If complete tumor excision is uncertain, initial reconstruction may be performed by the use of skin grafts with final reconstruction performed approximately 2 years later when there is no further evidence of recurrence. An alternative method of therapy is the use of a prosthetic device constructed by a prosthetic specialist following granulation healing. Again, following a 2-year period without evidence of recurrence, the patient may elect to undergo surgical reconstruction of the defect.

TABLE 49–7. Flaps Used in Reconstructive Surgery for Skin Tumors of the Head and Neck

Local Flap
1. Indications
   a. Tumors—high probability of complete excision
   b. Defect
      (1) Any location and depth
      (2) Tissue availability may limit size
2. Advantages
   a. Excellent cosmesis
   b. Reconstruction—rapid and high success
   c. Provides large volume of vascularized tissue
3. Disadvantages
   a. Additional scarring
      (1) Flap donor site
      (2) Subcutaneous area adjacent to defect and donor site
   b. Closure of donor defect
   c. Greater surgical expertise necessary
   d. Occasional limited availability of adjacent tissue

Regional and Distant Flaps
1. Indications
   a. Tumor—high probability of complete excision
   b. Defect size and depth—no limitations
2. Advantages
   a. Reconstruction of massive defects
   b. No additional scar adjacent to defect
3. Disadvantages
   a. Cosmesis (color) may be poorer than adjacent tissue
   b. Staged procedure may be required

REFERENCES

1. Albright SD: Treatment of skin cancer using multiple modalities. J Am Acad Dermatol 7:143, 1982.
2. Anderson RL, Ceilley RI: A multispecialty approach to the excision and reconstruction of eyelid tumors. Arch Ophthalmol 85:1150, 1978.
3. Andrade R, et al: Observations on the treatment of skin cancer. In Andrade R, Gumport SL, Popkin GL, et al (eds): Cancer of the Skin. Philadelphia, W. B. Saunders Co., 1976.
4. Aurora AL, Blodi FC: Reappraisal of basal cell carcinoma of the eyelids. Am J Ophthalmol 70:329, 1970.
5. Birge HL: Cancer of the eyelids: I. Basal cell and mixed basal cell and squamous cell epithelioma. Arch Ophthalmol 19:700, 1938.
6. Bumsted RM, Ceilley RI, et al: Auricular malignant neoplasms. Arch Otolaryngol 107:721, 1981.
7. Bumsted RM, Ceilley RI: Auricular malignant neoplasms: Identification of high-risk lesions and selection of method of reconstruction. Arch Otolaryngol 108:225, 1982.
8. Bumsted RM, Ceilley RI, Panje WR: Delayed skin grafting. J Dermatol Surg Oncol 9:288, 1983.
9. Bumsted RM, Panje WR, Ceilley RI: Delayed skin grafting in facial reconstruction—When to use and how to do. Arch Otolaryngol 109:178, 1983.
10. Ceilley RI, Anderson RL: Microscopically controlled excision of malignant neoplasms on and around eyelids followed by immediate surgical reconstruction. J Dermatol Surg Oncol 4:55, 1978.
11. Epstein E, Epstein E Jr: Techniques in Skin Surgery. Philadelphia, Lea & Febiger, 1979.
12. Goldschmidt H, Sherwin WK: Office radiotherapy of cutaneous carcinomas I and II. J Dermatol Surg Oncol 9:31, 1983.
13. Gottheil WS: Illustrated Skin Diseases: An Atlas and Textbook. New York, EB Treat and Co., 1897.
14. Henkind P, Friedman A: Cancer of the lids and ocular adnexa. In Andrade R, Gumport SL, Popkin GL, et al (eds): Cancer of the Skin. Philadelphia, W. B. Saunders Co., 1976, pp 1345–1371.
15. Jackson R: Basic principles of electrosurgery: A review. Can J Surg 13:354, 1970.
16. Kopf AW, Bart RS, Schrader D, et al: Curettage electrodesiccation treatment of basal cell carcinomas. Arch Dermatol 113:439, 1977.
17. Kwitko ML, Boniuk M, Zimmerman LE: Eyelid tumors with reference to lesions confused with squamous cell carcinoma: I. Incidence and error in diagnosis. Arch Ophthalmol 69:693, 1963.
18. Mohs FE: Chemosurgery: Microscopically controlled method of cancer excision. Arch Surg 42:279, 1941.
19. Mohs FE: Chemosurgical treatment of cancer of the ear: A microscopically controlled method of excision. Surgery 21:605, 1947.
20. Mohs FE: Chemosurgery for skin cancer: Fixed tissue and fresh tissue techniques. Arch Dermatol 112:211, 1976.
21. Mohs FE: Chemosurgery: Microscopically Controlled Surgery for Skin Cancer. Springfield, Ill., Charles C Thomas, 1978, pp 262–267.
22. Mohs FE, Lathrop TG: Modes of spread of cancer of the skin. Arch Dermatol 66:427, 1952.
23. Orton CI: The treatment of basal cell carcinoma by radiotherapy. Clin Oncol 4:317, 1978.
24. Panje WR, Ceilley RI: The influence of embryology of the midface on the spread of epithelial malignancies. Laryngoscope 89:14, 1979.
25. Payne JW, Duke JR, Dutner R, et al: Basal cell carcinoma of the eyelids: A long-term follow-up study. Arch Ophthalmol 81:538, 1969.

26. Popkin GL: Electrosurgery. *In* Epstein E Jr (ed): Skin Surgery. 4th ed. Springfield, Ill., Charles C Thomas, 1977, pp 285–309.

27. Reymann F, Kopp H: Treatment of basal cell carcinoma of the skin with ultrasoft x-rays. Dermatologica *156*:40, 1978.

28. Shiffman NJ: Squamous cell carcinomas of the skin of the pinna. Can J Surg *18*:279, 1975.

29. Stewart RH, Graham GF: Complications of cryosurgery in a patient with cryofibrinogenemia. J Dermatol Surg Oncol 4:743, 1978.

30. Tromovitch TA, Stegman SJ: Microscopically controlled excision of skin tumors: Chemosurgery (Mohs): Fresh tissue technique. Arch Dermatol *110*:231, 1974.

31. Tromovitch TA, Stegman SJ: Microscopic controlled excision of cutaneous tumors. Cancer *41*:653, 1978.

32. Zacarian SA: Cryosurgical Advances in Dermatology and Tumors of the Head and Neck. Springfield, Ill., Charles C Thomas, 1977, pp 672–679.

CHAPTER 50

Radiation Therapy of Tumors of the Skin of the Head and Neck

Peter J. Fitzpatrick, M.B., B.S., F.R.C.P.(C), F.R.C.R.

Tumors of the skin are the commonest of all cancers. They usually arise from damaged skin or from existing lesions. Basal and squamous cell carcinomas are the most common, melanoma is the most serious, and the keratoacanthoma is the most puzzling. Most occur on the head and neck. The majority grow slowly, and being readily visible, they can be diagnosed at an early stage. They are disfiguring, but rarely fatal, and can be managed in a variety of ways. Radiotherapy is an efficient and cost-effective in situ method of treatment, but it is not the only treatment. Fortunately, there are alternatives in surgery, chemosurgery, cryotherapy, electrodesiccation, and chemotherapy. Some cases are better treated by these methods. Others benefit from combined treatments, with the final result superior to that which can be obtained by any one method alone. The selection of optimal treatment is best made by a multidisciplinary oncologic team with decisions based on the probability of cure, cosmesis, function, and the relative comfort, time, and cost of treatment. The patient's wishes must also be considered. The parameters concerned in determining optimal treatment include the patient's general condition, age, complexion, occupation, and location of residence and whether the skin shows signs of damage or other lesions are present. Tumor factors to be considered include the site, size, degree of invasion, multifocal neoplasms, and previous treatment.

Some controversy exists as to whether radiotherapy or surgery is best for lesions at particular sites. In general, radiotherapy is contraindicated when post-treatment complications may be significant. Radiosensitive organs such as the eye usually can be protected from radiation, and so most contraindications relate to the possibility of the radiation scar becoming unstable. These include tumors in young people when the scar will worsen with time, those developing in severely actinically damaged skin, tumors in fair-skinned people and in others who have an excessive exposure to sunlight, and lesions arising at sites of friction or in areas with a poor blood supply. In addition, if the radiation scar would be unsightly and difficult to hide, such as an epilated patch on the scalp, alternative treatment should be considered. Surgery is preferred for most tumors that recur following irradiation. Every patient's treatment should be individualized, and if the preceding parameters are considered by the multidisciplinary team, a consensus can be reached as to optimal care.

The skin essentially consists of three main layers. The epidermis is a stratified squamous epithelium that covers a connective tissue dermis and an underlying fatty layer. Its thickness varies from site to site, and on the head and neck the epidermis varies from 0.06 mm on the eyelid to 1 mm on the nape of the neck. At special sites its anatomic, functional, and biologic characteristics give the sites the status of regional organs. The behavior of some tumors and the radiotolerance of the tumor bed present special problems. Basal and squamous cell carcinomas are both radiosensitive and radiocurable. Tumors developing at embryologic junctional sites must be treated with great care because of their tendency to deeper invasion along tissue planes. Overall, 95 per cent of skin carcinomas can be controlled by irradiation, usually with a good cosmetic and functional result.[10]

The Princess Margaret Hospital is a tertiary referral center and a major radiotherapy institute. Patients are preselected for treatment at other hospitals, and most are referred for radiation therapy. About one quarter of our skin cancer patients are first treated by surgery, and the other three quarters are primary cases. All patients are assessed in a multidisciplinary clinic staffed by dermatologists, surgeons, and radiation oncologists. After treatment is prescribed and carried out, the patients are followed in the same multidisciplinary clinic.

RADIOTHERAPY

Soon after Röntgen's discovery of x-rays in 1896, the first cases of radiation dermatitis were reported. By 1899 the first report on the apparent cure of a cancer appeared with the description of a basal cell epithelioma treated by this new modality.[2] The radiation would have been relatively superficial because the maximum energies produced would have been between 50 and 100 kv. The radiosensitivity of skin cancers and their dramatic response to irradiation led to the belief that a cancer cure had finally been discovered. This was followed by disillusionment when tumors recurred and damage to normal tissues began to appear. The discovery of radioactivity by Becquerel and of radium by the Curies led to the development of surface applicators and interstitial implants for skin tumors. Until the 1950s, interstitial implants with radium, radon seeds and other isotopes, or surface or sandwich molds utilizing radium were commonly used. Since then, with advances in radiation technology and the development of better machines, most skin tumors have been treated with superficial or orthovoltage x-rays. Today, the electron beam generated from linear accelerators with its specific physical characteristics is becoming the treatment of choice. In new departments it is often the only treatment modality for skin cancers. The effectiveness of superficial and orthovoltage x-rays is so well established that, where available, they will be used for many years to come.

General Considerations

Basal and squamous cell carcinomas of the skin have similar radiosensitivities, and most are radiocurable. All lesions should have histologic confirmation. The radiotherapeutic techniques and doses are many and varied; the methods described here are those that have been found to be reliable, although there are others, no doubt of equal efficacy and applicability. Each center must develop its own methods according to need and the technical resources available. Today, with a good understanding of the biologic effects of irradiation on tumors and normal tissues, local control rates exceed 90 per cent, usually with a good cosmetic result and few complications. In general, only one curative course of treatment is given.

Most cutaneous cancers are readily accessible and can be treated en bloc with a single direct beam of radiation. For big tumors, techniques using angled beams and wedges may be required. The gross tumor must be measured accurately in order to select the appropriate radiation energy to obtain homogeneity of radiation throughout the tumor volume. Tomography and computed tomographic (CT) scans are of value in assessing the extent of destruction caused by infiltrating lesions. The area to be irradiated includes the tumor with a margin of normal skin. This should be 0.5 cm in width for tumors up to 2 cm, 1.0 cm for lesions 2 to 5 cm in width, and 2 cm or more for large tumors. The radiotolerance of the tumor bed must be known and not exceeded, and the dose and depth of penetration must be carefully calculated so as not to complicate surgery should it be required. A course of treatment varies from one to 30 daily sessions treating five times weekly with the total dose depending on the fractionation. For most tumors, fractionated treatment is preferred because it increases the radiotolerance of the surrounding tissues and reduces the late high-dose effects, especially the necrosis that may follow the trauma. Cosmesis is also improved for all but small tumors. The field edges become blurred by minor changes in positioning each day, and so the punched-out appearance of a single exposure is avoided. However, for selected cases, a single radiation fraction constitutes optimal treatment. These include some tumors in old or infirm patients or those whose residence is far away and some lesions that are less than 1 cm in diameter. For large tumors, the field is often reduced as treatment progresses, and this also enhances the final appearance. The major goals of treatment are to preserve the normal anatomy and function and to achieve a good cosmetic result. Radiotherapy is equally effective in treating primary tumors and those that are residual or recurrent following surgery. Surgery is the preferred treatment for most tumors that recur after radiotherapy.

TABLE 50–1. Dose-Time Relationships Used to Treat Basal Cell and Squamous Cell Carcinomas*

cGy	Fractions	Days
2000	1	1
2250	1	1
3500	5	5
4000	5	7
4250	10	12
4500	10–15	12–19
5000–6000	20–30	26–38

*The maximum dose is prescribed at the skin surface. It includes backscatter for superficial and orthovoltage x-rays and allows for build-up when bolus is used with high energy electrons.

Radiation Dose

The radiation time-dose relationships necessary to destroy skin tumors without producing necrosis of normal tissues is well established.[3, 11–13] A single dose of 2150 cGy has a 99 per cent probability of curing a basal cell carcinoma or a squamous cell carcinoma and a 3 per cent chance of late skin damage. The choice of dose, time, number of fractions, and technique vary with the clinical problem. Common schedules that have proved to be effective are shown in Table 50–1. In general, the dose is increased and the treatment time is extended for large tumors. The preferred dose-time schedule for most tumors up to 2 cm is 3500 cGy in five daily fractions, and for 3 cm lesions the dose is 4250 to 4500 cGy in ten fractions in 12 days.

Higher cure rates can be obtained but at the expense of increased complications and poorer cosmesis. Tumor doses are calculated at the skin surface, and the minimum dose should be at least 90 per cent of the maximum.

Superficial and Orthovoltage X-rays

At the Princess Margaret Hospital, most skin tumors are treated with x-rays of energies between 100 and 250 kv. Their characteristics are shown in Figure 50–1. If a short 20-cm source-skin distance (SSD) is used, adjustments must be made if the whole tumor is not equidistant from the source or underdosage will result (Fig. 50–2). The simplest method is to take advantage of the inverse square law to increase the percentage depth dose by using a longer SSD. When a tumor covers an irregular surface, such as the bridge of the nose, a compensator should be used (Fig. 50–3). At short SSDs the radiation dose at the edge of a field is 20 per cent less than at the center (Fig. 50–4). This problem is solved by using a radiation field larger than the lead cut-out so that only the central rays are used. For 100 kv radiation, the field is delineated by a lead cut-out 1 mm thick and an open-ended applicator is used. For more penetrating x-rays up to a half-value layer (HVL) 1.1 mm Cu, the lead cut-out is made 2 mm thick, and the field is outlined with a treatment cone or light device. The absorption of radiation by bone is 2.4 times greater than in soft tissue at 100 kv HVL 0.7 mm Al and 1.7 times that at 250 kv HVL 1.1 mm Cu. Bone necrosis, however, because of increased dose has never been a clinical problem. The densities of cartilage and soft tissue are similar, and both absorb similar amounts of radiation. Cartilage necrosis is rare and probably only

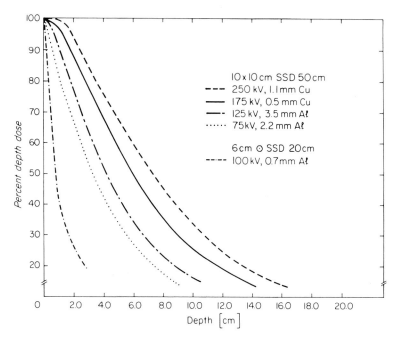

Figure 50–1. Depth-dose characteristics for superficial and orthovoltage radiation.

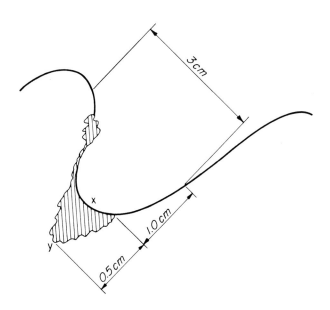

Figure 50–2. A common problem is giving irradiation to a tumor covering an irregular surface such as that at the inner canthus of the eye. The percentage depthdose can be increased by using a higher energy and a longer source-skin distance.

100 KV HVL 0.7 mm Al 20 cm SSD

Dose at X : $100 \times \left(\dfrac{20}{21}\right)^2 = 91\%$

Dose at Y : $1814 \times \left(\dfrac{21.0}{21.5}\right)^2 \times 63\% = 1090$ cGy

cGy	1 Tx
GD	2000
Dx	1814
Dy	1090

% DD @ 0.5 cm = 63%

125 KV HVL 3.5 mm Al 50 cm SSD

$100 \times \left(\dfrac{50}{51}\right)^2 = 96\%$

$1922 \times \left(\dfrac{51}{51.5}\right)^2 \times 95\% = 1790$ cGy

cGy	1 Tx
GD	2000
Dx	1922
Dy	1791

% DD @ 0.5 cm = 95%

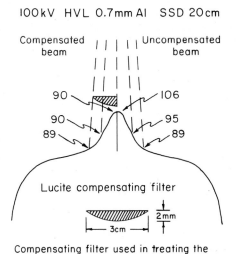

100 kV HVL 0.7 mm Al SSD 20 cm

Compensated beam | Uncompensated beam

90 — 106
90 — 95
89 — 89

Lucite compensating filter

2 mm
3 cm

Compensating filter used in treating the bridge and dorsum of nose

Figure 50–3. A compensator ensures homogeneity of radiation when using a short source-skin distance.

occurs when excessive damage is done to the surrounding tissues. This follows because cartilage is avascular and dependent for nourishment from the periphery.

The Electron Beam

Electron beams are now obtained from linear accelerators and are increasingly used in the treatment of skin cancer.[4, 5] Most linear accelerators have a range of fixed energies, and beams with characteristics intermediate between these energies may be obtained by using the nearest higher energy in conjunction with appropriate thickness of bolus. Monoenergetic electrons have a defined depth of penetration in tissues. They provide uniform irradiation to about one half of the penetration

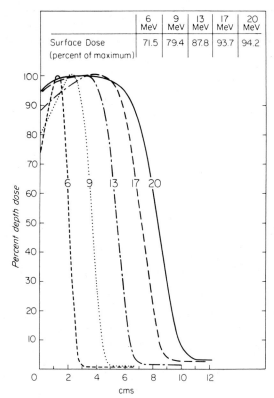

	6 MeV	9 MeV	13 MeV	17 MeV	20 MeV
Surface Dose (percent of maximum)	71.5	79.4	87.8	93.7	94.2

Figure 50–5. Central axis depth-dose curves for electron beams obtained from a Therac-20 AECL linear accelerator.

depth of the beam, after which there is a quick fall-off (Fig. 50–5). Because of the electron build-up the maximum dose is below the surface, and so a bolus of varying thickness must be used to increase the surface dose (Fig. 50–6). The beam characteristics have a distinct advantage in treatment with a relative biologic effect (RBE) that is almost the same as for high-energy pho-

5 MeV Electron Beam with 1.0 cm Tissue Equivalent Bolus

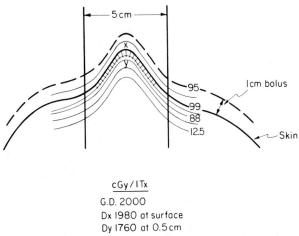

5 cm

95
99
88
12.5

1 cm bolus

Skin

cGy / 1 Tx
G.D. 2000
Dx 1980 at surface
Dy 1760 at 0.5 cm

Figure 50–6. Bolus must be used to bring the maximum dose to the surface.

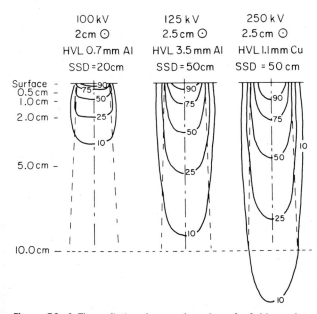

100 kV	125 kV	250 kV
2 cm ⊙	2.5 cm ⊙	2.5 cm ⊙
HVL 0.7 mm Al	HVL 3.5 mm Al	HVL 1.1 mm Cu
SSD = 20 cm	SSD = 50 cm	SSD = 50 cm

Surface
0.5 cm
1.0 cm
2.0 cm

5.0 cm

10.0 cm

Figure 50–4. The radiation dose at the edge of a field may be 20 per cent less than at the center.

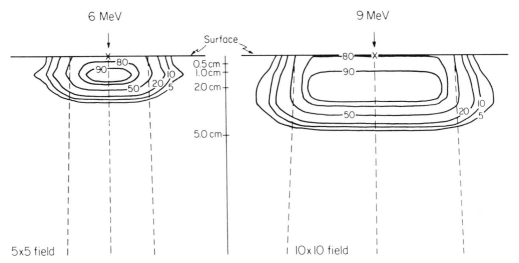

Figure 50–7. Isodose curves for 6- and 9-MeV electron beams. The characteristics of the curves vary with field size and energy.

tons. Necrosis in cartilage and bone is neither a theoretical nor a practical problem. To correct for the lower RBE of the electron beam with respect to superficial and orthovoltage x-rays, the dose is increased by 10 per cent.[5]

An important characteristic of the electron beam that must be considered in treatment planning is the decreased surface area due to scatter (Fig. 50–7). For example, a 6-cm circular field is effectively a 4.5-cm circle at the surface. Tissue heterogeneities that affect high-energy electron distributions must be considered in planning. The absorption of electrons in bone is similar to that for soft tissues; 1 cm of bone attenuates the beam to the same degree as 1.65 cm of muscle. Sloping surfaces and asymmetric contours produce significant changes in dose because of the changing SSD. In assessing the appropriate electron energy, the maximum penetration of the beam can be approximated by dividing the peak energy by 2 and the therapeutic range by 3.5. For each extra centimeter of air that the beam travels, the dose is decreased by approximately 4 per cent. Lead cut-outs are used to delineate the treatment field. Ninety-five per cent of 7- and 18-MeV beams are absorbed by 2.3 mm and 1 cm of lead, respectively.

Radiation Reactions in Skin and Tumor

Following irradiation a series of changes occur in both the normal skin and tumor. These vary in degree and are dependent upon the type of skin, field size, and dose. Therapeutic doses cause a bright erythema, which appears about the seventh day after a single exposure, 1 to 2 weeks after a 5-day course of treatment, and during the second and third weeks of protracted therapy. The erythema fades over 2 to 3 weeks with a dry desquamation. The hyperpigmented patch that is left disappears over several weeks, although a circumferential ring of pigmentation from scattered radiation may persist for some time. In about one half of patients a moist reaction occurs, and in another 10 per cent the tissue reactions are minimal and barely noticeable. Epilation follows 300 cGy and is often permanent after 1000 cGy.

A tumor starts to regress following the first dose of radiation, with the rate depending upon its radiosensitivity. This is not usually visible until the end of the second week, at which time the surrounding skin shows that a brisk erythema or a moist desquamation is commencing. At 1 month the average tumor is flat with the

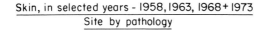

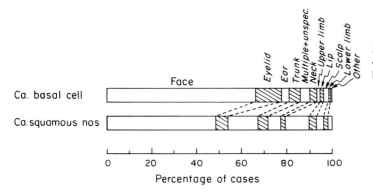

Figure 50–8. The majority of basal cell carcinomas and squamous cell carcinomas develop on the exposed surfaces of the head and neck.

surrounding skin, and complete disappearance is usual within 8 weeks. Occasionally a ghost outline will remain for several weeks before total disappearance. Any tumor detectable at 3 months is unlikely to be cured, and further management should be considered.

Care of Reactions

In general, irradiated tissues are best left exposed to the air and kept dry. Cornstarch, not talcum powder, which may contain heavy metals, can be used for this purpose. If a moist desquamation develops, the application of a 1 per cent solution of aqueous gentian violet will coagulate the serum and provide protection for the healing tissues. Wet saline soaks help to remove crusts. Dressings are best avoided except for lesions covered by clothing where they may be used to prevent friction. They are also used for cosmetic reasons to hide exposed lesions during the acute reaction. Greasy ointments should be avoided because they cause maceration of the superficial layers of the skin. If the irradiated tissues start to itch and this becomes a problem, the application of 0.5 per cent hydrocortisone cream will provide relief. Infection, which is rare, should be treated with the appropriate antibiotic.

A late complication that may follow injury months or years after treatment is tissue necrosis. This presents as a painful, inflamed, non-healing ulcer. Most of these soft-tissue ulcers heal if they are protected from further trauma, and healing can be hastened with the application of steroid and antibiotic creams. A persistent ulcer should be excised.

Follow-up

After radiotherapy, patients are followed in order to assess the results of treatment and to detect the onset of other lesions. In general, patients are seen at 1, 2, and 3 months following treatment in order to evaluate the response and advise on the care of reactions. Further visits are scheduled at 3-month intervals for 2 years, and then every 6 months until 5 years, and then annually. For some patients, many of whom are elderly, follow-up of these comparatively minor cancers is best carried out by the family physician once the tumor has disappeared and the reactions have healed. Most recurrences occur within 2 years.

CLINICAL EXPERIENCE AND RESULTS OF TREATMENT

Basal and squamous cell carcinomas behave in a similar manner and, with comparable radiosensitivities, can be considered together. Between 1958 and 1974 11,493 cases of basal cell carcinoma (BCC) and squamous cell carcinoma (SCC) were seen. The majority were on the exposed areas of the head and neck (Fig. 50–8). The median age at which patients were referred for treatment was 68.5 (males 67.8, females 69.5) years with a range of 14 to 96 years. For both sexes BCC was more common than SCC with an overall ratio of 3.3 to 1, but SCC had a 2.1 to 1 advantage in males. Multiple tumors developed in approximately three quarters of the patients, with a second lesion appearing in 25 per cent within 1 year.

Basal cell carcinoma arises from the basal layer of the epidermis and has a predilection for the skin of the head above a line joining the earlobe to the angle of the mouth. At embryologic junctional sites, these tumors

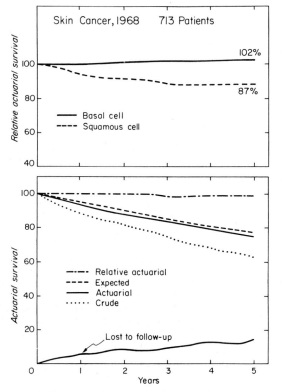

Figure 50–9. Basal cell carcinomas and squamous cell carcinomas have little effect on overall survival.

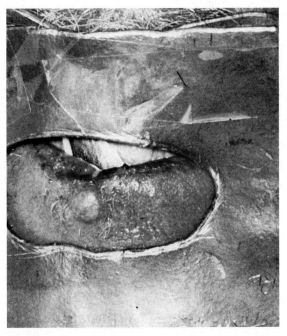

Figure 50–10. Lead cut-outs are used to delineate the tumor and to protect the underlying tissues.

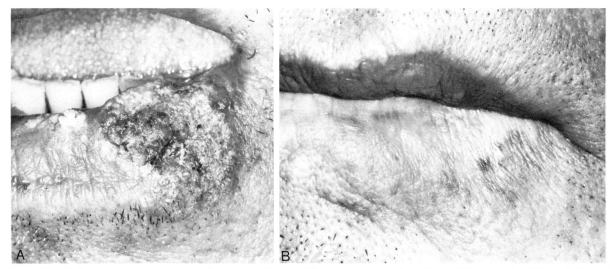

Figure 50–11. Squamous cell carcinoma of the lower lip in a 55-year-old man before (A) and 5 years after (B) irradiation. He received a dose of 5000 cGy at 250 kV half-value layer 11.1 mm Cu delivered in 20 fractions in 1 month with the field reduced in size at 3500 cGy.

tend to burrow deeply and can cause hideous deformity. The different clinical types are all responsive to radiotherapy. The average tumor had a diameter of 19 mm and a growth rate of 5 mm per year. The average duration of symptoms prior to diagnosis was 3.5 years.

Squamous cell carcinoma arises from squamous cells of the epidermis or its appendages in skin that usually shows other lesions. Most are well differentiated, and only about 1 per cent metastasize to the regional nodes. Bowen's disease is the in situ phase of intraepidermal carcinoma. At diagnosis the average tumor was also 19 mm in diameter but had been present for a shorter period of 14 months.

In order to obtain an overview of skin cancer on the head and neck, 713 patients seen in 1968 were selected for study and 308 were analyzed in detail. A pathology review of 592 tumors showed 464 BCC and 128 SCC, a ratio of 3.6 to 1, which is similar to that of our overall experience. There were 411 males and 301 females with median ages of 67.26 and 68.96 (30 to 97) years. Approximately one quarter (174) of the patients had been treated initially by surgery, with the other three quarters (539) being primary untreated cases. The tumor was

smaller than 2 cm in size in 245 (65 per cent) of 377 patients in whom measurements were available. These tumors had little effect on mortality, and the apparent anomaly in the relative actuarial survival curves reflects that these tumors develop in a healthier outdoors population (Fig. 50–9). Among 308 patients, only three were known to have died from skin cancer, two with BCC and one with a SCC. One third (74) of 229 primary cases were irradiated with a single fraction, and this achieved a 92 per cent 5-year disease-free rate. For 155 primary cases irradiated with multiple fractions, the 5-year disease-free rate was 95 per cent. Fifteen (5 per cent) of 229 primary tumors, which included nine BCC and six SCC, were not cured by radiotherapy. These patients had median ages of 74 and 84 years, respectively. In two patients the tumor did not resolve following treatment, and in 10 others recurrence was apparent within 2 years. This was central in three and marginal in nine, and one SCC metastasized to the regional nodes. Five patients had been treated with a single fraction, and ten were treated with multiple fractions. Further treatment was surgery in five cases and irradiation in three, and seven received no further treatment.

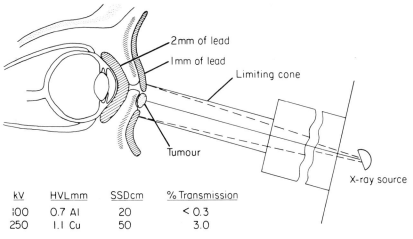

Figure 50–12. The dose of radiation received by the eye can be reduced by a simple lead shield. (Reprinted with permission from Int J Radiat Oncol Biol Phys *10:*451, 1984; Fitzpatrick PJ, et al: Basal and squamous cell carcinoma of the eyelids and their treatment by radiotherapy. Copyright 1984, Pergamon Press, Ltd.)

kV	HVLmm	SSDcm	% Transmission
100	0.7 Al	20	< 0.3
250	1.1 Cu	50	3.0

TABLE 50–2. Clinical Experience with Carcinoma of the Lip in 1268 Patients (1958–1972)*

Site	Squamous Cell Carcinoma			Basal Cell Carcinoma		
	Males	*Females*	*Total*	*Males*	*Females*	*Total*
Upper lip	26	12	38	11	17	28
Lower lip	954	28	982	16	4	20
	980	40	1020	27	21	48

Age: Males, 63.9 years; females, 70.4 years. Median age: 64.3 years. Range: 24–97 years. *Five-year survival:* crude, relative, 71 per cent; actuarial, 97 per cent.

SPECIAL SITES

The Lip

Tumors arise from both the skin and mucosa (Table 50–2). Those arising from the skin are similar in behavior to other skin cancers and are treated in the same way. Only squamous cell carcinomas develop from the lip mucosa. The ratio of males to females is 24.5 to 1. Most arise from an unstable vermilion margin, which is an embryologic junctional area and is prone to actinic chelitis. One in three patients has a premalignant lesion. Tumors predominate on the lower lip in comparison to the upper lip with a ratio of 26 to 1.

Following assessment in our multidisciplinary clinic, most patients selected for radiotherapy were irradiated with a direct 250-kv photon beam. (However, a 7-Mev electron beam is being used increasingly.) A 2-mm lead cut-out with a 1-cm margin is shaped to delineate the field, and another is placed in front of the gums to protect the underlying structures (Fig. 50–10). The dose-time schedules were varied with the size and nature of the tumor. Commonly, doses of 4250 cGy were given in ten equal fractions over 12 days, or doses of 5000 cGy were given in 15 to 20 fractions delivered over 3 to 4 weeks. Massive tumors require doses up to 6500 cGy delivered in 30 fractions over 6 weeks. When the whole lip must be irradiated because of an unstable epithelium, the field is reduced when 70 per cent of the tumor dose has been given.

Because regional metastases developed in only 7 per cent of patients, prophylactic cervical node irradiation is not recommended. Metastases were more common with large tumors and especially if the lateral commissures were involved. The first-echelon nodes are the submental and submaxillary groups, and subsequently, there is spread to the deep cervical chain. The rich lymphatic plexus with cross-over drainage allows both ipsilateral and contralateral metastases. When present at diagnosis, both sides of the upper neck are irradiated in continuity with the primary tumor using parallel opposed supervoltage fields with wedges and compensators. For those patients who develop metastases following primary treatment, surgery, which includes a full neck dissection on the affected side and a suprahyoid dissection on the other, is usually recommended. Postoperative irradiation may be indicated, and some patients with minimal disease or who are in poor general condition may be treated by radiotherapy alone.

The mucosal radiation reactions tend to be more severe than those on the skin surface. They are managed in a similar way. Patients should be counseled to avoid trauma, especially that due to excessive sun exposure. Soft-tissue necrosis is uncommon and only occurred in 2 per cent of patients. Most ulcers heal with conservative care, but painful or persistent ones should be excised. The cosmetic and functional results of treatment are generally good and are readily accepted by the patients (Fig. 50–11). Among 1268 patients seen between 1958 and 1972, the 5-year local control and relative actuarial survival rates were 84 and 97 per cent, and these rates were the same for both lower and upper lip tumors. Only 3 per cent of patients died from this cancer.

TABLE 50–4. Dose-Time Relationships Used to Treat 1166 Eyelid Tumors (1958–1978)

cGy	Fractions	Days	Basal Cell Carcinoma	Squamous Carcinoma	Per Cent
2000–2250	1	1	276	20	25
3500–4000	5	5–7	499	25	45
4250–4500	10	12	225	35	22
4500–5000	15	19	30	15	8
5000–6000	20–30	26–40	32	9	
			1062	104	100

Source: Adapted from Fitzpatrick PJ, et al: Int J Radiat Oncol Biol Phys 10:451, 1984. Copyright 1984, Pergamon Press, Ltd.

TABLE 50–3. Clinical Experience with 1166 Eyelid Tumors Treated by Radiotherapy (1958–1978)*

	Primary Tumors	Recurrent Tumors	Total	Five-Year Control	Per Cent
Basal cell carcinoma	686	376	1062	1009	95
Squamous cell carcinoma	62	42	104	97	93.3
	748	418	1166	1106	94.8

*Most of the primary tumors were controlled and the few failures were salvaged by surgery. Of the 1166 tumors, 745 (64 per cent) were less than 2 cm in diameter.
Source: Adapted from Fitzpatrick PJ, et al: Int J Radiat Oncol Biol Phys 10:450, 1984. Copyright 1984, Pergamon Press, Ltd.

TABLE 50–5. Radiation Complications in 1166 Cases of Eyelid Tumors (1958–1978)*

Skin atrophy	64
Ectropion	36†
Entropion	6
Epiphora	27†
Keratinization conjunctiva	21
Keratitis	5
Cataract	11
Perforated globe	3
	173

*Complications resulting from radiotherapy were difficult to separate from those due to the tumor. Complications occurred in 112 (9.6 per cent) patients.
†Often present before treatment.

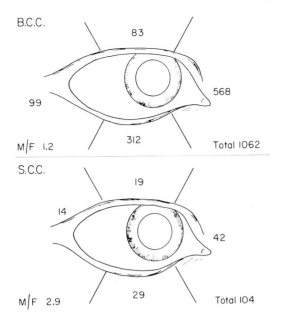

Figure 50–13. Sites of origin of 1166 eyelid tumors seen between 1958 and 1978.

TABLE 50–6. Cosmetic and Functional Results of Radiotherapy in Basal Cell and Squamous Cell Carcinoma of the Eyelids

Result	One Year		Five Years	
Excellent	346	(83%)	113	(77%)
Good	26	(6%)	25	(17%)
Fair	21	} (11%)	8	} (6%)
Poor	23		1	
	416	(100%)	147	(100%)

per cent owing to scatter. A similar technique can be used with the electron beam, but because of secondary x-ray emission the dose to the eye is about 15 per cent of the tumor dose.[1]

Our 20-year experience with 1166 tumors is outlined in Table 50–3. Nearly one third of the patients were first treated by surgery, and in two thirds the tumors were less than 2 cm in diameter. Most tumors were near the inner canthus or on the lower lid; this reflects the measure of difficulty associated with surgical excision at these sites (Fig. 50–13). Approximately one quarter of the patients were treated with a single fraction, one half with five fractions, and the others (because of their complexity) over longer periods and to higher doses (Table 50–4). It was difficult to differentiate the complications resulting from radiation from those resulting from the tumor. Most were related to large tumors with extensive damage to the eyelids. Complications were recorded in 112 (9.6 per cent) patients (Table 50–5). In a random survey of 147 patients carried out 5 years after radiotherapy concerning the cosmetic and functional results of treatment, 138 (94 per cent) patients considered the results to be good to excellent (Table 50–6 and Fig. 50–14*A* and *B*). For small tumors 1 cm or less in diameter, we could not distinguish on a cosmetic basis whether they had been irradiated with a single fraction or five fractions of radiation. Also, for the average tumor, the results were similar for those treated with five or ten fractions. The 5-year primary tumor control rates were 95 and 93.5 per cent for basal and squamous cell carcinomas, respectively. Five patients with squamous cell carcinomas developed regional node metastases, and three had cancer-related deaths.

The Eyelids and Periorbital Skin

The importance of tumors arising in the eyelid or periorbital skin lies in their ability to penetrate all layers of the eyelids. These destructive lesions, by involving the lid margin or lacrimal system, can produce severe functional disability and, in addition, can be very disfiguring. Because of the specialized function of the eyelids and the proximity to the eye, treatment presents many technical problems.[1, 6] The eye is a radiovulnerable organ, and every attempt must be made to limit the radiation that it receives, especially to its anterior segment. For most patients treated with photon radiation, the dose to the eye can be reduced by the insertion of a 2-mm acrylic-coated lead-equivalent shield into the conjunctival sac (Fig. 50–12). The percentage of radiation that is transmitted is low and only increases by a few

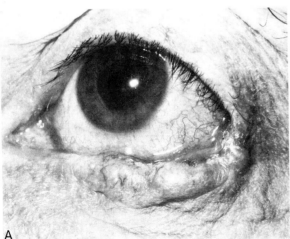

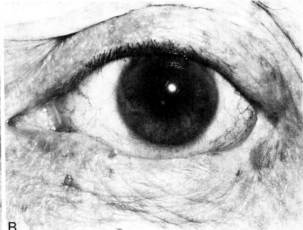

Figure 50–14. Extensive basal cell carcinoma of the lower eyelid in a 62-year-old man before (*A*) and 5 years after (*B*) irradiation. He received 4250 cGy delivered in ten fractions in 12 days at 125 kV HVL (half-value layer) 3.5 mm Al.

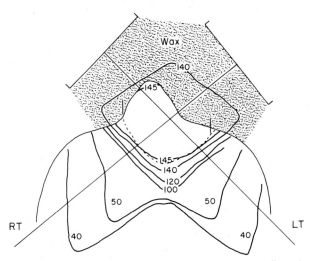

^{60}Co. Wedge pair 6W·5cm

R$_x$ 5000/15 at 145% / 3/52

Figure 50–15. Treatment plan for a large squamous cell carcinoma deeply invading the nose.

The Nose

In our records tumors arising from the skin of the nose were classified among those on the face. Between 1958 and 1978, a total of 10,387 tumors were registered. Accordingly, 320 cases, including 216 BCC and 104 SCC, that were treated by irradiation were randomly selected from our records for review (Table 50–7). Fifty-seven (18 per cent) patients had received previous treatment. Tumors arising in the nasolabial fold were separated

TABLE 50–7. Results of 320 Cases of Nasal Carcinoma Treated by Radiation*

Site	Primary	Recurrent Tumor	Total	Five-Year Control No.	Five-Year Control Per Cent
Nose					
Basal cell carcinoma	80	20	100	93	93
Squamous cell carcinoma	57†	17	74	70	94.6
Ala nasi					
Basal cell carcinoma	100	16	116	98	85
Squamous cell carcinoma	26	4	30	24	80
	263	57	320	285	89

*In this random selection of 320 cases of basal cell and squamous cell carcinoma, a total of 89 per cent of the primary lesions were controlled and surgical treatment salvaged most of the failures.
†One positive node DD (died of disease).

from those elsewhere on the nose. The irradiation techniques and doses were similar to those used at other sites; compensators or bolus were necessary to treat tumors on the bridge of the nose (see Figs. 50–3 and 50–6). Higher energies with greater penetration were used for lesions in the ala nasal region, and wax blocks and jigs were needed to treat large tumors when the whole nose was irradiated (Figs. 50–15 and 50–16A and B).

The overall 5-year local control rate was 89 per cent (Table 50–7). Soft-tissue or cartilage necrosis developed in eight (3.0 per cent) cases in whom the tumor was controlled. One patient died from metastatic carcinoma.

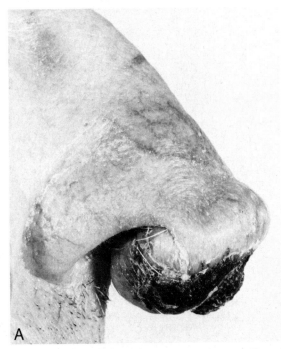

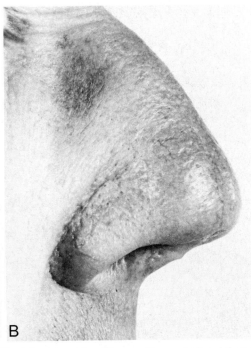

Figure 50–16. Large squamous cell carcinoma (Keratoacanthoma?) of the nose of a 67-year-old man before (A) and 3 years following (B) a dose of 4500 cGy delivered in 15 fractions in 3 weeks.

The Ear

From among 1168 patients with tumors on the ear, 743 who were treated by radiotherapy were available for review (Table 50–8). These included 349 patients with BCC and 323 with SCC. Tumors arising around the external auditory meatus (EAM) were reviewed separately from the others. Previous treatment had been given to 221 (30 per cent) patients. The overall 5-year control rate was 90.4 per cent, and the cosmetic results were usually good (Fig. 50–17A and B). Necrosis of soft tissue or cartilage, usually manifest by a painful non-healing ulcer, developed in 28 (4 per cent) patients and was mostly associated with large tumors. The skin of the ear is adherent to the cartilage and has little subcutaneous tissue, especially on its lateral surface. This paucity of soft tissue limits the radiotolerance of cartilage. However, this complication was only a minor problem and was readily corrected by surgery. Regional metastases developed in 14 (3.9 per cent) patients with SCC, including five patients with tumors involving the EAM. Four deaths were attributable to uncontrolled tumors.

OTHER TUMORS

Melanoma

For nodular and superficial spreading melanomas, an adequate surgical excision is the treatment of choice. Radiotherapy is used as postoperative treatment when

TABLE 50–8. Clinical Experience with 743 Cases of Carcinoma Arising from the Skin of the Ear and Treated by Radiotherapy*

Site	Primary Tumor	Recurrent Tumor	Total	Five-Year Control No.	Five-Year Control Per Cent
Ear					
Basal cell carcinoma	265	113	378	340	90
Squamous cell carcinoma	230†	92	322	293	91
External auditory meatus					
Basal cell carcinoma	6	3	9	9	100
Squamous cell carcinoma	21‡	13	34	30	90
	522	221	743	672	90.4

*The primary tumor control rate was 90.4 per cent, and most of the recurrences were salvaged by surgery.
†Nine positive nodes.
‡Five positive nodes, four DD (died of disease).

excision is incomplete and to palliate recurrent tumors.[8] There appears to be an advantage in using large fractions, and we recommend giving 5000 cGy in ten treatments in 12 days. Another schedule for palliation is to deliver 2400 cGy in three fractions at 0, 7, and 21 days.

Lentigo maligna and lentigo maligna melanoma

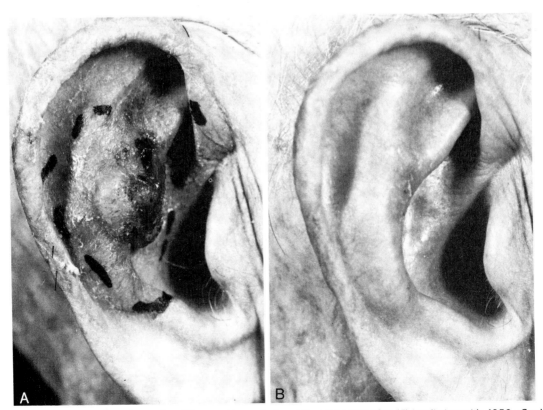

Figure 50–17. Squamous cell carcinoma in a 72-year-old man before (A) and 5 years after (B) irradiation with 4250 cGy delivered in 10 fractions in 12 days at 250 kV HVL (half-value layer) 1.1 mm Cu.

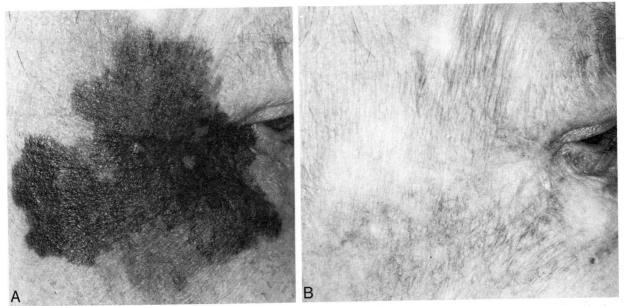

Figure 50–18. Lentigo maligna melanoma in a 69-year-old man before (*A*) and 5 years after (*B*) irradiation at 100 kV half-value layer 0.7 mm Al to a dose of 5000 cGy delivered in 20 fractions in 1 month.

(LMM) are both radiosensitive, and nodular melanomas developing from them are radiocurable (Fig. 50–18*A* and *B*).[7] Twenty-one of 23 patients with LMM on the head or neck had their tumor controlled from 1 month to 7 years following irradiation. Two tumors recurred locally,

and both were salvaged by excision. None of these patients developed regional or distant metastases. Following irradiation, lesions may take up to 24 months before final disappearance. All patients were treated with superficial or orthovoltage radiotherapy equipment

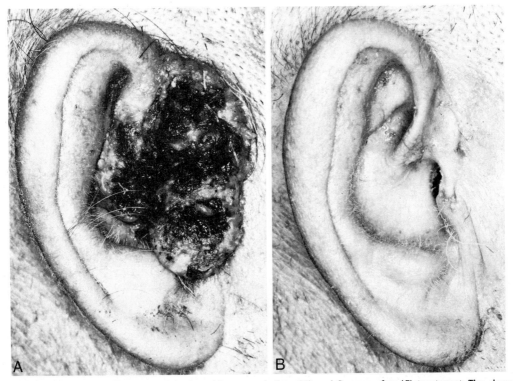

Figure 50–19. Large keratoacanthoma in an 82-year-old woman before (*A*) and 3 years after (*B*) treatment. The dose was 5100 cGy in 17 fractions delivered in 23 days.

with doses ranging from 3500 cGy in five fractions to 4500 or 5000 cGy in ten to 15 fractions.

Keratoacanthoma

This pseudocancer, also known as a "self-healing epithelioma," has an unpredictable clinical course. Many tumors heal spontaneously if left alone or spurred by biopsy. Others cause tremendous tissue destruction and may undergo malignant transformation with fatal results. These tumors should not be underestimated, and sometimes the term "acute epithelial carcinoma" is preferred. Small tumors under 15 mm in diameter can be excised or treated with curettage and diathermy. Most others can be cured by radiotherapy, with large tumors requiring higher doses and more penetrating radiation similar to that used to treat SCC (Fig. 50–19*A* and *B*). Radiotherapy controlled 59 (91 per cent) of 65 tumors. The median time for the tumor to completely disappear was 8 weeks.

The term keratoacanthoma denotes a benign lesion. However, the capricious nature of some of these tumors and our inability to detect which ones may undergo malignant degeneration should cause us to view them with caution. They should be treated rather than left alone in the hope that they will undergo spontaneous regression if their clinical behavior arouses suspicion.

REFERENCES

1. Asbell SO, Siu J, Lightfoot A, Brady LW: Individualized eye shields for use in electron beam therapy as well as low-energy photon irradiation. Int J Radiat Oncol Biol Phys 6:519, 1980.
2. Case JT: History of radiation therapy. *In* Buschke F (ed): Progress in Radiation Therapy. New York, Grune & Stratton, 1958.
3. Cohen L: The statistical prognosis in radiation therapy. Am J Roentgen 84:471, 1960.
4. du V Tapley N, Fletcher GH: Applications of the electron beam in the treatment of cancer of the skin and lips. Radiology 109:423, 1973.
5. du V Tapley N, Almond PR: Treatment planning and techniques with the electron beam. *In* Bleehan NM, Glatstein E, Haybittle JL (eds): Radiation Therapy Planning. New York, Marcel Dekker, 1983, pp. 343–392.
6. Fitzpatrick PJ, Jamieson DM, Thompson GA, Allt WEC: Tumours of the eyelids and their treatment by radiotherapy. Radiology 104:661, 1972.
7. Harwood AR: Conventional radiotherapy in the treatment of lentigo maligna and lentigo melanoma. J Am Acad Dermatol 6:310, 1982.
8. Harwood AR, Dancuart F, Fitzpatrick PJ, Brown T: Radiotherapy in non-lentiginous melanomas of the head and neck. Cancer 48:2599, 1981.
9. Lederman M: Radiation treatment of cancer of the eyelids. Br J Ophthalmol 60:794, 1976.
10. Moss WT, Brand WN, Baltifora H: Radiation Oncology, Rationale, Technique, Results. St. Louis, C. V. Mosby Co., 1979, pp 52–82.
11. Strandqvist M: Time-dose relationship. Acta Radiol suppl 55, 1944.
12. Von Essen CF: A spatial model of time-dose-area relationship in radiation therapy. Radiology 81:881, 1963.
13. Von Essen CF: A practical time-dose formula for x-ray therapy of skin cancer. Br J Radiol 42:474, 1969.

CHAPTER 51

Controversy in the Management of Tumors of the Skin

John E. Woods, M.D.

This chapter deals primarily with controversies in the treatment of malignant tumors of the skin, particularly as they relate to the head and neck, with the exception of one benign condition, port-wine stain (nevus flammeus), which continues to escape completely satisfactory treatment. Of the malignant conditions, attention will be focused on basal cell and squamous cell carcinoma and malignant melanoma because numerically they constitute the overwhelming majority of skin lesions in the head and neck area. A brief discussion of keratoacanthoma is included.

PORT-WINE STAIN

Nevus flammeus is seen in the newborn, occurring usually on the face in the sensory distribution of the trigeminal nerve. The true port-wine stain may be distinguished from the pale nevus flammeus neonatorum, which usually disappears within 6 months. The classical lesion does not spontaneously regress and, in fact, may develop wart-like excrescences in adulthood.[33]

Associated conditions include Sturge-Weber syndrome with intracranial hemangioma and ipsilateral glaucoma, which is seen in conjunction with nevus flammeus, occurring in the distribution of the first and second branches of the trigeminal nerve. These conditions are not discussed in this chapter.

Therapy

Treatments employed at present include (1) excision and reconstruction with skin grafts or flaps, (2) tattooing, (3) irradiation, (4) cryotherapy, (5) electrocoagulation, and (6) argon laser therapy. Throughout the years, each of these methods has had its advocate, with enthusiasm waxing and waning according to the experience of the individual surgeon.

Surgery

Among those advocating a surgical approach are Snyderman and Wynn-Williams[29] and Clodius.[8] These authors have indicated that with port-wine stains involving large areas of the face, excision of the involved areas and replacement with appropriate skin grafts may offer the best result. Certain guidelines and points of technique have been emphasized.

Snyderman advocates that the graft replacement of various areas of the face be done as units at separate operations and that the surgery be delayed until the patient is well past puberty.[29] The cheeks and temple areas may be dealt with in one operation and the eyelids and lips at another. He suggests that full-thickness postauricular grafts be used for the lower eyelids and that the entire lid be resurfaced, even though only a third might be involved with hemangioma. Thin grafts are best for the upper eyelids. If available, postauricular skin may also be used in grafting of the upper lip. When the nose is extensively involved, use of a forehead or arm flap is advocated. Free full-thickness scalp grafts may be used for the eyebrows. The interval between operations depends on tissue softening and is usually 3 to 4 months. Excision of scars at graft junctions after all grafting has healed may improve the final appearance.

Other donor graft sites include the supraclavicular skin and skin from the dorsum of the foot. Points of technique presented by Clodius include local infiltration with vasoconstrictive agents for better hemostasis and meticulous care in the depth of excision of the involved areas.[8] Under magnification, the lesion is sharply excised, taking about four fifths of the thickness of the dermis, leaving intact a layer of dermis and the underlying subdermal plexus. This provides for less bleeding and a better graft take and final appearance. Extreme care is exercised in immobilization of the grafts, even to the point of intermaxillary fixation and suturing of the lips. Tie-over dressings, sponge rubber, and elastic bandages are used.

These authors have presented some very acceptable results in patients with severe problems, and these results should be reproducible if guidelines and attention to detail are carefully observed. Such procedures are not for every patient, of course, and may be less frequently applicable, especially in females, in whom makeup may provide quite good camouflage.

Tattoos

Tattooing has been enthusiastically advocated by Conway and associates, who have published extensively on this technique.[9] In a report on their experience with 1022 cases treated by intradermal injection of insoluble pigments, they provide the rationale for this approach. Lesions most suitable for treatment are those in which the involvement is deep dermal or subdermal. Pigment, which is deposited into a layer of uninvolved dermis over the abnormal capillary dilatations, serves to mask the underlying pigmented areas.

The procedure is carried out under local or general anesthesia with a motor-driven dermajector under sterile operative conditions. Eschar formation follows and separates spontaneously. Evaluation is possible after 4 weeks to allow desquamation of pigment from the dermis. Multiple treatments are usually necessary, with five being the average for a satisfactory result. It is stressed that superficial lesions do not respond well to this approach.

Results as assessed by the authors in the preceding large series were 84 per cent satisfactory and the remainder unsatisfactory. A few patients required radical surgery, and about one fifth underwent some type of minor surgical procedure. Complications encountered were cellulitis and, more commonly, multiple small cavernous hemangioma formation.

Less sanguine about the results of tattooing were Thomson and Wright, who detailed the complications to a greater extent and subjected the results of treatment to independent analysis as well as their own.[34] The small group of patients presented were categorized as to the degree of involvement, whether mild, medium, or severe. Although patients and an independent panel were more generous in their assessment, the authors judged that none of their mild category patients were quite a bit better, and only 40 to 55 per cent in the medium and severe groups experienced this degree of improvement. Whether repeated treatments were utilized as in the Conway series is not clear. At any rate, judgment as to final results is to a significant degree subjective, and to date this technique is not widely employed.

Radiation

Radiation therapy is mentioned here only to be condemned, with its sometimes disastrous consequences of radiation dermatitis, less than satisfactory results, and the late appearance of basal and squamous cell carcinomas.

Cryotherapy

Although cryotherapy has been employed in the treatment of port-wine stains, the results have been classified as generally unsatisfactory, and further discussion here is not warranted.[1]

Laser

The argon laser currently probably enjoys the greatest popularity among active forms of treatment. Since 1976, when Apfelberg and associates reported their preliminary experience in argon laser management of cutaneous vascular deformities, considerable experience has accrued.[2] In a subsequent publication, the same author and his colleagues described the histologic appearance of port-wine stains following laser treatment.[3] The changes occurring include blister formation immediately after treatment, with coagulation necrosis of the entire epidermis and the uppermost collagen. Small-vessel thrombosis extended more deeply, and sweat glands, hair follicles, and sebaceous glands were affected superficially. A crust then formed for 7 to 14 days with histologic changes limited to the upper 1 mm of the dermis. Small vessels were decreased in number, and there was variable proliferation of collagen. The epidermis was essentially normal after healing, and sweat glands and pilosebaceous structures usually persisted. Similar changes were seen 7 years after treatment. The conclusion was that lesions with aberrant vessels largely confined to the upper 1 mm of the dermis may be expected to respond favorably while deeper lesions may persist.

Experience with argon laser therapy has also been reported by Noe and associates[23] and Cosman.[10] The former, in a series of 62 patients covering 2 to 95 per cent of the facial area, achieved a desirable result in 73 per cent of patients, with hypertrophic scarring occurring in 11 per cent. Lesions responded similarly whether associated with a systemic abnormality or not. A more favorable response rate (90 per cent) was observed in patients over 37 years of age and in lesions having a purple color, a vascular area of 5 per cent or greater, a mean vessel area of 2500 mm or greater, and a fullness

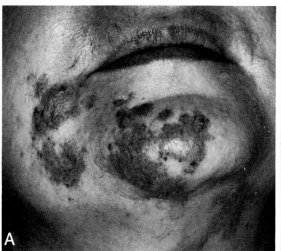
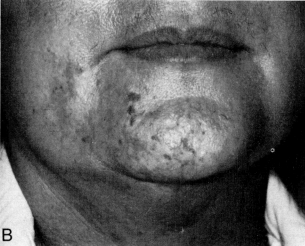

Figure 51–1. Port-wine stain before (*A*) and after (*B*) treatment with argon laser. (Courtesy of Dr. Michael Messenger, St. Paul, Minn.)

of 15 per cent or more. All these characteristics were found to be predictors of response with varying degrees of accuracy. Percentage of fullness appeared to be the best histologic discriminator of response.

In experience with 132 patients who were spot-tested, 54 patients received a total of 85 treatments in the series reported by Cosman.[10] Of those followed for 4 months or more, in 60 to 65 per cent of patients good to excellent results were achieved. Approximately 10 per cent of patients experienced scarring. Secondary treatment appeared to be beneficial in some patients. Lesions were rarely eliminated, but considerable improvement was usually observed, and scarring was not a prohibitive problem (Fig. 51–1).

Controversies in Treatment

The preceding differing views of treatment are not necessarily contradictory. Physicians not directly involved in a particular type of treatment tend to be somewhat less enthusiastic about results than those using a particular modality. It would appear, if one accepts the response rates reported by the various authors, that tattooing, especially when performed repeatedly and for lesions with an overlying layer of dermis, will yield reasonably good results in a majority of patients. Those reporting less favorable results place little emphasis on re-treatment. This technique is not widely practiced at the present time.

For more superficial lesions involving the upper 1 mm of the dermis, the argon laser may offer considerable improvement in a majority of patients, with consideration of re-treatment again as of some value.

If excisional therapy with grafting is deemed the only acceptable treatment in large deep lesions, attention to the sparing of the deep layer of the dermis is important, and meticulous attention to detail in graft immobilization is essential to a satisfactory result.

No one treatment is acceptable for all forms of the lesion.

BASAL CELL EPITHELIOMA

The chief points of controversy with basal cell epitheliomas again relate to preferred modes of therapy. The most widely accepted modes of treatment are (1) surgery, (2) radiotherapy, (3) Mohs' chemotherapy or a modification thereof, and (4) topical application of cytotoxic drugs. Each of these modalities has advantages and disadvantages, and each has its strong proponents.[16]

Therapy

Surgery

Surgery offers certain advantages in the treatment of primary basal cell carcinomas. Cure rates of 98 per cent are commonly achieved, and the treatment is usually in the form of a brief single operation with generally good cosmetic results and minimal scarring (due in large part to the age group in which these lesions commonly occur). Also, as with Mohs' approach, the diagnosis and adequacy of excisional margins may be confirmed by histopathologic examination.

Radiation

Radiation therapy also offers an acceptable cure rate in competent hands and satisfactory cosmetic results in most cases. It also exposes patients to the hazards of radiation, including radiation necrosis and radiation dermatitis, which when present is associated with a 20 per cent incidence of development of malignant tumor.[31] In addition, unless separate biopsies are taken, there is no histopathologic confirmation of diagnosis or adequacy of treatment. Treatment may be carried out over several days to weeks.

The most devastating problems that have followed radiation therapy in the past have been the development of burrowing or boratrizing basal cell carcinomas that extend subcutaneously to involve deeper tissues, which may require many mutilating procedures (in the author's experience one patient has undergone more than 80 procedures), are rarely cured, and may result in the death of the patient. It is hoped that with better understanding and newer techniques, this occurrence will be seen only very rarely in the future.

Although radiation therapists may disagree with the preceding perspective, there should be general agreement that radiation necrosis is more likely to occur in those areas where cartilage or tendon lies superficially under the skin.

When radiation therapy is considered, certain guidelines seem appropriate:

1. Radiation should be avoided in the treatment of lesions of the inner canthus, eyelids, tip of the nose and alar regions, base of the ala nasi, preauricular region, external ear, and auditory canal.

2. Radiation therapy should not be employed to treat lesions that have recurred after radiation treatment.

The preference for radiation therapy in some areas may have been occasioned by fear of mutilating surgical procedures performed by surgeons inexperienced in reconstruction or at a time prior to the development of many of the techniques currently available.

Moh's Chemosurgery

Since Frederic Mohs introduced his classic description of chemotherapy, the method has been slow to gain wide acceptance for reasons that will be described.[21] With modification in recent years, it has gained increasing favor.

Although the technique will not be described here in detail, it involves preliminary treatment of the area in question with a keratolytic agent, such as dichloroacetic acid, until the surface becomes white. This is necessary in order to render the keratin layer permeable to zinc chloride. The latter, which is the fixative agent, is applied to the cancer in a thickness varying from less than 1 to 3 mm or more, depending on the depth of penetration required.[22] A cotton and gauze dressing, reinforced with tape, is applied and after 24 hours the first excision is carried out through killed and fixed tissue with little accompanying bleeding or pain. On the undersurface of the specimen, which is carefully divided into sections and numbered, the fixed cancerous tissue with its dead-white color is usually distinguishable from the normal fixed tissue, which is gray in color. Specimens for histopathologic examination need be taken only from the areas of obvious involvement. If obvious cancer remains after the first excision, further zinc chloride is applied, and after another 24 hours re-excision is carried out, and the areas of the specimen are again marked out for accurate determination of involved sites and the possibility of need for further fixation and treatment. Each time after initial excision, only the cancerous areas are fixed and re-excised. After achievement of a completely cancer-free layer of tissue, the wound is covered with a petroleum gauze dressing and 3 days later the final layer of fixed tissue may be removed by cutting the holding strands of fibrous tissue with scissors. If preferred, the layer may be allowed to separate spontaneously in another day or two.

This leaves a smooth, highly vascular, germ-resistant granulation tissue that allows rapid growth of epithelium across the defect.

Acceptance of this technique has been limited because it requires an enormous amount of time and effort with mapping, staining, and examination by a physician trained in this special form of histopathology. As many as 75 slides may be required over several days for assurance that all cancer is removed. Few physicians have been trained in this technique, and the original technique required delay of reconstruction because of the several weeks necessary for granulations to heal the defect.[6]

Controlled Microscopic Excision

Mohs' technique underwent major modification by Tromovitch in a report published in 1974.[32] Controlled microscopic excision, which omits the use of zinc chloride, is otherwise similar to Mohs' technique, less painful, and much less time-consuming.

Lidocaine, 1 per cent solution, is injected in the clinically suspicious area and the areas of suspected tumor and is curetted. Hemostasis is achieved with spot desiccation or full-strength dichloroacetic acid, which is followed by curettement of any areas of suspected residual tumor, and excision of tissue 3 to 5 mm thick is carried out to include the entire defect with additional tissue around the periphery. Careful marking and mapping of sections is carried out so that all areas of the excised tissue may be accurately identified. Appropriate fixing and staining follow, and the slides are ready for examination within 30 min.

In a series of over 100 basal cell epitheliomas, many of which were recurrent, there were three recurrences—two in previously recurrent eschars, which were among those primarily treated. All were re-treated and none recurred. The follow-up for the total series was 3 to 8 years.[32] An example is shown in Figure 51–2.

The authors in comparing their method, which they

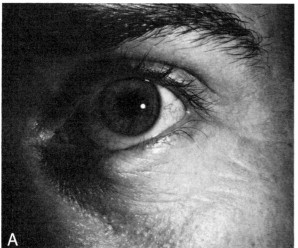

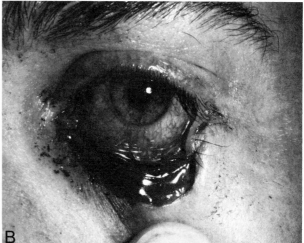

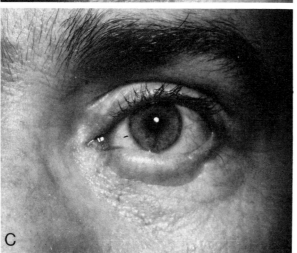

Figure 51–2. (*A*) Preoperative view of basal cell epithelioma extensively involving lower eyelid. (*B*) Defect after microscopically controlled excision. (*C*) Eyelid after reconstruction. (Courtesy of A. Callahan, G. D. Monheit, and M. A. Callahan, Birmingham, Ala.)

call microscopically controlled excision (MCE), with the original Mohs technique, emphasize certain definite advantages:

1. It eliminates the patient discomfort associated with the use of zinc chloride fixation.

2. The fixation beyond the surgical margins which is standard with Mohs' technique does not occur with MCE. This results in sparing of tissue, especially in the nose, where fewer perforations are encountered.

3. This technique is usually a much quicker procedure. With Mohs' technique requiring 24 hours after each application, if three different cuttings are required, 4 days may be necessary. With MCE, three and sometimes four cuttings can be made during the same morning, this markedly shortens the time required.

The disadvantages are increased bleeding and a greater tendency to cut uneven specimens compared with that seen with Mohs' chemosurgery.

Local Application of 5-Fluorouracil

Topical chemotherapy has been employed in the treatment of skin tumors using a number of agents as reported by Ryan and Krementz.[25] These same authors and other colleagues have subsequently reported experience in the treatment of basal cell and other malignant and premalignant skin lesions with 5-fluorouracil.[18]

The technique employs the use of 5, 10, or 20 per cent 5-fluorouracil in an aquaphor cream base. This was applied on a daily basis for periods ranging from 6 to 16 weeks after establishment of diagnosis by biopsy. Patients not responding to lower concentrations after 2 weeks were switched to a higher concentration of the cream.

The usual course noted has been one of initial inflammation, gradual regression, disappearance, and healing. In an initial series of 47 patients with basal cell or squamous cell carcinomas, or actinic or senile keratoses, all lesions treated were healed with no recurrence after 6 months to 2 years. When lesions were superficial, there was essentially no post-treatment eschar, and minimal scarring occurred with larger lesions extending through the dermis. The obvious disadvantages of this method of therapy are the time required and difficulties with patient compliance.

The microscopic response to this treatment was infiltration of the involved tissue by large numbers of lymphocytes and monocytes developing in 10 days to 2 weeks in most patients. Subsequent work suggests a relationship between the development of delayed hypersensitivity to 5-fluorouracil and therapeutic cure.[20]

Controversies in Treatment

The various methods of treatment of basal cell skin cancer discussed here may each have their place with areas of definite overlap. For the surgeon with thorough training and experience in both extirpative and reconstructive techniques, in the overwhelming majority of instances excision plus immediate reconstruction is the treatment of choice when good routine frozen section control is available. It has the distinct advantage of speed, rapid healing, and less expense and generally yields an excellent cure and follows the lines of classic en bloc excision of cancer.

In my opinion, radiotherapy has the least to recommend it, with the lack of histopathologic control, time consumption, and hazards of radiation, although the hazards are diminishing with improved techniques.

Mohs' chemosurgery has made its contribution in a pioneering effort, but is being increasingly displaced by microscopically controlled excision, which is much less time-consuming and less painful.[6] It, too, however, suffers from the disadvantage of being much more laborious, time-consuming, and demanding with respect to histopathologic technique. Its special place is probably for difficult lesions, which do not lend themselves to straightforward surgical excision and reconstruction by virtue of anatomic site or involvement of important structures.

The use of topical 5-fluorouracil, which to the present has not gained a large number of adherents, if carefully employed in varying concentrations, as described by Mansell and co-workers,[20] may very well have its place in extensive and deep lesions and for patients refusing surgery. Like any other form of cancer therapy, even in the best of hands it is not universally successful.[26] It suffers from the disadvantage of the time required and requires a cooperative and responsible patient.

SQUAMOUS CELL CARCINOMA

The same modalities of treatment employed in basal cell carcinoma are used in the management of squamous cell carcinoma, and many of the same arguments in favor of or against the various methods apply. Squamous cell cancer differs significantly from basal cell cancer, however, in that it has a much greater propensity for rapid and wider local spread. It also may spread to other parts of the body by blood stream or lymphatics.

Therapy

Insofar as local treatments are concerned, surgical excision, electrocoagulation, radiation, and chemosurgery are all employed.

Although dermatologists express considerable enthusiasm for *electrocoagulation* (electrosurgery),[30] it is my view that for squamous cell carcinoma excisional therapy is distinctly superior, except perhaps in the patient with multiple lesions in an already badly scarred area, probably secondary to radiation damage, where excision is not practical. In most other situations, *surgery* is preferable, with its rapid resolution of the problem with histopathologic control and minimal deformity, even for larger lesions, when there is experience with and knowledge of reconstructive techniques.

Radiation may be employed but, again, suffers from lack of histopathologic control and lengthy treatment and is often inadvisable or contraindicated because of previous radiation therapy and its accompanying risk of radiation necrosis. In previously untreated large lesions, it may play a useful role in operative or postoperative adjunctive therapy, and in some situations it is curative with less deformity than that occasioned by any other form of treatment except chemosurgery.

Chemosurgery may have its greatest usefulness in certain special circumstances, more specifically where the peripheral limits of the lesion are difficult to define.

Those epitheliomas that are considered in this category, as suggested by Stoll,[30] may fall into five groups:

1. Residual carcinoma following previous treatments.
2. Multiple carcinomas.
3. Carcinomas arising in late radiation change.
4. Large ill-defined carcinoma previously untreated.
5. Carcinoma invading bone and cartilage.

Controversies in Treatment

None of these treatments enjoys universal success, and the mode of therapy selected is undoubtedly strongly influenced by the training and experience of the treating physician. In the area of lymphatic metastases, however, treatment is almost always by either surgery or radiation therapy. If the disease is significant, nodal dissection with possible postoperative adjunctive radiation is preferred. Functional neck dissection may be performed rapidly with minimal morbidity or deformity and minimal disability, as has been the case at our institution.

A more critical and controversial question is: When should prophylactic node dissection be performed at the time of excision of a squamous cell carcinoma of the skin? Is close observation adequate?

In a study of skin carcinomas, Immerman and associates found that noninvasive squamous cell epitheliomas did not experience recurrence or metastatic spread.[17] Among invasive lesions, there was a 20 per cent incidence of recurrence after excision, and, more important, when the depth of lesions was determined, only those extending to Clark's level IV or V had the potential for recurrence or regional lymph node metastasis. Thus, depth of invasion may be helpful in determining the extent of treatment for squamous cell carcinoma of the skin, as it is in malignant melanoma.

Other factors influencing the likelihood of metastasis from squamous cell skin cancers, and hence the need for regional node dissection, are those lesions related to antecedent problems such as burns, scars, chronic ulcers, arsenical drainage, or x-ray injury.[19] Increasing degrees of dedifferentiation also increase the risk of metastatic spread, making more likely the advisability of regional node dissection.

KERATOACANTHOMA

The controversy with regard to keratoacanthoma, which is a papular lesion usually appearing on the face, hands, or fingers, relates to both its pathologic status and its treatment. The lesion most commonly regresses, beginning 6 to 8 weeks after onset with completion of involution by 4 to 6 months.

I consider the arguments as to whether it is benign or malignant to be academic. For accurate diagnosis, the specimen should be submitted to the pathologist in its entirety. Submission of only a portion of the lesion may result in the mistaken diagnosis of squamous cell carcinoma. Removal of the entire lesion for diagnosis amounts to curative resection, rendering the question of treatment moot.

Perhaps the true nature of the lesion is in accord with the view of Bremer, who concludes that keratoacanthoma is a true squamous cell carcinoma of very low

malignancy with a very high potential for the production of keratin. The keratin, acting as a foreign body, causes inflammatory changes in the tissue under and around the lesion, and these changes in turn cause extrusion of the tumor before metastasis occurs.[5]

MALIGNANT MELANOMA

There is, perhaps, no other malignancy surrounded by as much controversy as malignant melanoma. Although understanding of the disorder has increased significantly in the past decade, arguments as to the best form of treatment persist. Support in the literature for almost any therapeutic stance in all probability can be found.

Classification

The classification of malignant melanoma in its varying forms is now nearly universally accepted. *Lentigo maligna* is a noninvasive lesion, not to be confused with *lentigo maligna melanoma*, which though invasive, does not usually penetrate deeply. *Superficial spreading* and *nodular* melanomas are the other two common forms, with the latter demonstrating only a vertical growth component in contrast with the former, which demonstrates first a radial growth phase before invading vertically. Two other forms of melanoma, which are uncommon but are seen more frequently in the head and neck area than elsewhere in the body, are *melanoma of the mucous membranes* with its very grim prognosis and *desmoid*, or *desmoplastic*, melanoma. The latter is a very rare variant of spindle cell melanoma that occurs most commonly in the head and neck area as a subcutaneous tumor. It is locally recurrent, frequently metastatic, and commonly fatal.

Among the most significant contributions with respect to prediction of the metastatic potential of a given malignant melanoma have been Clark's classification of levels of penetration[7] and Breslow's classification by thickness.[4] It is assumed that the reader is familiar with these classifications, so they will not be detailed here except to indicate that there is almost universal acceptance that metastatic potential correlates directly to a significant degree with increasing depth of penetration or thickness of lesion.

Day and his colleagues have suggested different dividing points in thickness of lesions,[12] and they claim these points represent more natural dividing points on the basis of a study of a large group of patients with malignant melanoma. The categories they suggest are (1) <0.85 mm, (2) 0.86 to 1.69 mm, (3) 1.70 to 3.64 mm, and (4) >3.64 mm.

These authors further subdivide risk factors according to categories of thickness. In lesions 0.76 to 1.69 mm thick, the majority of deaths occurred in patients with lesions in the anatomic areas that have been designated as BANS, or upper *b*ack, posterior *a*rm, posterior *n*eck or posterior *s*calp. A mortality rate of 16 per cent was noted in these areas with relatively thin lesions as compared to a <1 per cent mortality rate when the lesion occurred in other areas.[13] Confirmation of this risk factor is yet to be forthcoming from other centers.

The variables of importance in lesions 1.51 to 3.99

mm thick affecting prognosis unfavorably were findings of >six mitoses per mm[2], presence of microscopic satellites, ulcerations >3 mm, and location in a site other than the forearm.[14] In lesions >3.56 mm thick, those factors that bore most unfavorably on prognosis were absent or minimal lymphocyte response; nodular melanoma; location on hands, trunk, or feet; and the presence of nodal metastases.

The presence or absence of nodal metastases is without question the single most important factor influencing outcome. In the head and neck region, the nodal areas of importance are the preauricular and cervical nodes for the head and face and the cervical (anterior and posterior) and supraclavicular nodes for the neck.

Controversies in Treatment

With the preceding factors in mind, it is appropriate to turn to the principal controversies in treatment. The two areas of difference of opinion are with respect to tumor-free margins of resection and prophylactic node dissection. The once nearly sacrosanct 5-cm tumor-free margins suggested by Sampson-Hadley, which often were inapplicable to head and neck melanomas, although still adhered to by some, are rapidly being discarded on the basis of more recent experience.[27] Not only are there important facial structures that preclude or influence against wide margins of resection, but more conservative margins have been found to produce results equivalent to those seen with radical treatment.[12] Thus, in our own practice, 2.0-cm margins are considered acceptable for lesions up to 1.50 mm in thickness. It should be noted here that even thin lesions may metastasize on occasion.[35] If a lesion is adjacent to a nodal drainage bed, the margins may be skewed toward the node-bearing area in a skewed or elliptical fashion.

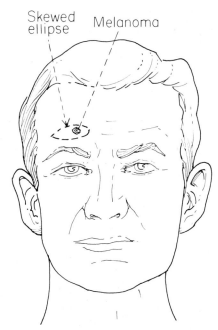

Figure 51–3. Diagrammatic representation of skewed excision of melanoma. The margin is "wide" only in the direction of regional lymph node drainage.

Thus, a 4- or 5-cm ellipse that is two cm wide may be oriented toward the regional nodes where spread is most likely to occur and will allow at the same time for direct skin closure (Fig. 51–3).

For thicker lesions, especially on the scalp, 3- to 4-cm margins of *resection* are routinely employed in our practice. This usually requires *skin grafting* for reconstruction.

Insofar as elective *node dissection* is concerned, the head and neck area differs in some respects from other areas of the body in that a much larger proportion of lesions in this area are located in relatively close proximity to regional nodes. Hence, though in a prospective randomized study of trunk and extremity lesions, prophylactic regional node dissection was found to be of no benefit,[28] in the head and neck area it is commonly employed because our previous experience has suggested that it may be of benefit.[36] Elective regional node dissection is performed whenever a lesion as thin as 0.75 mm lies directly over a node-bearing area or when thicker lesions lie within a few centimeters of such nodes.

A more recent review of our experience in melanoma of the head and neck has suggested that less extensive node dissections may be carried out than those formerly employed, inasmuch as skip nodes were rarely encountered.[24] In other words, if positive nodes were not found in the upper neck, they were very unlikely to be found in the middle or lower neck. On this basis, for example, in the presence of a high preauricular lesion, superficial parotidectomy and supraomohyoid (or upper jugular and digastric triangle) dissection may be carried out, and if all nodes are negative on frozen section, the dissection is carried no further. Final or conclusive data in support of this concept are not yet available.

Another trend has been the lessened use of the time-honored classical neck dissection with its often unnecessary sacrifice of important structures (such as spinal accessory nerve, internal jugular vein, and sternocleidomastoid muscle) in favor of functional neck dissection, except in the presence of extensive metastatic nodal involvement. To the present day, this has not resulted in any significant change in outlook in patients undergoing the more conservative procedure, although, again, conclusive data are not yet available.

The final controversial area in the treatment of malignant melanoma is the use of *radiation therapy*. An initial enthusiasm for radiation as postoperative adjunctive therapy to areas where extensive disease was removed has given way to a less sanguine view with regard to its efficacy.[11] Because of the lack of other good alternatives, however, and because of the occasional, anecdotal spectacular response seen, its use is continued in situations in which the risk of local or regional recurrence is high.[37]

The most recent addition to the treatment armamentarium, *interferon*, is used primarily for disseminated disease and has not yet been established as a consistently therapeutically reliable agent.

REFERENCES

1. Agris J: Vascular tissue tumors. *In* Dermatological Plastic Surgery. Houston, Texas, 1982.
2. Apfelberg DB, Maser MR, Lash H: Argon laser management of

cutaneous deformities: A preliminary report. West J Med *124*:99, 1976.

3. Apfelberg DB, Kosek J, Maser MR, Lash H: Histology of port wine stains following argon laser treatment. *In* McCoy FJ (ed): Year Book of Plastic and Reconstructive Surgery. Chicago, Year Book Medical Publishers, 1981, p 27.
4. Breslow A: Thickness, cross-sectional areas and depth of invasion in the prognosis of cutaneous melanoma. Ann Surg *172*:902, 1970.
5. Bruner JM: Keratoacanthoma. Plast Reconstr Surg *31*:281, 1963.
6. Callahan A, Monheit GD, Callahan MA: Cancer excision from eyelids and ocular adnexa: the Mohs fresh tissue technique and reconstruction. CA *32*:322, 1982.
7. Clark WH Jr, From L, Bernardino EA, Mihm MC: The histogenesis and biologic behaviour of primary human malignant melanoma of the skin. Cancer Res *29*:705, 1969.
8. Clodius L: Excision and grafting of extensive facial hemangiomas. Br J Plast Surg *30*:185, 1977.
9. Conway H, McKinney P, Climo M: Permanent camouflage of vascular nevi of the face by intradermal injection of insoluble pigments (tattooing): Experience through twenty years with 1022 cases. Plast Reconstruct Surg *40*:457, 1967.
10. Cosman B: Experience in argon laser therapy of port wine stains. *In* McCoy FJ (ed): Year Book of Plastic and Reconstructive Surgery. Chicago, Year Book Medical Publishers, 1981, p 30–31.
11. Creagan ET, Cupps RE, Ivins JC, et al: Adjuvant radiation therapy for regional nodal metastases from malignant melanoma: A randomized, prospective study. Cancer *42*:2206, 1978.
12. Day CL Jr, Lew RA, Mihm MC Jr, et al: The natural break points for primary-tumor thickness in clinical stage I melanoma. N Engl J Med *305*:1155, 1981.
13. Day CL Jr, Mihm MC Jr, Sober AJ, et al: Prognostic factors for melanoma patients with lesions 0.76–1.69 mm in thickness: An appraisal of "thin" level IV lesions. Ann Surg *195*:30, 1982.
14. Day CL Jr, Mihm MC Jr, Lew RA, et al: Prognostic factors for patients with clinical stage I melanoma of intermediate thickness (1.51–3.99 mm): A conceptual model for tumor growth and metastasis. Ann Surg *195*:35, 1982.
15. Day CL Jr, Lew RA, Mihm MC Jr, et al: A multivariate analysis of prognostic factors for melanoma patients with lesions >3.65 mm in thickness: The importance of revealing alternative Cox models. Ann Surg *195*:44, 1982.
16. Gibson EW, Lopez-Garcia J: Basal cell and squamous cell carcinoma of the skin. *In* Grabb WC, Smith JW (eds): Plastic Surgery, 3rd ed. Boston, Little, Brown and Co., 1979, p 497–510.
17. Immerman SC, Scanlon EF, Christ M, Knox KL: Recurrent squamous cell carcinoma of the skin. Cancer *51*:1537, 1983.
18. Litwin MS, Ryan RF, Reed RJ, Krementz ET: Topical chemotherapy of cutaneous malignancy of the head and neck. South Med J *62*:556, 1969.
19. Lund HZ: How often does squamous cell carcinoma of the skin metastasize? Arch Dermatol *92*:635, 1965.
20. Mansell PWA, Litwin MS, Ichinose H, Krementz ET: Delayed hypersensitivity to 5-fluorouracil following topical chemotherapy of cutaneous cancers. Cancer Res *35*:1288, 1975.
21. Mohs FE: Chemosurgery: A microscopically controlled method of cancer excision. Arch Surg *42*:279, 1941.
22. Mohs FE: Chemosurgical treatment of cancer of the lip: A microscopically controlled method of excision. Arch Surg *48*:478, 1944.
23. Noe JM, Barsky SH, Geer DE, Rosen S: Port wine stains and response to argon laser therapy: Successful treatment and predictive role of color, age, and biopsy. *In* McCoy FJ (ed): Year Book of Plastic and Reconstructive Surgery. Chicago, Year Book Medical Publishers, 1981, p 28.
24. Olson RM, Woods JE, Soule EH: Regional lymph node management and outcome in 100 patients with head and neck melanoma. Am J Surg *142*:470, 1981.
25. Ryan RF, Krementz ET: Cancericidal drugs: Indications and applications. *In* Irvine WT (ed): Modern Trends in Surgery, 2nd ed. London, Butterworth & Co., 1966.
26. Ryan RF, Litwin MS, Reed RJ: Topical use of 5-fluorouracil cream for skin cancer. *In* Irvine WT (ed): Modern Trends in Surgery, 3rd ed. London, Butterworth & Co., 1971, p 284–296.
27. Sampson-Handley W: The pathology of melanotic growths in relation to their operative treatment. Lancet *1*:966, 1907.
28. Sims FH, Ivins JC, Taylor WP, et al: A preoperative randomized study of the efficacy of routine prophylactic lymphadenectomy in the management of malignant melanoma: Preliminary results. Cancer *41*:948, 1978.
29. Snyderman RK, Wynn-Williams D: Complete replacement of port wine stains. NY State J Med *66*:1905, 1966.
30. Stoll HL Jr: Invasive squamous cell carcinoma (electrosurgery). *In* Helm F Jr (ed): Cancer Dermatology. Philadelphia, Lea & Febiger, 1979, p 126.
31. Texier M, Preaux J: Skin Cancer in Radiodermatitis. Transactions of the Sixth International Congress of Plastic and Reconstructive Surgery. Paris, Masson, 1976.
32. Tromovitch TA, Stegeman SJ: Microscopically controlled excision of skin tumors. Chemosurgery (Mohs): Fresh tissue technique. Arch Dermatol *110*:231, 1974.
33. Thomson HG: Hemangioma, lymphangioma, and arteriovenous fistula. *In* Grabb WC, Smith JW (eds): Plastic Surgery, 3rd ed. Boston, Little, Brown and Co., 1979, p 518–529.
34. Thomson HG, Wright AM: Surgical tattooing of the port wine stain: Operative technique, results, and critique. Plast Reconstr Surg *48*:113, 1971.
35. Woods JE, Soule EH, Creagan ET: Metastasis and death in patients with thin melanomas (<0.76 mm). Ann Surg *198*:63, 1983.
36. Woods JE, Soule EH, Borkowski JJ: Experience with malignant melanoma of the head and neck. Plast Reconstr Surg *61*:64, 1978.
37. Woods JE: The case for therapeutic positivism in head and neck malignancy. Ann Plast Surg *5*:273, 1980.

PART IX

Tumors of the Neck

CHAPTER 52

Clinical Evaluation of Tumors of the Neck

David E. Schuller, M.D.

The clinical evaluation of neck tumors is a diverse and expansive topic. When one considers the numerous benign and malignant processes that present as a neck tumor and add to that the congenital and inflammatory causes, it becomes apparent that a systematic approach to this subject is essential. Not only are there a great number of possible diagnoses for neck tumors, there are also numerous diagnostic procedures and approaches that have recently been developed to aid the clinician. Therefore, the potential for confusion is substantial.

There has been somewhat of a change in the approach to evaluating neck tumors over the past several years. Whereas incisional and excisional biopsies were previously the predominant means of evaluation, the development of the noninvasive radiographic imaging procedures, such as computed tomography (CT), and the microinvasive techniques, such as fine-needle aspiration, have decreased the frequency of the other procedures. The oft-mentioned warnings by Hayes Martin regarding the dangers of excisional biopsy when evaluating neck tumors takes on even added implications now that less dangerous meaningful alternatives have been developed. However, it is apparent that even in this age of high technologic advancement in medicine, the clinician still can effectively rely on the information obtained from a detailed history and physical examination to arrive at an accurate differential diagnosis that includes just a few possibilities.

BASIC ANATOMIC CONSIDERATIONS

Any discussion of neck tumors demands a better than average understanding of the neck nodal anatomy. This lymphatic system has a rich capillary network that becomes confluent to form lymphatic vessels. Although there are no lymphatics in the central nervous system and no lymphatics directly in muscular tissue, these vessels are present in the fascial planes of the neck muscles and are also involved with blood vessels that supply those muscles. These lymphatic vessels that interconnect the cervical nodal chain terminate in larger collecting trunks that ultimately enter the blood stream via the venous system. This usually occurs at the junction of the internal jugular vein with the subclavian vein. It is not unusual for these main collecting trunks to be multiple. The anatomic position of entrance into the venous system is quite variable.

The deep lateral nodes of the neck represent the group that has the greatest significance for neoplastic involvement. Although there is variability, these nodes can basically be divided into three major nodal groups (Fig. 52–1): (1) internal jugular, (2) spinal accessory, and (3) transverse cervical. The chain that is most frequently involved with metastatic disease is the internal jugular vein. The spinal accessory nodal group can contain as many as 20 nodes.[23] The transverse cervical chain connects the internal jugular with the spinal accessory group.

CLASSIFICATION AND STAGING

Classification and staging relate exclusively to those neck tumors that are malignant. The only classification system that exists relates to those cervical masses that are metastatic nodes from primary sites arising in the head and neck area. A grouping technique is critically important to permit the clinician an opportunity to analyze and compare results of different treatment programs not only on an intra-institutional but also on an interinstitutional basis. Such retrospective analyses can subsequently have input into what therapeutic approach should be planned for the future. This staging also provides a similar opportunity in a prospective fashion to plan treatment programs according to the extent of disease.

However, there are obvious potential weaknesses because of the lack of strict objectivity when one tries to measure a biologic system. The thickness of the patient's neck skin, the amount of subcutaneous fat, and the width and mass of the sternocleidomastoid muscle are all variables that could potentially lead to lack of agreement if measurements were taken by multiple individuals. As imperfect as the system may be, the potential benefits far outweigh these drawbacks, and those oncologists involved with treatment of head and neck malignancies are strongly encouraged to make classification and staging a mandatory part of their clinical evaluation.

In 1959, several medical societies and institutions collaborated to develop a viable staging system. The National Cancer Institute, the American College of Surgeons, the American College of Physicians, the American College of Radiology, the Cancer Control Program of the National Center for Chronic Disease, the American College of Pathologists, and the American Cancer

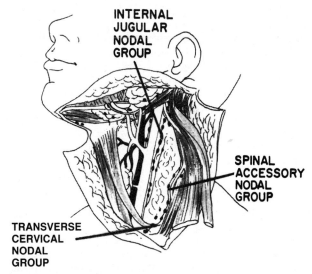

INTERNAL
JUGULAR
NODAL
GROUP

SPINAL
ACCESSORY
NODAL
GROUP

TRANSVERSE
CERVICAL
NODAL
GROUP

Figure 52–1. The internal jugular, transverse cervical, and spinal accessory nodal chains represent the major lymphatic drainage pathways on each side of the neck.

Society formed the Joint Committee for Cancer Staging and End Results Reporting. The system that has evolved is a function of information obtained by physical examination, diagnostic tests, and biopsies.

It is critically important to understand that this staging is based on pretreatment information. The staging is not changed as a result of information found during the course of treatment, such as a preoperatively unrecognized metastatic neck node. The staging system that does include post-treatment information is referred to as the "PNM" system, with the letter "P" referring to that information derived from the pathologic examination of the surgically removed tissue, rather than the "TNM" system, which is based on pretreatment information. However, because some head and neck cancer patients do not undergo surgery as part of their therapeutic program, the PNM system is rarely used. Also, it should be apparent that the intent of a staging system is to help the clinician plan appropriate therapy. Therefore, the system chosen has to rely on information obtained from pretreatment assessments.

The classification system that is currently being used by the American Joint Committee for Cancer Staging and End Results Reporting for head and neck malignancies was revised in 1980. The primary tumor (T) staging is a function of the individual anatomic site and is not discussed in this chapter. The regional cervical lymph node (N) classification is listed in Table 52–1. There are other staging systems that currently exist. The Union Internationale Contre le Cancer (UICC) is used by most European institutions. However, the American Joint Committee system is being used by most major cancer institutions and agencies in the United States.

It is imperative to have an understanding of those parameters that affect the particular stage of a cervical lymph node(s). The current nodal staging system emphasizes the prognostic impact of the size and number of those cervical nodes which are presumed to be metastatic. The system also takes into account the clinical significance of the position of a positive node, but not as heavily as size or number. There is no question that metastatic nodal disease in a patient with a head and neck malignancy unequivocably does worsen the prognosis.[22] There is evidence in the literature to support the prognostic importance of the number and size of metastatic nodes. Cachin and coworkers[4] did confirm the previous observations of others that survival appeared to be proportional to the size and the number of metastatic nodes. A report by Sancho and associates[20] in 1977 also found that size and the degree of histologic differentiation in squamous cell carcinoma did correlate with the patient's survival.

However, there have indeed been recent studies that have not found as much correlation of nodal size and numbers with prognosis. Sessions'[24] study of cancers of the hypopharynx and larynx demonstrated several clinical situations in which this correlation did not exist. Schuller and associates[22] reported on 244 patients with metastatic nodal disease from the University of Iowa and showed no correlation between prognosis in numbers or percentages of positive nodes, solitary versus multiple nodes, or size of the largest metastatic node in the surgical specimen. This study did identify certain features of nodal location that appeared to correlate with survival. Patients with positive nodes in the posterior triangle nodal chain had an extremely poor prognosis, and any patients who had positive nodes in noncontiguous anatomic areas or in multiple areas also had a poor prognosis.

However, some reports have hinted that there are other features that may also affect the prognosis that the current staging system does not even consider. Cachin in 1972[3] hinted at the possible effect on survival of extracapsular extension of nodal disease. The study demonstrated that the best survival rates occurred in patients whose lymph nodes had an intact capsule. The lowest survival rate was associated with rupture of the capsule and extension of tumor into the soft tissue of the neck. This finding was consistent regardless of the primary tumor site. Cachin and coworkers[4] continued to assess other parameters in a subsequent study and were able to evaluate survival as it relates to the presence of cancerous emboli within cervical lymphatics.

TABLE 52–1. Cervical Node Classification for Head and Neck Malignancies*

N0 No clinically positive node
N1 Single clinical positive homolateral node less than 3 cm in diameter
N2 Single clinically positive homolateral node 3 cm to 6 cm in diameter or multiple clinically positive homolateral nodes, none over 6 cm in diameter
   N2a: Single clinically positive homolateral node 3 cm to 6 cm in diameter
   N2b: Multiple clinically positive homolateral nodes, none over 6 cm in diameter
N3 Massive homolateral node(s), bilateral nodes, or contrateral node(s)
   N3a: Clinically positive homolateral node(s), one over 6 cm in diameter
   N3b: Bilateral clinically positive nodes (In this situation each side of the neck should be staged separately; that is, N3b - - - right N2a, left N1.)
   N3c: Contralateral clinically positive node(s) only

*American Joint Committee for Cancer Staging and End Results Reporting. Chicago, 1976.

They found a relationship between the presence of these emboli and capsular rupture.

The consideration of capsular rupture of lymph nodes has usually been felt to have a negative impact on survival. However, this rupture was felt to be associated with lymph nodes that were large and fixed to underlying cervical tissues. Metastatic cervical nodes less than 3 cm in diameter have not previously been considered to have a high possibility of extracapsular tumor extension. In 1981, Johnson and coworkers[15] from the University of Pittsburgh challenged this generalization. They reviewed the neck specimens of 177 patients who underwent radical neck dissection and found a disturbingly high incidence of extracapsular rupture in small lymph nodes. Sixty-five per cent of the nodes in this study that were smaller than 3 cm in diameter were found to have extracapsular tumor spread. This finding correlated with survival and showed a difference between those with and without extracapsular spread. Another report studying the same topic by Annyas and associates[1] showed a similarly high frequency of extracapsular rupture in small lymph nodes. The current nodal staging system does not have the capabilities of identifying this apparently important prognostic indicator.

Information continues to mount regarding evaluations of the clinical significance of current immune assessment techniques and how they relate to prognosis.[7, 8, 10, 11, 12, 14] The study by Berlinger and associates in 1976,[2] in which they were able to correlate lymph nodal histologic changes as they related to immunoreactivity with the prognosis of certain head and neck cancers, gave a hint at what may be in the future. The possibility of immunostaging, as techniques are refined and their value is established, will also have to be a matter of consideration that is not currently included in the nodal staging system.

Whereas there is no question that the current staging system may well have some potential prognostic loopholes, that does not minimize the importance of using this staging system. When enough information has been collected to substantiate these new findings and techniques have proved to be clinically reliable and reproduceable, it is inevitable that the current staging system of neck nodal disease in head and neck malignancies, once again, will be revised as it was in 1976.

PATIENT EVALUATIONS

The evaluation of the patient with a neck tumor should proceed initially by obtaining historical information and then proceeding with the physical examination. With such a variety of diagnostic possibilities that could range anywhere from a carotid body tumor, sebaceous cyst, lipoma, thyroglossal duct cyst, or numerous others, it is important that the clinician have a mechanism for grouping and prioritizing this information.

History

The first major aid is to establish diagnostic priorities based on the *patient's age*. A reasonable generalization can be made regarding the frequencies of certain types of neck tumors based on age. In the pediatric population, neck tumors most frequently represent an inflammatory etiology, with malignancies being relatively rare. Congenital tumors are even more common than malignancies in children. However, in adults, this order of frequency is just reversed and neoplastic disease represents the most common cause, followed then by inflammatory, and finally congenital etiologies. It is not the purpose of this chapter to discuss pediatric tumors, which are covered in Chapter 70. Therefore, the following discussion will relate only to adults. Obtaining certain critical pieces of information during the history will, in the majority of cases, allow the physician to be able to determine whether indeed the neck mass has a neoplastic, infectious, or congenital origin.

When one considers that neoplastic disease probably represents the most common etiology of adult neck tumors, it is helpful to determine whether the patient is part of that segment of the population which is at an increased risk for this problem. Therefore, questions pertaining to the patient's *use of tobacco and alcohol* are important.

The recently documented increased incidence of thyroid cancer following *previous exposure to radiation* therapy for benign disease is now well established, and this historical information should be obtained from every patient. A recent report[25] has further added to this fund of knowledge about the risks of radiation therapy for benign disease in that a disturbingly high incidence of neural tumors has been discovered in patients who have undergone radiation therapy for benign disease. The medical literature has included reports of radiation-induced tumors related to the thyroid gland, parotid gland, and now neural origin following treatment for benign disease. This fact documents the critical importance of questioning the patient about previous radiation therapy. It is oftentimes helpful to use what the lay public considers interchangeable terms, such as "cobalt" or "x-ray treatment," for radiation therapy in an effort to be thorough. The patient should also be questioned regarding exposure to pollutants that may be associated with an increased incidence of a head and neck malignancy.

Another important determination that can be discovered in the history is the *chronology of the neck mass*. The time of onset of the neck mass and how long it has persisted are important. For example, congenital neck tumors, which have been present since birth, have been found in adults.

The patient should be questioned about the *association of pain* with the neck tumor. Most inflammatory disease causes pain of varying degrees, but is especially exacerbated with pressure over the mass. Congenital cysts are infrequently painful. Neoplastic disease that involves a sensory root can also cause pain. However, it also can result in an area of anesthesia or paresthesia. Questioning for any sensory disturbance is important.

It is also imperative to question the patient to determine whether there has been some exposure to an etiologic agent, such as an *infectious process* present in another family member. The patient should also be questioned about the presence of any other *associated symptoms*. A concomitant sore throat may indeed be indicative of a tonsillar carcinoma with nodal metastases, or it may be nothing more than a pharyngitis.

Just as pharyngeal infections may result in cervical adenopathy, infections of the scalp or infected areas of facial skin can result in cervical adenopathy. Therefore, the answers to questions directed at the patient's awareness of any such conditions occurring in the recent past should be sought by the clinician.

Neck tumors can be associated with *trauma* as a result of hematomas in the deep tissues or even within the sternocleidomastoid muscle. Muscle tears can occur which result in healing by fibrosis and development of an area of induration that can be mistaken for a neck tumor. Therefore, the patient should be questioned about any recent or remote trauma to the neck.

An important historical item is the *growth pattern of the neck tumor*. If the mass has had a rather steady progressive growth, one should be thinking more of neoplastic disease, as contrasted with a neck tumor that suddenly appeared and then decreased in size, as would be more consistent with an inflammatory node. Often the patient has undergone an empirical course of antibiotics prior to referral to the otolaryngologist–head and neck surgeon. One should question the patient about whether or not antibiotics have been administered and whether any decrease in size of the mass has occurred as a result of the antibiotic therapy. This sequence of events is again consistent with an inflammatory rather than neoplastic etiology.

It is apparent that taking a thorough history can provide useful information to help narrow the number of possible diagnoses. Of course, the clinician must be aware that exceptions to the generalizations are a possibility. However, the coupling of thorough historical information with an exacting head and neck examination will minimize the possibility of making inaccurate conclusions.

Physical Examination

The physical examination provides an opportunity for obtaining further information and can be performed without the need for any specialized equipment. The recent development of the rigid and the flexible fiberoptic laryngopharyngoscopes, however, now provides the opportunity for non-otolaryngologic head and neck surgeons to examine the previously inaccessible anatomic areas, such as the nasopharynx, hypopharynx, and larynx.

It is not within the scope of this book to describe the specific techniques associated with the head and neck examination. The reader is referred to other excellent sources for that information.[5, 21] However, there are certain features of the neck examination which I have found useful to help increase accuracy. Although anatomy texts document the presence of lymph nodes intimately associated with the platysma muscle, the majority of neck tumors will be deep to substantial layers of musculature, such as the sternocleidomastoid laterally and the strap muscles medially, in addition to the overlying sheet of platysma. Whenever the examiner has the clinical impression of a superficial mass, one should be suspicious of a lipoma or sebaceous cyst. Whereas a lipoma is usually not adherent to the overlying neck skin, sebaceous cysts not only are adherent but also sometimes have an identifiable sinus tract. The majority of neck tumors will be in the deep tissues and,

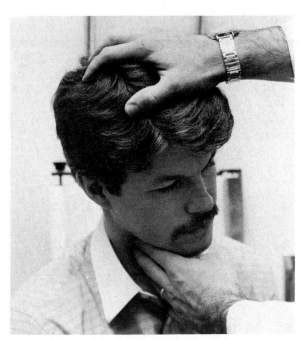

Figure 52–2. Flexing the patient's neck and turning it toward the side to be examined relaxes the tissue and facilitates a more thorough examination.

therefore, require expertise in palpation. The first important requirement is for the examiner to have an understanding of these anatomic landmarks in order to then position the patient in such a way as to permit a more accurate examination.

During the examination, the patient will invariably try to help by extending the neck and turning the head away from the physician's examining hand in an effort to provide more space for the physician. This posturing subsequently results in tensing of the platysma, sternocleidomastoid, and strap muscles and then makes the examination more difficult. This can be eliminated by placing one hand on top of the patient's head and holding the head in a straightforward position that is slightly flexed and tilted toward the shoulder on the side of the examiner (Fig. 52–2). These maneuvers then put all of the previously mentioned muscles at rest and make them flaccid and will hopefully result in facilitating a more accurate examination of the deep tissues.

Observation and palpation are the two most valuable techniques in the physical examination. A patient with a visible mass should be observed to see if this mass changes during the Valsalva maneuver to indicate continuity with the upper aerodigestive tract, such as with a laryngocele, or if there is any pulsation in the mass. One should be aware that tortuous carotid arteries (Fig. 52–3) are not at all uncommon in the elderly and infrequently are mistaken for an abnormal neck mass. After the mass has been observed for any changes with Valsalva or any pulsations, the primary important feature is the palpation of the mass.

The *position of the mass in the neck*, especially when correlated with the information obtained from the remaining portion of the head and neck examination, will often help determine whether indeed a mass is a probable malignancy. It is well known that head and neck

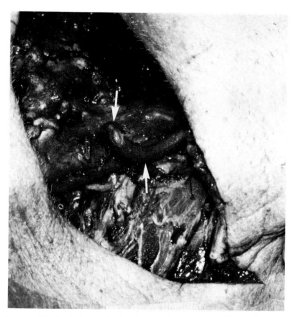

Figure 52–3. This patient undergoing a neck dissection was found to have an unusually tortuous internal carotid artery (arrow), which can be difficult to distinguish clinically from an aneurysm or other pulsatile neck tumor without the aid of angiography.

cancers have somewhat predictable nodal metastatic patterns. This topic has been studied in detail by Lindberg.[16] His exhaustive study involving approximately 2000 patients with previously untreated squamous cell cancer of the head and neck documented the frequency of anatomic sites of involvement. This important information (Figs. 52–4 to 52–12) helps a clinician to correlate any symptoms so that he or she could thoroughly examine a particular anatomic area in the upper aerodigestive tract. For example, a midjugular hard node is frequently associated with pyriform sinus malignancies and would tip off the clinician aware of that fact to completely and thoroughly examine the ipsilateral pyriform sinus.

The *mobility of a mass* is important because it affects the subsequent treatment. Although there are some rare occasions in which congenital or inflammatory masses have decreased mobility, immobility is usually an indication of fixation to the deep structures such as the transverse process of a cervical vertebra or scalene musculature. However, it is critically important to determine whether the neck tumor is indeed fixed to these underlying structures. There is no uniform agreement on the definition of "fixation." A strict definition is that the neck tumor cannot be moved without moving the patient. It is my impression that the designation of "fixation" is often not confirmed at the time of surgical resection. This determination has important clinical implications and demands a meticulous examination.

The physical examination should also provide information about whether or not a neck tumor is *tender to palpation*. Those which are exquisitely tender often are indeed inflammatory in origin. However, there is a margin of error in that some congenital cysts, such as a thyroglossal duct cyst, can become infected and subsequently become tender. Also, metastatic nodes can become secondarily infected and tender. If they are large enough and create tension of the surrounding structures, palpation will also precipitate pain. But generally speaking, the association of tenderness is most frequently seen with a neck tumor that is inflammatory in origin.

The *size of a tumor* should also be determined and recorded. This provides the opportunity for serial examinations to evaluate response to therapy. The relationship of the neck tumor to critical anatomic structures, once again, can provide meaningful information that has clinical significance. The major determination is the relationship of the mass to the carotid artery system. If the mass is near the carotid artery, one should also evaluate whether or not a Horner's syndrome exists by noting the presence of ptosis, enophthalmus, or miosis, which would indicate involvement of the cervical sympathetic chain.

One should auscult over the neck mass to determine whether there are any *alterations in the hemodynamics* that could produce a bruit. This might indicate the possibility of a vascular tumor such as a carotid body tumor or aneurysmal dilatation of some portion of the carotid artery system. However, it is important to realize that the absence of a bruit does not entirely exclude the diagnosis of a vascular abnormality.

The information obtained by a thorough history and physical examination does not require a large time commitment and usually results in a considerable reduction in the number of possibilities listed in the differential diagnosis. The history and physical examination should be the foundation for the remaining clinical evaluation that may involve radiographic or other diagnostic studies.

RADIOGRAPHIC EVALUATION

In the past, clinical evaluations of neck tumors were not especially enhanced by existing plain roentgenograms. *Nuclear imaging,* such as thyroid scans, occasionally were helpful. *Ultrasound echography* could sometimes support the diagnosis of a cystic tumor such as an abscess or congenital cyst. However, in the majority of instances, the standard available *radiographic studies* consistently failed to provide additional information that had already been determined or suspected from the history and physical examination.

The recent major technologic advancements in radiology have indeed provided techniques that are useful to the clinician..

Computed Tomography

Computed tomography has extended the capabilities of identifying detailed relationships within the deep tissues that previously have not been possible with other techniques. The differences in tissue densities can be readily identified with the CT scan, and not only can

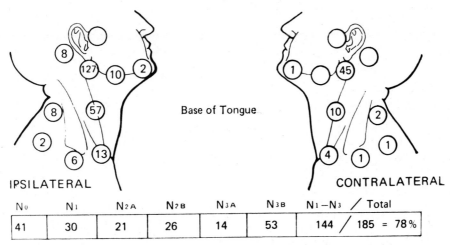

N₀	N₁	N₂A	N₂B	N₃A	N₃B	N₁–N₃ / Total
41	30	21	26	14	53	144 / 185 = 78%

Figure 52–4. Distribution of metastatic cervical nodes for tumors of the base of the tongue.

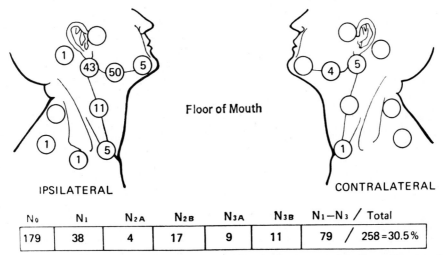

N₀	N₁	N₂A	N₂B	N₃A	N₃B	N₁–N₃ / Total
179	38	4	17	9	11	79 / 258 = 30.5%

Figure 52–5. Distribution of metastatic cervical nodes for tumors of the floor of the mouth.

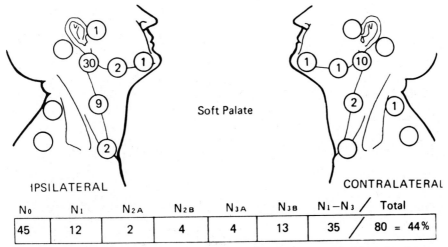

N₀	N₁	N₂A	N₂B	N₃A	N₃B	N₁–N₃ / Total
45	12	2	4	4	13	35 / 80 = 44%

Figure 52–6. Distribution of metastatic cervical nodes for tumors of the soft palate.

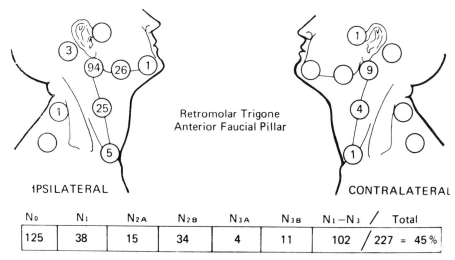

Figure 52–7. Distribution of metastatic cervical nodes for tumors of the retromolar trigone and anterior faucial pillar.

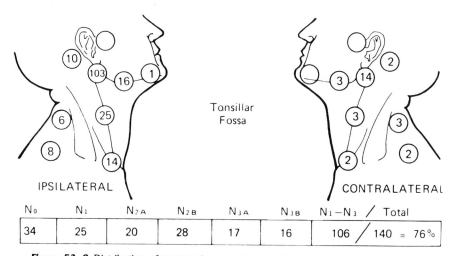

Figure 52–8. Distribution of metastatic cervical nodes for tumors of the tonsillar fossa.

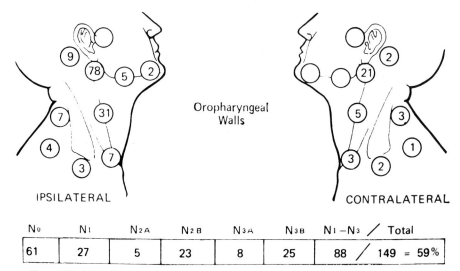

Figure 52–9. Distribution of metastatic cervical nodes for tumors of oropharyngeal walls.

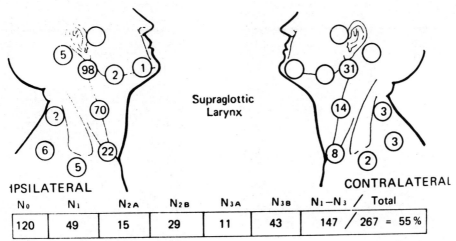

N₀	N₁	N₂ₐ	N₂ᵦ	N₃ₐ	N₃ᵦ	N₁–N₃ / Total
120	49	15	29	11	43	147 / 267 = 55%

Figure 52–10. Distribution of metastatic cervical nodes for tumors of the supraglottic larynx.

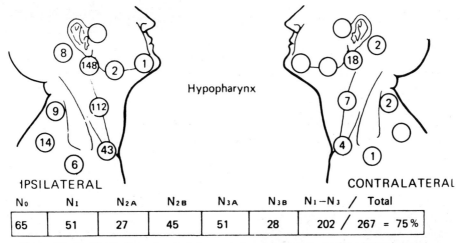

N₀	N₁	N₂ₐ	N₂ᵦ	N₃ₐ	N₃ᵦ	N₁–N₃ / Total
65	51	27	45	51	28	202 / 267 = 75%

Figure 52–11. Distribution of metastatic cervical nodes for tumors of the hypopharynx.

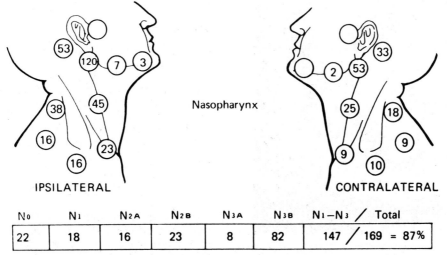

N₀	N₁	N₂ₐ	N₂ᵦ	N₃ₐ	N₃ᵦ	N₁–N₃ / Total
22	18	16	23	8	82	147 / 169 = 87%

Figure 52–12. Distribution of metastatic cervical nodes for tumors of the nasopharynx.

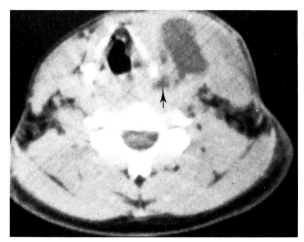

Figure 52–13. Large congenital neck cyst diagnosed with computed tomography, which also illustrates a tract (arrow) leading to the pyriform sinus.

even lymph nodes (Fig. 52–13) be identified but their relationship to the surrounding structures can be distinguished as well.

The use of CT scans in the evaluation of metastatic nodal disease has been especially helpful as it relates to involvement of surrounding normal structures. There is no question that cervical nodes of even moderate size can be readily identified (Fig. 52–14) with CT scanning techniques, especially useful in the evaluation of a large node felt to be fixed to deep structures (Fig. 52–15). The newer-generation CT technology will invariably increase the specificity and the capabilities of this valuable diagnostic tool.

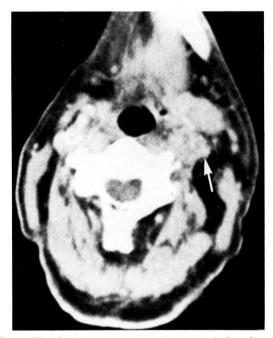

Figure 52–14. Patient with necrotic metastatic lymph node (arrow) deep to the sternocleidomastoid muscle.

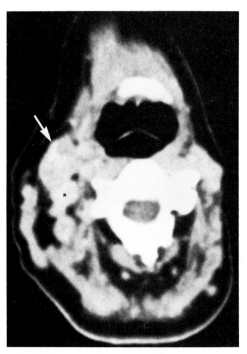

Figure 52–15. Computed tomogram demonstrates large metastatic node (arrow), which is fixed to surrounding deep structures, such as the internal jugular vein (asterisk).

Angiography

When it is necessary to evaluate the arterial system of the neck, angiography represents a valuable radiographic tool. Information obtained by the history and physical examination can indeed point to the possibility of a vascular tumor. But it is the angiogram that confirms that diagnosis. Although angiography represents a valuable diagnostic tool for those selected cases in which vascular tumors are suggested or the arterial system must be evaluated with respect to the relationship to certain neck tumors, it still is associated with a certain risk of morbidity and possibly even of death (Fig. 52–16).

Sialography

Parotid or submandibular sialography is only rarely used. In instances in which a neck tumor is located near the angle of the mandible, the parotid sialogram may provide useful information to delineate whether or not it is adjacent to or arising from within the gland. Occasionally a mass in the submandibular triangle can be differentiated from being extra- or intraglandular, once again with a submandibular sialogram.

DIAGNOSTIC TECHNIQUES

One needs to consider when it is necessary to obtain a histologic diagnosis prior to definitive treatment of a neck tumor and then to determine which is the preferred technique for a given clinical situation. The issue of

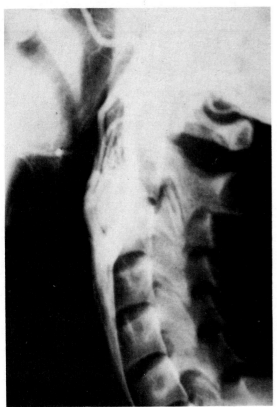

Figure 52–16. Carotid arteriogram showing highly vascular carotid body tumor located at the bifurcation and causing a bowing of the internal and external carotid arteries.

performing a biopsy on a neck tumor that is felt to be a metastatic cervical node has been frequently discussed in the medical literature for many years.[17, 18] The study of McGuirt and McCabe[18] in 1978 clearly documents that the morbidity and mortality rates are higher for patients undergoing excisional biopsy of a metastatic node. However, the increased acceptance of fine-needle aspiration[6, 19] has provided an opportunity to obtain some histologic information prior to any definitive therapeutic approach. The extensive experience of Frable and Frable[12, 13] has documented that there is only a minimal chance of tumor seeding with fine-needle aspiration.

Fine-Needle Aspiration Biopsy

The technique of fine needle aspiration involves the use of a narrow-gauge needle attached to a control syringe that permits a negative pressure after the needle is inserted into the neck tumor in an effort to aspirate cells from the mass; the cells are then immediately placed on glass slides, fixed, and then processed. The potential complications of the actual technique are minimal and are no different than for any other needle stick. However, the success of the procedure is clearly a function of the ability of the pathologist to read the relatively limited material that is submitted, and pathology expertise is essential.

Excisional Node Biopsy

In the clinical situation in which fine-needle aspiration biopsy fails to produce diagnostic material, or the clinician is suspicious of a malignancy other than a squamous carcinoma arising from the head and neck, then excisional node biopsy may be advisable. This technique is used primarily when non–squamous cell malignancies are suspected. It is important to remember that lymphomatous masses can involve cervical nodal chains. There is also the potential for neck tumors to represent metastases from primary tumor sites that are unrelated to head and neck sites. Malignancies arising in the genitourinary tract, breasts, and lungs can present as cervical neck masses. However, these usually are masses in positions that are somewhat different from metastatic squamous cancer, such as in the supraclavicular or low posterior triangle areas. Excisional biopsy can be used for those neck tumors when they present in patients who have the previously mentioned malignant diagnoses. Often such a procedure can be performed with local anesthesia. It is important for the surgeon to be aware of the relatively superficial course of the spinal accessory nerve in the posterior triangle after it exits the sternocleidomastoid muscle.

Incisional Biopsy

There are few indications for incisional biopsy. The rare circumstance may be in that patient with far advanced unresectable disease in which it is necessary to obtain a histologic diagnosis that can not be obtained by another technique such as a fine needle aspiration biopsy. The criticism of incisional biopsy relates to its propensity for seeding the wound with malignant cells.

REFERENCES

1. Annyas AA, Snow GB, VanSlooten EA: Prognostic factors of neck node metastasis: Their impact on planning and treatment regimen. Paper read before the American Society of Head and Neck Surgeons, Los Angeles, April 6, 1979.
2. Berlinger NT, Tsakraklides V, Pollak K, et al: Prognostic significance of lymph node histology in patients with squamous cell carcinoma of the larynx, pharynx, or oral cavity. Laryngoscope 86:792, 1976.
3. Cachin Y: Les Modalités et la Valeur Prognostique de l'Envahissement Ganglionnaire Cervical dans les Carcinomas des Voies Aérodigestives Supérieures. Vie Méd 4:46, 1972.
4. Cachin Y, Sancho-Garnier H, Micheau C, Marandas P: Nodal metastases from carcinomas of the oropharynx. Otolaryngol Clin North Am 12:145, 1979.
5. DeWeese DD, Saunders WH: Textbook of Otolaryngology, 6th ed. St. Louis, C. V. Mosby Co., 1982.
6. Einhorn J, Franzen S: Thin-needle biopsy in the diagnosis of thyroid disease. Acta Radiol 58:321, 1962.
7. Fisher B, Fisher ER: Studies concerning the regional lymph node in cancer: I. Initiation of immunity. Cancer 27:1001, 1971.
8. Ibid.; II. Maintenance of immunity. Cancer 29:1496, 1972.
9. Fisher ER, Reidbord HE, Fisher B: Studies concerning the regional lymph node in cancer: V. Histology and ultrastructural findings on regional and nonregional nodes. Lab Invest 28:126, 1973.
10. Fisher ER, Saffer E, Fisher B: Studies concerning the regional lymph node in cancer: VI. Correlation of lymphocyte transformation of regional node cells and some histopathologic discriminants. Cancer 32:104, 1973.
11. Fisher B, Wolmark N, Coyle J, et al: Studies concerning the regional lymph node in cancer: VIII. Effect of two asynchronous tumor faces on lymph node cell cytotoxicity. Cancer 36:521, 1975.
12. Frable MA, Frable WJ: Thin needle aspiration of the thyroid gland. Laryngoscope 90:1619, 1980.
13. Frable WJ, Frable MA: Thin needle aspiration biopsy. Cancer 43:1541, 1979.

14. Jenkins VK, Griffiths CM, Ray P, et al: Radiotherapy and head and neck cancer. Arch Otolaryngol *106*:414, 1980.
15. Johnson JT, Barnes EL, Myers EN, et al: The extracapsular spread of tumors in cervical node metastases. Arch Otolaryngol *107*:725, 1981.
16. Lindberg R: Distribution of cervical lymph node metastases from squamous cell carcinoma of the upper respiratory and digestive tracts. Cancer *29*:1446, 1982.
17. Martin H, Romieu C: The diagnostic significance of a "lump in the neck." Postgrad Med *11*:491, 1952.
18. McGuirt WF, McCabe BF: Significance of node biopsy before definitive treatment of cervical metastatic carcinoma. Laryngoscope *88*:594, 1978.
19. Persson PS: Cytodiagnosis of thyroiditis. Acta Med Scand (Suppl) *483*:7, 1968.
20. Sancho H, Hauss G, Sarvane D: Les Adénopathies Cervicales Métastatiques: Etude des Correlations Histo-cliniques. Conséquence sur le Plan Prognostique. Symposium International Adénopathies Cervicales Malignes (Milano). Nuovo Arch Ital Otol *12*:473, 1977.
21. Saunders WH: The physical examination. *In* Paparella MM, Shumrick DA (eds): Otolaryngology: Basic Sciences and Related Disciplines, vol. 1. Philadelphia, W. B. Saunders Co., 1973.
22. Schuller DE, McGuirt WF, McCabe BF, Young D: The prognostic significance of metastatic cervical lymph nodes. Laryngoscope *90*:557, 1980.
23. Schuller DE, Platz CE, Krause CJ: Spinal accessory lymph nodes: A prospective study of metastatic involvement. Laryngoscope *88*:439, 1978.
24. Sessions DG: Surgical pathology of cancer of the larynx and hypopharynx. Laryngoscope *86*:814, 1976.
25. Shore-Freedman E, Abrahams C, Recant W, Schneider AB: Neurilemomas and salivary gland tumors of the head and neck following childhood irradiation. Cancer *51*:2159, 1983.

CHAPTER 53

Pathology of Selected Soft Tissue Tumors of the Head and Neck

Michael Kyriakos, M.D.

This chapter describes some of the tumors that arise in the supporting tissues of the head and neck. These "soft tissues" include all the mesodermally derived, extraskeletal and nonepithelial tissues with the exception of the central nervous system glia and the components of the reticuloendothelial system.[13, 33] The tumors that arise in these tissues, therefore, include those that are composed of, or differentiate toward the development of, fat, fibrous tissue, smooth and skeletal muscle, blood vessels and lymphatics. Because of their frequent occurrence in the superficial soft tissues, tumors of peripheral nerves and the paraganglia, despite originating from the neuroectoderm, are also generally included in discussions of this system. Most of the tumors and tumor-like conditions of the supporting soft tissues also occur in the skin and viscera, but these usually reflect specific clinical problems and are dealt with in other chapters of this monograph.

Within the past decade, there has been a dramatic proliferation of newly described soft-tissue tumors or tumor-like conditions such that there are now well over 100 diagnostic entities with over 300 different synonyms.[13, 14, 20] Many of these entities, however, are so rare that they are outside the experience not only of most clinicians and radiologists but most pathologists as well. Even large medical centers may have only one or two examples of some of these lesions in their files. This chapter will touch on only a few of the conditions that might be of interest to the head and neck surgeon. Fortunately, recent monographs and papers devoted to the pathology of soft-tissue lesions present a broader and more intensive view of the subject than is possible here.[10–14, 20, 21, 25, 30, 41, 47]

GENERAL INFORMATION

Incidence and Origin

Tumors of the soft tissues are uncommon.[17, 33, 49] Reliable information on the incidence of benign lesions is difficult to find, as the emphasis in the literature has been on the malignant tumors and few institutions report their total experience with all soft-tissue lesions.[37] Enzinger and Weiss state that in a hospital population benign lesions outnumber the malignant in a ratio of 100:1.[14] At Columbia University, New York, a noted referral center for the diagnosis of soft-tissue tumors, there were 8700 of these tumors accessioned over a 45-year period. Of these, 7300 were benign and 1400 were malignant, a ratio of about 5:1.[47] Myhre-Jensen reported the occurrence of 1331 benign soft-tissue tumors in the 7-year period 1970 to 1977. During this same time there were only 72 malignant soft-tissue tumors, for a benign-to-malignant ratio of 18.5:1. These soft-tissue tumors comprised only 2 per cent of the total histopathologic examinations done during the same time span.[37] In the United States, approximately 4800 malignant soft-tissue tumors occur yearly, causing about 1600 cancer deaths.[1]

This should be viewed in the context of over 850,000 new cancers per year and 440,000 cancer deaths in the United States.[1] Although soft-tissue malignancies are relatively rare tumors, they are the fifth leading cause of cancer and cancer deaths in children under age 15.[1, 49, 52]

It is the rarity of these lesions that creates not only their fascination but their problems as well. Because few individual pathologists encounter a sufficient number of these tumors to become familiar with their variable histologic patterns, misdiagnoses with subsequent inadequate or improper therapy frequently occur.[12, 33] Perhaps in no other field of diagnostic pathology are so many errors made, frequently to the detriment of the patient. As an example, in a review of cases in the Swedish Tumor Registry that were diagnosed as sarcoma, 10 per cent were reclassified as benign reactive lesions.[9]

Many of these soft-tissue lesions have stimulated an interest that is out of proportion to their clinical occurrence. This is due, at least in part, to the fact that many affect children and young adults and require, at times, multilating surgical procedures for their removal. Fifty per cent of the sarcomas treated in the head and neck service at Memorial Hospital, New York, occurred in children.[16] Recent advances in chemotherapy and radiation therapy have also resulted in significantly improved cure rates for some sarcomas that had previously been almost uniformly fatal, and such results have naturally stimulated interest in the treatment of these tumors.[49]

Most patients with soft-tissue sarcomas have nonspecific symptoms, usually that of an enlarging, painless mass frequently located in an extremity. Few sarcomas occur with any frequency in the head and neck region, where over 80 per cent of the malignancies are epithelial in origin.[16] At Memorial Hospital during the 28-year period 1949 to 1977, only 285 sarcomas in children and adults were seen on the head and neck service.[16] Although sarcomas have developed subsequent to radiation therapy, the occurrence of such postradiation sarcomas in the head and neck area is also quite rare, despite the frequent use of large-dose radiation therapy in the treatment of epithelial malignancies of this region.[7]

In a study of malignant head and neck tumors seen at Boston Children's Hospital from 1960 to 1969, Jaffe reported 178 tumors, only 51 (28.7 per cent) of which were soft-tissue in origin.[22] In the same report, Jaffe also reviewed and summarized two previously reported series of head and neck tumors in children—one a 16-year experience at the M.D. Anderson Hospital in Texas and the other the 27-year experience of Dr. John Conley of New York. At the M.D. Anderson Hospital, there were 127 head and neck tumors, of which 43 (33.9 per cent) could be interpreted as arising from the soft tissues, while in Conley's series, 61 of 111 tumors (55 per cent) originated in the soft tissues. In a total of 416 such pediatric tumors, 155 (37.3 per cent) were soft-tissue malignancies.[22]

From the surgeon's viewpoint it must be remembered that as a general rule benign tumors arise from the dermis or superficial soft tissues, whereas sarcomas are usually deeply situated and rarely arise from these sites. In Myhre-Jensen's series, 73 per cent of the malignant tumors were deeply situated and only 12.5 per cent were superficial and freely movable in relation to the underlying fascia.[37]

The growth rates of sarcomas vary considerably and appear dependent on both the type of tumor and its differentiation. Some sarcomas may be present for several years before the patient seeks medical attention, or they may grow rapidly over a period of only a few weeks. Benign lesions, with some notable exceptions such as nodular fasciitis, usually grow slowly.

Clinical inspection of the tumor, or its appearance at the time of operation, usually produces few clues as to its nature or cell type. Benign proliferative lesions such as nodular fasciitis or desmoid tumor have an infiltrative growth pattern suggestive of malignancy. Sarcomas, however, usually appear well circumscribed or even encapsulated such that the surgeon assumes the tumor to be benign and attempts to "shell out" or locally excise it without sufficient margins.[13, 18] Microscopically, however, sarcomas lack a true capsule and always infiltrate the adjacent normal tissue. Necrosis, cystic degeneration and hemorrhage may be found in both benign and malignant lesions. With the exception of tumors noted to be arising within a large nerve trunk; the yellow, greasy appearance of some fat tumors; and the grape-like clusters of botryoid rhabdomyosarcoma, there is such an overlap in the appearance of soft-tissue lesions that the diagnosis of a specific tumor type is not possible from their gross appearance. Benign tumors tend to be small (<5 cm), and malignant tumors tend to reach a large size.[37] The surgeon, however, should consider every deeply located soft-tissue mass to be malignant until proved otherwise by microscopic examination.

Diagnosis

Because the type of therapy used for soft-tissue tumors very much depends upon the histologic nature of the tumor, a well-planned biopsy is usually mandatory.[28, 31, 43, 45] This may consist of an *incisional biopsy* or, with small superficial lesions, a wide *excisional biopsy*.[43] The biopsy incision should be so placed that it avoids creating possible future problems if subsequent radiation therapy is a possibility.[31, 48] The biopsy should include material from the periphery of the tumor, at the interface of the tumor and normal tissue, so as to avoid central necrotic foci.[43, 45] *Frozen section* examination may be useful in order to assure that adequate tumor tissue has been obtained, but the surgeon should realize that it may not be possible with frozen section material to accurately diagnose the specific tumor type.[43, 45] Biopsies of only a few millimeters from tumors that are several centimeters in size are to be avoided if possible.[43, 45] Many tumors or tumor-like conditions of the soft tissues contain a fibroblastic component and, if improperly sampled, may be misdiagnosed as fibrosarcoma.[12] Furthermore, many sarcomas contain a variety of cellular components and may have a variety of histologic patterns not only from tumor to tumor but even from area to area within the same tumor,[13, 14, 20] hence the requirement for as generous a biopsy specimen as possible. We feel that *core-needle biopsy* has only limited value in head and neck tumors, as for instance in confirming the presence of a metastatic epithelial neoplasm in a cervical lymph node or tissues of the neck, or for confirming recurrences of previously diagnosed lesions. We see no advantage of needle aspiration biopsy over core-needle biopsy in soft-tissue growths.[43, 45] Needle biopsies of any type may even be contraindicated in highly vascular tumors such as paragangliomas. Such closed biopsies yield insufficient tissue for diagnosis in up to one third of cases.[48] We prefer open biopsies for most head and neck tumors.

With some tumors, many sections may have to be cut, and a variety of stains employed, before a definitive histologic diagnosis is reached. Indeed, in some cases it may be possible for the pathologist to determine, on the basis of the biopsy material, only that the lesion is malignant, with the final tumor type being dependent upon examination of the entire tumor. However, even here, experienced pathologists find that for approximately 10 to 15 per cent of soft-tissue sarcomas it is not possible to assign a specific cell type.[13, 14, 32, 33] This stems from the fact that as lesions become less differentiated there may remain no clues, by light microscopy, as to the tissue of origin or direction of differentiation.[23] Indeed, tumors such as spindle cell epidermoid carcinoma, malignant melanoma, kidney carcinoma, granulocytic sarcoma, and pleomorphic lymphoma may histologically mimic sarcoma.[43] It is of obvious clinical importance to differentiate between a primary sarcoma and a metastasis from some other primary tumor.

Electron microscopy of such lesions may be helpful; however, it is just such tumors that are so difficult to diagnose at the light microscopic level for which electron microscopy, with its inherent sampling problems, may also be noncontributory because of the lack of tumor-specific cytologic structures.[19, 23, 27, 43, 51] Among some clinicians there is a belief that electron microscopy is more accurate than light microscopy—this is untrue. Electron microscopy is an ancillary tool, at times a very valuable and useful tool, but its use does not guarantee success in the diagnosis of difficult lesions.[27, 51] Electron microscopy may contribute to a specific diagnosis in from 1 to 8 per cent of cases.[19, 43] In one series, the diagnosis was determined by electron microscopy alone in 3 per cent of the cases.[19]

Recently, the use of immunohistologic techniques, using immunoperoxidase or avidin-biotin techniques, to demonstrate specific intermediate cell filaments and various other proteins offers hope that some sarcomas, now in the "unclassified" category, may be more accurately identified.[5, 15, 35, 36, 39, 50] The demonstration of such substances as cytokeratin, desmin, vimentin, glial fibrillary acidic protein, S-100 protein, laminin and myoglobin has been successful in not only distinguishing carcinomas from sarcomas but also identifying tumors as being of specific cell types.[4, 34, 36, 38] Soft-tissue lesions also produce specific types of collagen and mucosubstances, and techniques for their identification have also been applied to tumor diagnosis.[24, 29, 46]

Metastases

Sarcomas grow along fascial planes, nerve trunks, and tendon sheaths and spread via the blood stream, with the lungs, bones, and liver being common sites of involvement by metastases.[14, 33, 47] With few exceptions, such as in embryonal rhabdomyosarcoma and synovial sarcoma, lymph nodes are rarely involved.[18] The majority of metastases occur within 2 years of treatment, although with some sarcomas 10 to 20 years may elapse before metastases become evident.[18, 26, 33]

Treatment

Surgical therapy remains the mainstay for the treatment of both benign and malignant soft-tissue tumors.[6] Although local excision, even incomplete local excision, may be curative for some benign tumors, the recurrence rate for sarcomas is very much dependent upon the type of surgical therapy employed. Purely local excisions yield recurrences in from 75 to 90 per cent of cases, and even wide radical excision may yield local recurrence in from 25 to 30 per cent of patients.[26, 33] Absence of local recurrence, however, is no guarantee of cure, as approximately one quarter of patients will develop metastases that are unassociated with local recurrence.[26] In the head and neck region, radical surgical procedures may not be practical owing to their mutilating effects, especially in children. Compromise surgical excisions with subsequent radiation and chemotherapy may be necessary. This program has fortunately been quite successful in the treatment of rhabdomyosarcoma, the most common sarcoma to occur in the head and neck region. Although the use of adjuvant chemotherapy to eliminate micrometastases has proved successful in the treatment of rhabdomyosarcoma, effective chemotherapeutic agents for most soft-tissue sarcomas are still being developed.[2, 3, 40, 42, 49]

The preceding statements are generalizations, and sarcomas cannot, any more than can carcinomas, be grouped together in terms of their behavior. Each tumor type has its own clinical presentation, predilection for certain anatomic sites, age range of host, and prognosis.

Classification and Staging

The classification of soft-tissue tumors, both benign and malignant, is based upon the type of tissue they contain or toward which they have differentiated.[10, 14, 26, 33] An encapsulated tumor composed of mature adipose cells is designated as a lipoma. Its malignant counterpart, the liposarcoma, contains malignant-appearing lipoblasts but may lack any significant amount of mature adipose tissue. This is not to imply that sarcomas arise from their benign counterparts or from mature, fully differentiated normal cells.[12, 13] With few exceptions, sarcomas apparently arise de novo and not through malignant degeneration of a previously benign lesion.

Staging systems have been proposed for soft-tissue sarcomas, most based principally upon the pathologist's evaluation of the grade or differentiation of the tumor.[8, 44] Since no well-established or published grading criteria exist for the majority of sarcomas, we do not believe that such systems are of much practical value in their current state of development.[41, 43]

FIBROSARCOMA

Fibrosarcoma was formerly considered to be the most common sarcoma, but with better definition of such lesions as the benign fibromatoses and malignant fibrous histiocytoma, the number of tumors now diagnosed as fibrosarcoma has been considerably reduced. In reviews of cases previously diagnosed as fibrosarcoma, it was found that from one third to one half belonged in other diagnostic categories.[62, 66] Today, fibrosarcomas make up only 5 to 10 per cent of all sarcomas.[59, 63, 66]

Whereas fibrosarcoma occurs in patients of all ages, it most commonly affects adults between 40 and 70 years of age, with male patients accounting for approximately 60 per cent of cases.[55, 62, 66, 68] Fibrosarcomas in children usually develop during the first year of life with about one half being congenital.[25, 55, 68] In the two largest series of head and neck fibrosarcomas, there was a total of 94 patients with an equal sex incidence.[57, 69] The 54 patients reported by Conley and associates included six patients less than 15 years old, and three between 15 and 21 years of age.[57] In the series of 40 patients reported by Swain and coworkers, 20 patients were less than age 40, 11 of whom were less than age 9.[69]

Fibrosarcoma usually arises in the extremities, especially the lower extremities.[10, 14, 66] The head and neck region is not a common location, being the site of origin in only 10 to 20 per cent of cases.[10, 54, 55, 62, 68, 70] In infantile or congenital fibrosarcoma, the head and neck has been involved in 13.2 and 18.2 per cent of reported cases.[55, 68] The commonest locations in the head and neck area are the soft tissues of the face, followed by those of the neck, the scalp, paranasal sinuses, mandible, larynx, and in rare cases the nasal cavity, nasopharynx, pharynx, and intraoral sites.[10, 54, 57, 58, 69]

Fibrosarcoma usually develops as a slowly growing painless mass that may be present for several years. The tumors tend to be superficially located with origin from the fascial connective tissue or deep subcutaneous tissue, although those in the head and neck may be deeply situated.[66, 69] On gross inspection, they are firm, gray-white, lobulated, well-circumscribed tumors.[14, 66] The tumors in infants and young children tend to be more friable and less well circumscribed.[55, 62] The poorly differentiated fibrosarcomas may contain visible areas of necrosis and hemorrhage. Tumor size is dependent on location; superficial tumors are usually in the range of 3.0 to 4.0 cm, whereas deeply situated tumors may be many centimeters larger.[55, 62, 66, 68]

Histologically, fibrosarcomas are composed of spindle-shaped fibroblasts arranged in intersecting fasicles that give rise to the typical "herringbone" pattern.[14, 62, 66, 68] Nuclei have tapered ends and are usually uniform without great atypia (Fig. 53–1). The cytoplasm tends to be ill-defined, with poorly formed cell borders. In poorly differentiated tumors there is increased cellularity with crowding of the cells and a decrease in reticulin and collagen production.[14, 62, 68] The cells also assume a more rounded or plump shape with greater cell to cell

variation in size and shape, and there is increased mitotic activity. Reticulin and collagen production is best seen in the well-differentiated tumors.[14, 62, 68] Congenital or infantile fibrosarcomas are histologically similar to those in adults, although there is a greater tendency for such lesions to be less differentiated, with loss of the herringbone pattern, and more vascular than their adult counterparts.[55, 61, 62] The presence of many large and atypical bizarre tumor giant cells in a spindle cell tumor excludes the diagnosis of fibrosarcoma.[41, 66] Unfortunately, several reported series of fibrosarcomas use the term "undifferentiated fibrosarcoma."[57] At the light microscope level, such a diagnosis is untenable. Electron microscopic studies have shown the presence of occasional myofibroblasts in fibrosarcomas.[56, 64]

Fibrosarcoma is the sarcoma that lends itself best to histologic grading based on its differentiation. Tumors may be classified as well-, moderately, or poorly differ-

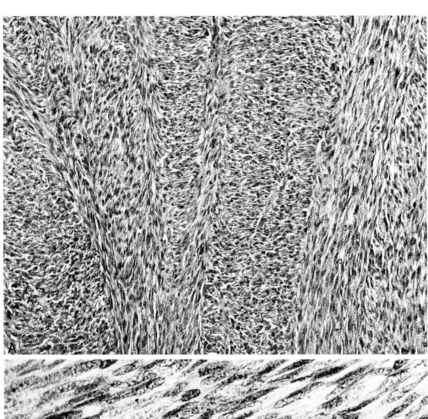

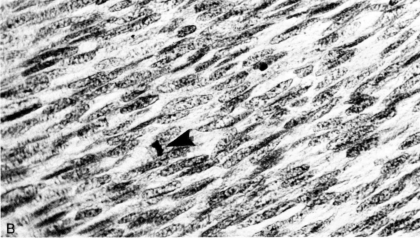

Figure 53–1. Fibrosarcoma. (*A*) Herringbone pattern produced by interlacing fascicles of spindle-shaped fibroblasts. (*B*) Elongated nuclei of the fibroblasts of fibrosarcoma. Cells show only minimal variability. A mitotic figure (arrowhead) is present.

entiated, or they may be designated by a numerical grade, I to IV, with grade IV being the least differentiated. Most fibrosarcomas tend to be moderately differentiated (grades II to III).[62, 66, 68] In adults, this grading system has prognostic implications, as it correlates closely with local recurrence, metastases, and survival. The lower the grade, the better the prognosis.[10, 14, 41, 54, 66]

Caution should be observed when the diagnosis of fibrosarcoma is made from a small biopsy sample because other sarcomas, notably synovial sarcoma, neurosarcoma, malignant fibrous histiocytoma, and rhabdomyosarcoma, may contain fibroblastic or spindle cell foci that mimic fibrosarcoma. We also caution against the use of the term "fibroma" for any deeply situated fibrous tumor. Such lesions will usually prove to be fibrosarcomas or one of the fibromatoses, both of which are capable of aggressive local growth, which the term fibroma does not imply.[65]

A major problem in the diagnosis of fibrosarcoma is its separation from the more common benign fibromatoses and reactive fibroblastic lesions. This problem is especially acute with the fibrous lesions that occur in children. The distinction between a very cellular fibromatosis and a well-differentiated fibrosarcoma may be quite difficult and at times impossible. The terminology used in some older publications on head and neck fibrosarcoma is confusing in this respect by their equating of infiltrative fibromatosis with low-grade fibrosarcoma.[53, 57] Unlike fibrosarcomas, fibromatoses do not metastasize.

Surgical management, with wide local excision, is the therapy of choice for fibrosarcoma. Recurrence rates range from 30 to 75 per cent, with the higher rates noted in tumors treated by local resection and in poorly differentiated tumors. Approximately 50 per cent of patients develop distant metastases, almost all of which are blood-borne.[66] Regional lymph node involvement occurs in less than 10 per cent of patients, with some large series containing no examples of lymph node metastases.[10, 14, 57, 66, 69] Prophylactic radical lymph node dissection has no place in the treatment of fibrosarcoma.

In the two largest series of head and neck fibrosarcomas, distant metastases occurred in 20 to 25 per cent of cases.[57, 69] Overall 5- and 10-year survival rates for fibrosarcomas of all sites are in the 50 to 60 per cent range, patients with the better differentiated tumors having the best survival.[10, 14, 66] In their study of head and neck fibrosarcomas, Conley and associates found 31 per cent of their patients had died or were living with incurable disease. The "undifferentiated" fibrosarcomas had a poor prognosis, with 67 per cent of the patients dying of tumor.[57] Swain and coworkers found that in those patients correctly treated for cure, 12 of 16 (75 per cent) with well-differentiated tumors survived, but only one of five with poorly differentiated tumors survived. They also found that patients with more superficially located tumors, which also tended to be better differentiated, also had the best prognosis.[69] Care, however, should be exercised in the interpretation of these reports. In Conley's series, fibrosarcomas were combined with infiltrative fibromatosis, and 23 per cent of the 54 cases were interpreted as "undifferentiated" fibrosarcoma. In the series by Swain, the definition of what the authors interpreted as poorly differentiated fibrosarcoma indicated that at least some of these fibro-

sarcomas would today probably be considered malignant fibrous histiocytomas. Therefore, neither of these two series deals with pure fibrosarcoma, and the data should be viewed with this in mind. In another report, which includes 20 fibrosarcomas in the head and neck, the 5-year survival rate was given as 36 per cent and the 10-year survival rate as 15 per cent.[70] In a small, but more recent series, Das Gupta reported 5-year survival in 8 of 13 patients (62 per cent).[10] Compared with fibrosarcomas of the extremities, those in the head and neck appear to have a poorer prognosis despite the fact that most are well-differentiated tumors.[10, 70] This may reflect the limitation on the type of operative excision that is possible in the head and neck area.

Unlike adult fibrosarcomas, the prognosis for those in children cannot be predicted on the basis of their histology.[55, 68] In general, fibrosarcomas in children have a more favorable prognosis, with 5-year survival rates as high as 80 per cent despite local recurrence rates of approximately 50 per cent after wide local excision.[25, 47, 55, 68] Few patients with childhood fibrosarcoma have died of metastatic disease.[47, 53, 55, 67, 68] The younger the child, the more favorable is the prognosis.[42] However, this may reflect the inclusion of some locally aggressive nonmetastasizing fibromatoses that are difficult to distinguish from fibrosarcoma in this age group. Older children have the less favorable adult survival rates.[68]

FIBROMATOSES

The fibromatoses consist of a diverse group of nonmetastasizing, locally invasive fibroblastic or myofibroblastic lesions, many of which tend to recur after resection.[71, 80, 82] Despite the lack of metastases, these lesions may prove fatal owing to their local aggressiveness, especially those situated in the head and neck region close to vital structures.[71]

In general, the fibromatoses arise in a wide variety of anatomic locations and in all age groups. However, some are found either exclusively or predominantly in infants and young children, and others occur more frequently in adults. This has led to the broad division into the infantile, or juvenile, fibromatoses and the adult fibromatoses.[71, 81] In the former category are such lesions as fibrous hamartoma of infancy, fibromatosis colli, diffuse infantile fibromatosis, aggressive infantile fibromatosis (congenital fibrosarcoma-like fibromatosis), juvenile aponeurotic fibroma, digital fibrous tumor of childhood, congenital generalized and solitary fibromatosis, hereditary gingival fibromatosis, juvenile nasopharyngeal angiofibroma, and fibromatosis hyalin multiplex juvenalis.[71, 75, 85] Some of these entities are histologically quite cellular, being composed of primitive-appearing mesenchymal cells. This, combined with their infiltrative growth pattern, has, unfortunately, led to a diagnosis of sarcoma in some cases with disastrous consequences. Furthermore, even experienced pathologists may have great difficulty in distinguishing between an "aggressive" fibromatosis, or congenital fibrosarcoma-like fibromatosis, and a true fibrosarcoma that is fully capable of metastasis.[85] Fibromatosis may, as can fibrosarcoma, develop secondary to radiation therapy.[84]

Among the adult lesions are the Dupuytren's-type fibromatoses—that is, palmar and plantar fibromatoses and Peyronie's disease—and the various types of the desmoid fibromatoses.[71, 81] As a group, the adult varieties are more common than the juvenile forms, some of which are so exceedingly rare that they are outside the experience of most pathologists. Whereas the head and neck region has its share of these lesions, indeed being site-specific for fibromatosis colli, some fibromatoses do not occur in this area. We describe here only some of the fibromatoses, and the reader is referred to the excellent reviews and articles on fibromatoses, which are listed in the bibliography, for more comprehensive coverage.[71, 75, 81, 82, 85]

As mentioned in the previous section on fibrosarcoma, care should be taken not to consider these fibrous soft-tissue lesions to be "fibromas."[65] Use of the term "fibroma" in the same manner that "adenoma" is used to designate benign glandular tumors is to be avoided.[81] Most fibromatoses arise from the muscular and musculoaponeurotic tissues of the body and hence are for the most part deeply situated lesions.[14, 83] Unlike well-circumscribed and self-limited adenomas that may be locally excised without much fear of recurrence, a well-circumscribed soft-tissue lesion composed of bland, well-differentiated fibroblasts may behave as a highly invasive and destructive lesion with a propensity to recur following simple excision. We agree with those who avoid the term "fibroma" as a designation for deeply situated soft-tissue lesions.[65, 81]

Desmoid Fibromatosis (Desmoid)

The desmoid fibromatoses are arbitrarily divided into those that arise in the anterior abdominal wall and those located elsewhere, the "extra-abdominal" desmoids also known as musculo-aponeurotic fibromatoses, or "aggressive" fibromatoses.[71, 76, 78, 81] Regardless of their site of origin, the lesions are histologically similar. The extra-abdominal lesions are more common than the abdominal wall type.

Desmoids occur in infants as well as in patients in the eighth decade of life, but most occur in the third and fourth decades.[14, 71-74, 76, 81, 83] Unlike abdominal desmoids, which are unusual in patients under 20 years of age, extra-abdominal lesions do occur in children.[71, 72, 82] In Masson and Soule's series of 34 head and neck desmoids, the youngest patient was 18 months old and the oldest was 72 years of age.[83] Thirty of the 34 patients had developed a lesion by age 50. In the series of 40 fibromatoses of the head and neck reported by Conley and associates, the youngest patient was a newborn and the oldest was age 70, with 25 per cent of the patients being under age 15.[73] Although abdominal desmoids occur more frequently in women, especially parous women,[82] the extra-abdominal lesions do not show such a dramatic sex difference, and in some series men have been equally affected.[14, 71, 76, 81, 82] In Masson and Soule's series there was a female-to-male ratio of 3:2, and in Conley's series there was an equal sex distribution.[73, 83]

The head and neck region accounts for roughly 10 to 20 per cent of all the extra-abdominal lesions.[10, 14, 71, 74, 79, 82, 83] In Das Gupta's review of seven series, totaling 187 patients, 26 (13.9 per cent) were located in the head and neck area.[10] Among 367 patients with desmoids at the Armed Forces Institute of Pathology (AFIP), 35 (9.5 per cent) had head and neck lesions.[14] Of the desmoid fibromatoses that are located in the head and neck area, 40 to 85 per cent are situated in the neck. Other sites include the face, scalp, oral cavity, nasal cavity, and paranasal sinuses.[14, 60, 73, 83, 87] The supraclavicular fossa is a common location, either as a primary site of origin, or from secondary involvement by desmoids arising in the shoulder-girdle area.[14, 76, 83]

Clinically, desmoids are usually slowly growing, firm to hard masses that may be tender or painful, although most are painless.[73, 74, 76, 79] Desmoids in the head and neck may develop rapidly unlike their usual slow growth at other sites.[73, 83] Twenty-one of the 34 patients (62 per cent) reported by Masson and Soule were aware of the lesion for less than 1 year.[83] Desmoids have also developed in surgical scars and in sites that have received radiation therapy.[14, 71, 72] Rare familial cases have been reported.[88] There is an increased incidence of desmoid tumors in patients with Gardner's syndrome, in which the desmoids may develop either prior to or after the appearance of the intestinal polyps.[71, 82]

Desmoids vary considerably in size, with lesions often exceeding 20 cm.[14, 74, 76, 79] Grossly, they are gray-white, whorled or trabeculated masses, usually with ill-defined margins[71, 73, 74, 76] that develop within the muscle, aponeurosis, or fascia.[14, 74, 79] They infiltrate the muscle, usually developing along its long axis, and at times extend along the fascia beyond the muscle.[74, 76, 79] The actual histologic extent of the lesion may be several centimeters beyond the grossly visible margins.[82] The lesion resembles scar tissue and this is, for surgeons dealing with recurrent lesions, its most treacherous aspect, as it may be impossible to distinguish true scar tissue from the proliferating fibrous tissue of the desmoid, making it difficult to define the lesion's true extent. It is not uncommon for the surgeon to believe that the margins of the resection were well beyond the boundaries of the desmoid, only to have the pathologist report the surgical margins to be involved.

Microscopically, there is invasion of muscle and tendon by mature, uniform spindle-shaped fibroblasts that are arranged in interlacing bands and fascicles. These are surrounded and separated by varying amounts of collagen.[71, 74, 76, 79, 83] The process separates and pushes aside the muscle fibers, many of which eventually atrophy and disappear (Fig. 53–2). Residual isolated muscle fibers are seen within this stroma, which varies from hypocellular hyalinized foci to compact cellular regions.[76, 83] The cells lack pleomorphism, and mitoses are rare.[71, 74, 76, 79, 83] It is this lack of pleomorphism and mitotic activity that helps distinguish desmoids from fibrosarcoma. However, it must be admitted that at times a cellular fibromatosis that contains a few mitotic figures may be difficult to separate from a well-differentiated fibrosarcoma.[81] Electron microscopic studies have shown myofibroblasts in these lesions, and at times these may be the dominant cells.[77]

Local recurrence rates following excision have varied from 19 to 77 per cent, with multiple recurrences not uncommon.[71, 72, 76, 79, 82, 83] Extra-abdominal desmoids, especially those in the head and neck, are more aggressive than their abdominal counterparts.[54] Masson and Soule reported that 70 per cent of their traced patients with head and neck desmoids had recurrences, whereas 50 per cent of their patients with desmoids in other loca-

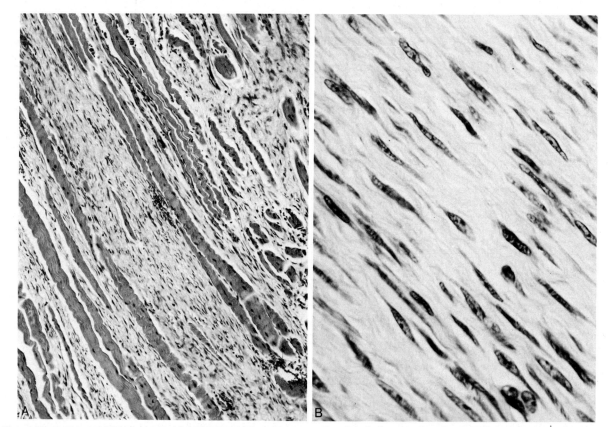

Figure 53–2. Desmoid fibromatosis. (*A*) Infiltration and replacement of muscle by bands of mature fibrous tissue. Muscle fibers show atrophy and degeneration. (*B*) Fibroblasts of desmoid fibromatosis are widely separated by collagenous stroma. Note uniformity of nuclei. Compare this appearance with that shown in Figure 53–1 *B*.

tions developed recurrences.[83] In Conley's series, almost one half of the patients developed local recurrences, and 15 per cent were living with unresectable lesions.[73] Four of the six patients with head and neck lesions reported by Das Gupta and associates were free of disease at 5 years.[74] Most recurrences manifest themselves within a few months of the original operation.[14, 76] Recurrence rates, as would be expected, depend upon the adequacy of the original operation, with wide local resections yielding lower recurrence rates than when the lesion is simply locally excised. Analysis of recurrent lesions indicates that in most patients the initial operative procedure had been inadequate with incomplete removal of the affected muscle.[72, 73, 79, 83] However, even with wide resections, recurrences are reported in 19 to 40 per cent of cases.[73, 74]

Radical surgery, including radical neck dissection, has been advocated by some, regardless of the size of the lesion, for desmoids in the head and neck region.[79, 83] However, mutilating operations for nonmetastasizing lesions are not to be undertaken lightly. This must be balanced by the fact that, although quite rarely, patients have died of locally invasive tumors that have involved vital structures in the neck and caused tracheal compression.[60, 71, 72, 74, 83] Three of the 34 patients reported by Masson and Soule died of extensive local disease.[83] Among the 52 determinate patients with extra-abdominal desmoids reported by Das Gupta and associates, two died of disease, one due to a massive lesion in the neck.[74] One of 11 patients reported by Cole and Guiss

died of a desmoid that had originated in the sternocleidomastoid muscle and extended into the mediastinum.[72] One of the six patients with fibromatoses of the nasal cavity and paranasal sinuses reported by Fu and Perzin died of recurrent tumor.[60] However, it should be noted that local excisions have also been curative.[71] In the series of shoulder-girdle lesions reported by Enzinger and Shiraki, 13 of 30 patients (43 per cent) were cured by simple excision.[76]

Radiation therapy may also be beneficial.[83] In the series reported by Wara and associates there were 16 patients referred for radiation therapy, 12 of whom had recurrent lesions and four who had not been previously treated. Thirteen of the lesions were controlled, without any recurrence during follow-up intervals of 2 to 6 years, by radiation doses of 4500 to 6100 rads.[86] Desmoids have also been noted to stabilize in their growth, and some have even spontaneously regressed, although this latter event is quite unusual.[71, 76]

Juvenile Fibromatoses

Congenital Fibromatosis

The occurrence of some form of fibromatosis, mainly fibromatosis colli or plantar fibromatosis, is not uncommon in children. Kauffman and Stout claim that the fibromatoses are second in incidence only to vascular tumors in the newborn period.[93] Fifty per cent of the solitary fibromatoses in their study of congenital mesenchymal tumors arose in the head and neck area. However, the lesions designated as congenital generalized or congenital solitary fibromatoses are exceedingly rare, with probably less than 100 well-documented cases reported in the English language literature[85, 92] since first described by Stout in 1954.[98]

These lesions, which usually arise in the subcutaneous tissue or muscle, may occur as solitary lesions; as multiple lesions widely distributed over the body, including the bones, but without visceral involvement; or in a generalized form that involves visceral organs as well.[85, 91] Some authors have used the terms "multiple," "diffuse," or "generalized" to refer either to cases in which more than one lesion is present or to those in which there is visceral involvement. We prefer the classification used by Rosenberg and coworkers, who divided their cases into multiple and visceral forms. The multiple types included tumors of the skin, subcutaneous tissue, muscle, and bone, and the visceral forms had some visceral organ involved.[85] This lesion has recently been designated as "infantile myofibromatosis" because of its content of myofibroblasts.[92]

As the name implies, these lesions are almost always present at birth or are noted shortly thereafter, although new lesions may develop after birth.[85, 91] As the experience with their histopathology has increased, similar lesions have been found in older children and, rarely, in adults.[71, 85, 91, 94] Enzinger and Weiss mention a 24-year-old patient with a solitary lesion.[14] Visceral lesions, however, apparently occur only in newborns or neonates.[14] Familial cases have been reported.[75] Boys are more commonly affected than girls in ratios up to 3:1.[71, 85, 90-92]

The superficially located lesions involve the skin and subcutaneous tissue and appear as firm to rubbery, well-delimited nodules, which may be solitary or up to 100 in number and may be widely distributed over the body surface.[71, 85] The more superficial nodules may have a purplish hue and simulate a hemangioma.[92] They are small, usually less than 3.0 cm, but nodules up to 7.5 cm have been reported.[14, 90-92] Intramuscular lesions also tend to be well circumscribed and may even shell out easily at the time of operation, but occasionally they appear grossly to invade the soft tissue.[71, 85, 89, 92] Both types of lesion may contain central necrotic foci.[71, 85, 91, 92, 94] Intraosseous lesions, which may affect any bone, produce a lucent appearance on roentgenograms. Bone involvement is quite common in both the multiple and visceral forms of the disease, occurring in over 60 per cent of those with multiple lesions and in almost half of those with visceral lesions.[85]

The lesions are located in any area of the body, with a predilection for the trunk, extremities, shoulder girdle, and head.[71, 85, 91, 95] Within the head and neck region, the scalp, orbit, skull, parotid region, tongue, and larynx have been involved.[89, 90-92, 96] Any visceral organ, including the central nervous system, may be involved, with the lungs, heart, and gastrointestinal system being involved most frequently.[14, 71, 85, 92, 99] At the AFIP, the head and neck region was involved in 16 of 45 solitary lesions (36 per cent), with the scalp and skull involved in six, the forehead and orbit in five, the cheek-parotid region in two, and the neck in three patients. At least four of 16 patients with multicentric lesions also had head and neck involvement, and four other patients with "gen-

eralized" disease had lesions widely distributed over the body surface, presumably including the head and neck region.[92] In the series of 18 solitary lesions reported by Briselli and associates, four were in the head and neck, with the scalp involved in two patients and the tongue and eyelid/orbit involved in one patient each.[91] Roggli and associates reported on 16 patients with pulmonary involvement. Five of these patients had some head and neck area involved, with the tongue involved in all five; one patient also had an orbital lesion, and in two patients the larynx was involved.[96] About an equal number of patients with and without visceral lesions have been reported.[85]

Unlike the desmoid fibromatoses, the spindle-shaped mesenchymal cells of these lesions have an immature appearance. Plump oval cells with an abundant eosinophilic cytoplasm may also be found.[14, 71, 75, 85, 94] Depending on location, the cells are arranged in bands, fascicles, or ball-like clusters, the latter being common in pulmonary lesions.[85, 91] The cells may assume a smooth muscle appearance.[71, 76, 85, 91, 92] These fibromatoses are quite vascular and in areas may histologically simulate a hemangiopericytoma, especially in the more central portions of the nodules.[14, 91, 92, 94] Collagen may be abundant.[85] The occurrence of hyaline-like or chondroid areas is claimed to be a helpful histologic clue to the diagnosis.[91] Mitoses are quite common, and the central portions of the lesion may contain polyhedral cells having slightly pleomorphic nuclei.[85] The central regions may also have bland calcified necrosis, such necrosis being unique among the fibromatoses.[71, 91]

Most infants with visceral involvement die shortly after birth, although survival for as long as 4 months has been reported.[71, 85] Chung and Enzinger, however, had one patient who had visceral lesions and was alive and well at 5 years.[92] Patients with pulmonary lesions have an especially grim prognosis.[96] In a review by Rosenberg and associates, two of four patients without lung involvement survived, but only two of 11 with pulmonary lesions survived. In contrast, only one of 16 patients without visceral lesions died, and that single patient had a cervical lesion that expanded into the spinal canal.[85] Most of the nonvisceral solitary or multiple lesions, including the bone lesions, eventually undergo spontaneous regression.[85, 91]

Fibromatosis Colli (Sternocleidomastoid Tumor)

Fibromatosis colli is the most common of the juvenile fibromatoses. In the series of fibromatoses from the Texas Children's Hospital, 20 of the 76 patients with fibromatoses in infancy or childhood had a sternocleidomastoid tumor.[85] This lesion is unique among the fibromatoses not only in its selectivity for a specific muscle but also for its lack of extension beyond the muscle. Because of this, some do not include it among the fibromatoses but consider it separately as some form of fibrous proliferation.[14, 54]

Clinically, this lesion may produce a torticollis ("wryneck"). There are several types of torticollis including congenital and acquired varieties. These types vary from simple postural torticollis to those caused by neurologic, anatomic, traumatic, infectious, or neoplastic conditions. Fibromatosis colli is only one such cause. All too often in the literature torticollis is equated with fibromatosis colli when it is only the clinical result of that condition, and even here, not all examples of fibromatosis colli result in a torticollis. Hulbert reported the incidence of a sternocleidomastoid tumor in congenital torticollis as from 14 to 23 per cent.[105]

Clinically, fibromatosis colli is rarely found at birth but usually develops within the following several weeks.[100, 101, 103, 105, 107, 109, 110] The mean time reported by Coventry and Harris in their 35 patients was 3.5 weeks, similar to the 3.0 weeks reported by Macdonald in his series of 50 patients.[102, 109]

The lesion develops as an "olive-shaped" or oval tumor mass in the lower third of the sternocleidomastoid muscle within either the sternal or clavicular heads, frequently both.[75, 110] In 52 patients with muscular torticollis reported by Macdonald, eight were mainly in the sternal head, 19 were in the clavicular head, and both heads of the muscle were involved in 25 patients.[109] The mastoid insertion rarely is involved.[85, 103] Boys are more frequently involved than girls,[100, 105, 107, 109] although in some reports there is no particular sex dominance.[85, 101, 102] There is a high incidence of difficult labor and breech presentation in this condition (40 to 50 per cent), although whether trauma secondary to difficult delivery is involved in the pathogenesis of the lesion is unknown.[101, 102, 105, 109] Cases are reported of fibromatosis colli in children delivered by caesarean section.[101, 109] Although multiple possible explanations for the histogenesis of sternocleidomastoid tumor have been proposed, an acceptable explanation is still not available.[105, 108] Coventry and Harris reported the condition in 30 of 7835 (0.4 per cent) infants born in Rochester, Minnesota.[102]

The sternocleidomastoid lesion may be so inconspicuous that it is overlooked by the child's parents and is discovered only during a well-baby examination.[102] The tumor slowly increases in size over 2 to 3 months and then gradually regresses to disappear, in most cases, in 4 to 6 months.[85, 102, 104, 106] It is usually movable, may be somewhat tender, and may be associated with a torticollis. In the series of 46 cases reported by Kiesewetter and associates 17 had a sternocleidomastoid tumor without associated torticollis, 15 had tumor with torticollis, and 14 had torticollis without a gross tumor.[107] In 12 of 50 babies with sternocleidomastoid tumor, Macdonald found a transient torticollis that subsided with disappearance of the tumor.[109] Enzinger and Weiss state that only one fourth to one third of patients develop a torticollis initially, and that it is usually mild and transient.[14] If torticollis is present, the head is tilted toward the side of the involved muscle, which in most cases is on the right side. Rarely, the condition is bilateral. As the tumor grows, asymmetry of the face and head may develop.[100, 102, 105] Japanese workers noted a 14 per cent incidence of ipsilateral congenital dislocation of the hip in patients with muscular torticollis.[106]

In about 20 per cent of cases, the sternocleidomastoid tumor does not regress, producing a gradually increasing torticollis that requires operation.[105] In patients in whom there is spontaneous regression, a torticollis may subsequently develop several years later.[85, 103, 105] Although this torticollis is not associated with a sternocleidomastoid tumor mass, most believe that such cases probably are the result of a previously overlooked sternocleidomastoid tumor that had regressed and, over the course of time, progressive fibrous replacement of the muscle produces a torticollis when the child begins to grow rapidly.[102, 103–105] Fitzsimmons, who believes that torticollis in an older child is the end stage of a previous sternocleidomastoid tumor, reported that in 36 cases, 25 had a known history of such a lesion shortly after birth, followed in 5 to 6 years by the onset of torticollis.[103] In 41 patients with sufficient information to evaluate, Macdonald found subsequent torticollis developed in seven (17 per cent) during an average follow-up period of 6 years. However, in one third the follow-up had been 1 year or less.[109]

Older children who develop torticollis due to fibromatosis colli are usually in the first decade of life, with occasional patients being adolescents, although about one third of Macdonald's older children began to develop their torticollis in the first year of life.[105, 109] Ten of 52 patients in this latter series (19 per cent) had a history of proven or probable sternocleidomastoid tumor at birth.

In children who require operation, either as infants or later, the tumor consists of a firm, spindle-shaped, 0.5- to 3.0-cm mass that has a glistening, white, tendon-like appearance within the belly of the muscle.[85, 101, 103, 107, 110] Microscopically, there is replacement of the muscle fibers, which are in various stages of degeneration, by immature-appearing cellular fibrous tissue (Fig. 53–3A).[85, 101, 103, 107] Mitoses are rare.[85] Hemosiderin pigment, although noted by Kiesewetter and associates in 25 per cent of cases,[107] is never prominent and has been noted to be absent by other authors.[85, 101, 103] This is a point against the thesis that the lesion results from trauma and hemorrhage into the muscle during birth. In older children, the fibrous tissue is usually replaced by a mature-appearing noncellular collagenous scar-like tissue in which are scattered remnants of muscle fibers (Fig. 53–3B).[85, 108, 110] The muscle fibers in the older lesions are claimed to lack degenerative changes.[110]

The fibrosis is focal or diffuse within the muscle, but it does not extend beyond the confines of the muscle.[85] The process resembles a desmoid tumor,[100] although some have noted qualitative differences with that lesion.[14, 54, 107]

The proper treatment for sternocleidomastoid tumor has been debated in the literature between those who advocate early surgical intervention in infants and those who advise conservative stretching exercises for the lesion.[100, 101, 104, 105] Because over 80 per cent of the tumors that develop in infants will spontaneously regress, operative management is usually not required.[102, 105] Surgical intervention may be reserved for those with persistent and deforming torticollis or for children who develop progressive torticollis at an older age.[109]

PSEUDOSARCOMAS

Because of their cellularity, content of atypical cells, and high mitotic activity, a group of benign reactive fibrous lesions exist that may be misdiagnosed as sarcomas by the inexperienced pathologist. These "pseudosarcomas" include nodular fasciitis, proliferative fasciitis, and proliferative myositis. Only nodular fasciitis, however, occurs with any significant frequency in the head and neck region.

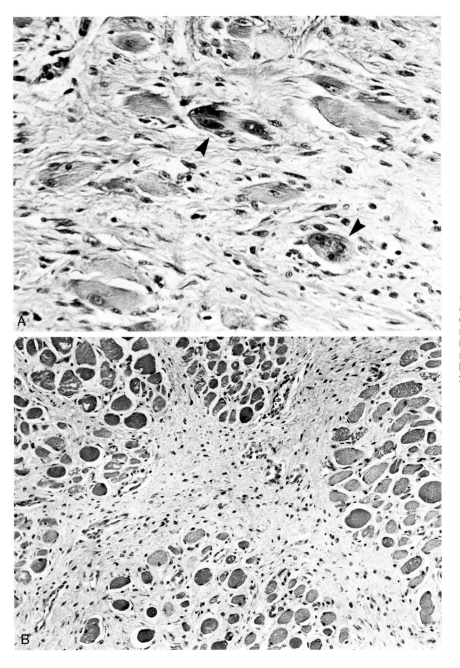

Figure 53–3. Fibromatosis colli. (A) Muscle fibers entrapped by proliferating fibrous tissue. Degenerating muscle fibers are present (arrowheads). (B) Mature lesion of fibromatosis colli. Muscle is divided into lobules by dense fibrous tissue. Some muscle fibers are atrophic.

As pathologists have become familiar with these entities, their misdiagnosis has become less frequent. However, we still receive consultation cases in which radical surgery is contemplated for what proves to be one of these reactive lesions. The problem is illustrated by the fact that in one large national cancer registry, slightly over 10 per cent of the lesions histologically classified as sarcomas were, upon review, reclassified as benign, and in this latter group approximately 60 per cent of the cases consisted of one of these pseudosarcomatous fibrous lesions.[9]

Nodular Fasciitis

Nodular fasciitis has had a variety of names applied to it, from the original, "subcutaneous pseudosarcomatous fibromatosis,"[121] to "infiltrative fasciitis," "pseudosarcomatous fasciitis," and "proliferative fasciitis."[11, 14, 124] Because the latter term has also recently been used to designate another type of pseudosarcoma, we prefer the appellation "nodular fasciitis" for the lesion discussed here.

Nodular fasciitis is the most frequent of the pseudosarcomatous fibrous lesions. Although it occurs in patients from newborns to those over 80 years of age, most are adults in the third and fourth decades of life, with mean or median ages between 38 to 44 years.[115, 116, 118, 120, 124, 128] In 843 cases at the AFIP, just over one half occurred in patients between 20 and 40 years of age,[111] and in the review by Kleinstiver and Rodriquez of 314 reported cases, 43 per cent occurred in this age range.[120] Eighty-five per cent of the 114 patients reported by Bernstein and Lattes were younger than 50 years of age.[112] Male patients are more commonly affected than female patients, although the difference is not great. Meister and coworkers reported 100 cases of nodular fasciitis and reviewed seven other series. Of the 537 patients in whom the sex was reported, 53 per cent were males.[124]

Although first described as a subcutaneous lesion, nodular fasciitis may involve any portion of the body, including the deep soft tissues and visceral organs, being reported in such locations as the parotid gland, breast, esophagus, trachea, vagina, and the labia.[111, 128] However, approximately one half of the cases are found in the upper extremities, the forearm being the single most common site.[9, 111, 112, 116, 118, 120, 124, 128] The head and neck region accounts for approximately 10 to 20 per cent of cases. In the review by Meister and associates, 191 of 1269 cases (15.1 per cent) were in the head and neck region, with the range in reported series from 0 to 19.4 per cent.[124] In Allen's review of 829 cases at the AFIP, 163 (20 per cent) were in the head and neck, with 51 located in the neck, 49 in the face, 21 in the forehead, 13 in the scalp, 13 in the orbit, nine in the conjunctiva, five in the eyelid, and two in the buccal mucosa.[111] Such intraoral lesions are extremely rare, Lumerman and associates having reported the first such case in the English literature in 1972.[123] In 45 cases reported by Kleinstiver and Rodriquez, six were in the head and neck, four in the jaw and cheek, and one each in the neck and occiput.[120] Twenty of 134 cases reported by Bernstein and Lattes were in the head and neck, with ten in the face, three in the parotid, four in the neck, and three in the occiput.[112] Hutter and associates found three cases in the neck and one in the submental region in their total of 66 cases at Memorial Hospital, New York.[118] In children, it is claimed that the head and neck region is the most commonly involved site, accounting for about half of the cases.[14, 116] However, in Stout's series of 123 cases of fasciitis, 15 were in children less than 16 years old and no case arose in the head or neck.[129]

The recently described "cranial fasciitis" involves the deep layers of the scalp and the underlying bone and develops in children from 3 months to 6 years of age (median 18 months).[122] Small to medium-sized arteries and veins have also been the sites of origin of nodular fasciitis. Five of 17 such cases were in the head and neck region, with the face involved in three and the neck and scalp in one case each.[126]

Nodular fasciitis usually manifests itself as a rapidly growing, occasionally painful or tender nodule present for less than 1 month in over half the patients.[111, 116, 124] Although some slowly growing lesions are occasionally encountered, it is uncommon for symptoms to be present for more than a year.[111, 118, 124, 127] The vast majority of lesions arise from the superficial fascia from which they grow into the subcutaneous tissue as round to oval, well-circumscribed nodules, although at times they may grossly appear to be poorly delimited and infiltrative. Occasional examples grow primarily along the fascia, whereas others extend into the underlying muscle.[14, 116, 124] They are usually small, rarely exceeding 5.0 cm; most are between 1.0 and 3.0 cm in maximum dimension.[111, 124]

Histologically, nodular fasciitis has a wide range of morphologic patterns, one report listing 11 different histologic varieties.[111] Most lesions, however, have a mixture of these patterns and all share certain features. These consist of spindle-shaped fibroblast-like cells that are arranged in long fascicles that are described as curved, whorled, or S-shaped (Fig. 53–4A). A storiform pattern may also be present.[25, 112] The fascicles are loosely arranged, being separated by a myxoid stroma that gives the lesion a characteristic edematous or "feathery" appearance.[14, 111, 113, 116] Cells with prominent nucleoli and a more oval to round shape may also be present (Fig. 53–4B). Although cellular atypia does occur, and a rather high mitotic rate is common, bizarre pleomorphic cells are not found and the mitotic figures are not atypical.[25, 111, 113, 116] A frequent finding is the presence of extravasated red blood cells that either diffusely insinuate themselves between the stromal cells or are arranged in clusters within microscopic spaces that contain a hyaluronidase-sensitive acid mucopolysaccharide.[25, 111, 116, 124] Despite its name, inflammatory cells, mainly lymphocytes, are never numerous. Multinucleated giant cells may be found.[112] Nodular fasciitis is quite vascular, frequently with capillaries arranged in a fan-like or radial array at the periphery of the nodules.[111] Electron microscopy has demonstrated that these spindle cells are myofibroblasts.[129]

Depending on the cellularity and the amount of myxoid stroma, nodular fasciitis may simulate fibrous histiocytoma, a desmoid fibromatosis, or fibrosarcoma.[25, 112, 127] Bernstein and Lattes emphasize four histologic features that distinguish nodular fasciitis from malignant tumors of soft tissue. The nuclei in nodular fasciitis are never hyperchromatic; the lesion is typically

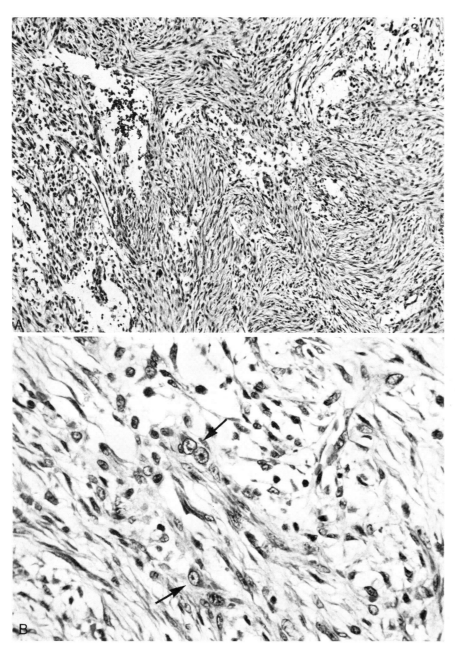

Figure 53–4. Nodular fasciitis. (*A*) Fibroblasts (myofibroblasts) are shown arranged in a whorled pattern. Microcystic spaces are present with extravasated red blood cells. These spaces also contain hyaluronic acid. At this magnification there is little, if any, cellular atypia seen. (*B*) Scattered atypical nuclei are seen (arrows), some with nucleoli. The background stroma is loose and edematous.

subcutaneous without extension into the skin; plasma cells are uncommon; and the mitotic index rarely exceeds one mitotic figure per high-power field.[112]

Local excision, even at times incomplete excision, is curative in almost all cases. Recurrences are reported in less than 5 per cent of cases.[111, 124] In 134 patients reported by Bernstein and Lattes, 18 had recurrences, 15 of which recurred within 2 years of therapy. However, upon review of the original lesions in these cases, none were confirmed as being nodular fasciitis. Eleven of the 18 were reclassified as some form of malignancy, the most frequent being malignant fibrous histiocytoma, especially the inflammatory variant. The authors were of the opinion that recurrence of a true nodular fasciitis is an exceedingly rare event.[112]

Proliferative Myositis and Proliferative Fasciitis

Because their histologic features frequently overlap, these two benign lesions are discussed together. They are both closely related in a histologic sense to nodular fasciitis and may be considered as variants of that lesion.[125] Indeed, areas with the histomorphologic appearance of nodular fasciitis may also be found within these two lesions.[115] The term proliferative fasciitis was previously used as a synonym for nodular fasciitis but should now be restricted to the lesion described here.[114] Both proliferative myositis and proliferative fasciitis occur less often than nodular fasciitis.

Although nodular fasciitis frequently occurs in young adults and children, neither proliferative fasciitis nor proliferative myositis has been reported in children.[114, 115, 117] The average age of patients with these lesions is older than that for patients with nodular fasciitis, being between 50 and 60 years.[114, 115, 117] As with nodular fasciitis, both have a rapid clinical onset, evolving over a period of a few weeks.[114, 115, 117] Pain and tenderness may occur, especially in proliferative fasciitis.[114, 117]

Proliferative myositis is located within muscles, usually those of the upper arm and shoulder.[115, 117] The lesion varies from 1.0 to 6.0 cm and appears as poorly demarcated scar-like tissue within the muscle.[117] The head and neck is an uncommon site, with only four of the 33 cases (12.1 per cent) reported from the AFIP located in this area. Three of these were within the sternocleidomastoid muscle, and the fourth case was within the neck. The three intramuscular lesions varied from 2.0 to 3.0 cm, and the neck lesion was 6.0 cm.[117]

Proliferative fasciitis is also only rarely found in the head and neck, with the extremities, especially the forearm and thigh, being the most common sites of origin.[114] One of the 53 cases reported from the AFIP involved the head,[114] and the face was involved in one of the eight cases reported by Kitano and associates.[119] Grossly, the lesion is situated between the muscle and the subcutaneous tissue. It proliferates along the superficial fascia, in an infiltrative fashion, as well as along fibrous septa that extend into the subcutaneous tissue. Mixed forms exist where muscle, fascia, and subcutaneous tissue are all involved.[114, 115]

Histologically, these lesions show a proliferation of spindle-shaped cells as seen in nodular fasciitis. The distinguishing feature, which separates these lesions from conventional nodular fasciitis, is the presence of large cells with abundant basophilic cytoplasm and one to two prominent nucleoli, giving them the appearance of ganglion cells (Fig. 53–5).[114, 115, 117] Nissl substance, however, is absent. These cells may also be confused with rhabdomyoblasts, but their lack of striations and their basophilic, rather than eosinophilic, cytoplasm

serves to separate them. A myxoid background, as in nodular fasciitis, is also present. As with nodular fasciitis, cartilaginous and osseous tissue may be present.[112, 115] In the series by Kitano and associates, their eight patients were culled from 159 cases that had previously been diagnosed as nodular fasciitis.[119]

Despite their histologic appearance and infiltrative character, these lesions are self-limited with no tendency to recur following local excision.

NEUROGENOUS TUMORS

The term "schwannoma" has been used as the appellation for the two commonest benign tumors of peripheral nerves—neurilemoma and neurofibroma. Although the Schwann cell is thought by most authors to be the cell of origin for both these tumors,[130, 134, 155, 176] they are sufficiently distinctive both clinically and pathologically that they are usually easily separable. In our hands, the term "schwannoma" is used only as a synonym for neurilemoma. The tumors of the sympathetic nervous system—neuroblastoma, ganglioneuroblastoma, and ganglioneuroma—are not described in this chapter.

Because neurilemoma and neurofibroma are thought to have Schwann cells as their major cellular component, they are considered to be derived from the neuroectoderm. Some authors, however, believe that the mesodermally derived perineural fibroblasts are the cells principally involved in the formation of these tumors or at least that these fibroblasts share equally with Schwann cells in their formation.[130, 134, 162, 163] In either case, the tumor cells are believed to have the capacity to form a variety of tissues including bone, cartilage, fat, muscle, collagen, and even glands.[130, 180] Such a diversity of tissues is seen most commonly in the malignant neurogenous tumors.

Neurilemoma and neurofibroma should not be con-

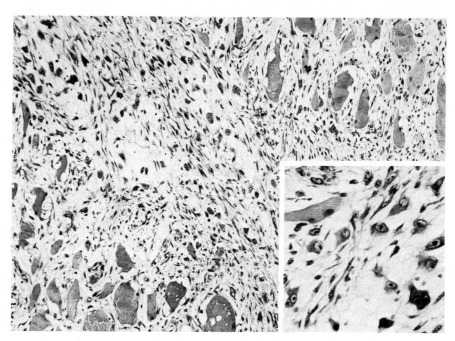

Figure 53–5. Proliferative myositis. Muscle fibers are separated by a pale myxoid stroma in which stellate cells are present. Inset shows that some of these stellate cells are multinucleated, and some have prominent nucleoli.

fused with the "traumatic" neuroma that develops following some form of tissue injury.[130, 155] These firm, rubbery, tender or painful masses result from an exaggeration of the normal repair process and are not true tumors. They are composed of a tangle of regenerating axons interwoven with Schwann cells in a fibrous stroma. They rarely produce symptoms until they assume sufficient size to be clinically evident.

The head and neck region is the most common location for both neurilemoma and neurofibroma. In Das Gupta's combined Memorial Hospital and University of Illinois series, 151 of 359 (42 per cent) "solitary benign schwannomas" arose in the head and neck, with the remainder in the extremities, trunk, and mediastinum.[10] Unfortunately, Das Gupta did not separate neurilemoma from neurofibroma in this series, using "schwannoma" to designate both lesions.

Neurilemoma

Neurilemomas develop from the neural sheath of peripheral motor, sensory, sympathetic and cranial nerves, the exceptions being the optic and olfactory cranial nerves that lack Schwann cell sheaths.[138, 139, 153, 155] In reports that distinguish neurilemoma from neurofibroma, approximately 25 to 45 per cent of the neurilemomas occur in the head and neck region.[138, 144, 153, 167, 178] In the series by Gore and coworkers from Presbyterian Hospital, New York, 251 of 389 neurilemomas (65 per cent) arose in the "central nervous system," with 228 of these in the acoustic nerve. Of the 138 neurilemomas outside the central nervous system area, 52 (37.6 per cent) were in the head and neck region.[153] Neurogenous tumors of the head and neck are, however, not common. Oberman and Sullenger report the incidence at two large medical centers, the University of Michigan and the Mayo Clinic, as only two to four cases per year.[165]

Daly and Roesler divided these tumors into medial and lateral groups.[145] The lateral tumors arise from the cervical nerve trunks, and the cervical and brachial plexus; the medial tumors arise from the last four cranial nerves and the cervical sympathetic chain. These latter tumors frequently manifest clinically as "parapharyngeal" tumors.[145] However, any nerve, small or large, may be involved.

The lateral cervical region of the neck is the commonest location.[54, 146, 159, 165] At the Mayo Clinic, 80 of 148 head and neck neurilemomas (54.1 per cent) arose in this region.[159] The exact nerve of origin, however, may be impossible to determine, as in only 22 of these 80 neurilemomas was a specific nerve recognized. Of the 22 tumors, seven arose in the sympathetic chain, seven from cervical nerves, five from the vagus nerve, one from the hypoglossal nerve, and two from the brachial plexus. In 90 neurogenous tumors of the head and neck, which included 76 neurilemomas and 14 malignant neural tumors, reported by Conley and Janecka, only one half the tumors could be localized to a specific nerve trunk, and the others arose in the soft tissues of the head and neck.[139] In the neck, the vagus nerve and the nerves of the cervical and brachial plexus are the ones most commonly affected when the nerve can be recognized.[153, 158, 159, 178] In the paper by Conley and Janecka, there were 45 tumors within the neck, with 11 arising

in the cervical plexus, eight in the vagus nerve, six in the brachial plexus, and two in the sympathetic chain.[139] In 25 head and neck neurilemomas reported by Whitaker and Droulias, the nerve was specified in 16, with four each in the brachial plexus and vagus nerve, two each in the cervical plexus, cervical sympathetic chain, and hypoglossal nerve, and one each in the facial and great occipital nerves.[178] In the head, the facial nerve was the site in 15 of the 41 neurilemomas in the series by Conley and Janecka.[139] In a separate study these authors reported their experience with 23 neurilemomas (two malignant) of the facial nerve in 17 patients.[140] Almost every anatomic site in the head and neck has been involved by neurilemoma, including the soft tissues of the face, especially the preauricular region, the forehead, orbit, scalp, lip, maxilla, mandible, floor of mouth, tongue, paranasal sinus, nasal fossa, nasopharynx, and larynx.[10, 139, 147, 159, 165, 166] In the Mayo Clinic series, there were 12 intraoral lesions, five in the tongue, four in the floor of the mouth, two in the cheek, and one in the mandible; there were 13 facial tumors, with 10 in the preauricular area and one each in the chin, upper lip, and bridge of the nose; there were 16 parapharyngeal tumors, five nasal fossa tumors, eight forehead/scalp tumors, seven orbital tumors, three middle ear/mastoid tumors, and two laryngeal tumors.[159] Tumors that arise from the cervical nerve trunks may extend through the spinal foramen into the spinal cord,[145, 159] and the parapharyngeal lesions may present as bulging tonsillar or retrotonsillar masses.[159]

Patients are usually in the third to fourth decades of life,[130, 134, 139, 144, 147, 153, 158, 159] but no age group is exempt, from infants to patients over 80 years of age. Women are affected more often than men in ratios of 2:1 to 3:2,[134, 147, 159, 167] although in the series by Conley and Janecka there was no significant sex difference.[139]

Most patients complain of a painless mass without neurologic symptoms.[54] The tumors may produce pressure symptoms as they enlarge, especially those within the confined anatomic regions of the head and neck.[134, 138, 139, 147, 153] Vocal cord dysfunction, hoarseness, cough, breathing difficulty, and rarely a Horner's syndrome may be produced because of the specific anatomic region affected by the tumor.[145, 153] In the 90 patients reported by Conley and Janecka, only eight had pain, while in Das Gupta's series only 12 of 303 patients complained of pain radiating along the course of the nerve.[139, 147] The tumor may be present for several years before the patient seeks medical attention. In Kragh's series of 77 patients with cervical neurilemoma, 22 had a mass for over 5 years, one patient for over 30 years.[159] A correct preoperative diagnosis of neurilemoma is rarely made.[139, 178]

Neurilemomas, in contrast to neurofibromas, are usually sharply circumscribed and encapsulated tumors with an oval, round, or fusiform shape.[130, 134, 155] When in a large nerve trunk, they may be pedunculated or even bulbous. In the soft tissues, a nerve may not be recognizable. The tumors are usually small—most are less than 5.0 cm—but lesions up to 10.0 cm have occurred in the head and neck region.[138, 139, 144, 147, 159] Important in the management of these tumors is the fact that for neurilemomas that arise in a major nerve trunk, the surgeon may be able to dissect the tumor free without impairing the nerve. Nerve fibers are not part of the tumor, which arises from the nerve sheath and pushes the nerve axons aside. The tumors are tangray to white and frequently have a watery or slimy consistency. Cystic degeneration and hemorrhage are not uncommon.[134, 155] Multiple neurilemomas may occur, and such patients are frequently found to have associated multiple neurofibromas.[155, 157] Bilateral acoustic nerve neurilemomas are also found in such patients.

The typical neurilemoma has a biphasic histologic pattern composed of compact cellular regions, the Antoni A areas, mixed with loosely arranged hypocellular regions, the Antoni B areas (Fig. 53–6).[130, 134, 155] The relative proportions of these regions varies from tumor to tumor, and tumors are found in which one of these regions may form the entire lesion. Most neurilemomas, however, will contain Antoni A and Antoni B foci in some areas. The Antoni A regions are composed of bipolar spindle-shaped Schwann cells that have oval to elongate nuclei and fibrillar eosinophilic cytoplasm that may fuse to form hyaline masses. These cells characteristically are aligned into interweaving fascicles or are so arranged that their nuclei are juxtaposed into rows, creating the classic palasading pattern of this tumor. However, a similar palasading pattern may be found in other lesions, such as smooth muscle tumors, and although highly suggestive of a neurogenous lesion, it is not in itself diagnostic. The Schwann cells may also

group themselves to create organoid structures, the Verocay bodies that are similar in appearance to tactile corpusules (Fig. 53–7). Mitotic figures are either absent or rare.

The cells within the Antoni B regions are separated by a watery matrix that stains poorly, if at all, with stains for acid mucopolysaccharide in contrast to the strong positive reaction that is given by the stroma of neurofibromas. Microcystic areas are also present in these hypocellular regions, along with lymphocytes and macrophages.

Neurilemomas are quite vascular, accounting for the large hemorrhagic foci noted in some. Large blood vessels with densely hyalinized walls are quite common and are characteristic of neurilemomas. Neurites are not present within the substance of the tumor. Occasional neurilemomas are found in which the cells are hyperchromatic and take on bizarre nuclear configurations. These have been termed "ancient" neurilemomas, with the cell changes reflecting degeneration.[131, 143] Cellular atypia in neurogenous tumors is not evidence of malignancy. An unsettled issue is the relationship between the Schwann cells and the perineural fibroblasts in the formation of these tumors, with some authors believing that these are actual functional variants of the same cell.[163]

Neurilemomas stain strongly with antibodies to S-100

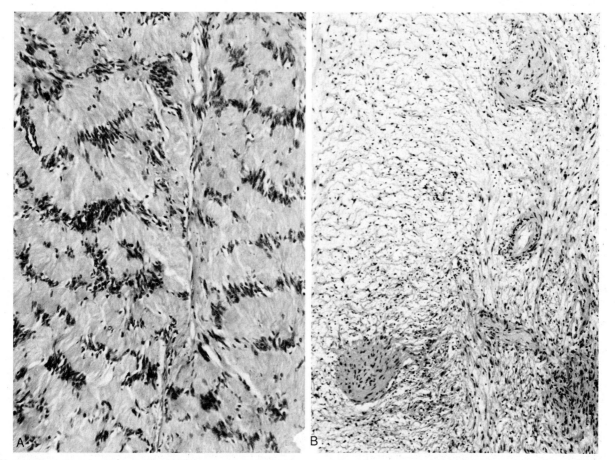

Figure 53–6. Neurilemoma. (A) Antoni A region with alignment of tumor cell nuclei in palisading pattern. (B) Mixture of cellular Antoni A areas with loose, edematous Antoni B region that is best seen in the upper left of the figure.

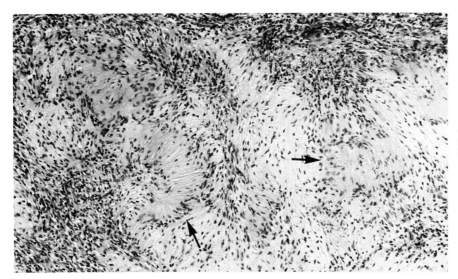

Figure 53–7. Neurilemoma. Antoni A region with Verocay bodies (arrows).

protein. This stain may be used to distinguish the more cellular neurilemomas from smooth muscle tumors, with which they may be confused, but which are negative for S-100 protein.[171, 177]

Following simple local excision, neurilemomas rarely recur.[130, 134, 159, 165] In Conley's 76 patients, only two developed a recurrence.[139] Neurilemomas do not undergo malignant degeneration.

Woodruff and coworkers have recently described two varieties of neurilemoma that they designated as "cellular schwannoma" and "plexiform (multinodular) schwannoma."[181, 182] Of their 14 cellular schwannomas, two occurred in the neck, one in the face, and one in the supraclavicular area. The lesions were characterized by predominantly compact cells arranged in a whorled pattern without the formation of Verocay bodies or palisades; a moderate degree of mitotic activity and nuclear atypia; and in some, the presence of perivascular neural whorls. Cellular schwannoma has been confused with other tumor types and has been misdiagnosed as malignant in some cases. To date, it has had a benign course.[181]

The plexiform schwannoma was described in a single case, its distinction being its resemblance to plexiform neurofibroma and the possibility of confusing it with a malignant neurogenic tumor because of its high mitotic activity.[182]

Neurofibroma

Neurofibromas tend to occur earlier than do neurilemomas, usually in patients from 20 to 40 years of age,[14] with an approximately equal sex incidence. Neurofibromas are also somewhat more common, but this probably reflects the inclusion within reports of patients with multiple neurofibromatosis (von Recklinghausen's disease). Solitary neurofibromas that are limited to the head and neck area are rare.[138, 153] Among 13 neurogenous tumors of the face and neck reported by Katz and associates, 11 were neurilemomas and two were neurofibromas.[158] In the report by Oberman and Sullenger, there were 16 neurofibromas and 15 neurilemomas in the head and neck region,[165] and Perzin and associates found six neurofibromas and two neurilemomas in their

study of neurogenous tumors of the nasal cavity, nasopharynx, and paranasal sinuses.[166]

In the skin, neurofibromas are usually solitary but elsewhere they tend to be multiple and part of the von Recklinghausen's disease complex. Of 328 patients with von Recklinghausen's disease seen at the Mayo Clinic, 47 had neurofibromas removed from the head and neck. During the same time, only 21 patients without von Recklinghausen's disease had a solitary neurofibroma removed from this area.[160] Nine of the 16 neurofibromas of the head and neck described by Oberman and Sullenger were associated with von Recklinghausen's disease; the mean age in this group was 15 years, seven patients being less than age 10 years, reflecting the generally young age of patients with multiple neurofibromatosis.[165]

Neurofibromas generally arise in the subcutaneous tissue as small 2.0- to 4.0-cm nodules. In the skin they may produce protuberant, sagging, disfiguring masses.[160] Within the head and neck region, they are more frequently seen in the head area, unlike neurilemomas, for which the lateral cervical area is the most common site.[165] In patients with multiple neurofibromatosis, the neurofibromas that occur in the head and neck are most commonly located in the orbital region and midlateral aspect of the neck.[149] As with neurilemomas, neurofibromas also take origin from a variety of locations in the head and neck, including the nasopharynx, paranasal sinuses, hypopharynx, larynx, tongue, floor of mouth, vagus nerve, salivary gland, and buccal area.[158, 165, 166] In the tongue, which is a common site, macroglossia may result from infiltration by the neurofibroma.[54, 165] Neurofibromas have also developed in areas that received radiation therapy.[130]

When located in the superficial soft tissues, neurofibromas are usually ill-defined and unencapsulated, but when located within the deeper soft tissues or arising in a major nerve, they are better circumscribed and appear encapsulated.[130, 134, 155, 165] In large nerve trunks they may also form irregular fusiform swellings, creating a tangled "worm-like" mass. The finding of such a plexiform neurofibroma is tantamount to a diagnosis of von Recklinghausen's disease.[155]

On gross examination, neurofibromas tend to be

softer than neurilemomas and, on cut surface, have a gray-white glistening appearance. The tumor feels slimy, and may be quite gelatinous. This gelatinous quality may be so exaggerated as to suggest the diagnosis of myxoma.[132, 155] When found associated with a large nerve, the nerve is seen to course through the tumor and is such an integral part of it that it cannot be dissected free of the tumor.[134]

Histologically, neurofibroma contains a mixture of cells, which vary from spindle-shaped to stellate, and whose nuclei tend to be elongated and at times wavy or twisted.[130, 132, 134, 135] Scattered lymphocytes and mast cells are also present, the mast cells being far more common than in neurilemomas. Short collagen fibers are present and are arranged in bundles or nodular arrays (Fig. 53–8). Unlike neurilemomas, neurites are present within the substance of the tumor, although without special stains, they may be difficult to see. The tumor matrix is loose and appears edematous, with the cells being widely separated within it. This matrix stains strongly for acid mucopolysaccharide, unlike the weak or negative reaction given by the matrix of neurilemomas.[132, 155] Plexiform neurofibromas may contain large areas of normal nerve lying within the mucoid matrix and between the spindle-shaped tumor cells. The biphasic pattern of Antoni A and Antoni B areas is usually absent, as is the conspicuous vascularity of neurilemoma. However, some neurofibromas contain areas that resemble neurilemoma to such a degree that a clear distinction between the two tumors is not always possible.[132, 155]

Mitoses are scarce in the usual neurofibroma. Indeed, the presence of more than an occasional mitotic figure in several high-power fields should suggest the possibility of malignancy. Focal cellular pleomorphism, which may occur in these tumors, is not an indication of malignancy when it is unassociated with mitotic activity.[132, 155] Neurofibromas, like neurilemomas, also stain positively for S-100 protein, although the intensity of the reaction and the number of cells that stain is not as great as in neurilemomas.[171, 177] Rare and unusual neurofibromas have been described with a variety of different histologic patterns and content, which are described in detail elsewhere.[14, 155, 168]

Solitary neurofibroma, like solitary neurilemoma, has a low incidence of recurrence following local excision.[147, 155] Among 13 head and neck neurofibromas with follow-up information reported on by Oberman and Sullenger, three patients had a local recurrence and one tumor caused death from respiratory obstruction caused by invasion of the hypopharynx into the superior mediastinum.[165] Malignant development in a solitary neurofibroma is not common; however, patients with multiple neurofibromatosis do have a significant risk of developing malignant neurogenous tumors. This is discussed in the next section.

Neurosarcoma ("Malignant Schwannoma")

Malignant tumors of peripheral nerve are most commonly designated as malignant schwannomas. This is somewhat confusing in that "schwannoma" is used as a synonym for neurilemoma, a tumor that virtually never becomes malignant. Furthermore, some of these malignant neurogenous tumors histologically resemble fibrosarcoma, for which the term "neurofibrosarcoma" has been used.[172] However, because many of the malignant tumors that arise in peripheral nerves tend to be undifferentiated or pleomorphic tumors with little to suggest either Schwann cell differentiation or fibrosarcoma, we prefer the term neurosarcoma to designate those peripheral nerve tumors that have a sarcomatous pattern.

A soft-tissue tumor that microscopically has a spindle-cell or pleomorphic pattern, and which does not conveniently fit into one of the well-established sarcoma categories is, unfortunately, far too often diagnosed by the pathologist as neurogenous. We restrict the diagnosis of neurosarcoma to tumors that either clearly arise within a nerve, contain histologic areas of neurofibroma, or develop in a patient with von Recklinghausen's disease. When such criteria are used, neurosarcoma is

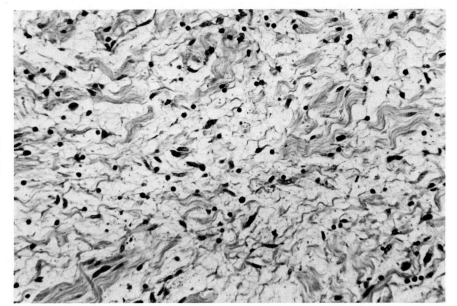

Figure 53–8. Neurofibroma. Loosely arranged Schwann cells are seen within a myxoid stroma. Short, thick, wavy collagen bundles are present.

not common, making up no more than 5 to 10 per cent of all sarcomas.[59, 63] They are far less frequent than benign peripheral nerve tumors, making up only about 2 to 12 per cent of neural sheath tumors.[152, 174] In the series from the Massachusetts General Hospital, there were 607 patients with neurilemomas or neurofibroma seen from 1962 to 1979. During the same time there were only 24 patients with neurosarcoma.[174] At the Mayo Clinic, from 1910 to 1957, there were 148 cases of neurilemoma of the head and neck, but only four malignant neurogenous tumors were reported during the same time.[159] Rosenfeld and associates reported seven malignant neurogenous tumors in the lateral neck, while at the same time there were 17 neurilemomas and four neurofibromas.[169] Among the 90 neural tumors in the series by Conley and Janecka,[139] 14 were malignant, and among 40 neurogenous head and neck tumors seen by Oberman and Sullenger, three were malignant.[165]

Neurosarcomas arise in patients with and without von Recklinghausen's disease.[141, 142] In large series, neurosarcomas that are found in patients without associated von Recklinghausen's disease are somewhat more common, although this is dependent on the criteria used to establish the clinical diagnosis of von Recklinghausen's disease. Patients with this disease have a higher risk of developing a malignant neurogenous tumor than do patients in the general population. The magnitude of this risk, however, is not well established because long-term prospective studies of patients with von Recklinghausen's disease have not been reported. Furthermore, many patients with only minor degrees of the disease complex may never come to medical attention. In those reports in which incidence figures are given, the percentage of patients with von Recklinghausen's disease who develop a malignant neurogenous tumor has ranged from 5 to 30 per cent.[142, 148] In the series reported by Das Gupta and Brasfield, 19 per cent of patients born with multiple neurofibromatosis developed a malignant tumor by age 40, and 53 per cent (8 of 15) of those who developed evidence of neurofibromatosis between the ages of 16 to 25 subsequently developed a malignant neural tumor within 5 to 8 years.[148] Malignant degeneration in a solitary neurofibroma is rare.

Malignant neural tumors found in association with von Recklinghausen's disease develop in patients 20 to 50 years of age (mean age approximately 30 years), but patients who develop spontaneous neurosarcomas are about 10 to 15 years older.[141, 142, 152, 170, 175] Women are somewhat more commonly affected than men, although in the large series by Das Gupta and Brasfield, 56 per cent of the patients were men.[141, 142, 146, 152, 170, 175] Sordillo and associates reported an equal sex incidence in patients without von Recklinghausen's disease and a slight female preponderance in those with the disease.[170] Women have been more commonly affected in those few reports that mention neurosarcomas in the head and neck, but the number of patients in these reports is not large.[141, 142, 159, 165]

The most common clinical complaint in patients with neurosarcoma is the presence of a swelling or mass that is painful in about one half of the cases.[141, 142, 154, 175] Paresthesia, muscle atrophy, and weakness may be present, depending on whether or not a major nerve trunk is involved.[141, 142, 154] Patients with von Reckling-

hausen's disease may indicate that the lesion had been present for many years prior to its sudden enlargement.[142] Rapid growth in a known neurofibroma or the spontaneous development of a rapidly growing soft-tissue mass, associated with pain, in a patient with von Recklinghausen's disease is highly suggestive of malignancy.

Most neurosarcomas develop in the extremities or the trunk.[25, 142, 152, 154, 175] Despite being a frequent site for benign neurogenous tumors, the head and neck region is not a common location for these malignant tumors, accounting for only 6 to 17 per cent of all cases.[10, 25, 141, 142, 146, 152, 154, 175] In most series, less than 10 per cent of neurosarcomas are in this area. The tumors that develop in patients with von Recklinghausen's disease tend to be centrally located in the trunk, pelvic, and shoulder regions, with fewer tumors in the extremities or head and neck.[154, 170]

Neurosarcomas of the head and neck are found in a variety of locations, including the brachial plexus, vagus and other cranial nerves, lateral and posterior neck, cheek, pharynx, larynx, supraclavicular area, maxilla, mandible, upper lip, parotid region, nose, parapharyngeal area, paranasal sinuses, and nasopharynx.[54, 137, 139, 146, 159, 165, 166] Of 14 head and neck malignant neurogenous tumors studied by Conley and Janecka, 13 were in the head and one was in the neck,[139] but in 18 cases reported by Das Gupta and Brasfield, the neck was involved in 17.[146]

When a major nerve is affected, the tumor frequently forms a fusiform or nodular swelling that diffusely infiltrates the nerve.[25, 141, 142, 154, 175] It also extends into the surrounding soft tissue and contains areas of hemorrhage and necrosis. Few neurosarcomas are small[146, 152, 154]; over one third were greater than 10.0 cm and 30 per cent were between 5.0 and 10.0 cm in the series reported by Ghosh and associates.[152] In patients with von Recklinghausen's disease the tumors have arisen not only in major nerve trunks but in areas from which neurofibromas had been previously removed; from areas adjacent to major nerves; and in areas where a major nerve could not be identified.[142]

Many neurosarcomas have fields composed of spindle cells that are arranged in interlacing fascicles with a herringbone pattern as in fibrosarcoma.[141, 154, 155, 175] Nuclei show various degrees of pleomorphism and hyperchromasia and are either round or elongated. The stroma is fibrotic or myxomatous. Mitoses are frequent, usually one or more per high-power field (Figs. 53–9 and 53–10). Foci of hemorrhage and necrosis are also common.[25, 152, 154, 155, 175] On a purely histologic basis, these "neurofibrosarcomas" are indistinguishable from the usual soft-tissue fibrosarcoma. Undifferentiated pleomorphic sarcomas may also arise within peripheral nerves. These contain bizarre giant cells and polygonal mononuclear cells with hyperchromatic nuclei.[142, 152, 170] Pleomorphic tumors are noted by some to develop more frequently in patients with von Recklinghausen's disease, but others report them to be more common in patients without von Recklinghausen's disease.[142, 152, 170] Neurosarcomas have developed in areas that have received radiation therapy, and these are usually of the pleomorphic type.[170]

Metaplastic elements such as malignant osteoid and cartilage, as well as areas of liposarcoma and rhabdo-

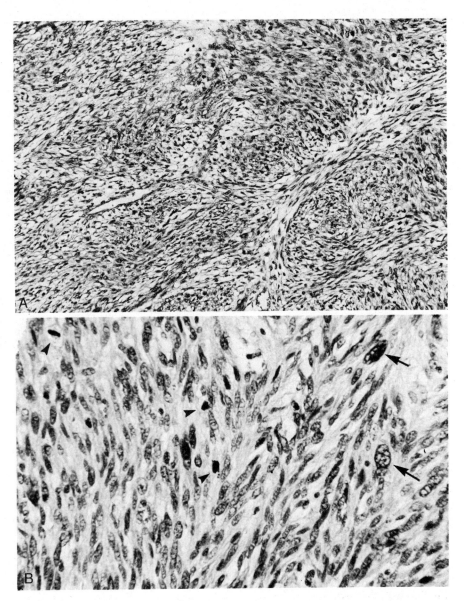

Figure 53–9. Neurosarcoma. (*A*) Fascicles and nodules of spindle-shaped tumor cells with a loose-textured stroma. (*B*) Spindle cells similar to those of fibrosarcoma. Some larger, rounded, and more pleomorphic tumor cells are seen (arrows). Several mitotic figures are present (arrowheads).

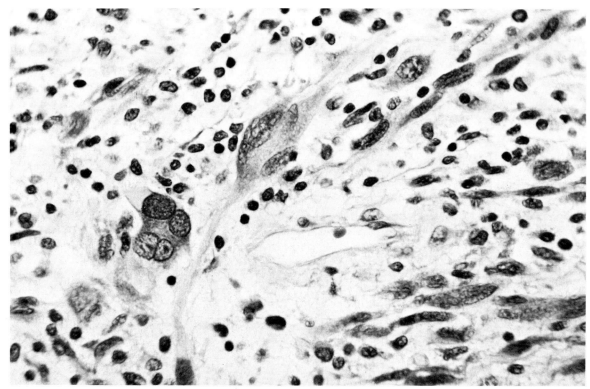

Figure 53–10. Neurosarcoma. Large pleomorphic tumor cells are present. Such atypical cells may occasionally be found within benign neural tumors.

myosarcoma may also occur in neurosarcomas.[142, 152, 154, 155] Tumors with rhabdomyosarcomatous differentiation have been termed malignant "triton" tumors.[136, 180] In the three cases described by Woodruff and associates, two were located in the neck, one in the vagus nerve and the other in the brachial plexus. Two of seven previously reported cases reviewed by these authors were also located in the neck.[180] In a recent review of 23 cases, Brooks and associates found that the most common single location was the neck, which was involved in six cases.[136] Benign peripheral nerve tumors with striated muscle also occur, and these have been variously called neuromuscular hamartoma, benign triton tumor, or neuromuscular choristoma.[135, 164] One of the two patients reported by Bonneau and Brochu had the lesion in the supraclavicular fossa. In their review of the literature, they found six cases, three of which arose in the brachial plexus and, with the exception of one patient, age 14 years, all the tumors were in children under 2 years of age.[135]

A "glandular" schwannoma has also been reported by Woodruff.[179] These tumors consist of benign-appearing glands within a spindle cell stroma. This stroma appeared malignant in four of the five cases reported. Two of the tumors were in the neck. Krumerman and Stingle also reported such a tumor in the neck of an 8-year-old girl with congenital neurofibromatosis. This was also malignant.[161]

Although stains for S-100 protein are positive in almost all benign neural tumors, the malignant tumors are less commonly positive. Approximately half of these tumors will be positive for S-100 protein, but the inten-sity of the reaction is not great, and usually only a few tumor cells are stained.[171, 177] Because of the poorly differentiated nature of many of these tumors, electron microscopy has not been very successful in differentiating them from other soft-tissue spindle cell tumors,[171, 177] although some tumors with the light microscopic features of malignant fibrous histiocytoma have been successfully diagnosed as malignant neural tumors by electron microscopy.[156]

Neurosarcomas are highly malignant lesions with recurrences following local excision in from 50 to 80 per cent of patients.[141, 142, 152, 170, 175] Patients with von Recklinghausen's disease who develop neurosarcoma have a poor prognosis, with 5-year survival rates of 15 to 30 per cent, in contrast to patients without von Recklinghausen's for which the 5-year survival rates have been from 50 to 75 per cent.[133, 141, 142, 152, 154, 170] Recurrences and metastases from these tumors may occur as late as 5 and 10 years after therapy.[152, 154] Local recurrence of neurosarcoma in patients with von Recklinghausen's disease is indicative of a grave prognosis, with almost all such patients dying of their disease.[170] Small tumors, less than 5.0 cm, have a better prognosis than larger lesions.[150] There is no apparent correlation of survival with the grade of the tumor or the mitotic rate. Malignant "triton" tumors and glandular schwannomas have a poor prognosis, and radiation-induced neurosarcomas are almost always fatal.[136, 170, 179, 180] In Conley and Janecka's series of 14 patients with head and neck malignant neural tumors, 12 died within 3 years, and the other two patients were alive and free of disease at 1 year and 4 years after therapy.[139] In D'Agostino's seven patients with head and neck neural malignancies, four died, one had a local recurrence, and the other two patients were alive at 43 months and 16 years after therapy.[141, 142] Two of the four patients mentioned by Kragh and associates died at 1 year and 3 years, with the other two patients alive after 1 and 3 years.[159] Two of the three patients reported by Oberman and Sullenger died of tumor, but the other patient was alive at 5 years.[165] Patients with head and neck neurosarcomas are said to have a poorer prognosis than those with extremity tumors.[150]

PARAGANGLIOMAS

Paraganglionic tissue of the head and neck embryologically derives from the neural crest, develops in the paravertebral region in association with the arterial vessels and cranial nerves of the ontogenetic gill arches, and is associated with the autonomic nervous system.[188, 203] Cells of the paraganglia are capable of producing and storing vasoactive and neurotransmitter substances, such as the catecholamines norepinephrine and epinephrine, as well as a variety of hormones, including serotonin, gastrin, and somatostatin, that are found in peripheral nerves. The catecholamines are stored in neurosecretory granules that may be seen by electron microscopy. Catecholamines can be oxidized by solutions of chromic acid to form brown polymers. This "chromaffin" reaction has long been used to identify catecholamine-containing tissue, most notably that of the adrenal medulla and its tumor, the pheochromocytoma. However, the chromaffin reaction is a relatively insensitive method for the identification of catecholamines and is usually positive only in the presence of large quantities of these substances.[188, 189] Tumors of extra-adrenal paraganglionic tissue usually do not give a positive chromaffin reaction and therefore were termed, "nonchromaffin paragangliomas."[189, 203] It is now well established, by the use of more sensitive methods such as formaldehyde-induced fluorescence, that extra-adrenal paraganglionic tumors do contain catecholamines and the term "nonchromaffin" should no longer be used as a prefix for these tumors.[188, 189, 203]

The term "glomus tumor," frequently used in the past as an appellation for tumors of the paraganglionic system, is to be avoided. True glomus tumors are mainly located in the skin and superficial soft tissues of the extremities and have no relationship to the tumors of the paraganglia.[54, 189, 214]

Through the work of Glenner and Grimley, a practical classification of the paraganglionic system has been established to clarify an area previously noted for its diverse terminology. This classification is based on location, and it divides the paraganglia into branchiomeric, intravagal, aortico-sympathetic and visceral-autonomic groups.[188] The branchiomeric group, some tumors of which directly concern the otolaryngologist, includes the jugulotympanic, intercarotid, orbital, subclavian, laryngeal, coronary, corticopulmonary and pulmonary paraganglia. Although not associated with arterial vessels in the same manner as these branchiomeric paraglanglia, tumors of the intravagal paraganglia are usually included with this group for the sake of discussion.

Several locations in the head and neck have been the sites for paragangliomas, including the nose,[190, 194, 197] nasopharynx,[206] orbit,[194, 213] and larynx[194, 212, 216]; however, in this section we deal only with the tumors of the carotid body and intravagal paraganglia. The clinically important jugulotympanic tumors are more correctly discussed as part of the tumors of the inner ear.

Carotid Body Paraganglioma (Carotid Body Tumor)

The normal carotid body is found at the bifurcation of the common carotid artery as an adherent, 5.0-mm to 6.0-mm pink mass on the adventitia of the medial side of the vessel.[188, 203, 207] It is supplied by blood vessels of the external carotid artery and has a sensory nerve supply via the glossopharyngeal nerve.[203, 207] The carotid body monitors and responds to changes in blood oxygen, carbon dioxide, and pH levels,[189, 207] and tumors of this organ have previously been termed "chemodectomas." The function of the other paraganglia, such as the intravagal or jugulotympanic, has, however, not been defined, and because no chemoreceptor function is known for these, chemodectoma is not an accurate general designation for tumors of this system.[189]

The normal carotid body is composed of epithelial cells, the chief cells, which originate from the neural crest.[188, 189, 203, 207] These cells are arranged in clusters forming the so-called "Zellballen." They have a finely granular eosinophilic cytoplasm, and the cell nests are surrounded by thin, richly vascular fibrous septa, which are best demonstrated by reticulin stains. Between the chief cells are the Schwann-like sustentacular cells that are difficult to identify by light microscopy but are found by electron microscopy.[189] The function of these sustentacular cells is not yet established, but they are intimately associated with the chief cells. The chief cells contain the argyrophilic neurosecretory granules that contain the catecholamines.[188]

Carotid body tumors, namely, carotid body paragangliomas, are the most common tumors of the head and neck paraganglia, composing between 60 and 67 per cent of the total.[14, 191, 194] Despite over 600 cases having been reported,[186] it should be remembered that these are still rare lesions. Lack and associates found only 69 paragangliomas of the head and neck in over 600,000 operations (0.12 per cent) at Memorial Hospital, New York, and only one in 13,400 autopsies.[194] Crowell and associates found an incidence, over an 8-year period, of only one paraganglioma in the head and neck for every 6000 adult surgical specimens.[184] They are thought to be more common in patients who live at high altitudes.[188, 205] They occur at all ages, from children to patients in the ninth decade of life, but the mean patient age is between 45 and 50 years.[187, 194-196, 198, 201, 207] Sex ratios have varied. Sixty-two of 90 patients (69 per cent) reported by Shamblin and associates were male,[207] whereas in the study by Parry and associates of 222 patients from 10 institutions, 146 (66 per cent) were females.[201] This female dominance has also been found in other series,[187, 199] whereas others have found an almost equal sex incidence.[194-196] Enzinger and Weiss[14] claim that the male-to-female incidence is about equal, except for a higher female incidence in patients living at high altitudes.

Carotid body paragangliomas manifest themselves as slowly growing, painless neck masses located beneath the anterior edge of the sternocleidomastoid muscle just lateral to the tip of the hyoid bone.[191, 194, 195, 199, 201, 203, 207] They may expand upward into the neck or, occasionally, bulge into the pharynx.[54, 203] Owing to compression of adjacent cranial or sympathetic nerves, hoarseness, vocal cord paralysis, and dysphagia are noted.[188, 194, 195, 203, 207] Patients have usually noted their lesion for a long time, with an average of from 2 to 8 years, some for as long as 47 years.[187, 194, 198, 201, 207] Occasionally, however, symptoms may be present for only a few weeks.[187, 194]

Between 2 and 10 per cent of patients have bilateral tumors, either initially or subsequently.[196, 201, 204, 207] Parry and associates state that such patients are younger than those with unilateral tumors.[201] Carotid body paragangliomas are rarely functional[184, 186, 191, 194, 203] but may occur along with paragangliomas of the jugulotympanic or intravagal paraganglia, or with pheochromocytoma.[186, 196, 202, 204] They have also been noted in association with medullary carcinomas of the thyroid and in patients

with neurofibromatosis.[188] Occasional cases occur in families and appear to be transmitted as an autosomal dominant trait. Up to one third of familial tumors are bilateral.[201, 204]

On physical examination, the carotid body tumor may be movable from side to side, but not in a vertical direction, and may transmit the arterial pulse.[191, 195, 203] The diagnosis may almost always be established preoperatively by selective angiography, which shows a vascular mass at the carotid artery bifurcation.[186, 195, 199] We do not believe that preoperative biopsy of such a mass has any place in the management of these lesions.[54, 191, 186, 199]

Grossly, the tumors vary from 2.0 to 9.0 cm, with most being about 4.0 cm.[187, 194–196, 198, 203, 207] They are well circumscribed and appear encapsulated. They are firm, reddish gray to brown, and quite vascular. Shamblin and associates divided them into three groups depending upon the size of the tumor and its relationship to

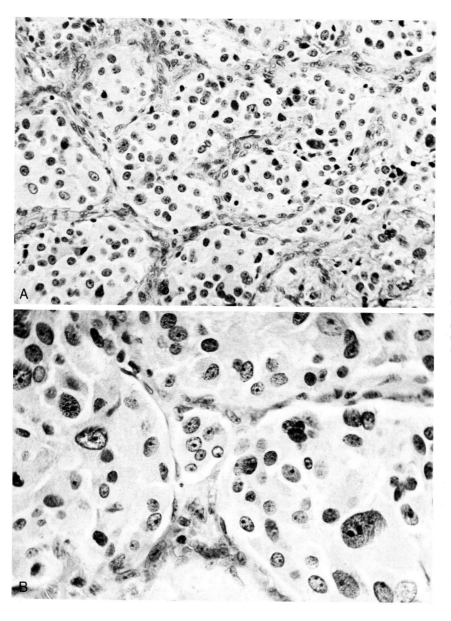

Figure 53–11. Paraganglioma of carotid body. (*A*) Tumor cells (chief cells) are arranged in ball-like configurations. (*B*) Tumor cells have abundant cytoplasm. Nuclei show a moderate degree of atypia. This is not a reliable criteria of malignancy.

the carotid artery.[207] In group I are small tumors that were only loosely adherent to the adventitia of the artery and which could be easily removed. Group II tumors are somewhat larger and more densely adherent to the artery and even infiltrate the vessel wall. These required sharp adventitial dissection for their removal. In group III are very large tumors that encircle or encompass the artery to such an extent that a portion of the vessel must be resected for complete removal of the tumor. Group II tumors were the most common, accounting for 45 per cent of the cases, although the group I and II tumors were about equal in incidence in this study.[207] Lees and associates, in a series of 41 patients, classified 18 of the tumors as group II, 15 as group III, and 8 as group I.[195] Any surgeon treating carotid body tumors must be prepared not only for extensive bleeding, due to this tumor's great vascularity, but also to perform vascular surgery if necessary.

Histologically, carotid body paragangliomas closely replicate the morphology of the normal carotid body (Figs. 53–11 and 53–12).[188, 203, 207] The nests of chief cells tend to be somewhat larger than normal,[193, 203] and areas may be found where the cells are spindle-shaped ("sarcomatoid" foci) (Fig. 53–12A); other areas are so highly vascular that they are suggestive of an angioma or hemangiopericytoma.[193, 203, 207] Most tumor cells have a bland appearance, but it is not uncommon to find scattered large pleomorphic cells with hyperchromatic nuclei (Fig. 53–11A).[193, 203, 207] Mitotic activity is not com-

mon and is usually absent. The tumor cells have an abundant clear to finely granular eosinophilic cytoplasm, and the cell nests are set off by reticulin fibers (Fig. 53–12B).[14, 188, 198] The lesion is highly vascular.[188, 198, 203] Occasionally, the cells are arranged in short ribbons or cords that are divided and compressed by extensive fibrous bands.[14, 193] A capsule may not be present, and infiltration of the tumor cells into the adventitia of the adjacent artery is seen.[198] By electron microscopy, the tumor cells can be seen to contain neurosecretory granules[184, 188, 189, 193, 196, 205] and at the light microscope level are found to be argyrophilic but argentaffin-negative by silver staining.[14, 194, 205] Some electron microscopic studies have also shown the presence of sustentacular cells, but in most such studies these cells have been lacking.[14, 184, 189, 193, 205] This supports the general view that these carotid body lesions are true tumors rather than hyperplasias, in which more than one cell type would be expected.[205]

In an immunohistochemical study of 11 head and neck paragangliomas, nine of which were carotid body tumors, Warren and associates found that all stained intensely for neuron-specific enolase and some contained a variety of hormones such as serotonin, leuenkephalin, substance P, vasoactive intestinal peptide, gastrin, somatostatin, vasopressin, melanocyte-stimulating hormone (MSH), and calcitonin.[215]

The histologic differential diagnosis includes metastatic medullary carcinoma, hemangiopericytoma, angiosarcoma, melanoma, and epidemoid carcinoma.[193, 198]

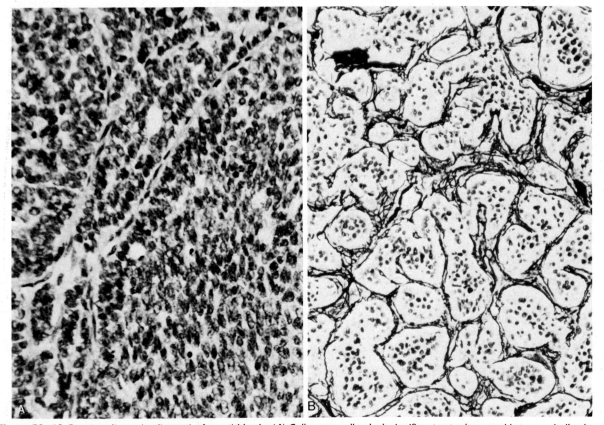

Figure 53–12. Paraganglioma (malignant) of carotid body. (*A*) Cells are smaller, lack significant cytoplasm and have a spindle shape, creating a "sarcomatoid" appearance. Such areas have also been found in benign paragangliomas. (*B*) Reticulin stain shows that the nests of tumor cells are surrounded by reticulin fibers in which capillaries course.

In a series reported by Oberman and coworkers, 18 tumors previously diagnosed as "chemodectoma" were reclassified upon review as melanoma, squamous cell carcinoma, thyroid and salivary gland tumors, malignant lymphoma, and metastatic adenocarcinoma.[198] In addition, biopsy material in 11 of their 40 head and neck paragangliomas, including carotid body tumor, was initially misdiagnosed as some other tumor type.[198]

Surgical therapy is the essential method of treatment for carotid body tumors. If the tumor is completely removed, recurrences are rare and occur in about 10 per cent of cases.[194, 207] None of 49 completely resected tumors reported by Shamblin and associates recurred,[207] and only four of 39 patients reported by Lack and associates had a recurrence.[194] Local recurrence may take place in any partially excised benign tumor, and such an occurrence is not in itself an indication of malignancy.[198, 203] Even partially resected tumors may take a long time to recur as evidenced by a patient who developed a local recurrence 17 years after partial excision.[198] Oberman and associates reported three patients who remained well for 7 to 17 years after only partial resection of their tumors.[198] The operative mortality rate has decreased over the years with improved techniques for grafting and bypass procedures. The rate of occurrence of cerebrovascular accidents following operation has been dramatically reduced by these techniques.[199, 207] The operative mortality rate is now less than 2 per cent.[54] Further problems may also develop owing to the necessity to sacrifice branches of the vagus and glossopharyngeal nerves in some of the larger tumors.[186, 194, 195, 199, 207] Radiation therapy should not be used as a primary mode of treatment, as most have reported these tumors to be radioresistant.[207] One patient treated with radiation therapy died 26 years later of unrelated causes and at autopsy still had residual tumor in the neck.[194] Radiation therapy may be useful as a palliative method for those rare paragangliomas uncontrolled by surgical means.

The incidence of carotid body tumors that are malignant has varied in the literature from 1.5 to 50 per cent.[187, 194, 196, 198, 199, 201, 205, 207] Such a wide discrepancy in incidence is caused by the variable criteria that are used to determine malignancy in these tumors. The higher figures were based on the histologic presence of pleomorphic cells and local invasion, criteria that have proved unreliable in predicting malignant behavior. The only reliable criteria for establishing the malignancy of a paraganglioma is the actual presence of either local lymph node involvement, distant metastases, or extensive local invasion as into the brain stem. When these more stringent guidelines are used, less than 10 per cent of paragangliomas are reported as malignant and most likely the true rate is less than 5 per cent.[196, 199, 201, 207] The evolution of metastatic disease, however, may be quite slow, with metastases developing from 3 to 16 years after diagnosis, with some patients developing metastases 35 years after the original therapy.[188, 195, 201, 203] In the review by Shamblin and associates of approximately 500 reported carotid body tumors, 16 patients had local metastases, and another 16 had distant metastases, with the lung and bone being the most common sites of involvement.[207] In the series of 222 patients with carotid body paragangliomas reported by Parry and associates, there were nine with metastatic disease, four with regional lymph node involvement, four with bone metastases, and one with pulmonary metastases during intervals of from 6.1 to 8.2 years.[201]

Intravagal Paraganglioma

Intravagal paragangliomas arise from nests of paraganglionic tissue located within or adjacent to the vagus nerve, most commonly at the level of the ganglion nodosum, which may itself be replaced by tumor.[54, 183, 185, 188] However, intravagal paragangliomas may be located at any point along the cervical path of the vagus nerve.[188]

Women are more commonly affected than men, and patient ages parallel those for carotid body lesions, with the mean age being approximately 50 years, with a range of 18 to 71 years.[54, 188, 194, 198] The tumors usually manifest themselves as a painless neck mass located behind the angle of the mandible, and they not infrequently bulge into the pharynx and produce dysphagia.[14, 188, 198, 200, 208, 210] Tumor compression of the ninth and twelfth cranial nerves may produce neurologic symptoms such as weakness of the tongue, vocal cord paralysis, hoarseness, or even Horner's syndrome.[14, 191, 194, 200, 210, 211] Angiography shows a vascular mass situated above the carotid bifurcation, and such a finding is virtually diagnostic of this tumor.[194, 200]

As with carotid body tumors, the duration of symptoms is usually long, about 4 years.[194, 200, 210] In the series of 13 patients reported by Lack and associates, the duration of symptoms ranged from 3 months to 14 years.[194] Only one functional intravagal paraganglioma has been reported.[183]

Intravagal paragangliomas are less common than either carotid body or jugulotympanic paragangliomas, with less than 100 cases reported in the literature. A review by Chaudhry and associates in 1979 yielded only 72 previously reported cases.[183] Intravagal paragangliomas have been found in association with other head and neck paragangliomas.[183, 192, 209] Although familial examples have been reported, these are much rarer than familial cases of carotid body tumors. Kahn reported only the second such case in 1976,[192] and Chaudhry and associates found only four such cases in 1979.[183]

Grossly, intravagal paragangliomas appear well circumscribed, but they may extend upward into the base of the skull and range in size from 2.0 to 6.0 cm.[194, 198] Histologically, intravagal paragangliomas differ only slightly from carotid body paragangliomas, with perhaps more abundant fibrous septa that compress the chief cells.[188, 208] Nerve fibers and ganglion cells may be seen owing to the tumor's close association with the vagus nerve and the ganglion nodosum.[188] Only a few of these tumors have been examined by electron microscopy, with sustentacular cells seen in some studies and not in others.[183, 192]

As with carotid body tumors, surgical excision is the treatment of choice for intravagal paraganglioma. In Lack's series of 13 cases, surgery was done in 12, with follow-up available in 11 cases. Of these, eight patients were alive and well for an average of 7 years (range 6 months to 16 years). Two patients were alive with residual tumor, 2 and 15 years later, and one patient died of unrelated causes 14 years after therapy.[194]

Malignant vagal paragangliomas are reported to be

more frequent than malignant carotid body tumors.[183, 185, 192, 193, 208] In the review by Chaudhry, 13 of the 72 intravagal paragangliomas (18 per cent) had metastasized, only four of these to distant sites, whereas the remainder involved only the regional lymph nodes.[183]

SYNOVIAL SARCOMA

Synovial sarcoma accounts for approximately 3 to 10 per cent of all sarcomas.[20, 48, 59, 218, 232] It is a tumor that predominantly affects young adults, two thirds of the patients being under age 40 years, most in their thirties.[47, 218, 219, 224] Male patients are affected more commonly than females in ratios of 2:1 to 3:2.[47, 218, 219, 233, 234]

Despite its name, synovial sarcoma rarely arises directly from synovial membranes, with only about 10 per cent of the tumors actually involving joint spaces.[41, 47, 238] More commonly, the tumor is found in the vicinity of large joints and bursae, with 75 to 95 per cent of cases located in the extremities, the lower extremity being affected in 40 to 70 per cent of cases. The most common sites of origin are about the hip joint, knee, ankle, shoulder, and wrist.[14, 25, 47, 218, 219]

The tumor has also been found in areas anatomically devoid of synovioblastic tissue such as the abdominal wall, pelvis, and the head and neck region.[218, 237, 238] Location in the latter site is uncommon. The first such case was reported by Jernstrom in 1954, with the tumor located in the left hypopharynx.[231] Since that time there have been several individual case reports but few series that contain an appreciable number of patients. Many of the larger reported series of synovial sarcomas have either no cases in the head or neck region or only a few examples. In 1965 Cadman and associates reported 134 synovial sarcomas from the Mayo Clinic, only one of which was in the head and neck.[218] Cameron and Kostuik had no head and neck cases among 39 synovial sarcomas at the Toronto General Hospital,[219] and Evans had none among 40 patients seen at the M.D. Anderson Hospital.[224] Krall and associates reported one synovial sarcoma, of the neck, in a series of 26 such tumors.[232] In a 1982 report updating the Mayo Clinic experience with synovial sarcoma, five of 185 cases (2.7 per cent) were in the head and neck.[242]

In a 1961 review, Harrison and associates found only four previously reported head and neck cases and added one of their own.[229] In 1967, Batsakis and associates added three more cases, for a total of only eight cases in the literature at that time.[217] In 1974, Jacobs and Weaver found 10 cases in the literature and added one of their own.[230] Roth and associates reported 24 patients on file at the AFIP with synovial sarcoma of the neck.[238] A review by Lockey, in 1976, discovered 19 previously reported head and neck synovial sarcomas, and he added two further cases.[233] These did not include the cases reported by Roth and associates. In a more recent publication from the AFIP, Enzinger and Weiss had 31 cases in the head and neck region in a total of 345 synovial sarcomas (9 per cent) from all sites.[14] This higher percentage of cases in the head and neck region may reflect the referral pattern of unusual cases that are sent to the AFIP in consultation.[14] A recent report on orofacial synovial sarcoma, from the same institution, included 11 such cases from over 600 synovial sarcomas on file, and an additional 11 cases in the literature.[240]

Patients with synovial sarcomas of the head and neck have a mean age of approximately 25 years, with an age range of from 7 to 63 years.[230, 233, 238, 240] This appears to be somewhat lower than the ages for patients with synovial sarcomas at other sites. Lockey found that the average age of 411 patients with synovial sarcomas of the trunk and extremities was 37.9 years versus 24.8 years in 21 patients with head and neck sites.[233] In the series by Roth and associates, one half of the 24 patients were less than 20 years of age, with a median of 19 years.[238] As with synovial sarcomas at other sites, men are more frequently affected than women in approximately the same ratios.[233, 238, 240]

In the head and neck, the tumors may be located high in the superior aspect of the neck just beneath the mandible,[217, 229] in the prevertebral area from the base of the skull to the hypopharynx, in the retropharyngeal and parapharyngeal areas, and in the anterior neck along the borders of the sternocleidomastoid muscle, as well as in orofacial and laryngeal sites.[217, 229, 237, 238, 240] In the 24 cases reported from the AFIP, ten were in the hypopharynx, three in the anterior or posterior hyoid region, three were retropharyngeal, six were in the neck, and one each in the mastoid and supraclavicular areas.[238] Lockey listed 21 cases, with six in the cervical region (one posterior); four in the hypopharynx; two each in the tongue, submandibular region, and the clavicular area; and one case each in the temporomandibular joint, retromolar, temporal, and cheek areas.[233] Synovial sarcomas taking origin from the orofacial region included six in the cheek; five in the tongue (four in the base, one dorsal); two each in the parotid and tonsillar areas; and one each in the buccal, infraorbital, submental, temporal, palate, retromolar, and temporomandibular joint areas.[240] In the 31 head and neck synovial sarcomas mentioned by Enzinger and Weiss, 26 had a specific location mentioned—12 in the neck, seven in the pharynx, and seven in the larynx.[14]

In the extremities, synovial sarcoma, unlike most sarcomas, not infrequently causes pain, which is either localized or referred. In about 25 per cent of cases this pain may not be associated with any recognizable mass, in another 25 per cent of cases a painless mass is present, and in the remaining patients a painful mass is present.[219] Patients with head and neck synovial sarcomas usually come to medical attention because of a painless mass; only about 20 per cent of the patients complain of pain.[229, 233, 238] However, occasionally dysphagia, dyspnea, or hoarseness may be the initial complaints owing to the pressure effects of the tumor on the hypopharynx and larynx.[229, 230, 238, 240] Unlike patients with synovial sarcomas located elsewhere, whose symptoms may be present for several years,[47, 218] most patients with head and neck lesions seek medical attention within a year of onset of their symptoms.[233, 238] Lockey reported the average duration of symptoms in patients with head and neck synovial sarcomas as 6.3 months versus 26.3 months in patients with trunk and extremity involvement.[233]

Synovial sarcomas of the head and neck vary in size from 2.0 cm to 10 cm with an average size of about 5.0 cm.[233, 238] Those in the neck are somewhat larger than those in the orofacial region, where the mean size is 3.8 cm.[240] They are usually firm to rubbery well-circumscribed, spherical or micronodular tumors with a pseudocapsule. Cystic and hemorrhagic foci may be present.[14, 238] Tumor calcification is noted radiologically in 30 to 40 per cent of synovial sarcomas in the extremities.[47, 257, 258] This may be so extensive as to justify the appellation of "calcifying synovial sarcoma."[241] However, none of the 32 patients recently reported under this designation had tumors in the head and neck.[241]

Synovial sarcomas are histologically characterized by the presence of a "biphasic" pattern consisting of a background stroma, composed of tightly compacted fibroblast-like spindle cells, in which is scattered pale epithelial-like cells arranged in glandular formations, compact nests, or cleft-like spaces (Fig. 53–13).[25, 47, 234] The spindle cell areas resemble those of fibrosarcoma, although it is claimed by some that these cells are plumper and have more rounded nuclei than the usual fibroblasts of fibrosarcoma.[218, 226, 234] Mast cells may be quite numerous in this tumor.[224, 238] Hyalinized scar-like areas may be quite prominent, and microcalcification is found in from 30 to 60 per cent of cases.[218, 238] Such calcification was found in two of 11 orofacial lesions reported by Shmookler and associates[240] and in 14 of the 24 cases of the neck analyzed by Roth and coworkers.[238] Synovial sarcomas may be quite vascular and at times histologically mimic a hemangiopericytoma, the tumor with which they are most easily confused.[25, 223, 224, 228]

The epithelial-like cells may be cuboidal or tall and columnar in shape and form papillary projections into the cleft-like spaces. The glandular formations may be so well differentiated that they simulate the glands of metastatic adenocarcinoma.[225] The epithelioid cells are set off from the surrounding stromal spindle cells by a basement membrane. Pleomorphism of either cell type is not a feature of these tumors.[218] Special stains show reticulin fibers in the spindle cell areas but not in the epithelial clusters.[25] The gland-like spaces and clefts contain a mucin-like material that stains with periodic acid–Schiff (PAS), mucicarmine, and alcian blue stains and is resistant to hyaluronidase digestion.[224, 228, 238] The spindle cells also elaborate a stromal mucin, the staining of which is eliminated by prior treatment with hyaluronidase.[238] The relative proportion of spindle cells to epithelial cells varies from case to case and even within the same lesion.[234] The fibrosarcomatous areas are preponderant in most lesions, and many sections may have to be examined before the epithelial-like cells are found. Reticulin stains are quite useful in such tumors, as they may help to distinguish more easily the epithelial cells from the spindle cells. It is therefore easy to understand that a small biopsy of such a lesion could miss the epithelial-like foci and the tumor interpreted as a fibrosarcoma.

Some pathologists insist that there exists a "monophasic" form of synovial sarcoma, which consists entirely of either spindle cells or epithelial-like cells, and that the classic biphasic pattern is present in only a minority of cases.[224, 228, 232] It is our view, however, that for a diagnosis of synovial sarcoma a biphasic pattern

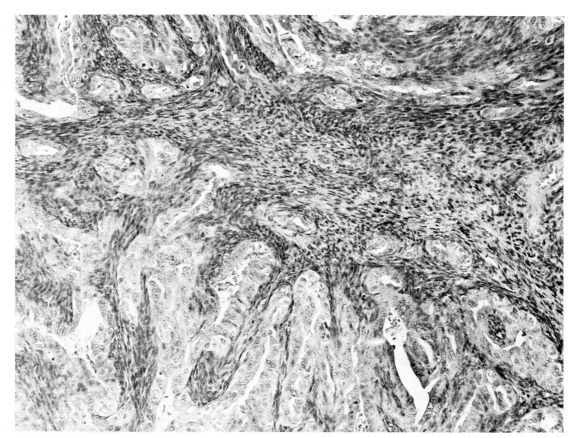

Figure 53–13. Synovial sarcoma. Biphasic pattern is present, consisting of pale glandular areas, composed of cuboidal to columnar cells, within a spindle cell stroma.

must be recognized somewhere in the tumor.[25, 47, 226, 234, 239] This problem may yield to newer diagnostic methods. Immunohistologic techniques for the demonstration of cytokeratin have recently been used to study synovial sarcoma. Miettinen and associates found staining of the epithelial cells in four cases of biphasic synovial sarcoma but found no reaction in the spindle cells.[236] Corson and coworkers, however, found that both cell types stained for cytokeratin in all eight of their biphasic tumors and in 11 of 16 monophasic spindle cell lesions. In total, 19 of their 24 tumors gave positive reactions, although the number of spindle cells that stained positively was small.[220, 221] Significantly, the cells of normal synovium failed to stain for cytokeratin.[220, 236] These immunohistologic methods may therefore prove helpful in dealing with tumors that the pathologist, on the basis of the clinical, radiologic, and microscopic pattern, believes are synovial sarcomas that lack the classic biphasic pattern. The histologic appearance of head and neck synovial sarcomas does not differ from those arising in other sites, with most having the usual biphasic pattern.

Electron microscopic studies have yielded conflicting interpretations as to whether or not the spindle cells are true fibroblasts.[227, 232, 235, 243] However, there is general agreement that they are unlike those of normal synovial cells, adding some evidence that these tumors do not derive directly from synovial cells despite their synovial-like appearance by light microscopy.[222, 235, 239] These tumors probably originate from undifferentiated or pluri-potential cells that have the capacity to differentiate either toward fibroblast-like or epithelial-like cells.[237, 238] This serves to explain the occurrence of these tumors in such locations as the cheek, base of tongue, neck, and retropharyngeal areas that are devoid of normal synovial tissue.[235, 237, 238] The situation is analogous to the occurrence of rhabdomyosarcoma in areas devoid of skeletal muscle.

In general, synovial sarcomas pursue a protracted course with some patients developing metastases 20 years following initial therapy.[25, 47, 218, 232] Average survival is approximately 5 to 6 years, and long survival is possible even in the presence of metastases.[14, 25, 218] Five-year survival rates have ranged from 3 to 69 per cent with most series reporting survival rates of 40 to 50 per cent, with lower 10-year survival rates that reflect the late appearance of metastases.[10, 14, 25, 218, 219, 228, 232, 234, 238, 242] Some believe that all patients, if followed for a sufficient time, will develop metastatic disease.[47] Except for those who divide their cases into monophasic and biphasic categories, there does not appear to be any correlation between histologic features and survival except that calcifying synovial sarcoma appears to have a much better prognosis than the usual synovial sarcoma.[241] Those who do divide their cases into mono- and biphasic forms report that the monophasic variety has an increased local recurrence rate and a lower 5-year survival rate.[228, 232] Tumor size is probably the most important single prognostic determinant, with tumors of less than 5.0 cm having a better prognosis.[224, 228, 238, 242]

Recurrence rates vary from 30 to 65 per cent following local excision.[14, 219, 224, 232, 234] Although most metastases are blood-borne, about 10 to 20 per cent of patients have lymph node metastases.[10, 41, 218, 242] Metastases from biphasic tumors may have either a biphasic or monophasic pattern, and metastases from a monophasic tumor are also monophasic.[224, 228, 232] Five-year survival figures for head and neck lesions do not differ significantly from those for synovial sarcomas at other sites.[238, 240]

Roth and associates had a 47 per cent 5-year survival rate among their 24 head and neck synovial sarcomas. Ten patients developed pulmonary metastases, but lymph nodes were involved in only one of eight cases that were examined.[238] None of the 11 patients reported by Jacobs and Weaver had lymph node metastases.[230] In nine patients with orofacial tumors reported by Shmookler and associates, three died of tumor at intervals of 2.1, 2.6, and 2.9 years. Two of these patients had pulmonary metastases, and all three patients had facial lesions. Two of the 11 patients reported in the literature also died, and both had facial tumors.[240]

The best mode of treatment for these tumors is still evolving. Surgical excision is still the first choice, but the necessary wide and radical procedures required may be difficult to accomplish in head and neck tumors. Routine radical lymph node dissection is not advocated in the absence of lymphadenopathy. Das Gupta has reported encouraging results in patients with synovial sarcoma who received adjuvant chemotherapy, with a 5-year survival in seven of his eight patients (87.5 per cent) with "high-grade" lesions so treated.[10]

LYMPHANGIOMA AND CYSTIC HYGROMA

Of lesions of the lymphatic system, only lymphangioma and cystic hygroma are encountered frequently in the head and neck region. Whether these are true tumors or represent malformations or hamartomas is still debated, but this issue is of no clinical consequence, and the lesions are treated here as true tumors.[14, 255]

In relation to tumors of the arterial and venous systems, lymphangioma and cystic hygroma are not common. The largest single series is that reported by Watson and McCarthy, who studied 1363 tumors of blood and lymphatic vessels of all types. There were a total of only 55 lymphatic tumors (4 per cent) consisting of 41 lymphangiomas and 14 hygromas.[259] Bill and Sumner reported on 61 patients with lymphangioma and cystic hygroma seen at a children's hospital during a 25-year period. The frequency of these tumors was on an average of only five cases for every 3000 admissions per year.[245] Van Cauwelaert and Gruwez state that lymphangiomas account for 6 per cent of benign tumors in childhood and 5 per cent of vascular tumors. In a series of 152 benign tumors in the neck, only four lymphangiomas were found (2.6 per cent).[258]

The terminology of these lesions has caused some confusion in the past, but basically they may be divided into three morphologic types—capillary (lymphangioma circumscriptum), cavernous (lymphangioma cavernosum), and cystic (cystic hygroma).[14, 245, 259]

Lymphangioma circumscriptum is clinically the least significant and usually is confined to the superficial skin, forming small vesicle-like lesions.[10, 247, 254] They are usually asymptomatic, although they may cause symptoms by being irritated by clothing. They are cutaneous tumors and will not be further considered here except to say that they may be seen in conjunction with the other two forms of lymphangioma.

The separation of cavernous lymphangioma from cystic hygroma is valid only in the clinical sense, as histopathologically the lesions are similar.[10, 252] The distinctive gross pattern that separates the two is primarily based on the location and the quality of the surrounding soft tissue.[245, 251] If the surrounding soft tissue, as in the neck, is loose and permits expansion of the lesion, the lymphatic tumor will expand into the typical multicystic appearance of the hygroma.

Approximately two thirds of lymphangiomas are present or noted shortly after birth, and 80 to 95 per cent are present by the end of the second year of life.[245, 249, 250, 253, 255, 257, 259] In most series there has been either no significant sex difference, or only a slight male prevalence. Ninh and Ninh found a male predominance in a ratio of 4:3 in a series of 126 cases of cystic hygroma,[253] and in a series of 177 cases Saijo and associates found 56 per cent were in male patients.[255] Peachey and Whimster reported that 43 of 65 cutaneous lymphangiomas were in female patients.[254]

Lymphangiomas occur in a variety of body locations including the retroperitoneum, mesentery, groin, extremities, chest wall, mediastinum, and within viscera.[250, 255, 258] The head and neck region, however, accounts for between 40 and 70 per cent of all lesions. Das Gupta lists four series of cavernous lymphangiomas, totaling 151 cases, with 61 involving the head and neck (40.4 per cent).[10] Van Cauwelaert and Gruwez reviewed 453 reported cases of lymphangioma in which the neck was involved in 39 per cent and the head in 20 per cent.[258] In the series by Bill and Sumner, 35 tumors were in the head, eight in the tongue, seven in the cheek, seven in the floor of the mouth, five in the parotid region, two each in the lip and nose, and one each in the larynx, scalp, eyelid, and preauricular region. In the same series, there were 25 lymphangiomas in the neck.[245] In the 14 head and neck lesions reported by Harkins and Sabiston, four each were in the neck and tongue, two in the floor of the mouth, and one each in the lip, and parotid, preauricular, and postauricular regions.[250] In the 126 cases of cystic hygroma reviewed by Ninh and Ninh, 76 (60.3 per cent) were in the head and neck, with the anterior and lateral neck alone involved in 55, the neck and axilla in six, the posterior neck in one, the face in 11, and the tongue and sublingual region in three patients.[253] Saijo and associates found 70 per cent of 177 lymphangiomas were in the head and neck, with 91 in the neck, 19 in the face, five in the tongue, six in combined tongue, mouth, and neck, and one case in the mouth.[255] Of the 32 cystic lymphangiomas described by Singh and associates, 12 were in the neck, and one each was in the cervicomediastinum, neck and larynx, and parotid, with the remainder of cases outside the head and neck region.[256]

The cavernous form is found most frequently in sites such as the tongue, cheek, floor of mouth, lips, and nose. Cystic hygroma is most common in the neck,[245, 250, 259] frequently located in the posterior triangle lying behind the sternomastoid muscle. It is less common in the anterior cervical triangle.[249] However, as it enlarges it may extend into the anterior compartment, upward into the cheek or parotid region, or down into the mediastinum or axilla.[252] The tongue is the most frequently involved intraoral site, and most of the tumors arise in the anterior two thirds, although the base of the tongue may occasionally be involved.[246, 251] In the tongue, it produces macroglossia and is the single most common cause of that condition.[246] Lymphangiomas of the tongue have also been associated with cystic lymphangiomas located at other sites.[246, 251]

Most children with lymphangioma are brought to the physician's attention because the parents notice a mass that has slowly enlarged.[245, 252, 259] Occasionally, however, because of the marked size that some of these tumors may attain, especially cystic hygromas, the child may have signs of respiratory distress, difficulty in swallowing, or difficulty in nursing, with regurgitation.[245, 248, 249, 252, 255, 257] In Stromberg's series of 58 patients, 20 per cent had dysphagia or respiratory difficulty.[257] However, in most series these problems are rare, with most patients being asymptomatic.[249, 253] Patients with lesions of the tongue may have such an enlarged and protruding tongue that it cannot be placed within the mouth because of its size.[246, 251]

Cavernous lymphangiomas vary from millimeter-sized lesions to those of several centimeters.[250, 251, 254] They may be well circumscribed or diffusely invasive, involving subcutaneous tissue and underlying muscle. These are prone to extend by budding along fascial planes, great vessels, or nerve trunks to form ill-defined spongy and compressible masses.[14, 54, 250] When the skin is involved, they may produce bluish bulges.[10] Cystic hygromas vary from a single soft mass with a smooth round contour to lobulated, multicystic masses.[249, 259] Their walls are quite thin and, unless there has been previous infection, they will transilluminate.[54, 249] The individual cysts communicate with each other such that accidental rupture of any one of them will cause collapse of the entire mass, thus masking the limits of its extension.[252] Cystic hygromas in the neck have room to expand, owing to the loose areolar type connective tissue in this region, and like the cavernous lymphangioma, also extend along the great vessels and nerves, and between muscle groups by finger-like projections.[245, 249, 250] These may be easily overlooked at surgery and may serve as a focus for recurrence. Cystic hygromas vary from 1.0 cm to 30.0 cm; the mean size in Stromberg's series was 8.0 cm.[257] They usually contain clear, serous type fluid.[249, 259] In the tongue, lymphangiomas vary from localized pinhead single vesicles to extensive and diffuse infiltration of the entire tongue, causing nodularity of the surface with vesicle-like projections.[246, 251]

As mentioned, cavernous lymphangioma and cystic hygroma are histologically very similar and consist of dilated, thin-walled sinuses that are filled with eosinophilic, acellular lymph fluid.[245, 247] These spaces are lined by flat endothelial cells.[249, 252, 259] The spaces vary in size from capillary to cavernous, much in the same way as a hemangioma may contain capillary- or cavernous-sized channels.[245] The intervening stroma may be quite scanty, with closely packed channels, or it may be more abundant, with the spaces separated by stroma. This stroma varies from a loose myxomatous lace-like material to areas with dense hyalinization.[245, 247, 249] When there has been previous infection, the stroma is markedly increased.[253] Scattered lymphoid aggregates are also found, occasionally in the form of germinal follicles, and wisps of smooth muscle fibers may also be present (Figs. 53–14 and 53–15).[14, 259] In 61 tumors described by Bill and Sumner, 21 appeared without cystic spaces, 23

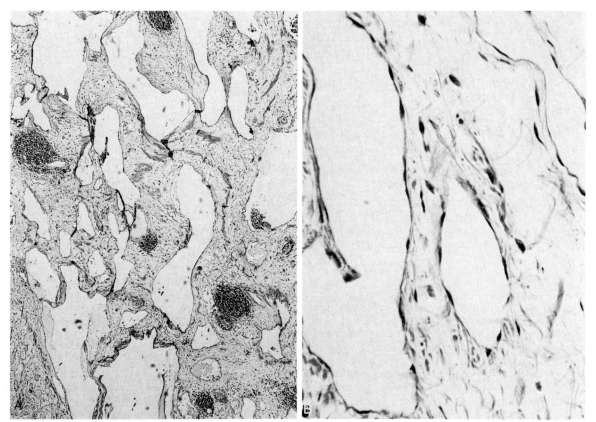

Figure 53–14. Cavernous lymphangioma. (*A*) Dilated lymphatic channels are separated by fibrous bands, creating a Swiss-cheese pattern. Lymphoid aggregates are also present. (*B*) Higher magnification of a lymphangioma shows the lymphatic channels lined by flat endothelial cells.

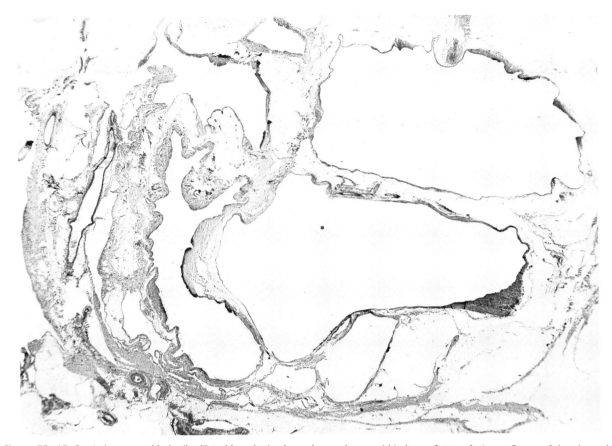

Figure 53–15. Cystic hygroma. Markedly dilated lymphatic channels are shown within loose fatty soft tissue. Some of the channels have smooth muscle in their walls.

were composed of large cysts only, and 17 had a combination of small cavernous spaces and large cysts.[245]

Surgical therapy, with as wide an excision as possible while preserving cosmetic function, appears to be the best approach to these lesions.[245, 248, 250, 252, 255] They are radioresistant, and the use of such therapy in infants and young children is to be avoided whenever possible.[253, 257, 259] Despite their benign nature, surgical management is difficult, especially for the cavernous lymphangioma, because of its tendency to spread along vital structures and the subsequent high incidence of recurrence. Harkins and Sabiston[250] reported 88 operations required in 27 patients with cavernous lymphangioma, and Watson and McCarthy[259] reported a 41 per cent recurrence rate (17 of 41 patients) in their series of cavernous lymphangiomas, while only one of their 14 cystic hygromas recurred (7 per cent). Stromberg and associates reported a success rate in 13 of 14 cystic hygromas completely excised (93 per cent) versus only a 17 per cent cure rate (3 of 18) when only partial excision was done.[257] Saijo and associates reported a 61.4 per cent cure rate (27 of 44) for all lymphangiomas, including cystic hygromas, with the least successfully treated tumors being located on the head and face, and the best results for those tumors in the neck. There was no recurrence in any case thought to be completely excised.[255] In their 21 cases of cystic hygroma with follow-up information, 19 were excised, and of these, 14 (73.7 per cent) had a successful result after one or

two operations.[255] Most recurrences appear within 1 year, many within 6 months.[248, 257]

Mortality rates are between 3 and 7 per cent, with the largest lesions having the higher mortality rates.[245, 248–250, 253, 255, 256, 259] In Barrand and Freeman's series of nine "massive" infiltrating hygromas, four of eight patients operated upon died.[244] Most deaths have been postoperative.

Examples of spontaneous regression of lymphangiomas or regression subsequent to infection are occasionally reported as part of a large series of cases,[249, 253] but many authors have never seen such an occurrence.[245, 255, 257] Therapy should not be predicated upon the hope that regression will occur. Lymphangiomas, especially intraoral ones, are prone to becoming infected and may suddenly increase in size because of this, with life-threatening consequences.[10, 253] Surgical therapy, with as wide an excision as possible, with care taken to avoid rupturing the lesion, is the treatment of choice. Staged excisions may be necessary in order to avoid mutilating surgery for these benign, but troublesome, tumors.

LIPOMA

Lipoma is the commonest soft-tissue tumor,[14, 263] but its true incidence is difficult to assess, as many patients have small asymptomatic masses and never seek medical attention. In a series of 1331 benign soft-tissue tumors, lipomas made up 48.1 per cent of the total cases.[37] It is only when the tumor reaches such a size that it either is cosmetically distracting or impinges on vital structures that the patient seeks attention. There are few published reports in which large numbers of patients with adipose tumors are described,[260, 270] as pathologists and clinicians have not been stimulated by this prosaic tumor, and usually only individual case reports are published when the lipoma arises in unusual locations. Allen's recent excellent monograph on adipose tumors, however, describes over 40 varieties of benign mesenchymal lesions in which fat is a prominent or major component.[261] In addition, recent descriptions of lipomas with histologic features that may mimic or may be confused with liposarcoma have stimulated a renewed interest in the common lipoma.

Lipomas tend to occur in obese patients or those with recent weight gain.[14, 260] Approximately 60 to 75 per cent of these patients are women[260, 261, 271, 280] in the fifth to sixth decades of life.[260, 261, 266, 271, 280] However, in his extensive review of lipomas of the oral cavity, Hatziotis found that of 125 recorded cases in which the sex of the patient was mentioned, 68 were males (54.4 per cent).[271] The tumor is uncommon in the first two decades of life and is rarely found in children.[14, 47, 260, 261, 263, 270, 280] The tumor usually manifests as a solitary, painless mass that gradually increases in size or becomes stationary after a period of growth.

Most lipomas are between 1.0 cm and 5.0 cm in maximum dimension.[14, 261] However, depending on location, they may reach enormous size, 50 to 60 cm, and may weigh many kilograms.[14, 261, 270, 272] Lipomas are usually soft, freely movable masses that almost always arise in the subcutaneous tissue.[261, 264, 280] The most common sites include the shoulder, arms, and trunk.[14, 261, 263, 266, 280] The head and neck region accounts for approximately 15 to 20 per cent of all lipomas, with the neck being more commonly affected than the head; the face and scalp are rarely involved.[14, 260, 264] In a review of 195 lipomas in 179 patients, Dixon and coworkers found the head and neck involved in 21.5 per cent, the upper extremity in 22.1 per cent, the lower extremity in 11.8 per cent, the chest and back in 16.9 per cent, and the abdomen in 7.7 per cent.[266] Of the 109 patients with lipomas in Allen's series, in which an anatomic site was known, 19.3 per cent were in the head and neck region, with nine tumors in the head and 12 in the neck.[261] Oral cavity lipomas are rare, accounting for only 1 to 2 per cent of all benign tumors in this site.[271] In 26 oral cavity lipomas reported by Seldin and associates[277] the cheek was involved in 11, the gingiva in four, the lip in three, and two each were in the buccal fold in the region of the mental foramen, the lower buccal fold, the palate, and the floor of the mouth. The cheek was the most common site in the 145 oral lipomas reported by Hatziotis, accounting for 46 cases, whereas the tongue was the site in 28, the floor of the mouth in 21, the buccal sulcus and vestibule in 18, the palate in 13, the lips in nine, and eight in the gingiva, with two sites not stated.[271] Wakeley and Somerville[280] list 180 lipomas in 170 patients, with 30 (16.5 per cent) in the head and neck (14 in the head and 16 in the neck). Pharyngeal lipomas are equally rare; Toppozada and associates reviewed the literature in 1973 and found 48 reported

cases and added four more.[279] In the neck and oral cavity, the tumor may be pedunculated or sessile.[264, 271] Lipomas have also been found in the larynx, tonsil, and maxillary antrum.[269, 277]

It should be remembered that lipomas are usually superficially located, in contrast to the malignant tumor of adipose tissue, liposarcoma, which arises from the deep soft tissue and which is rarely superficial. This is an important clinical point for distinguishing between these two tumors. Intra- and intermuscular lipomas, however, do occur, but these are usually found in the distal extremities and shoulder region and are quite rare in the muscles of the head and neck.[261, 265, 267, 274]

Grossly, lipomas are smooth, well-circumscribed, round to oval encapsulated masses. The cut surface varies from yellow to orange and is greasy to the touch. The tumors may be lobulated.[14, 261] Microscopically, there is a thin fibrous capsule from which delicate fibrous septa extend into the substance of the tumor, separating it into lobules that are composed of mature adipose cells (Fig. 53–16). The presence of a fibrous capsule serves to distinguish a lipoma from a simple aggregation of fat.[261] Scattered myxoid areas may be found, and small foci of fat necrosis, probably the result of minor trauma, may also occasionally be seen within the lobules. Electron microscopic studies have shown that the cells of the lipoma are morphologically similar to the cells of normal mature adipose tissue.[268, 273]

Multiple lipomas occur in from 1 to 7 per cent of cases, at times in patients with a family history of multiple lipomas. Multiple lipomas have also been reported in patients with neurofibromatosis and in those with the multiple endocrine adenoma syndrome.[261, 263] These multiple fatty tumors must be distinguished from the more common angiolipoma, which is frequently multiple but rarely occurs in the head and neck.

True lipomas rarely recur (1 to 2 per cent) after adequate local excision.[14, 261, 264] Such an occurrence should raise the clinical suspicion of liposarcoma, especially if the tumor is not superficially located. Two subvariants of lipoma, spindle cell lipoma and pleomorphic (atypical) lipoma, have been described; they are frequently found in the posterior neck and histologically may be confused with liposarcoma.

Unlike the more common subcutaneous lipomas, there are deeper soft tissue infiltrating lipomas that either exist between muscle groups (intermuscular lipoma) or are confined within muscle (intramuscular lipoma).[261, 264, 265, 267, 274] This is largely a tumor of adults, with patients usually in the fifth to seventh decades of life, 80 per cent of all patients being over age 40.[261, 265, 267, 274]

Unlike their subcutaneous counterparts, these infiltrating lipomas are more common in male patients.[261, 267] They present as painless masses that may only become obvious upon contraction of the involved muscle, when they may become round and firm.[261, 264, 267, 274] Despite at times reaching very large size, up to 35 cm, they rarely produce actual dysfunction of the involved muscle.[265, 274] Approximately two thirds of these tumors are located in the thigh and shoulder regions and, less commonly, in the upper arm, chest wall, and head and neck area.[261, 267, 274] None of the 43 intermuscular or intramuscular lipomas described by Kindblom and associates[274] were in the head or neck region, nor were any of the

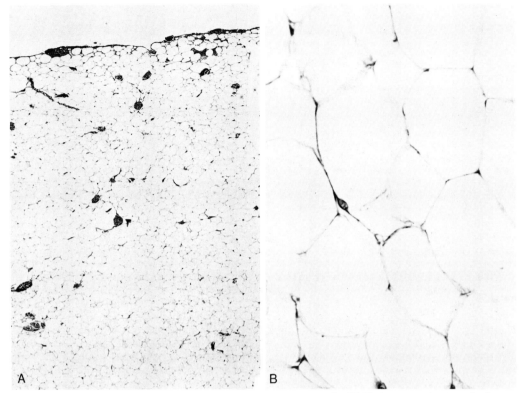

Figure 53–16. Lipoma. (A) Thin fibrous capsule (top) encloses mature adipose cells. (B) Higher magnification of adipose cells shown in (A). Nuclei are compressed against their cell borders by single large cytoplasmic fat vacuoles.

13 infiltrating lipomas listed by Dionne and Seemayer.[265] However, three of the 78 patients mentioned by Enzinger had intramuscular lipomas in the head and neck region.[267]

Roentgenograms may show a sharply circumscribed radiolucent defect within the muscle, and angiographic studies show that these tumors, unlike soft-tissue sarcomas, are poorly vascularized.[274]

On gross examination, the tumor is noted either to infiltrate and replace large portions of the muscle or to extend and infiltrate the tendons and fascia between muscles.[267] Histologically, most tumors are composed of mature, normal-appearing fat cells that lack atypicality or mitotic activity.[267, 274] The cells infiltrate between the muscle fibers, replacing them and causing pressure atrophy and degeneration. Some intramuscular lipomas do have cells that show a significant degree of cytologic atypia. These pleomorphic or atypical lipomas are described later in this chapter.

Recurrence rates following local excision of these infiltrating lipomas have ranged widely, from 3 to 62.5 per cent,[261, 266, 267] with some patients having multiple recurrences. These recurrence rates more than likely reflect the adequacy of the initial excision, rather than any inherent aggressive propensity of these tumors. In the series by Kindblom and associates,[274] only one of 33 excised tumors recurred, the single exception being a tumor that had been previously incompletely resected. In the AFIP series, 85 per cent of the patients with follow-up information were well without recurrence following excision of the tumor. In three of seven patients with recurrences, the tumor recurred more than once.[267] No metastases have been reported, and patients have remained well on extended follow-up study. As with any deep fatty tumor, the distinction from liposarcoma is important. The infiltrative growth pattern of the lipoma, rather than the gross expansile pattern of liposarcoma, as well as the absence of lipoblasts and the bland nature of the fat cells in the lipoma, serve to differentiate it from well-differentiated liposarcoma.

A peculiar distribution of fatty tissue about the cervical region may be encountered by the head and neck surgeon. This entity, termed Madelung's disease, cervical lipomatosis, or symmetric cervical lipomatosis, is a striking condition that causes gross deformity of the head and neck region by producing a "horse-collar" cervical distribution of fat.[262, 276, 278] It is characterized by the gradual deposit of nontender fat tissue in a superficial location about the neck, postauricular area, and suboccipital and parotid regions.[261, 276, 278] These subcutaneous deposits of fat are nonencapsulated and poorly circumscribed, with tongue-like extensions of the fat between muscle groups. The deposits consist of mature fat with an increased amount of fibrous tissue.[261]

Patients are middle-aged men frequently with a history of alcoholism and liver disease.[261, 262, 276, 278] They usually complain of the gross cosmetic deformity, although some patients have sought medical attention because of respiratory distress caused by airway compression by the fatty masses.[261, 262, 278] The larynx has been involved by extension of the fat through the thyrohyoid membrane into the false cord.[275]

Excision of the fatty masses may be necessary, although the lack of clearly defined surgical tissue planes makes dissection difficult.[274, 276, 278] The condition may improve with abstinence from alcohol.[14, 261]

Spindle Cell Lipoma

Unlike the usual lipoma, spindle cell lipoma is far more common in men than women, with over 90 per cent of the reported cases occurring in men. In the 114 patients reported from the AFIP, 104 (91 per cent) were men[283]; 12 of the 14 patients in the series by Angervall and associates were men,[281] as were all five of the patients reported by Bolen and Thorning.[282] Allen reported 10 patients, eight of whom were men.[261] It is uncommon in patients younger than age 40, the mean age being between 55 to 60 years, with a range of 24 to 81 years.[281, 282, 283] Almost all these tumors are located in the subcutaneous tissue of the upper back, shoulder, or neck. In the large series by Enzinger and Harvey, of 114 cases, 41 (36 per cent) were located in the posterior neck, and 53 (47 per cent) were in the shoulder or back. Two other tumors were located in the head, eight in the extremities, and six in the trunk.[283] In Angervall's series of 14 patients, seven tumors were in the posterior neck; one each in the forehead, upper back, and thigh; and four in the shoulder.[281] In Bolen and Thorning's cases, two each were in the posterior neck and upper back, and one was located behind the ear.[282] A spindle cell lipoma of the perianal region has been reported,[284] as well as examples in the foot and hand.[261] Some of the spindle cell lipomas have extended from the deep subcutaneous tissue to involve the fascia and underlying muscle.[281, 283]

Spindle cell lipomas range in size from 1 cm to 13 cm with a median size between 4.0 cm and 5.0 cm.[261, 281–283] Grossly, they resemble an ordinary lipoma, being circumscribed and encapsulated, although the deeper situated lesions may appear to be infiltrative.[267, 281, 283] They may at times have gray-white gelatinous foci.[261, 267, 281, 283] Microscopically, the lesion consists of varying proportions of bland-appearing, elongated, spindle cells; fat cells; bundles of birefringent collagen; and a myxoid stroma (Fig. 53–17). Mast cells may also be quite common. In some tumors the spindle cells make up almost the entire lesion, with only a few scattered fat cells seen, but others may show the usual pattern of a conventional lipoma with only a few small foci of spindle cells. The spindle cells and the collagen bands may at first suggest a diagnosis of neurilemoma, neurofibroma, hemangiopericytoma, or smooth muscle tumor.[267, 281–283] At times, scattered multivacuolated cells having hyperchromatic and atypical nuclei are present. These, combined with the mucoid matrix, may simulate a sclerosing or myxoid liposarcoma.[261, 281, 282] Mitotic activity, however, is rare in spindle cell lipomas, and the superficial location of the spindle cell lipoma should serve as a clue to the benign nature of the lesion. Spindle cell lipomas also lack lipoblasts, pools of mucinous material, and a diffuse plexiform capillary network, as is found in some liposarcomas.[261, 281, 283] The atypical cells may reflect a transitional-type lesion from a pure spindle cell lipoma to the closely related entity, pleomorphic (atypical) lipoma.[261, 267, 281, 282]

Electron microscopic studies have been done on only a few examples of spindle cell lipoma, with the spindle cells thought to represent fibroblasts or fibroblast-like cells analogous to the stellate mesenchymal cells seen in primitive fat lobules.[273, 282, 283]

None of the 63 cases reported by Enzinger and Harvey,[283] for which adequate follow-up information was available, had recurrences following surgical excision, and neither did any of the 14 patients reported by Angervall and associates.[281] Allen, however, noted a recurrence 3 years after therapy in one of his 10 patients.[261] The concern for spindle cell lipoma is, as for atypical lipoma, that it not be confused with liposarcoma.

Pleomorphic (Atypical) Lipoma

This benign tumor of adipose tissue is histologically the most likely to be misdiagnosed as liposarcoma because of its content of atypical lipoblasts.[267, 287] Although some differences of opinion exist as to what type of lesion should be designated as a pleomorphic or atypical lipoma,[285, 287] its general histologic features have been well described.[285–287]

The age and anatomic distribution of pleomorphic lipoma are similar to those for spindle cell lipoma, a finding that is not surprising because transitional histologic forms containing elements of both lesions exist.[261, 267, 281, 282] Pleomorphic (atypical) lipoma occurs almost exclusively in adults, with the mean patient age between 50 and 70 years.[261, 266, 285, 287] They are rare in patients less than age 40, with only two of Shmookler and Enzinger's 48 patients in that age group.[287] However, one of Allen's nine patients was 23 years old,[261] and four of the 21 patients reported by Kindblom and associates were in their twenties.[286] In four publications, the percentage of male patients has ranged from 57 to 89 per cent.[261, 285–287]

In most instances, patients complain of a slowly growing mass that may have been present for many years. In some, however, the mass rapidly enlarges within only a few weeks.[267, 287] Approximately 80 per cent of the lesions occur in the neck, shoulder, and upper back. In Shmookler and Enzinger's series of 48 patients, the neck was the site of origin in 24 patients, with 15 of these in the posterior neck, and the head was involved in three other patients. Other sites included the extremities and shoulder region in seven patients each, the back in six, and the chest wall in one patient.[287] Evans and associates divided their cases into subcutaneous (nine) and intramuscular (13) tumors. There was one neck and one posterior scalp lesion among the subcutaneous tumors and one neck and one facial lesion among the intramuscular tumors.[285] Among the 21 cases of atypical lipoma reported by Kindblom and associates, only one was in the posterior neck, the others were located outside the head and neck region, most commonly in the thigh.[286] Two of Allen's nine cases were in the neck, with the others in the thigh, elbow, forearm, shoulder, and trapezius.[261]

The tumors arise from the subcutaneous tissue as well as within muscle, with the former being more common. The intramuscular lesions are more common in the extremities, especially in the thigh.[286] The subcutaneous lesions are usually well circumscribed, being partially or completely encapsulated, whereas the intramuscular tumors may have an infiltrative appearance. In either location, tumors as large as 29 cm have been

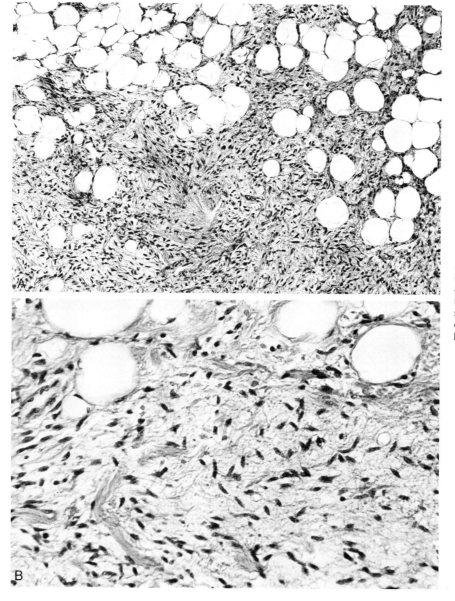

Figure 53–17. Spindle cell lipoma. (A) Mixture of mature adipose cells and spindle cells. (B) Higher magnification shows widely separated spindle cell nuclei and a few bundles of thick collagen in the lower left of the field.

recorded, although most are in the 5.0-cm to 10.0-cm range.[267, 285–287] Subcutaneous tumors are usually smaller than the intramuscular lesions.

Histologically, atypical lipomas are characterized by the presence of pleomorphic cells, consisting of multivacuolated lipoblasts with atypical nuclei, mixed with hyperchromatic, multinucleated cells (Fig. 53–18). These latter cells have their nuclei arranged in a peripheral wreath-like pattern about a central core of eosinophilic cytoplasm and have been called "floret-like" cells.[267, 287] The nuclei of these cells tend to overlap each other and may blend together (Fig. 53–19). The number of floret cells varies from case to case, being abundant in some and rare in others.[287] Whether their presence is essential to the diagnosis[261] is debated, with Evans and associates noting them in only one third of their cases.[285] In addition to floret cells, mononuclear cells of various sizes, with hyperchromatic and atypical nuclei, are also found. Between these atypical cells are mature fat cells and bands of birefringent collagen.[267, 287] In up to one quarter of the cases focal areas may be found with the features of spindle cell lipoma.[287] Myxoid areas within the collagen bands, or between the cells, are also common. Mast cells and lymphocytes are also present. Mitoses are uncommon.

The histologic distinction between pleomorphic lipoma and sclerosing liposarcoma may be difficult to make.[267, 285, 287] Indeed, at the AFIP 65 per cent of the pleomorphic lipomas that were received in consultation were diagnosed as liposarcoma by the submitting pathologists.[287] The site of the lesion may well be the deciding factor in determining whether one is dealing with a liposarcoma or a benign fat tumor. Apparently, those atypical lipomas arising in the subcutaneous tissue do well, with only rare recurrences reported despite even less than adequate excision.[285, 287] There is some difference of opinion about whether the intramuscular lesions should be designated as benign. Although Evans and associates reported a local recurrence rate of close

to 70 per cent for the intramuscular lesions, no tumor recurred after total excision.[285] Shmookler and Enzinger, however, claim that some recurrences are less differentiated than the initial tumor and are fully malignant, and they prefer to regard the intramuscular tumors as low-grade liposarcomas.[287] In Kindblom's series, nine of the 21 tumors recurred during follow-up intervals of 6 months to 25 years. Five of these nine were subcutaneous, and the other four were inter- or intramuscular tumors. The single lesion in the neck recurred four times.[286]

LIPOSARCOMA

Liposarcoma is probably the most common adult soft-tissue sarcoma, although the reported incidence varies greatly from institution to institution.[25] It has been reported to make up from 5 per cent to about 30 per cent of all soft-tissue sarcomas.[39, 63, 297] With the establishment of malignant fibrous histiocytoma as a distinct entity, this tumor has, in some institutions, equaled or surpassed liposarcoma as the most common sarcoma in adults.[14, 59] Furthermore, with the recent descriptions of spindle cell lipoma and pleomorphic (atypical) lipoma, benign tumors of fat that may be histologically confused with liposarcoma, some lesions previously diagnosed as liposarcoma will no doubt, upon review, be reclassified as one or the other of these tumors.[285, 287] Indeed, in some series, one half of the lesions previously designated as liposarcoma were, upon review, placed in some other diagnostic category.[297, 299] It should be remembered that liposarcomas are still relatively rare tumors and are estimated to be approximately 100 times less common than lipomas.[261] In the series of "lipoid" tumors reported by Geshickter, there were 478 lipomas and only 12 liposarcomas.[270] During the years 1970 to 1977, Myhre-Jensen found 640 soft-tissue lipomas and only 10 liposarcomas.[37] For all practical purposes,

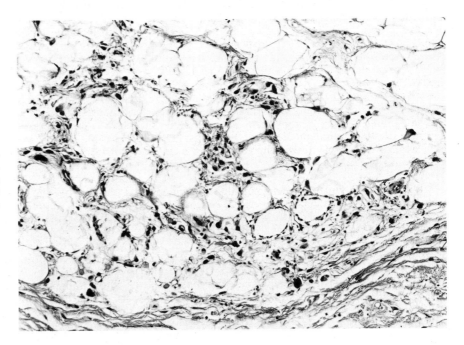

Figure 53–18. Pleomorphic (atypical) lipoma. Numerous large hyperchromatic adipose cells. There is increased fibrosis. Compare with the lipoma shown in Figure 53–16.

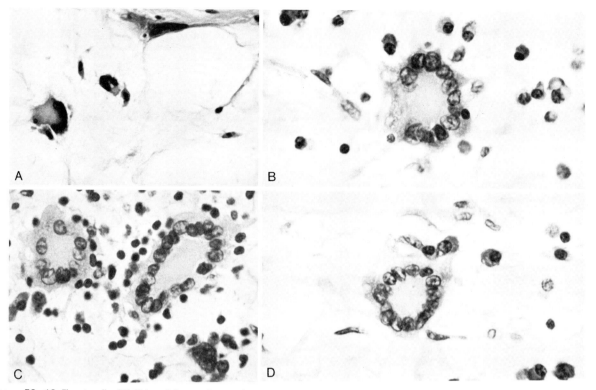

Figure 53—19. Floret cells. (*A*) This cell has an incomplete ring of nuclei, which are also "smudged" together. (*B, C, D*) These cells show a wreath-like arrangement of nuclei enclosing a central core of cytoplasm.

liposarcomas arise de novo and not from pre-existing lipomas.

Most patients with liposarcoma are adults in the fourth to sixth decades of life, with a mean patient age of about 50 years.[47, 291, 296, 299] However, in two reports that review head and neck liposarcoma, the patients were younger, with mean ages of 38 and 42.8 years with a range of from 2 to 90 years.[288, 302] Owing to the lack of a large number of patients in these reports, this difference in mean ages between liposarcomas of the head and neck and those of other sites may not be significant. Children are rarely involved. In a recent survey from the AFIP, Shmookler and Enzinger found only 17 examples in children in their collection of 2500 liposarcomas, and they found only 29 previously reported cases, not all of which they accepted as documented.[303] Only two of the AFIP tumors occurred in patients under 10 years of age. Many cases reported as liposarcoma in children probably represent benign lipoblastoma.[292, 303] A diagnosis of liposarcoma in a child less than age 5 years should be viewed with skepticism.[25, 261, 296]

Unlike lipomas, which are more common in women, men account for roughly 55 to 60 per cent of cases.[47, 291, 296, 299] This male prevalence also holds true for liposarcomas of the head and neck region, where almost two thirds of the patients have been males.[288, 302]

In general, liposarcomas originate from the deep soft tissues and, unlike lipomas, rarely arise in the subcutaneous tissue.[14, 261, 301] They usually occur between major muscle groups, with the most frequent locations being the thigh, retroperitoneum, inguinal region, shoulder area, and buttocks.[14, 25, 47, 291, 296] The head and neck region

is involved in only 2 to 6 per cent of all cases, and in some series no cases are mentioned as originating in this area. In a combined series of 335 liposarcomas, Das Gupta lists only nine (1.8 per cent) within the head and neck region.[10] Only three of 122 cases of liposarcoma from a Swedish national series were in the neck (2.5 per cent).[298] In this national series, the authors had previously reported their head and neck liposarcomas in combination with those of the trunk and listed a total of 12 in this combined region.[299] In Allen's study of 126 confirmed liposarcomas, eight (6.3 per cent) were in the head and neck.[261] At the AFIP, 60 of 1067 liposarcomas (5.6 per cent) were in this region.[14] None of Evan's 55 liposarcomas were in the head and neck.[297] Baden and Newman, in a review of the literature in 1977, found 40 reported head and neck liposarcomas, 35 of which contained sufficient data that could be analyzed.[288] In 1978, Kindblom and associates included only 17 cases from the literature and added four new cases, but did not include the new cases added by Baden and Newman.[298] In 1979, Saunders and associates also reviewed the literature and listed 25 previous reports and added four new cases.[302] This series neglected the cases described by Kindblom and associates and Baden and Newman. Stoller and Davies reported an incidence of only four liposarcomas of the head and neck in a population of 8.5 million people in southern England, although how this figure was established was not stated.[305]

Most liposarcomas in the head and neck have been located in the neck, with other sites including the cheek, forehead, scalp, orbit, floor of mouth, soft palate, pharynx, meninges, larynx, nasopharynx, paranasal sinuses, nasal cavity, supraclavicular fossa, maxilla, and mastoid.[269, 288, 298, 302, 303] In a tabulation of 60 cases at the AFIP, the neck was involved in 36, the face in 17, and the scalp in four.[14]

As with other soft-tissue sarcomas, liposarcomas are usually nodular masses that appear well circumscribed. In the head and neck area they are usually smaller than those in such areas as the thigh or retroperitoneum, where lesions weighing many thousands of grams may be found,[47, 296] although liposarcomas as large as 15.0 cm have been reported in the head and neck region.[302] In Allen's eight head and neck liposarcomas, the tumors ranged in maximum dimensions from 2.0 cm to 12 cm with a mean of 5.9 cm.[261] In the listing of cases by Saunders and associates there were 14 tumors for which the size was given. These ranged from 1.0 cm to 15.0 cm, with a mean of 5.2 cm.[302]

Depending on the histologic variety of liposarcoma, the tumors may vary grossly from those that resemble a benign lipoma, being soft, greasy, and bright yellow, to myxoid tumors with a white-gray translucent surface that feels "slimy."[261, 299] Mucoid material may freely drip from the surface of such tumors. Other liposarcomas, however, may have a gross appearance that does not differ from other types of sarcomas.

Histologically, liposarcoma is considered to be a tumor that is composed of lipoblasts. However, the number of lipoblasts present may vary considerably among the various histologic subtypes of liposarcoma. Furthermore, the presence of lipoblasts per se does not establish a tumor as a liposarcoma because these cells, or cells that simulate them, are also found in reactive conditions involving fat and in benign lipoblastoma of childhood.[261, 292] In addition, other malignant tumors such as malignant fibrous histiocytoma and osteosarcoma may also contain cells that are indistinguishable from lipoblasts.[14] The correct diagnosis depends upon the finding of other cellular constituents as well as the overall pattern of the lesion.

Lipoblasts are divided into univacuolated and multivacuolated types (Fig. 53–20).[261] In the univacuolated form, the cells are smaller than mature adipose cells and have a signet-ring appearance produced by a single, large, and sharply delimited cytoplasmic fat vacuole that pushes the nucleus against the cell membrane and deforms it into a demilune shape.[25, 261] These univacuolated lipoblasts may be confused with the cells of a signet-ring lymphoma or, more commonly, with the cells of a mucin-producing adenocarcinoma. Multivacuolated lipoblasts have a central hyperchromatic nucleus that is frequently large and bizarre in shape. The cytoplasm contains several large or small fat vacuoles that are characteristically well defined and that indent or scallop the nucleus.

Liposarcomas have been divided into four major histologic varieties: a well-differentiated type, which is further classified into a lipoma-like and sclerosing forms; a myxoid type; a round cell type; and a pleomorphic type. There are also mixed tumors that contain various combinations of the four types.[296, 299] A dedifferentiated form of liposarcoma has recently been described that consists of well-differentiated liposarcoma in association with undifferentiated spindle-cell areas.[297]

Myxoid liposarcoma is the commonest histologic type, accounting for 35 to 50 per cent of liposarcomas at all sites.[261, 296, 297] It is characterized by widely separated, monomorphic fusiform or stellate cells residing in a mucoid stroma rich in hyaluronic acid (Fig. 53–21). Pools or lakes of this material are frequently present. A diagnostically important feature is the presence of a delicate plexiform capillary network that serves to separate liposarcoma from the essentially avascular soft-tissue myxoma, with which it may be confused.[261, 296, 297] Cell pleomorphism and significant mitotic activity are not part of myxoid liposarcoma, and lipoblasts may at times be difficult to find in some of these tumors.

Well-differentiated liposarcoma accounts for 20 to 30 per cent of cases.[261, 297, 299] The lipoma-like variety, as its name implies, histologically closely resembles a simple lipoma except for the focal occurrence of regions in which hyperchromatic and bizarre lipoblasts are found. It is this form of liposarcoma that may be underdi-

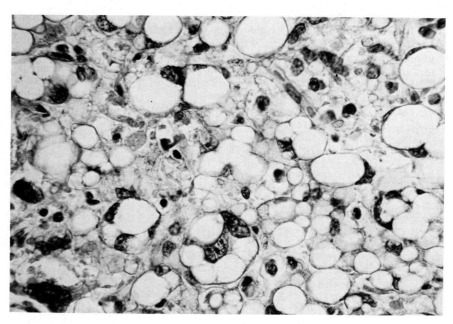

Figure 53–20. Liposarcoma. Numerous univacuolated and some multivacuolated lipoblasts are shown. Note the signet-ring appearance of the univacuolated cells and the scalloping of the nuclei in the multivacuolated cells.

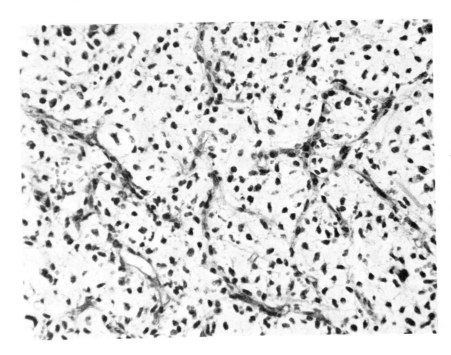

Figure 53–21. Myxoid liposarcoma. Widely separated small stellate tumor cells are embedded in a myxoid stroma. There is a well-formed plexiform capillary network. Well-defined lipoblasts are not present.

agnosed as a lipoma if sufficient sampling of the lesion is not done. The true nature of the "lipoma" may become evident only when it recurs despite what was thought to be adequate local excision. In Kindblom's series, 10 of the 26 well-differentiated liposarcomas were originally diagnosed as lipoma until microscopic examination of the recurrent tumors established the correct diagnosis.[298, 299] On the other hand, some well-differentiated liposarcomas probably would today be included among the spindle-cell or pleomorphic (atypical) lipomas for which the head and neck region is a common location.[281, 283, 285, 287] The diagnosis of a subcutaneous well-differentiated liposarcoma in the head and neck area should be viewed with some skepticism.

Pleomorphic liposarcoma is the most anaplastic of the liposarcomas and accounts for 10 to 25 per cent of cases.[261, 296, 299] It contains an abundant mix of tumor giant cells that have a dense, glassy eosinophilic cytoplasm and bizarre lipoblasts (Fig. 53–22). Numerous abnormal mitotic figures are present throughout the tumor. Pleomorphic liposarcoma may be difficult or impossible to distinguish from pleomorphic rhabdomyosarcoma or malignant fibrous histiocytoma (fibroxanthosarcoma).[14, 25, 295] Malignant fibrous histiocytoma may even contain lipoblasts, and there may be such an overlap between these two tumor entities that they are not distinguishable at the light microscopic level.

Round cell liposarcoma is considered by some to be a variant of the myxoid type, although foci of myxoid liposarcoma are noted in less than half the cases.[297] The tumor is composed of round to oval cells that have a fine, multivacuolated cytoplasm and a central round nucleus that may be hyperchromatic but usually is not markedly atypical (Fig. 53–23). Mitoses are not common. Round cell liposarcoma makes up about 10 to 15 per cent of all liposarcomas.[261, 296, 299]

Recurrent liposarcomas may have a histologic appearance that differs from the original primary tumor. These tumors may contain components of the other liposarcoma subtypes or, more important from a diagnostic standpoint, features of other sarcomas such as malignant fibrous histiocytoma, hemangiopericytoma, or unclassified spindle cell sarcoma.[304]

Electron microscopic studies of liposarcoma have dealt mainly with the myxoid variety. Here, the prevailing view is that the tumor roughly recapitulates the embryonic development of white fat,[268, 289, 290, 293, 306] although some have suggested an origin from brown fat.[300]

The myxoid liposarcoma is the commonest variety found in the head and neck region. In the 35 cases reported by Baden and Newman, 71.4 per cent were myxoid, 14.2 per cent were round cell, and 8.5 per cent were mixed liposarcomas.[288] Among the 29 liposarcomas listed by Saunders and associates, nine were myxoid, eight were well-differentiated, four were round cell, two were pleomorphic, and six were of unknown type.[302] In Allen's eight cases, three were myxoid, three were well-differentiated, and two were of the round cell type.[261] Two of the four cases of liposarcoma of the neck reported by Kindblom and associates[298] were well-differentiated, one was pleomorphic, and one was round cell. Among the four head and neck juvenile liposarcomas listed in the report from the AFIP, one was of mixed type, two were well-differentiated, and one was "poorly differentiated."[303]

Prognosis for liposarcoma is directly correlated with the histologic appearance of the tumor.[261, 296, 299] The overall 5-year survival rate is roughly 45 to 65 per cent for all liposarcomas. The well-differentiated and myxoid tumors have excellent 5-year survival rates of 75 to 100 per cent despite local recurrence rates that have ranged between 50 and 100 per cent in some series.[261, 296, 297, 299] Pleomorphic liposarcoma has a much poorer prognosis, with 5-year survival rates of from 0 to 21 per cent. Round cell liposarcoma has only a slightly better prognosis with 18 to 27 per cent 5-year survival rates. Local recurrence rates for these latter two liposarcomas have been between 75 and 80 per cent.[261, 296, 297, 299] The well-

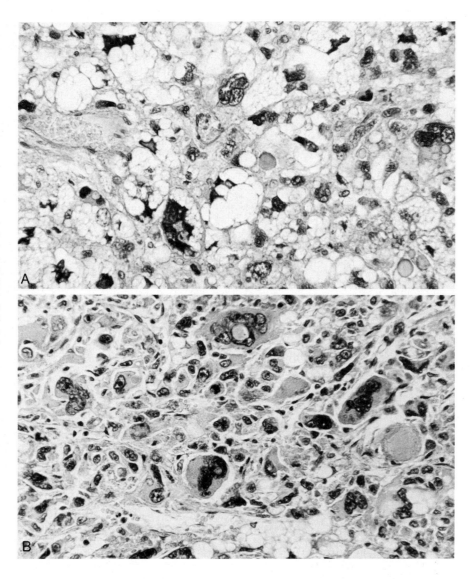

Figure 53–22. Pleomorphic liposarcoma. (*A*) Numerous bizarre-appearing multivacuolated lipoblasts are shown. Note the scalloping of the tumor cell nuclei by the cytoplasmic fat vacuoles. (*B*) Another field in a highly pleomorphic liposarcoma where the tumor cells are large, with an abundant amount of cytoplasm. Most of these cells lack cytoplasmic fat vacuoles.

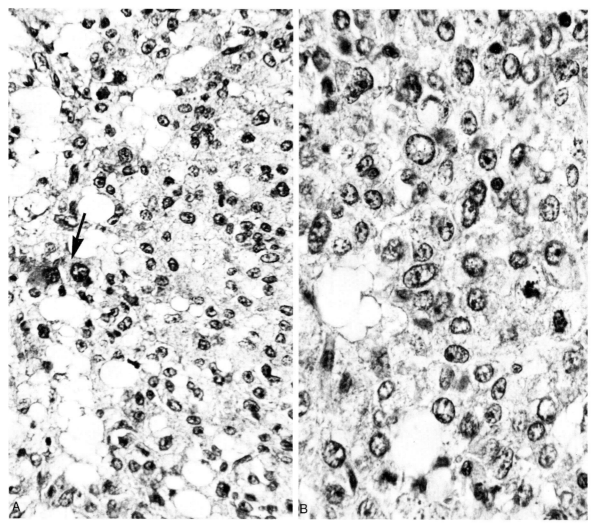

Figure 53–23. (*A*) Round cell liposarcoma. Tumor cells with and without fat vacuoles are shown. Some tumor cell nuclei (arrow) are atypical and large. (*B*) Closer view shows round to oval tumor cells with some variability in size and shape of nuclei. Cytoplasm is granular with ill-defined borders. Small fat vacuoles are seen in some cells.

differentiated tumors tend to recur locally before there is evidence of distant metastases. Indeed, metastases from a well-differentiated liposarcoma are extremely rare. Metastases from the other liposarcomas are usually via the blood stream, with the lungs being the most commonly involved site. Lymph nodes are only rarely involved. Of the 35 patients with head and neck liposarcomas listed by Baden and Newman, 10 were lost to follow-up. In the remaining 25 cases, two patients died of causes unrelated to their tumor at 15 months and 3 years after therapy; 14 patients died of their tumor; 8 were alive with tumor. In the eight patients free of tumor, six had a "well-differentiated myxoid" type and two had a mixed liposarcoma. The patient alive with tumor also had a well-differentiated myxoid tumor.[288] In Saunder's review, six of seven patients with well-differentiated liposarcomas were alive and free of tumor, as were three of seven with myxoid liposarcomas, two of four with round cell, and one of two with pleomorphic liposarcomas. Those liposarcomas located outside the neck area had a poor prognosis.[302]

Surgical therapy remains the main form of treatment, although postoperative radiation therapy may be beneficial, especially for the well-differentiated and myxoid variants that appear to respond best to such therapy.[291, 294]

RHABDOMYOMA

Rhabdomyoma of the soft tissue is a benign tumor that accounts for only 1 to 2 per cent of tumors with skeletal muscle differentiation, the remainder being rhabdomyosarcomas.[313] Rhabdomyomas are uncommon, with less than 100 cases being reported in the literature.[314, 318] During the years 1970 to 1977, Myhre-Jensen encountered 1331 benign soft-tissue tumors, none of which were rhabdomyomas.[37] Konrad and coworkers had only one rhabdomyoma among 5844 soft-tissue tumors diagnosed in the interval 1960 to 1969.[323] Despite this rarity, rhabdomyomas are discussed here not only because they have a predilection to occur in the head and neck but also because they must be differentiated from the more common, and more clinically significant, rhabdomyosarcoma that also occurs frequently in the head and neck.

The glycogen-containing lesion of the heart, also designated as "rhabdomyoma," is most likely a hamartoma and bears no relationship to the tumors described here. The cardiac lesion is associated with the tuberous sclerosis syndrome, but the soft-tissue rhabdomyoma is not.[325]

Rhabdomyomas are divided into two histologic forms, the adult and fetal varieties, the latter only recently well described.[313] Roughly an equal number of cases of each have been reported. In a 1980 review, di Sant'Agnese and Knowles[314] listed 25 patients previously reported with adult rhabdomyomas and 28 with fetal rhabdomyomas, the latter including eight patients with vulvovaginal lesions, which some consider to be different from the usual soft-tissue rhabdomyomas.[319, 323] These authors added 15 new cases, three adult and 12 fetal tumors, four of which were vulvovaginal tumors.[314] Konrad and associates reviewed the literature in 1982 and found 49 published cases of the adult form, 33 of the fetal type, and 16 genital tract fetal rhabdomyomas.

This tabulation did not include the new cases added by di Sant'Agnese and Knowles. They added five new cases—two adult, two fetal, and one genital tract fetal tumor.[323]

Adult rhabdomyoma occurs principally in patients with a mean age between 50 and 55 years.[310, 314, 320, 323, 329, 333] The mean age of the 28 patients with adult rhabdomyoma reported by di Sant'Agnese and Knowles, 26 of whom had head and neck lesions, was 52 years (range of 8 to 82 years). Twenty of the patients (71 per cent) were older than 40 years, and only two (7 per cent) were younger than age 20. Nineteen of the 26 head and neck rhabdomyomas were in patients over age 40.[314]

Fetal rhabdomyoma occurs over a broader age span than the adult type, from newborns to patients over age 60.[314, 320, 323] However, the patients are usually younger than those with adult rhabdomyomas, with a mean age of 22 to 26 years.[314, 323] Excluding the patients listed by di Sant'Agnese and Knowles with female genital tract rhabdomyoma, whose mean age was 38.1 years (range of 8 to 52 years), only seven of 28 (25 per cent) fetal rhabdomyomas occurred in patients over age 40, and 17 of 28 (60.7 per cent) were in patients 20 years of age or younger. Thirteen of the patients (46.4 per cent) were 3 years of age or younger. Among the 22 patients who had head and neck tumors, six were older than age 40 (27.2 per cent); 12 (54.5 per cent) were age 20 or less; and nine (40.9 per cent) were 3 years of age or younger.[314]

Adult rhabdomyoma is found four to five times more frequently in male patients as compared with female patients. Approximately 80 per cent of the patients with adult rhabdomyoma (23 of 28) listed by di Sant'Agnese and Knowles were males.[314] Almost an equal number of male and female patients with fetal rhabdomyoma have been reported; however, this includes women with genital tract lesions. If these are excluded, there is a male prevalence in fetal rhabdomyomas and it is similar to that in the adult variety, and this also holds true for fetal rhabdomyomas of the head and neck.[314]

Adult rhabdomyomas occur almost exclusively in the head and neck.[314] In the review by Konrad and associates, only three of 49 reported cases arose outside the head and neck area.[323] The most common sites include the pharynx (including the nasopharynx, oropharynx, and hypopharynx), larynx, soft tissues of the neck, and intraoral sites including the lip, tongue, base of tongue, submandibular and sublingual areas, floor of mouth, tonsil, soft palate, buccal mucosa, and orbit.[307–311, 314–318, 321–323, 325–337] In contrast to the common occurrence of rhabdomyosarcoma in the orbit, Knowles and Jakobiec reported the first documented example of orbital rhabdomyoma in 1975, and rejected, as undocumented, five previously reported cases.[322] Few rhabdomyomas have actually been found within skeletal muscle such as the sternocleidomastoid and sternohyoid muscles.[321, 327] A total of eight multicentric adult rhabdomyomas have been reported. These may be simultaneous or may develop asynchronously several years apart. All these multicentric lesions have been in the head and neck and were found in patients older than 50 years, all but one of whom have been men.[318, 328]

Fetal rhabdomyomas are also principally found in the head and neck, but as stated above, they also occur in the female genital region.[25, 313, 314, 329] Excluding these, between 70 and 75 per cent of fetal rhabdomyomas are in the head and neck,[314, 319] with other sites including the axilla, chest wall, stomach, anus, abdominal wall, and thigh.[310, 312–314, 319, 323, 324] Within the head and neck, the posterior auricular region is the commonest location; other sites include the orbit, nose, tongue, soft palate, base of tongue, parotid region, larynx, and nasopharynx. Rare examples of multicentric fetal rhabdomyomas are also reported.[312, 313]

Rhabdomyomas are slowly growing lesions that may be present for many years, some patients having noted a mass for up to 50 years.[307, 314, 321, 325, 328] Labeling studies by Scrivner and Meyer suggest that it would take approximately 10 years for a rhabdomyoma to reach 1.0 cm, confirming the long clinical history given by some patients.[329]

Grossly, the adult form appears to be well circumscribed or even encapsulated,[312] but the fetal type may be less well defined and may even appear infiltrative.[14, 313, 314, 320, 322] The adult variety varies from a few millimeters to tumors up to 15 cm,[307, 314, 323, 333] whereas fetal rhabdomyomas tend to be somewhat smaller, ranging from 1.5 to 8.0 cm.[313, 314]

Histologically, the adult tumor is more easily recognized. It consists of a uniform aggregation of large oval to round cells that have an abundant granular eosino-philic cytoplasm that contains an abundant amount of glycogen that causes it to be vacuolated in routine sections, creating spider-web cells.[14, 311, 325] Nuclei are uniform and either centrally or eccentrically located (Fig. 53–24). Intracytoplasmic crystalline-like or rod-shaped bodies are also found.[311, 314, 320, 321, 325] Electron microscopic studies have shown these to be hypertrophic Z-band material that resembles that seen in nemaline myopathy. Thick and thin myofilaments and large mitochondria are also found.[14, 307–309, 311, 323, 332, 334, 337] Despite the apparent mature differentiation of the cells, cross striations are difficult to find, but a careful search will yield at least some cells with striations. Mitotic figures are rare. Owing to the granularity of their cytoplasm, these cells have been confused with those of granular cell myoblastoma. However, the cells of this latter tumor lack cross striations, and although they contain intracytoplasmic PAS-positive material, this is diastase-resistant and not glycogen. They also lack the thick and thin myofilaments of skeletal muscle cells.[309, 311, 325] The cells of granular cell myoblastoma also stain positively with antibodies to S-100 protein, while those of rhabdomyoma do not.[38, 171, 177]

Fetal rhabdomyomas are histologically less uniform than the adult tumors. They tend to arise in the subcutaneous tissue or within the superficial soft tis-

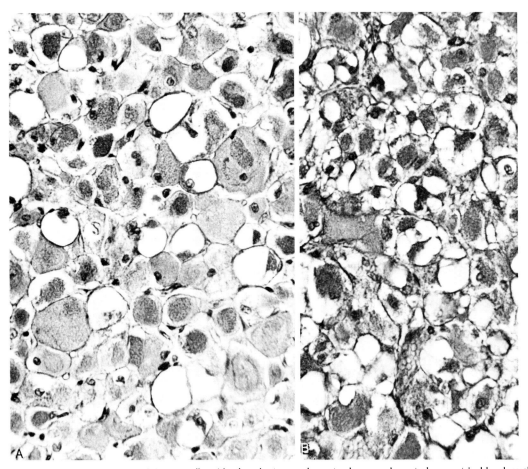

Figure 53–24. Adult rhabdomyoma. (*A*) Large cells with abundant granular cytoplasm and central eccentric bland nuclei. Cross striations are not present. (*B*) Another field from adult rhabdomyoma. Cells have highly vacuolated cytoplasm due to the presence of abundant cytoplasmic glycogen.

sues.[312, 313] They are composed of immature-appearing skeletal muscle fibers, in various stages of differentiation, mixed with mesenchymal-type cells that vary from small oval to round cells to larger cells with bipolar tapering cytoplasmic extensions.[312-314] Cross striations are present, but, like the adult form, the number of cells with striations varies considerably. The most mature cells are found at the periphery of the lesion.[313] Both cell types are loosely arranged in bands that are haphazardly arranged within a myxoid stroma that contains hyaluronic acid and gives the lesion an overall "edematous" appearance.[313, 314] Mitoses are scarce. di Sant'Agnese and Knowles divide fetal rhabdomyomas into two groups—a "fetal myxoid" type, which is the same as the tumor originally described by Dehner and Enzinger,[313] and a "fetal cellular" variant. They found a total of four such cellular tumors among the 28 fetal rhabdomyomas in the literature, and six of their own 15 new cases were of this type. In this variety, the myxoid stroma is either lacking or sparse, and there is a preponderance of thin, elongate spindle cells that are arranged in a herringbone or palisading pattern.[314] Mild nuclear pleomorphism may be seen in the cells of this cellular form. Occasional ribbon- and strap-shaped cells are also present, but cross striations are difficult to find. Gardner and Corio question whether the myxoid stroma must be present in the so-called "fetal myxoid" variant and feel that there are cases, one of which they report, in which the patterns of both forms of fetal rhabdomyoma blend with each other.[319]

Few cases of fetal rhabdomyoma have been studied by electron microscopy, but the cells of these tumors also show skeletal muscle differentiation, as in the adult form[312, 313, 323]; however, they lack the Z-band hypertrophy seen in the latter.[134]

Although adult rhabdomyoma is histologically easily separated from rhabdomyosarcoma, the fetal variety may be confused with this malignant tumor. Indeed, as suggested by Dehner and Enzinger,[313] this distinction may be quite "subtle." The superficial location of rhabdomyoma, versus the usually deeply situated rhabdomyosarcoma; the lack of necrosis and significant cell pleomorphism; the maturation of the tumor cells toward the periphery; and the scarcity of mitotic activity are all points in favor of the diagnosis of rhabdomyoma.[14, 312-314]

Local recurrences of adult rhabdomyoma are rare after excision,[310, 311, 317, 322, 323, 329, 336] but some patients have had several recurrences.[310, 336] Only one fetal rhabdomyoma has been reported to recur, and this tumor was located in the neck.[323] Metastases have never been reported from rhabdomyomas.

Dahl and coworkers believe that the fetal rhabdomyoma is in reality a malformation and is not a true tumor. This conclusion was based on their finding of two rhabdomyomas in a patient with the basal cell nevus syndrome.[312] Dehner and Enzinger, in their original description of fetal rhabdomyoma, also raised the possibility that it could be hamartomatous.[313]

RHABDOMYOSARCOMA

Within the past 10 to 15 years, rhabdomyosarcoma has been the sarcoma that has received the most clinical interest as evidenced by the extensive number of publications on the subject that have appeared during this time. Among the factors that contribute to this interest is the highly aggressive nature of rhabdomyosarcoma and its propensity to affect children and young adults, with all the emotional impact that such a situation engenders among physicians and parents alike. In addition, rhabdomyosarcoma is the sarcoma that has responded best to improved methods in radiation therapy and chemotherapy to the extent that its previous poor prognosis has been replaced by the hope that the majority of patients may now be cured.[403] The various reports from the Intergroup Rhabdomyosarcoma Study group (IRS) that are referred to in this chapter serve as models of what a cooperative effort among pathologists, surgeons, radiation therapists, and oncologists can accomplish.

Rhabdomyosarcoma is the commonest sarcoma in children, accounting for approximately one half of the malignant soft-tissue tumors in this group and 4 to 8 per cent of all malignant lesions in those younger than 15 years.[342, 377, 380, 381, 403] Overall, rhabdomyosarcoma accounts for 8 to 20 per cent of sarcomas in patients of all ages.[59, 63, 369, 379-381, 400, 403]

There are four principal histologic varieties of rhabdomyosarcoma—embryonal, botryoid, alveolar, and pleomorphic. The botryoid variety, however, is only a variant of embryonal rhabdomyosarcoma with a characteristic gross appearance.[365] Because the embryonal, botryoid, and alveolar tumors occur predominantly in children, while the pleomorphic tumor is most common in elderly adults, the general term "juvenile rhabdomyosarcoma" has been used by some to designate the former three tumors, and "adult rhabdomyosarcoma" has been used as a synonym for the pleomorphic tumors.[47, 341] However, although it is true that these tumors are more common in certain age groups, any one of them may occur in patients of any age.

Approximately two thirds of patients with childhood rhabdomyosarcoma are younger than 10 years of age.[403] At the AFIP, the median age for 440 patients with embryonal rhabdomyosarcoma was 8 years and for 118 patients with alveolar rhabdomyosarcoma, it was 16 years.[14] Of the 95 patients with juvenile rhabdomyosarcomas reported by Bale and associates, 86 per cent were less than age 8; the average age was 4.5 years.[341] In the series of 75 rhabdomyosarcomas analyzed by Mahour and coworkers, the average age was 5.8 years.[377] Most reported age figures for rhabdomyosarcoma are influenced by the preponderance of the embryonal tumors that account for approximately two thirds of all rhabdomyosarcomas and usually occur in patients younger than age 10 years.[14, 379] Alveolar rhabdomyosarcoma tends to occur in slightly older patients, with a mean age of 15 to 20 years.[353] Less than 10 per cent of the pleomorphic rhabdomyosarcoma are in children[369]; the mean age for this rhabdomyosarcoma is 50 to 55 years.[365, 391] Newborns account for 2 to 3 per cent of patients with rhabdomyosarcoma.[14]

Males account for roughly 55 to 70 per cent of patients.[341, 350, 358, 359, 367, 391] In the IRS group, the male-to-female ratios are from 1.27 to 1.47:1.[384, 403] In some reports, however, there were no significant sex differences.[358, 366] Black patients may be less commonly affected than white patients.[350, 358, 367, 379, 389, 392]

The distribution of tumor types depends on the anatomic region involved. In children, the head and neck accounts for 30 to 50 per cent of cases, whereas the genitourinary tract and the extremities each account for about 20 per cent of the total.[342, 381, 403, 404] Within the head and neck region, embryonal rhabdomyosarcoma is most common,[349, 350, 367, 381, 389, 392, 411] whereas alveolar and pleomorphic tumors are more common in the extremities.[353, 355, 369, 375, 400]

In the IRS, 57 per cent of the rhabdomyosarcomas were embryonal, 19 per cent were alveolar, 6 per cent were botryoid, and 1 per cent were pleomorphic.[361] These figures closely parallel the distribution noted at the AFIP, an institution that has a large number of consultation cases involving patients of all ages. Here, 69 per cent of the rhabdomyosarcomas were embryonal, 19 per cent were alveolar, and 11 per cent were pleomorphic.[313] In addition to the classic varieties of rhabdomyosarcoma, the IRS distinguished a special group of tumors, called type I and II, that histologically resemble extraskeletal Ewing's sarcoma.[361] These accounted for about 7 per cent of the total tumors accessioned. Finally, another 10 per cent of the cases consisted of undifferentiated mesenchymal tumors that did not fit within the other categories and were called "type undeterminate." In other reports, such tumors have been called "sarcoma of undetermined histogenesis" and have accounted for slightly over 25 per cent of cases previously diagnosed as rhabdomyosarcoma.[364]

This points out the difficulty that may exist in the diagnosis of the "small cell" tumors, such as neuroblastoma, Ewing's sarcoma, and malignant lymphoma, that are prone to develop in children.[341, 406] Pathologists vary in the criteria they use to make a diagnosis of rhabdomyosarcoma. Some are quite liberal and diagnose almost any small cell undifferentiated tumor that occurs in a child as a rhabdomyosarcoma. Others are more stringent, insisting on the presence of skeletal maturation, with cross striations in the tumor cells, before they make the diagnosis. In the former situation many cases will be overdiagnosed and in the latter many will be underdiagnosed. Although the finding of cross striations in tumor cells in a malignant-appearing soft-tissue tumor is unequivocal evidence of rhabdomyosarcoma, whether or not a tumor is determined to have such cells very much depends upon the diligence and skill of the pathologist. An extensive search of many sections may be required before striated tumor cells are found.[402] Furthermore, the likelihood of misinterpretation of cytoplasmic artifacts for actual striations increases with the pathologist's desire to prove that the tumor is a rhabdomyosarcoma.[14]

The problem is highlighted by the figures from the literature, in which striated cells have been reported in 15 to 67 per cent of embryonal types, 23 to 50 per cent of alveolar types, and 7 to 100 per cent of the pleomorphic rhabdomyosarcomas.[14, 317, 341, 342, 368, 376, 379, 392] Such a wide range of results emphasizes not only the difficulty of finding striated cells in these tumors, even by experienced pathologists, but also that the diagnosis of rhabdomyosarcoma does not depend on the presence of such cells.[14, 349, 382, 391] The clinical situation, the location of the tumor, and the histologic pattern may be so characteristic that, given a tumor composed of cells with the proper features, a diagnosis of rhabdomyosarcoma may be made in the absence of striated cells. Electron

microscopic examination may be helpful in making a specific diagnosis in those situations in which the light microscopic diagnosis is in doubt.[344, 382] The presence of both the thick and thin myofilaments, myosin and actin, or actual Z-band material is diagnostic of skeletal muscle differentiation.[382, 386] However, even these studies may fail to provide the evidence needed for a diagnosis of rhabdomyosarcoma.[51, 364, 386] Owing to the inherent sampling problems associated with electron microscopy, the area of tumor that is most differentiated may be missed. Furthermore, the tumor cells may be so primitive that they do not contain morphologic features of skeletal muscle differentiation. In an electron microscopic study of 31 rhabdomyosarcomas, Mierau and Favara found 13 that contained specific morphologic features, either myofilaments or Z-bands, to establish a diagnosis. However, in 17 tumors even the most differentiated cells lacked specific myoblastic characteristics. In a survey of the literature, these authors found that in only about one half of the tumors considered to be rhabdomyosarcomas did electron microscopy verify the diagnosis.[382]

Immunohistochemical techniques are now being applied to the diagnosis of these tumors. The demonstration, by these methods, of such cell constituents as desmin, myosin, or myoglobin has allowed tumors to be categorized as having myogenous differentiation. Desmin, one of the cytoplasmic intermediate filaments, is present in both smooth and skeletal muscle fibers. In three cases of alveolar rhabdomyosarcoma, Miettinen and associates were able to demonstrate the presence of desmin despite the fact that the cells lacked myogenous features by electron microscopy.[383] Significantly, however, only some of the tumor cells stained. Altmannsberger and associates reported similar results in four cases of embryonal rhabdomyosarcoma as well as in one case of an undifferentiated sarcoma thought, by light microscopy, to probably represent a rhabdomyosarcoma. All five tumors stained for desmin.[338] Tsokos and associates reported the results in 23 rhabdomyosarcomas, 11 alveolar and 12 embryonal, immunologically stained for myosin, myoglobin, and several isoenzymes.[407] Myosin was found in a higher percentage of the tumors, being present in all 11 alveolar lesions and 10 of the 12 embryonal lesions, whereas myoglobin was found in 10 of 11 alveolar tumors and five of the 11 embryonal tumors tested. Because myosin is also found in smooth muscle cells, myoglobin was considered to be the more specific marker for skeletal muscle differentiation. Mukai and associates also found myoglobin in rhabdomyosarcomas and noted that even in positive cases not all tumor cells stained.[388] Of 65 childhood rhabdomyosarcomas, 53 embryonal and 12 alveolar, Kahn and associates found myoglobin in 30 per cent of the embryonal and 67 per cent of the alveolar tumors versus the presence of striated cells in 23 per cent of the embryonal tumors and 33 per cent of the alveolar tumors.[368] Again, even in the positive cases, not all tumor cells could be stained. The presence or absence of staining was not correlated with the presence or absence of cells with cross striations, as some striated cells stained while others did not. In this study, there was positive immunologic staining for myoglobin, or electron microscopic evidence of skeletal muscle differentiation, in 16 of 25 embryonal rhabdomyosarcomas (64 per cent) and seven of nine alveolar rhabdomyosarcomas (78 per cent). Bale and associates reported similar findings.[341] Here, 11 of 12 rhabdomyosarcomas stained for myoglobin; the single exception was an embryonal rhabdomyosarcoma that contained striated cells. Eusebi and associates warn against the overinterpretation of the results of these immunohistochemical methods.[356] They found that some nonmyogenous tumor cells that infiltrated skeletal muscle, such as cells from breast carcinoma, melanoma, and lymphoma, also stained for myoglobin, as did other cells identified as histiocytes. These spurious results were thought to be due to nonspecific adsorption or ingestion of released myoglobin from the damaged normal muscle cells, or to represent some form of fixation artifact.

Mukai and associates have described the use of immunohistochemical methods to demonstrate Z-protein, a protein recently isolated by Japanese workers from skeletal muscle Z-bands, and which is an excellent marker for muscle differentiation.[387] Using immunoperoxidase techniques, 15 of 18 rhabdomyosarcomas (83 per cent) were positive for Z-protein (five of five pleomorphic tumors, seven of nine embryonal tumors, and three of four alveolar tumors). Of these 18 tumors, only four contained striated cells.

Embryonal Rhabdomyosarcoma

Embryonal rhabdomyosarcoma is the most common of the rhabdomyosarcomas and occurs mainly in children less than 12 years of age.[341, 358, 372, 403, 404] Embryonal rhabdomyosarcomas of the head and neck have the same age distribution as those that arise elsewhere in the body, with a mean patient age of from 4.5 to 8.0 years.[340, 350, 358, 367, 385, 392, 402] Adults are, however, occasionally affected.[350, 358, 379, 390] Approximately 10 per cent of the 170 rhabdomyosarcomas of the head and neck reviewed by Dito and Batsakis were in patients older than age 30.[350]

These tumors are quite cellular, with a nonspecific gross appearance of a soft, fleshy, gray-white and ill-defined mass that may contain areas of hemorrhage and necrosis.[358, 391, 392, 402] The most common locations are the head and neck region, the urogenital tract, and the retroperitoneum.[47, 342, 350, 354, 380, 403, 404] The extremities are not commonly involved,[14, 341, 354, 377] although in one series the extremities and shoulder girdle region were involved in 20 to 25 per cent of cases.[400] In general, adults with embryonal rhabdomyosarcoma more commonly have them in the extremities or trunk rather than in the head and neck.[376]

The botryoid variety of rhabdomyosarcoma grows beneath mucosal surfaces of hollow viscera or body cavities and forms edematous, smooth, polypoid masses that, as the name implies, have a grape-like appearance.[14, 47, 365, 391] This rhabdomyosarcoma is commonly found in the urogenital tract, common bile duct, and, in the head and neck, in the nasal cavity, paranasal sinuses, nasopharynx, and auditory canal.[14, 317, 341, 345, 349, 358, 365, 379, 393]

Most embryonal rhabdomyosarcomas have no direct association with skeletal muscle but arise instead from between muscle groups or directly from the deep connective tissue. For the most part, they grow rapidly, such that symptoms are usually present for less than 1 year,[350, 365, 367, 372, 385, 400, 402] although isolated cases have been encountered in which it is claimed that symptoms were present for several years.[379]

Histologically, embryonal rhabdomyosarcomas vary considerably, from very primitive-appearing lesions with virtually no evidence of muscle differentiation, to those tumors that contain numerous strap-shaped cells having cross striations.[14, 47, 364, 365, 391, 400] The overall pattern has been likened to the embryologic stage of normal muscle development found between the third and tenth weeks of gestation.[391] Most tumors consist of small, spindle-shaped cells with tapering bipolar cytoplasmic extensions, mixed with small, round to oval cells, which are not much larger than lymphocytes or small monocytes, with little or no visible cytoplasm. With further maturation, these latter cells accumulate an intensely eosinophilic cytoplasm (Fig. 53–25). Such "rhabdomyoblasts" may be scarce, but, if present, they are an

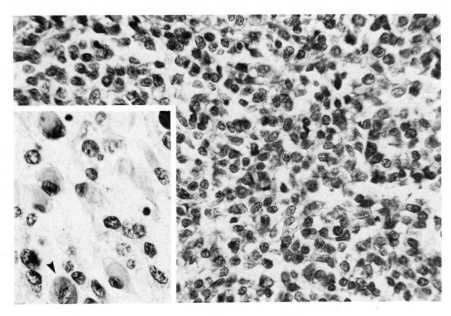

Figure 53–25. Embryonal rhabdomyosarcoma. Small, undifferentiated tumor cells with little or no visible cytoplasm. Inset shows larger tumor cells with abundant cytoplasm. These rhabdomyoblasts are helpful in identifying the tumor as a rhabdomyosarcoma. One of these cells contains cross striations (arrowhead).

important diagnostic feature. Trichrome stains may be helpful in locating these cells, as their cytoplasm will stain brightly with these stains.[14] Mitoses are common in embryonal rhabdomyosarcomas.

The tumor commonly has a loose myxoid matrix, which contains acid mucopolysaccharide, in which the tumor cells are widely dispersed. In some embryonal rhabdomyosarcomas, however, the tumor cells are closely packed, have spindle forms, and are arranged in fascicles or bands such that the tumor resembles a leiomyosarcoma or fibrosarcoma.[342] The cells, like those of all rhabdomyosarcomas, contain glycogen, although not every cell will stain using the PAS method. The cells located at the periphery of the tumor will most consistently stain for glycogen. The presence of cytoplasmic glycogen in small, oval to round tumor cells is similar to what is found in extraskeletal Ewing's sarcoma.[339] Indeed, by light microscopy and routine stains, the differential diagnosis between embryonal rhabdomyosarcoma and Ewing's sarcoma may be impossible to make.[363] Fortunately, this may only be an academic problem, as both tumors appear to respond to the same therapeutic measures with similar overall results.[401, 406] In general, striated cells are found in approximately one third of embryonal rhabdomyosarcomas, with reported figures from 15 to 60 per cent.[14, 317, 341, 365, 368, 372, 376, 379, 391, 392]

Some embryonal rhabdomyosarcomas have been termed "well-differentiated" because they contain numerous spindle-shaped or tubular cells with cross striations (Fig. 53–26).[392] Still others describe "pleomorphic" foci, within otherwise typical embryonal tumors, that contain cells with large, irregular, and atypical nuclei, as would be seen in an adult pleomorphic rhabdomyosarcoma.[14] In the botryoid rhabdomyosarcomas, there is an exaggeration of the myxoid matrix such that it comes to form the major component of the tumor. The central portions of these tumors are characteristically hypocellular, and there is a tendency of the tumor cells to aggregate in a narrow band at their periphery just beneath the overlying mucosa or body cavity lining (Fig. 53–27). This "cambium layer" is distinctive to this form of rhabdomyosarcoma.[14, 47, 365]

Alveolar Rhabdomyosarcoma

This variety of rhabdomyosarcoma tends to occur in somewhat older patients than do embryonal rhabdomyosarcomas, with the mean patient age being between 15 and 20 years. Although occasionally also found in older adults, it is rare after age 50.[14, 25, 353, 355, 391] Unlike the embryonal tumor, alveolar rhabdomyosarcoma is more commonly located in the extremities and not infrequently arises within skeletal muscle.[353, 355, 400] The tumor accounts for from 3 to 21 per cent of all rhabdomyosarcomas.[341, 361, 365, 368] The head and neck region has been involved in 2 to 20 per cent of cases.[25, 317, 340, 350, 355, 361, 367, 378, 379, 389, 392]

In its fully developed form, alveolar rhabdomyosarcoma is histologically characterized by tumor cells arranged in ill-defined groups or nests separated by fibrous bands. Within the center of these nests, the cells are loosely cohesive, forming spaces which, under low-power microscopic examination, mimic pulmonary alveolar spaces (Fig. 53–28).[14, 353, 355, 364] The peripheral cells of these nests rest upon the fibrous trabeculae, being attached by tapered strands of cytoplasm. Free-floating tumor cells, 15 to 30 μm in diameter, are found within the alveolar spaces, along with smaller cells similar to those in embryonal rhabdomyosarcoma. Large, multinucleated giant cells, up to 200 μm in diameter, with a wreath-like arrangement of their nuclei and a granular eosinophilic cytoplasm, are also commonly found floating within these spaces. In other portions of the tumor, the cells may be either compact or loosely arranged but without evidence of space formation, creating regions indistinguishable from embryonal rhabdomyosarcoma. Strap-shaped and tadpole-shaped rhabdomyoblasts, and spider-web cells produced by cytoplasmic vacuolization, may also be found in these tumors but are less common than in the embryonal form. Striated cells are

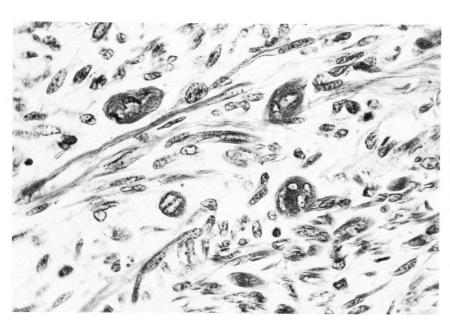

Figure 53–26. Embryonal rhabdomyosarcoma. In this area there has been further differentiation with long spindle cells containing cross striations. Other oval to round rhabdomyoblasts with cross striations are also present.

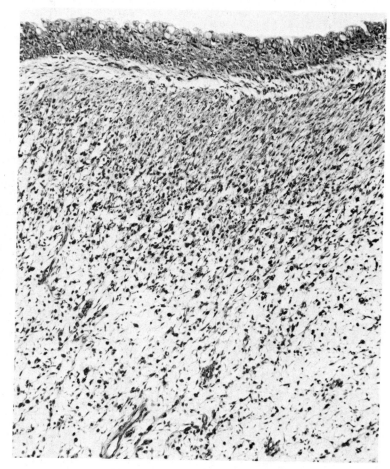

Figure 53–27. Botryoid rhabdomyosarcoma. Note concentration of tumor cells beneath the overlying mucosa (top), creating the cambium-layer characteristic of this tumor. Central portion of the tumor shows separation of the cells by the myxoid matrix.

found in about 30 per cent of cases but may be difficult to find.[14, 25, 353, 355, 368] Mitotic figures are usually plentiful.

As would be expected from their microscopic description, rhabdomyosarcomas are found that contain varying proportions of both alveolar and embryonal patterns.[25, 341, 353] Such tumors are either diagnosed as mixed rhabdomyosarcomas or designated by the preponderant pattern.

Pleomorphic Rhabdomyosarcoma

This rhabdomyosarcoma, which is uncommon in the head and neck area,[10, 369, 389] was formerly considered to be the most common rhabdomyosarcoma. However, with the increasing awareness by pathologists of the histologic parameters of both the embryonal and alveolar types, pleomorphic rhabdomyosarcoma is now the least frequent of the rhabdomyosarcomas. Furthermore, many pleomorphic tumors previously diagnosed as rhabdomyosarcoma probably are examples of malignant fibrous histiocytoma,[409] a tumor that frequently has a pleomorphic and anaplastic microscopic appearance and that occurs in similar patients, namely elderly adults,[369, 375, 391] and in similar locations, the extremities, as does pleomorphic rhabdomyosarcoma.[14, 25, 409] The diagnosis of pleomorphic rhabdomyosarcoma should be restricted to those tumors in which cells show unequivocal cross

striations, contain myoglobin, or by electron microscopy show thick and thin myofilaments or Z-bands.[409] Because this tumor arises within large muscle groups in the extremities,[10, 47, 354, 369, 375] care must be exercised not to confuse degenerating and abnormal-appearing muscle cells, which still retain their striations, with actual tumor cells. If pleomorphic rhabdomyosarcoma actually exists, it is a rare tumor.[409]

Based on older descriptions, these tumors are composed of numerous anaplastic cells, many with irregular bizarre configurations.[369, 375] Numerous large, multinucleated tumor giant cells, which have a bright eosinophilic glassy cytoplasm, are present. Tadpole-shaped, racquet-shaped, and strap-shaped cells are seen. Mitotic figures are common, many of which have abnormal shapes, and necrosis is common. Striated cells are reported in the literature in 7 to 100 per cent of cases.[341, 365, 369, 375]

As alluded to in the discussion of embryonal rhabdomyosarcoma, juvenile rhabdomyosarcomas tend to mimic the embryologic development of striated muscle, which originates from a proliferation of undifferentiated mesenchymal cells.[386, 391] As such cells may be located anywhere in the soft tissues, this helps explain the occurrence of rhabdomyosarcoma, in areas of the body where skeletal muscle is not normally found, such as the bladder, middle ear, prostate, bile ducts, and brain

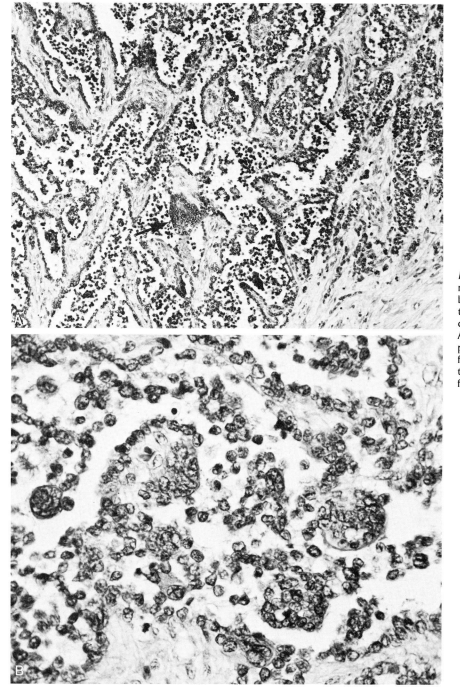

Figure 53–28. Alveolar rhabdomyosarcoma. (*A*) Spaces, formed by thick fibrous septa, are lined by tumor cells. Free-floating tumor cells are noted within the spaces. A large multinucleated tumor cell is present (arrow). (*B*) Higher magnification shows small, undifferentiated tumor cells arranged along fibrous septa and within the spaces.

as well as the occurrence of tumor cells with skeletal muscle differentiation in heterologous tumors of the uterus and kidney.[10, 14, 399]

In the head and neck region, the orbit is the single most common site for these tumors. Of 246 rhabdomyosarcomas of the head and neck at the AFIP, 44.3 per cent were located in the orbit, and this site accounted for almost 20 per cent of all rhabdomyosarcomas on file, being second only to paratesticular lesions in occurrence. The remaining head and neck rhabdomyosarcomas involved the nasal cavity, nasopharynx, palate, mouth, and pharynx in 29.7 per cent; the paranasal sinuses, cheek, and neck in 19.1 per cent; and the ear and mastoid in 6.9 per cent.[14] In a more detailed survey of the nonorbital rhabdomyosarcomas at the AFIP, Feldman lists 32 in the nasal cavity, 16 in the paranasal sinus, 16 in the nasopharynx, 12 in the ear, three in the larynx, two in the pharynx, two in the soft palate, and one in the tonsil.[358] In other series, the incidence of orbital involvement has varied from 10 to 47 per cent of those within the head and neck.[10, 341, 350, 374, 377, 379, 381, 385, 389, 403]

Although the orbit is a common site for rhabdomyosarcoma, in overall incidence such tumors make up only a small portion of all orbital tumors. At Columbia University, New York, they accounted for only 3 per cent of the total orbital tumors on file,[367] and Porterfield and Zimmerman found only 55 orbital rhabdomyosarcomas in 1000 orbital tumors accessioned at the AFIP.[392] In Das Gupta's list of nonorbital sites, the most common locations were the nasopharynx, involved in 19 per cent; the nose in 17 per cent; and the parotid and mandibular regions in 8 per cent each.[10] Of the 88 cases in the head and neck reported by Masson and Soule, the commonest sites were the orbit, involved in 22 cases, the nasopharynx (in 15), the nose (in 14), and the antrum (in seven).[379] In the review by Dito and Batsakis of 170 rhabdomyosarcomas of the head and neck, the orbit and eyelids were involved in 54 cases; the soft tissues of the face, neck, and temple in 40; intraoral, intranasal, and pharyngeal sites in 49 (nasopharynx 16, tongue 12, palate/uvula 12, hypopharynx 3, tonsil 3); the ear/mastoid and maxillary sinus in 15; and 12 cases distributed in the mandible, salivary gland, and occipital regions.[350] Of 38 head and neck childhood rhabdomyosarcomas reported from the Mayo Clinic, 11 involved the nasopharynx; 11 the soft tissues, presumably of the neck; six were in the nose; four in the orbit; two each in the tonsil and tongue; and one each in the larynx and antrum.[377] In a recent series of 95 juvenile rhabdomyosarcomas, which included 33 in the head and neck, the orbit was involved in 14, the eyelid in four, the nose in four, the nasopharynx in three, the palate in one, the neck, salivary gland, cheek, and lip in four, and the ear, mastoid, and mandible in three cases.[341]

In the head and neck, embryonal rhabdomyosarcoma is the commonest rhabdomyosarcoma, accounting for approximately 75 per cent of cases. Of the 155 head and neck rhabdomyosarcomas in the IRS, 114 (73.5 per cent) were embryonal, 18 (11.6 per cent) were alveolar, six were botryoid (3.9 per cent), 14 were "undifferentiated" (9.0 per cent), and three were type I or II lesions (1.9 per cent). Of their 55 orbital tumors, 44 (80 per cent) were embryonal, three (5.5 per cent) were alveolar, seven were "undifferentiated" (12.7 per cent), and one was a type I or II lesion (1.8 per cent).[361] Pleomorphic rhabdomyosarcomas are uncommon in the head and neck.[10, 341, 345, 361, 365, 367, 369, 379, 389, 411] In the report by Newman and Rice of 26 head and neck rhabdomyosarcomas, 21 were embryonal, four were alveolar, and only one was pleomorphic.[389] Of the 204 cases of pleomorphic rhabdomyosarcoma reported by Keyhani and Booher, only 15 (7.4 per cent) were in the head and neck.[369] This distribution of rhabdomyosarcoma tumor types in the head and neck is that which is generally noted, with minor variations, regardless of the specific anatomic location, such as the ear, nasopharynx, or larynx.[317, 343, 345, 347, 349, 352, 366, 378, 411]

Li and Fraumeni found some evidence of a familial association of malignancies in patients with rhabdomyosarcomas.[373] They found a higher incidence of soft-tissue sarcomas in siblings of these patients, as well as a higher incidence of breast cancer and other tumors, which tended to occur at a young age, in their relatives. An increased incidence of brain tumors and adrenocortical carcinoma has also been noted by others in relatives of those with rhabdomyosarcomas, as well as a purported incidence of rhabdomyosarcoma in patients with neurofibromatosis.[380, 384]

Patients with head and neck rhabdomyosarcomas demonstrate a variety of presenting symptoms that are dependent on the anatomic location of the tumors. Patients with orbital tumors almost always have exophthalmos that is of rapid onset and progressive.[350, 367, 392] Middle ear tumors may manifest as otitis media with pain and ear drainage, at times bloody, or the presence of granulation-type tissue or polyp in the external auditory canal.[347, 350, 352, 366, 379, 397] Nasal and nasopharyngeal tumors may cause breathing difficulty, nasal stuffiness or nasal bleeding.[317, 345] Polypoid masses may be found in these locations.[393] Neurologic symptoms, including facial nerve paralysis, may be produced by lesions arising in the mastoid and nasopharynx.[360] The duration of symptoms is usually less than 1 year, most less than 6 months.[350, 365, 385, 389, 402] In the series reported by Masson and Soule, only six of 88 patients had symptoms for longer than 1 year; one patient had symptoms for 5½ years.[379]

The IRS developed a clinical grouping or staging classification that is both simple and useful in coordinating reports and end results from various institutions. This consists of four groups and is based on the extent of the tumor and whether or not it is totally resected.[380, 381] Patients in group I are those with localized tumors that are completely resected; group II includes patients whose tumors have been completely resected grossly but in whom there is microscopic residue; group III contains patients in whom gross tumor is still present after resection, or in whom only a biopsy is done; and group IV is used to designate patients with distant metastases. It should be emphasized that the group in which a patient is placed may very much depend on the aggressiveness, or lack of it, of the surgeon. For instance, a patient with an orbital tumor for which a resection is done may be placed into group I or II. However, if the surgeon decides only to biopsy the tumor and treat the patient with chemotherapy and radiation therapy, such a patient would be categorized as a group III patient. Despite this potential for variability, survival correlates with this clinical grouping;

group I patients have the best prognosis, and those in group IV have the least favorable outlook. In reported series, roughly 15 per cent of patients are in group I, 25 per cent are in group II, 40 per cent are in group III, and 20 per cent are in group IV.[380, 403]

In the past, rhabdomyosarcoma carried an extremely poor prognosis, with usually only 10 to 15 per cent of patients surviving,[342, 377, 379, 391, 403, 405] although some reports indicated better survival rates of about 30 to 35 per cent, depending upon the type of rhabdomyosarcoma involved.[359, 369, 404] Alveolar rhabdomyosarcoma had the worst prognosis, with a 5-year survival rate of only 5 per cent and most patients dying within a year of diagnosis.[353-355, 379, 400, 404] Embryonal rhabdomyosarcoma had a slightly better prognosis with 5-year survival rates of 10 to 20 per cent.[354, 372, 400] Pleomorphic rhabdomyosarcomas had a better prognosis than the childhood cases, with 5-year survival rates of approximately 30 to 35 per cent.[354, 369, 375]

This overall poor prognosis applied equally to rhabdomyosarcomas of the head and neck, with the exception of the orbital tumors, which tended to remain localized, had a lower rate of local recurrence, and a relatively low incidence of lymph node metastases.[350, 371, 380, 381, 395, 404] In the review by Dito and Batsakis, local recurrence developed in 85 of 116 patients (73.3 per cent) with nonorbital head and neck rhabdomyosarcomas but in only 25 of 54 (46.3 per cent) with orbital tumors. Twelve of the patients with orbital tumors were alive for longer than 3 years. The overall 3-year survival rate in their patients was 15.8 per cent, but the 5-year survival rate was only 5.9 per cent. The average survival for all patients was 16.6 months.[350] Of the 37 patients with embryonal rhabdomyosarcomas of the head and neck analyzed by Moore and Grossi, 92 per cent died.[385] In Porterfield and Zimmerman's study of 33 orbital tumors, 20 patients died and nine were alive from 3 to 15 years,[392] and in the series of 34 orbital tumors reported by Ashton and Morgan, 16 patients died, five others were alive with tumor, five were lost to follow-up, and eight were alive and free of tumor.[340] At the Mayo Clinic, 69 of the 88 patients with head and neck rhabdomyosarcomas died, eight were alive and free of tumor, one was alive with tumor, and 10 were lost to follow-up. Almost one half of those who died did so within 1 year.[379]

Most patients who die of rhabdomyosarcoma do so within 2 years; thus, survival beyond this time is a good indication of potential cure.[379, 380, 388] Distant metastases, especially to the lungs, liver, bones, and the central nervous system are common in those who die.[350, 365, 380] The incidence figures for lymph node metastases from head and neck primary tumors have been widely disparate. Although the IRS reported that only 3 per cent of their patients had positive lymph nodes at the time of diagnosis,[370, 371, 380] other studies have reported a much greater incidence of nodal involvement, with figures up to 36 per cent.[10, 351, 374, 379, 389] The reason for this dramatic difference is not clear.

The poor survival statistics noted previously have dramatically changed since the introduction and use of radiation therapy and multidrug chemotherapy for treatment so that survival figures in the 85 to 95 per cent range are now being reported. Prognosis has been found to depend less upon tumor type than on its extent,[341, 342, 351, 361, 389] with the possible exception of the so-called "solid variant" of alveolar rhabdomyosarcoma.[408] An analysis of 36 patients with poor survival reported from the National Cancer Institute found that 27 of the 36 patients had alveolar tumors. A histologic solid variant, identified by these authors, was characterized by a poor prognosis and advanced stage.[408]

Radical and mutilating surgery for the treatment of head and neck rhabdomyosarcoma has been largely replaced by the use of radiation and chemotherapy. Surgical therapy is used to excise small, readily accessible tumors or to reduce tumor bulk.[380] This is followed by intense treatment with the other two treatment modalities.[396] Chemotherapy itself can reduce tumor size to an extent that a large nonresectable tumor may become amenable to resection.[357]

An important finding of the IRS was the fact that tumors originating in so-called parameningeal sites, which include the ear and mastoid, nasopharynx, paranasal sinuses, and parapharyngeal areas, have a propensity to extend into the central nervous system.[362, 394, 398, 405] Tefft and associates reported that in 57 tumors originating in these areas, 20 (35 per cent) developed meningeal extension that, despite therapy, is almost uniformly fatal.[362, 405] Proper therapy for these parameningeal tumors is still in the process of being defined.

The most recent overall survival data from the IRS give projected survival rates for patients in group I as approximately 90 per cent; for those in group II as 70 to 75 per cent; for group III as 60 to 65 per cent; and for group IV 30 per cent. The overall 2-year tumor-free survival rate is estimated to be 54 per cent.[380] Sutow reported an 86 per cent 5-year survival rate for rhabdomyosarcomas of the head and neck treated with three-drug chemotherapy.[403] Raney and associates reported that orbital lesions still have the best prognosis, with a 77 per cent survival rate versus a 51 per cent survival for nonorbital head and neck lesions.[396] Nasopharyngeal, paranasal, and nasal tumors still have a poor prognosis, with an approximately 20 per cent survival rate.[317, 345, 349]

Similar poor survival is associated with rhabdomyosarcomas of the ear and mastoid. These tumors are not common, and there is no great experience in their management. In a 1972 review of rhabdomyosarcomas of the ear, Edland was able to find only 42 previously published cases.[352] Deutsch and Felder added five new cases in 1974 and reviewed 73 previous cases.[347] These rhabdomyosarcomas were highly aggressive. Deutsch and Felder had only five long-term survivors among the 78 patients in their report, and there was only one survivor among the 40 patients whose cases were reported by Jaffe and associates, the average survival time being 7.2 months.[366]

Raney and associates[397] studied 24 patients with aural rhabdomyosarcomas accessioned as part of the IRS group. These patients make up 12 per cent of the head and neck sarcomas and 4 per cent of the total IRS sarcomas. All the aural tumors were of embryonal or botryoid type. Patients were treated with radiation therapy and chemotherapy. Cranial nerve palsy, especially involving the facial nerve, was present at the time of diagnosis in 14 of the 22 (65 per cent) patients with available data. Fourteen patients died, 13 of their tumor; nine were alive and free of tumor for 2.2 to 6.5 years after diagnosis; and one patient was alive with local recurrence after 6.5 years. The median survival for those who died was 10 months (range of 5 to 25 months). These survival results were better than previously reported, but the high incidence of meningeal extension by these tumors is still a major obstacle to their adequate treatment.[347, 397]

Laryngeal rhabdomyosarcomas are quite rare. In their single case report in 1970, Batsakis and Fox accepted only five previous cases in the literature and concluded that rhabdomyosarcoma might be the least common sarcoma to affect the larynx.[343] Winther and Lorentzen added two further cases in 1978 and accepted only seven previous cases as being well documented.[411] Canalis and associates in 1976 found 24 cases in the literature, half of which occurred in children.[346] In a review in 1984, Diehn and coworkers added one case and analyzed five cases on file at the AFIP.[348] They also found 28 cases in the literature, only 15 of which were well documented. They concluded that rhabdomyosarcoma is the rarest laryngeal sarcoma. The patients ranged in age from the newborn period to 72 years, with the majority in the first two decades of life. Of the 21 tumors analyzed, 14 were embryonal, three were pleomorphic, two were alveolar, and two were botryoid. Of the 20 patients listed, nine died, two were lost to follow-up, and nine were alive without tumor from 8 months to 5 years after therapy, five for longer than 3 years. Canalis and associates thought that laryngeal rhabdomyosarcomas might have a slightly better prognosis than rhabdomyosarcomas at other sites in the head and neck.[346]

Another important finding that has emerged from the IRS is that the presence of metastases at the time of diagnosis, or the development of recurrence or metastases while the patient is on therapy, bodes for an extremely poor prognosis.[380, 389, 395, 403] Raney and associates reported relapse in 115 of 341 (33.7 per cent) IRS patients. Of the patients with remission who were treated, a second complete relapse was obtained in 37 per cent, but only 5.5 per cent remained tumor-free. Orbital lesions had the lowest rate of recurrence (11 per cent) versus 29 per cent for other head and neck tumors.[395] Wharam and associates estimate that the risk for relapse for lesions in the neck is six times higher than for other nonorbital and nonparameningeal tumors.[410] Of the patients with local recurrence in the head and neck reported by Newman and Rice, 82 per cent subsequently died of their disease.[389] Maurer and associates report a median survival of only 20 weeks for such patients.[380] Therefore, all possible attempts to eradicate and treat the primary tumor adequately are mandatory.

Although 2- and 5-year survival rates are now being reported, the longer term results are still to be determined. The long-term effects of these radiation and chemotherapy regimens, especially in young children, await future evaluation. However, that such questions are even asked is a tribute to the successful efforts made in the treatment of this aggressive and formerly highly fatal tumor.

REFERENCES

INTRODUCTION AND GENERAL INFORMATION

1. American Cancer Society: Cancer statistics, 1983. CA 33:9, 1983.
2. Benjamin RS, Baker LH, O'Bryan RM, et al: Advances in the chemotherapy of soft tissue sarcomas. Med Clin North Am 61:1039, 1977.
3. Benjamin RS, Baker LH, Rodriguez V, et al: The chemotherapy of soft tissue sarcomas in adults. *In* Management of Primary Bone and Soft Tissue Tumors. Chicago, Year Book Medical Publishers, 1977, pp 309–315.
4. Brooks JJ: Immunohistochemistry of soft tissue tumors: Myoglobin as a tumor marker for rhabdomyosarcoma. Cancer 50:1757, 1982.
5. Brooks JJ: Immunohistochemistry of soft tissue tumors: Progress and prospects. Hum Pathol 13:969, 1982.
6. Chang P: Management of soft tissue sarcomas: Current status. Am J Med Sci 273:244, 1977.
7. Coia LR, Fazekas JT, Kramer S: Postirradiation sarcoma of the head and neck: A report of three late sarcomas following therapeutic irradiation for primary malignancies of the paranasal sinus, nasal cavity, and larynx. Cancer 46:1982, 1980.
8. Costa J, Wesley RA, Glatstein E, et al: The grading of soft tissue sarcomas. Results of a clinicohistopathologic correlation in a series of 163 cases. Cancer 53:530, 1984.
9. Dahl I, Angervall L: Pseudosarcomatous lesions of the soft tissues reported as sarcoma during a 6-year period (1958–1963). Acta Pathol Microbiol Scand 85:917, 1977.
10. Das Gupta TK: Tumors of the Soft Tissues. Norwalk, Connecticut, Appleton-Century-Crofts, 1983.
11. Enjoji M, Hashimoto H: Diagnosis of soft tissue sarcomas. Pathol Res Pract 178:215, 1984.
12. Enterline HT: Histopathology of sarcomas. Semin Oncol 8:133, 1981.
13. Enzinger FM, Lattes R, Torloni H: Histological typing of soft tissue tumours. International Histological Classification of Tumors, No. 3. Geneva, World Health Organization, 1969.
14. Enzinger FM, Weiss SW: Soft Tissue Tumors. St. Louis, The C. V. Mosby Co., 1983.
15. Falini B, Taylor CR: New developments in immunoperoxidase techniques and their application. Arch Pathol Lab Med 107:105, 1983.
16. Farr HW: Soft Part sarcomas of the head and neck. Semin Oncol 8:185, 1981.
17. Ferrell HW, Frable WJ: Soft part sarcomas revisited. Cancer 30:475, 1972.
18. Fine G, Ohorodnik JM, Horn RC Jr: Soft-Tissue Sarcomas: Their Clinical Behavior and Course and Influencing Factors. Seventh National Cancer Conference Proceedings. Philadelphia, J. B. Lippincott Co., 1973, pp 873–882.
19. Gyorkey F, Min K-W, Krisko I, et al: The usefulness of electron microscopy in the diagnosis of human tumors. Hum Pathol 6:421, 1975.
20. Hajdu SI: Pathology of Soft Tissue Tumors. Philadelphia, Lea & Febiger, 1979.
21. Hajdu SI: Soft tissue sarcomas: Classification and natural history. CA 31:271, 1981.
22. Jaffe BF: Pediatric head and neck tumors: A study of 178 cases. Laryngoscope 83:1644, 1973.
23. Kaye GI: The futility of electron microscopy in determining the origin of poorly differentiated soft tissue tumors. Prog Surg Pathol 3:171, 1981.
24. Kindblom L-G, Angervall L: Histochemical characterization of mucosubstances in bone and soft tissue tumors. Cancer 36:985, 1975.
25. Lattes R, Enzinger FM: Soft Tissue Tumors. Proceedings of the thirty-ninth annual anatomic pathology slide seminar of The American Society of Clinical Pathologists, Chicago, 1973.
26. Lindberg RD, Martin RG, Romsdahl MM, et al: Conservative surgery and postoperative radiotherapy in 300 adults with soft-tissue sarcomas. Cancer 47:2391, 1981.
27. Mackay B: Electron microscopy of soft tissue tumors. *In* Management of Primary Bone and Soft Tissue Tumors. Chicago, Year Book Medical Publishers, 1977, pp 259–269.
28. Mackay B, Ordoñez NG: The role of the pathologist in the evaluation of poorly differentiated tumors. Semin Oncol 9:396, 1982.
29. Mackenzie DH: The myxoid tumors of somatic soft tissues. Am J Surg Pathol 5:443, 1981.

30. Management of Primary Bone and Soft Tissue Tumors. Chicago, Year Book Medical Publishers, 1977.
31. Mankin HJ, Lange TA, Spanier SS: The hazards of biopsy in patients with malignant primary bone and soft-tissue tumors. J Bone Joint Surg (Am) 64:1121, 1982.
32. Martin RG, Butler JJ, Albores-Saavedra J: Soft tissue tumors: Surgical treatment and results. *In* Tumors of Bone and Soft Tissue. Chicago, Year Book Medical Publishers, 1965, pp 333–366.
33. Martin RG, Lindberg RD, Sinkovics JG, et al: Soft tissue sarcomas. *In* Clark RL, Howe CD (eds): Cancer Patient Care at M.D. Anderson Hospital and Tumor Institute, The University of Texas. Chicago, Year Book Medical Publishers, 1976, pp 473–483.
34. Miettinen M, Foidart J-M, Ekblom P: Immunohistochemical demonstration of laminin, the major glycoprotein of basement membranes, as an aid in the diagnosis of soft tissue tumors. Am J Clin Pathol 79:306, 1983.
35. Miettinen M, Lehto V-P, Bradley RA, et al: Expression of intermediate filaments in soft-tissue sarcomas. Int J Cancer 30:541, 1982.
36. Mukai K, Rosai J: Applications of immunoperoxidase techniques in surgical pathology. Prog Surg Pathol I:15, 1980.
37. Myhre-Jensen O: A consecutive 7-year series of 1331 benign soft tissue tumours. Acta Orthoped Scand 52:287, 1981.
38. Nakajima T, Watanabe S, Sato Y, et al: An immunoperoxidase study of S-100 protein distribution in normal and neoplastic tissues. Am J Surg Pathol 6:715, 1982.
39. Osborn M, Weber K: Biology of disease. Tumor diagnosis by intermediate filament typing: A novel tool for surgical pathology. Lab Invest 48:372, 1983.
40. Presant CA, Lowenbraun S, Bartolucci AA, et al: Metastatic sarcomas: Chemotherapy with Adriamycin, cyclophosphamide, and methotrexate alternating with actinomycin D, DTIC, and vincristine. Cancer 47:457, 1981.
41. Rosai J: Ackerman's Surgical Pathology, 6th ed. St. Louis, The C. V. Mosby Co., 1981, pp 1407–1479.
42. Rosenberg SA, Tepper J, Glatstein E, et al: Prospective randomized evaluation of adjuvant chemotherapy in adults with soft tissue sarcomas of the extremities. Cancer 52:424, 1983.
43. Ross J, Hendrickson MR, Kempson RL: The problem of the poorly differentiated sarcoma. Semin Oncol 9:467, 1982.
44. Russell WO, Cohen J, Enzinger F, et al: A clinical and pathological staging system for soft tissue sarcomas. Cancer 40:1562, 1977.
45. Simon MA: Biopsy of musculoskeletal tumors. J Bone Joint Surg (Am) 64:1253, 1982.
46. Stern R: Current concepts in the diagnosis of human soft tissue sarcomas. Hum Pathol 12:777, 1981.
47. Stout AP, Lattes R: Tumors of the Soft Tissues. Atlas of Tumor Pathology, second series, fascicle I. Washington, D.C., Armed Forces Institute of Pathology, 1967.
48. Suit HD: Sarcoma of soft tissue. CA 28:284, 1978.
49. Sutow WW: Malignant Solid Tumors in Children. A Review. New York, Raven Press, 1981.
50. Taylor CR: Immunoperoxidase techniques. Practical and theoretical aspects. Arch Pathol Lab Med 102:113, 1978.
51. van Haelst, UJGM: General considerations on electron microscopy of tumors of soft tissues. Prog Surg Pathol 2:225, 1980.
52. Young JL Jr, Miller RW: Incidence of malignant tumors in U.S. children. J Pediatr 86:254, 1975.

FIBROSARCOMA

53. Balsaver AM, Butler JJ, Martin RG: Congenital firbrosarcoma. Cancer 20:1607, 1967.
54. Batsakis JG: Tumors of the Head and Neck. Clinical and Pathological Considerations. 2nd ed. Baltimore, Williams & Wilkins Co., 1979.
55. Chung EB, Enzinger FM: Infantile fibrosarcoma. Cancer 38:729, 1976.
56. Churg AM, Kahn LB: Myofibroblasts and related cells in malignant fibrous and fibrohistiocytic tumors. Hum Pathol 8:205, 1977.
57. Conley J, Stout AP, Healey WV: Clinicopathologic analysis of eighty-four patients with an original diagnosis of fibrosarcoma of the head and neck. Am J Surg 114:564, 1967.
58. Davies DG: Fibrosarcoma and pseudosarcoma of the larynx. J Laryngol Otol 83:423, 1969.
59. Enjoji M, Hashimoto H, Tsuneyoshi M, et al: Malignant fibrous histiocytoma. A clinicopathologic study of 130 cases. Acta Pathol Jpn 30:727, 1980.
60. Fu Y-S, Perzin KH: Nonepithelial tumors of the nasal cavity, paranasal sinuses, and nasopharynx. A clinicopathologic study. VI. Fibrous tissue tumors (fibroma, fibromatosis, fibrosarcoma). Cancer 37:2912, 1976.
61. Gonzalez-Crussi F, Wiederhold MD, Sotelo-Avila C: Congenital fibrosarcoma. Presence of a histiocytic component. Cancer 46:77, 1980.
62. Iwasaki H, Enjoji M: Infantile and adult fibrosarcomas of the soft tissues. Acta Pathol Jpn 29:377, 1979.
63. Krall RA, Kostianovsky M, Patchefsky AS: Synovial sarcoma. A clinical, pathological, and ultrastructural study of 26 cases supporting the recognition of a monophasic variant. Am J Surg Pathol 5:137, 1981.
64. Lagacé R, Schürch W, Seemayer TA: Myofibroblasts in soft tissue sarcomas. Virchows Arch (Pathol Anat) 389A:1, 1980.
65. Mackenzie DH: Fibroma: A dangerous diagnosis. A review of 205 cases of fibrosarcoma of soft tissue. Br J Surg 51:607, 1964.
66. Pritchard DJ, Soule EH, Taylor WF, et al: Fibrosarcoma—a clinicopathologic and statistical study of 199 tumors of the soft tissues of the extremities and trunk. Cancer 33:888, 1974.
67. Rosenberg HS, Stenback WA, Spjut HJ: The fibromatoses of infancy and childhood. *In* Rosenberg HS, Bolande RP (eds): Perspectives in Pediatric Pathology, Vol. 4. Chicago, Year Book Medical Publishers, 1978, pp 269–348.
68. Soule EH, Pritchard DJ: Fibrosarcoma in infants and children. Cancer 40:1711, 1977.
69. Swain RE, Sessions DG, Ogura JH: Fibrosarcoma of the head and neck: A clinical analysis of forty cases. Ann Otol 83:439, 1974.
70. van der Werf-Messing B, van Unnik JAM: Fibrosarcoma of the soft tissues: A clinicopathologic study. Cancer 18:1113, 1965.

FIBROMATOSES (DESMOID TUMOR)

71. Allen PW: The fibromatoses: A clinicopathologic classification based on 140 cases. Am J Surg Pathol 1:255; 305, 1977.
72. Cole NM, Guiss LW: Extra-abdominal desmoid tumors. Arch Surg 98:530, 1969.
73. Conley J, Healey WV, Stout AP: Fibromatosis of the head and neck. Am J Surg 112:609, 1966.
74. Das Gupta TK, Brasfield RD, O'Hara J: Extra-abdominal desmoids: A clinicopathological study. Ann Surg 170:109, 1969.
75. Enzinger FM: Fibrous tumors of infancy. *In* Tumors of Bone and Soft Tissue, University of Texas, M.D. Anderson Hospital and Tumor Institute. Chicago, Year Book Medical Publishers, 1965, pp 375–396.
76. Enzinger FM, Shiraki M: Musculo-aponeurotic fibromatosis of the shoulder girdle (extra-abdominal desmoid). Analysis of thirty cases followed up to ten or more years. Cancer 20:1131, 1967.
77. Goellner JR, Soule EH: Desmoid tumors. An ultrastructural study of eight cases. Hum Pathol 11:43, 1980.
78. Griffiths HJ, Robinson K, Bonfiglio TA: Aggressive fibromatosis. Skeletal Radiol 9:179, 1983.
79. Hunt RTN, Morgan HC, Ackerman LV: Principles in the management of extra-abdominal desmoids. Cancer 13:825, 1960.
80. Lipper S, Kahn LB, Reddick RL: The myofibroblast. Pathol Annu 15 (PART 1):409, 1980.
81. Mackenzie DH: The Differential Diagnosis of Fibroblastic Disorders. Oxford, Blackwell Scientific Publications, 1970.
82. Mackenzie DH: The fibromatoses: A clinicopathological concept. Br Med J 4:277, 1972.
83. Masson JK, Soule EH: Desmoid tumors of the head and neck. Am J Surg 112:615, 1966.
84. Pettit VD, Chamness JT, Ackerman LV: Fibromatosis and fibrosarcoma following irradiation therapy. Cancer 7:149, 1954.
85. Rosenberg HS, Stenback WA, Spjut HJ: The fibromatoses of infancy and childhood. *In* Rosenberg HS, Bolande RP (eds): Perspectives in Pediatric Pathology, Vol. 4. Chicago, Year Book Medical Publishers, 1978, pp 269–348.
86. Wara WM, Phillips TL, Hill DR, et al: Desmoid tumors—treatment and prognosis. Radiology 124:225, 1977.
87. Wilkins SA Jr, Waldron CA, Mathews WH, et al: Aggressive fibromatosis of the head and neck. Am J Surg 130:412, 1975.
88. Zayid I, Dihmis C: Familial multicentric fibromatosis—desmoids: A report of three cases in a Jordanian family. Cancer 24:786, 1969.

CONGENITAL FIBROMATOSIS

89. Baer JW, Radkowski MA: Congenital multiple fibromatosis: A case report with review of the world literature. AJR 118:200, 1973.
90. Baird PA, Worth AJ: Congenital generalized fibromatosis: An autosomal recessive condition? Clin Genet 9:488, 1976.
91. Briselli MF, Soule EH, Gilchrist GS: Congenital fibromatosis: Report of 18 cases of solitary and 4 cases of multiple tumors. Mayo Clin Proc 55:554, 1980.

92. Chung EB, Enzinger FM: Infantile myofibromatosis. Cancer 48:1807, 1981.
93. Kauffman SL, Stout AP: Congenital mesenchymal tumors. Cancer 18:460, 1965.
94. Kindblom L-G, Termén G, Säve-Soderbergh J, et al: Congenital solitary fibromatosis of soft tissue, a variant of congenital generalized fibromatosis. Acta Pathol Microbiol Scand 85:640, 1977.
95. Plaschkes J: Congenital fibromatosis: Localized and generalized forms. J Pediatr Surg 9:95, 1974.
96. Roggli VL, Kim H-S, Hawkins E: Congenital generalized fibromatosis with visceral involvement. A case report. Cancer 45:954, 1980.
97. Shnitka TK, Asp DM, Horner RH: Congenital generalized fibromatosis. Cancer 11:627, 1958.
98. Stout AP: Juvenile fibromatoses. Cancer 7:953, 1954.
99. Walts AE, Asch M, Raj C: Solitary lesion of congenital fibromatosis. A rare cause of neonatal intestinal obstruction. Am J Surg Pathol 6:255, 1982.

STERNOCLEIDOMASTOID TUMOR (FIBROMATOSIS COLLI)

100. Armstrong D, Pickrell K, Fetter B, et al: Torticollis: An analysis of 271 cases. Plast Reconstr Surg 35:14, 1965.
101. Chandler FA: Muscular torticollis. J Bone Joint Surg (Am) 38:566, 1948.
102. Coventry MB, Harris LE: Congenital muscular torticollis in infancy. Some observations regarding treatment. J Bone Joint Surg (Am) 41:815, 1959.
103. Fitzsimmons HJ: Congenital torticollis. Review of the pathological aspects. N Engl J Med 209:66, 1933.
104. Gruhn J, Hurwitt ES: Fibrous sternomastoid tumor of infancy. Pediatrics 8:522, 1951.
105. Hulbert KF: Congenital torticollis. J Bone Joint Surg (Br) 32:50, 1950.
106. Iwahara T, Ikeda A: On the ipsilateral involvement of congenital muscular torticollis and congenital dislocation of the hip. J Jpn Orthop Assoc 35:1221, 1962.
107. Kiesewetter WB, Nelson PK, Palladino VS, et al: Neonatal torticollis. JAMA 157:1281, 1955.
108. Lidge RT, Bechtol RC, Lambert CN: Congenital muscular torticollis. Etiology and pathology. J Bone Joint Surg (Am) 39:1165, 1957.
109. Macdonald D: Sternomastoid tumour and muscular torticollis. J Bone Joint Surg (Br) 51:432, 1969.
110. Middleton DS: The pathology of congenital torticollis. Br J Surg 18:188, 1930.

PSEUDOSARCOMATOUS FIBROUS LESIONS (NODULAR FASCIITIS, PROLIFERATIVE MYOSITIS, PROLIFERATIVE FASCIITIS)

111. Allen PW: Nodular fasciitis. Pathology 4:9, 1972.
112. Bernstein KE, Lattes R: Nodular (pseudosarcomatous) fasciitis, a nonrecurrent lesion: Clinicopathologic study of 134 cases. Cancer 49:1668, 1982.
113. Butler JJ: Fibrous tissue tumors: Nodular fasciitis, dermatofibrosarcoma protuberans, and fibrosarcoma, grade I, desmoid type. In Tumors of Bone and Soft Tissue. The University of Texas, M.D. Anderson Hospital and Tumor Institute. Chicago, Year Book Medical Publishers, 1965, pp 397–413.
114. Chung EB, Enzinger FM: Proliferative fasciitis. Cancer 36:1450, 1975.
115. Dahl I, Angervall L: Pseudosarcomatous proliferative lesions of soft tissue with or without bone formation. Acta Pathol Microbiol Scand 85:577, 1977.
116. Enzinger FM: Recent trends in soft tissue pathology. In Tumors of Bone and Soft Tissue. Chicago, Year Book Medical Publishers, 1965, p 315.
117. Enzinger FM, Dulcey F: Proliferative myositis. Report of thirty-three cases. Cancer 20:2213, 1967.
118. Hutter RVP, Stewart FW, Foote FW Jr: Fasciitis: A report of 70 cases with follow-up proving the benignity of the lesion. Cancer 15:992, 1962.
119. Kitano M, Iwasaki H, Enjoji M: Proliferative fasciitis. A variant of nodular fasciitis. Acta Pathol Jpn 27:485, 1977.
120. Kleinstiver BJ, Rodriquez HA: Nodular fasciitis: A study of forty-five cases and review of the literature. J Bone Joint Surg (Am) 50:1204, 1968.
121. Konwaler BE, Keasbey L, Kaplan L: Subcutaneous pseudosarcomatous fibromatosis (fasciitis). Am J Clin Pathol 25:241, 1955.
122. Laver DH, Enzinger FM: Cranial fasciitis of childhood. Cancer 45:401, 1980.
123. Lumerman H, Bodner B, Zambito R: Intraoral (submucosal) pseudosarcomatous nodular fasciitis: Report of a case. Oral Surg 34:239, 1972.
124. Meister P, Buckmann F-W, Konrad E: Nodular fasciitis (analysis of 100 cases and review of the literature). Pathol Res Pract 162:133, 1978.
125. Meister P, Konrad EA, Buckmann FW: Nodular fasciitis and proliferative myositis as variants of one disease entity. Invest Cell Pathol 2:277, 1979.
126. Patchefsky AS, Enzinger FM: Intravascular fasciitis: A report of 17 cases. Am J Surg Pathol 5:29, 1981.
127. Price EB Jr, Silliphant WM, Shuman R: Nodular fasciitis: A clinicopathologic analysis of 65 cases. Am J Clin Pathol 35:122, 1961.
128. Stout AP: Pseudosarcomatous fasciitis in children. Cancer 14:1216, 1961.
129. Wirman JA: Nodular fasciitis, a lesion of myofibroblasts: An ultrastructural study. Cancer 38:2378, 1976.

NEUROGENOUS TUMORS (NEURILEMOMA, NEUROFIBROMA, NEUROSARCOMA)

130. Abell MR, Hart WR, Olson JR: Tumors of the peripheral nervous system. Hum Pathol 1:503, 1970.
131. Ackerman LV, Taylor FH: Neurogenous tumors within the thorax: A clinicopathological evaluation of forty-eight cases. Cancer 4:669, 1951.
132. Allen PW: Myxoid tumors of soft tissues (part 1). Pathol Annu 15:133, 1980.
133. Ariel IM: Tumors of the peripheral nervous system. CA 33:282, 1983.
134. Asbury AK, Johnson PC: Pathology of peripheral nerve. Philadelphia, W. B. Saunders Co., 1978, pp 206–226.
135. Bonneau R, Brochu P: Neuromuscular choristoma: A clinicopathologic study of two cases. Am J Surg Pathol 7:521, 1983.
136. Brooks J, Rhodes H, Freeman M, et al: Malignant "Triton" tumors: Natural history of seven new cases with literature review (abstract). Lab Invest 48:10A, 1983.
137. Clairmont AA, Conley JJ: Malignant schwannoma of the parapharyngeal space. J Otolaryngol 6:28, 1977.
138. Conley JJ: Neurogenous tumors in the neck. Arch Otolaryngol 61:167, 1955.
139. Conley J, Janecka IP: Neurilemmoma of the head and neck. Trans Am Acad Ophthalmol Otol 80:459, 1975.
140. Conley J, Janecka I: Schwann cell tumors of the facial nerve. Laryngoscope 84:958, 1974.
141. D'Agostino AN, Soule EH, Miller RH: Primary malignant neoplasms of nerves (malignant neurilemomas) in patients without manifestations of multiple neurofibromatosis (von Recklinghausen's disease). Cancer 16:1003, 1963.
142. D'Agostino AN, Soule EH, Miller RH: Sarcomas of the peripheral nerves and somatic soft tissues associated with multiple neurofibromatosis (von Recklinghausen's disease). Cancer 16:1015, 1963.
143. Dahl I: Ancient neurilemmoma (schwannoma). Acta Pathol Microbiol Scand 85:812, 1977.
144. Dahl I, Hagmar B, Idvall I: Benign solitary neurilemoma (schwannoma). Acta Pathol Microbiol Immunol Scand 92:91, 1984.
145. Daly JF, Roesler HK: Neurilemmoma of the cervical sympathetic chain. Arch Otolaryngol 77:262, 1963.
146. Das Gupta TK, Brasfield RD: Solitary malignant schwannoma. Ann Surg 171:419, 1970.
147. Das Gupta TK, Brasfield RD, Strong EW, et al: Benign solitary schwannomas (neurilemomas). Cancer 24:355, 1969.
148. Das Gupta TK, Brasfield RD: Von Recklinghausen's disease. CA 21:174, 1971.
149. Davis WB, Edgerton MT, Hoffmeister SF: Neurofibromatosis of the head and neck. Plast Reconstruct Surg 14:186, 1954.
150. Ducatman BS, Scheithauer BW, Piepgras DR, et al: Malignant peripheral nerve sheath tumor: A clinicopathologic review of 120 cases (abstract). Lab Invest 50:17A, 1984.
151. Erlandson RA, Woodruff JM: Peripheral nerve sheath tumors: An electron microscopic study of 43 cases. Cancer 49:273, 1982.
152. Ghosh BC, Ghosh L, Huvos AG, et al: Malignant schwannoma: A clinicopathologic study. Cancer 31:184, 1973.
153. Gore DO, Rankow R, Hanford JM: Parapharyngeal neurilemmoma. Surg Gynecol Obstet 103:193, 1956.
154. Guccion JG, Enzinger FM: Malignant schwannoma associated with von Recklinghausen's neurofibromatosis. Virchows Arch (Pathol Anat) 383A:43, 1979.
155. Harkin JC, Reed RJ: Tumors of the peripheral nervous system. Atlas of Tumor Pathology, second series, fascicle 3. Washington, D.C., Armed Forces Institute of Pathology, 1969.
156. Herrera GA, Reimann EF, Salinas JA, et al: Malignant schwannomas presenting as malignant fibrous histiocytomas. Ultrastruct Pathol 3:253, 1982.

157. Izumi AK, Rosato FE, Wood MG: Von Recklinghausen's disease associated with multiple neurolemmomas. Arch Dermatol 104:172, 1971.
158. Katz AD, Passy V, Kaplan L: Neurogenous neoplasms of major nerves of face and neck. Arch Surg 103:51, 1971.
159. Kragh LV, Soule EH, Masson JK: Benign and malignant neurilemmomas of the head and neck. Surg Gynecol Obstet 111:211, 1960.
160. Kragh LV, Soule EH, Masson JK: Neurofibromatosis (von Recklinghausen's disease) of the head and neck: Cosmetic and reconstructive aspects. Plast Reconstruct Surg 25:565, 1960.
161. Krumerman MS, Stingle W: Synchronous malignant glandular schwannomas in congenital neurofibromatosis. Cancer 41:2444, 1978.
162. Lassmann H, Jurecka W, Lassmann G, et al: Different types of benign nerve sheath tumors. Light microscopy, electron microscopy and autoradiography. Virchows Arch (Pathol Anat) 375(A):197, 1977.
163. Lazarus SS, Trombetta LD: Ultrastructural identification of a benign perineural cell tumor. Cancer 41:1823, 1978.
164. Markel SF, Enzinger FM: Neuromuscular hamartoma—a benign "Triton tumor" composed of mature neural and striated muscle elements. Cancer 49:140, 1982.
165. Oberman HA, Sullenger G: Neurogenous tumors of the head and neck. Cancer 20:1992, 1967.
166. Perzin KH, Panyu H, Wechter S: Nonepithelial tumors of the nasal cavity, paranasal sinuses and nasopharynx: A clinicopathologic study. XII: Schwann cell tumors (neurilemoma, neurofibroma, malignant schwannoma). Cancer 50:2193, 1982.
167. Putney FJ, Moran JJ, Thomas GK: Neurogenic tumors of the head and neck. Laryngoscope 74:1037, 1964.
168. Reed RJ, Harkin JC: Tumors of the Peripheral Nervous System, second series, fascicle 3 (supplement). Washington, D.C., Armed Forces Institute of Pathology, 1983.
169. Rosenfeld L, Graves H Jr, Lawrence R: Primary neurogenic tumors of the lateral neck. Ann Surg 167:847, 1968.
170. Sordillo PP, Helson L, Hajdu SI, et al: Malignant schwannoma—clinical characteristics, survival, and response to therapy. Cancer 47:2503, 1981.
171. Stefansson K, Wollmann R, Jerkovic M: S-100 protein in soft-tissue tumors derived from schwann cells and melanocytes. Am J Pathol 106:261, 1982.
172. Storm FK, Eilber FR, Mirra J, et al: Neurofibrosarcoma. Cancer 45:126, 1980.
173. Taxy JB, Battifora H, Trujillo Y, et al: Electron microscopy in the diagnosis of malignant schwannoma. Cancer 48:1381, 1981.
174. Trojanowski JQ, Kleinman GM, Proppe KH: Malignant tumors of nerve sheath origin. Cancer 46:1202, 1980.
175. Tsuneyoshi M, Enjoji M: Primary malignant peripheral nerve tumors (malignant schwannomas): A clinicopathologic and electron microscopic study. Acta Pathol Jpn 29:363, 1979.
176. Waggener JD: Ultrastructure of benign peripheral nerve sheath tumors. Cancer 19:699, 1966.
177. Weiss SW, Langloss JM, Enzinger FM: Value of S-100 protein in the diagnosis of soft tissue tumors with particular reference to benign and malignant schwann cell tumors. Lab Invest 49:299, 1983.
178. Whitaker WG, Droulias C: Benign encapsulated neurilemoma: A report of 76 cases. Am Surg 42:675, 1976.
179. Woodruff JM: Peripheral nerve tumors showing glandular differentiation (glandular schwannomas). Cancer 37:2399, 1976.
180. Woodruff JM, Chernik NL, Smith MC, et al: Peripheral nerve tumors with rhabdomyosarcomatous differentiation (malignant "triton" tumors). Cancer 32:426, 1973.
181. Woodruff JM, Godwin TA, Erlandson RA, et al: Cellular schwannoma. A variety of schwannoma sometimes mistaken for a malignant tumor. Am J Surg Pathol 5:733, 1981.
182. Woodruff JM, Marshall ML, Godwin TA, et al: Plexiform (multinodular) schwannoma. A tumor simulating the plexiform neurofibroma. Am J Surg Pathol 7:691, 1983.

PARAGANGLIOMA

183. Chaudhry AP, Haar JG, Koul A, et al: A nonfunctioning paraganglioma of vagus nerve: An ultrastructural study. Cancer 43:1689, 1979.
184. Crowell WT, Grizzle WE, Siegel AL: Functional carotid paragangliomas: Biochemical, ultrastructural, and histochemical correlation with clinical symptoms. Arch Pathol Lab Med 106:599, 1982.
185. Druck NS, Spector GJ, Ciralsky RH, et al: Malignant glomus vagale: Report of a case and review of the literature. Arch Otolaryngol 102:634, 1976.
186. Farr HW: Carotid body tumors: A 40-year study. CA 30:260, 1980.
187. Gaylis H, Mieny CJ: The incidence of malignancy in carotid body tumours. Br J Surg 64:885, 1977.
188. Glenner GG, Grimley PM: Tumors of the extra-adrenal paraganglion system (including chemoreceptors). Atlas of Tumor Pathology, second series, fascicle 9. Washington, D.C., Armed Forces Institute of Pathology, 1974.
189. Grimley PM, Glenner GG: Histology and ultrastructure of carotid body paragangliomas: Comparison with the normal gland. Cancer 20:1473, 1967.
190. Himelfarb MZ, Ostrzega NL, Samuel J, et al: Paraganglioma of the nasal cavity. Laryngoscope 93:350, 1983.
191. Irons GB, Weiland LH, Brown WL: Paragangliomas of the neck: Clinical and pathologic analysis of 116 cases. Surg Clin North Am 57:575, 1977.
192. Kahn LB: Vagal body tumor (nonchromaffin paraganglioma, chemodectoma, and carotid body-like tumor) with cervical node metastasis and familial association: Ultrastructural study and review. Cancer 38:2367, 1976.
193. Lack EE, Cubilla AL, Woodruff JM: Paragangliomas of the head and neck region: A pathologic study of tumors from 71 patients. Hum Pathol 10:191, 1979.
194. Lack EE, Cubilla AL, Woodruff JM, et al: Paragangliomas of the head and neck region: A clinical study of 69 patients. Cancer 39:397, 1977.
195. Lees CD, Levine HL, Beven EG, et al: Tumors of the carotid body: Experience with 41 operative cases. Am J Surg 142:362, 1981.
196. Merino MJ, Livolsi VA: Malignant carotid body tumors: Report of two cases and review of the literature. Cancer 47:1403, 1981.
197. Moran TE: Nonchromaffin paraganglioma of the nasal cavity. Laryngoscope 72:201, 1962.
198. Oberman HA, Holtz F, Sheffer LA, et al: Chemodectomas (nonchromaffin paragangliomas) of the head and neck: A clinicopathologic study. Cancer 21:838, 1968.
199. Padberg FT Jr, Cady B, Persson AV: Carotid body tumor: The Lahey Clinic experience. Am J Surg 145:526, 1983.
200. Palacios E: Chemodectomas of the head and neck. AJR 110:129, 1970.
201. Parry DM, Li FP, Strong LC, et al: Carotid body tumors in humans: Genetics and epidemiology. J Natl Cancer Inst 68:573, 1982.
202. Pritchett JW: Familial concurrence of carotid body tumor and pheochromocytoma. Cancer 49:2578, 1982.
203. ReMine WH, Weiland LH, ReMine SG: Carotid body tumors: Chemodectomas. Curr Probl Cancer 11:1, 1978.
204. Resler DR, Snow JB Jr, Williams GR: Multiplicity and familial incidence of carotid body and glomus jugulare tumors. Ann Otol Rhinol Laryngol 75:114, 1966.
205. Robertson DI, Cooney TP: Malignant carotid body paraganglioma: Light and electron microscopic study of the tumor and its metastases. Cancer 46:2623, 1980.
206. Schuller DE, Lucas JG: Nasopharyngeal paraganglioma. Arch Otolaryngol 108:667, 1982.
207. Shamblin WR, ReMine WH, Sheps SG, et al: Carotid body tumor (chemodectoma): Clinicopathologic analysis of ninety cases. Am J Surg 122:732, 1971.
208. Someren A, Karcioglu Z: Malignant vagal paraganglioma: Report of a case and review of literature. Am J Clin Pathol 68:400, 1977.
209. Spector GJ, Ciralsky R, Maisel RH, et al: IV. Multiple glomus tumors in the head and neck. Laryngoscope 85:1066, 1975.
210. Spector GJ, Ciralsky RH, Oqura JH: Glomus tumors in the head and neck: III. Analysis of clinical manifestations. Ann Otol Rhinol Laryngol 84:73, 1975.
211. Spector GJ, Gado M, Ciralsky R, et al: Neurologic implications of glomus tumors in the head and neck. Laryngoscope 85:1387, 1975.
212. Stearns MP: Chemodectoma of the larynx. J Laryngol Otol 96:1181, 1982.
213. Thacker WC, Duckworth JK: Chemodectoma of the orbit. Cancer 23:1233, 1969.
214. Tsuneyoshi M, Enjoji M: Glomus tumor: A clinicopathologic and electron microscopic study. Cancer 50:1601, 1982.
215. Warren WH, Memoli VA, Gould VE: Immunohistochemical and ultrastructural analysis of paragangliomas of the head and neck. Lab Invest (abstract) 50:66A, 1984.
216. Wetmore RF, Tronzo RD, Lane RJ: Nonfunctional paraganglioma of the larynx: Clinical and pathological considerations. Cancer 48:2717, 1981.

SYNOVIAL SARCOMA

217. Batsakis JG, Nishiyama RH, Sullinger GD: Synovial sarcomas of the neck. Arch Otolaryngol 85:327, 1967.
218. Cadman NL, Soule EH, Kelly PJ: Synovial sarcoma: An analysis of 134 tumors. Cancer 18:613, 1965.

219. Cameron HU, Kostuik JP: A long-term follow-up of synovial sarcoma. J Bone Joint Surg (Br) 56:613, 1974.
220. Corson JM, Weiss LM, Banks-Schlegel SP, et al: Keratin proteins in synovial sarcoma. Am J Surg Pathol 7:107, 1983.
221. Corson JM, Weiss LM, Banks-Schlegel SP, et al: Keratin proteins in synovial sarcomas: An immunohistochemical study of 24 cases (abstract). Lab Invest 48:17A, 1983.
222. Dische FE, Darby AJ, Howard ER: Malignant synovioma: Electron microscopical findings in three patients and review of the literature. J Pathol 124:149, 1978.
223. Enzinger FM, Smith BH: Hemangiopericytoma. An analysis of 106 cases. Hum Pathol 7:61, 1976.
224. Evans HL: Synovial sarcoma: A study of 23 biphasic and 17 probable monophasic examples (part 2). Pathol Annu 15:309, 1980.
225. Farris KB, Reed RJ: Monophasic, glandular, synovial sarcomas and carcinomas of the soft tissues. Arch Pathol Lab Med 106:129, 1982.
226. Fechner RE: Neoplasms and neoplasm-like lesions of the synovium. In Ackerman LV, Spjut HJ, Abell MR (eds): Bones and Joints, Baltimore. Williams & Wilkins Co., 1976, pp 157–186.
227. Gabbiani G, Kaye GI, Lattes R, et al: Synovial sarcoma: Electron microscopic study of a typical case. Cancer 28:1031, 1971.
228. Hajdu SI, Shiu MH, Fortner JG: Tendosynovial sarcoma: A clinicopathological study of 136 cases. Cancer 39:1201, 1977.
229. Harrison EG Jr, Black BM, Devine KD: Synovial sarcoma primary in the neck. Arch Pathol 71:137, 1961.
230. Jacobs LA, Weaver AW: Synovial sarcoma of the head and neck. Am J Surg 128:527, 1974.
231. Jernstrom P: Synovial sarcoma of the pharynx: Report of a case. Am J Clin Pathol 24:957, 1954.
232. Krall RA, Kostianovsky M, Patchefsky AS: Synovial sarcoma: A clinical, pathological, and ultrastructural study of 26 cases supporting the recognition of a monophasic variant. Am J Surg Pathol 5:137, 1981.
233. Lockey MW: Rare tumors of the ear, nose and throat: Synovial sarcoma of the head and neck. South Med J 69:316, 1976.
234. Mackenzie DH: Monophasic synovial sarcoma—a histological entity? Histopathology 1:151, 1977.
235. Mickelson MR, Brown GA, Maynard JA, et al: Synovial sarcoma. An electron microscopic study of monophasic and biphasic forms. Cancer 45:2109, 1980.
236. Miettinen M, Lehto V-P, Virtanen I: Keratin in the epithelial-like cells of classical biphasic synovial sarcoma. Virchows Arch (Cell Pathol) 40B:157, 1982.
237. Nunez-Alonso C, Gashti EN, Christ ML: Maxillofacial synovial sarcoma: Light- and electron-microscopic study of two cases. Am J Surg Pathol 3:23, 1979.
238. Roth JA, Enzinger FM, Tannenbaum M: Synovial sarcoma of the neck: A follow-up study of 24 cases. Cancer 35:1243, 1975.
239. Schmidt D, Mackay B: Ultrastructure of human tendon sheath and synovium: Implications for tumor histogenesis. Ultrastruct Pathol 3:269, 1982.
240. Shmookler BM, Enzinger FM, Brannon RB: Orofacial synovial sarcoma. Cancer 50:269, 1982.
241. Varela-Duran J, Enzinger FM: Calcifying synovial sarcoma. Cancer 50:345, 1982.
242. Wright PH, Sim FH, Soule EH, et al: Synovial sarcoma. J Bone Joint Surg (Am) 64:112, 1982.
243. van Haelst UJGM: General considerations on electron microscopy of tumors of soft tissues. Prog Surg Pathol 2:225, 1980.

LYMPHANGIOMA

244. Barrand KG, Freeman NV: Massive infiltrating cystic hygroma of the neck in infancy. Arch Dis Child 48:523, 1973.
245. Bill AH Jr, Sumner DS: A unified concept of lymphangioma and cystic hygroma. Surg Gynecol Obstet 120:79, 1965.
246. Dinerman WS, Myers EN: Lymphangiomatous macroglossia. Laryngoscope 86:291, 1976.
247. Flanagan BP, Helwig EB: Cutaneous lymphangioma. Arch Dermatol 113:24, 1977.
248. Galofré M, Judd ES, Pérez PE, et al: Results of surgical treatment of cystic hygroma. Surg Gynecol Obstet 115:319, 1962.
249. Gross RE, Goeringer CF: Cystic hygroma of the neck. Report of twenty-seven cases. Surg Gynecol Obstet 69:48, 1939.
250. Harkins GA, Sabiston DC: Lymphangioma in infancy and childhood. Surgery 47:811, 1960.
251. Litzow TJ, Lash H: Lymphangiomas of the tongue. Mayo Clinic Proc 36:229, 1961.
252. Lynn HB: Cystic hygroma. Surg Clin North Am 43:1157, 1963.
253. Ninh TN, Ninh TX: Cystic hygroma in children: A report of 126 cases. J Pediatr Surg 9:191, 1974.
254. Peachey RDG, Whimster IW: Lymphangioma of skin. A review of 65 cases. Br J Dermatol 83:519, 1970.
255. Saijo M, Munro IR, Mancer K: Lymphangioma. A long-term follow-up study. Plast Reconstr Surg 56:642, 1975.
256. Singh S, Baboo ML, Pathak IC: Cystic lymphangioma in children: Report of 32 cases including lesions at rare sites. Surgery 69:947, 1971.
257. Stromberg BV, Weeks PM, Wray RC Jr: Treatment of cystic hygroma. South Med J 69:1333, 1976.
258. Van Cauwelaert PH, Gruwez JA: Experience with lymphangioma. Lymphology 11:43, 1978.
259. Watson WL, McCarthy WD: Blood and lymph vessel tumors. A report of 1,056 cases. Surg Gynecol Obstet 71:569, 1940.

LIPOMA

260. Adair FE, Pack GT, Farrior JH: Lipomas. Am J Cancer 16:1104, 1932.
261. Allen PW: Tumors and Proliferations of Adipose Tissue. A Clinicopathologic Approach. New York, Masson Publishing USA, 1981.
262. Birnholz JC, Macmillan AS Jr: Advanced laryngeal compression due to diffuse, symmetric lipomatosis (Madelung's disease). Br J Radiol 46:245, 1973.
263. Brasfield RD, Das Gupta TK: Soft tissue tumors: Benign tumors of adipose tissue. CA 19:3, 1969.
264. Das Gupta TK: Tumors and tumor-like conditions of the adipose tissue. Curr Probl Surg (March) 1, 1970.
265. Dionne GP, Seemayer TA: Infiltrating lipomas and angiolipomas revisited. Cancer 33:732, 1974.
266. Dixon AY, McGregor DH, Lee SH: Angiolipomas: An ultrastructural and clinicopathological study. Hum Pathol 12:739, 1981.
267. Enzinger FM: Benign lipomatous tumors simulating a sarcoma. In Management of Primary Bone and Soft Tissue Tumors. Chicago, Year Book Medical Publishers, 1977, pp 11–24.
268. Fu YS, Parker FG, Kaye GI, et al: Ultrastructure of benign and malignant adipose tissue tumors (part 1). Pathol Annu 15:67, 1980.
269. Fu Y-S, Perzin KH: Non-epithelial tumors of the nasal cavity, paranasal sinuses and nasopharynx: A clinicopathologic study. VIII. Adipose tissue tumors (lipoma and liposarcoma). Cancer 40:1314, 1977.
270. Geschickter CF: Lipoid tumors. Am J Cancer 21:617, 1934.
271. Hatziotis JC: Lipoma of the oral cavity. Oral Surg 31:511, 1971.
272. Hirshowitz B, Goldan S: Giant lipoma of the back and neck: Case report. Plast Reconstr Surg 52:312, 1973.
273. Kim YH, Reiner L: Ultrastructure of lipoma. Cancer 50:102, 1982.
274. Kindblom L-G, Angervall L, Stener B, et al: Intermuscular and intramuscular lipomas and hibernomas: A clinical, roentgenologic, histologic, and prognostic study of 46 cases. Cancer 33:754, 1974.
275. Moretti JA, Miller D: Laryngeal involvement in benign symmetric lipomatosis. Arch Otolaryngol 97:495, 1973.
276. Schuler FA III, Graham JK, Horton CE: Benign symmetrical lipomatosis (Madelung's disease): Case report. Plast Reconstr Surg 57:662, 1976.
277. Seldin HM, Seldin DS, Rakower W, et al: Lipomas of the oral cavity: Report of 26 cases. J Oral Surg 25:270, 1967.
278. Taylor LM, Beahrs OH, Fontana RS: Benign symmetric lipomatosis. Mayo Clinic Proc 36:96, 1961.
279. Toppozada HH, Shehata MA, Maher AI: Lipoma of the pharynx (a report of four cases). J Laryngol Otol 87:787, 1973.
280. Wakeley C, Somerville P: Lipomas. Lancet 2:995, 1952.

SPINDLE CELL LIPOMA

281. Angervall L, Dahl I, Kindblom L-G, et al: Spindle cell lipoma. Acta Pathol Microbiol Scand 84:477, 1976.
282. Bolen JW, Thorning D: Spindle-cell lipoma: A clinical, light- and electron-microscopical study. Am J Surg Pathol 5:435, 1981.
283. Enzinger FM, Harvey DA: Spindle cell lipoma. Cancer 36:1852, 1975.
284. Robb JA, Jones RA: Spindle cell lipoma in a perianal location. Hum Pathol 13:1052, 1982.

PLEOMORPHIC (ATYPICAL) LIPOMA

285. Evans HL, Soule EH, Winkelmann RK: Atypical lipoma, atypical intramuscular lipoma, and well differentiated retroperitoneal liposarcoma: A reappraisal of 30 cases formerly classified as well differentiated liposarcoma. Cancer 43:574, 1979.
286. Kindblom L-G, Angervall L, Fassina AS: Atypical lipoma. Acta Pathol Microbiol Immunol Scand 90:27, 1982.
287. Shmookler BM, Enzinger FM: Pleomorphic lipoma: A benign tumor simulating liposarcoma. A clinicopathologic analysis of 48 cases. Cancer 47:126, 1981.

LIPOSARCOMA

288. Baden E, Newman R: Liposarcoma of the oropharyngeal region: Review of the literature and report of two cases. Oral Surg 44:889, 1977.
289. Battifora H, Nunez-Alonso C: Myxoid liposarcoma: Study of ten cases. Ultrastruct Pathol 1:157, 1980.
290. Bolen JW, Thorning D: Benign lipoblastoma and myxoid liposarcoma: A comparative light- and electron-microscopic study. Am J Surg Pathol 4:163, 1980.
291. Brasfield RD, Das Gupta TK: Liposarcoma. CA 20:3, 1970.
292. Chung EB, Enzinger FM: Benign lipoblastomatosis. An analysis of 35 cases. Cancer 32:482, 1973.
293. Desai U, Ramos CV, Taylor HB: Ultrastructural observations in pleomorphic liposarcoma. Cancer 42:1284, 1978.
294. Edland RW: Liposarcoma: A retrospective study of fifteen cases, a review of the literature and a discussion of radiosensitivity. AJR 103:778, 1968.
295. Enzinger F: Management of Primary Bone and Soft Tissue Tumors. Chicago, Year Book Medical Publishers, 1977, pp 454–455.
296. Enzinger FM, Winslow DJ: Liposarcoma: A study of 103 cases. Virchows Arch 335:367, 1962.
297. Evans HL: Liposarcoma: A study of 55 cases with a reassessment of its classification. Am J Surg Pathol 3:507, 1979.
298. Kindblom L-G, Angervall L, Jarlstedt J: Liposarcoma of the neck: A clinicopathologic study of 4 cases. Cancer 42:774, 1978.
299. Kindblom L-G, Angervall L, Svendsen P: Liposarcoma: A clinico-pathologic, radiographic and prognostic study. Acta Pathol Microbiol Scand (Suppl) 253:1, 1975.
300. Lagacé R, Jacob S, Seemayer TA: Myxoid liposarcoma. An electron microscopic study: Biologic and histogenetic considerations. Virchows Arch (Pathol Anat) 384A:159, 1979.
301. McKee PH, Lowe D, Shaw M: Subcutaneous liposarcoma. Clin Exp Dermatol 8:593, 1983.
302. Saunders JR, Jaques DA, Casterline PF, et al: Liposarcomas of the head and neck: A review of the literature and addition of four cases. Cancer 43:162, 1979.
303. Shmookler BM, Enzinger FM: Liposarcoma occurring in children: An analysis of 17 cases and review of the literature. Cancer 52:567, 1983.
304. Snover DC, Sumner HW, Dehner LP: Variability of histologic pattern in recurrent soft tissue sarcomas originally diagnosed as liposarcoma. Cancer 40:1005, 1982.
305. Stoller FM, Davies DG: Liposarcoma of the neck. Arch Otolaryngol 88:419, 1968.
306. Wetzel W, Alexander R: Myxoid liposarcoma: An ultrastructural study of two cases. Am J Clin Pathol 72:521, 1979.

RHABDOMYOMA

307. Albrechtsen R, Ebbesen F, Pedersen SV: Extracardiac rhabdomy-oma: Light and electron microscopic studies of two cases in the mandibular area, with a review of previous reports. Acta Otolaryngol 78:458, 1974.
308. Bagby RA, Packer JT, Iglesias RG: Rhabdomyoma of the larynx. Arch Otolaryngol 102:101, 1976.
309. Battifora HA, Eisenstein R, Schild JA: Rhabdomyoma of larynx. Ultrastructural study and comparison with granular cell tumors (myoblastoma). Cancer 23:183, 1969.
310. Corio RL, Lewis DM: Intraoral rhabdomyomas. Oral Surg 48:525, 1979.
311. Czernobilsky B, Cornog JL, Enterline HT: Rhabdomyoma: Report of a case with ultrastructural and histochemical studies. Am J Clin Pathol 49:782, 1968.
312. Dahl I, Angervall L, Säve-Söderbergh J: Foetal rhabdomyoma: Case report of a patient with two tumors. Acta Pathol Microbiol Scand 84:107, 1976.
313. Dehner LP, Enzinger FM: Fetal rhabdomyoma: An analysis of nine cases. Cancer 30:160, 1972.
314. di Sant'Agnese PA, Knowles DM II: Extracardiac rhabdomyoma: A clinicopathologic study and review of the literature. Cancer 46:780, 1980.
315. Eveson JW, Merchant NE: Sublingual rhabdomyoma. Int J Oral Surg 7:27, 1978.
316. Ferracini R, Cavina C, Morrone B: Rhabdomyoma (adult type) of the sublingual region. Tumori 63:43, 1977.
317. Fu Y-S, Perzin KH: Nonepithelial tumors of the nasal cavity, paranasal sinuses, and nasopharynx: A clinicopathologic study. V. Skeletal muscle tumors (rhabdomyoma and rhabdomyosarcoma). Cancer 37:364, 1976.
318. Gardner DG, Corio RL: Multifocal adult rhabdomyoma. Oral Surg 56:76, 1983.

319. Gardner DG, Corio RL: Fetal rhabdomyoma of the tongue, with a discussion of the two histologic variants of this tumor. Oral Surg 56:293, 1983.
320. Gold JH, Bossen EH: Benign vaginal rhabdomyoma: A light and electron microscopic study. Cancer 37:2283, 1976.
321. Goldman RL: Multicentric benign rhabdomyoma of skeletal muscle. Cancer 16:1609, 1963.
322. Knowles DM II, Jakobiec FA: Rhabdomyoma of the orbit. Am J Ophthalmol 80:1011, 1975.
323. Konrad EA, Meister P, Hübner G: Extracardiac rhabdomyoma: Report of different types with light microscopic and ultrastructural studies. Cancer 49:898, 1982.
324. Misch KA: Rhabdomyoma purum: A benign rhabdomyoma of tongue. J Pathol Bacteriol 75:105, 1958.
325. Moran JJ, Enterline HT: Benign rhabdomyoma of the pharynx: A case report, review of the literature, and comparison with cardiac rhabdomyoma. Am J Clin Pathol 42:174, 1964.
326. Olofsson J: Extracardiac rhabdomyoma. Acta Otolaryngol 74:139, 1972.
327. Ross CF: Rhabdomyoma of sternomastoid. J Pathol Bacteriol 95:556, 1968.
328. Schlosnagle DC, Kratochvil FJ, Weathers DR, et al: Intraoral multifocal adult rhabdomyoma: Report of a case and review of the literature. Arch Pathol Lab Med 107:638, 1983.
329. Scrivner D, Meyer JS: Multifocal recurrent adult rhabdomyoma. Cancer 46:790, 1980.
330. Silseth C, Veress B, Bergstrom B: A case of adult rhabdomyoma in the tonsillar region. Acta Pathol Microbiol Immunol Scand 90:1, 1982.
331. Solomon MP, Tolete-Velcek F: Lingual rhabdomyoma (adult variant) in a child. J Pediatr Surg 14:91, 1979.
332. Tandler B, Rossi EP, Stein M, et al: Rhabdomyoma of the lip: Light and electron microscopical observations. Arch Pathol 89:118, 1970.
333. Tanner NSB, Carter RL, Clifford P: Pharyngeal rhabdomyoma: An unusual presentation. J Laryngol Otol 92:1029, 1978.
334. Warner TFCS, Goell W, Sundharadas M, et al: Adult rhabdomy-oma: Ultrastructure and immunocytochemistry. Arch Pathol Lab Med 105:608, 1981.
335. Weitzner S, Lockey MW, Lockard VG: Adult rhabdomyoma of soft palate. Oral Surg 47:70, 1979.
336. Winther LK: Rhabdomyoma of the hypopharynx and larynx: Report of two cases and a review of the literature. J Laryngol Otol 90:1041, 1976.
337. Wyatt RB, Schochet SS, McCormick WF: Rhabdomyoma: Light and electron microscopic study of a case with intranuclear inclusions. Arch Otolaryngol 92:32, 1970.

RHABDOMYOSARCOMA

338. Altmannsberger M, Osborn M, Treuner J, et al: Diagnosis of human childhood rhabdomyosarcoma by antibodies to desmin, the structural protein of muscle specific intermediate filaments. Virchows Arch (Cell Pathol) 39:203, 1982.
339. Angervall L, Enzinger FM: Extraskeletal neoplasm resembling Ewing's sarcoma. Cancer 36:240, 1975.
340. Ashton N, Morgan G: Embryonal sarcoma and embryonal rhab-domyosarcoma of the orbit. J Clin Pathol 18:699, 1965.
341. Bale PM, Parsons RE, Stevens MM: Diagnosis and behavior of juvenile rhabdomyosarcoma. Hum Pathol 14:596, 1983.
342. Bale PM, Reye RDK: Rhabdomyosarcoma in childhood. Pathology 7:101, 1975.
343. Batsakis JG, Fox JE: Rhabdomyosarcoma of the larynx: Report of a case. Arch Otolaryngol 91:136, 1970.
344. Bundtzen JL, Norback DH: The ultrastructure of poorly differentiated rhabdomyosarcomas: A case report and literature review. Hum Pathol 13:301, 1982.
345. Canalis RF, Jenkins HA, Hemenway WG, et al: Nasopharyngeal rhabdomyosarcoma: A clinical perspective. Arch Otolaryngol 104:122, 1978.
346. Canalis RF, Platz CE, Cohn AM: Laryngeal rhabdomyosarcoma. Arch Otolaryngol 102:104, 1976.
347. Deutsch M, Felder H: Rhabdomyosarcoma of the ear-mastoid. Laryngoscope 84:586, 1974.
348. Diehn KW, Hyams VJ, Harris AE: Rhabdomyosarcoma of the larynx: A case report and review of the literature. Laryngoscope 94:201, 1984.
349. Dito WR, Batsakis JG: Intraoral, pharyngeal and nasopharyngeal rhabdomyosarcoma. Arch Otolaryngol 77:123, 1963.
350. Dito WR, Batsakis JG: Rhabdomyosarcoma of the head and neck: An appraisal of the biologic behavior in 170 cases. Arch Surg 84:582, 1962.
351. Donaldson SS, Castro JR, Wilbur JR, et al: Rhabdomyosarcoma of

head and neck in children: Combination treatment by surgery, irradiation and chemotherapy. Cancer 31:26, 1973.

352. Edland RW: Embryonal rhabdomyosarcoma of the middle ear. Cancer 29:784, 1972.

353. Enterline HT, Horn RC Jr: Alveolar rhabdomyosarcoma: A distinctive tumor type. Am J Clin Pathol 29:356, 1958.

354. Enzinger FM: Recent trends in soft tissue pathology. In Tumors of Bone and Soft Tissue. Chicago, Year Book Medical Publishers, 1965, pp 315–332.

355. Enzinger FM, Shiraki M: Alveolar rhabdomyosarcoma: An analysis of 110 cases. Cancer 24:18, 1969.

356. Eusebi V, Bondi A, Rosai J: Immunohistochemical localization of myoglobin in nonmuscular cells. Am J Surg Pathol 8:51, 1984.

357. Exelby PR: Surgery of soft tissue sarcomas in children. Natl Cancer Inst Monogr 56:153, 1981.

358. Feldman BA: Rhabdomyosarcoma of the head and neck. Laryngoscope 92:424, 1982.

359. Flamant F, Hill C: The improvement in survival associated with combined chemotherapy in childhood rhabdomyosarcoma: A historical comparison of 345 patients in the same center. Cancer 53:2417, 1984.

360. Fleischer AS, Koslow M, Rovit RL: Neurological manifestations of primary rhabdomyosarcoma of the head and neck in children. J Neurosurg 43:207, 1975.

361. Gaiger AM, Soule EH, Newton WA Jr: Pathology of rhabdomyosarcoma: Experience of the Intergroup Rhabdomyosarcoma Study, 1972–78. Natl Cancer Inst Monogr 56:19, 1981.

362. Gerson JM, Jaffe N, Donaldson MH, et al: Meningeal seeding from rhabdomyosarcoma of the head and neck with base of the skull invasion: Recognition of the clinical evolution and suggestions for management. Med Pediatr Oncol 5:137, 1978.

363. Gillespie JJ, Roth LM, Wills ER, et al: Extraskeletal Ewing's sarcoma: Histologic and ultrastructural observations in three cases. Am J Surg Pathol 3:99, 1979.

364. Gonzalez-Crussi F, Black-Schaffer S: Rhabdomyosarcoma of infancy and childhood: Problems of morphologic classification. Am J Surg Pathol 3:157, 1979.

365. Horn RC Jr, Enterline HT: Rhabdomyosarcoma: A clinicopathological study and classification of 39 cases. Cancer 11:181, 1958.

366. Jaffe BF, Fox JE, Batsakis JG: Rhabdomyosarcoma of the middle ear and mastoid. Cancer 27:29, 1971.

367. Jones IS, Reese AB, Krout J: Orbital rhabdomyosarcoma: An analysis of sixty-two cases. Trans Am Ophthalmol Soc 63:223, 1965.

368. Kahn HJ, Yeger H, Kassim O, et al: Immunohistochemical and electron microscopic assessment of childhood rhabdomyosarcoma: Increased frequency of diagnosis over routine histologic methods. Cancer 51:1897, 1983.

369. Keyhani A, Booher RJ: Pleomorphic rhabdomyosarcoma. Cancer 22:956, 1968.

370. Lawrence W Jr, Hays DM: Surgical lessons from the Intergroup Rhabdomyosarcoma Study. Natl Cancer Inst Monogr 56:159, 1981.

371. Lawrence W Jr, Hays DM, Moon TE: Lymphatic metastasis with childhood rhabdomyosarcoma. Cancer 39:556, 1977.

372. Lawrence W Jr, Jegge G, Foote FW Jr: Embryonal rhabdomyosarcoma: A clinicopathological study. Cancer 17:361, 1964.

373. Li FP, Fraumeni JF Jr: Rhabdomyosarcoma in children: Epidemiologic study and identification of a familial cancer syndrome. J Natl Cancer Inst 43:1365, 1969.

374. Liebner EJ: Embryonal rhabdomyosarcoma of head and neck in children: Correlation of stage, radiation dose, local control, and survival. Cancer 37:2777, 1976.

375. Linscheid RL, Soule EH, Henderson ED: Pleomorphic rhabdomyosarcomata of the extremities and limb girdles. A clinicopathological study. J Bone Joint Surg (Am) 47:715, 1965.

376. Lloyd RV, Hajdu SI, Knapper WH: Embryonal rhabdomyosarcoma in adults. Cancer 51:557, 1983.

377. Mahour GH, Soule EH, Mills SD, et al: Rhabdomyosarcoma in infants and children: A clinicopathologic study of 75 cases. J Pediatr Surg 2:402, 1967.

378. Makishima K, Iwasaki H, Horie A: Alveolar rhabdomyosarcoma of the ethmoid sinus. Laryngoscope 85:400, 1975.

379. Masson JK, Soule EH: Embryonal rhabdomyosarcoma of the head and neck. Report on eighty-eight cases. Am J Surg 110:585, 1965.

380. Maurer HM, Donaldson M, Gehan EA, et al: Rhabdomyosarcoma in childhood and adolescence. Curr Probl Cancer 2:1, 1978.

381. Maurer HM, Moon T, Donaldson M, et al: The Intergroup Rhabdomyosarcoma Study: A preliminary report. Cancer 40:2015, 1977.

382. Mierau GW, Favara BE: Rhabdomyosarcoma in children: Ultrastructural study of 31 cases. Cancer 46:2035, 1980.

383. Miettinen M, Lehto V-P, Badley RA, et al: Alveolar rhabdomyosarcoma: Demonstration of the muscle type of intermediate filament protein, desmin, as a diagnostic aid. Am J Pathol 108:246, 1982.

384. Miller RW: Contrasting epidemiology of childhood osteosarcoma, Ewing's tumor, and rhabdomyosarcoma. Natl Cancer Inst Monogr 56:9, 1981.

385. Moore O, Grossi C: Embryonal rhabdomyosarcoma of the head and neck. Cancer 12:69, 1959.

386. Morales AR, Fine G, Horn RC Jr: Rhabdomyosarcoma: An ultrastructural appraisal. Pathol Annu 7:81, 1972.

387. Mukai M, Iri H, Torikata C, et al: Immunoperoxidase demonstration of a new muscle protein (Z-protein) in myogenic tumors as a diagnostic aid. Am J Pathol 114:164, 1984.

388. Mukai K, Rosai J, Hallaway BE: Localization of myoglobin in normal and neoplastic human skeletal muscle cells using an immunoperoxidase method. Am J Surg Pathol 3:373, 1979.

389. Newman AN, Rice DH: Rhabdomyosarcoma of the head and neck. Laryngoscope 94:234, 1984.

390. O'Day RA, Soule EH, Gores RJ: Embryonal rhabdomyosarcoma of the oral soft tissues. Oral Surg 20:85, 1965.

391. Patton RB, Horn RC Jr: Rhabdomyosarcoma: Clinical and pathological features and comparison with human fetal and embryonal skeletal muscle. Surgery 52:572, 1962.

392. Porterfield JF, Zimmerman LE: Rhabdomyosarcoma of the orbit: A clinicopathologic study of 55 cases. Virchows Arch (Pathol Anat) 335:329, 1962.

393. Prior JT, Stoner LR: Sarcoma botryoides of the nasopharynx. Cancer 10:957, 1957.

394. Raney RB: Spinal cord "drop metastases" from head and neck rhabdomyosarcoma: Proceedings of the Tumor Board of the Children's Hospital of Philadelphia. Med Pediatr Oncol 4:3, 1978.

395. Raney RB Jr, Crist WM, Maurer HM, Foulkes MA: Prognosis of children with soft tissue sarcoma who relapse after achieving a complete response: A report from the Intergroup Rhabdomyosarcoma Study—I. Cancer 52:44, 1983.

396. Raney RB Jr, Donaldson MH, Sutow WW, et al: Special considerations related to primary site in rhabdomyosarcoma: Experience of the Intergroup Rhabdomyosarcoma Study, 1972–1976. Natl Cancer Inst Monogr 56:69, 1981.

397. Raney RB Jr, Lawrence W Jr, Maurer HM, et al: Rhabdomyosarcoma of the ear in childhood: A report from the Intergroup Rhabdomyosarcoma Study—I. Cancer 51:2356, 1983.

398. Shimada H, Newton WA Jr, Soule EH, et al: Pathology of fatal rhabdomyosarcoma: Intergroup Rhabdomyosarcoma Study IRS I and II. Lab Invest 50:12P, 1984.

399. Smith MT, Armbrustmacher VW, Violett TW: Diffuse meningeal rhabdomyosarcoma. Cancer 47:2081, 1981.

400. Soule EH, Geitz M, Henderson ED: Embryonal rhabdomyosarcoma of the limbs and limb-girdles: A clinicopathologic study of 61 cases. Cancer 23:1336, 1969.

401. Soule EH, Newton W Jr, Moon TE, Tefft M: Extraskeletal Ewing's sarcoma: A preliminary review of 26 cases encountered in the Intergroup Rhabdomyosarcoma Study. Cancer 42:259, 1978.

402. Stobbe GD, Dargeon HW: Embryonal rhabdomyosarcoma of the head and neck in children and adolescents. Cancer 3:826, 1950.

403. Sutow WW: Childhood rhabdomyosarcoma. In Malignant Solid Tumors in Children. A Review. New York, Raven Press, 1981, pp 129–147.

404. Sutow WW, Sullivan MP, Ried HL, et al: Prognosis in childhood rhabdomyosarcoma. Cancer 25:1384, 1970.

405. Tefft M, Fernandez C, Donaldson M, et al: Incidence of meningeal involvement by rhabdomyosarcoma of the head and neck in children: A report of the Intergroup Rhabdomyosarcoma Study (IRS). Cancer 42:253, 1978.

406. Triche TJ, Askin FB: Neuroblastoma and the differential diagnosis of small-, round-, blue-cell tumors. Hum Pathol 14:569, 1983.

407. Tsokos M, Howard R, Costa J: Immunohistochemical study of alveolar and embryonal rhabdomyosarcoma. Lab Invest 48:148, 1983.

408. Tsokos M, Miser A, Pizzo P, et al: Histologic and cytologic characteristics of poor prognosis childhood rhabdomyosarcoma (abstract). Lab Invest 50:61A, 1984.

409. Weiss SW, Enzinger FM: Malignant fibrous histiocytoma. An analysis of 200 cases. Cancer 41:2250, 1978.

410. Wharam MD Jr, Foulkes MA, Lawrence W Jr, et al: Soft tissue sarcoma of the head and neck in childhood: Nonorbital and nonparameningeal sites. A report of the Intergroup Rhabdomyosarcoma Study (IRS)—I. Cancer 53:1016, 1984.

411. Winther LK, Lorentzen M: Rhabdomyosarcoma of the larynx. Report of two cases and a review of the literature. J Laryngol Otol 92:417, 1978.

CHAPTER 54

Radiation Therapy of Tumors of the Neck

Gilbert H. Fletcher, M.D. · Robert D. Lindberg, M.D.

EPITHELIAL TUMORS

The initial labeling of different types of cancers as being either radiosensitive or radioresistant was based on clinical observations made in the 1930s and 1940s. Primary squamous cell carcinoma of the oral cavity was considered radiosensitive because a significant percentage of control could be obtained with interstitial implants. Nodal metastases were considered radioresistant because, using 250 Kv, irradiation control of clinically positive neck nodes was practically never obtained. Elective irradiation of the neck was not done because at that time the concept was that of an "all or none" radioresistance or radiosensitivity linked with histologic type, for control rates had not yet been correlated with the volume of cancer and doses of irradiation. If clinically positive nodes were not controlled, any size of cancer aggregates would not be controlled.

With the availability in the mid-1950s of megavoltage irradiation, elective irradiation of clinically negative lymphatics was started at the University of Texas M. D. Anderson Hospital. The first analysis was published in 1963 and showed that in excess of 90 per cent of expected occult deposits were controlled with 4500 to 5000 rad.[25] The effectiveness of this dose range on subclinical disease has repeatedly been confirmed by analyses done for all the anatomic sites of the respiratory and digestive tracts, both at the M. D. Anderson Hospital and at other institutions.[4, 22, 26]

With megavoltage irradiation, much higher doses could be given than the original 250 Kv given to positive neck nodes from primary tumors originating in the nasopharynx or in the oropharynx treated by irradiation alone, and a significant percentage of nodes were permanently controlled.

The basic indications for combining surgery and irradiation in the management of neck disease came from a detailed analysis made at Memorial Sloan-Kettering Cancer Center in New York City of the failures in the radically dissected neck according to the extent of disease in the surgical specimen.[29] There have been several publications showing the effectiveness of the combined treatment in the management of neck disease.[2]

This investigation was supported in part by grants CA06294 and CA16672 awarded by the National Cancer Institute, Department of Health and Human Services.

Today there is a scientific rationale substantiated by clinical data for using irradiation in the management of metastatic neck disease, either as elective treatment of clinically negative lymphatic areas, as the sole treatment of clinically positive nodes in specific situations, or as an adjuvant to neck dissection.

Topographic Distribution on Admission of Clinically Positive Neck Nodes

By recording the topographic location of clinically positive nodes at the time of the patient's admission, it has been shown that the location of involved nodes is usually predictable for a given primary tumor site.[18] The initial metastasis from well-differentiated squamous cell carcinoma is usually limited to the first node level for a specific site, but with advanced disease, spread to other levels is common. Metastatic cancer from anaplastic squamous cell carcinoma or lymphoepithelioma more frequently involves multiple levels of lymph nodes. Spread to the contralateral neck area is usually to the corresponding first level, that is, the opposite subdigastric nodes.

Oral Tongue (Fig. 54–1). The subdigastric nodes are most commonly involved, followed by the submaxillary triangle nodes and the midjugular nodes. The submental, low jugular, and posterior cervical nodes are seldom involved.

Floor of the Mouth (Fig. 54–1). The subdigastric nodes are most commonly involved, followed by the nodes of the submaxillary triangle. The submental nodes are rarely affected in spite of the anterior location of the tumors. The low jugular and posterior cervical nodes are seldom involved.

Retromolar Trigone–Anterior Faucial Pillar (Fig. 54–2). The most commonly involved node is the node at the angle of the jaw, followed by the midjugular nodes. The posterior cervical nodes are rarely involved.

Soft Palate (Fig. 54–2). Because the soft palate is a midline structure, the incidence of bilateral subdigastric nodes is high.

Tonsillar Fossa (Fig. 54–2). The node at the angle of the jaw is almost always the first to be involved. The incidence of involvement of mid- and low jugular nodes is also significant. Metastasis to the posterior cervical nodes is common, both ipsilaterally and contralaterally. The parapharyngeal nodes can be involved.

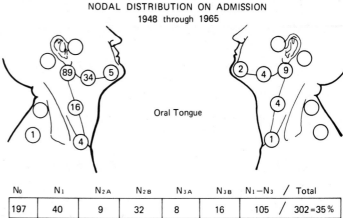

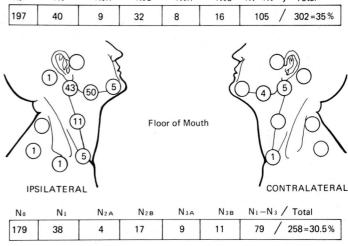

NODAL DISTRIBUTION ON ADMISSION
1948 through 1965

Oral Tongue

N₀	N₁	N₂ₐ	N₂ᴮ	N₃ₐ	N₃ᴮ	N₁–N₃ / Total
197	40	9	32	8	16	105 / 302=35%

Floor of Mouth

IPSILATERAL   CONTRALATERAL

N₀	N₁	N₂ₐ	N₂ᴮ	N₃ₐ	N₃ᴮ	N₁–N₃ / Total
179	38	4	17	9	11	79 / 258=30.5%

Figure 54–1. Locations of clinically positive nodes at the time of admission for tumors of the oral tongue and floor of mouth. (From Lindberg RD: Cancer *29*:1446, 1972.[18])

Base of the Tongue (Fig. 54–3). Because the base of the tongue is a midline structure, bilateral metastases are common. The midjugular nodes are often involved, but posterior cervical nodes are rarely involved. Low jugular nodes are involved if there is extensive nodal disease in the subdigastric and midjugular lymphatics.

Oropharyngeal Walls (Fig. 54–3). The subdigastric nodes are involved most commonly. This is followed by involvement of the midjugular nodes and of the posterior cervical nodes. The parapharyngeal nodes can be involved.

Supraglottic Larynx (Fig. 54–4). The subdigastric nodes are most commonly involved, followed by the midjugular nodes. The incidence of bilateral metastases is significant. The posterior cervical nodes seldom are involved.

Hypopharynx (Fig. 54–4). The majority of metastases are to the jugular chain—upper, mid-, and low in decreasing order of frequency. Because most lesions arise in the pyriform sinus, the frequency of bilateral metastases is low. Ipsilateral posterior cervical nodes occasionally are involved.

Nasopharynx (Fig. 54–4). Nasopharyngeal lesions have the greatest incidence of bilateral metastases and of posterior cervical chain involvement of any anatomic site. The incidence of low jugular or supraclavicular metastasis is significant.

Paranasal Sinuses. If the lesion is located in the suprastructure of the maxillary antrum or ethmoids, the involved nodes are usually subdigastric, often bilater-

ally. If the lesion is located in the infrastructure of the maxillary antrum, the first nodes involved are located in the submaxillary triangle.

Parotid Gland. The ipsilateral neck nodes can be involved in the high-grade tumors.

Skin. Squamous cell carcinoma of the temples, forehead, and canthi spread to the preauricular nodes and the nodes inside the parotid.

Vestibule and Ala Nasi. The submaxillary triangle nodes are involved first. Transit metastases, that is, nodules within the cheek (involvement of the buccal nodes), are not uncommon.

Sequential Spread

Not only is the topographic location of involved nodes predictable for the various anatomic sites, but the sequential spread from one echelon to the other is also predictable. If the first echelon of lymphatics is not involved, the probability of involvement of the next echelon is low. In lateralized lesions, the probability of contralateral metastases is low when the ipsilateral side of the neck is clinically negative. The probability increases as the extent of ipsilateral metastases increases.

Staging System

The staging system shown in Table 54–1 has been used at M. D. Anderson Hospital and is based on the experience that the size and number of node(s) have a

NODAL DISTRIBUTION ON ADMISSION
1948 through 1965

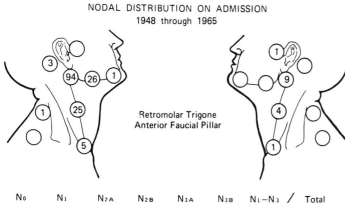

Retromolar Trigone
Anterior Faucial Pillar

N₀	N₁	N₂ₐ	N₂ᵦ	N₃ₐ	N₃ᵦ	N₁–N₃ / Total
125	38	15	34	4	11	102 / 227 = 45%

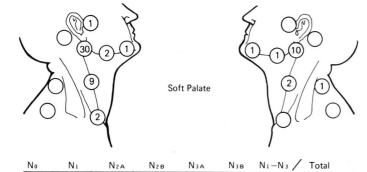

Soft Palate

N₀	N₁	N₂ₐ	N₂ᵦ	N₃ₐ	N₃ᵦ	N₁–N₃ / Total
45	12	2	4	4	13	35 / 80 = 44%

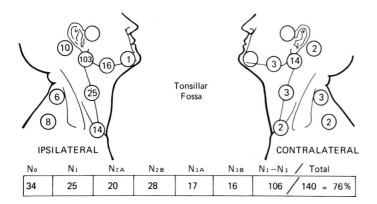

Tonsillar
Fossa

IPSILATERAL   CONTRALATERAL

N₀	N₁	N₂ₐ	N₂ᵦ	N₃ₐ	N₃ᵦ	N₁–N₃ / Total
34	25	20	28	17	16	106 / 140 = 76%

Figure 54–2. Locations of clinically positive nodes at the time of admission for tumors of the retromolar trigone, anterior faucial pillar, soft palate, and tonsillar fossa. (From Lindberg RD: Cancer *29*:1446, 1972.[18])

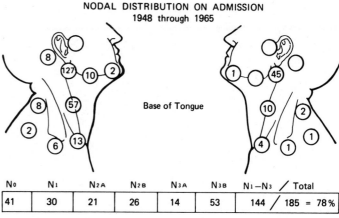

NODAL DISTRIBUTION ON ADMISSION
1948 through 1965

Base of Tongue

N0	N1	N2A	N2B	N3A	N3B	N1–N3	Total
41	30	21	26	14	53	144 / 185 = 78%	

Figure 54–3. Locations of clinically positive nodes at the time of admission for tumors of the base of the tongue and oropharyngeal walls. (From Lindberg RD: Cancer 29:1446, 1972.[18])

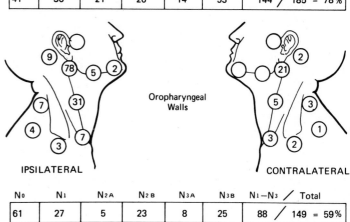

Oropharyngeal Walls

IPSILATERAL   CONTRALATERAL

N0	N1	N2A	N2B	N3A	N3B	N1–N3	Total
61	27	5	23	8	25	88 / 149 = 59%	

direct bearing on the failure rates and require different management. It is similar to the system adopted by the American Joint Committee in 1977.[19]

Table 54–2 shows the correlation between clinical and pathologic staging in patients having had a neck dissec-

tion at M. D. Anderson Hospital between 1964 and 1978. A positive correlation increases with the size of the nodes. With nodes larger than 3 cm in diameter, the incidence of a clinically false positive finding is less than 3 per cent.

There is a correlation of neck staging with the later appearance of distant metastases as shown in a series of patients having had their primary lesion and initial neck node(s) controlled (Fig. 54–5).[5] In patients with lesions of the pyriform sinus, the incidence of distant metastases is 16 per cent in patients with N0 and N1 neck disease and 28 per cent in patients with N2 and N3 neck disease.[7]

Evolution of Neck Disease

The incidence of occult deposits in patients with a clinically negative neck has been documented by either elective neck dissections or observation of patients with an N0 neck left untreated. Table 54–3, which is a composite of analyses from multiple institutions, shows the frequency of clinically positive neck and of occult deposits for all anatomic sites of the upper respiratory and digestive tracts. The incidence of neck disease developing later in patients with squamous cell carcinoma of the oral tongue and an N0 neck increases with the size of the primary lesion (Table 54–4).

The percentage of patients who die of cancer increases sharply with later appearance of neck disease. A 3 per cent incidence of distant metastases was found in patients with remaining N0 neck versus 11 per cent in

TABLE 54–1. Staging System Used at the University of Texas M. D. Anderson Hospital for Cervical Lymph Node Metastases*

Stage	Description
N0	No clinically positive node.
N1	Single, clinically positive, homolateral node less than 3 cm in diameter.
N2	Single, clinically positive homolateral node 3 to 6 cm in diameter; or multiple, clinically positive, homolateral nodes, none over 6 cm in diameter.
N2A	Single, clinically positive, homolateral node 3 to 6 cm in diameter.
N2B	Multiple, clinically positive, homolateral nodes, none over 6 cm in diameter.
N3	Massive homolateral node(s), bilateral nodes, contralateral node(s).
N3A	Clinically positive, homolateral node(s), one node 6 cm or more in diameter.
N3B	Bilateral, clinically positive nodes. (In this situation each side of the neck should be staged separately; for example, N3B: right N2A, left N1.)
N3C	Contralateral, clinically positive node(s) only.

*Similar to 1977 staging of the American Joint Committee.[19]

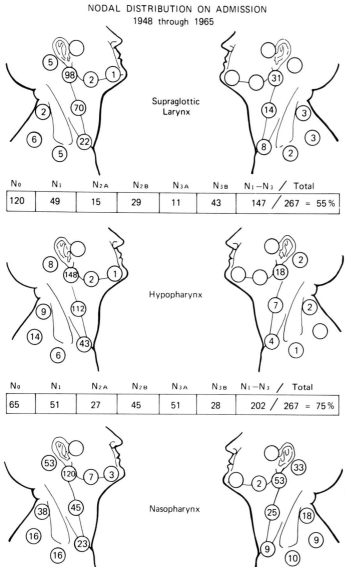

NODAL DISTRIBUTION ON ADMISSION
1948 through 1965

Figure 54–4. Locations of clinically positive nodes at the time of admission for tumors of the supraglottic larynx, hypopharynx, and nasopharynx. (From Lindberg RD: Cancer 29:1446, 1972.[18])

TABLE 54–2. Percentage of Lack of Correlation of Clinical with Pathologic N Staging: Neck Dissections (1964 through 1978)

Clinical N Stage	Pathologic Status	Oral Cavity	Oropharynx	Supraglottic	Glottic	Hypopharynx
N0	+	24.5 (47/192)	43.2 (35/81)	53.4 (31/58)	28.1 (16/57)	63.3 (31/49)
N1	−	23.7 (41/173)	18.2 (16/88)	17.3 (9/52)	19.0 (4/21)	12.3 (7/57)
N2A	−	7.9 (3/38)	0 (0/25)	0 (0/17)	0 (0/5)	0 (0/28)
N2B	−	14.0 (7/50)	12.5 (5/40)	12.0 (3/25)	20.0 (2/10)	1.6 (1/62)
N3A	−	0 (0/10)	0 (0/11)	20.0 (1/5)	0 (0/6)	0 (0/22)
N3B	−	9.5 (2/21)	0 (0/23)	3.6 (1/28)	0 (0/2)	0 (0/17)

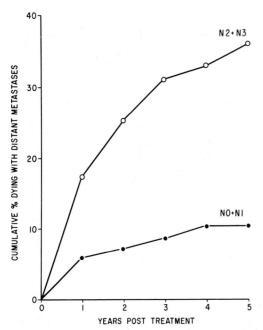

Figure 54–5. Cumulative percentage of patients dying with distant metastases by initial N stage. The primary and the initial neck disease were controlled. (From Berger DS, Fletcher GH: Radiology *100*:141, 1971.[5])

those who become N+.[16] In another study with controlled N1 or N2 disease in the ipsilateral side of the neck, the incidence of distant metastases is 12 per cent if the contralateral side of the neck stays N0 and 24 per cent if it becomes involved.[27] Elective irradiation of the clinically negative lymphatics in patients with supraglottic lesions reduced from 29 per cent to 4 per cent the incidence of regional failures and reduced tumor-related deaths from 35 to 5 per cent.[15]

Radiation Control of Neck Disease Correlated with Dose and Volume of Cancer

Elective Irradiation of Subclinical Disease

With elective irradiation of 4500 to 5000 rad, the control rate of occult deposits in surgically untampered lymphatics is almost 100 per cent (Tables 54–5 and 54–6). This has been confirmed in other series.[22, 26] There is not an "all-or-none" response to irradiation, and with doses less than 5000 rad, such as 3000 to 4000 rad, the control rate is approximately 70 to 80 per cent (Tables 54–6 and 54–7). With doses lower than 3000 rad, the control rate is much lower. In a series of patients with pyriform sinus lesions who received preoperatively 3000 rad to the midline through the ipsilateral side of the neck, approximately 2000 to 2500 rad is delivered to the contralateral side of the neck. After total laryngectomy–partial pharyngectomy and ipsilateral radical neck dissection, 23 per cent of the patients developed contralateral metastases,[20] whereas with 5000 to 6000 rad given postoperatively, there was less than 2 per cent appearance of contralateral metastases (Tables 54–6 and 54–8).

Clinically Positive or Proven by Biopsy Positive Nodes

Increasing doses are necessary to control neck nodes of increasing sizes. Table 54–9 relates the failure rates with both the size of the nodes and doses of irradiation given in patients with squamous cell carcinoma of all sites treated with external irradiation alone.[28] Table 54–10 correlates in a series of patients with pyriform sinus lesions the control of neck nodes with external irradiation with the size of the nodes and the doses of irradiation given.[3] For nodes less than 3 cm in diameter, a high control rate is obtained with 5500 rad, but for more than 3 cm, it requires 6500 rad or more. Even with these high doses, the failure rate is significant.

TABLE 54–3. Incidence of Lymph Node Metastasis by Site of Primary Lesions in Squamous Cell Carcinomas of the Head and Neck

Site	Percentage of Patients*		
	N + at Presentation	N0 Clinically, N + Pathologically	N0 Clinically Initially, N + Later with No Neck Treatment
Floor of mouth	30–59	40–50	20–35
Gingiva	18–52	19	17
Hard palate	13–24		22
Buccal mucosa	9–31		16
Oral tongue	34–65	25–54	38–52
Nasopharynx	86–90		19–50†
Anterior tonsillar pillar/retromolar trigone	39–56		10–15
Soft palate/uvula	37–56		16–25
Tonsillar fossa	58–76		22‡
Base of tongue	50–83	22	
Pharyngeal walls	50–71	66	
Supraglottic larynx	31–54	16–26	33
Hypopharynx	52–72	38	

*The numbers indicate the range from various series.
†T1 N0 patients only.
‡Patients received preoperative radiation.
Source: Mendenhall WM, et al: Head Neck Surg 3:15, 1980. Courtesy of John Wiley & Sons, New York.[22]

TABLE 54–4. Incidence of Neck Disease Developing in Patients with Squamous Cell Carcinoma of the Oral Tongue and N0 Neck

Total Number of Patients	Stage of Primary Tumor	Patients with Neck Disease (Number/Percentage)
95	T1	28/29.5
77	T2	33/42.9
13	T3	10/77.0

Note: More than 60 per cent of the patients died of uncontrolled neck disease after a radical neck dissection.

Source: Strong EW: Otolaryngol Clin North Am 12:107, 1979.[30]

Technique of Irradiation of the Lymphatics

Figure 54–6 shows the surface coverage of the lymphatics of the neck used for planning the irradiation portals.

Subdigastric and Midjugular Lymphatics

In the patients in whom the posterior subdigastric nodes were not covered there was a significant appearance of marginal failures, and to include adequate coverage of the posterior subdigastric nodes, the bodies of the vertebrae must be seen on the simulator films (Fig. 54–7).[23] Also the nodes at the junction of the subdigastric and the midjugular lymphatics must be covered. Electively, 5000 rad is given if the primary is treated by a surgical excision or an interstitial implant. When the primary site is treated with external irradiation only, the dose is higher and is determined by the dose given to the primary site.

Lower Neck Irradiation

Irradiation to the lower neck is administered through an anterior field with the larynx shielded (Fig. 54–8). Usually, 5000 rad is the given dose, delivered in 5 weeks. If there is advanced disease in the upper neck, the dose to the lower neck may be 5500 or even 6000 rad.

Employing a ^{60}Co unit or 4 MeV, the tumor dose to the low jugular, supraclavicular, and posterior cervical triangle nodes is the same as the given dose because the nodes are all located immediately under the skin; for the midjugular nodes, approximately 2 cm deep, the tumor dose is about 90 per cent of the given dose (Fig. 54–8).

TABLE 54–5. Results of Elective Irradiation (5000 rad) in Two Series of Patients with Squamous Cell Carcinoma of the Head and Neck Having Initially N0 Neck with Primary Tumor Controlled*

Site	No. Failures/ No. Patients Treated
Oral cavity and oropharynx (whole neck irradiated) 1970–1973: Analysis July 1976	1/45
Supraglottic larynx (subdigastric and midjugular nodes irradiated) 1948–1970: Analysis 1980	0/108

*From Fletcher GH: Cancer 53:1274, 1984.

Front and Back Portals

In some situations, usually in patients with a tumor of the nasopharynx, front and back portals are used (Fig. 54–9). Figure 54–10 shows the dosimetry for various doses desired.

Elective Irradiation of Clinically Uninvolved Lymphatic Areas

Although irradiation with 5000 rad in 5 weeks does not produce detectable fibrosis, it should be used only when there is significant probability of occult disease because both subdigastric areas cannot be irradiated without including the mucosa of the oral cavity and oropharynx (5000 rad will produce some dryness). Irradiation of the lower neck may interfere with treatment to the supraclavicular areas for possible future carcinomas of the lung or breast as well as other sites of the head and neck.

Irradiation of just the first echelon is advisable only in lesions with low potential to metastasize. Treatment of the entire neck is indicated for an N0 neck when the primary lesion is in the nasopharynx, base of the tongue, tonsillar fossa, or pyriform sinus.

Oral Cavity

With an initially N0 neck, patients with squamous cell carcinomas of the buccal mucosa and upper and lower gum have a low risk of later developing neck disease. Furthermore, the appearance of contralateral metastases is negligible. Therefore, for small lesions, assuming that the primary tumor will be treated by

TABLE 54–6. Appearance of Contralateral Node Metastases in Squamous Cell Carcinoma According to the Dose of Irradiation Delivered to the Contralateral Side of the Neck

Site	No Irradiation*		With Irradiation†	
Oral tongue	27%	(8/30)	9% (2/22)	3000–4000 rad
Floor of mouth	47%	(9/19)	11% (3/28)	
Total	34.5%	(17/49)	10% (5/50)	
Faucial arch	30%	(3/10)	0% (0/72)	≥ 5000 rad
Supraglottic larynx and pyriform sinus	20%	(26/128)	1.5% (1/65)	
Total	21%	(29/138)	<1% (1/137)	

*Primary lesion and initial ipsilateral neck disease controlled.
†All treatment 1000 rad per week, five fractions per week.
Source: Adapted from Fletcher GH: Elective irradiation of subclinical disease in cancers of the head and neck. Cancer 29:1450, 1972.[8]

TABLE 54–7. Percentage of Eradication of Expected Occult Infestation* in the Lymphatics of the Neck As Function of Dose†

Dose	Percent of Eradication
3000–4000 rad (50 patients)	60–70%
5000 rad (356 patients)	>90%

*Squamous cell carcinoma of the upper respiratory and digestive tracts.
†1000 rad per week, 5 days a week.
Source: Adapted from Fletcher GH: Elective irradiation of subclinical disease in cancers of the head and neck. Cancer 29:1450, 1972.[8]

TABLE 54–8. Site of Recurrence above the Clavicles in Patients with Lesions of the Pyriform Sinus—1949 through 1976 (Analysis, 1981)

Site of Recurrence*	Postoperative Irradiation (125 Patients)	Surgery Alone (203 Patients)
Contralateral nodes	2	35
Ipsilateral nodes	1	13
Along pharyngeal wall	3	11
Parapharyngeal nodes	3	11
Base of skull	1	2
Stoma	3	6
Not specified	6	25
Total sites of recurrence	19 (14)†	103 (80)†

*A patient may have more than one site of recurrence.
†Number of patients with recurrence.
Source: Adapted from El Badawi SA, Goepfert H, Herson J, et al: Laryngoscope 92:357, 1982.[7]

either surgery or interstitial irradiation, there is no real indication for elective treatment of the neck. In larger lesions, even if the neck is N0, treatment of the ipsilateral side of the upper neck is indicated. In patients with squamous cell carcinomas of the oral tongue or floor of the mouth with an N0 neck who have a high risk of later developing neck disease, including bilateral neck metastases, irradiation of both subdigastric areas is indicated. Even in lesions located anteriorly on the mobile tongue or the floor of the mouth, the posterior subdigastric nodes must be included.

Faucial Arch

In patients with an N0 neck, the appearance of contralateral metastases is extremely rare. The ipsilateral subdigastric nodes must be covered generously and the hyoid bone must be seen on the simulator film. With larger lesions, the ipsilateral mid- and low jugular nodes should be irradiated (Fig. 54–11).

Oropharynx

With the exception of patients with small, well-differentiated tumors, the entire neck is irradiated. For lesions of the tonsillar fossa, the spinal accessory and parapharyngeal nodes are irradiated (Fig. 54–8).

Supraglottic Larynx

In patients with lesions of the supraglottic larynx and pyriform sinus, the subdigastric nodes must be irradiated, in addition to the midjugular nodes (Fig. 54–12).

Nasopharynx, Pharyngeal Walls, and Pyriform Sinus

In lesions of the paranasal sinuses, the incidence of cancer developing later in nodes is significant with T3 and T4 lesions. In lesions of the ethmoid sinuses and upper structure of the maxillary antrum, the subdigastric nodes should be irradiated bilaterally. If the infrastructure of the maxillary antrum only is involved, the submaxillary triangle lymphatics must also be irradiated because of the anterior lymphatic drainage of the skin of the cheek.

Vestibulum of the Nose

The incidence of nodes appearing later is significant, and they are usually located anteriorly in the submaxillary triangle lymphatics. In addition, an incidence of metastases has been observed in the thickness of the cheek between the nose and neck. A strip, moustache-like, is irradiated (Fig. 54–13).

Radiation Only for Clinically Positive Neck Nodes

The decision to treat palpable neck nodes by irradiation only rests on the following criteria:

1. *Site of origin.* In tumors of the nasopharynx and

Text continued on page 1311

TABLE 54–9. Failures in Irradiated Fields*—Primary Tumor Controlled, Minimum 4-Year Follow-Up January 1948 through December 1967 (Analysis, January 1972)

N Stage	Total Patients	Fast Treatment (400 rad × 5)	Conventional Treatment (200 rad × 5 weekly)		
			Marginal Coverage or Uncertain Dose	*5500 rad*	*≥ 6500 rad*
N1	100	3/6	11†	1/8 (12.5%)	6/75 (8%)
N2	83	—	13‡	2/3 (66%)	13/67 (20%)

*Failures per total number treated.
†Of the 18 N1 failures.
‡Of the 28 N2 failures.
Source: Adapted from Schneider JJ, Fletcher GH, Barkley HT Jr: AJR 123:42, 1975.[28]

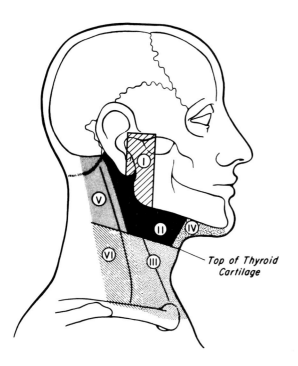

Figure 54–6. Lymphatic areas outlined for planning of radiation portals.

Area I: Parapharyngeal lymphatics to the base of the skull.

Area II: Subdigastric nodes. The field is bounded posteriorly by a line bisecting the sternocleidomastoid muscle, inferiorly by a line drawn at the upper border of the thyroid cartilage, anteriorly by the posterior border of the submaxillary gland, and superiorly by a line extending over the lower border of the mandible.

Area III: Mid- and low jugular nodes. The field is bounded anteriorly by the midline, posteriorly by a line following the posterior border of the sternocleidomastoid muscle, superiorly by the upper border of the thyroid cartilage, and inferiorly by the clavicle.

Area IV: Submaxillary triangle and submental nodes. The field is bounded by the chin superiorly and the upper border of the thyroid cartilage inferiorly, and it has a common boundary with Area II laterally.

Area V: Upper spinal accessory nodes.

Area VI: Posterior cervical triangle nodes that are a continuation of the upper spinal accessory nodes.

(Adapted from Fletcher GH: Textbook of Radiotherapy. 3rd ed. Philadelphia, Lea & Febiger, 1980.)

Top of Thyroid Cartilage

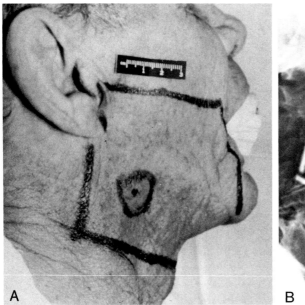

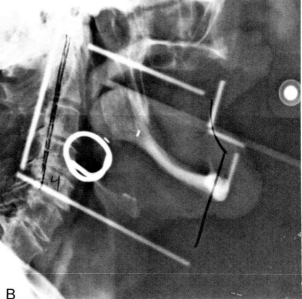

A   B

Figure 54–7. Patient with a T2 lesion of the oral tongue and 2-cm palpable node in the right subdigastric area. A lead marker was placed over the node to show the relationship of the node to the field edges (*A*). To cover the subdigastric nodes adequately, the vertebral bodies must be seen on the simulator film (*B*).

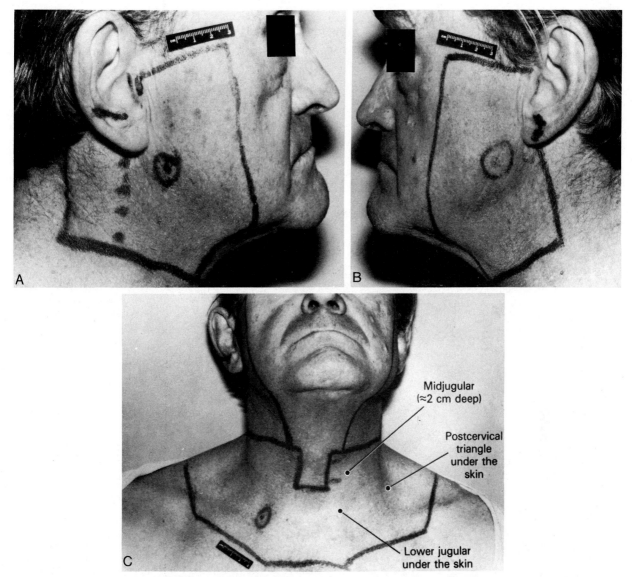

Figure 54–8. This 58-year-old patient presented in January 1980 with a 3 × 3.5 cm mass in the right tonsillar fossa with extension to the anterior faucial arch, glossopalatine sulcus, and lateral pharyngeal wall. There were no palpable nodes. Stage T3N0.

(A) Ipsilateral portal covering the parapharyngeal and subdigastric lymphatics. Because tumors of the tonsillar fossa can spread to the spinal accessory chain of nodes, the posterior neck was irradiated with 6 MeV electron beam.

(B) Contralateral portal covering also the parapharyngeal and the subdigastric lymphatics. Through these two portals a dose of 5000 rad was given to the tumor using a 2:1 loading in favor of the involved side. The right posterior lymph nodes received 5000 rad. Through a reduced field, an additional 2000 rad was given to the primary lesion using a combination of 18 MeV electrons and photons.

(C) Irradiation of the lower neck through an anterior portal with shielding of the larynx. With a given dose of 5000 rad the lower jugular nodes, supraclavicular nodes, and the nodes in the posterior cervical triangles, which are under the skin, receive the same dose. The midjugular nodes, which are approximately 1 to 2 cm deep, receive approximately 4500 rad.

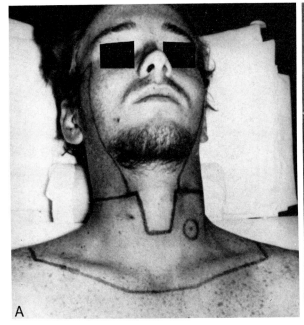

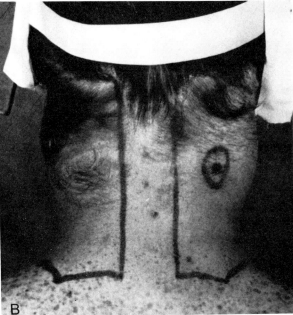

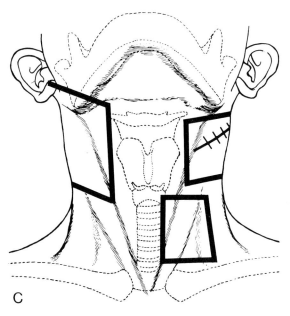

Figure 54–9. Patient seen in August 1971 with a lymphoepithelioma of the nasopharynx with extensive bilateral neck disease.

(A) Anterior field used to irradiate the lower neck. The larynx and cricoid are blocked.

(B) A posterior split field is used to supplement the dose to the upper neck nodes. The lower margin is at the level of the trapezius, as the supraclavicular and low jugular nodes can be irradiated entirely from an anterior field.

(C) Reduced size glancing fields are used for boosting residual disease. If there has been an excisional biopsy of a node, the scar is a potential site of recurrence and should also receive additional irradiation. The patient developed distant metastases within 6 months, received chemotherapy, and died from disease in December 1974.

(From Fletcher GH: Textbook of Radiotherapy. 3rd ed. Philadelphia, Lea & Febiger, 1980.)

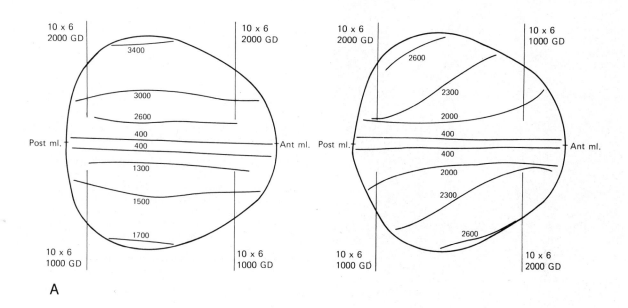

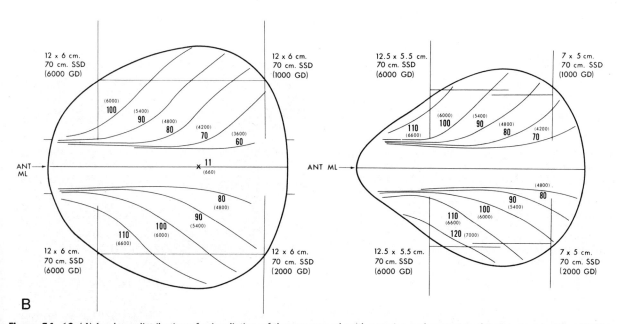

Figure 54–10. (A) Isodose distributions for irradiation of the upper neck with anterior and posterior glancing portals. After 4500 to 5000 rad to the upper neck by lateral portals, additional irradiation to neck nodes is given through opposed anterior and posterior portals. The medial border of these portals is usually 2 cm from the midline. Depending upon the clinical situation, the respective loading of the anterior and posterior portals varies, taking into consideration the original size and location of the palpable node(s). (B) Volume distribution in two patients with different neck sizes. When 6000 rad given dose has been delivered through the anterior portal, by adding 1000 or 2000 rad given dose to the posterior portal, one raises the dose to the spinal accessory chain nodes. (From Fletcher GH: Textbook of Radiotherapy. 3rd ed. Philadelphia, Lea & Febiger, 1980.)

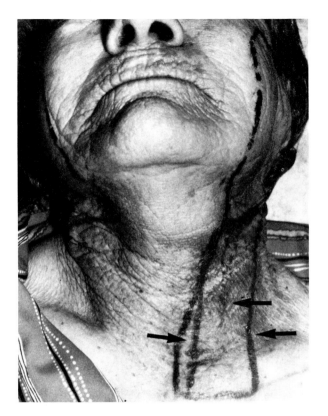

Figure 54–11. This 81-year-old patient presented in July 1982 with a T3 ulcerated lesion centered on the left retromolar trigone with involvement of the soft palate to the midline and of the lower alveolar ridge. No nodes were palpated. After 5000 rad was delivered to the primary and subdigastric nodes, the lower margin of the field was moved up. The total dose to the primary site was 6800 rad in 6½ weeks at a 4-cm depth. Although the ipsilateral subdigastric nodes were negative, because of the extensive primary tumor, the mid- and low jugular nodes were irradiated to 5000 rad through an anterior appositional portal. The central arrow indicates the course of the jugular vein, the lateral arrows show the margins of the portal after a correction. The patient showed no evidence of disease in June 1983.

Figure 54–12. This 53-year-old patient was seen in August 1980 with a squamous cell carcinoma of the suprahyoid epiglottis, stage T2N0. Because of the N0 staging, only the subdigastric and midjugular nodes were irradiated to a dose of 5000 rad; then through small circular fields an extra 1600 rad was given to the primary site, avoiding irradiating the arytenoids. The patient showed no evidence of disease in March 1982, and had a good voice. (From Fletcher GH, Goepfert H: Role of irradiation in treatment of laryngeal cancer. *In* Ferlito A (ed): Cancer of the Larynx, Vol. III. Boca Raton, CRC Press, 1985, pp. 69–114.)

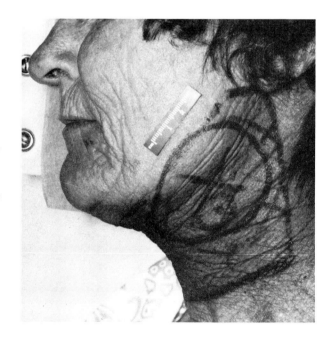

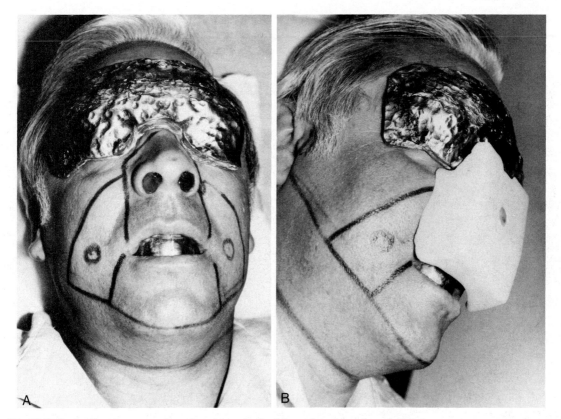

Figure 54–13. Patient with squamous cell carcinoma, grade II, of the columella and nasal septum.

(*A*) In 25 fractions, 5000 rad tumor dose was delivered to the nose through a field extending to the upper lip, using a combination of 15 MeV electrons and ⁶⁰Co, in the ratio of 4:1, electrons to photons. The vermilion border of the upper lip was blocked. A lead shield blocked the eyes and a lead stent was used to avoid irradiating the mouth, and custom-made beeswax was placed in each naris during treatment. A beeswax bolus was placed over the nose during treatment. The field was then reduced to include only the lower two thirds of the nose, and 2000 rad in 10 fractions was added, using the same combination of beams. The right and left moustache areas each received 5000 rad in 25 fractions using 7 MeV electrons.

(*B*) The upper neck received 5000 rad tumor dose in 25 fractions using lateral parallel opposed fields with ⁶⁰Co. The lower neck received a 4500-rad dose given in 18 fractions through a single anterior field with ⁶⁰Co. The larynx was blocked. The overall treatment time was 7½ weeks.

tonsillar fossa, even large neck nodes can be controlled by irradiation (Fig. 54–14).

2. *Size of the neck nodes.* From Tables 54–9 and 54–10, it can be seen that with irradiation a high percentage of nodes less than 3 cm in diameter is controlled.

3. *Location of the node(s).* A node from a primary tumor in the oropharynx is usually located at the angle of the jaw, and if the primary site is treated with external irradiation, the node will be in the reduced field giving a boost to the primary lesion and will get at least 7000 rad. However, unless the primary tumor is in the tonsillar fossa for a node more than 3 cm in diameter, a neck dissection is indicated despite its clinical disappearance.

Marginal coverage or uncertain dosage results in a high failure rate.

Boost

The complications become more frequent and more severe with large doses delivered to large volumes. Because tolerance is related to the volume irradiated, one must use the shrinking field technique; that is, after

a basic dose to the lymphatic area of interest, a "boost" dose of 1000 to 2000 rad is given to the palpable masses through reduced portals (Fig. 54–15). An interstitial implant with ¹⁹²Ir or ¹⁹⁸Au may be used in selected situations.

TABLE 54–10. Control Rates* As a Function of the Size of the Node(s) and Radiation Dose in the Squamous Cell Carcinomas of the Laryngopharynx

Size	Dose		Control Rate
< 3 cm	≤ 65 Gy	}>0.001	15/26 (58%)
	> 65 Gy		86/95 (91%)
3–5 cm	≤ 70 Gy	}<0.005	3/9 (33%)
	> 70 Gy		11/13 (85%)
> 5 cm	≤ 70 Gy	}<0.002	1/9 (11%)
	> 70 Gy		11/15 (73%)

*Determinate group.
Source: Data from Bataini JP, et al: *In* Pinel J, Leroux-Robert J (eds): Adenopathies Cervicales les Malignes. Paris, Masson Publishers, 1982. pp 129–135.[3]

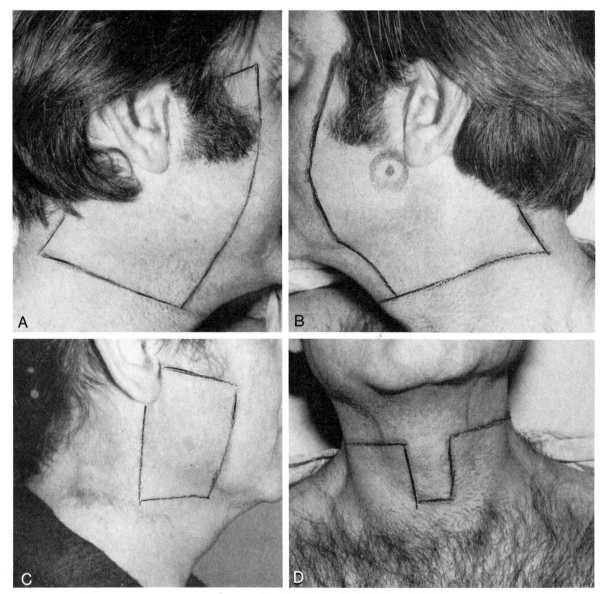

Figure 54–14. This 42-year-old male was seen on November 20, 1974, with a T3N2B poorly differentiated squamous cell carcinoma of the right tonsillar fossa. The lesion extended anteriorly to involve the anterior faucial pillar and retromolar trigone, and inferiorly to involve the glossopharyngeal sulcus. In the right side of the neck, a 4.5 × 4.5 cm node was in the subdigastric region and another smaller node was in the posterior triangle. The left side of the neck was negative for disease. The primary lesion received 5300 rad with ^{60}Co to the midline through parallel opposed portals (A and B), with daily doses of 200 rad, with an added 1700 rad through a reduced portal (C) utilizing half 18-MeV photons and 18-MeV electrons to give a total dose of 7000 rad in 7 weeks. The right posterior neck received 5000 rad with ^{60}Co with an added 1500 rad with 7-MeV electrons. The anterior two thirds of the subdigastric node received 7000 rad, and the posterior one third received 6500 rad. The left posterior neck received 4100 rad. The lower neck received 5000 rad with ^{60}Co in 5 weeks (D).

By the last week of treatment, the large right subdigastric node and the primary tumor had completely disappeared. The patient showed no evidence of disease in July 1982. There is a small area of exposed bone behind the last molar on the right. (From Fletcher GH: Semin Oncol 4:375, 1977. Courtesy of Grune & Stratton, Inc., New York.[9])

Figure 54–15. (A) The whole neck receives 5000 rad (1000 rad per week), or 5500 rad (900 rad per week). (B) For the tumor 1500 to 2000 rad is given through a field treating the primary site, or if not, with glancing fields or electron beam. (C) For very large nodes to be treated by external irradiation only, an additional 500 to 1000 rad is given with electron beam or glancing fields, for 7500 to 8000 rad total dose. (From Fletcher GH: Textbook of Radiotherapy. 3rd ed. Philadelphia, Lea & Febiger, 1980.)

SHRINKING FIELD TECHNIQUE

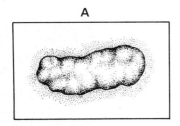

A
B
C

Field-within-a-Field

It is not uncommon for neck nodes to grow under treatment of 900 to 1000 rad per week. In that situation an extra dose is given concomitantly through an appositional portal, using an electron beam of energy, depending on the thickness of the nodes (Fig. 54–16), or front and back glancing portals. Usually 150 rad, three times a week, is delivered after an interval of 3 hours after the first treatment.

Unresectable Nodes

Unresectable nodes (Fig. 54–17) are treated with irradiation with very high doses presently using twice-a-day treatment at 3-hour intervals. The total dose can be as high as 8000 rad, and a modified neck dissection can still be done. A significant percentage of control has been obtained using the twice-a-day treatment technique.[24]

An interstitial implant can be added to external beam irradiation if the node(s) does not become resectable after external irradiation. Total doses of 8000 to 9000 rad are an effective method of treatment.

Combined Treatment

Figure 54–18 shows the incidence of failures in the radically dissected neck by extent of nodal involvement.[32] To evaluate the prognostic significance of cervical lymph node invasion, a meticulous and detailed study of the type and extent of nodal disease was carried out in a series of patients who had had a radical neck dissection for squamous cell carcinoma of the upper respiratory and digestive passages.[6] The survival at 3

Figure 54–16. The patient was seen on April 18, 1983, with a history of recurrent squamous cell carcinoma of the skin of the left facial region. There is a large defect on the left side of the face, the orbit and maxillary sinus having been removed. A 1.5-cm hard node is palpable at the angle of the left mandible. Postoperatively 5000 rad tumor dose was given to the primary site in 5 weeks. The left upper neck nodes received 5000 rad, plus a boost of 2500 rad with 10-MeV electron beam given through a small field (double arrows) 3 hours later to the node at the left angle of the mandible, which kept growing under treatment to 3 to 4 cm, becoming attached to the skin. The total dose to the node was 7500 rad. The left lower neck received 5000 rad dose given with anterior portal in 25 fractions in 5 weeks using ^{60}Co. At completion of irradiation the node at the angle of the mandible was less than 2 cm in size. Six weeks later a residual mass was dissected. There was no delay in wound healing. *Pathology report: tail of parotid*—foreign body reaction to keratin debris and microscopic focus of atypical cells in salivary gland. The cells are degenerated with enlarged but poorly visualized nuclei. Although not diagnostic, the morphologic appearance of the atypical cells suggests radiated tumor cells.

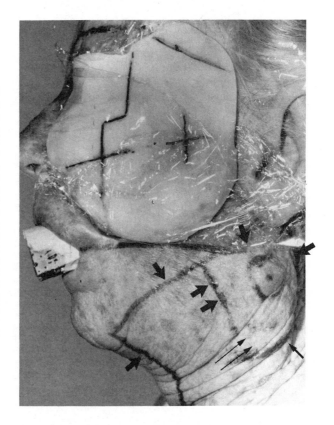

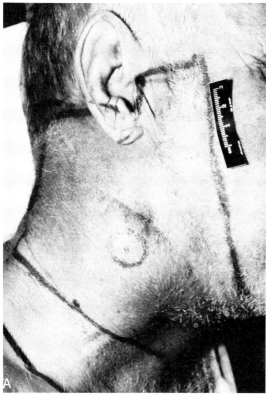

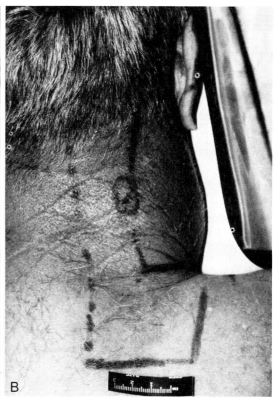

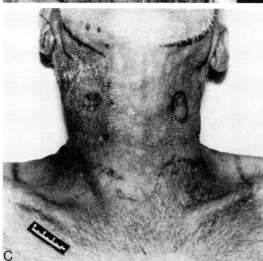

Figure 54–17. This 58-year-old male was seen in November 1979, with approximately a 2-month history of swelling in the right side of the neck that at first grew slowly and then increased rapidly in size. Biopsy of the 10 × 10 cm mass showed metastatic squamous cell carcinoma. Examination revealed a small exophytic lesion in the right midpyriform sinus. Irradiation was started with parallel opposed portals covering the neck mass, with 180 rad tumor dose per day at midpharynx (A). Three hours after the first treatment, 120 rad was given through front and back tangential portals (B). The lower neck was treated with 200 rad per day, for a total of 5000 rad. In 6 weeks, the primary lesion received 6460 rad, and the node received 8460 rad. At the end of treatment, the patient had only a brisk erythema with small patches of moist desquamation (C). Six weeks later the patient had a modified neck dissection followed by normal wound healing.

The surgical specimen report read as follows: "No viable appearing tumor is present. The larger nodule may represent total tumor replacement of a lymph node, with extensive calcification and necrosis. Many scattered, separate small nests of degenerated cells are present in connective tissue and skeletal muscle, which are extensively calcified and which have elicited a marked tissue foreign body reaction. Degenerated cells of squamous cell carcinoma are identifiable within some of these."

In September 1980, the patient showed no evidence of disease above the clavicles but had lung metastases. Despite chemotherapy, the patient died on July 14, 1981 with no evidence of disease above the clavicles. (From Fletcher GH: Radiation boost or added limited surgery as a means of improving local-regional control. *In* Fletcher GH, Nervi C, Withers HR (eds.): Biologic Bases and Clinical Implications of Tumor Radioresistance. New York, Masson Publishing USA, Inc., 1983, pp. 269–279.[11])

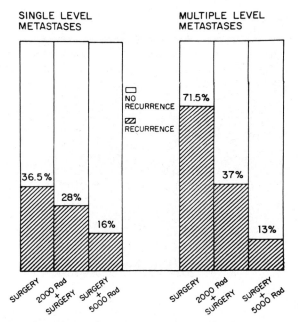

SINGLE LEVEL METASTASES

MULTIPLE LEVEL METASTASES

☐ NO RECURRENCE

▨ RECURRENCE

71.5%

36.5%

28%

16%

37%

13%

SURGERY

2000 Rad + SURGERY

SURGERY + 5000 Rad

SURGERY

2000 Rad + SURGERY

SURGERY + 5000 Rad

Figure 54–18. Comparison of the rates of recurrences in the neck among patients treated by surgery alone or surgery with 2000 rad preoperative irradiation (historically derived from Strong[29]) and patients treated by surgery and 5000 to 6000 rad postoperative irradiation. Almost all the recurrences were in patients with a delay of more than 6 weeks to start of irradiation. (From Vikram B, Strong EW, Shah JP, Spiro R: Head Neck Surg, 6:724, 1984. Courtesy of John Wiley & Sons, New York.[32])

years was correlated with several parameters of the neck disease in the surgical specimen. The data show clearly that the single most important feature is the presence or absence of rupture of the node capsule. Rupture of the capsule was strongly associated with the presence of tumor emboli in the lymphatic vessels. The survival rate at 3 years decreased sharply in those patients with rupture of the node capsule, even in those with early T1 lesions and well-differentiated tumors. Disease present in connective tissue in the radical neck dissection specimen is indicative of aggressive disease with a great potential for local regrowth.

The indication for postoperative irradiation is very strong if (1) a node is over 3 cm, (2) connective tissue is invaded, or (3) several nodes are positive for cancer.

In irradiation combined with neck dissection, the density of infestation must be considered because as the number of clonogens increases more irradiation is needed to eradicate the disease. The density of residual infestation increases with staging. Table 54–11 shows in

TABLE 54–11. Recurrences after Radical Neck Dissection According to Clinical or Histologic Staging and Doses of Irradiation

Stage	Dose of <4500 rad	Dose of ≥4500 rad
N0 (clinical *or* histologic)	20%	0%
N+ (clinical *and* histologic)	50%	20%

Source: Adapted from Arriagada R, Eschwege F, Cachin Y, Richard JM: Cancer 51:1819, 1983.[1]

TABLE 54–12. Recurrences in the Head and Neck of Patients Electively Irradiated Postoperatively for Stages III and IV Epidermoid Carcinoma of the Head and Neck

	Delay up to 6 Weeks		Delay over 6 Weeks*	
	Number of Patients	*Per-centage*	*Number of Patients*	*Per-centage*
Nodes negative	0/5	0	0/3	0
Nodes positive at one level	0/18	0	3/11	27
Nodes positive at multiple levels	2/25	8	12/32	37
Total	2/48	4	15/46	32.5

*In the patients with a delay over 6 weeks there was no palpable disease at the time of the initiation of irradiation.

Source: Vikram B, Strong EW, Shah JP, Spiro R: Am J Surg 140:580, 1980.[31]

one series[1] and Figure 54–18 in another series[32] the correlation of failures in the radically dissected neck with extent of neck involvement and dose levels.

Table 54–12 indicates that delay in the start of irradiation beyond 6 weeks decreased the likelihood of local control, and every effort should, therefore, be made to start irradiation as soon as possible after surgery.[31] Although delay might be due to unavoidable reasons in some cases, in others the likelihood of delay could be reduced by the elimination of unnecessary extensive surgery or by careful selection of the reconstructive procedure. For instance, no recurrences were seen in this series in the clinically negative contralateral side of the neck; therefore, elective neck dissections of a clinically negative contralateral side of the neck when postoperative irradiation is planned would not only be unlikely to increase the control rate, but might prove counterproductive by increasing the likelihood of delay in the start of irradiation.[31]

In the University of Texas M. D. Anderson Hospital series when 6000 rad to the upper neck and 5000 rad to the lower neck were given, either preoperatively or postoperatively, the incidence of recurrences was 7.6 per cent.[2] With N2 or more stage neck disease, the upper neck, and in some situations also the lower neck, should receive 6000 rad and perhaps 6500 rad in selected areas.

Figures 54–19, 54–20, and 54–21 are examples of postoperative irradiation for various anatomic sites. The entire surgical area must be covered.[13]

Nodes Appearing Secondarily

Figure 54–22 shows that there is a fast growth rate because the failures above the clavicles appear rapidly. The management of nodes appearing secondarily depends on how the neck was treated initially. If there had been no treatment to the neck, the same guideline applies. In the appearance of contralateral neck nodes if only a neck dissection has been done on the ipsilateral side of the neck, the same guidelines apply. The results are poor in patients with tumors of the pyriform sinus developing contralateral neck nodes and having had no postoperative irradiation (Table 54–12). Of the 35 pa-

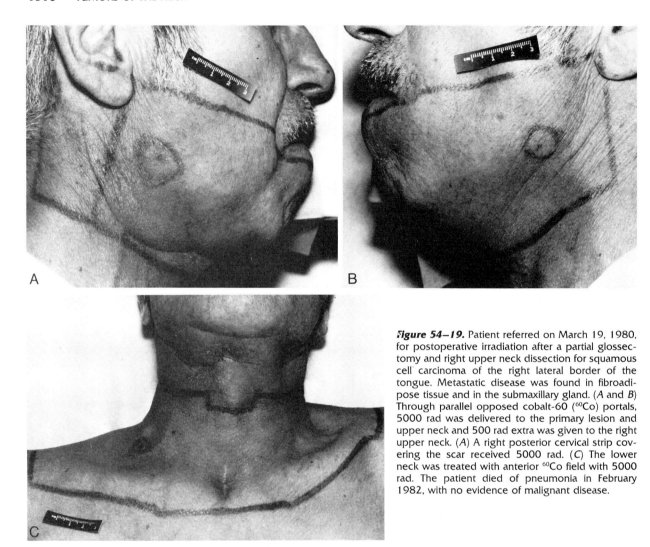

Figure 54–19. Patient referred on March 19, 1980, for postoperative irradiation after a partial glossectomy and right upper neck dissection for squamous cell carcinoma of the right lateral border of the tongue. Metastatic disease was found in fibroadipose tissue and in the submaxillary gland. (*A* and *B*) Through parallel opposed cobalt-60 (^{60}Co) portals, 5000 rad was delivered to the primary lesion and upper neck and 500 rad extra was given to the right upper neck. (*A*) A right posterior cervical strip covering the scar received 5000 rad. (*C*) The lower neck was treated with anterior ^{60}Co field with 5000 rad. The patient died of pneumonia in February 1982, with no evidence of malignant disease.

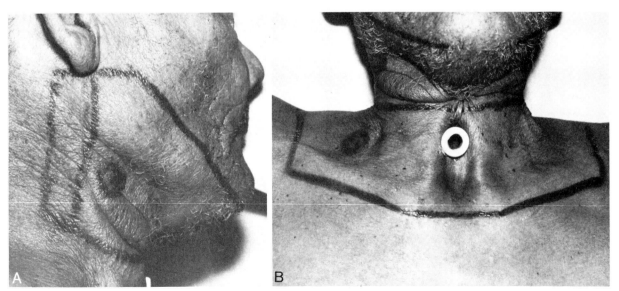

Figure 54–20. This 71-year-old patient was seen on September 22, 1980, and following work-up underwent total laryngectomy and bilateral modified neck dissection on October 21, 1980. None of 53 nodes was positive for tumor. On October 28, 1980, he was referred for radiation therapy with the diagnosis of grade II, T4N0 squamous cell carcinoma of the infrahyoid epiglottis, extending inferiorly into the anterior pre-epiglottic space with destruction of the thyroid cartilage.

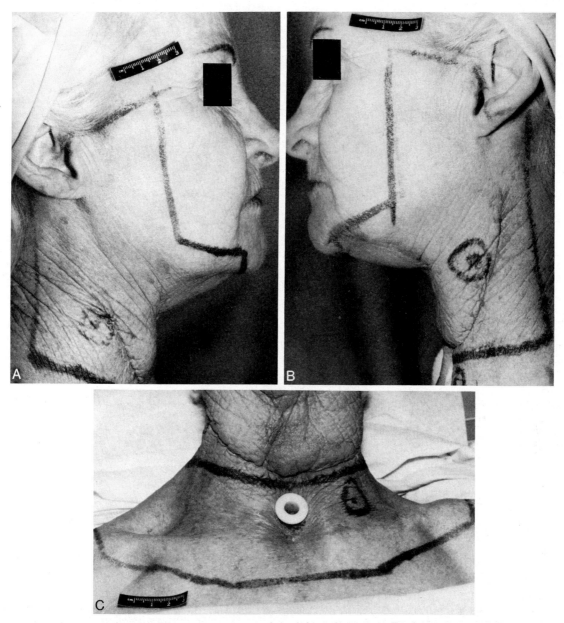

Figure 54–21. Biopsy revealed squamous cell carcinoma of the left pyriform sinus. The lesion was stage T4N0. A wide-field laryngectomy was performed. The margins of resection were free; one area showed a focus of marked squamous dysphagia. There was no tumor in 16 lymph nodes recovered. (*A* and *B*) The patient received through parallel opposed portals 6000 rad to the upper neck and 5000 rad to the parapharyngeal lymphatics. At 5000 rad the lateral portals were moved forward and the posterior aspects of the neck were treated with 6 MeV electrons. (*C*) The lower neck, including the stoma because of extensive subglottic disease, received through an appositional portal 5000 rad in part cobalt 60 and in part 9 and 6 MeV electrons to minimize the dose to the spinal cord. A plastic tracheostomy tube was used during irradiation to bring up the surface dose. The patient developed lung metastases in January 1980, but had no evidence of disease above the clavicles. (From El Badawi SA, Goepfert H, Fletcher GH, et al: Laryngoscope 92:357, 1982.[7])

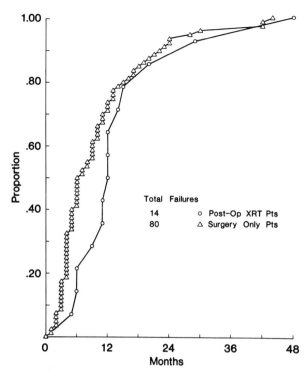

Figure 54–22. Cumulative appearance rates of failures above the clavicles. Almost half of the failures in the surgery only group have appeared by 6 months. (From Fletcher GH, Goepfert H: Role of irradiation in treatment of laryngeal cancer. *In* Ferlito A (ed): Cancer of the Larynx, vol III. Boca Raton, CRC Press, 1985, pp. 69–114.)

tients having developed contralateral neck nodes, only five did not die from cancer, four of them being treated with a contralateral neck dissection and one by irradiation (Table 54–13).

The sooner the recurrence, the worse the prognosis because an early recurrence is rarely isolated (Fig. 54–23).

Salivary Gland Tumors

Because of the propensity of high-grade tumors to metastasize to cervical lymph nodes, the appropriate lymphatic areas are electively irradiated to 5000 rad.

TABLE 54–13. Management of Postsurgical Recurrences in 80 Patients with Squamous Cell Carcinoma of the Pyriform Sinus

Too advanced (no treatment)	8
Refused treatment	2
Surgery (16 contralateral nodes):	28
4 patients with contralateral nodes	
(NED at 48, 52, 72, and 116 months)	
Radiation therapy	27
Pharyngeal wall, 87 mos NED	
Contralateral node, 78 mos NED	
Chemotherapy	5
Surgery + radiation therapy	9
Radiation therapy + chemotherapy	1

Key: NED = No evidence of disease.
Source: Fletcher GH, Goepfert H: *In* Ferlito A (ed): Cancer of the Larynx, vol III. Boca Raton, Florida, CRC Press, 1985, pp 69–114.

Previous analyses have shown that subclinical disease of the salivary gland tumors has the same radiosensitivity, regardless of the histologic type.[21] In tumors of the parotid or submaxillary glands or in a lateral location of an ectopic salivary gland tumor, only the ipsilateral side of the neck is irradiated (Fig. 54–24). In lesions originating inside the oral cavity or oropharynx, the appropriate lymphatic drainage is irradiated. For instance, if the lesion is located in the soft or hard palate, both subdigastric areas are irradiated.

Unknown Primary Site

Between 1948 and 1968, 210 patients were seen with neck disease without a known primary lesion.[17] In 26 patients the location was in the supraclavicular area, and in 184 patients the location was in the other lymphatic areas of the neck. The staging system used is the same as in Table 54–1, and previously excised node(s) were staged NX.

The diagnosis of cancer in the cervical nodes was made by biopsy or excision before admission to M. D. Anderson Hospital in 114 (52 per cent) of the patients. If the initial examination at M. D. Anderson Hospital failed to determine the primary site, almost all patients had, under general anesthesia, a direct examination of the mucosal surfaces of the upper respiratory and alimentary tracts. Biopsies were performed of any mucosal areas that were slightly abnormal. Random biopsy samples of apparently normal mucosa were usually taken from the nasopharynx, the base of the tongue, tonsillar area, and pyriform sinus.

The histologic diagnosis of the node(s) was squamous cell carcinoma in 62 per cent, undifferentiated carcinoma in 28 per cent, and glandular carcinoma of salivary origin in 10 per cent of the patients.

Surgical Operation

At the M. D. Anderson Hospital 104 patients underwent a surgical procedure as the initial treatment. Of the 104 patients, 29 had secondary treatment later for disease appearing at the primary site, recurrence in the treated side of the neck, or new disease in the untreated contralateral side of the neck.

Radiation Therapy

Radiation therapy was the initial treatment in 52 patients, 45 of whom had portals covering the nasopharynx, tonsil, base of the tongue, and the entire neck. If the clinically positive lymph nodes were high jugular nodes under the sternocleidomastoid muscle or in the posterior cervical chain, a high probability of a nasopharyngeal primary site existed, and 6000 rad was given to the nasopharynx.

Results

In all stages, the combination of radiation therapy and surgical operation was superior to either modality alone. Surgical therapy or radiation therapy were equally effective in controlling early cervical disease. Some superiority of radiotherapy over the surgical procedure was demonstrated in those patients with nodal

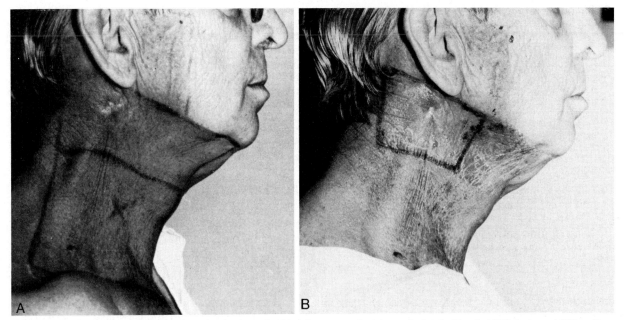

Figure 54–23. The patient had an intraoral resection of a T1 right retromolar trigone lesion in March 1973. In June 1973, a 2-cm right subdigastric node was found, and a right radical neck dissection was performed. Only one of 54 nodes recovered was positive for tumor. In August 1973, the patient developed a mass in the area of the right mastoid tip, and biopsy of necrotic material revealed squamous cell carcinoma.

(A) It was felt that the parotid bed should be irradiated to 5000 rad at a 5-cm depth. The upper neck was irradiated with 11 MeV electrons to 6000 rad in 5 weeks and an additional 1000 rad to the mass through a reduced field.

(B) The lower neck received 5000 rad in 4 weeks. On October 29, 1973, a lump was found in the right lower neck just above the sternoclavicular joint. Biopsy showed squamous cell carcinoma in connective tissue. In addition to extensive neck disease and widespread metastases, the patient developed intractable pain due to involvement of the brachial plexus. The patient received chemotherapy without alleviation of his symptoms; he died in March 1974.

Figure 54–24. The patient presented on December 14, 1982, with a 5 × 3 cm lesion in the right buccal mucosa extending from the maxillary gingival buccal sulcus down into the mandibular sulcus and within 2 cm from the oral commissure and extending posteriorly to the retromolar trigone. The lesion was not fixed to the mandible. On December 16, 1982, the patient underwent an excision of the right buccal mucosa lesion with a partial mandibulectomy, and resection of the superficial lobe of the parotid. Pathologic examination showed high-grade adenoid cystic carcinoma in fibromuscular tissue with involvement of perineural spaces of several nerves, and the tumor was extremely close to the margins of the resection. Postoperatively, the parotid area was treated with a mixture of 17 MeV electrons and 18 MeV photons delivering 5500 rad tumor dose at 5 cm in 28 fractions in 5½ weeks. At 4500 rad at 4-cm depth, the field was removed from the spinal cord. The anterior buccal mucosa was treated with 13 MeV electrons delivering 5600 rad given dose in 28 fractions in 5½ weeks. The lower neck was treated with 9 MeV electrons delivering 5000 rad in 25 fractions in 5 weeks.

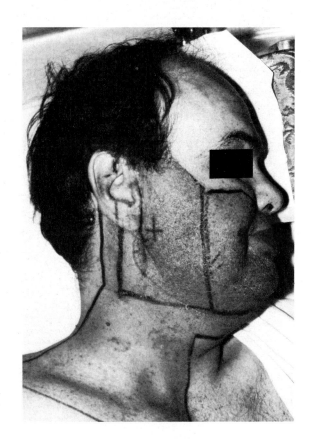

TABLE 54–14. Location of Primary Lesions Appearing after Treatment of 37 Patients (3 Years to Unlimited Follow-Up)

Location	Surgery	Irradiation
Nasopharynx	2	—
Maxillary antrum	—	—
Tonsil or faucial arch	4	—
Base of tongue, valleculum	4	—
Oral cavity, salivary glands	2	2
Aryepiglottic fold, epiglottis	1	—
Hypopharynx	6	1
Cervical esophagus	1	—
Thyroid	1	—
Total head and neck	21/104	3/52
New primary tumors	20%	6%
Primary tumors below clavicles	5	3

Source: Adapted from Jesse RH, Perez CA, Fletcher GH: Cervical lymph node metastasis: Unknown primary cancer. Cancer *31*:854, 1973.[17]

disease in the advanced stages. If initial treatment to the neck failed, additional therapy was not effective in producing a further disease-free interval.

Only patients having had a unilateral neck dissection as their initial therapy developed nodes in the contralateral side of the neck. In contrast, no patient having radiation alone or as a part of the treatment developed contralateral metastases because the entire neck was included in the initial radiation portals.

Thirty-seven patients developed a primary lesion at some time after the initial treatment to the neck (Table 54–14). The hypopharynx and oropharynx were the most common sites. The majority of the patients who developed primary cancers in the head and neck sites were in the surgically treated group.

Patients who developed a primary lesion above the clavicle had only a 31 per cent chance of living 3 years, as opposed to 58 per cent for those who never developed a primary lesion in the head and neck area.

Present Policies

Radical or modified neck dissection appears to be an adequate treatment for a single node less than 3 cm located in the submaxillary triangle and the low subdigastric node(s).

Irradiation covering the nasopharynx, tonsillar fossa, base of the tongue, and the entire lymph node–bearing area of the neck through fields that spare the larynx and hypopharynx is preferred as the only treatment for patients with small, high jugular–spinal accessory nodes and those who have posterior cervical nodes. For other locations of the node(s), usually subdigastric and midjugular, the pharyngeal walls and the pyriform sinus are also included (Fig. 54–25).

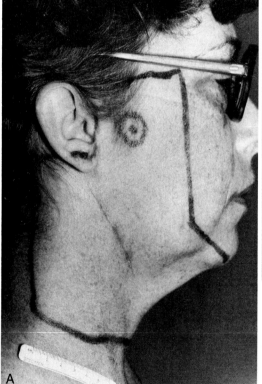

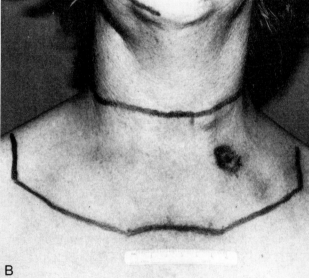

Figure 54–25. This 42-year-old white female presented in September 1977 with a scar in the right subdigastric area. A node had been excised at another institution in May 1977 showing poorly differentiated squamous cell carcinoma. A nasopharynx tumor survey was compatible with a lesion on the roof of the nasopharynx, but multiple biopsies showed no tumor. Through lateral parallel opposed fields using ⁶⁰Co, the patient received 5500 rad tumor dose in 28 fractions to the nasopharynx, tonsillar fossa, base of tongue, and pyriform sinus. (*A*) The lower neck received 5000 rad in 25 fractions with ⁶⁰Co through a single anterior field. (*B*) The parallel opposed fields were moved "off cord" after 4500 rad tumor dose and irradiation of the posterior aspects of the neck was continued to 5500 rad with 7 MeV electrons. The overall treatment time was 6 weeks. In 1981, the patient became clinically hypothyroid, requiring hormonal replacement. She had no evidence of disease in August 1983. Because of the location of the subdigastric node at the angle of the jaw, the pharyngeal walls and pyriform sinus were included in the field of irradiation.

Postoperative irradiation is usually reserved for those patients originally selected for surgery, but in whom the specimen shows more than one small node involved or disease in connective tissue.

Supraclavicular Nodes

Few of the 26 patients with disease in the supraclavicular nodes survived, regardless of the treatment. The incidence of later appearance of a primary lesion anywhere in the body is high. Palliative irradiation alone is usually indicated.

LYMPHOMAS

Lymphomas are divided into two basic categories: Hodgkin's disease (HD) and non-Hodgkin's lymphoma (NHL). In Hodgkin's disease the pathologic criteria for diagnosis are well recognized, whereas in non-Hodgkin's lymphoma the histologic classification continues to change.[33] This constant change causes problems for the clinician, first, in understanding the similarities and differences of the classification systems and, second, in assessing the published results. Hodgkin's disease is primarily nodal with predictable patterns of spread, whereas patients with non-Hodgkin's lymphoma present in advanced stages with generalized involvement of both nodal and extranodal sites. The majority of patients with Hodgkin's disease have involvement of the cervical lymph nodes.[35] The high incidence of extranodal involvement in stages I and II of non-Hodgkin's lymphoma is well documented.[36, 39, 44, 49] The majority of the extranodal sites are limited to the head and neck area.[46, 49]

The treatment of lymphomas has changed drastically during the past three decades. Gilbert in 1939[37] laid the foundation for principles of modern-day radiation therapy in the treatment of Hodgkin's disease. Using Gilbert's technique, Peters in 1950[43] reported the curability of Hodgkin's disease, and Easson and Russell in 1963[34] reported the curability of both Hodgkin's disease and non-Hodgkin's lymphoma. This was followed by systematic use of aggressive treatment led by the group at Stanford.[40] Since then there have been many studies on lymphomas reported from single institutions and cooperative groups stressing the use of single or multimodality treatment depending upon the stage of the disease.

Diagnosis and Evaluation

Correct assessment of the extent of the disease is crucial in lymphomas. It starts with an adequate biopsy to properly define the histologic subtypes. The staging classification for both Hodgkin's disease and non-Hodgkin's lymphoma is the Ann Harbor Staging Classification.[33] In Hodgkin's disease the workup includes the routine laboratory evaluation, chest x-ray, lymphangiogram or computerized tomographic (CT) scan of the abdomen, and bone marrow biopsy. Other tests such as chest tomograms, intravenous pyelogram, or bone scan may be indicated. An exploratory laparotomy should be considered on all patients with clinical stage I, II, or III disease if the treatment regimen will change

with the findings at laparotomy. In non-Hodgkin's lymphoma, laboratory workup is the same; however, roentgenographically, more emphasis is placed on the CT scan of the abdomen instead of lymphangiography. A bone marrow biopsy is indicated on all patients. Those patients with clinical stage I or II non-Hodgkin's lymphoma should be considered for an exploratory laparotomy.

Treatment and Results

Hodgkin's Disease

The curative treatment of Hodgkin's disease can consist of radiotherapy alone, chemotherapy alone, or a combination of both. The discussion will be limited to patients with stage I Hodgkin's disease with cervical presentation. In general, these patients are treated by radiation therapy alone. For small to moderate-sized lesions, less than 6 cm in diameter, Thar and associates[48] recommended 3500 rad at 150 to 170 rad fractions. Analysis of their results showed only a 7 per cent infield recurrence. Doses up to 4000 rad may be required for tumors larger than 6 cm. Doses over 4000 rad do not significantly improve the control rate but may increase the complication rate.[48] The actual treatment of the individual patient depends upon a number of factors and should be decided by a multimodality team approach.

The results of treatment of Hodgkin's disease are usually presented by stage and treatment technique rather than by anatomic location of the disease. In stage IA and IIA patients, Helman and Mauch[38] reported an 80 per cent relapse-free survival of 10 years and a 95 per cent overall survival rate. The initial studies from the Stanford group[40] have shown that total nodal irradiation in stages IA and IIA Hodgkin's disease improved the relapse-free survival over involved field irradiation, but the overall survival rate was not improved. In patients with stage I disease, total nodal irradiation is not necessary.[38]

Non-Hodgkin's Lymphomas

Although extranodal non-Hodgkin's disease is common in the head and neck area, less than 10 per cent of the patients have the disease limited to the neck. The most common sites of solitary neck involvement are the thyroid and submandibular glands.[41, 45, 49] Most patients with head and neck NHL have disease in Waldeyer's ring.[41, 45, 49] One of the highest incidences of nodal disease (16 per cent) was reported by Fierstein and Thawley in 1978.[35] This discussion will be limited to stage I disease with cervical presentation.

The treatment of choice for patients with stage I NHL is radiation therapy. There is a debate about whether involved field or extended field radiotherapy gives better cure rates. NHL can be divided into favorable and nonfavorable histologic subtypes for treatment purposes.[41, 47] The favorable lymphomas include the nodular lymphomas, except for nodular histiocytic and diffuse well-differentiated lymphocytic lymphoma. The remaining histologic subtypes, including diffuse poorly differentiated lymphocytic, diffuse histiocytic, diffuse undifferentiated, and nodular histiocytic lymphoma are in the unfavorable group. A dose recommended for the favorable NHL is 3000 rad at the rate of 150 to 170 rad per fraction. The dose of radiotherapy required for local control of unfavorable histologic types is 4500 to 5500 rad at the rate of 180 rad per fraction. The radiotherapeutic technique used in localized treatment of stage I NHL is similar to that used for the treatment of the neck in squamous cell carcinoma of the various head and neck sites. Wong and associates[49] pointed out that thyroid presentations were treated with an anterior extended field to cover the neck and the mediastinum. A posterior field was used to augment the tumor dose calculated at midplane of the mediastinum. They report a 58 per cent disease-free survival at 5 years for stage I disease of the head and neck. They also pointed out that dissemination is common in extranodal stage I and stage II diffuse lymphomas and, therefore, recommend staging celiotomy and a clinical trial using multiagent chemotherapy in addition to radiation therapy. Reddy and associates[46] in 1980 reported a 5-year recurrence-free survival for a stage I extranodal NHL of 77 per cent. They also recommended prospective trials of multiagent chemotherapy and radiation therapy in stage II extranodular NHL. Recently, Mill and associates[41] reported their results with stages I and II extranodal NHL of the head and neck: a 5-year survival rate of 100 per cent in the favorable group and 52 per cent in the unfavorable group. The overall disease-free survival rate for a stage I disease at 5 years is 49 per cent. They point out that the major problem is not local control of tumor but eradication of occult disseminated disease. In 1978, Fierstein and Thawley[35] reported on 88 patients with NHL of the head and neck. Interestingly, 12 of the 55 patients with stage I disease presented with nodal sites. In general, the patients with stage I disease were treated by radiation therapy alone, with doses ranging from 4000 to 5500 rad. Two of the 43 patients with non-nodal stage I disease failed, whereas five of the 12 patients with nodal stage I disease failed. This is one of the two reports showing that patients presenting with nodal disease in the head and neck area have a poor prognosis as compared with the extranodal sites. This report also recommended combined chemotherapy and radiation in all except stage I disease. Thus, the consensus is that stage I NHL can be adequately treated with radiation therapy alone, whereas in more advanced disease combined chemotherapy and radiation therapy should be used.

The sequelae and complications of radiation therapy for lymphoma arising in the neck are similar to those for the treatment of squamous cell carcinoma metastatic to neck nodes. In general, the late sequelae are minimal owing to the limited dose of 3000 to 5000 rad usually given at 180 rad per fraction or less. When the entire neck is treated, however, patients must be evaluated for potential dental sequelae of the mandibular teeth. Many of the problems can be prevented with proper care. Full neck irradiation will usually cause some degree of xerostomia, especially at rest, because the majority of resting saliva is produced by the submaxillary glands, which are included in the field. Patients are also at risk for hypothyroidism. Although this is usually not clinically manifest, proper testing with T_4 and thyroid-stimulating hormone (TSH) determinations may detect subclinical hypothyroidism. Patients are potentially at

risk for spinal cord damage, including Lhermitte's sign; therefore, the tumor dose to the spinal cord should be kept below 4500 rad in 5 weeks.

SOFT-TISSUE SARCOMAS

Soft-tissue sarcomas are relatively rare malignant tumors arising from the connective tissues throughout the body. According to the American Cancer Society statistics,[51] there are approximately 4800 new cases per year. About 55 per cent of the cases arise in the extremities, 40 per cent being in the lower extremity. Average patient age is 45 years, and the male-to-female ratio is almost the same, being 53 per cent and 47 per cent, respectively. Soft-tissue sarcomas are named according to their tissue of origin. The most common histologic types are liposarcoma, fibrosarcoma, neurofibrosarcoma, and malignant fibrohistiocytoma.[56]

The treatment of soft-tissue sarcomas, especially those arising in the extremities, has changed over the past two decades. Twenty years ago the treatment of choice was radical surgery. The extensive local invasion of soft-tissue sarcomas has resulted in a high incidence of local recurrence, varying with the type of surgical procedure: 80 to 100 per cent after local excision,[50, 66] 39 per cent after wide excision,[66] 25 to 28 per cent after soft part resection,[53, 67] and 7 to 18 per cent after amputation.[52, 68] As the clinical behavior of the soft-tissue sarcomas became better appreciated, the overall incidence of local recurrence decreased from 30 per cent in the mid-1960s[52, 60] to approximately 20 per cent by 1980.[67, 68] Historically, radiation therapy was not considered in the treatment of soft-tissue sarcomas because they were considered to be radioresistant.[64] Recently, several investigators have advocated the use of limb-sparing surgery in the treatment of extremity soft-tissue sarcomas.[54, 58, 62, 63, 69] The limb-sparing surgery has been combined with radiation therapy, with or without adjunctive chemotherapy.[54, 62, 63] Rosenberg and associates[63] have shown in a prospective randomized trial that there is no statistically significant difference in disease-free or overall survival in patients treated by limb-sparing surgery plus radiation therapy or amputation. These conservative approaches are now being applied to the soft-tissue sarcomas arising in the head and neck region.

Diagnosis and Evaluation

A cervical mass should be considered metastatic epidermoid carcinoma from a primary lesion in the upper aerodigestive tract until proved otherwise. Thus, the workup proceeds along the line of an "unknown primary site," with the diagnosis of a primary soft-tissue sarcoma arising in the neck made by exclusion. When the workup does not show an obvious "primary tumor," the diagnosis of soft-tissue sarcoma may be made by a core biopsy, but more commonly an excisional biopsy of the mass is performed.

Once the diagnosis has been established, the next step is to stage the disease. Recently, the American Joint Committee[65] published a staging system for soft-tissue sarcomas that incorporates the grade of the lesion, in addition to the TNM system. Although some investigators have used the AJC Staging System, recently pathologists have questioned the reproducibility of grading the soft-tissue sarcomas.* Therefore, the very essence of the AJC System is being questioned. The incidence of nodal metastasis in soft-tissue sarcomas is usually less than 5 per cent.[70] Therefore, special studies, other than a routine physical examination, are usually not fruitful. This is especially true for the soft-tissue sarcomas arising in the neck. The major question in staging is the presence or absence of distant metastasis. Because the initial site of distant metastasis is the lung in approximately 90 per cent of the patients with soft-tissue sarcomas, some investigators advocate lung tomograms or CT scan, whereas others believe that routine chest x-rays are adequate. We do not recommend lung tomograms or CT scan of the lung in well-differentiated or low-grade lesions because incidence of metastasis is only 5 to 10 per cent. Some investigators also advocate liver scan and bone scan as part of the routine workup.[63] The yield from these tests is so low that they cannot be recommended as routine studies.

Treatment and Results

The main part of the treatment of soft-tissue sarcomas is surgical resection. The small to moderate-sized soft-tissue sarcomas arising in the neck can usually be widely excised with minimal functional defect. Owing to the invasiveness of the disease and the anatomic limitations of the dissection, we recommend postoperative radiation therapy. We deliver 6000 rad tumor dose in 6 weeks for low-grade lesions and give 6500 rad tumor dose in 6½ weeks for intermediate and high-grade lesions, with field reduction after 5000 rad. The volume to be irradiated, of course, varies with the anatomic location in the neck. It is generous enough to cover the entire surgical bed and increases as the grade of the tumor increases. Usually the involved side of the neck from the mandible to the clavicle is treated.

Occasionally patients may present with massive disease in the neck. Extrapolating from our experience with soft-tissue sarcomas of the extremities,[61] we advocate preoperative radiation therapy followed by conservative excision. The preoperative radiation therapy consists of 5000 rad tumor dose in 5 weeks, utilizing appropriate field arrangements to deliver a uniform dose. Patients with unresectable lesions can be treated by radiation therapy alone; however, based on data from other sites, the chance of local control by radiation therapy alone is low (37 per cent).[57] The role of adjuvant chemotherapy in localized soft-tissue sarcomas is undecided, and there have been conflicting reports in the literature.[59, 62] Any recommendations regarding adjuvant chemotherapy must await further clarification.

Owing to the rarity of soft-tissue sarcomas in the head and neck area, there are few reports in the literature, making it difficult to properly evaluate treatment. One exception, however, is the report by Farr[55] in 1981 of 285 patients with soft-tissue sarcomas of the head and neck treated at Memorial Sloan-Kettering Cancer Center in New York. Their overall 5-year absolute cure rate is 32 per cent, but they point out that if children were eliminated, the 5-year cure rate would rise to 50 per cent. From their report the 5-year disease-free survival with four of the more common tumors—fibrosarcoma, neurofibrosarcoma, liposarcoma, and leiomyosarcoma—is 59.2 per cent (58 of 98). Thirty of the 98 lesions arose in the neck, and this is an unusually high proportion. Unfortunately, they do not give the 5-year cure rate for localized sarcomas arising in the neck.

A recent review of 550 patients with localized soft-tissue sarcoma treated by radiotherapy alone or in conjunction with surgery at M. D. Anderson Hospital showed that only 11 lesions (2.0 per cent) arose in the neck (unpublished data). Eight patients were treated by surgery and postoperative radiation therapy. Four of the patients are living free of disease from 24 to 69 months, one died at 11 months with recurrence in the neck, and the remaining three patients have died of distant metastasis. Two patients who received preoperative radiation therapy are dead of distant metastases at 10 and 11 months. The final patient was treated by radiation therapy alone for a massive unresectable fibrosarcoma and is living free of disease at 16 years. Although there have been no complications and only one local recurrence, there are too few patients to draw significant conclusions.

REFERENCES

EPITHELIAL TUMORS

1. Arriagada R, Eschwege F, Cachin Y, Richard JM: The value of combining radiotherapy with surgery in the treatment of hypopharyngeal and laryngeal cancers. Cancer 51:1819, 1983.
2. Barkley HT Jr, Fletcher GH, Jesse RH, Lindberg RD: Management of cervical lymph node metastases in squamous cell carcinomas of the tonsillar fossa, base of tongue, supraglottic larynx and hypopharynx. Am J Surg 124:462, 1972.
3. Bataini J-P, Bernier J, Brugere J, Et al: Approche radiotherapique des adenopathies cervicales secondaires aux cancers epidermiques du larynx et du pharynx. In Pinel J, Leroux-Robert J (eds): Adenopathies Cervicales les Malignes. Paris, Masson, 1982, pp 129–135.
4. Berger DS, Fletcher GH, Lindberg RD, Jesse R Jr: Elective irradiation of the neck lymphatics for squamous cell carcinomas of the nasopharynx and oropharynx. AJR 111:66, 1971.
5. Berger DS, Fletcher GH: Distant metastases following local control of squamous cell carcinoma of the nasopharynx, tonsillar fossa, and base of the tongue. Radiology 100:141, 1971.
6. Cachin Y: Les modalities et la valeur pronostique de l'envahissement ganglionnaire cervical dans les carcinomes des voies aerodigestives superieures. Vie Med Can Fr 1:48, 1972.
7. El Badawi SA, Goepfert H, Herson J, et al: Squamous cell carcinoma of the pyriform sinus. Laryngoscope 92:357, 1982.
8. Fletcher GH: Elective irradiation of subclinical disease in cancers of the head and neck. Cancer 29:1450, 1972.
9. Fletcher GH: Place of irradiation in the management of head and neck cancer. Semin Oncol 4:375, 1977.
10. Fletcher GH: Textbook of Radiotherapy. 3rd ed. Philadelphia, Lea & Febiger, 1980.
11. Fletcher GH: Radiation boost or added limited surgery as a means of improving local-regional control. In Fletcher GH, Nervi C, Withers HR (eds): Biological Bases and Clinical Implications of Tumor Radioresistance. New York, Masson Publishing, 1983, pp 269–279.
12. Fletcher GH: Lucy Wortham James Lecture: Subclinical disease. Cancer 53:1274, 1984.
13. Fletcher GH, Evers WT: Radiotherapeutic management of surgical recurrences and postoperative residuals in tumors of the head and neck. Radiology 95:185, 1970.
14. Fletcher GH, Goepfert H: Role of irradiation in the treatment of laryngeal cancer. In Ferlito A (ed): Cancer of the Larynx, vol III. Boca Raton, Florida, CRC Press, 1985, pp 69–114.
15. Harwood AR, Beal FA, Cummings BJ, et al: Supraglottic laryngeal carcinoma: An analysis of dose-time-volume factors in 410 patients. Int J Radiat Oncol Biol Phys 9:311, 1983.
16. Jesse RH, Barkley HT Jr, Lindberg RD, Fletcher GH: Cancer of the oral cavity. Is elective neck dissection beneficial? Am J Surg 120:505, 1970.

---

*A. C. Ayala: Personal communication.

17. Jesse RH, Perez CA, Fletcher GH: Cervical lymph node metastasis: Unknown primary cancer. Cancer 31:854, 1973.
18. Lindberg RD: Distribution of cervical lymph node metastases from squamous cell carcinoma of the upper respiratory and digestive tract. Cancer 29:1446, 1972.
19. Manual for Staging of Cancer, 1977. American Joint Committee Staging and End-Results Reporting. Chicago, 1977.
20. Marks JE, Kurnik B, Powers WE, Ogura JH: Carcinoma of the pyriform sinus: An analysis of treatment results and patterns of failure. Cancer 41:1008, 1978.
21. McNaney D, McNeese M, Guillamondegui OM, et al: Postoperative irradiation in malignant epithelial tumors of the parotid. Int J Radiat Oncol Biol Phys 9:1289, 1983.
22. Mendenhall WM, Million RR, Cassisi NJ: Elective neck irradiation in squamous-cell carcinoma of the head and neck. Head Neck Surg 3:15, 1980.
23. Meoz RT, Fletcher GH, Lindberg RD: Anatomical coverage in elective irradiation of the neck for squamous cell carcinoma of the oral tongue. Int J Radiat Oncol Biol Phys 8:1881, 1982.
24. Meoz RT, Fletcher GH, Peters LJ, et al: Twice-daily fractionation schemes for advanced head and neck cancer. Int J Radiat Oncol Biol Phys 10:831, 1984.
25. Million RR, Fletcher GH, Jesse RH: Evaluation of elective irradiation of the neck for squamous cell carcinoma of the nasopharynx, tonsillar fossa, and base of tongue. Radiology 80:973, 1963.
26. Million RR: Elective neck irradiation for TX N0 squamous carcinoma of the oral tongue and floor of the mouth. Cancer 34:149, 1974.
27. Northrop M, Fletcher GH, Jesse RH Jr, Lindberg RD: Evolution of neck disease in patients with primary squamous cell carcinomas of the oral tongue, floor of mouth, and palatine arch and clinically positive neck nodes neither fixed nor bilateral. Cancer 29:23, 1972.
28. Schneider JJ, Fletcher GH, Barkley HT Jr: Control by irradiation alone of nonfixed clinically positive lymph nodes from squamous cell carcinoma of the oral cavity, oropharynx, supraglottic larynx, and hypopharynx. AJR 123:42, 1975.
29. Strong EW: Preoperative radiation and radical neck dissection. Surg Clin North Am 49:271, 1969.
30. Strong EW: Carcinoma of the tongue. Otolaryngol Clin North Am 12:107, 1979.
31. Vikram B, Strong EW, Shah J, Spiro RH: Elective postoperative radiation therapy in stages III and IV epidermoid carcinoma of the head and neck. Am J Surg 140:580, 1980.
32. Vikram B, Strong EW, Shah JP, Spiro R: Failure in the neck following multimodality treatment in advanced head and neck cancer. Head Neck Surg 6:724, 1984.

LYMPHOMAS

33. Carbone PP, Kaplan HS, Musshoff K, et al: Report of the Committee on Hodgkin's Disease Staging Classification. Cancer Res 31:1860, 1971.
34. Easson EC, Russell MH: The cure of Hodgkin's disease. Br Med J 1:1704, 1963.
35. Fierstein JT, Thawley SE: Lymphoma of the head and neck. Laryngoscope 88:582, 1978.
36. Fuller LM, Banker FL, Butler JJ, Gamble JF: Natural history of non-Hodgkin's lymphoma stages I and II. Br J Radiol 31:270, 1975.
37. Gilbert R: Radiotherapy in Hodgkin's disease (malignant granulomatosis) anatomic and clinical foundations: Governing principles: Results. AJR 41:198, 1939.
38. Helman S, Mauch P: Role of radiation therapy in the treatment of Hodgkin's disease. Cancer Treat Rep 66:915, 1982.
39. Johnson RE, Chretien PB, Oconor GT, et al: Radiotherapy implications of prospective staging in non-Hodgkin's lymphoma. Radiology 110:655, 1974.
40. Kaplan HS: Hodgkin's Disease. 2nd ed. Cambridge, Harvard University Press, 1980.
41. Mill WB, Lee FA, Franssila KO: Radiation therapy treatment of Stage I and II extranodal non-Hodgkin's lymphoma of the head and neck. Cancer 45:653, 1980.
42. National Cancer Institute sponsored study of classifications of non-Hodgkin's lymphomas. Summary and description of a working formulation for clinical usage. Cancer 49:2112, 1982.
43. Peters MV: A study of survival of Hodgkin's disease treated radiologically. AJR 63:299, 1950.
44. Peters MV, Hasselback R, Brown TC: Natural history of lymphoma related to clinical classification. In Zarafonetis C (ed): Proceedings of the International Conference on Leukemia-Lymphoma. Philadelphia, Lea & Febiger, 1968.
45. Plantenga KF, Hart G, van Heerde P, Tierie AH: Non-Hodgkin's malignant lymphomas of the upper digestive and respiratory tracts. Am J Radiat Oncol Biol Phys 7:1419, 1981.
46. Reddy S, Bellettiere E, Saxena V, Hendrickson FR: National non-Hodgkin's lymphoma. Cancer 46:1925, 1980.
47. Thar TL: Lymphomas and related diseases presenting in the head and neck. In Million RR, Cassissi NJ (eds): Textbook of Head and Neck Cancer. Philadelphia, J. B. Lippincott Co., 1983.
48. Thar TL, Million RR, Housner RJ, McKetty MHB: Hodgkin's disease Stage I, II: Relationship of recurrence to size of disease, radiation dose, and number of sites involved. Cancer 43:1101, 1979.
49. Wong DS, Fuller LM, Butler JJ, Shullenberger CC: Extranodal non-Hodgkin's lymphomas of the head and neck. AJR 123:123, 1975.

SOFT-TISSUE SARCOMAS

50. Cadman J, Soule FH, Kelley JP: Synovial sarcoma: An analysis of 134 patients. Cancer 18:613, 1957.
51. Cancer Statistics 1983. CA 33:16, 1984.
52. Cantin J, McNeer GB, Chu FC, Booker RJ: The problem of local recurrence after treatment of soft tissue sarcomas. Ann Surg 168:47, 1968.
53. Castro EB, Hajdu SI, Fortner JG: Surgical therapy of fibrosarcoma of extremities. Arch Surg 107:284, 1973.
54. Eilber FR, Mirra JJ, Grant TT, et al: Is amputation necessary for sarcomas? A seven year experience with limb salvage. Ann Surg 192:431, 1980.
55. Farr HW: Soft tissue sarcomas of the head and neck. Semin Oncol 8:185, 1981.
56. Hajdu SI: Pathology of Soft Tissue Sarcomas. Philadelphia, Lea & Febiger, 1979.
57. Lindberg RD: The role of radiation therapy in the treatment of soft tissue sarcoma in adults. In Proceedings of the Seventh National Cancer Conference. Philadelphia, J. B. Lippincott Co., 1973.
58. Lindberg RD, Martin RG, Romsdahl MM, Barkley HT: Conservative surgery in postoperative radiation therapy in 300 adults with soft tissue sarcomas. Cancer 47:2391, 1981.
59. Lindberg RD, Murphy WK, Benjamin RS, et al: Adjuvant chemotherapy in the treatment of primary soft tissue sarcomas: A preliminary report. In Martin RG, Ayala AG (eds): Management of Primary Bone and Soft Tissue Tumors. Chicago, Year Book Medical Publishers, 1977, pp 342–352.
60. Martin RG, Butler JJ, Albores-Saavadra J: Soft tissue tumors: Surgical treatment and results. In Copeland MM, et al (eds): Tumors of Bone and Soft Tissue. Chicago, Year Book Medical Publishers, 1965, pp 333–347.
61. Martin RG, Lindberg RD, Russell WO: Preoperative radiotherapy and surgery in the management of soft tissue sarcoma. In Martin RG, Ayala AG (eds): Management of Primary Bone and Soft Tissue Tumors. Chicago, Year Book Medical Publishers, 1977, pp 299–307.
62. Rosenberg SA, Tepper J, Glatstein E, et al: Prospective randomized evaluation of adjuvant chemotherapy in adults with soft tissue sarcomas of the extremities. Cancer 52:424, 1983.
63. Rosenberg SA, Tepper J, Glatstein E, et al: The treatment of soft tissue sarcomas of the extremities. Prospective randomized evaluations of (1) limb-sparing surgery plus radiation therapy compared with amputation, and (2) the role of adjuvant chemotherapy. Am J Surg 196:305, 1982.
64. Rostock P: Indikationsstelking und daueretoig der rontgenbestrahlung ber sarkomen. Fortschr Therap 4:24, 1928.
65. Russell WO, Cohn J, Enzinger F, et al: A clinical and pathological staging for soft tissue sarcomas. Cancer 40:1562, 1977.
66. Shieber W, Graham P: An experience with sarcoma of soft tissue in adults. Surgery 52:295, 1962.
67. Shiu MH, Castro EB, Hajdu SI, Fortner JG: Surgical treatment of 297 soft tissue sarcomas of the lower extremity. Ann Surg 182:597, 1975.
68. Simon MA, Spanier SS, Enneking WF: Management of adult soft tissue sarcomas in extremities. Ann Surg 11:363, 1979.
69. Suit HD, Proppe KH, Monkin HJ, Wood WC: Preoperative radiation therapy for sarcoma of soft tissue. Cancer 47:2269, 1981.
70. Weingard DN, Rosenberg SA: Early lymphatic spread of osteogenic and soft tissue sarcomas. Surgery 84:231, 1978.

CHAPTER 55

Surgical Management of Tumors of the Neck

MALIGNANT TUMORS

Raleigh E. Lingeman, M.D. • Robert H. Shellhamer, Ph.D.

Neck dissection for removal of cancer metastatic to the regional cervical lymphatic system from primary malignant lesions of the head and neck has been done by a variety of operations. Since the early 1900s, radical neck dissection has been accepted as a most effective means of treatment of head and neck cancer, and the technique of this has become well standardized. It is done in a relatively short period of operating time and with an operative mortality rate for a unilateral procedure of less than 1 per cent. The classic en bloc procedure has stood the test of time as the basic operation for control of metastatic cervical cancer and for the training of head and neck surgeons, but there are surgical schools of thought that favor more conservative operations. These operations range from simple sparing of the accessory nerve with radical neck dissection to modified neck dissection with preservation of the sternocleidomastoid muscle, internal jugular vein, and the spinal accessory nerve. This discussion reviews the history of head and neck dissection, surgical anatomy of the neck, surgical technique, the complications of neck dissection, and the results.

HISTORICAL REVIEW

Prior to the early and mid-1800s, there was no mention made of surgical procedures capable of controlling metastatic cancer to the cervical glands, the name given to cervical lymph nodes at that time. Surgeons in this period were inclined to include with the cervical glands the salivary glands, the thyroid, and the nodes of the lymphatic system. Chelius (1847) stated that when the neighboring glands and lymphatics became hard and painful and once cancer from a primary lesion in the head and neck had spread to the cervical glands, control of the disease is impossible. In 1847, Warren of Boston attempted removal of metastatic cancer of the neck through use of an incision made from the masseter to the clavicle. In 1880, Kocher described an operation in which the tongue was removed through a submandibular approach after first dissecting the lymphatic glands. Several years later, Kocher devised a surgical procedure that involved cervical lymph node removal and introduced the Kocher incision, a Y-shaped incision with a

long arm running from the mastoid process to the level of the clavicle along the anterior border of the sternocleidomastoid muscle and a short arm running at right angles to the submandibular area. In 1900, Henry Butlin[4] recommended dissection of the cervical lymphatics using the Kocher incision and also discussed elective excision of lymph nodes for cancer of the oral cavity. Von Bergmann and von Bruns (1904) advised removal of lymph nodes of the neck involved with cancer from primary lesions in the oral cavity. Their operation was not a systematic procedure but was described as an extensive removal of these glands.

Credit for the first description given of a well-standardized anatomic dissection of the cervical lymphatics goes to George Crile, Sr., of Cleveland. A report in the Journal of the American Medical Association on December 1, 1906 cited his results with planned dissection of 132 operations.[10] He noted that up until this time treatment of metastatic cancer to the neck had received little attention and had not kept pace with progress for surgical treatment of other conditions in the cervical region. Crile was a pioneer in surgery of the head and neck and for years had made a study of surgery of the neck in clearing the cervical lymph nodes involved with metastases from primary head and neck disease. He recognized that anything less than radical surgery was not effective in control of cervical metastatic disease and reasoned that the proximity of the cervical lymph nodes to the internal jugular vein and to other adnexal structures, which included the sternocleidomastoid muscle and the spinal accessory nerve, made it imperative to carry out an en bloc dissection for removal of these structures. Crile advocated bilateral removal of the jugular veins when necessary and postulated that the vertebral plexus and other deep veins of the neck were adequate to serve the cranial and cervical venous return. For anesthesia, Crile recommended the use of two nasal tubes to the level of the epiglottis with packing of the oropharynx and hypopharynx, which is close to the technique as practiced today with the use of the endotracheal tube.

Hayes Martin[21] reported on experiences at Memorial Hospital in New York with the en bloc radical neck dissection as described by Crile and emphasized that anything less than this en bloc resection would hamper the excision of the cervical lymphatic system and compromise control of the cancer. John Conley[8] described his experiences with posterior neck dissection, which was a more anatomic en bloc neck dissection. His procedure began along the anterior margin of the trapezius muscle, and the dissection continued deep, medially and cranially, while identifying the important neurovascular structures. His was a monobloc dissection that included removal of the prevertebral fascia, internal jugular vein, sternocleidomastoid muscle, and the spinal accessory nerve.

In 1966, Bocca published the results of his experiences with conservative neck dissection for control of metastatic cancer of the neck. He compared 100 cases of a conservation neck dissection with 100 cases in which the classic radical neck dissection had been performed; end result studies demonstrated no differences in the salvage of the two groups of patients. Bocca's procedure[2, 3] entailed careful dissection of the cervical fascias and the removal of all fibrofatty tissue in the neck containing the lymphatic system, but with preservation of the sternocleidomastoid muscle, internal jugular vein, spinal accessory nerve, the cervical plexus, and usually the submandibular gland.

At about the same time at the M. D. Anderson Hospital in Houston, Texas, Jesse and co-workers[18] were doing conservation neck dissection that was similar to that described in detail by Bocca and associates,[3] with excellent results in selected cases. What was for them a change in philosophy toward neck dissection for the control of metastatic cervical cancer was based on the question as to why certain important structures (such as the carotid artery; vagus, phrenic, hypoglossal, and lingual nerves; and the supraclavicular trunks of the brachial plexus) could be spared and yet other structures (such as the sternocleidomastoid muscle, spinal accessory nerve, and jugular vein) could or should not be salvaged in order to eradicate the disease and still retain an adequate degree of function. At about the same time, at the Indiana University Medical Center, modified neck dissection for sparing of the spinal accessory nerve, jugular vein, and sternocleidomastoid muscle was done in selected cases, and the modified neck procedure has been done in greater numbers over the last 15 years.[20] The advantages of electing to do modified neck dissection as practiced by the group at M. D. Anderson[18] and at other centers throughout the United States and elsewhere are as follows:

1. Preservation of neck and shoulder girdle function.
2. Better cosmetic contour of the neck.
3. Protection of the internal carotid artery.
4. Capability of performing bilateral procedures with lessened concern of complications.
5. The procedure's use as a staging operation for determining the prognosis, the need for a more extensive procedure, and the need for postoperative x-ray therapy.

The rationale of doing this less-than-radical neck dissection for control of metastatic cervical cancer is that one can obtain control of neck disease in selected situations, such as in N0 and N1 staged necks, as with radical neck dissection but with significantly less disease.

All surgeons who are interested in head and neck cancer at the present time agree that the purpose of neck dissection, radical or modified, should focus on the complete excision of all metastatic disease in the neck and must include in the removal the less essential structures, the associated lymph nodes, cervical fascias, and fibrofatty connective tissue. If necessary, other structures remaining should be sacrificed if their removal will make possible more complete excision of metastatic cancer.

SURGICAL ANATOMY OF THE NECK

A rational plan for surgery of cancer of the cervical lymphatics is based upon a thorough understanding of the details of anatomy of the neck including the cervical lymphatic system, the deep cervical fascias, and the relation of these to the important muscles and neurovascular structures of the anterior and lateral neck.

Anterior, Lateral, and Posterior Neck: Anatomic Overview

Whether the surgeon is electing to do radical or modified neck dissection, the surgery actually becomes a dissection of the anterior or lateral neck, and more rarely the posterior neck, for the purpose of removing metastatic tumor involving lymph-bearing tissues. The sternocleidomastoid muscle divides the cervical region into anterior neck (anterior triangle) and lateral neck (lateral triangle). The part of the neck covered by the trapezius muscle in continuity with the posterior cervico-occipital region is the posterior neck (Fig. 55–1).

The anterior neck contains the cervical parts of the aerodigestive tract: larynx and trachea, hypopharynx and esophagus, thyroid and parathyroid glands, the carotid sheath and the large neurovascular structures contained therein, the supra- and infrahyoid strap muscles, as well as a host of associated neurovascular and lymphatic structures. The anterior neck extends cranially to the mandibular margin and caudally to the chest at the thoracic outlet (cervicothoracic isthmus) and can be divided into the right and left anterior triangles by the plane of the ventral midline. The inferior margin of the mandible along with the digastric-stylohyoid-mylohyoid muscle complex outlines the submandibular area (submandibular triangle). The submandibular area contains the submandibular gland, associated fascias, lymphatic structures, parts of the anterior facial vein and facial artery, and the marginal mandibular branch of the facial nerve. It also is the area from which anatomic and surgical access can be gained to the floor of the mouth.[24]

The position of the most lateral of the infrahyoid muscles, the omohyoid muscle, demarcates the upper part of the anterior neck as the *carotid triangle*, where the carotid sheath structures are relatively superficial in their location, and the lower and anterior part of the neck as the *muscular triangle*, containing the infrahyoid muscle strap muscles, the aerodigestive tract, and the thyroid gland complex.

The lateral neck, or lateral triangle of the neck, is often less appropriately referred to as the posterior triangle and is bounded by the borders of the sternocleidomastoid and trapezius muscles and the middle of the clavicle. The area of the lateral neck, indeed, takes

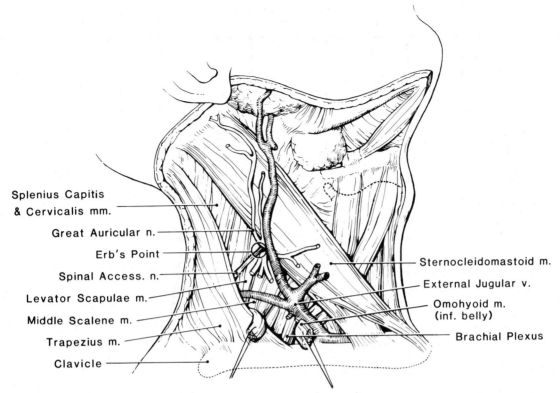

Figure 55–1. Anatomy of the neck. As the inferior belly of the omohyoid muscle is sectioned and retracted, the deep neuromuscular structures are visible.

on the geometric form of a triangle. The contents of the triangle include fibrofatty lymphatic-containing tissue, the eleventh cranial nerve, the superficial and cutaneous components of the cervical nerve plexus, and a host of small vascular bundles, the presence of which at surgery has in the past lead to the appellation of this surgical area as "bloody gulch." The presence of the lower muscle belly of the omohyoid muscle in the triangle just above the clavicle demarcates a small subclavian triangle in the lateral neck, carrying with it important surgical implications because in the depths of the subclavian triangle are found the cervical and thoracic outflow of nerves and vessels into the axilla: the brachial plexus from the interscalene muscle interval and the subclavian vessels arching over the first rib from the thorax to the axilla (Fig. 55–1).

Cervical Lymphatics

Present-day descriptions of the lymphatic system refer to the earlier descriptions of Rouviere[23] and have been put into the perspective of their application to head and neck cancer by Haagensen and associates.[17] Confirmation of the validity of the descriptions of Rouviere on the anatomy of the lymphatics in the head and neck has been presented by Fisch and Sigel,[14] who prior to surgery selectively identified in patients retroauricular and subcutaneous lymphatics by using a patent blue-violet dye for the purpose of visualizing and cannulation of a lymphatic vessel. Fisch then injected the lymphatic system using Ultra Fluid Lipiodol contrast and was able

thereby to identify the lymph nodes. Radiographic demonstration of the lymphatic system enhanced his ability to identify and remove all tissues desired and also facilitated the identification of lymphatic structures in the specimen by the pathology staff following surgery. Various adaptations of descriptive patterns of lymph nodes and vessels have been given by others, and because an estimated one third of all lymph nodes in the body are concentrated in the head and neck region, it is important to adopt a useful working description of the cervical lymphatics. We have adopted a combination of those descriptions given by Rouviere and Fisch.

Lymph nodes are either superficial, suprafascial, subfascial, or deep; that is, they are perivascular, intraglandular, submuscular, retropharyngeal, and so on. Superficial (subcutaneous) lymphatics perforate the superficial layer of deep cervical fascia to communicate with deep cervical lymph nodes. Although the superficial lymph nodes are frequently involved in cervical metastasis, especially during the late stages of cancer, the superficial nodes in a subcutaneous tissue, such as those found along the external jugular vein and the anterior jugular vein, are nevertheless of little significance from a practical standpoint of surgical treatment. If superficial lymphatics are involved with cancer, they cannot be removed without resection of large areas of skin.

At the junction between the head and the neck are groups of nodes named appropriately from their locations: occipital (suboccipital), retroauricular (mastoid), parotid, submandibular, submental, lingual, and retropharyngeal. Collectively, these groups of lymph nodes form a pericervical collar, or ring, with the lingual and retropharyngeal nodes found very deep within the outline of the ring. These are first echelon nodes, and lymphatic vessels are efferent to the pericervical collar of nodes from superficial areas of the scalp and face as well as from deeper mucous membranes of the upper aerodigestive tract.

Lymph nodes of the lateral neck are largely confined to the fibrofatty tissue of the lateral triangle and follow the course of the spinal accessory nerve. They are sometimes referred to as spinal nodes. From the point where the accessory nerve crosses the deep aspect of the sternocleidomastoid muscle and across the fibrofatty tissue of the lateral triangle of the neck, lymph nodes can be found along the course of the nerve. The upper nodes in this group are in the anterior neck and represent a coalescence of the nodes of both the upper jugular group and the spinal accessory group. This represents a most important surgical area and defines a group of nodes referred to as junctional nodes by Rouviere[23] and Fisch and Sigel.[14] These nodes drain the uppermost part of the aerodigestive tract, including the nasopharynx and choanal areas.

Cervical lymph nodes in the anterior neck, except for those bordering on being microscopic and situated along the aerodigestive tract or in association with the thyroid gland, are located along the internal jugular vein from the level of the posterior belly of the digastric muscle to the root of the neck where the internal jugular vein joins the subclavian vein. Those that are most cranial in their position are deep at the level of the posterior belly of the digastric muscle and drain the deep face and anterior neck. One of these nodes commonly is referred to as the jugulodigastric node, emphasized so often because it is the first-echelon node draining the posterior faucial region, including the tonsil.[19]

Middle jugular nodes are located in the neck to the level where the omohyoid muscle crosses the carotid sheath; these nodes drain the middle parts of the aerodigestive tract in the neck and the thyroid gland. Inferior nodes are found along the internal jugular vein from the level of the omohyoid to the root of the neck where the jugular vein joins the subclavian vein. These nodes drain the thyroid and the lower cervical parts of the aerodigestive tract, that is, the trachea and esophagus. The lowest of the jugular nodes are confluent with the medial extent of the transverse cervical nodes of the lateral neck and usually constitute what are referred to as the prescalene nodal masses so importantly located at the interface between body regions: low neck, apex of the axilla, and the thoracic outlet. Nodes of the jugular group are found in the loose connective tissue of the carotid sheath and lie anterior, lateral, and posterior to the internal jugular vein in the sheath. The possibility of lymphatic efferents from the nodes low in the neck communicating with lymph nodes in the superior mediastinum is very real and of serious concern to the head and neck surgeon.

Efferent lymphatic vessels in the cervical region on the left and right sides are confluent with vessels of varying caliber, achieving ultimate lymphovenous communication with the great veins. On the left side, a singularly large lymph vessel, the thoracic duct, receives lymphatic tributaries from the neck and is a major lymphatic vessel from the mediastinum and abdomen.

The thoracic duct enters the jugulosubclavian venous junction on the left side at the root of the neck. From the mediastinum, the course of this vessel describes an upward and left lateral arch behind the carotid sheath, receives lymphatic tributaries from the neck, and enters the venous junction in the angle between the left internal jugular and subclavian veins. Injury to this vessel in any surgery performed on the left side of the neck should be carefully avoided in order to prevent a chylous fistula from developing. No singular or large lymph vessel is found on the right side of the root of the neck. Rather, multiple lymph vessels are seen, although one vessel may be identified and termed the right lymphatic duct. Such vessels on the right, single or multiple, will join the jugulosubclavian venous junction as on the left side.

By whatever surgical technique described, en bloc dissection should entail removal of the loose areolar connective tissue that contains lymphatic tissue. If the capsules of the nodes are effaced by disease, tumor will involve the fascias of adjacent muscles, viscera, or vessels. If this be the case, judgmentally it requires of the surgeon a revision of the game plan from a modified or conservative procedure to a more radical one in order to remove all disease, even at the expense of sacrificing major structures, rather than salvage of muscles, vessels, or nerves at the risk of leaving disease behind.

Cervical Fascias and Fascial Cleavage Planes and Spaces

The fascias and fascial planes of the head and neck were described in detail in the 1930s by Coller and Yglesius[7] and by Grodinsky and Holyoke.[16] These authors emphasized cervical fascial spaces and addressed infections that invaded these spaces as localized processes, which allowed spread to occur from one locale to another. The fascial spaces were described as being within the boundaries of fascial envelopes about muscles, around cervical viscera, or around vascular structures and as loose areolar tissue spaces between the fascias or fascial planes.

Cleavage planes are identified at surgery and are equated with the loose connective tissue described as cervical fascial spaces by Coller and Yglesius and by Grodinsky and Holyoke. As such, cleavage planes aid in developing a rapid surgical exposure.

Lymphatic tissue is found in loose tissue, and as such, the bulk of tissue removed in a radical or conservative neck procedure contains much areolar connective tissue and with it lymphatic structures. Although the lymph nodes can lie close to muscle fascias, and to the fascias of visceral or neurovascular structures, the nodes are not normally directly related to or intimate with arteries or to muscles covered by them. Invasion into muscles or vessels by metastatic cancer of the lymph nodes of the neck may occur by extension after the capsule of diseased lymph nodes has been effaced. Radical dissection of the lymphatic system of the neck implies resection of all structures contained in the anterior and lateral triangles of the neck. This, of course, means removal of a number of important structures whose only relationship with the lymphatic system is one of proximity. By contrast, in the modified neck dissection, the fascias of the muscles and vessels are carefully stripped away, and the loose and fatty connective tissue containing lymphatic tissue is removed en bloc after the essential structures such as nerves, vessels, and muscle have been identified and preserved.

The superficial fascia of the anterior and lateral neck contains the platysma muscle. A plane can be developed superficial to the platysma, or a skin flap can be raised to include the platysma muscle in it. Invasion of this plane by disease can be problematic because surgery may then require extensive removal of cutaneous layers and requires careful determination of the boundaries of the surgical removal of the disease.

Deep to the superficial fascia lies a discrete fascial lamina, the superficial layer of the deep cervical fascia. Intimately related to muscle, the deep fascia in the neck attaches to bone superiorly to the hyoid bone and mandible, posteriorly to the spines of the cervical vertebrae, inferiorly to the thoracic cage and clavicle (Fig. 55–2):

1. *From anterior to posterior*—the fascia invests the sternocleidomastoid and trapezius muscles. In the lateral neck the fascia loses the distinct laminar characteristic of the anterior neck and becomes a very dense fibrofatty meld of connective tissue that harbors lymphatic structures, small vessels, the spinal accessory nerve, and cutaneous branches of the cervical nerve plexus.

2. *Superiorly*—before attaching to the mandible the deep cervical fascia splits to invest the submandibular gland, thereby creating a fascial compartment for the gland and contained lymphatic structures and vessels. The cervical fascia also splits to invest the parotid gland to thereby create a compartment for the parotid and the many structures located in that gland; such structures include the facial nerve, terminal branches of the external carotid artery, retromandibular vein, and lymphatic structures.

3. *Inferiorly*—the superficial layer of deep cervical fascia continues inferiorly to attach to the sternum and clavicle. Just above the sternum, the fascia splits and attaches to the anterior and posterior surfaces of the sternum, thereby creating an interlaminar space, the suprasternal space of Burns. In the space of Burns are found lymphatic and venous communication across the midline between the two anterior jugular veins occupying a position along the anterior margin of the sternocleidomastoid muscles.

Fascias deeper in the anterior neck invest the strap muscles (the middle layer of deep cervical fascia) and the aerodigestive tract and thyroid gland (visceral fascial layer). Clearly, each fascial lamina is separated from the next by a readily definable areolar connective tissue cleavage plane.

More laterally in the anterior neck, fascial laminae contribute to the carotid sheath, a discrete fascial investment of the internal jugular vein, carotid artery, and vagus nerve. According to Grodinsky and Holyoke,[16] the carotid sheath "is made up primarily of alar fascia reinforced in the neck by layers of sternothyroid fascia anteromedially and sternocleidomastoid fascia anterolaterally, making the carotid sheath wall double in these portions. Within the sheath are separate individual sheaths for each of its main constituents." The carotid sheath is continuous with laminae of the neighboring fascias, such as that of the pharyngeal wall (buccopharyngeal fascia), that of the prevertebral muscles (prevertebral fascia), that of the infrahyoid muscles (middle fascial layer), and that of the sternocleidomastoid muscle (superficial layer of the deep cervical fascia). Areolar connective tissue external to the carotid sheath contains lymph nodes on the anterior, lateral, and posterior aspects of the sheath.

In or on the carotid sheath lies an unusual nerve entity, the ansa cervicalis. The superior limb of the ansa cervicalis is a branch of the hypoglossal nerve and contains C1 and C2 nerve fibers. The inferior limb of the nerve ansa emerges from behind the internal jugular

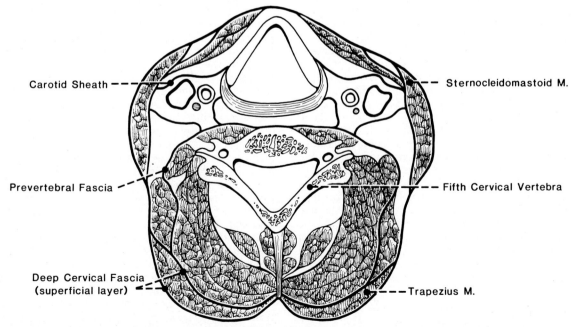

Figure 55–2. Superficial layer of the deep cervical fascia and the deep layer or prevertebral fascia of the deep cervical fascia. Note contributions to the carotid sheath and the sternocleidomastoid and trapezius muscles.

vein and contains fibers from C2 and C3. The two limbs unite on the carotid sheath and constitute the nerve supply to the infrahyoid strap muscles as nerve branches from the ansa distribute to these muscles.

Internally the carotid sheath is somewhat partitioned by connective tissue septa and is, thereby, compartmentalized to contain the jugular vein, the carotid vessels, and the vagus nerve. On the posterior aspect of the carotid sheath, but more fully incorporated in the fascia of the prevertebral muscle, lies the cervical part of the sympathetic trunk.

The deepest fascial lamina of the neck, and readily separated from the other fascias by a cleavage plane, is the prevertebral fascia. This fascia invests the cervical vertebral column and its associated prevertebral muscles: the splenius capitis; levator scapulae; anterior, middle, and posterior scalenes; longus capitis and cervicis muscles; and the small ventrally placed atlanto-occipital muscles. Intrafascial or subfascial lymphatics or nodes have not been described in the prevertebral fascia, and this leads one to question the need to include this fascial lamina when doing an en bloc radical neck procedure. The consequences of elevating prevertebral fascia in doing a neck dissection, beyond merely increasing the devastation wrought by the surgical exercise, can be severe. If this fascia is raised, there is risk of involving what lies deep to the fascia, notably the cervical and brachial plexuses, the sympathetic trunk, and the phrenic nerve. The cervical plexus emerges from between the scalene muscle bundles. The brachial plexus emerges from the interscalene interval between anterior and middle scalene muscles, as does the subclavian artery at the level of the first rib, and together these neurovascular structures descend into the axilla. An infundibular ensheathment of these structures, the axillary sheath, occurs as an attenuation of the prevertebral fascia accompanying nerves and vessels into the axilla. The phrenic nerve crosses obliquely on the anterior surface of the anterior scalene muscle from lateral to medial and lies deep to the prevertebral fascia. It originates from C3–5 and descends into the mediastinum to supply the diaphragm.

Calearo and Teatini[5] reviewed 265 cases of functional neck dissections. The procedure included stripping the prevertebral fascia in an en bloc dissection of nodes and connective tissues. They listed among their iatrogenic complications five cases of section of the phrenic nerve and four cases of section of the sympathetic trunk. They cited no injuries to the brachial plexus. It is advisable to remember that if the surgical procedure denudes prevertebral muscles of their investing fascias, the nerves that lie deep to the prevertebral fascia are put at risk. It is better to consider avoiding these structures and thereby obviate loss of shoulder function because of injury to the brachial plexus, of diaphragmatic respiratory function because of section of the phrenic nerve, or of sympathetic disturbances in the head and neck and upper limb because of injury to the sympathetic trunk. Surgically, an adequate cleavage plane can be developed superficial to the prevertebral fascia.

Sternocleidomastoid Muscle and Spinal Accessory Nerve

The sternocleidomastoid muscle is attached cranially to the lateral surface of the mastoid of the temporal bone and to the lateral part of the superior nuchal line of the occipital bone. Caudally, it divides into sternal and clavicular heads to attach on the sternum and clavicle. It is invested by the superficial layer of deep cervical fascia, split into two laminae to cover the superficial and deep surfaces of the muscle. At the anterior margin of the sternocleidomastoid muscle, thickened fascia attaches to the fascia at the angle of the mandible, thereby creating the angular band, or Charpy's band. The presence of this band can make it difficult to open the interval between the sternocleidomastoid muscle, the angle of the mandible and the parotid gland.

Crossing the outer surface of the sternocleidomastoid in its upper half is the external jugular vein, marking out its course from the angle of the mandible to the midpoint of the posterior margin of the sternocleidomastoid muscle. Within one fingerbreadth cranial to and parallel to the vein, the great auricular nerve also crosses the outer surface of the muscle from Erb's point (the midpoint along the posterior margin of the sternocleidomastoid muscle), coursing to cutaneous distribution in the region of the auricle and over the parotid gland. From Erb's point, one or more other nerves derived from the cervical plexus also cross the outer surface of the sternocleidomastoid muscle and distribute to cutaneous areas of the anterior neck and submental region. These are the anterior cutaneous nerves of the neck.

The spinal accessory nerve lies deep to the sternocleidomastoid muscle, somewhat paralleling the more superficial course of the external jugular vein. The accessory nerve divides deep to the sternocleidomastoid muscle to supply it and to continue through the lateral neck to distribute to the trapezius muscle. Cranial nerve XI has rootlets of origin from the brain stem (bulbar fibers) and from the cervical cord (spinal fibers) originating from the cord as low as C5 or C6. The spinal rootlets contribute to a nerve that rises alongside the cord to enter the cranium at the foramen magnum and to be joined in the posterior fossa by the bulbar fibers. The combined fibers exit from the cranium by way of the jugular foramen, and the accessory nerve crosses ventral to the internal jugular vein deep to the posterior belly of the digastric muscle. Fibers of bulbar origin join the vagus in the jugular foramen and distribute to pharyngolaryngeal muscles. Fibers of spinal origin distribute to girdle muscles, such as the sternocleidomastoid and trapezius.

The accessory nerve can be identified entering the deep surface of the sternocleidomastoid muscle 4 cm or more below the mastoid. It can be located at Erb's point just superior to where the great auricular nerve surfaces from the deep neck. The spinal accessory nerve can also be located readily in the lateral neck at the point where it disappears on the deep surface of the trapezius muscle, roughly two fingerbreadths superior to the clavicle at the anterior margin of the trapezius muscle. Deep to the sternocleidomastoid muscle the spinal accessory nerve may in its course invade the muscle bundle on its way to the lateral neck, in which case care must be exercised to isolate the nerve from muscle in clearing the area of connective tissue and lymphatic tissue in doing a modified neck procedure.

Blood supply to the sternocleidomastoid muscle is extensive. Multiple vascular bundles are given to the muscle on its deep surface along its length from cranial to thoracic attachments: branches from the occipital artery, from the posterior auricular artery, from the superior thyroid artery, from superficial and transverse cervical arteries, and from the transverse scapular artery.

Functionally, the sternocleidomastoid muscle acts in elevation of the thoracic cage and shoulder girdle or, with fixation of the limb, acts in lateral flexion of the head to the shoulder on the same side and rotate the head to direct the chin upward to the opposite side. The trapezius muscle is one of several muscles that elevate the shoulder girdle and retract the girdle dorsally. It assists the sternocleidomastoid muscle in rotation of the head and in lateral flexion of the neck.

Internal Jugular Vein

From the skull base in the jugular foramen to the root of the neck and junction there with the subclavian vein, the internal jugular vein receives venous tributaries from the parotid, from the floor of mouth, from the occipital region, and from thyroid areas. Each tributary may need to be contained by ligature in the removal of the internal jugular vein in radical or modified neck procedures. At the skull base, the spinal accessory nerve crosses in front of the internal jugular vein at the level of the transverse process of the atlas. Related to this area in the anterior neck, lymph nodes associated with the accessory nerve and those of the superior jugular group lie in the loose connective tissue and are identified there as junctional lymph nodes. These are first- or second-echelon nodes draining primary tumor sites high in the aerodigestive tract, that is, the nasopharyngeal areas. Nodal tissue can be found on the anterior, lateral, and posterior aspects of the connective tissue sheath of the internal jugular vein. Coller and Yglesias[7] refer to the lymph space posterolateral to the carotid sheath. It is the connective tissue of this space closely associated with the internal jugular vein that is removed en bloc in preserving the vein in conservation procedure.

Carotid Arteries and the Hypoglossal Nerve

In the carotid sheath at or just below the level of the tip of the hyoid bone, the common carotid artery bifurcates into the internal and external carotid arteries. The internal carotid artery typically takes a straight and unbranched course to the skull base to its entrance into the carotid canal and the petrous bone. In about 15 per cent of cases, the internal carotid artery can vary from normal and may be somewhat redundant, may be aneurysmic, or can take on the form of being frankly kinked or coiled at some point from the bifurcation to the skull base.[11] Any direct association between these occurrences and either intramural or intraluminal disease of the carotid is not yet fully understood.

The hypoglossal nerve descends from the occipital skull base to enter the floor of mouth just above the tip of the hyoid bone. In its descent between the internal jugular vein and the internal carotid artery, the hypoglossal nerve crosses the lateral aspect of both arteries in a gentle downward curve dictated by the nerve being locked into its curvilinear position by the branching of the occipital artery from the external carotid artery. At this point of potential entrapment there has been de-

scribed (1) constrictive compression of the hypoglossal nerve by the occipital artery and (2) occurrence of an aneurysm of the internal carotid artery just medial to the hypoglossal nerve.[6]

Two branches of the hypoglossal nerve contribute to the motor supply of supra- and infrahyoid muscles: (1) direct branches from cranial nerve XII to the thyrohyoid and geniohyoid muscles, nerve fibers thought to be mixed in origin from the hypoglossal nucleus in the brain stem and from C1 level of the spinal cord, and (2) the superior limb of the ansa cervicalis (descendens hypoglossi). This latter branch represents C1–3 origin of the motor fibers to the infrahyoid strap muscles by way of the nerve ansa that is found on the carotid sheath.

The hypoglossal nerve passes deep to the stylohyoid, digastric, and mylohyoid muscles, and on the lateral surface of the hyoglossus muscle it passes into the floor of the mouth deep to the submandibular gland. The nerve is accompanied by the largest tributary of the lingual vein, the vena comitans of the hypoglossal nerve. Cranial nerve XII is the motor nerve to tongue muscles and provides for all motor supply to the tongue with the exception of the palatoglossus muscle supplied by the vagal complex.

The ventrally disposed branches of the external carotid artery distribute to the thyroid (superior thyroid artery), facial regions (external maxillary artery), tongue and tonsil (lingual artery), deep face and nose (internal maxillary artery), and superficial scalp (superficial temporal artery). Dorsally directed branches of the external carotid artery pass superficially across the internal jugular vein and go to occipital and auricular areas (occipital and posterior auricular arteries), or are muscular branches to the sternocleidomastoid muscle, branching either directly from the external carotid artery or as branches of the occipital, posterior auricular, or superior thyroid artery. These arteries may need to be secured in the course of oncologic neck surgery. The ascending pharyngeal artery arises in the bifurcation of the common carotid artery and from that point courses straight to the occipital skull base as a major contributor of vascular supply to the pharyngeal wall, including the tonsil, and to the cranial dura in the posterior cranial fossa. This artery ordinarily does not become visible during the usual course of neck dissection.

Infrahyoid Strap Muscles

Ranging from cranial attachments on the hyoid bone and thyroid ala to more caudal attachments on the sternum and scapula are muscles of the anterior neck lying anterior and lateral to the thyroid gland and referred to as the infrahyoid strap muscles. They are described by Fink[13] as accessory muscles of respiration. Functionally, they are a part of a longitudinal motor complex that ranges in attachment from the base of the tongue to the superior mediastinum and regulates the luminal dimension of the laryngeal part of the airway in respiration. Thus, the sternothyroid and sternohyoid muscles are described as being involved in increasing the dimension of the glottic segment of the airway in inspiration.

The omohyoid muscle, the most lateral of the infrahyoid group, is like the digastric, a two-bellied muscle. Its superior belly is attached to the hyoid bone, and its inferior belly is attached to the superior margin of the scapula just posterior to the lesser scapular notch. The two bellies are joined together by a tendon located deep to the sternocleidomastoid muscle and having fascial continuity with the fascias of the overlying sternocleidomastoid muscle and clavicle and the underlying carotid sheath. The omohyoid muscle becomes somewhat of a surgical landmark, for the carotid sheath lies deep to its superior belly in the anterior neck. The brachial plexus and subclavian vessels lie deep to the inferior belly of the omohyoid in the lower part of the lateral neck just above the clavicle (Fig. 55–1).

The ansa cervicalis, draped across the carotid sheath, is the nerve supply to the infrahyoid strap muscles and is noticeably at risk in any surgical procedure done in the anterior neck. At worst, some degree of inspiratory disturbance of respiratory function could be anticipated, being transitory in nature, following interruption of these nerves. Only the external jugular vein lies superficial to the posterior belly of the omohyoid in the lateral neck. All important neurovascular structures lie deep to the muscle belly.

Digastric, Stylohyoid, and Mylohyoid Muscles

The key to understanding continuity of anatomy or in planning surgical techniques in the area of junction between the head and neck is the digastric-stylohyoid-mylohyoid muscle complex. The digastric muscle is attached to the deep surface of the mastoid in the digastric groove as a posterior muscle belly, to the lesser cornu of the hyoid bone as a tendon slip, and to the deep surface of the mandible in the mental region as an anterior muscle belly. Associated with the tendinous attachment of the digastric to the hyoid bone is the stylohyoid muscle, which splits into two muscle bundles to permit the digastric tendon to pass between them. The posterior belly of the digastric and the stylohyoid have become landmarks that are junctional in position between the head and neck. Certain anatomic axioms can apply to the surgical anatomy of this area:

1. All major structures coursing between the head and neck do so by passing deep to the digastric-stylohyoid complex. This includes the hypoglossal and vagus nerves, the carotid arteries, and the internal jugular vein. Only the marginal mandibular branch of the facial nerve, the anterior facial vein, and the posterior facial vein lie superficial to the digastric-stylohyoid complex. The usual relationship of the marginal mandibular branch of the facial nerve to the anterior facial vein is that the nerve lies superficial to the vein. Advantage can be taken of this anatomic relationship in doing a dissection of the submandibular area by ligating the vein and elevating it along with the marginal mandibular nerve cranially and over the mandible in order to protect the nerve against injury. By not doing so, there is risk of injury to this nerve and consequent facial disfigurement owing to loss of depressor functions of the lower lip and corner of the mouth.[9, 22]

2. Branches of nerves that descend and distribute to the aerodigestive tract, that is, pharyngeal and laryngeal branches of the vagus nerve and even the recurrent laryngeal nerves, course on the deep surfaces of the great vessels of the neck.

3. The facial nerve emerges from the stylomastoid

foramen of the temporal bone and before entering the parotid compartment is located briefly in loose connective tissue. This occurs just above the anterior margin of the posterior belly of the digastric muscle and inferior to the tip of the mastoid process.

The suprahyoid muscles lying between the hyoid bone and the body of the mandible constitute a muscular framework of the floor of the mouth referred to by Didio and Anderson[12] as the oral diaphragm. This includes the anterior belly of the digastric muscle, the mylohyoid muscle, and the geniohyoid muscle arranged from superficial to deep in the suprahyoid area. Each is a masticator muscle, a jaw depressor by function, since each attaches to the mandible. Collectively, they contribute to the muscular support of the floor of the mouth and provide the tension needed, much like a springboard, to allow the backward thrust of the tongue in the oral cavity in the first phase of swallowing. The mylohyoid muscle is a sheet of muscle contributing to the floor of the mouth. It is attached to the mylohyoid line on the inner surface of the mandible bilaterally and to the hyoid bone and to the muscle of the opposite side by way of a midline muscular raphe. The deep parts of the submandibular gland and duct enter the floor of mouth by passing around the posterior free margin of the mylohyoid muscle. Hence, the deep part of the submandibular gland and the sublingual gland lie in the loose connective tissue superior to the mylohyoid muscle. Also found in the loose connective tissue is the submandibular duct and the lingual and hypoglossal nerve.[24]

The nerve to the anterior belly of the digastric and mylohyoid muscles, the mylohyoid branch of the trigeminal nerve, is quite superficially placed in the suprahyoid region between the two muscles and can be injured or interrupted in doing a dissection in the area of the submandibular compartment. The risk of injury to this nerve involves loss of muscular support of the floor of mouth and reduced tongue thrust in the first phase of swallowing.

A rational plan for surgical management of cancer that involves the cervical lymphatic system is based upon a correct and thorough understanding of the anatomy of the neurovascular and muscular structures, cervical lymphatics, and cervical fascias of the anterior and lateral neck. Whether one practices en bloc radical dissection or some form of conservation or functional neck dissection, thorough knowledge of the anatomy of the head and neck is essential.

CERVICAL METASTASIS FROM AN UNKNOWN PRIMARY TUMOR

A metastatic malignancy within a cervical lymph node may indicate metastasis from a known primary tumor or a primary lesion that is occult or unknown to the physician. An occult or unknown primary is defined as histologic evidence of malignancy in the cervical lymph nodes with no apparent site of origin for the metastatic tumor. These are difficult cases, both for diagnostic and therapeutic decisions. The number of patients with unknown primary lesions is a small percentage of the total number of patients seen with head and neck malignancies. The majority of patients presenting with a cervical mass have evidence of a primary lesion that can be located following an intensive evaluation.

Over two thirds of patients who present with a metastatic cervical node are discovered to have primary lesions above the clavicles; therefore, the evaluation for these unknown primary lesions should be intensified to that area.[33] The routine work-up of patients with unknown primary cervical tumors may consist of (1) a history; (2) physical examination, including indirect nasopharyngoscopy and laryngoscopy; (3) palpation of the nasopharynx and base of tongue and floor of mouth; (4) sinus films; (5) sputum cytologic specimen; and (6) complete panendoscopy, with blind biopsies of the nasopharynx; oropharynx, including base of tongue; hypopharynx; larynx; esophagus; and major bronchi. Bronchial washings may also be performed.

A cervical lymph node should not be excised for diagnostic purposes until the other evaluations have revealed no evidence of a primary lesion. A study from the University of Iowa indicates that surgical disruption of lymphatic drainage and manipulation of the cervical metastasis is more apt to worsen the chances for a clean surgical extirpation and cure unless that disruption is performed at the time of definitive resection.[41] In that study, patients who had undergone previous biopsy had a higher incidence of complication, such as distant metastasis, local recurrences, and wound necrosis. Other studies indicate that initial biopsy may not influence overall survival.[44] However, most head and neck surgeons follow the recommendation that an open biopsy not be performed until a search for the primary lesion is completed. A fine-needle biopsy of a cervical lymph node is considered appropriate.[31]

From various studies, the success rate of finding the primary lesion ranges from 10 to 75 per cent.[27, 29, 32, 36, 39, 43] In patients who initially present with a metastatic cervical lymph node, the incidence in which the primary lesion is not found after appropriate evaluation is generally less than 5 to 8 per cent. The region of Waldeyer's ring provides nearly 50 per cent of the sites of origin of carcinomas originally considered as occult in the cervical area.[25] The tonsil and base of tongue area are the most common sites, followed by the nasopharynx. The next most common site is the hypopharynx and cervical esophagus.[33, 37, 38, 45] After those areas, other sites in the head and neck are associated with a much lower incidence of harboring a primary cancer. These areas include the nasal cavity, buccal mucosa, palate, paranasal sinuses, larynx, floor of mouth, salivary glands, and thyroid gland. The most common primary sites below the clavicles, in order of frequency, are the lung; gastrointestinal tract, including colon, stomach, and gallbladder; breast; pancreas; prostate gland; ovary; bladder; testes; and uterus.[27, 28, 34, 35, 42]

The location of the cervical node within the neck may provide a clue to the location of the primary unknown lesion. Most occult primary disease located inferior to the clavicle will have nodes that are in the lower portions of the cervical area. Cervical metastasis from the thyroid gland may present either in the middle or lower portions of the neck. Primary lesions more superior in the mouth and nasopharynx will generally present with higher neck nodes, whereas primary lesions in the oropharynx and hypopharynx will present with high or middle cervical adenopathy. The majority of patients presenting with only supraclavicular nodes almost always have primary neoplasms below the clavicle. The majority of patients with cervical metastasis from an unknown primary have unilateral high cervical nodes. Multiple adenopathy is found in 16 to 20 per cent, whereas 30 to 40 per cent have nodes larger than 4 cm. The majority of patients have epidermoid carcinoma. Less frequent are undifferentiated tumors and adenocarcinoma.[25]

If thorough evaluation fails to reveal a primary tumor in the area above the clavicles, a biopsy should be done. If histologic studies of the cervical lymph nodes suggest a primary tumor in an area below the clavicles, appropriate diagnostic evaluation should be performed in those areas. When histologic study and biopsy of the node show undifferentiated tumor, it frequently will resemble primary lesions found in the nasopharynx, base of tongue, and pyriform fossa, although the primary lesion may not be demonstrable in each case.

Irradiation alone is generally used to control neck masses smaller than 3 cm. Radiation is effective in approximately 80 per cent of these patients, and the cure rate for tumors greater than 3 cm or for fixed nodes is about 35 per cent with this modality. The addition of surgery for this stage of disease is likely to increase local neck control. The area of radiation should encompass the nasopharynx, oropharynx, hypopharynx, and neck area. The treatment doses generally are 6000 rad in the midplane or, with boosting of the gross disease, 7000 to 7500 rad. The primary site is discovered after treatment in 20 to 40 per cent of patients with cervical lymph nodes from originally occult primary disease.[25] In surgery-only patients, the failure rate is approximately 20 per cent in either the nasopharynx, oropharynx, or hypopharynx, areas that would be encompassed in the typical radiotherapy portal. In those patients treated with radiation alone or a combined approach, the incidence of primary tumor appearance in the head and neck area is reduced to 4 to 14 per cent.[46] Approximately 15 per cent of patients will eventually manifest disease in the irradiation fields. Of the patients for whom control fails, approximately 50 per cent will demonstrate uncontrolled disease in the neck or primary lesion; the remaining 50 per cent of these patients have distant metastasis.

The prognosis for a patient with a subsequently located primary neoplasm after the initial therapy is completed is generally worse than for those patients in whom the primary cancer remains indeterminate.[28, 37, 43] A cervical metastasis from a poorly differentiated squamous cell carcinoma carries a better prognosis than that from a well-differentiated squamous cell carcinoma.[25] The possibility of a subsequent presentation of a hidden primary tumor decreases with increasing time. If tumors above the clavicle become manifest, they will usually do so within the first two years. Most of the primary lesions below the clavicles become apparent during the first year. The worst prognosis is generally associated with those patients who have lower neck nodes, especially in the supraclavicular area; multiple or bilateral nodes; nodes greater than 3 cm; or fixed nodes.

Any discussion concerning cervical metastasis from occult primaries should include the lesion known as *branchiogenic carcinoma*. This controversial lesion was first described in 1882 as carcinoma that develops in branchial cleft remnants. Many pathologists and surgeons today consider this entity either nonexistent or at best extremely rare. The criteria before the diagnosis of branchiogenic carcinoma is acceptable are:

1. The cervical tumor must occur along a line extending from a point just anterior to the tragus along the anterior border of the sternocleidomastoid muscle to the clavicle.

2. The histologic appearance of the neoplasm must be consistent with an origin from tissue known to be present in the vestiges of the branchial apparatus.

3. No primary source of the carcinoma should be discovered during at least a 5-year follow-up. [39, 40]

The best criterion is the histologic demonstration of a carcinoma arising in the wall of a structure consistent with a branchial cyst. [25] Most of the reported examples of branchiogenic carcinoma do not meet these criteria. [26, 47, 48] All of the reported branchiogenic carcinomas have been squamous tumors varying from well-differentiated to poorly differentiated and from keratinizing to non-keratinizing carcinomas. If the nodal lesion is a nonkeratinizing carcinoma, percentages strongly favor the anatomic region of Waldeyer's ring as a primary site. The hypopharynx also ranks high if the lesion in the neck is a keratinizing squamous cell carcinoma. [30]

Presence of a cystic component in combination with a lymphoid matrix has led to the presumed diagnosis of a branchiogenic carcinoma; however, neither the cystic component nor the lymphoid tissue should lead one to make such a diagnosis. Cystic changes are not unusual for metastasis from primary carcinomas in the region of Waldeyer's ring, especially the tonsil. Metastases from squamous cell carcinomas are not usually associated with pseudocystic changes produced by necrosis or central liquefactive degeneration. The presence or absence of lymphatic tissue should not be a criterion for either eliminating or suggesting a branchiogenic carcinoma or metastasis to a lymph node. Metastasis to cervical nodes can obscure the architecture of a lymph node, whereas branchial cleft cysts often lie within lymph nodes. Batsakis believes that the probability of a branchiogenic carcinoma is remote and that the lesions should always be considered as a metastasis. [25]

SURGERY OF NECK DISSECTION

Surgeons doing neck dissection (radical or modified) must regard the indications for these operations from a broad perspective based on three basic principles:

1. There should be definite clinical evidence that cancer is present in the cervical lymphatics or that the primary lesion is accompanied with high risk of metastasis to the cervical lymphatics and first-echelon nodes.

2. The primary lesion should have been controlled clinically, or if not controlled, should be removed at the time neck dissection is carried out.

3. There should be no clinical evidence of distant disease.

In addition to the basic indications for both procedures as noted above, there are specific indications and contraindications for the modified neck dissection. The indications are as follows:

1. N0 neck in which the primary tumor is to be treated surgically and carries a significant risk of recurrent metastasis.

2. N1 neck disease.

3. Papillary and follicular adenocarcinoma of the thyroid.

4. Malignant melanoma when the neck is N0.

The contraindications to the modified neck dissection are as follows:

1. N2 and N3 neck disease.

2. Nodal and primary disease that are treatable with radiation therapy, including primary sites and nodal metastases from the (a) nasopharynx and (b) selected tonsil lesions.

Specific contraindication to radical neck dissection in the absence of distant metastases is fixation of the metastatic mass to the deep neck muscles or to the carotid artery. Often it is difficult to be certain of this prior to surgery. Determination of the problem of fixation to the carotid artery and to muscle depends upon the experience of the surgeon. More often than not, the surgeon will find the disease is, in fact, operable.

Decision as to when to perform an en bloc radical neck dissection or a modified neck dissection will depend upon the staging of the neck. If the primary tumor involving the oral cavity, oropharynx, or larynx is staged at a level of II or III with high risk of metastases and if it is decided that surgery is the treatment of choice for the primary tumor, then even if the neck is staged N0, modified neck dissection should be carried out. There are situations in which radical dissection for N0 neck disease could be recommended, but in most cases N0 necks should be treated with a modified neck dissection with the expectancy that salvage will be just as effective as might be expected for a more radical procedure. The basic objective of neck dissection, whether it be radical neck dissection or modified neck dissection, is to remove all cancer, and no modification of the basic operation should change this. If all lymph-bearing tissue can be excised with sparing of certain anatomic structures, this will maintain a greater degree of shoulder function and yet not compromise control of cancer. This is the desire and objective of surgery of neck dissection.

The experiences at Indiana University[20] and at the M. D. Anderson Hospital[18] indicate that with the neck staged at N0 the chance of error from negative to positive is 10 to 20 per cent. Based upon this important information, it is recognized that in the N0 neck, eight of 10 patients having radical neck dissection will not have positive nodes and that there is a price paid for sacrifice of important structures such as the spinal accessory nerve. The resultant incapacitating shoulder syndrome, causing persistent pain due to the strain placed on supporting shoulder muscles with drooping of the shoulder and loss of shoulder girdle function, is related to the absence of trapezius function and is completely unnecessary.

Patients who are staged at N1 will have a chance of error from positive to negative of approximately 37 per cent. Patients who are staged at N2 and N3 have an error from positive to negative of 6 per cent. If bilateral neck procedures are done for N2 and N3 neck disease, an attempt should be made to preserve one internal jugular vein. It is recommended that if radical neck dissection is done and the spinal accessory nerve is sacrificed, the accessory nerve should be reconstructed with a cable graft. The result has been satisfactory for partial or complete return of function over a period of many months.

Preoperative preparation is important. The preoperative work-up mainly will be concerned with the investigation of uncovering any systemic abnormalities that might be corrected or improved in order to minimize postoperative complications. There are no medical contraindications to surgery as stated by Martin,[21] and this is entirely reasonable because the cancer itself is always fatal if left untreated. If surgery would offer the best chance of control, it is more reasonable to accept the operative risk than the inevitable death from uncontrolled cancer. It is best that patients who are being considered for neck dissection be reviewed by the Medicine Service with the understanding that the decision is to be made when the operation is to be done rather than whether it should be done at all. The medical work-up should include a review of the cardiovascular, renal, pulmonary, and hematopoietic systems.

EN BLOC STANDARD RADICAL NECK DISSECTION

For either radical neck dissection or modified neck dissection, the incision described by Jesse and associates[18] provides adequate exposure and is especially ideal for use in the irradiated neck, in which case maximal preservation of blood supply to the flaps is required. The incision adopted by Jesse begins slightly below the mastoid process and continues in a downward and horizontal direction toward the ventral midline. This incision can be converted into a horizontal T if necessary and can be incorporated in a lower lip-splitting incision or as a part of an incision for exposure of the parotid compartment. Superior and inferior skin flaps, which include the platysma muscle, are raised (Fig. 55–3).

The dissection begins along the anterior border of the trapezius muscle, clearing the lateral triangle of the fibrofatty lymphatic tissue, with no attempt made to preserve the accessory nerve. The mastoid attachments of the sternocleidomastoid muscle are detached, and the mastoid attachment of the posterior belly of the digastric muscle and the upper part of the jugular vein is identified. Dissection is then started in the inferior part of the neck with ligation of the lower part of the external jugular vein. Just beneath the external jugular vein, the omohyoid muscle is identified, and deep to it, the brachial plexus. By sweeping the fibrofatty lymphatic tissue in an upward and medial direction, the brachial plexus can be identified.

The dissection continues from the lateral part of the neck medially and upward to the third and fourth spinal nerves, which are key landmarks for identifying the carotid sheath. At this time the common carotid artery in the carotid sheath is only a few millimeters medial to the roots of the cervical plexus. Dissection is then carried to the internal jugular vein. The sternal and clavicular attachments of the sternocleidomastoid muscle are cut, and the omohyoid muscle is avulsed from the scapula and reflected medially and upward. The phrenic nerve is identified and preserved intact. The internal jugular vein is clamped, cut, ligated, and transfixed, and the dissection is carried along the carotid sheath to the upper neck. The internal jugular vein with the deep jugular chain of nodes is dissected from the vagus nerve and internal carotid artery, and is clamped, cut, and transfixed. The dissection continues into the subman-

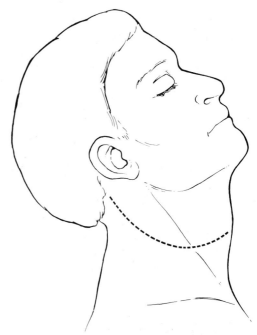

Figure 55–3. Standard radical neck dissection. Horizontal incision as described by Jesse. Vertical arm along the anterior border of the trapezius muscle to the clavicle will provide additional exposure for dissection of the lateral triangle of the neck if necessary.

dibular area with clearing of the nodes in the submandibular triangle together with the submandibular salivary gland. At the conclusion of the procedure, the nodes of the lateral neck—the superior, middle, and inferior jugular nodes and the supraclavicular group of nodes—together with nodal groups of the submandibular and submental area have been removed with the sternocleidomastoid muscle, the internal jugular vein, and the submandibular salivary gland (Figs. 55–3 to 55–12).

STANDARD NECK DISSECTION WITH SPARING OF THE SPINAL ACCESSORY NERVE

A modification of the en bloc radical neck dissection but with the important feature of conservation of the spinal accessory nerve is frequently the procedure of choice by many surgeons. After elevation of the skin flaps as described previously, the spinal accessory nerve is identified in the anterior neck in its relation to the internal jugular vein and the posterior belly of the digastric muscle and followed inferiorly to determine whether it enters the muscle or passes deep to the sternocleidomastoid muscle. In most cases, the nerve passes directly through the muscle, emerging at Erb's point along the posterior border of the sternocleidomastoid muscle at its upper and middle thirds (see Figure 55–14). The accessory nerve is then followed in a downward direction until it passes under the anterior border of the trapezius muscle.

With the nerve identified (see Figure 55–15), it is carefully dissected away from the surrounding muscle fibers of the sternocleidomastoid muscle and the muscle is separated from its attachment to the mastoid process

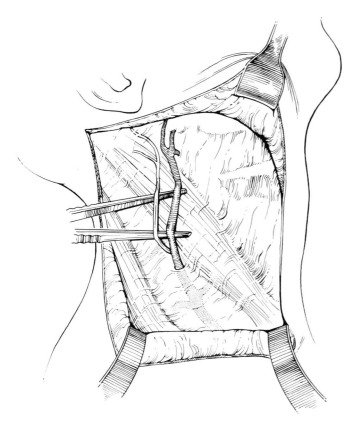

Figure 55–4. Standard radical neck dissection. Relation of the external jugular vein and the great auricular nerve as it emerges from the posterior border of the sternocleido-mastoid muscle is the most accurate guide for identification of the spinal accessory nerve.

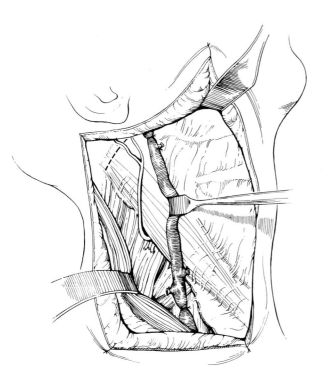

Figure 55–5. Standard radical neck dissection. The external jugular vein has been ligated superiorly and inferiorly, spinal accessory nerve has been cut, and dissection along the anterior borders of the trapezius muscle has been started.

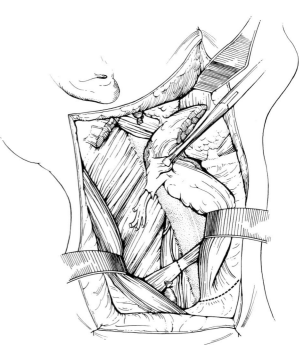

Figure 55–6. Standard radical neck dissection. Mastoid attachments of the sternocleidomastoid muscle have been separated, and the omohyoid muscle is identified.

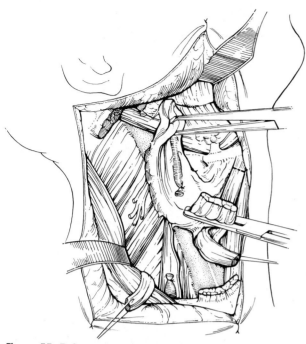

Figure 55–7. Standard radical neck dissection. The omohyoid muscle has been cut as well as the sternal and clavicular attachments of the sternocleidomastoid muscle; brachial plexus and phrenic nerve are identified in the lateral neck.

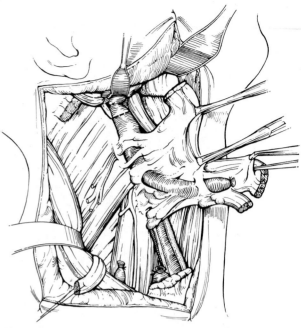

Figure 55–9. Standard radical neck dissection. Dissection of deep jugular chain of nodes to the upper neck; internal jugular vein has been ligated and cut beneath posterior belly of digastric muscle.

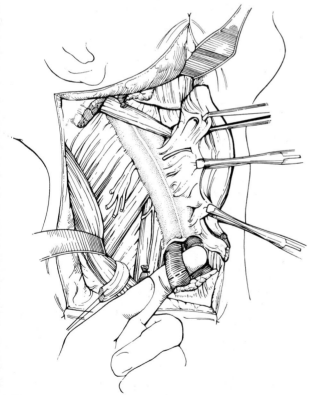

Figure 55–8. Standard radical neck dissection. Dissection carried from the lateral triangle medially and superiorly, and dissection of the internal jugular vein from the vagus nerve and common carotid artery. Internal jugular vein has been ligated and cut, and the dissection of the carotid sheath and deep jugular nodes carried into the upper neck.

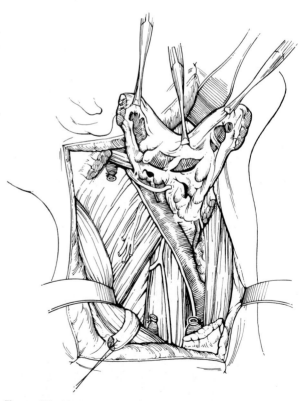

Figure 55–10. Standard radical neck dissection. The internal jugular vein is ligated beneath the posterior belly of the digastric muscle, dissection of the carotid sheath and deep jugular nodes is completed, and dissection is carried into the submandibular triangle.

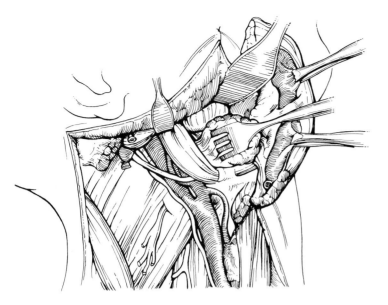

Figure 55–11. Standard radical neck dissection. Dissection of the nodes of the submandibular triangle with identification of the hypoglossal nerve.

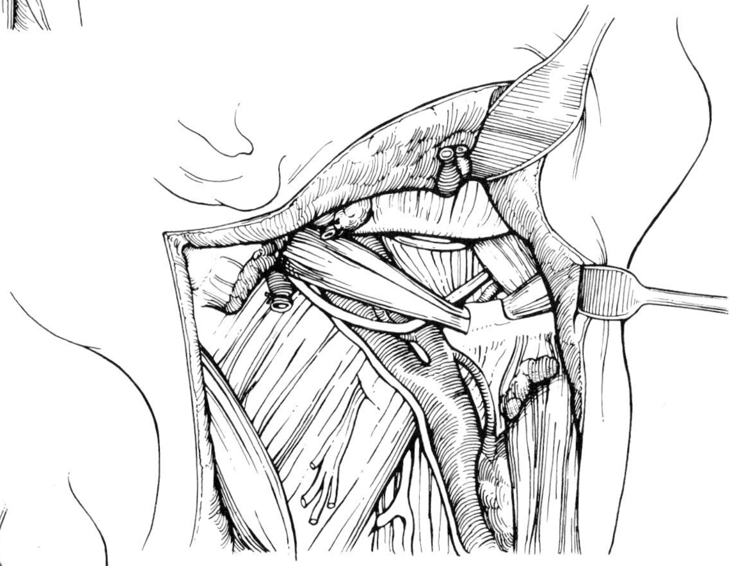

Figure 55–12. Completion of standard radical neck dissection, with removal of nodes of the lateral triangle, supraclavicular lymphatics, deep jugular nodes, and submandibular nodes. The carotid artery, vagus, and hypoglossal nerves are preserved. The internal jugular vein, the 12th cranial nerve, and the sternocleidomastoid muscle have been removed.

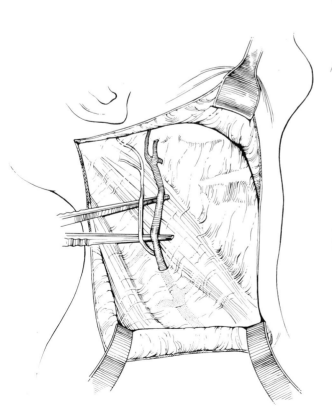

Figure 55–13. Standard neck dissection with sparing of spinal accessory nerve. Exposure of anterior and lateral neck with identification of external jugular vein and great auricular nerve.

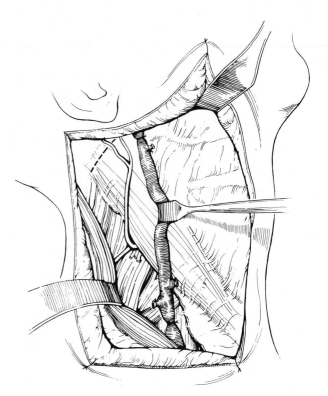

Figure 55–14. Standard neck dissection with sparing of spinal accessory nerve. Identification of the spinal accessory nerve in the lateral triangle of the neck as it relates to the great auricular nerve at Erb's point.

and is reflected downward (see Figure 55–16). After the sternocleidomastoid muscle is severed from its mastoid attachments, the internal jugular vein and relation of the nerve to this vessel is identified. The remainder of the dissection is as described previously, beginning along the anterior border of the trapezius muscle and carried in a careful dissection medially and upward with clearing of the posterior cervical group of nodes together with the supraclavicular nodes. The omohyoid muscle is avulsed from beneath the clavicle; the sternal and clavicular attachments of the sternocleidomastoid mus-

cle are cut; the brachial plexus and phrenic nerve are identified and preserved. The internal jugular vein is dissected from the vagus nerve; the common carotid artery is clamped, cut, ligated, and transfixed; and the dissection of the deep jugular nodes is carried into the upper neck where the internal jugular vein is ligated, cut, and transfixed beneath the posterior belly of the digastric muscle after the accessory nerve is identified and preserved. Dissection is then carried into the submandibular area with clearing of the submandibular and submental group of nodes (Figs. 55–13 to 55–22).

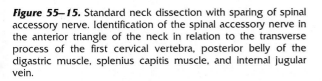

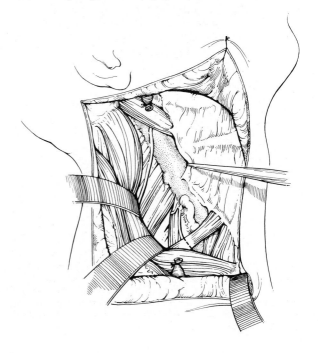

Figure 55–15. Standard neck dissection with sparing of spinal accessory nerve. Identification of the spinal accessory nerve in the anterior triangle of the neck in relation to the transverse process of the first cervical vertebra, posterior belly of the digastric muscle, splenius capitis muscle, and internal jugular vein.

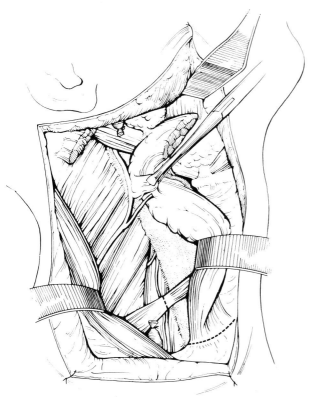

Figure 55–16. Standard neck dissection with sparing of spinal accessory nerve. Mastoid attachment of sternocleidomastoid muscle cut after the spinal accessory nerve has been dissected through or beneath the muscle.

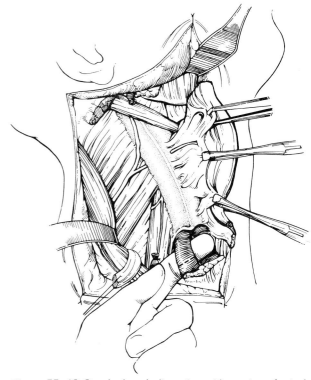

Figure 55–18. Standard neck dissection with sparing of spinal accessory nerve. The internal jugular vein is ligated and cut in the inferior neck, and the dissection is carried from the lateral triangle of the neck medially and upward with dissection of the deep jugular lymph nodes.

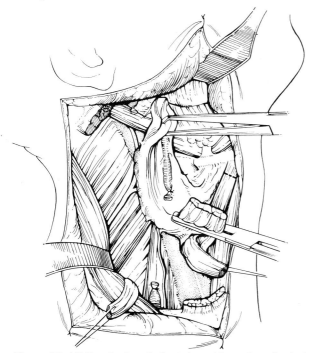

Figure 55–17. Standard neck dissection with sparing of spinal accessory nerve. Omohyoid muscle and the clavicular and sternal attachment of sternocleidomastoid muscle cut with exposure of the brachial plexus between the medial and anterior scalene muscles and the phrenic nerve lying on the anterior scalene muscle.

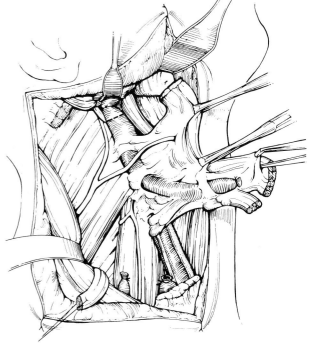

Figure 55–19. Standard neck dissection with sparing of spinal accessory nerve. Further dissection of the deep jugular nodes, with dissection again being carried medially and upward to the superior part of the neck.

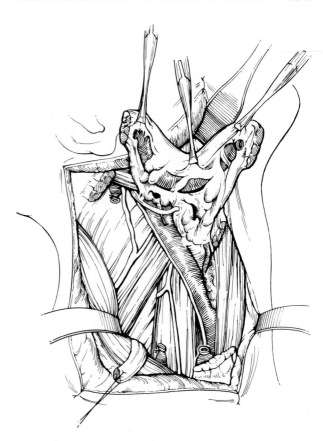

Figure 55–20. Standard neck dissection with sparing of spinal accessory nerve. The internal jugular vein is ligated beneath the posterior belly of the digastric muscle with preservation of the spinal accessory nerve. Dissection of the deep jugular nodes is carried into the upper neck.

ANTERIOR MODIFIED NECK DISSECTION

A modification of the en bloc neck dissection is a procedure that ablates all the lymph-bearing tissue that is removed in the classic operation, but with the important feature of preservation of the spinal accessory nerve and sternocleidomastoid muscle, with or without sparing of the internal jugular vein. If the dissection includes only the anterior triangle of the neck, the external jugular vein is ligated high and low, and the superior fascia that has been preserved is now interrupted along the upper border of the submandibular compartment and following along the anterior border of the sterno-cleidomastoid muscle to the clavicle.

The spinal accessory nerve is identified in the upper part of the anterior triangle of the neck in relation to the internal jugular vein, the posterior belly of the digastric muscle, and the bony prominence of the trans-

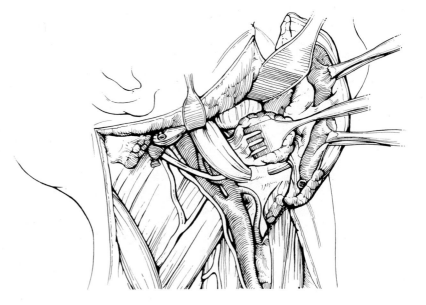

Figure 55–21. Standard neck dissection with sparing of spinal accessory nerve. Dissection is carried into the submandibular triangle with identification of the hypoglossal nerve.

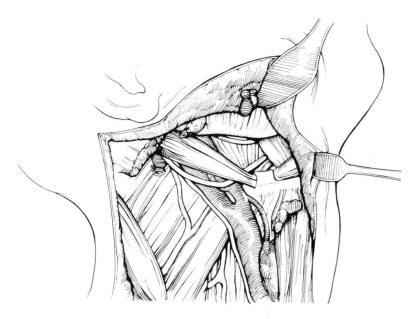

Figure 55–22. Standard neck dissection with sparing of spinal accessory nerve. Completion of dissection of the submandibular triangle with removal of lymph nodes of the lateral neck and supraclavicular area. Dissection of the deep jugular nodes and lymphatics of the submandibular triangle with preservation of the spinal accessory nerve.

verse process of the first cervical vertebra. At this time it is necessary to dissect the group of lymph nodes beneath the posterior belly of the digastric muscle—the superior deep jugular nodes—which are the nodes most commonly involved in metastatic cancer of the head and neck. This is done by retracting the sternocleidomastoid muscle laterally, identifying the splenius capitis muscle, and carefully dissecting the fibrofatty lymphatic tissue in this area from beneath the sternocleidomastoid muscle and from the spinal accessory nerve. It must be accented that this is without question the most important part of the modified neck dissection.

With the sternocleidomastoid muscle retracted laterally from the underlying fibrofatty lymphatic tissue, dissection is carried to the deep prevertebral muscles and their fascias beginning in the middle and lower part of the neck. The omohyoid muscle is avulsed from beneath the clavicle and is reflected medially and anteriorly with identification and preservation of the brachial plexus and the phrenic nerve. The dissection is now similar to the posterior radical neck dissection: dissection is carried medially and anteriorly to the roots of cervical nerves 3 and 4, which are cut. Dissection is then carried to the carotid sheath; the internal jugular

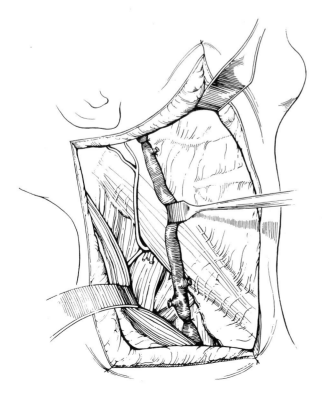

Figure 55–23. Anterior modified neck dissection. Relations of the structures at Erb's point, spinal accessory nerve, and the great auricular nerve.

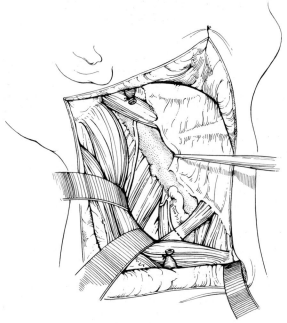

Figure 55–24. Anterior modified neck dissection. Exposure of the spinal accessory nerve in the superior-anterior neck as it relates to the posterior belly of the digastric muscle, splenius capitis muscle, and internal jugular vein.

vein is identified, and the deep jugular nodes are dissected in an upward direction from the lateral, posterior, and anterior aspects of the jugular vein. The upper nodes already have been cleared so that when the dissection reaches the upper part of the neck, the

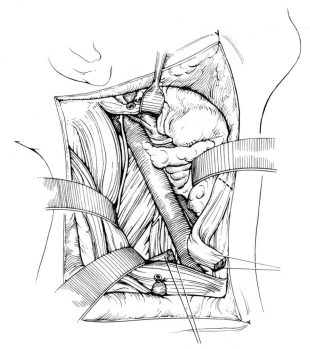

Figure 55–26. Anterior modified neck dissection is carried medially and upward, including the deep jugular nodes.

operator identifies and preserves the hypoglossal nerve descending between the jugular vein and the internal carotid artery. The contents of the submandibular triangle in the submental area are cleared of these nodes, and the procedure is completed (Figs. 55–23 to 55–28).

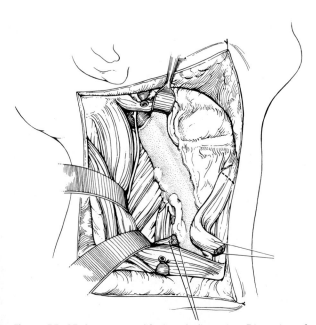

Figure 55–25. Anterior modified neck dissection. Dissection of the spinal accessory nerve in the superior-anterior neck as it relates to the splenius capitis muscle, internal jugular vein, and posterior belly of the digastric muscle, with complete dissection of the superior jugular nodes in the subdigastric area.

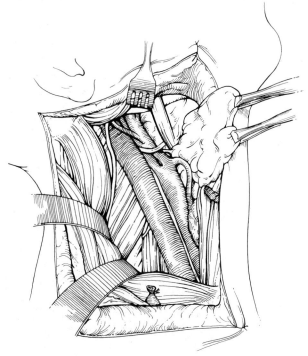

Figure 55–27. Completion of anterior modified neck dissection of the deep jugular nodes, with dissection carried into the submandibular triangle of the anterior neck.

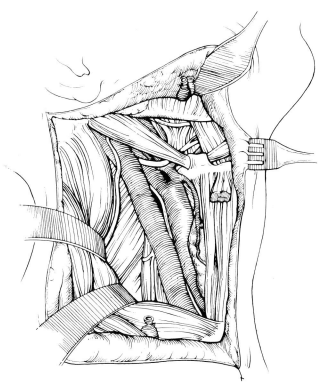

Figure 55–28. Completion of anterior modified neck dissection, with preservation of spinal accessory nerve, sternocleidomastoid muscle, and internal jugular vein and removal of the supraclavicular lymph nodes, deep jugular lymph nodes, and lymphatics of the submandibular triangle.

ANTERIOR AND LATERAL MODIFIED NECK DISSECTION

If a decision is made to include the lateral cervical nodes in the dissection, the dissection is much the same as that just described except that the spinal accessory nerve is identified not only in the anterior triangle but also as it emerges in relation to Erb's point along the posterior border of the sternocleidomastoid muscle. From this point dissection of the nerve is carried in a downward direction to its innervation of the trapezius muscle. The fascia enclosing the sternocleidomastoid muscle is cut anteriorly and posteriorly, and the sternocleidomastoid is elevated from underlying structures from the mastoid process to the clavicle. Careful dissection of the subdigastric or superior group of deep jugular nodes is done as mentioned previously, exposing the splenius capitis muscle, the accessory nerve, and the internal jugular vein, and the dissection is carried forward and medially.

Dissection is then started from the anterior border of the trapezius muscle and is carried anteriorly and medially. The omohyoid muscle is avulsed beneath the clavicle, identifying and preserving the brachial plexus and phrenic nerve deep to the prevertebral fascia and carrying the dissection to the roots of the third and fourth cervical nerve roots. These roots are cut, the dissection is carried to the carotid sheath, and the lower and middle group of deep jugular nodes are cleared from the lateral, posterior, and anterior aspects of the jugular vein. The dissection is carried into the upper neck, and again, the submandibular and submental

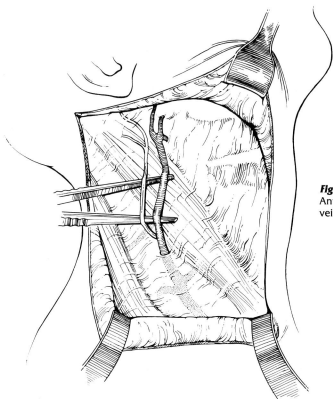

Figure 55–29. Anterior and lateral modified neck dissection. Anterior and lateral neck with relations of the external jugular vein and the great auricular nerve at Erb's point.

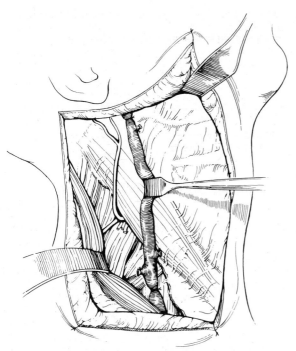

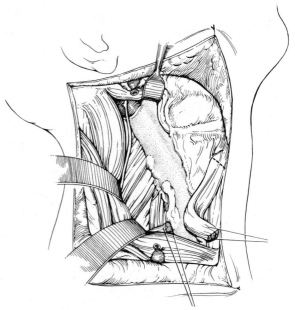

Figure 55–30. Anterior and lateral modified neck dissection. Exposure of the spinal accessory nerve as it emerges from the posterior border of the sternocleidomastoid muscle at Erb's point.

Figure 55–32. Anterior and lateral modified neck dissection. Further dissection of the spinal accessory nerve either beneath or through the sternocleidomastoid muscle.

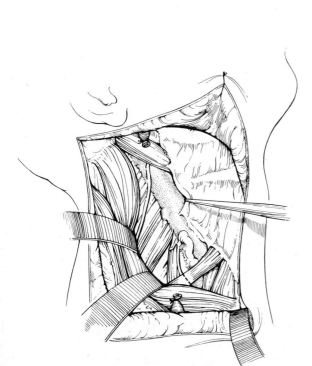

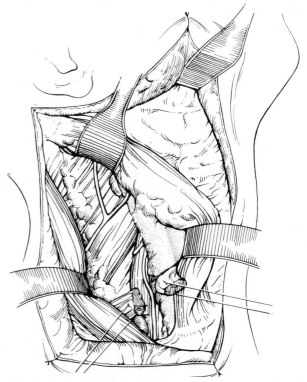

Figure 55–31. Anterior and lateral modified neck dissection of the spinal accessory nerve in the anterior-superior neck and relation of the nerve to the internal jugular vein, posterior belly of the digastric muscle, and splenius capitis muscle. Dissection of the lymph nodes of the superior jugular chain beneath the digastric muscle.

Figure 55–33. Anterior and lateral modified neck dissection of the spinal accessory nerve in the lateral triangle of the neck where it passes under the anterior border of the trapezius muscle. The omohyoid muscle is cut in the inferior neck, the brachial plexus and phrenic nerve are identified, and the dissection is carried forward beneath the sternocleidomastoid muscle.

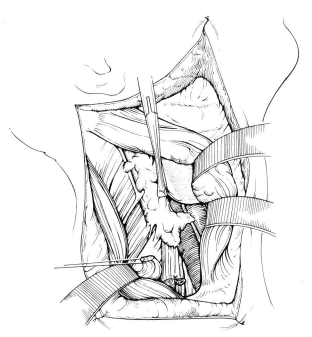

Figure 55–34. Anterior and lateral modified neck dissection. Further dissection from the anterior border of the trapezius muscle clearing the lymphatic system of the lateral neck and the superior, middle, and inferior lymph nodes. Dissection of the supraclavicular group of nodes is done, and dissection is carried medially and upward, removing the inferior and middle lymph nodes of the deep jugular chain from the internal jugular vein.

areas are cleared of this group of nodes. The procedure is now complete.

The procedure just described is the most that is done in a conservative modified type of neck dissection, and at completion of the surgery is the same picture one would see with an en bloc neck dissection but with the preservation of the sternocleidomastoid muscle, the spinal accessory nerve, and the internal jugular vein along with the brachial plexus, phrenic nerve, sympathetic trunk, carotid arterial system, and the hypoglossal nerve (Figs. 55–29 to 55–38).

POSTEROLATERAL NECK DISSECTION

In order to complete this chapter on neck dissection, mention must be made of the posterolateral neck dissection as described by Goepfert, Jesse, and Ballantyne of the M. D. Anderson Hospital in Houston, Texas.[15] Their procedure is done for patients with squamous cell carcinoma of the skin of the posterior part of the scalp or for melanoma with metastatic disease confined to the lymph nodes in the posterior and lateral neck. There are two distinct groups of lymph nodes in the upper posterior part of the neck: retroauricular nodes, which are located behind the mastoid, and suboccipital nodes. The latter nodes consist of three subgroups: superficial occipital nodes, subfascial or deep occipital nodes, and one lymph node associated with the splenius muscle and along the occipital artery.

Metastasis from melanoma or squamous cell carcinoma on the scalp may drain primarily into the posterior

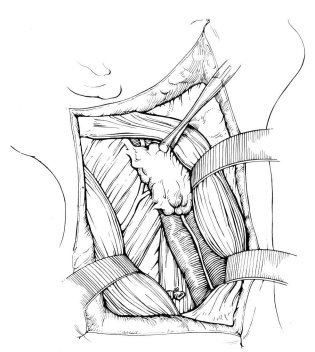

Figure 55–35. Anterior and lateral modified neck dissection into the upper lateral anterior neck, with reflection of the sternocleidomastoid muscle forward and further exposure of the contents of the carotid sheath.

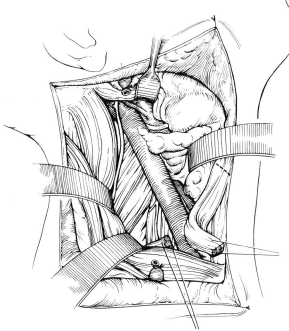

Figure 55–36. Anterior and lateral modified neck dissection is completed in the anterior neck with removal of the inferior and middle deep jugular lymph nodes. The dissection is carried into the submandibular area.

auricular or suboccipital nodal groups. Secondary and tertiary nodes of the spinal accessory chain and upper internal jugular nodal groups receive efferent vessels from the occipital nodes. Whenever a regional node dissection is indicated for these lesions, an adequate surgical procedure includes a posterolateral neck dissection, often a parotid compartment dissection and either a radical or modified neck dissection. The technique as described by Goepfert and associates[15] is a dissection of the posterior and lateral group of nodes as has been described. If the primary lesion lies close to the limits of the posterolateral neck dissection, the primary lesion should be incorporated in the dissection with adequate margins. Thin skin flaps are developed to the posterior edge of the sternocleidomastoid and to the posterior midline. The cranial attachment of the trapezius is separated from the nuchal line, and its vertebral attachments are resected down to the level of the spines of the third or fourth cervical vertebrae. The occipital artery is identified, and any nodes associated with it are removed. Large veins are usually encountered close to the midline and deep to the trapezius muscle. The upper portions of the splenius capitis, levator scapulae, and semispinalis capitis muscles become visible during this part of the dissection.

In a neck with clinically negative nodes, the spinal accessory nerve is preserved throughout its course, and this forms the inferior margin of the dissection. If the nodes are clinically positive along the accessory nerve, no attempt is made to preserve the nerve. By retracting the sternocleidomastoid muscle anteriorly, the junc-

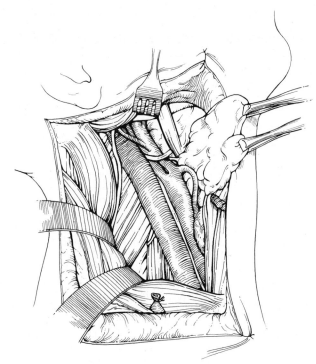

Figure 55–37. Anterior and lateral modified neck dissection. Completion of the dissection of the anterior triangle of the neck. The hypoglossal nerve is identified, and dissection is carried into the submandibular triangle.

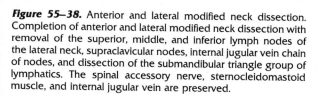

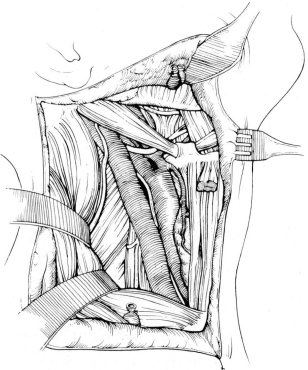

Figure 55–38. Anterior and lateral modified neck dissection. Completion of anterior and lateral modified neck dissection with removal of the superior, middle, and inferior lymph nodes of the lateral neck, supraclavicular nodes, internal jugular vein chain of nodes, and dissection of the submandibular triangle group of lymphatics. The spinal accessory nerve, sternocleidomastoid muscle, and internal jugular vein are preserved.

tional lymph nodes and nodes of the upper extent of the jugular group are dissected. In the regional posterolateral neck dissection, the lymph nodes to be included will be retroauricular, suboccipital, upper and middle jugular, and the contents of the lateral triangle of the neck down to the level of the spinal accessory nerve. Such procedures cause minimal deformity.

The author has not had experience with this procedure as described previously by the M. D. Anderson Hospital surgeons, but it is a sensible procedure and should be considered a part of the control of cancer arising from primary lesion in the posterior scalp.

COMPLICATIONS OF NECK DISSECTION

Recovery from neck dissection, whether it be the en bloc radical neck dissection or modified neck dissection, usually extends over a period of 1 to 2 weeks. The majority of the wounds heal without serious complications. The operative mortality rate is less than 1 per cent. The most serious complication of neck dissection is pneumothorax occurring as a result of pleural injury during the course of neck dissection, especially in clearing the root of the neck of bulky metastatic disease behind the clavicle. The most frequently occurring complications of neck dissection are wound breakdown, hemorrhage, and fistula formation. During the course of a radical neck dissection, or any of the variety of conservation procedures, numerous vessels are ligated, and the surgeon must be meticulously careful in order to prevent postoperative hemorrhage. Manipulation of and dissection around the common and internal carotid arteries must be done with great care because injury to these vessels may cause stroke or death, especially in patients with known or suspected peripheral vascular disease.

In clearing the lower neck, lymph vessels that communicate with the thoracic cavity must be carefully identified and ligated in order to minimize the possibility of the occurrence of a chylous fistula. The brachial plexus is seldom injured; however, the phrenic nerve is particularly prone to injury that can result in paralysis of the diaphragm. Injury to the vagus nerve in the upper neck in the older patient causes marked disability in swallowing and in speech. The operator also needs to be aware of the possibility of sympathetic disturbances associated with trauma to the cervical part of the sympathetic trunk.

DISCUSSION AND RESULTS

The overview of the relative values placed upon standard and modified neck dissection techniques must be presented not only with respect to the control of metastatic cancer of the neck but also with respect to the education of young surgeons who will be doing oncologic surgery of the head and neck with desirability of preservation of function of the shoulder girdle by salvage of the spinal accessory nerve. It must be emphasized that radical neck dissection is still the basic operation of choice for control of head and neck cancer and should continue to be taught to young surgeons in training as a standard procedure. It is our opinion that

the modified neck dissection should be a part of their training for head and neck surgery, but it should be recognized that the modified neck dissection is more difficult and more time-consuming than the standard radical en bloc neck dissection.

The radical neck dissection can be done more rapidly, and technically, it is easier to accomplish. If the young surgeon can master the technique of modified neck dissection, the surgeon is then able to deal with any disease that may be treated by surgery in the head and neck. To perform a modified neck dissection effectively and safely, a surgeon must have a thorough working knowledge of the anatomy of the neck, and more specifically, the anatomy of the cervical connective tissues and lymphatics. On the other hand, if the surgeon is not familiar with the modified neck dissection and does only a limited number of major procedures in the head and neck each year, it is our recommendation that the en bloc neck dissection be practiced rather than to undertake a procedure that may compromise the control of cancer in the hands of an inexperienced surgeon.

An incapacitating shoulder syndrome results from sacrifice of the spinal accessory nerve as a part of the standard en bloc neck dissection. Significant alteration of shoulder girdle function is present in 80 per cent of patients having the standard en bloc neck dissection operation. Loss of the spinal accessory nerve causes persistent pain owing to the strain placed on supporting shoulder muscles, with drooping of the shoulder and loss of shoulder girdle function, related to the absence of trapezial activity. All patients who have had sparing of the accessory nerve either with the standard radical neck dissection or with the modified operation will have some pain and limitation of shoulder function, but this is expected to be temporary in nature. In our experience, the patients who have had the accessory nerve spared as part of their neck dissection ultimately will have good function of the shoulder girdle.

Cosmetic deformity is of no great concern unless the patient has been subjected to a bilateral procedure. Patients having had bilateral necks done will demonstrate progressive atrophy of the trapezius muscles on each side with increasingly more severe cosmetic disfigurement (marked thinning of the neck) and dysfunction disability. Cutaneous anesthesia from either procedure is an annoying symptom that improves over the first 6 to 12 months following surgery. In the hands of some surgeons who practice the modified neck dissection with preservation of the cervical plexus, the prospect of postoperative cutaneous anesthesia is totally eliminated.

An analysis by us of the control of metastatic cancer of the neck with standard en bloc neck dissection as compared with modified neck dissection in the years 1966 to 1976 concluded that with N0 and N1 necks the control of disease was essentially the same. Comparing a small number of N2 staged necks treated by means of modified neck dissection with a larger number of cases treated with standard radical neck dissections, the conclusion was that the percentage of 5-year control of the disease was the same in both groups. Since 1976, most of the neck dissections that have been done for metastatic cancer at the Indiana University Medical Center have been modified procedures or standard neck dissections, but with sparing of the spinal accessory nerve. The majority of these were staged at N0, and the

TABLE 55–1. Experience with Radical Neck Dissection and Modified Neck Dissection (1966 to 1981): Recurrences of Disease in N0, N1, and N2 Necks

Description	Cases	Recurrences in Neck	Recurrence (%)
N0 disease			
Radical neck dissection	115	17	14
Modified neck dissection	235	27	11
N1 disease			
Radical neck dissection	138	21	15
Modified neck dissection	184	25	16
N2 disease			
Radical neck dissection	80	21	20
Modified neck dissection	8	2	25

incidence of recurrence in the neck was found to be much as reported in the cases reviewed from 1966 to 1976. With a smaller but significant number of patients staged as N1 the incidence of tumor recurrence was also the same (16 per cent) as had been previously reported in 1977.

We conclude that modified neck dissection, although a more difficult and more time-consuming procedure, is as effective in the N0 and N1 situations as the standard radical neck dissection. Based on our observations with the use of this operation since 1966, it is our opinion that this should be the procedure of choice to be used for N0 and N1 neck disease by the surgeon who is experienced and who does a significant number of head and neck surgeries each year (Table 55–1).

CURRENT PRACTICE

Our current practice is as follows: If the primary tumor is to be treated surgically and the neck is staged as N0 or N1, modified neck dissection is the treatment of choice. If the neck is staged at N2 or N3, radical neck dissection is done and, if possible, with sparing of the accessory nerve. If the spinal accessory nerve is sacrificed in the radical neck dissection, reconstruction of the nerve is done using a cable graft. Radiation therapy is given 3 weeks postoperatively if positive nodes are present. Radiation therapy is not given for metastatic melanoma or for well-differentiated thyroid cancer. If the primary lesion is treated with radiation therapy, 5000 rad are given to each side of the neck, and if the neck is staged at N0, no surgery is recommended. If the neck is staged N1, a modified neck dissection is done. If the neck is staged N2 or N3, radical neck dissection is necessary and, if possible, with sparing of the accessory nerve. If the nerve is sacrificed, a cable graft for reconstruction of the nerve is recommended.

We conclude that modified neck dissection is as effective in the N0 or N1 situations as radical neck dissection but caution that it is a more difficult and more time-consuming procedure. With the use of this operation and based on our review of experiences since 1966, it is our opinion that this is the procedure that should be done by the surgeon who is experienced and does a significant number of head and neck surgeries each year.

Table 55–1 reviews the experience of the surgeons at the Indiana University Medical Center during the years 1966 to 1981.

REFERENCES

1. Bocca E: Supraglottic laryngectomy and functional neck dissection. J Laryngol Otol 80:831, 1966.
2. Bocca E, Pignataro O: A conservation technique in radical neck dissection. Ann Otol 76:975, 1967.
3. Bocca E, Pignataro O, Sasaki CT: Functional neck dissection. A description of operative technique. Arch Otol 106:524, 1980.
4. Butlin HT: Diseases of the Tongue. Philadelphia, Lea Brothers & Co., 1885.
5. Calearo CV, Teatini G: Functional neck dissection. Anatomical grounds, surgical technique, clinical observations. Ann Otol 92:215, 1983.
6. Carney AL, Anderson EM: Diagnosis and treatment of brain ischemia. Adv Neurol 30:223, 1981.
7. Coller FA, Yglesias S: The relations of the spread of infection to fascial planes in the neck and thorax. Surgery 1:323, 1937.
8. Conley JJ: Concepts in Head and Neck Surgery. New York, Grune & Stratton, 1970.
9. Conley JJ: Paralysis of the mandibular branch of the facial nerve. Plast Reconstruct Surg 70:569, 1982.
10. Crile G: Excision of cancer of the head and neck. JAMA 47:1780, 1906.
11. Desai B, Toole JF: Kinks, coils and carotids. A review. Stroke 6:649, 1975.
12. Didio LJA, Anderson MC: The Sphincters of the Digestive System. Baltimore, Williams & Wilkins Co., 1968.
13. Fink BR: Folding mechanism of the human larynx. Acta Otol 78:124, 1974.
14. Fisch M, Sigel ME: Cervical lymphatic system as visualized by lymphography. Ann Otol 73:869, 1964.
15. Goepfert H, Jesse RH, Ballantyne AJ: Posterolateral neck dissection. Arch Otol 106:618, 1980.
16. Grodinsky M, Holyoke EA: The fasciae and fascial spaces of the head and neck and adjacent regions. Am J Anat 63:367, 1938.
17. Haagensen CE, Feind CR, Herter FP, et al: The Lymphatics in Cancer. Philadelphia, W. B. Saunders Co., 1972.
18. Jesse RH, Ballantyne AJ, Larson DL: Radical or modified neck dissection: Therapeutic dilemma. Am J Surg 136:516, 1978.
19. Lindberg R: Distribution of cervical lymph node metastases from squamous cell carcinoma of the upper respiratory and digestive tracts. Cancer 29:1446, 1972.
20. Lingeman RE, Helmus C, Stephens R, Ulm J: Neck dissection: Radical or conservative. Ann Otol 80:737, 1977.
21. Martin H, et al: Neck dissection. Cancer 4:441, 1951.
22. Moffett Ramsden RT: The deformity produced by a palsy of the marginal mandibular branch of the facial nerve. J Laryngol Otol 91:401, 1977.
23. Rouviere H: Anatomy of the Human Lymphatic System. Edwards Brothers, 1938.
24. Skandalakis JE, Gray SW, Rowe JS Jr: Surgical anatomy of the submandibular triangle. Am Surg 45:590, 1979.

CERVICAL METASTASIS

25. Batsakis JG: The pathology of head and neck tumors: The occult primary and metastases to the head and neck, part 10. Head Neck Surg 3:409, 1981.
26. Black B, Maran AGD: Branchiogenic carcinoma. Clin Otolaryngol 3:27, 1978.
27. Bridger GP, Reay-Young P: Metastatic neck nodes of unknown primary origin. Med J Aust 2:49, 1978.
28. Coker DD, Casterline PF, Chambers RG, Jaques DA: Metastases to lymph nodes of the head and neck from an unknown primary site. Am J Surg 134:517, 1977.
29. Comess MS, Beahrs OH, Dockerty MB: Cervical metastasis from occult carcinoma. Surg Gynecol Obstet 104:607, 1957.
30. Compagno J, Hyams VJ, Safavian M: Does branchiogenic carcinoma really exist? Arch Pathol Lab Med 100:311, 1976.
31. Davis GL, Sessions DG, Silverman RS: Needle biopsy in the diagnosis of head and neck lesions. Laryngoscope 77:376, 1967.
32. France CJ, Lucas R: The management and prognosis of metastatic neoplasms of the neck with an unknown primary. Am J Surg 106:835, 1963.

33. Fried MP, Diehl WH Jr, Brownson RJ: Cervical metastasis from an unknown primary. Ann Otol Rhinol Laryngol 84:152, 1975.
34. Greenberg BE: Cervical lymph node metastases from unknown primary sites: An unresolved problem in management. Cancer 19:1091, 1966.
35. Hendrick JW: Occult cancer with cervical lymph node metastasis. In Conley J (ed): Cancer of the Head and Neck. Washington, DC, Butterworths, 1967, pp 41–55.
36. Jesse RH, Neff LE: Metastatic carcinoma in cervical nodes with an unknown primary lesion. Am J Surg 112:547, 1966.
37. Jesse RH, Perez CA, Fletcher GH: Cervical lymph node metastasis: Unknown primary cancer. Cancer 31:854, 1973.
38. Marchetta FC, Murphy WT, Kovaric JJ: Carcinoma of the neck. Am J Surg 106:974, 1963.
39. Martin H, Morfit HM: Cervical lymph node metastasis as the first symptom of cancer. Surg Gynecol Obstet 78:133, 1944.
40. Martin H, Morfit HM, Ehrlich H: The case for branchiogenic cancer (malignant branchioma). Ann Surg 132:867, 1950.
41. McGuirt WF, McCabe BF: Significance of node biopsy before definitive treatment of cervical metastatic carcinoma. Laryngoscope 88:594, 1978.
42. Nordstrom DG, Tewfik HH, Latourette HB: Cervical lymph node metastases from an unknown primary. Int J Radiat Oncol Biol Phys 5:73, 1979.
43. Pico J, Frias Z, Bosch A: Cervical lymph node metastases from carcinoma of undetermined origin. Am J Roentgenol 111:94, 1971.
44. Razack MS, Sako K, Marchetta FC: Influence of initial neck node biopsy on the incidence of recurrence in the neck and survival in patients who subsequently undergo curative resectional surgery. J Surg Oncol 9:347, 1977.
45. Richard JM, Micheau C: Malignant cervical adenopathies from carcinomas of unknown origin. Tumori 63:249, 1977.
46. Silverman RS, Marks JE, Lee F, Ogura JH: Treatment of epidermoid and undifferentiated carcinoma from occult primary presenting with cervical lymph nodes. Laryngoscope 93:645, 1982.
47. Willis RA: The Spread of Tumours in the Human Body. London, J & A Churchill, 1934.
48. Wolff M, Rankow RM, Fleigel J: Branchiogenic carcinoma: Fact or fallacy? J Maxillofac Surg 7:41, 1979.

BENIGN TUMORS

Steven M. Sobol, M.D.

Although not well documented, it is often said that approximately 20 per cent of all masses occurring in the neck are benign. Indeed, the incidence is considerably different if one considers children and adults separately. The differential diagnosis may be arranged categorically into *congenital, inflammatory,* and *neoplastic* lesions. A selective and careful history and physical examination, which define the characteristics and location of the mass, often helps to narrow the long list of possible causes and at times will pinpoint the diagnosis. Selective use of noninvasive and invasive diagnostic studies also helps to establish the diagnosis and the extent of disease. Surgery plays a vital role in the diagnosis and management of virtually all congenital and neoplastic masses in the neck. Surgical treatment of many of these requires an understanding of embryologic concepts. The purpose of this section is to define and classify congenital cysts and benign tumors presenting in the neck, and to discuss the surgical management of each with attention to indications, techniques, alternatives, complications, and prognoses.

CYSTIC HYGROMA

Embryogenesis and History

First described by Redenbacher[7] in 1828, Wernher[11] is credited for giving this tumor its name—cystic hygroma. Borst[2] first suggested that these lesions arose from sequestered embryonal tissue. McClure and Sylvester[4] suggested that hygromas were derived from sequestration of lymphatic tissue of the developing jugular lymphatic sac. Ribbert[8] further postulated that lymphan-

giomas arose from developing lymphatic capillary buds derived from pinched-off cells of the developing venous system. These buds subsequently canalize, but their failure to reunite with the venous system sets the stage for cyst formation and the ultimate growth of a hygroma.

Histopathologically, a cystic hygroma is one of three types of lymphangioma[1]: lymphangioma simplex, cavernous lymphangioma, and cystic hygroma. These differ with respect to the size of the vascular spaces and thickness of the adventitia. The schema is somewhat artificial and indistinct, however, because aspects of each may be found in one tumor. Histologic variation seems to correlate best with tissue location; that is, noncystic varieties tend to arise most often in lips, cheeks, and tongue, whereas cystic forms arise predominantly in regions containing loose, nonrestrictive areolar tissue and fascial planes (for example, the neck). Eighty-five per cent of lymphangiomas arise in the neck, the bulk of which are more common in the posterior triangle. The extent is quite variable, but larger masses extend beyond the sternocleidomastoid (SCM) into the anterior compartment and often cross the midline. Posterior neck masses may reach up into the cheek or down into the mediastinum or axilla. There is no sex predominance and an even distribution as to the side of involvement.

Clinical Presentation

A review of several series indicates that about half are present at birth and 75 to 90 per cent are present by 3 years of age. In general, symptoms relate to pressure of a painless enlarging mass. Cystic hygromas or cervical

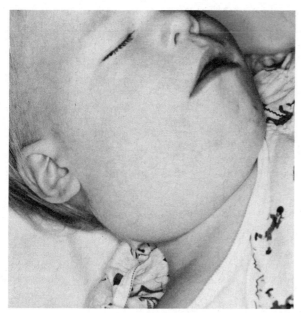

Figure 55–39. Cystic hygroma producing asymmetry of neck.

lymphangiomas may grow progressively at variable rates, remain static, or occasionally regress and even spontaneously disappear. Occasionally local trauma will precipitate an inflammatory reaction. Symptoms of neural encroachment, such as facial paresis, vocal cord paralysis, or shoulder weakness, are uncommon. Their size may vary considerably—at times being massive. Neck asymmetry is cosmetically disturbing (Fig. 55–39). Most lesions will be cystic or wormy to palpation. The overlying skin may be tense and at times discolored. Many tumors will transilluminate, except for those in which blood has filled the cystic spaces.

The differential diagnosis must include hemangioma, lipoma, branchial cleft cyst, and malignant diseases with cystic degeneration. Differentiating lymphangiomas from hemangiomas is not always possible on clinical grounds. Moreover, the histologic appearance of both may show a similar proliferation of endothelium-lined vascular spaces and fibrous stroma. Needle aspiration of the fluid may help in such cases but runs the risk of causing infection. With lipomas, their margins are often better defined than those of hygromas. Helpful ancillary diagnostic studies include sonography, soft-tissue xerography (looking for calcification), and computed tomographic (CT) scans. These studies must be used selectively.

Surgical Management: Indications and Considerations

The treatment of cystic hygromas and all lymphangiomas of the neck has varied from benign neglect to complete excision. Surgical advocates[1, 5, 10] claim that these tumors may grow relentlessly, producing unacceptable cosmetic distortion of the face and neck, and at times severe functional disability. Occasionally, they compromise vital structures, causing tracheal compression resulting in respiratory embarrassment, brachial plexus compression with pain, hypoesthesia, or altered motor function. Repeated trauma may predispose to infection. Therefore, procrastination in therapy only compromises one's ability to perform a complete resection.

Proponents of benign neglect submit that in many of these lesions, particularly the larger, more infiltrative ones, surgery poses the greatest risk. Recognizing the potential for incomplete excision in some, they cite the surgical sequelae of neural injury (to the eleventh cranial nerve, tenth cranial nerve, brachial plexus), persistent lymphedema, lymphocele, and persistent lymphorrhea as being worse than the presence of the tumor itself. With lymphangiomas of the tongue, for instance, radical excision would seem unwarranted in those patients whose tongue function is only minimally compromised. Because many of these will remain relatively static, observation (perhaps tempered with occasional conservative laser excision in those cases showing progressive signs of speech, deglutitory, or airway compromise) seems appropriate.

The surgical philosophy has perhaps been best summarized by Potts[6]:

> The objective in surgery of cystic hygroma is relief of obstruction upon vital structures and a good cosmetic result. Good judgement must control the extent of the operation. Inadequate operation is just as inexcusable as a daring operation, and nowhere does this maxim apply more forcefully than in the surgical treatment of large cystic hygromas of the neck.

The definite tendency of cavernous lymphangiomas to recur following local excision constitutes the most difficult problem in its management.[3] Complete excision should be successful in more than 80 per cent of cases. Partial excision results in high rates of recurrence. Relative recurrence rates, according to the number of surgical procedures necessary to complete the excision, varies with (1) *extent*—localized lesions, 1 to 1.5 procedures; extensive lesions, 3 to 4 procedures, and (2) *site*—neck, 1 to 1.5 procedures; cheek, 2 to 3 procedures; tongue, 3+ procedures. The optimal age for surgery has been said to be 18 months to 2 years; however, little objective data exists to support this concept. Watchful waiting until the child is older may be prudent in selected cases.

The adjunctive use of sclerosing agents may reduce or at least delay some recurrences, but this approach is fraught with the potential for sclerosing injury to adjacent neural structures. Injecting sclerosing agents alone has resulted in no cures.[10]

Aspiration of these masses except as a diagnostic tool is useful only to decompress those lesions compromising vital structures.

Lymphangiomas respond poorly to radiation therapy. Therefore, particularly because of the risk of delayed carcinogenesis, its use is condemned.

Surgical Approach

The surgical approach will depend, in large part, on the size and location of the lesion. For the majority located in the neck (not previously infected or operated), an incision in a natural horizontal or oblique skin crease overlying the mass is appropriate. Stepladder incisions may be necessary for larger lesions. Subplatysmal undermining of flaps should permit exposure of the region involved; sufficient exposure is necessary to allow complete mobilization of the tumor with identification and preservation of all adjacent neural and vascular structures. Hygromas may not always follow the natural planes of cleavage but may insinuate in and around adjacent vital structures. "Shelling out" these lesions is difficult and fraught with high rates of recurrence. If any point of dissection is obscure, the surgical plane is first developed beyond the hygroma in an uninvolved area. Nerves and vessels are then carefully identified before being traced through or around the lesion. A layer of "fascial" tissue (pseudocapsule) around the tumor should be preserved if possible while manipulating and dissecting the lesion. This will minimize the risk of incomplete excision. It is the author's preference not to grasp the lesion with clamps or forceps, but rather to manipulate it manually. On occasion, when the lesion infiltrates adjacent muscle, a cuff of muscular tissue must be excised to ensure complete excision.

Previous surgery or infection may hamper a clean anatomic dissection and may necessitate sacrifice of some overlying skin. Again, every attempt should be made to completely excise the lesion without compromising vital structures.

HEMANGIOMA

Classification

Hemangiomas of the face and neck are most often congenital "neoplasms." They have been classified according to the predominant vessel involved: capillary, cavernous, or mixed. In truth, this classification may be more myth because the majority have components of both. These lesions may occur intracutaneously, subcutaneously, or in both ways. In roughly three quarters of the patients, hemangiomas are present at birth, and in close to 90 per cent it has manifested itself by the first year of life. The biologic behavior of particular hemangiomas varies, making it appropriate to discuss the clinical characteristics of the lesions most often seen.[16, 19]

Cavernous hemangiomas may appear as globular, bright red or deep purple lesions that are compressible. They may temporarily increase in size when the patient strains or cries. More raised lesions may ulcerate and bleed; thus, it is advisable to cut a child's fingernails short during the period of observation. A visible lesion on the face or neck may signal the presence of another internal hemangioma. The cavernous hemangioma tends to predominantly involve deep and subcutaneous tissues but may occur with an overlying capillary lesion.

Capillary hemangiomas usually consist of bright red, or bluish red, slightly elevated plaque-like lesions that may also be compressible. Many capillary lesions also have cavernous components. Lesions tend to be more superficial than cavernous lesions, occurring predominantly at the dermal level; but many mixed lesions extend deeper.

Port-wine stain (nevus flammeus) is a flat predominantly capillary hemangioma that is present at birth. Most occur on the face and neck. Their color varies from pink to purple. Lesions are a diffuse plexus of arteries that ramify mostly in the dermis and less so in the subcutaneous and deeper tissues. As the patient becomes older, lesions grow only in relation to the growth of the affected area. They rarely regress spontaneously. Port-wine stains may be part of the Sturge-Weber syndrome and may be associated with glaucoma and encephalotrigeminal angiomatosis.

Strawberry marks are considered capillary hemangiomas by most, although they may have an associated cavernous component. They are seen at birth, often as fairly well circumscribed macules or nodules that may enlarge over the first several months of life. However, they usually undergo subsequent spontaneous involution.

Senile hemangiomas (cherry angiomas, ruby spots) are acquired capillary lesions that appear during adult life as elevated, circular ruby-red papules occurring anywhere on the body. They are perhaps the most common angiomatous lesions seen. They rarely exceed 3 mm. Treatment is rarely necessary.

Spider telangiectasis (starburst angioma, nevus araneus) have the appearance of a red spider—with an ascending central artery and fine radiating vessels. Although common on the face and neck, they may be seen in several locations and may occur in association with pregnancy, vitamin B deficiency, and cirrhosis. Treatment is rarely indicated.

Cirsoid aneurysms (angioma racemosum) are pulsatile, plexiform, cavernous hemangiomas that have multiple arteriovenous shunts. Although many locations are possible, many lesions appear on the skin near the carotid and may extend over the neck and scalp. They have a propensity to extend into deep tissues and muscle and may even penetrate the cranium. Their extent must be evaluated thoroughly prior to treatment.

Management

Treatment of hemangiomas of the face and neck requires a knowledge of their particular natural history. Much of the controversy concerning therapy stems in part from a failure to accurately classify the lesion—classification is often difficult because many hemangiomas are of a mixed variety.

The most significant advance in recent years has been the recognition that most hemangiomas disappear spontaneously through a process of gradual involution after the first year or two of life. During the first year of life they may undergo a period of growth. The trigger mechanism for involution remains unclear. However, it often occurs following superficial ulceration or inflammation of the lesions. Unfortunately, not all lesions will spontaneously involute—therefore, the difficulty lies in determining which will and which will not. It is often said that if by the age of 2 years there has been no sign of spontaneous regression or continued growth, surgical treatment may be indicated.[19]

Some feel that it is unwise to rely on the tendency toward spontaneous regression, because many lesions will grow, ulcerate, and distort features.[13] Clearly, although most hemangiomas are harmless vascular marks, proliferating lesions may destroy local tissue, compromise vital structures, or cause hemodynamic and coagulation disorders. Before their tendency toward spontaneous regression was appreciated, hemangiomas not easily camouflaged were assailed with silver nitrate, liquid nitrogen, carbon dioxide snow, electrodesiccation, sclerosing solutions, radon seeds, external irradiation, steroids, surgical excision, and tattooing.[19, 21]

Concerning *surgery*, excision of relatively small hemangiomas in conspicuous locations is justifiable, without waiting for involution, when immediate repair of the defect produces acceptable cosmetic results. The type of surgery required for extensive, invasive lesions depends on their size and location. Arteriography determines the nature of the feeding blood supply. Occasionally, ligation of an accessible dominant vessel(s) is helpful prior to *complete excision* of selected lesions. Arteriographic embolization with muscle, Gelfoam, or polymerizing substances has played an increasingly important role in the immediate preoperative treatment of large hemangiomas and arteriovenous (AV) malformations by substantially reducing the amount of blood loss at surgery.[20] However, occlusion of a predominant vascular supply followed by an *incomplete excision* may create disastrous results. It is well known that partial occlusion enhances collateralization and, at times, proliferation.

En bloc resection of aggressive hemangiomatous lesions of the head and neck has been the mainstay of therapy with or without the adjunctive use of preoperative embolization.[13, 19] Following excision, adjacent or regional skin flaps may be transposed for substantial defects, and full-thickness skin grafts may be used to resurface more superficial ones.

More recently, the argon laser has played an increasingly important role in the management of congenital and acquired hemangiomatous lesions of the head and neck.[12, 14-18] Reports from the past 10 years in the dermatologic,[12, 16] plastic surgical,[15, 17] and otolaryngologic[14] literature have documented the favorable response of vascular lesions to argon laser radiation (Figs. 55–40 and 55–41). Because the argon laser radiation is selectively absorbed by red tissues, such as vascular tissues and hemoglobin, the laser is capable of penetrating the

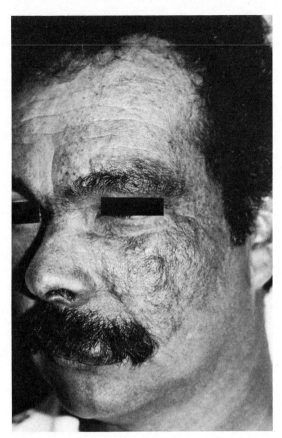

Figure 55–41. Patient in Figure 55–40 after treatment with the argon laser. (Courtesy of Dr. Joseph DiBartolomeo.)

keratin layer of skin, leaving it relatively unscathed, until it reaches underlying vascular tissue where most of its energy is absorbed. Optical energy is converted into thermal energy, and photocoagulation occurs instantly. Not all hemangiomas of the face and neck are amenable. Hemangioma depth and channel variegation are important relative to the laser's therapeutic value. It is most effective in ablating superficial channels. Noe and associates[18] and DiBartolomeo[14] have shown that the superficial ectatic vessels in port-wine stains are particularly suited to this form of therapy. Indeed, the argon laser is perhaps the best available treatment of the cosmetically deforming lesions. Unfortunately, many hemangiomas proliferate at a subcutaneous level beyond the effectiveness of the currently available argon laser beam.

After laser therapy, the skin is swollen for several months and by 1 year the epidermis becomes thin and atrophic and the dermis tight. The eventual skin color and texture is never as good as is the case after spontaneous involution. Cooling the skin during treatment may minimize thermal damage to the overlying epidermis and papillary dermis.[15] Overall, argon laser radiation appears to be a safe and relatively effective treatment for selective vascular lesions of the head and neck.

BRANCHIAL CLEFT REMNANTS

Branchial apparatus anomalies are lateral cervical lesions that result from congenital developmental defects

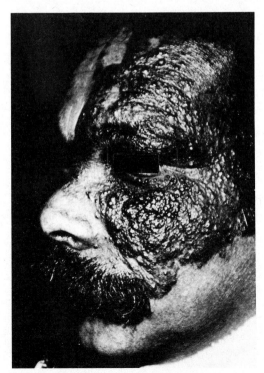

Figure 55–40. Facial hemangioma.

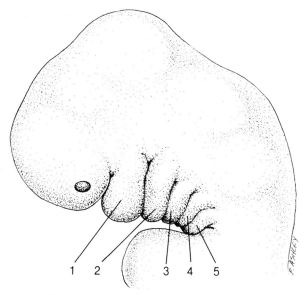

Figure 55–42. External configuration and location of branchial arches in a 4- to 5-week embryo. (Redrawn from Gage JF, Lipman SP, Meyers EN: Diagnosis and Management of Congenital Masses in the Neck: A Self-Instructional Package. Committee on Continuing Medical Education, American Academy of Otology, 1976.)

arising from the primitive branchial arches, clefts, and pouches.

Embryogenesis

The branchial apparatus develops during the third and fourth embryonic weeks and persists until the end of the sixth week. The branchial arches consist of five parallel bars of mesoderm, each with its own nerve supply and blood vessel. The external configuration and location of the branchial arches in the embryo after 4 to 5 weeks are seen schematically in Figure 55–42.

These unique structures account for the formation of the pharynx, neck, jaws, and middle and external ear. The branchial apparatus is marked *externally* by four ectodermal branchial *clefts* on each side of the embryo in the region of the pharynx. *Internally*, the embryonic pharynx, which begins at the stomadeal plate, is invaginated into five lateral pharyngeal *pouches*, of which the first four correspond to the external branchial clefts. Between each "cleft-pouch set" is a mesodermal branchial *plate*. Each branchial arch is anterior to its corresponding cleft and pouch. This relationship is retained throughout development. Within the mesoderm of the arch are a cartilaginous bar, a primitive arterial arch, and a nerve (Fig. 55–43). Of the four branchial clefts visible in the fifth week, only the most dorsal portion of the first cleft persists in adult life as the external auditory canal. The corresponding portion of the first pharyngeal pouch becomes the eustachian tube and middle ear space, and the corresponding branchial plate between the two is represented by the tympanic membrane.

The concept of the formation of the cervical sinus of His in which the second arch fuses with the fifth, closing both the third and fourth arches, remains controversial

with respect to humans. In humans it is likely that the cervical sinus consists of only the junction of the third and fourth clefts at the surface and has only a transitory existence. Isolated remnants of the fourth pouch persist only up to the eighth week. According to Frazer,[24] areas of the deep dorsal portions of the third and fourth clefts separate from the cervical sinus and obliterate separately. These constitute the epibranchial placodes and are said to contribute sensory nerve elements to the adjacent ganglia of the glossopharyngeal and vagus nerves.

A number of theories exist to explain the genesis of branchial cleft anomalies.[23, 25, 26] The most widely accepted theory is that the remnants result from incomplete obliteration of the branchial clefts, arches and pouches. Lesions may take the form of cysts, sinuses (internal or external), or fistulas. Cystic lesions presumably develop as a result of buried epithelial cell rests. Sinus anomalies have, by definition, a communication, with either the external skin surface or pharyngeal mucosa, and end as a blind tubular or saccular anomaly within mesenchymal tissue; they likely arise from incomplete obliteration of part of a branchial groove. Fistulas suggest complete communication from the ectodermal surface to the endodermal surface and presumably relate to incomplete formation of the closing branchial plate or rupture of the same (Fig. 55–44).

Despite this seemingly simple, cogent concept concerning embryogenesis, a wholly acceptable hypothesis

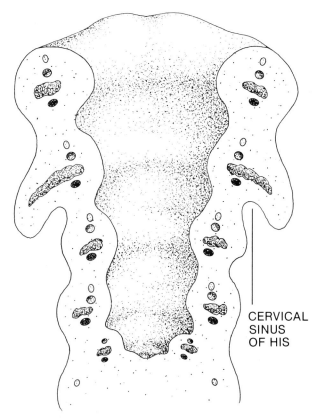

CERVICAL
SINUS
OF HIS

Figure 55–43. Schematic of developing branchial system denoting relationships of branchial pouches and clefts to mesodermal arches and plates (see text). (Courtesy of H. M. Tucker, M.D.)

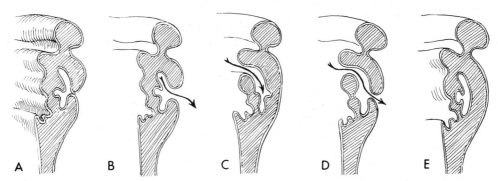

Figure 55–44. Series of diagrams to show how several kinds of tracts and cysts may arise through faulty development of the pharynx. (*A*) Normal pharynx showing closure of the cervical sinus. (*B*) Incomplete closure of the cervical sinus forming the basis for a tract opening externally upon the surface of the neck. (*C*) Rupture of the closing membrane leaving a permanent opening into the position of the second pouch. (*D*) Branchial fistula resulting from a combination of the conditions in *B* and *C*. (*E*) Cystic remnant of the cervical sinus. (From Brauer RO: Congenital cysts and tumors of the neck. *In* Converse JM (ed): Reconstructive Plastic Surgery, 2nd ed., vol. 5. Philadelphia, W. B. Saunders Co., 1977, p. 2910. Adapted with permission from Ward GE, Hendrick JW: Diagnosis and Treatment of Tumors of the Head and Neck. Copyright 1950, The Williams & Wilkins Company, Baltimore.)

of the origin of branchial anomalies has not been agreed upon. This stems from the lack of hard data and the conjectural explanations offered through the years.

Although Rathke (1828) may have provided the first description of branchial clefts, Lahey and Nelson[27] credited Hunczowski with the first description of a cervico-aural fistula in 1789. Von Asherson (1832) related fistulous tract anomalies in the cervico-aural region to the branchial apparatus. Bland-Sutton (1887) suggested that failure of obliteration of branchial clefts in animals resulted in persistent fistulas. Rabl (1907) first presented the notion that migration and invagination of the branchial arch system explained the formation and location of branchial anomalies that were being clinically observed. Fundamentally, his concept supported the theory of "failure of obliteration" and "trapped epithelial remnants" to explain the observed anomalies.

Wenglowski[33] put forth an entirely different hypothesis based on embryo and cadaver studies. He suggested that branchial anomalies arose from retained elements of the "thymopharyngeal duct"; this structure connects the pharynx with the third branchial entodermal evagination, which forms the thymus. Wenglowski contended that incomplete obliteration of the duct explained the persistence of epithelium-lined tracts associated with lymphoid tissue. A major problem with the theory is that more anomalies should be found at the lower end of the embryonic thymopharyngeal duct, that is, at the lower end of the neck and mediastinum, rather than cephalad near the hyoid bone.

Yet another even less tenable explanation was put forth by Bhaskar and Bernier,[23] who suggested that anomalies occurring above the hyoid bone were secondary to sequestered buds of parotid gland epithelium.

Regardless of the mechanism, the obliteration of all the branchial clefts to the exclusion of the first takes place during the sixth and seventh weeks. Because the changes in the neck region are so extensive, it is not easy to determine the location of the obliterated embryonic clefts and arches in the adult.

Specific adult structures are derived from each branchial arch and its related cleft and pouch. These are summarized for simplicity in the schematic shown in Figure 55–45.

Clinical Presentation

Branchial cysts, fistulas, and sinuses occur with equal frequency in males and females. They may be bilateral, and familial tendencies have been noted. Cysts are rarely diagnosed at birth but become apparent in late childhood or adulthood when they enlarge because of infection or for unknown reasons (Figs. 55–46 and 55–47). They may fluctuate in size without warning. Infected cysts may develop into abscesses, which may spontaneously rupture, forming a draining sinus. In many, there is a history of previous incision and drainage (Fig. 55–48), with extensive induration and scarring (Fig. 55–49).

Fistulas and sinuses usually present as a small opening along the anterior border of the sternocleidomastoid (Figs. 55–50 and 55–51). The pinhole orifice may discharge material, which may be milky, serous, mucoid, or purulent (Fig. 55–52). Cysts occur more often than sinuses, which occur more often than fistulas. The sinus or fistulous tract may occasionally be palpated as a fibrous cord. The precise location and course of these anomalies depends on the particular branchial pouch or cleft from which they are derived.

First Branchial Cleft Remnants. Belanky and Medina (1980) reviewed the history of first branchial cleft remnants in the literature. Virchow (1865) described a child with a fistula extending below and behind a microtic auricle communicating with the nasopharynx. Konig (1895) described an anomaly presenting with a fistulous tract opening in the upper neck anterior to the sternocleidomastoid and terminating in the external ear canal after passing through the parotid gland. Sulton (1898) described the first branchial cleft cyst. In 1929, Hyndman and Light reviewed 108 cases, of which they believed only one was derived from the first branchial apparatus.

Arnot[22] proposed the first classification for anomalies of the first branchial cleft. He designated *type I* as any cyst or sinus in the parotid presenting in early or midadult life and *type II* as a sinus or cyst developing during childhood presenting in the anterior triangle of the neck with a communication to the external auditory canal. He believed that type I anomalies were secondary

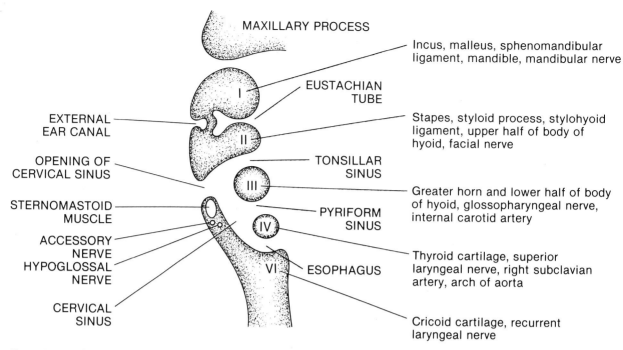

MAXILLARY PROCESS

Incus, malleus, sphenomandibular ligament, mandible, mandibular nerve

EUSTACHIAN TUBE

EXTERNAL EAR CANAL

Stapes, styloid process, stylohyoid ligament, upper half of body of hyoid, facial nerve

OPENING OF CERVICAL SINUS

TONSILLAR SINUS

Greater horn and lower half of body of hyoid, glossopharyngeal nerve, internal carotid artery

STERNOMASTOID MUSCLE

PYRIFORM SINUS

ACCESSORY NERVE

HYPOGLOSSAL NERVE

ESOPHAGUS

Thyroid cartilage, superior laryngeal nerve, right subclavian artery, arch of aorta

CERVICAL SINUS

Cricoid cartilage, recurrent laryngeal nerve

Figure 55–45. Summary of adult structures derived from each branchial arch and its related cleft and pouch. (With permission from Liston SL, Siegel LG: Branchial Cysts, Sinuses and Fistulas. ENT J *58*:9–17, 1979.[28])

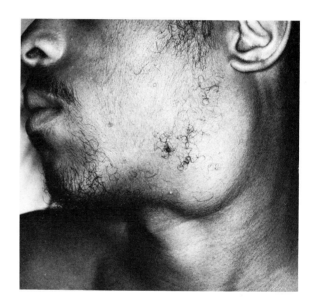

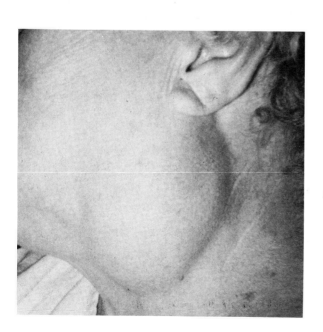

Figure 55–46. Branchial cleft cyst initially mistaken for a tail of parotid neoplasm.

Figure 55–47. Branchial cleft cyst present for 17 years.

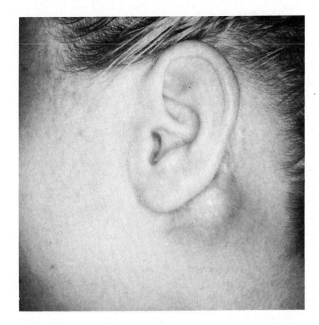

Figure 55–48. Fluctuant first branchial cleft cyst just prior to rupture.

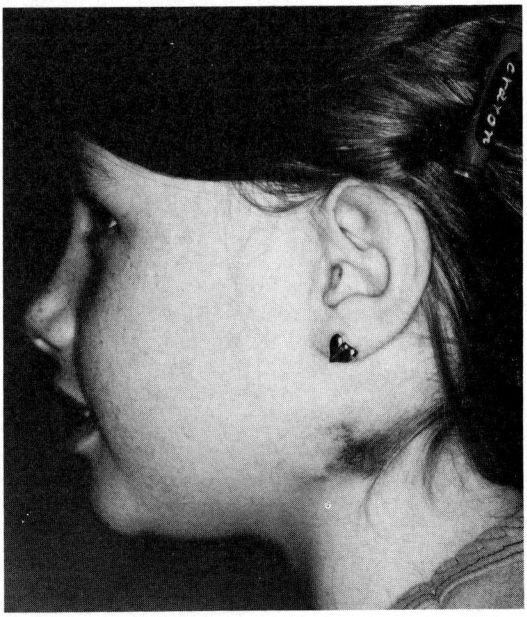

Figure 55–49. First branchial cleft cyst with postauricular scarring from multiple incision and drainage procedures.

Figure 55–50. Second branchial cleft remnant with pinhole opening along anterior border of sternocleidomastoid muscle.

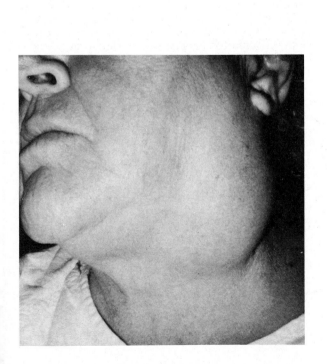

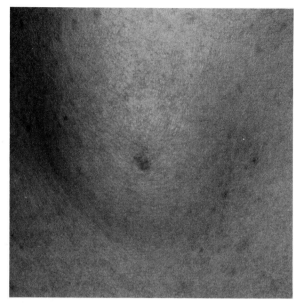

Figure 55–51. Close-up view of external orifice of branchial cleft remnant sinus tract.

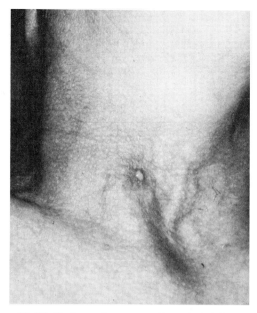

Figure 55–52. Discharge from second branchial cleft tract along anterior border of sternocleidomastoid muscle.

to epithelial rests and that type II were due to incomplete closure of the branchial apparatus.

Work[34] restructured this classification schema. Type I anomalies were considered duplications of the membranous external auditory canal ending in a cul-de-sac at the bony plate at the level of the mesotympanum; type II anomalies extended from near the angle of the mandible through the parotid substance (intimately related to the facial nerve) to the vicinity of the membranous external canal (Figs. 55–53 and 55–54).

Perhaps the most comprehensive review of these anomalies was published by Olson and associates[30]; they reviewed 460 branchial cleft anomalies at the Mayo Clinic; 38 (8 per cent) were of first branchial cleft origin. Two thirds of these were cysts without tracts. They postulated that these arose from buried cell rests. Sinus tracts with cysts occurred in a fifth of these cases. Most communicated with the external canal. Complete fistulas accounted for the remainder. Communications may exist between the postauricular region, lobule, angle of jaw, external auditory canal, and middle ear space.[32]

Second Branchial Cleft Remnants. These are by far the most common anomalies, accounting for up to 90 per cent in some series. The external opening, when present, is usually located along the anterior border of the sternocleidomastoid at the junction of its middle and lower thirds. The tract, if there is one, follows the carotid sheath crossing over the hypoglossal nerve and coursing between the internal and external carotid arteries, ending at the tonsillar fossa (Fig. 55–55). Cystic dilatation may occur anywhere along the course of the tract. The sinus or fistulous tract ascends through the subcutaneous tissue and platysmal muscle and the superficial investing fascia to reach the carotid sheath. Openings in the pharynx, although rare, usually occur in the region of the posterior pillar. Many external sinuses are not congenital but result from previous incision and drainage of an infected cyst.

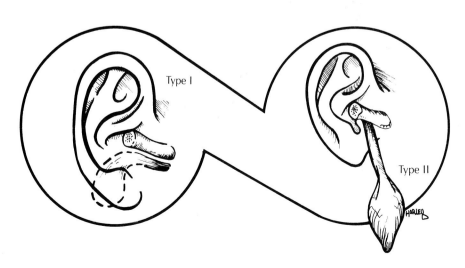

Figure 55–53. Classification of first branchial cleft remnants according to Work. (Redrawn from Gage JF, Lipman SP, Meyers EN: Diagnosis and Management of Congenital Masses in the Neck: A Self-Instructional Package. Committee on Continuing Medical Education, American Academy of Otology, 1976.)

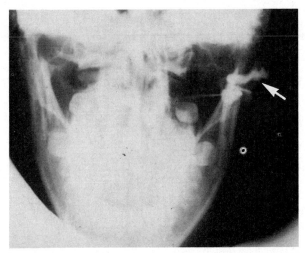

Figure 55–54. Opaque dye filling first branchial cleft tract parallel to external auditory canal and projecting medially (see arrow).

Proctor[31] classified second branchial cleft cysts into the following: type I—superficial cysts lying anterior to the sternocleidomastoid and adjacent to it; type II—cysts lying on the jugular vein and attached to the muscle; type III—those extending between the internal and external carotid arteries; and type IV—those lying near the pharyngeal wall (Fig. 55–56).

Third Branchial Cleft Anomalies. These anomalies are relatively rare. The external ostium of such lesions may be located in the same place as those of second branchial cleft anomalies. The tract and associated cyst extend along the carotid sheath behind the internal carotid artery (a third branchial arch derivative) over the hypoglossal nerve and follow the superior laryngeal

nerve to the region of the pyriform sinus (Fig. 55–55). Internal sinus tracts from the third branchial apparatus have been reported by Raven (1933). Fowler in 1962 reported what he thought was the eleventh case in the English literature. Cysts lying deep to the internal carotid and intimately associated with the vagus are probably remnants of the third cleft or pouch.

Fourth Branchial Cleft Anomalies. These anomalies remain more of a theoretical possibility than a reality, although one or two cases have been reported. Anomalies would have to have external openings along the anterior border of the sternocleidomastoid in the lower neck, and the tracts would have to descend along the carotid sheath into the chest, passing under either the arch of the aorta on the left or the subclavian on the right (both derived from the fourth branchial arch). They should then ascend in the neck, having their internal openings in the esophagus, a fourth branchial pouch derivative (Fig. 55–55).

Management Principles

Complete surgical excision is the only satisfactory method of treatment of these lesions, which are prone to recurrent infection and scarring, rendering dissection tedious and difficult. Any infection should be treated with antibiotics and drainage before surgical excision is attempted. Aspiration of an uninfected cyst is not indicated because this may predispose to infection and make dissection more hazardous. The wall of the cyst and tract may be extremely adherent to adjacent nerves and vessels.

The surgical principles are similar regardless of whether one is dealing with a first, second, or third cleft remnant, although the approach is different. When no sinus opening is present, a single transverse skin crease incision over the cyst is often adequate. The

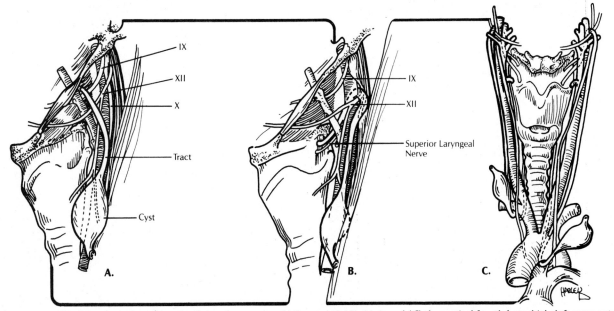

Figure 55–55. Schematic illustration depicting the course of (A) second, (B) third, and (C) theoretical fourth branchial cleft remnants and their relationship to neurovascular structures and the adult pharynx. (Redrawn from Gage JF, Lipman SP, Meyers EN: Diagnosis and Management of Congenital Masses in the Neck: A Self-Instructional Package. Committee on Continuing Medical Education, American Academy of Otology, 1976.)

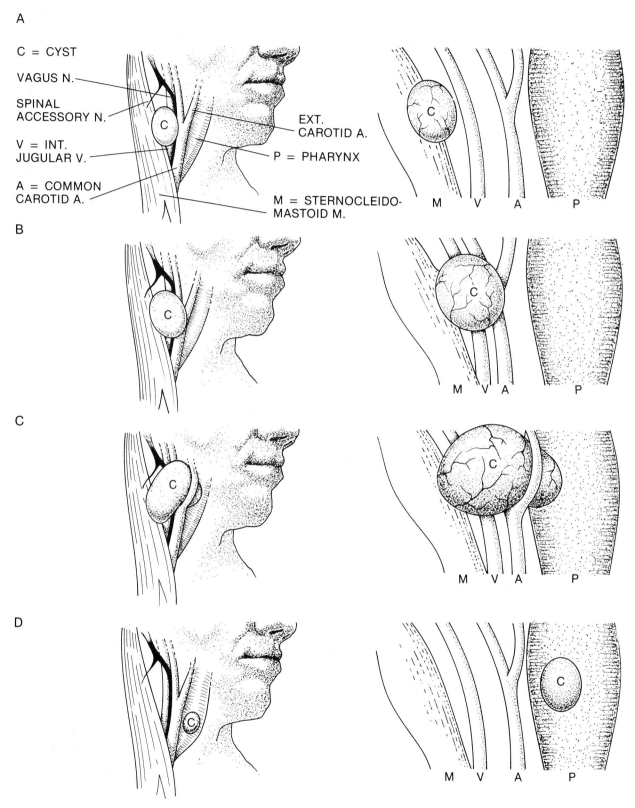

A

C = CYST

VAGUS N.

SPINAL
ACCESSORY N.

V = INT.
JUGULAR V.

A = COMMON
CAROTID A.

EXT.
CAROTID A.

P = PHARYNX

M = STERNOCLEIDO-
MASTOID M.

M   V   A   P

B

M   V   A   P

C

M   V   A   P

D

M   V   A   P

Figure 55–56. *See legend on opposite page.*

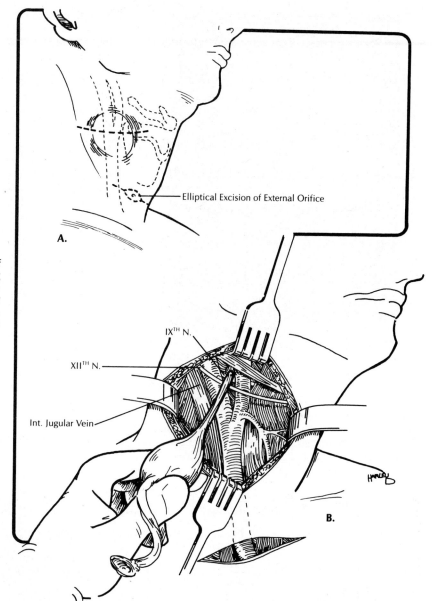

Figure 55–57. Technique for removal of second branchial cleft remnant utilizing step-ladder incision. (Redrawn with permission from Montgomery WW: Surgery of the Upper Respiratory System, Vol. II. Philadelphia, Lea & Febiger, 1973, pp 138–158.)

dissection is extended through the platysma, retracting the sternocleidomastoid laterally, exposing the region of the cyst. It is then sharply and delicately dissected away from vital structures. Despite absence of an external tract, an internal tract may be present and followed.

Second branchial anomalies, being most common, have their pinpoint or slit-like external orifice located below the hyoid, anterior to the sternocleidomastoid. An elliptic transverse incision is made about the orifice (Figs. 55–57 and 55–58), which is then grasped as the

Figure 55–56. Classification of second branchial cleft cysts. The branchial cleft is divided into four types based on their anatomic location.

(A) Type I is found superficially on the anterior border of the sternocleidomastoid muscle beneath the cervical fascia. It probably has its origin from a remnant of the external tract connecting the cervical sinus to the external surface.

(B) Type II, the most common type, lies deep to the investing fascia, is in contact with the great vessels, and may be adherent to the internal jugular vein. It probably originates from a persistent cervical sinus.

(C) Type III is similar to Type II except that it passes between the internal and external carotid arteries and extends to the pharyngeal wall. It probably originates from a dilated second external pharyngeal duct.

(D) Type IV is found adjacent to the pharyngeal wall medial to the great vessels. It probably has its origin from a remnant of the internal pharyngeal duct.

(With permission from Montgomery WW: Surgery of the Upper Respiratory System, Vol. II. Philadelphia, Lea & Febiger, 1973, pp 138–158.)

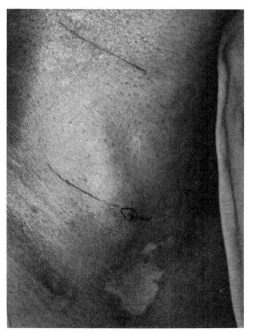

Figure 55–58. Step-ladder incisions designed for excision of second branchial cleft remnant with excision of external orifice in continuity.

tract is dissected sharply from adherent surrounding structures. This dissection is facilitated by injection of the tract gently with a solution of methylene blue. In its lower part the tract is usually superficial to the carotid sheath and omohyoid muscle. After the dissection is

extended cephalad, a stepladder incision is made (Figs. 55–58 and 55–59), and the tract is brought through this incision as the dissection continues. The tract and cyst are then traced along their course to complete excision (Figs. 55–60 and 55–61). Thorough knowledge of anatomy is essential. Identification of the internal and external carotid arteries and the vagus, hypoglossal, glossopharyngeal, and superior laryngeal nerves will avoid injury. Should the internal tract extend to the lateral pharynx, a small area is excised, and the rent is repaired primarily with absorbable suture.[28, 29]

First branchial remnants presenting at the angle of the jaw (Fig. 55–62) or in and around the parotid gland require a superficial parotid dissection with identification and preservation of the seventh cranial nerve (Fig. 55–63). The tract is traced through the gland, where it may lie medial, lateral, or between the branches of the facial nerve (Figs. 55–63 and 55–64). The tract should be traced to its junction with the external auditory canal. An elliptic incision of this orifice is made in continuity. A canal skin graft may be required to prevent subsequent canal stenosis.

THYROGLOSSAL DUCT CYSTS

Among the various developmental neck cysts, the thyroglossal duct cyst is most common, accounting for up to 70 per cent of such lesions.[48]

Embryogenesis

During the fourth week in utero, the thyroid anlage arises in an invagination of endodermal cells of the

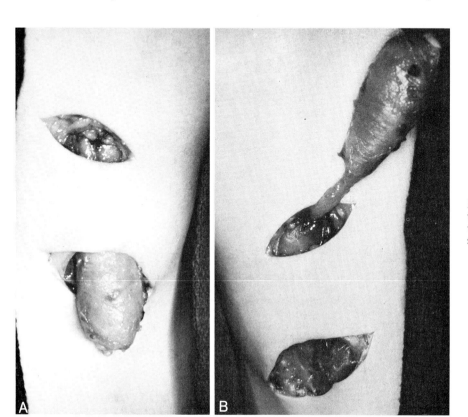

Figure 55–59. (A and B) Dissection of second branchial cleft cyst tract remnant through first incision into second incision.

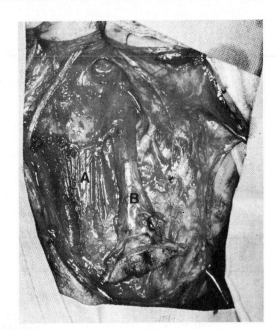

Figure 55–60. Second branchial cleft tract dissected in neck (A = sternocleidomastoid muscle; B = skin fistula of tract). (Note different approach in this case.)

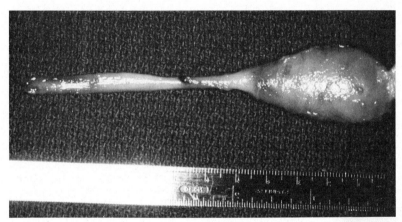

Figure 55–61. Completely excised second branchial cleft cyst tract remnant.

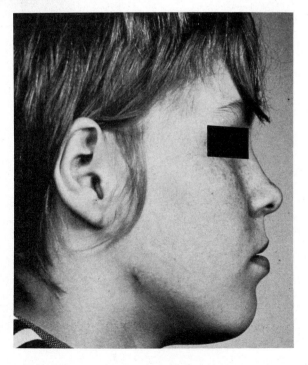

Figure 55–62. First branchial cleft remnant presenting at the angle of the jaw.

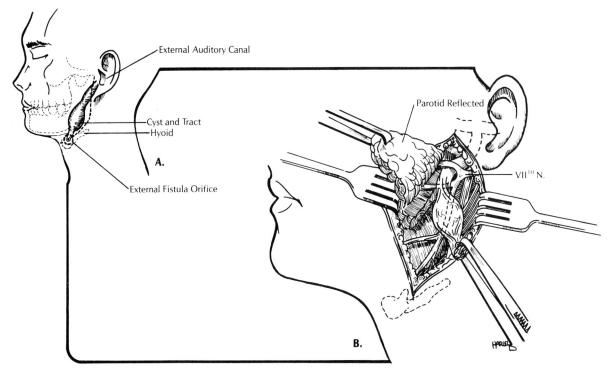

Figure 55–63. Schematic illustration depicting the recommended technique for excision of a first branchial cleft remnant. Note parotidectomy and dissection of tract through the branches of the seventh cranial nerve, as the remnant is traced to the external auditory canal. (From Montgomery WW: Surgery of the Upper Respiratory System, Vol. II. Philadelphia, Lea & Febiger, 1973, pp 138–158.)

ventral pharynx at the level of the tuberculum impar.[42] The tuberculum impar appears as a median eminence just behind the bilateral lingual swellings derived from the first branchial arch destined to become the anterior two thirds of the tongue. This outpouching enlarges

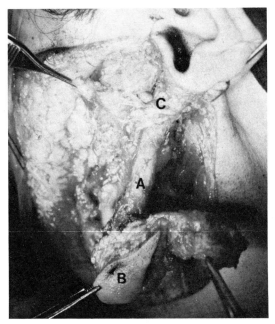

Figure 55–64. First branchial cleft remnant dissected beneath the branches of the seventh cranial nerve to the external auditory canal. (A) Tract. (B) External skin opening. (C) Facial nerve.

caudally as a bilobed diverticulum, staying ventral to all arch derivatives caudal to the first arch. This caudal migration leaves in its path a connecting tract between the thyroid gland (isthmus or pyramidal lobe) and the floor of the pharynx (foramen cecum, at the tongue base). This thyroglossal tract runs ventral to the developing hyoid bone, which rotates during maturation drawing the tract posteriorly and cranially at the inferior edge of the bone.[37] Because the hyoid anlagen join in the midline, the thyroglossal tract may become trapped, resulting in a tract lying within the substance or periosteum of the adult hyoid.[43] The thyroglossal tract usually atrophies and obliterates between the fifth and tenth weeks, with its caudal attachment often presenting as the pyramidal lobe. Persistence of the tract with an epithelial remnant results in formation of thyroglossal duct cysts (Figs. 55–65, 55–66, and 55–67). Controversy still exists whether the thyroglossal tract is a solid core of epithelial tissue, a hollow tube, or true duct that eventually becomes obliterated.[35] The stimulus responsible for triggering the epithelial rest or lining to encyst is not clear, but most likely it is either inflammation from adjacent reactive lymphoid tissue or perhaps secretion retention secondary to a blocked foramen cecum.[35]

Clinical Features

In a series of 1747 patients reviewed in the literature by Allard,[35] no sex predominance was noted. Allard noted that of 1316 analyzable cases, 31.5 per cent occurred in patients under the age of 10 years, 20.4 per cent occurred in the second decade, 13.5 per cent

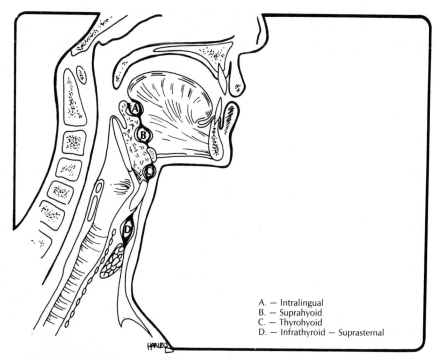

Figure 55–65. Potential sites for thyroglossal duct cysts to occur. (From Allard RHB: Head Neck Surg *1*:134, 1982.)

A. — Intralingual
B. — Suprahyoid
C. — Thyrohyoid
D. — Infrathyroid — Suprasternal

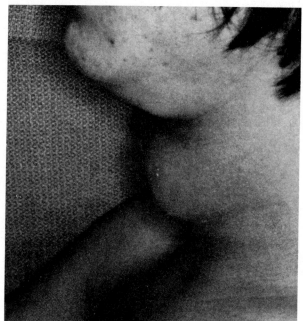

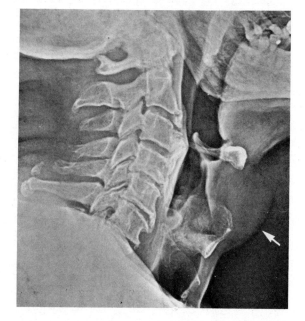

Figure 55–66. Infected thyroglossal duct cyst.

Figure 55–67. Xeroradiograph of thyroglossal duct cyst (see arrow).

TABLE 55–2. Distribution According to Age of Onset of Thyroglossal Duct Cysts

Age (years)	Incidence (%)
0–10	31.5
11–20	20.4
21–30	13.5
>30	34.6

Source: Based on 1316 cases reviewed by Allard RHB: Head Neck Surg 1:134, 1982.[35]

appeared in the third decade, and 34.6 per cent were found in patients older than 30 years (Table 55–2).

This analysis may not be completely reliable because some authors refer to age of onset as time of presentation, whereas others refer to the time of initial diagnosis.

Clinically, most cysts occur in the midline (90 per cent),[51] although some may occur paramedian, most often to the left.[47] The vertical location is such that approximately 60 per cent are over the thyrohyoid membrane, 24 per cent are suprahyoidal, 13 per cent occur between the thyrohyoid membrane and the suprasternal notch, and 2 per cent occur intralingually.[35] (Table 55–3 and Fig. 55–65).

Overall, 70 to 80 per cent occur below the hyoid bone. Cysts may fluctuate in size, but except for the presence of the mass, they are often asymptomatic unless they become infected[43, 46] (Fig. 55–66). When attached to the hyoid bone and tongue by a tract, they may retract on swallowing or tongue protrusion.[36, 39, 47] Intralingual cysts may cause choking spells, dysphagia, and cough.[35]

Fistulas may occur spontaneously or secondary to trauma, infection, drainage, or inadequate surgery. The incidence has been estimated from 15 to 34 per cent.[35, 49]

Thyroid scintiscans should probably be obtained on all patients undergoing surgical excision of thyroglossal duct cysts; despite the fact that a small amount of functioning thyroid tissue is found associated with the tract in 30 per cent of cases, it rarely, if ever, represents the only functioning thyroid tissue, as is often true with lingual thyroid cysts.[40]

Soft-tissue radiographs offer little diagnostic assistance, but ultrasound studies may assist in differentiating ill-defined or firm masses from true cysts (Fig. 55–67). Radiopaque substance injection is to be condemned because it may result in pain, rupture, delayed infection, and fistulas and offers little diagnostic assistance.

Surgical Management

The treatment of thyroglossal duct remnants—whether cyst, sinus, or fistula—is complete surgical

TABLE 55–3. Frequency of Location for Thyroglossal Duct Cysts

Location	Frequency (%)
Intralingual	2.1
Suprahyoidal	24.1
Thyrohyoidal	60.9
Suprasternal	12.9

Source: Allard RHB: Head Neck Surg 1:134, 1982.

excision. In 1920 Sistrunk[49] emphasized the importance of removing the central portion of the hyoid bone with the tract to prevent recurrence. This is because of the intimate relationship of the tract to the hyoid bone. In a large series of adult laryngeal sections, Ellis and Van Nostrand[41] found the thyroglossal tract constantly ventral to the hyoid bone (despite the serpentine course under and behind the body) and never found it coursing through the bone.

Surgery[35, 48, 49, 50] begins with the patient being positioned supine with the neck hyperextended (Fig. 55–68). Access to the mouth must be allowed for later palpation of the base of the tongue. A transverse skin crease incision is made over the cyst elliptically, excising a fistula if present (Fig. 55–69*A* to *C*). Subplatysmal flaps are created inferiorly and superiorly and are retracted. The investing facia is incised in the midline, the strap muscles are retracted laterally, and the cyst is exposed. Dissection of the mass and tract (which may be fragile and not easily recognized) is performed superiorly to the level of the hyoid, where the midportion of the hyoid bone is resected in continuity (Fig. 55–69*D*). Division of the midline aspects of the mylohyoid and geniohyoid muscles facilitates this process. With gentle traction on the cyst-tract-hyoid complex, dissection of a central core of genioglossus (presumably containing the delicate sinus tract) proceeds to the tongue base (Fig. 55–69*E*). With bimanual palpation, the tract is dissected to the foramen cecum where the tract is divided and ligated (Fig. 55–69*F*). The musculature of the tongue is repaired over this. The straps are reapproximated in the midline, as are the suprahyoid muscles, to eliminate dead space, and the incisions are closed in two layers after a small rubber drain is inserted (Fig. 55–69*G*). Although some discomfort in the neck and tongue on swallowing may occur at first, symptoms usually disappear within days.

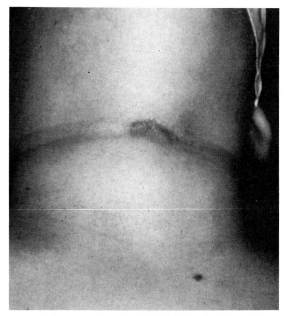

Figure 55–68. Thyroglossal duct fistula tract with neck hyperextended.

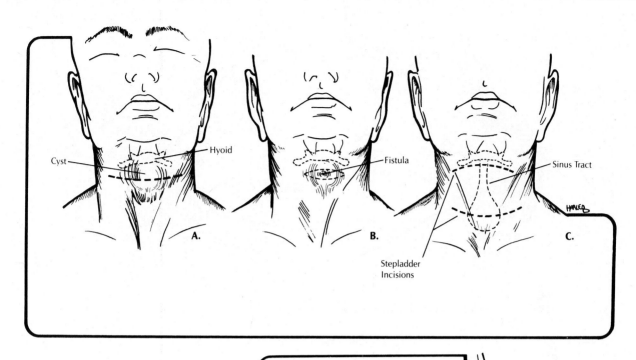

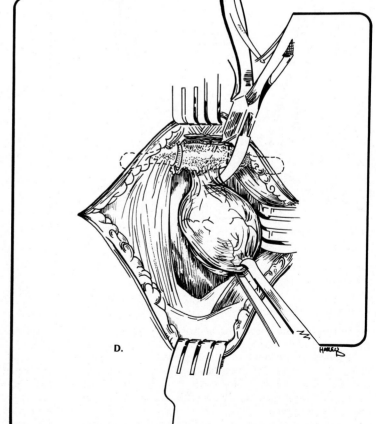

Figure 55–69. Surgical incisions for the simple thyroglossal duct cyst (A), including the external fistulous tract when present (B), and utilizing step-ladder incisions when necessary (C). Cyst dissected to body of hyoid, which is sectioned (D).
Illustration continued on following page

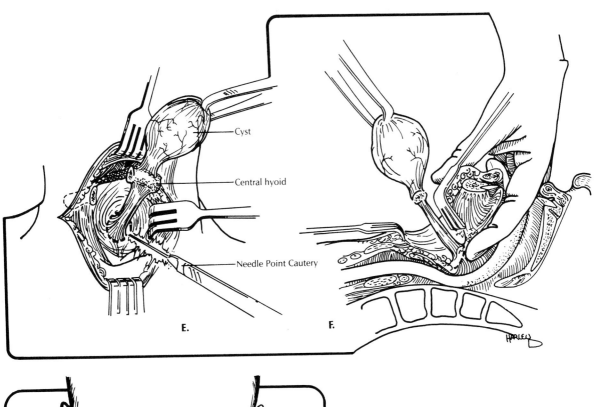

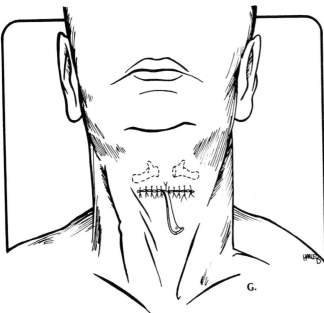

Figure 55–69 *Continued.* Bimanual palpation is used to remove the tract up to the foramen cecum (*E* and *F*). Closure of wound and drain inserted (*G*). (From Montgomery WW: Surgery of the Upper Respiratory System. Philadelphia, Lea & Febiger, 1973.)

Prior to routine use of the Sistrunk operation, recurrence rates were as high as 85 per cent,[50] whereas the recurrence rate is now less than 10 per cent and perhaps closer to 4 per cent.[45] Complications of the procedure are rare, although dissection off the midline may result in injury to the superior or internal laryngeal or even hypoglossal nerves.

Rare reports of malignancy in thyroglossal duct remnants are found in the literature. Most are papillary carcinomas, presumably arising in thyroid tissue in the remnant.[35] The incidence is less than 1 per cent,[38, 44] with a total of 91 cases reported.[35] Rarely is the diagnosis made or even entertained preoperatively. Because of the paucity of cases and the fact that the malignancy is not recognized until after complete pathologic examination of the remnant, it is difficult to delineate treatment and prognosis. Most agree, however, that (1) total thyroidectomy is not routinely indicated provided there are no palpable abnormalities in the gland or significant scintiscan findings, (2) thyroid hormone administration to suppress thyroid-stimulating hormone (TSH) secretion might be of value, and (3) the Sistrunk procedure probably offers a reasonable chance of cure.

DERMOIDS AND TERATOMAS

Arnold[52] described the most widely accepted terminology relating to teratoma-type lesions. Dermoids are composed of two germ layers, ectoderm and mesoderm, and are the most common teratoma-type lesion in the neck. Dermoid cysts are to be differentiated from simple epidermal inclusion cysts, in that with the former there is an epithelium-lined cyst with varying amounts of underlying skin appendages (hair follicles, sebaceous glands, connective tissue). Because many pathologists fail to study many of these benign lesions in detail, many are often simply labeled epidermal cysts when in reality the frequency of true dermoid cysts may be higher than appreciated.

True teratomas are composed of identifiable tissue from all three germ layers—ectoderm, mesoderm, and endoderm.[58] Varying degrees of differentiation and development may exist; for example, in epignathi the fetal limbs have already formed to a varying degree.

Embryopathogenesis

No all-encompassing totally adequate theory exists to explain all clinical presentations of dermoids and teratomas; however, three exist:[57]

1. *Acquired implantation* of epidermal and dermal elements, presumably following a traumatic cutaneous injury, would permit the subsequent development of an ectopic dermoid cyst.

2. *Totipotential rests* of cells derived from two or three germ layers may become anatomically isolated and ultimately grow in a disorganized fashion. This may occur from a pinching-off of a portion of the blastomere.

3. *Congenital inclusion* of germ layers into deeper tissues along lines of embryologic fusion may allow the subsequent growth of these sequestered cells, again in a somewhat disorganized fashion.

New and Erich[57] classified dermoids based on the preceding theories of embryopathogenesis. Congenital dermoids arising in and around the gonads most likely are secondary to the second theory noted, whereas those arising around the orbit, nose, and submandibular region presumably occur from inclusion (third theory). Classic periorbital dermoids may arise from inclusions occurring between the maxillary and mandibular processes in the naso-optic groove. Dermoids occurring around the nasal dorsum presumably arise from inclusion between the developing nasal bones, frontal bone, and dura. Teratomas and dermoids of the nasopharynx are well known and perhaps more common than other sites.[56]

Submental and submandibular dermoids (Fig. 55–70) may result from inclusion at the time of branchial arch fusion. In this region, they may occur above or below the mylohyoid, pushing the tongue upward or creating a double chin appearance.

Cervical dermoid cysts and teratomas have been associated with polyhydramnios.[54] Affected infants may

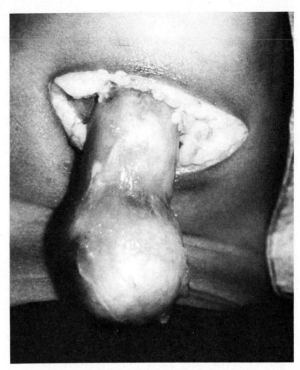

Figure 55–70. Large submental dermoid cyst.

be symptomatic at birth or may remain asymptomatic until later when these masses enlarge. Most true teratomas are present at birth, whereas dermoid cysts may present later in life. Most are semicystic, unattached to the overlying skin, and are mobile. Extremely large lesions may compress vital structures, causing dysphagia or airway compromise. Other compressive lesions must be differentiated, including cystic hygromas, branchial cleft cysts, and thyroglossal duct cysts. Katz[55] found that 25 per cent of midline lesions were dermoids.

True cervical teratomas may show evidence of calcification or the presence of teeth on soft-tissue radiography or even on prenatal pelvimetric radiographs. With midline lesions, thyroid scans rule out the presence of functioning tissue.

Surgical Management

Because this chapter deals solely with the neck, remarks concerning surgical treatment will be confined to lesions arising in the cervical region. A dermoid cyst in the neck, midline or lateral, may not always be diagnosed preoperatively. Complete surgical excision is therefore indicated both for diagnosis and to prevent subsequent recurrent infection, and on occasion to ameliorate a cosmetically deforming lesion.

With simple dermoid cysts, simple excision with attention to adjacent vital structures suffices. The incision is placed in an appropriately relaxed skin tension line. With previous infection or surgical drainage, overlying skin may require sacrifice. The surgeon must be prepared for the possibility of deeper attachments, particularly when the lesion is closely adherent to the mastoid or mandible. Erich has suggested that dermoid cysts are often densely adherent to surrounding structures, making their removal by blunt dissection difficult and the need for sharp dissection apparent.

With cervical teratomas, complete excision is recommended and should be performed as soon as is medically feasible in infants and neonates, because many of these lesions are quite large and may induce airway compromise. The main problem is failure to adequately secure the airway. Of 112 cervical teratomas reviewed by Hawkins and Park,[53] the surgical mortality rate was 9 per cent, although all those not treated died. Failure to perform a complete excision will result in recurrence.

MISCELLANEOUS BENIGN SOFT-TISSUE LESIONS IN THE NECK

Sebaceous Cysts

Sebaceous cysts may appear in any part of the neck but are commonly found in the infra-auricular region. They are often asymptomatic unless they become infected. Infected sebaceous cysts are treated with local heat, antibiotics, and if necessary, drainage. Definitive treatment requires simple elliptic excision, often including a small amount of the overlying skin. Rupture during dissection may give rise to local recurrence if all remnants of the cyst are not removed. This may be avoided by meticulous technique. If infection has occurred, the procedure should be delayed for a minimum of 6 weeks following the infectious process. All sebaceous cysts in the head and neck region probably should be excised because, given sufficient time, most will become infected. With the exception of attention to meticulous technique to avoid leaving a portion of the cyst behind, the only major surgical consideration relates to appropriate placement of the incision to produce minimal scarring. Properly placed linear incisions follow the relaxed skin tension lines.

Lipoma

Lipomas are benign tumors of fat and are found in any location where fat is normally present. They are soft and mobile and may occur superficially or deep to the platysma muscle. They may occur singly or in multiple masses linked together. Unless troublesome or cosmetically disturbing, they may be left untreated. They rarely enlarge rapidly, if at all, and do not appear related to liposarcomas. Infiltrating lipomas, although well recognized in other sites, are exceptionally rare in the neck, but have been reported.[64] Surgical excision, if performed, should adhere to proper cosmetic principles. Rather large lipomas can often be delivered through fairly small incisions.

Fibroma

It may be difficult to distinguish on clinical grounds or even histologically benign fibromas from nodular subcutaneous fibrosis, neurofibroma, sclerosing hemangioma, simple scars, and slow-growing well-differentiated fibrosarcomas. Many soft subcutaneous lesions are in fact fibrolipomas. Treatment of these benign soft tissue tumors is excision.

Nodular fasciitis falls into the category of fibrous lesions of the head and neck and represents more of a curious histopathologic entity than a clinical or therapeutic dilemma. It has been termed infiltrating fasciitis, aggressive fibromatosis, pseudosarcomatous fasciitis, and subcutaneous pseudosarcomatous fibromatosis. Although not common, roughly 15 per cent of these lesions present in the extramucosal soft tissues of the head and neck.[66, 67] An unusual intravascular variant that tends to involve small- to medium-sized vessels has a particular predilection for the head and neck. Clinically, nodular fasciitis presents with rapid onset (less than 3 months), a nodular growth pattern, a peak incidence in the third and fourth decades, and varying degrees of adherence and fixation to adjacent soft-tissue structures. Most lesions are 4 cm in diameter or less.[60] Complete surgical excision—for both diagnosis and definitive therapy—is indicated. Appropriate tissue for ultrastructural studies should be obtained in the event light microscopy proves unsatisfactory for distinguishing other histologically similar lesions, as well as malignancy, such as fibrous histiocytoma or fibrosarcoma.[59] Recurrence is rare with benign nodular fasciitis, but should it occur, the clinician and pathologist must be alerted to the likelihood that the original diagnosis was incorrect. Correct diagnosis is most often inflammatory fibrous histiocytoma or sarcoma.[60]

Neurogenic Tumors

Neurilemomas (schwannomas), derived from nerve sheath cells, and neurofibromas may arise from sensorimotor and sympathetic nerves in the neck. Neurofibromas are benign lesions occurring in the skin or soft tissue. When present as multiple nodules, associated with café-au-lait spots, it is called von Recklinghausen's disease (neurofibromatosis) (Fig. 55–71). Superficial benign neurofibromas do not become malignant. However, neurofibromas occurring deeper in the soft tissues are nonencapsulated, may become quite large and plex-

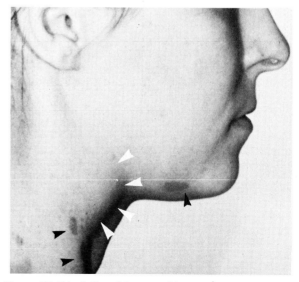

Figure 55–71. Café-au-lait spots (black arrows). Notice neck mass representing neurofibroma (white arrows).

iform, and occasionally undergo malignant degeneration. Conversely, neurilemomas are slow-growing, well-encapsulated lesions that are always attached to a defined nerve and never become malignant. Solitary lesions of either type presenting deep in the neck are difficult to differentiate from other solid neoplasms on clinical grounds alone and thus warrant proper evaluation prior to definitive excision (Fig. 55–72).

Treatment of superficial neurofibromas is surgical excision as required for cosmesis. Excision of deeper masses proceeds in a similar fashion as that for dermoid and branchial cleft cysts, with attention to adjacent vascular and neural structures. Neurilemomas often shell out easily by sharp dissection around the capsule, and the nerve of origin may be preserved in many cases—though not in all cases. Deep neurofibromas offer a more formidable surgical challenge, with dissection being more complex and tedious. Neurogenic tumors in the parapharyngeal space need special attention and are covered in that section.

Laryngocele

Laryngoceles are discussed in this section as they may present in a similar fashion to other benign neck tumors.

Laryngoceles were first described by Virchow[69] in 1863 as a tumor-like lesion consisting of an anomalous air sac communicating with the laryngeal ventricle. He used the term laryngocele ventricularis to describe the entity. Laryngoceles are intimately associated with the laryngeal saccule. This is an appendix of the laryngeal ventricle and consists of a membranous sac located between the false cord and the inner surface of the thyroid cartilage. Laryngoceles presumably result from an abnormally large saccule that extends up above the thyroid cartilage. These anomalies communicate freely with the laryngeal lumen and, as such, are filled with air. They may be congenital or acquired.

The saccule develops as an outpouching of the laryngeal cavity at the end of the second month of development. Although relatively large at birth, it regresses with time. Numerous mucus glands are located in the submucosal areolar tissue. It is lined by pseudostratified ciliated columnar respiratory epithelium.

Laryngoceles are to be differentiated from saccular cysts—the latter being filled with mucus and not communicating with the laryngeal lumen.[61] Saccular cysts are more common in infants, whereas laryngoceles tend to occur later in life.

Classification

Three types of laryngoceles have been described:
1. Internal laryngocele is confined to the interior of the larynx, extending into the paraglottic region of the false vocal cord and aryepiglottic fold (Fig. 55–73).
2. External laryngocele extends and dissects superiorly through the thyrohyoid membrane, intimately associated with the superior laryngeal nerve. It is labeled external as it frequently presents as a mass lateral to the thyrohyoid membrane (Fig. 55–74A).
3. A combined internal-external laryngocele has both internal and external components existing simultaneously (Fig. 55–74B).

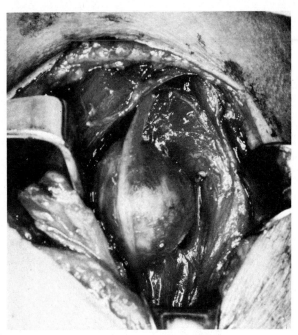

Figure 55–72. Neurofibroma in cervical area, note associated nerve.

Should the communication between a laryngocele and the laryngeal lumen become obstructed, fluid may accumulate within the sac. If mucus is found, a more appropriate term for the anomaly is a laryngomucocele, and if pus is found, it is called a laryngopyocele.[68] Should a laryngocele become completely filled with fluid, it is difficult to distinguish from a saccular cyst.

Pathophysiology

Factors that increase intralaryngeal pressure such as coughing, straining or blowing wind instruments are said to foster the development of laryngoceles. Presumably, the gradual weakening of the laryngeal tissues during aging is contributory. Laryngoceles are occupational hazards of professional glass blowers. Whether or not the neck of the saccule acts as a one-way valve, allowing the entrance of air but preventing its egress, is controversial. Clearly, such a mechanism might be operative when laryngoceles are associated with neoplastic or inflammatory processes, partially obstructing the ventricular opening.

Clinical Manifestations

Many laryngoceles are discovered incidentally when radiographs of the neck or endolaryngeal examinations are performed for related symptoms. When symptoms are present, they include hoarseness, cough, and the sensation of a foreign body in the throat. External or combined laryngoceles may present with a cervical mass adjacent to the thyrohyoid membrane (Fig. 55–75). If large enough, internal or combined laryngoceles may cause airway distress.

Diagnosis is most easily established by laryngoscopy

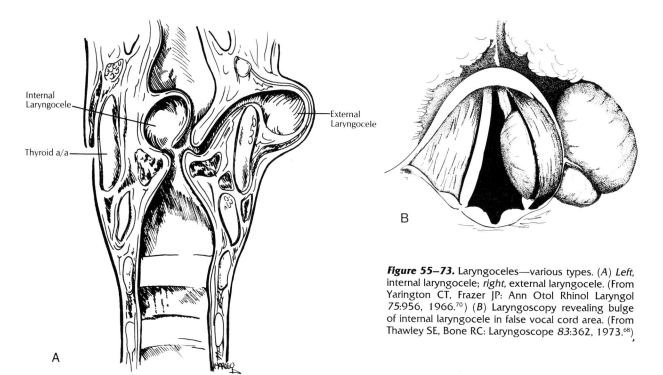

Figure 55–73. Laryngoceles—various types. (A) *Left,* internal laryngocele; *right,* external laryngocele. (From Yarington CT, Frazer JP: Ann Otol Rhinol Laryngol *75*:956, 1966.[70]) (B) Laryngoscopy revealing bulge of internal laryngocele in false vocal cord area. (From Thawley SE, Bone RC: Laryngoscope *83*:362, 1973.[68])

(indirect) and soft-tissue radiography. Internal and combined laryngoceles appear as submucosal masses in the region of the false cord and aryepiglottic fold. With the use of a flexible fiberoptic scope these masses may be seen to enlarge during the Valsalva maneuver.

Compression of the external or combined laryngocele may produce a hissing sound as air escapes endolaryngeally. This compressive maneuver is, however, dangerous, particularly in the combined laryngoceles, as air may be forced from the external component to the

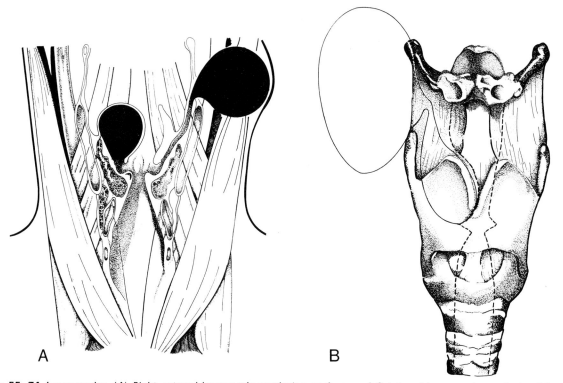

Figure 55–74. Laryngoceles. (A) *Right,* external laryngocele producing neck mass; *left,* internal laryngocele producing false cord mass. (B) Combined external and internal laryngocele. Notice external component exiting through the thyrohyoid membrane.

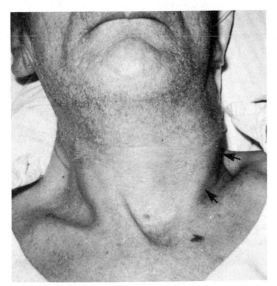

Figure 55–75. External laryngocele producing neck mass (arrows).

internal component, precipitating airway compromise. With purely external laryngoceles, the endolaryngeal examination may be normal.

The typical radiographic appearance of an air-filled, external or combined laryngocele is one of a well-defined radiolucent area protruding into the soft tissues of the neck lateral to the thyrohyoid membrane (Fig. 55–76). Internal laryngoceles are less well defined. Computerized tomographic (CT) scans in the transverse and, particularly, coronal planes may aid in defining the precise extent of the lesion.

Laryngoceles are rare in infants and, when they occur, are congenital. Hollinger and his colleagues,[62] in presenting their experience, found 10 cases of saccular cysts and only two of laryngoceles in children. Congenital laryngoceles have been managed conservatively when there has been no airway compromise, and most can be expected to resolve without surgical intervention. This is in contrast to the treatment of saccular cysts in infants; when they occur in infants, they should be aspirated or marsupialized endoscopically.

Carcinoma of the larynx has been associated with unilateral laryngoceles. In autopsy series the incidence varies from 2 to 18 per cent.[65] Laryngoceles may be bilateral with carcinoma of the larynx as well. This association mandates a careful examination of the larynx in all cases of adult laryngoceles to rule out the presence of a neoplasm.

Surgical Management

External Lateral Neck Approach. Many favor the external lateral neck approach for the surgical management of virtually all laryngoceles, citing the improved exposure, minimal morbidity, and reduced chance of recurrence associated with this approach.[63, 70] Internal laryngoceles may require removal of a minimal portion of the superior aspect of the thyroid cartilage to allow adequate surgical exposure. External and combined laryngoceles are dissected through the thyrohyoid membrane and rarely require cartilage sacrifice. Dissection of these masses proceeds in a fashion similar to that used during herniorrhaphy. The proximal opening of the laryngocele is closed on itself after complete dissection of the sac.

Laryngofissure Technique. This procedure has of course been well described. Utilizing this technique, access may be gained for resection, particularly of internal laryngoceles. A submucosal or transmucosal technique may be utilized via this approach. The laryngofissure approach runs the risk of blunting of the anterior commissure and subglottic stenosis.

Endoscopic Approach. In the past, Hollinger and others have advocated suspension microlaryngoscopy with marsupialization of the laryngocele endoscopically. Although this technique does serve to decompress large internal laryngoceles and saccular cysts, the drainage site rarely remains patent, and recurrence often occurs. Its major purpose is that of relieving impending airway obstruction. A definitive external lateral approach is preferable.

Technical Aspects of the External Approach for Resection of Laryngoceles. The surgeon creates a horizontal incision following a natural skin crease over the region of the thyrohyoid membrane, which is often overlying the mass (Figs. 55–77 and 55–78). (If the mass is compressed, a gurgling and hissing sound may occur; this is Bryce's sign.) Upper and lower subplatysmal skin flaps are elevated. The strap muscles are noted to bulge anteriorly, and if large enough, the carotid sheath is pushed posterolaterally. The strap muscles may be transected or parted for exposure. The ansa hypoglossi-cervicalis is often adherent and may be dissected free

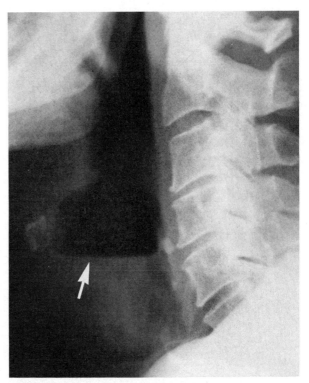

Figure 55–76. Soft-tissue radiograph of partially fluid-filled laryngocele. Note air-fluid level (arrow).

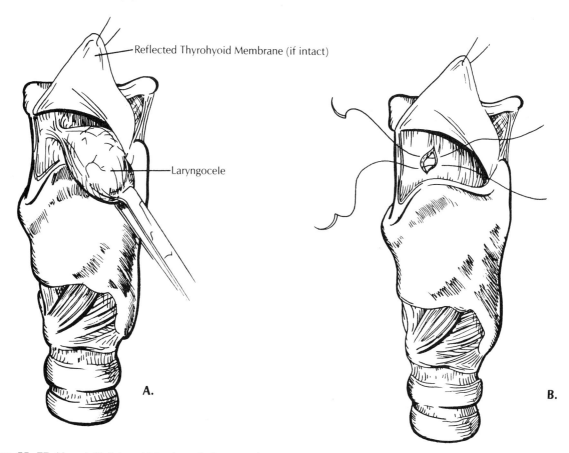

Figure 55–77. (A and B) External-lateral surgical approach to resection of external or combined laryngocele (as described by Yarington[70]) in which the sac is traced through the thyrohyoid membrane and its neck cut and oversewn.

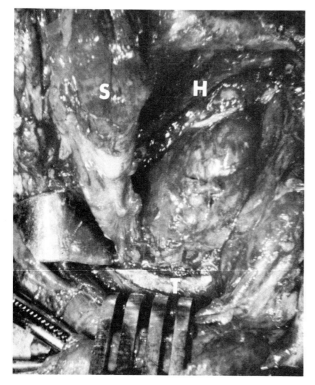

Figure 55–78. External and internal laryngocele with neck of sac dissected. (T = upper border of thyroid cartilage, H = hyoid bone, S = laryngocele sac.)

or transected as necessary. Gentle sharp and blunt dissection helps to further deliver the laryngocele. The neck of the mass is often at the level of the thyrohyoid membrane (Fig. 55–77A), which may be partially dehiscent. An attempt should be made to carefully identify and preserve the superior laryngeal nerve, which is often intimately related to the mass. Likewise, the superior laryngeal artery and vein arising from the superior thyroid vascular pedicle may be identified and ligated or preserved as necessary. The cyst may be traced into the larynx if required, as with combined laryngoceles (Fig. 55–78). When the sac has been completely dissected, it should be ligated and the cut ends of the mucosa and submucosa gently sutured with fine nonabsorbable material (Fig. 55–77B). If the dissection has proceeded gently and without excessive hemorrhage, the airway is rarely compromised and a tracheotomy need not be performed. With internal laryngoceles, the approach is similar. The strap muscles may be separated in the midline and retracted laterally, exposing the ipsilateral thyroid ala, thyrohyoid membrane, and hyoid bone. An incision may be made along the upper border of the thyroid ala through the thyrohyoid membrane, which may be elevated superiorly from the underlying adipose tissue of the pre-epiglottic space (Fig. 55–79A). The cyst or sac should be seen as a bulge in this region. Careful dissection now proceeds as above with appropriate transection and repair of the sac near the region of the laryngeal ventricle (Fig. 55–79B).

Potential complications include edema with airway

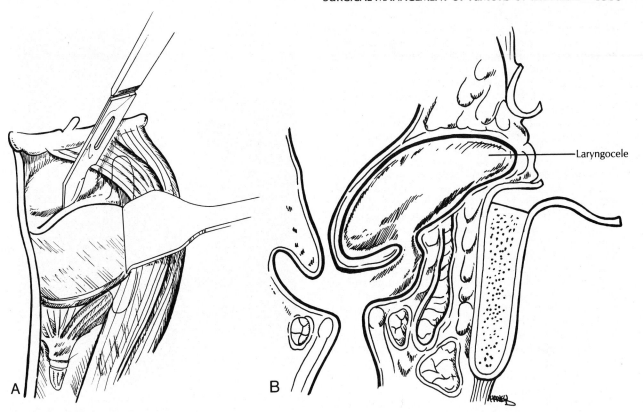

Figure 55–79. (*A* and *B*) Surgical approach to an internal laryngocele. The strap muscles and the perichondrium of the thyroid cartilage are reflected to allow resection of the upper portion of the thyroid ala and access to the sac. (From Tucker H: Surgery for Phonatory Disorders. New York, Churchill Livingstone, 1981.)

compromise, laryngocutaneous fistula, subcutaneous emphysema, injury to the superior or internal laryngeal nerve and recurrence of the lesion. Attention to meticulous technique should avoid these problems.

CAROTID BODY TUMORS

In regard to the surgical aspects of carotid body tumors, Matthews' words are still appropriate: "This rare tumor presents unusual difficulties to the surgeon and should he encounter it without having suspected the diagnosis, the experience will not soon be forgotten."[78]

Major controversies concerning management include (1) whether or not slow-growing lesions ever need to be removed, (2) whether or not preoperative angiography is essential, (3) the role of radiation therapy, (4) the criteria for malignancy, and (5) the indications for, and technique of, carotid artery replacement.

Historically, the carotid body was described in 1743 by VanHower.[83] The only major disease affecting this structure is neoplasia. Riegner's[80] attempt to resect a carotid body tumor resulted in death, but Maydl[79] successfully resected such a tumor, although his patient suffered a postoperative hemiplegia and aphasia. The first account of a carotid body tumor excised without ligating the vessels was by Albert in 1889, and the first one was accomplished in the United States by Scooter in 1903. To date, over 900 cases have been reported, and many more have not been reported.

Chemodectomas have engendered an inordinate amount of controversy regarding their natural history, biologic behavior, proper technique in excision, and risk of operative morbidity and mortality. They are classified as paragangliomas. However, carotid body tumors rarely secrete catecholamines, are nonchromaffin (that is, do not react with dichromate salts), and contain few if any nerve fibers. The word chemodectoma comes from the Greek words "chemieia," meaning infusion, "dechesthai," meaning to receive, and "oma," or tumor. The carotid body is ovoid, normally measures 3 to 6 mm, and is located on the posteromedial aspect of the common carotid artery near the bifurcation. The carotid body and sinus are often confused. The latter lies within the wall of the proximal internal carotid artery and is composed of complicated sensory nerve endings responding to alterations in pressure and, as such, is not a chemoreceptor. The carotid body responds to decreases in oxygen tension (not content), increases in blood acidity, and increases in CO_2 tension, resulting in an increase in blood pressure, cardiac rate, and depth and rate of respiration. The carotid body's role in overcoming the effects of hypoxia has been used to explain the recent suggestion that chemodectomas occur with an increased incidence in oxygen-deprived persons, such as those with cyanotic heart disease or those exposed to chronic hypoxia at high altitude.

A positive family history for carotid body tumors or chemodectomas is significant. In a review of over 900 such tumors, Grufferman and associates[73] suggest an autosomal-dominant genetic transmission. The overall familial incidence is approximately 10 per cent. As with other familial tumors, bilateral disease is more common in the familial form—30 vs. 4 per cent. In addition, 6 to 10 per cent of patients with cervical chemodectomas develop additional paragangliomas elsewhere, including glomus jugulares, glomus tympanicum and glomus vagalis, and pheochromocytomas. The controversy concerning the malignant potential of cervical chemodectomas continues. Several series quote different incidences, but most agree that it is probably less than 5 per cent and perhaps less than 3 per cent. Most carotid body tumors grow slowly; although cytologic alterations, such as pleomorphism, have been suggested to be correlated with malignant behavior, most surgeons and pathologists describe a poor correlation between histopathologic characteristics and ultimate biologic behavior. The presence of regional or distant metastasis clearly identifies those tumors that are malignant. Tumor size and symptoms on presentation appear to be the best prognostic index for future biologic behavior of this tumor. Many patients who have not undergone excision of cervical chemodectomas have done well for many years. Nevertheless, these tumors may cause severe disability or death. Locally aggressive lesions continue to grow relentlessly, invading adjacent structures including the base of skull, and often cause lower cranial neuropathies resulting in dysarthria, dysphagia, and at times, aspiration and death.

The history of a slowly growing mass in the neck at the level of the carotid bifurcation, particularly when associated with a bruit, should raise a strong suspicion and prompt appropriate radiographic evaluations (Figs. 55–80 to 55–86). Computerized tomographic scan with

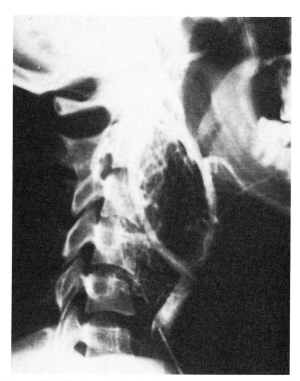

Figure 55–81. Carotid body glomus tumor separating the internal and external carotid arteries as seen during the arterial phase of the angiogram. (Courtesy of Gershon Spector, M.D.)

enhancement certainly clarifies the vascular nature of the tumor and determines its extent (Figs. 55–87 and 55–88). Angiography not only confirms the diagnosis but allows evaluation of the feeding blood supply in large tumors and of coexistent atherosclerotic occlusive disease. Digital subtraction angiography (DSA) has recently come into use for assessment of these lesions and promises to be a valuable tool in the future.

Surgical Management

Shamblin and associates[81] have described three classes of carotid body tumors: (1) *group I*—tumors that are small and easily dissected from the adjacent vessels, (2) *group II*—tumors that are more adherent and partially surround the vessel, and (3) *group III*—tumors that are large and adhere intimately to the entire circumference of the carotid bifurcation. In Group I patients, small, often asymptomatic lesions can usually be resected without injury to the underlying vessel. Group II patients have lesions that are less easily dissected and occasionally produce symptoms. They are amenable to careful surgical excision, but one needs to be prepared for a bypass should resection be necessary. Group III patients often have symptoms with lesions that incarcerate the carotids and mandate resection of the artery with replacement.

As these tumors grow, they push the internal and external carotid arteries apart and extend up either or both of the arteries for variable distances. The tumor may erode through the skull following the internal carotid artery cephalad. The size of these tumors varies from less than 1 cm to several centimeters. Their growth

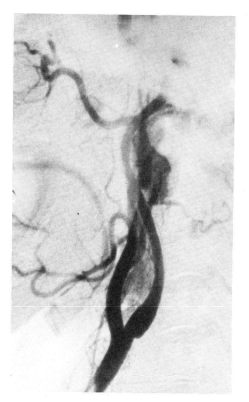

Figure 55–80. Arteriogram demonstrating glomus tumor extending from the base of the skull to the carotid bifurcation. (Courtesy of Gershon Spector, M.D.)

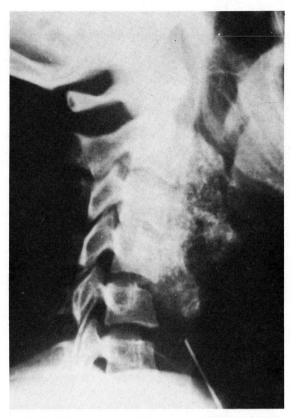

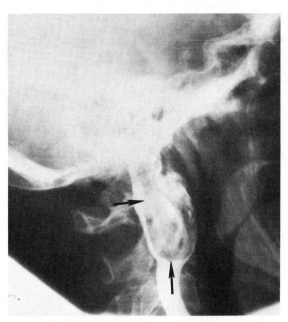

Figure 55–84. Glomus jugulare (arrows) filling internal jugular vein (venogram). (Courtesy of Gershon Spector, M.D.)

Figure 55–82. Carotid body glomus tumor in capillary phase of arteriogram. (Courtesy of Gershon Spector, M.D.)

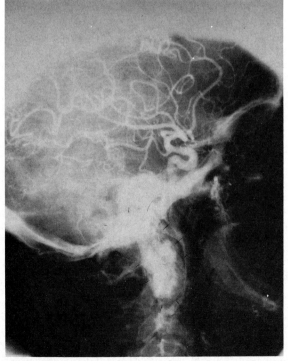

Figure 55–83. Glomus jugulare filling internal jugular vein. (Courtesy of Gershon Spector, M.D.)

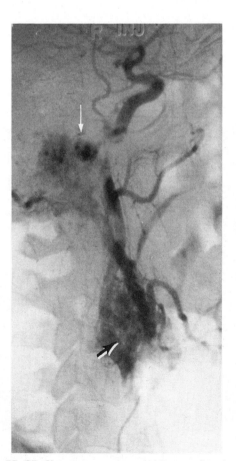

Figure 55–85. Glomus tympanicum (white arrow) and carotid body tumors (black arrow). (Courtesy of Gershon Spector, M.D.)

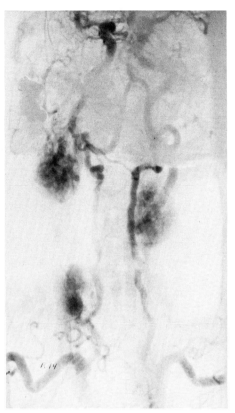

Figure 55–86. Multiple bilateral glomus tumors. (Courtesy of Gershon Spector, M.D.)

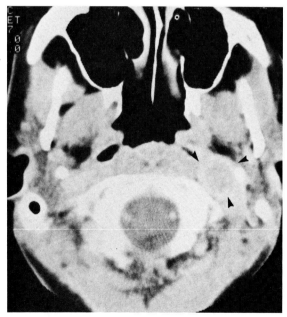

Figure 55–87. Computed tomographic (CT) scan with dye enhancement demonstrating mass at jugular foramen (arrowheads). (Courtesy of Gershon Spector, M.D.)

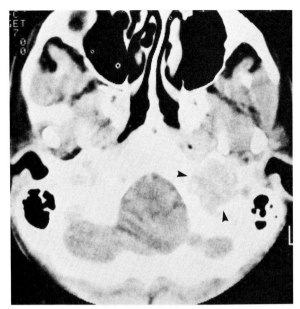

Figure 55–88. Computed tomographic scan demonstrating base of skull erosion (arrowheads). (Courtesy of Gershon Spector, M.D.)

rate has been estimated at 5 mm per year or approximately 2 cm in 5 years.[72] Although the tumors are well circumscribed, there is no microscopic capsule. These lesions may extend into the adventitia or even the media of the carotid artery but are most adherent at the bifurcation. Because of the rather slow growth rate, one of the controversies over the years has been whether or not these lesions need to be removed. Recognizing their tendency for relentless growth and improved technical aspects of their surgical resection favors surgical removal in the majority of cases.

Overall complication rates may be as high as 40 per cent. Mortality rates range from 5 to 13 per cent, stroke rates from 8 to 20 per cent, and postoperative cranial nerve deficits from 30 to 45 per cent.[71, 72, 74, 76, 82] These statistics underscore the importance of preoperative preparation and the cooperation and attendance of an experienced vascular surgeon.

Surgical Approaches

With group I and early group II lesions, recognition of the relatively avascular cleavage point between the artery and the tumor (white line) allows a meticulous subadventitial dissection that is crucial to the safe removal of these lesions (Fig. 55–89). Excessive bleeding may be avoided by ligating the small tumor-feeding vessels on the posterior aspect of the carotid bifurcation. Proximal and distal control of the common external and internal carotid arteries is essential in all cases.

With larger lesions (groups II and III), early ligation of the external carotid facilitates dissection by reducing tumor blood flow and provides a "handle" by which the tumor can be manipulated during mobilization.[76]

With more extensive tumors, partial or complete carotid resection may be necessary. Preoperative arteriography will have defined the cerebrovascular circula-

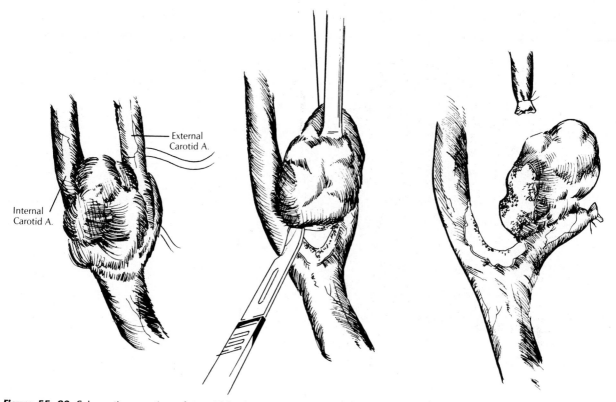

Figure 55–89. Schematic resection of carotid body tumor requiring ligation of external carotid artery and dissection from the adventitia of the internal carotid artery. (From Dent TL, Thompson NW, Fry WJ: Surgery *80:*365, 1976.[71])

tion and the contralateral carotid circulation; carotid stump pressures may be measured, and if less than 50 mm Hg, a temporary indwelling[75] shunt should be placed. Many utilize these shunts routinely regardless of stump pressures. When resection is deemed required preoperatively, intraoperative EEG may also be beneficial in monitoring. Autogenous reconstruction is favored by most over synthetic grafting, although this concept is not cast in stone.[77]

BENIGN TUMORS OF THE PARAPHARYNGEAL SPACE

An understanding of the anatomy of the parapharyngeal space is essential to understanding the surgical approaches to this region. It is roughly a pyramid- or cone-shaped space with the apex directed inferiorly toward the greater cornu of hyoid bone. It is limited at this point by attachments to the submandibular fascia. Laterally, it is limited by the ascending ramus of the mandible and the medial pterygoid muscle, and posterolaterally it is limited by the fascia surrounding the parotid gland. The medial wall of the parapharyngeal space is formed by the visceral fascia investing the superior constrictor muscle, tensor veli palatini, and levator veli palatini. Although these tumors have been variably described in the literature, most authors identify the fascia surrounding the contents of the carotid sheath as the posterior limit of the space. From a surgical standpoint, however, the space may be extended posteriorly to the prevertebral fascia, with the styloid proc-

ess and its muscular attachments dividing it into anterior and posterior compartments.[88, 89, 90]

Growths and masses arising within the parapharyngeal space (Fig. 55–90) tend to enlarge medially and inferiorly, displacing medial structures such as the tonsil, soft palate, and lateral pharyngeal wall and creating retromandibular fullness. Tumors developing in the parapharyngeal space may arise from any of the tissues contained within it. This includes loose connective tissue, fat, muscle, lymphatics, blood vessels, nerves, and major or minor salivary glands. Parotid tumors will not be discussed in detail in this chapter because they have been covered in Chapter 44, Surgical Therapy of Tumors of the Salivary Glands.

Deep-lobe parotid tumors account for about 50 per cent of all parapharyngeal space neoplasms. Patey and Thackray[92] popularized the concept of the "stylomandibular tunnel" to describe the channel through which retromandibular parotid tumors extended into the parapharyngeal space. The opening is formed by the skull base above, the ascending mandibular ramus and medial pterygoids anteriorly, and the styloid process and stylomandibular ligament posterosuperiorly. Because the tunnel does not expand, tumors that extend from the parotid gland medially into the parapharyngeal space may become dumbbell-shaped, with wide medial and lateral portions joined with a narrow isthmus. The deep retromandibular portion of the parotid gland approximates the parapharyngeal space and is separated from it only by the parotid fascia. The histologic appearance and incidence of tumors of the deep lobe are

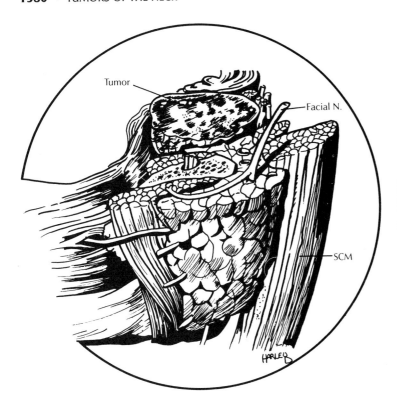

Figure 55–90. Three-dimensional illustration of parapharyngeal space neoplasm and its relationship to surrounding structures. (From Som PM, Biller HF, Lawson W: Ann Otol Rhinol Laryngol Suppl 80, *90*:3, 1981.)

similar to those for tumors originating in the superficial lobe and will be discussed in the section on salivary gland neoplasms.[92, 95]

Neurogenic tumors are the next most common primary tumor arising in the parapharyngeal space. They account for roughly 30 per cent of all neoplasms in the parapharyngeal space. Most arise from the vagus nerve. Histologically, these tumors include schwannomas (neurilemomas), neurofibromas, and paragangliomas. Paragangliomas arise from the chemoreceptor cells near the carotid bulb or from the glomus bodies located within the sheath of the carotid artery system or intimately associated with the vagus or glossopharyngeal nerves. Glomus vagale tumors arising from the glomus bodies of the inferior vagal ganglion are the most common form of paragangliomas arising in this region.

Other vascular neoplasms that occasionally arise in this area include *hemangiomas, lymphangiomas,* and *hemangiopericytomas,* or *hemangioendotheliomas.* Tumors of the minor salivary glands arising from the wall of the pharynx grow laterally into the parapharyngeal space. These are most often malignant, but occasionally are benign mixed pleomorphic adenomas. These will be discussed in more detail in the chapter on salivary gland neoplasms. Lymphomas may also arise in this space, as do inflammatory nodal conditions.[94]

Inflammation in the nasopharyngeal and tonsillar regions tends to involve nodes within the parapharyngeal space. Fortunately, these inflammatory processes, which may be suppurative, rarely affect traversing cranial nerves or large blood vessels. However, fatal erosion and hemorrhage from the carotid artery secondary to an inflammatory process have been described. Internal jugular vein thrombophlebitis is fortunately also a relatively rare event. Parapharyngeal space infections most often present as acute febrile illnesses associated with a fluctuant swelling and severe tenderness along the lateral pharyngeal wall intraorally and diffuse pain and swelling in the retromandibular region. Of importance is the notion that parapharyngeal space infections may spread to involve several other potential deep neck spaces, including the carotid sheath, retropharyngeal space, and mediastinum.[86, 87, 91, 93]

Metastatic tumors may also present as masses in the parapharyngeal space. Most commonly this involves neoplasms developing in the nasopharynx, oropharynx, paranasal sinuses, parotid gland, and mandible which have metastasized to the nodes of Rouviere. Metastatic or primary malignancies arising in the parapharyngeal space may cause paralysis of adjacent cranial nerves including the glossopharyngeal, vagus, and spinal accessory. At times, retrograde involvement of this node is seen in previously treated or irradiated carcinomas of the upper aerodigestive tract and neck.

Clinical Aspects

Symptoms of parapharyngeal space tumors are often minimal. Most often, patients incidentally note a bulge in the lateral pharyngeal wall, producing mild discomfort on swallowing or a mass at the angle of the jaw. Bimanual palpation should permit the examiner to differentiate these lesions from primary soft palate tumors with separate neck metastasis. With continued enlargement, a muffled hyponasal voice is produced and the airway may be compromised. Should the tumor encroach on the perieustachian tubal structures, a conductive hearing loss may also occur. In inflammatory conditions and malignant tumors, trismus may occur from impairment secondary to impairment of the pterygoid musculature or encroachment of the same. Paralysis of cranial nerves IX, X, XI, and XII is extremely rare with benign or inflammatory conditions but is occasionally seen with primary or metastatic malignancies. Erosion of the mucous membrane rarely occurs, and when present, a malignant process should be suspect.

Although plain sinus films and tomography of the base of skull help to delineate the presence and size of most neoplasms in the parapharyngeal space as well as indicate evidence of bony invasion, the CT scan is most valuable (Fig. 55–91). Using the combined CT-sialogram with enhancement allows differentiation of the deep lobe parotid tumor from an extraparotid parapharyngeal space neoplasm and determines whether a tumor is a vascular or avascular (enhancing vs. nonenhancing) mass. The sialographic contrast allows maximum visualization of the parotid gland margin. When a zone of decreased attenuation is seen on the scan between the posterolateral margin of the parapharyngeal mass and the contrast in the parotid, then the mass is extraparotid in origin. The line represents the fibrofatty supporting matrix of the parapharyngeal space as it is compressed between the mass and the deep lobe of the parotid gland. When no line is seen, the mass is in the deep lobe.

Most parapharyngeal lesions are salivary in origin, arising in the parotid or from minor salivary glands. These may be benign or malignant. Because none of these tumors enhance, even on angiography, a vascular blush is virtually never seen. Angiograms are not indicated in nonenhancing lesions. Lymphomatous, metastatic nodal lesions and a variety of miscellaneous tumors, including some neurogenic tumors, also produce nonenhancing masses. There is nothing unique or specific about their appearance on the scan and, as such, the scan is unable to make a histologic diagnosis. Occasionally, low-density parapharyngeal space masses that are nonenhancing are seen; these most commonly are lipomas, liposarcomas, or hybridomas. Their fat content shows as low attenuation on the CT scan. Dermoids and teratomas have also been reported.

The only deep-lobe tumor that enhances is a hemangioma. Enhancing lesions in the parapharyngeal space most often are extraparotid and include chemodectomas, schwannomas, and some neurofibromas. Occasionally, areas of hemorrhage or cystic degeneration within a tumor that normally enhances produce spotty areas of nonenhancement within it. Parapharyngeal glomus vagale tumors enhance and show a characteristic pattern of vascularity on carotid angiography. Meningioma is another rare enhancing lesion in the parapharyngeal space.

Enhancing lesions require subsequent angiography to delineate the pattern, extent, and nature of the vascularity as well as to clarify the status of the cerebral circulation. The CT scan gives a more accurate assessment of the actual tumor size and extent.

Even after a complete physical and radiographic evaluation, a diagnosis may not readily be made. Intraoral incisional biopsy should not be attempted, as this is fraught with potential complications including carotid laceration and hemorrhage, acute swelling of the mass with airway obstruction, and spread of benign pleomorphic adenomas with increased risk of recurrence in this particular lesion. Reports of needle biopsies performed intraorally have not occurred.

Surgical Management

Complete surgical excision is indicated for diagnosis and treatment of virtually all parapharyngeal space neoplasms—perhaps excluding *known* metastatic tumors. Untreated, benign lesions will continue to enlarge, compressing adjacent vital structures and ultimately involving the skull base and intracranium.[84, 85]

Surgical Approaches

The surgical approach best applied to tumors of the parapharyngeal space is an external one. Adequate visualization, control of bleeding and identification of major vessels and nerves can be accomplished through this approach. Internal approaches are to be discouraged except perhaps in the rare circumstance of extremely small lesions localized to the medial aspect of the space which can clearly be defined as such. The four external approaches that are available include the submandibular approach, total parotidectomy with retromandibular dissection, and a combination of the two with a lateral or a midline mandibulotomy.

Submandibular Approach (Cervical Approach). A relatively small extraparotid parapharyngeal space tumor (3 to 4 cm) occasionally may be removed through a submandibular approach. In this approach, an incision is made approximately two fingerbreadths below the angle of the mandible, and after identification and preservation of the margin mandibular nerve, the submandibular gland is removed, the parapharyngeal space is entered from below, and the lesion is dissected free and removed. Sharp and blunt dissection are often possible and allow, under direct visualization, the prevention of injury to major structures. Some prefer simply to retract the submandibular gland with the overlying nerve superiorly, using a transverse incision at the level of the hyoid bone. Cutting the digastric muscle and elevating the tail of parotid gland may give more

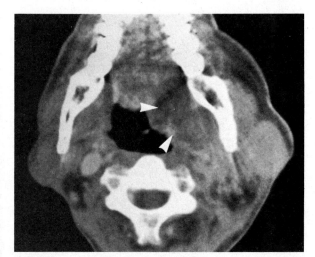

Figure 55–91. Computed tomographic scans demonstrating parapharyngeal mass (arrowheads).

exposure from below. Exposure in the parapharyngeal space is limited, but blunt finger dissection and limited sharp dissection are possible.

Disadvantages include limited exposure medially, superiorly, and posteriorly. Complete control of vascular structures particularly at the skull base is of course not possible. At times, the mandible may be dislocated anteriorly for a minimal amount of additional exposure. Should further exposure be necessary, osteotomy techniques must be utilized.

Transparotid-Cervical Approach. This approach is fundamentally reserved for deep lobe parotid tumors and, of course, involves routine isolation and preservation, when possible, of the facial nerve. Further discussion concerning this technique will be found in the section on salivary gland neoplasms.

Cervical-Transoropharyngeal with Mandibular Osteotomy Approach. This approach is fundamentally reserved for the majority of large extraparotid parapharyngeal space neoplasms, both vascular and nonvascular. This is especially helpful because of the maximum exposure at the base of skull required for both control of major vasculature and tumor removal. Combinations of this technique with the transparotid approach are of course possible in large deep lobe tumors as well.

A tracheotomy is required because of the degree of postoperative oropharyngeal edema and potential for airway obstruction. Exposure is accomplished through a transverse incision at the level of the hyoid bone, the medial limb of which extends superiorly to split the lip in the midline and the lateral limb of which extends posteriorly into the preauricular and occasionally retroauricular regions.

Lateral Osteotomy. When the transparotid approach has been used following a superficial parotidectomy and identification of the facial nerve, the lateral osteotomy is most often performed (Fig. 55–92). The osteotomy is performed in the region of the angle of the mandible after the masseter muscle has been cut from the mandible and retracted superiorly. The osteotomy transects the inferior alveolar nerve. The mandibular segments are distracted, and often a portion of the medial pterygoid muscle must be separated to increase exposure. Further distraction is limited by the attachments of the stylomandibular ligament and the ligaments surrounding the temporomandibular joint as well as the temporalis tendon attachment to the coronoid. Severing the attachments of the stylomandibular ligament often creates significantly increased exposure. With traction maintained to separate the mandibular fragments, the tumor can be both bluntly and sharply dissected with control of the major neurovascular structures. This technique may be utilized without previous superficial parotidectomy, although exposure is more limited. The submandibular gland may be removed or retracted, and the parotid can be deflected superiorly along with the masseter muscle from the inferior border of the mandible prior to osteotomy. The facial nerve may be temporarily paretic secondary to the retraction of adjacent soft tissues. The osteotomy is repaired using an osteosynthesis eccentric dynamic compression plate, thus averting the need for prolonged intermaxillary fixation.

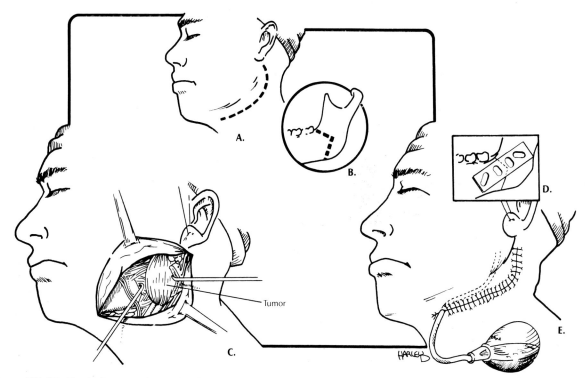

Figure 55–92. Surgical approach to the large parapharyngeal space neoplasm utilizing curvilinear incision (A) with lateral mandibulotomy (B), which exposes the tumor (C). Mandibular repair with wire or compression plate (D) and wound closure with suction drain in place (E). (From Som PM, Biller HF, Lawson W: Ann Otol Rhinol Laryngol Suppl 80, 90:3, 1981.[94])

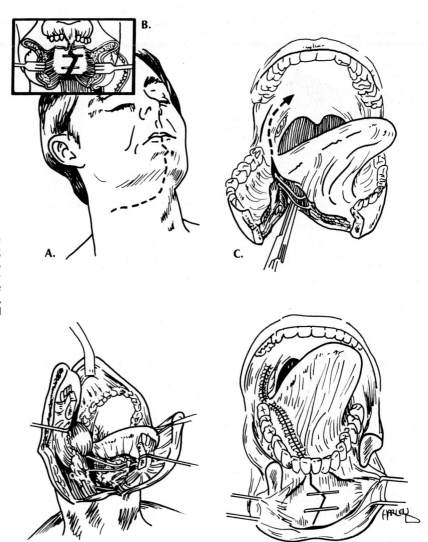

Figure 55–93. Surgical approach to the parapharyngeal space neoplasm utilizing midline (*A*), jaw-splitting approach (*B*), with mandibular swing (*C*). Tumor exposed (*D*) and after resection mandible repaired (*E*). (From Som PM, Biller HF, Lawson W: Ann Otol Rhinol Laryngol Suppl 80, *90*:3, 1981.[94])

Midline Mandibulotomy. A lip-splitting incision communicating with the previously described cervical incision is used (Fig. 55–93). The anterior lip flaps are not elevated more than 2 cm off the midline, following which a midline mandibular osteotomy is made. Drill holes are placed on either side of the planned osteotomy before it is made. The osteotomy cut is beveled in both the vertical and horizontal planes. The floor of the mouth is incised along the lateral gutter between the alveolus and the tongue. The incision may be extended to the superior aspect of the anterior tonsillar pillar. The lingual and hypoglossal nerves are identified and preserved. The mandible is then retracted laterally after severing the floor of mouth musculature. Severing the pterygoid attachments will also add in the exposure. The internal and external carotid arteries may then be identified and secured with vascular tapes if necessary. The facial nerve may be identified carefully from below without complete superficial parotidectomy in selected cases. Closure of the osteotomy following tumor removal is performed with a figure-of-8 wire, and intermaxillary fixation is rarely necessary. Major disadvantages of this technique include the need for tracheotomy and the cosmetically unappealing midline scar.

REFERENCES

CYSTIC HYGROMA

1. Batsakis JG (ed): Tumors of the Head and Neck. Baltimore, Williams & Wilkins Co., 1974, p 221.
2. Borst M: Die Lehre von den Deschwulstein. Wiesbaden, J. F. Bergman, 1902, p 191.
3. Harkins GA, Sabiston DC Jr: Lymphangioma in infancy and childhood. Surgery 47:811, 1960.
4. McClure CRW, Sylvester CF: Sequestration of lymphatic tissue of developing jugular lymphatic sac. Anat Rec 3:534, 1909.
5. Montgomery WW (ed): Surgery of the Upper Respiratory System. Philadelphia, Lea & Febiger, 1973, p 76.
6. Potts WJ: The Surgeon and the Child. Philadelphia, W. B. Saunders Co., 1959, p 245.
7. Redenbacher EH: De Ranula Sublingua: Speciale com Casa Congenito. Monachi Lindauer, 1828.
8. Ribbert H: Beschwulstehre für Arzte und Studrerende. Bonn, Cohen, 1914, p 226.
9. Sobol SM, Gogan RJ: Parotid lymphangioma—pathologic quiz. Arch Otolaryngol *107*:320, 1981.

10. Stromberg BV, Weeks PM, Wray RC Jr: Treatment of cystic hygroma. Southern Med J 69:1333, 1976.
11. Wernher A: Die Angeborenen Kysten-Hygrome und die Ihnen Verwondtem Berch-Wulste in Anatomscher, Diagnostester und Therapustischer Brezehung Giessen. Vatter, Sweden, G. G. Heyer, 1843, p 76.

HEMANGIOMA

12. Apfelberg DB, Maser MR, Lash H: Extended clinical use of the argon laser for cutaneous lesions. Arch Dermatol 115:719, 1979.
13. Brown JB, Fryer MP: Hemangioma: The role of surgery in early treatment for prevention of deformities. Plast Reconstruct Surg 71:197, 1953.
14. DiBartolomeo JR: Response of vascular lesions of the head and neck to argon laser radiation. Otolaryngol Head Neck Surg 91:203, 1983.
15. Gilchrest BA, Rosen S, Noe JM: Chilling portwine stains improves the response to argon laser therapy. Plast Reconstruct Surg 69:278, 1982.
16. Goldman L, Drefer R: Laser treatment of extensive mixed cavernous and port wine stains. Arch Dermatol 113:504, 1977.
17. Hobby LW: Further evaluation of the potential of the argon laser in the treatment of strawberry hemangiomas. Plast Reconstruct Surg 71:481, 1983.
18. Noe JM, Barsky SH, Beer DE, Rosen S: Port wine stains and response to argon laser therapy: Successful treatment and the predictive role of color, age and biopsy. Plast Reconstruct Surg 65:130, 1980.
19. Paletta FX: Tumors of the skin. In Converse JM (ed): Reconstructive Plastic Surgery. Vol. 5. Philadelphia, W. B. Saunders Co., 1977, pp 2865–2873.
20. Schrudde J, Petrovici V: Surgical treatment of giant hemangioma of the facial region after arterial embolization. Plast Reconstruct Surg 68:878, 1981.
21. Zarem HA, Edgerton MT: Induced resolution of cavernous hemangiomas following prednisolone therapy. Plast Reconstruct Surg 39:76, 1967.

BRANCHIAL CLEFT REMNANTS

22. Arnot RS: Detects of the first branchial cleft. South Afr J Surg 9:93, 1971.
23. Bhaskar SN, Bernier JL: Histogenesis of branchial cysts. Am J Pathol 35:407, 1959.
24. Frazer E: The disappearance of the precervical sinus. J Anat 61:132, 1926.
25. Gage JF, Lipman SP, Meyers EN: Diagnosis and Management of Congenital Masses in the Neck: A Self-Instructional Package. Washington, D.C., Committee on Continuing Medical Education, American Academy of Otology, 1976.
26. Gray SW, Skandalakis JE (eds): The pharynx and its derivatives. In Embryology for Surgeons, Philadelphia, W. B. Saunders Co., 1972, pp 15–58.
27. Lahey FH, Nelson HF: Branchial cysts and sinuses. Ann Surg 113:508, 1941.
28. Liston SL, Siegel LG: Branchial cysts, sinuses and fistulas. Ear Nose Throat J 58:9, 1979.
29. Montgomery WW: In Surgery of the Upper Respiratory System. Vol. II. Philadelphia, Lea & Febiger, 1973, pp 138–158.
30. Olson KD, Maragos NE, Weiland LH: First branchial cleft anomalies. Laryngoscope 90:423, 1980.
31. Proctor B: Lateral vestigal cysts and fistulas of the neck. Laryngoscope 65:355, 1955.
32. Randall P, Rayster HP: First branchial cleft anomalies: A not so rare and potentially dangerous condition. Plast Reconstruct Surg 31:497, 1963.
33. Wenglowski R: Ueber die Halsfisteln und Cysten. Arch Klin Chir 100:789, 1913.
34. Work WP: New concepts of first branchial cleft defects. Laryngoscope 82:1581, 1972.

THYROGLOSSAL DUCT CYST

35. Allard RHB: The thyroglossal duct cyst. Head Neck Surg 1:134, 1982.
36. Bertilli A, Freitas JPA: Thyroglossal cysts and fistulae. Ear Nose Throat Monthly 50:88, 1971.
37. Brintnall ES, Davies J, Huffman WC, Lierk DM: Thyroglossal ducts and cysts. Arch Otolaryngol 59:282, 1954.
38. Choy F, Ward R, Richardson R: Carcinoma of the thyroglossal duct. Am J Surg 108:361, 1964.
39. Clute HM, Catell RB: Thyroglossal cysts and sinuses. Ann Surg 92:57, 1930.
40. Dishe S, Berg PK: An investigation of the thyroglossal tract using the radioisotope scan. Clin Radiol 14:298, 1963.
41. Ellis TDM, Van Nostrand AWT: The applied anatomy of thyroglossal tract remnants. Laryngoscope 87:765, 1977.
42. Gray SW, Skandalakis JE (eds): The pharynx and its derivatives. In Embryology for Surgeons. Philadelphia, W. B. Saunders Co., 1972, pp 15–58.
43. Gross RE, Connerly ML: Thyroglossal cysts and sinuses: A study and report of 198 cases. N Engl J Med 223:616, 1962.
44. Keeling JH, Ochsner A: Carcinoma in thyroglossal duct remnants. Cancer 12:596, 1959.
45. Marshall SF, Becker WF: Thyroglossal cysts and sinuses. Ann Surg 129:642, 1949.
46. McClintock JC: Lesions of the thyroglossal tract. Arch Surg 33:890, 1936.
47. McDonald DM: Thyroglossal cysts and fistulae. Int J Oral Surg 3:342, 1974.
48. Montgomery WW: Surgery of the Upper Respiratory System. Philadelphia, Lea & Febiger, 1973.
49. Sistrunk WE: The surgical treatment of cysts of the thyroglossal tract. Ann Surg 71:121, 1920.
50. Thomas JR: Thyroglossal-duct cysts. Ear Nose Throat J 58:21, 1979.
51. Ward GE, Hendrick JW, Chambers RB: Thyroglossal tract abnormalities, cysts and fistulae. Surg Gynecol Obstet 89:727, 1949.

DERMOIDS AND TERATOMAS

52. Arnold J: Ein Fall von congenitalen zusammengesetzen Lipon der Zunge unter der Pharynx. Virchows Arch 51:482, 1880.
53. Hawkins DB, Park R: Teratoma of the pharynx and neck. Ann Otol Rhinol Laryngol 81:848, 1972.
54. Holt GR, Holt JE, Weaver RG: Dermoids and teratomas of the head and neck. Ear Nose Throat J 58:37, 1979.
55. Katz AD: Midline dermoid tumors of the neck. Arch Surg 109:822, 1974.
56. Macavoy JM, Zuckerbraun L: Dermoid cysts of the head and neck in children. Arch Otol 102:529, 1976.
57. New GB, Erich JB: Dermoid cysts of the head and neck. Surg Gynecol Obstet 65:48, 1937.
58. Weaver RG, Meyerhoff WL, Gates GA: Teratomas of the head and neck. Surg Forum 27:539, 1976.

MISCELLANEOUS BENIGN LESIONS

59. Batsakis JG, Rice DH, Howard DR: The pathology of head and neck tumors: Spindle cell lesions (sarcomatoid carcinoma, nodular fasciitis, and fibrosarcoma) of the aerodigestive tract. Head Neck Surg 1:499, 1982.
60. Bernstein KE, Lattes R: Nodular (pseudosarcomatous) fasciitis, a nonrecurrent lesion: Clinicopathologic study of 134 cases. Cancer 49:1668, 1982.
61. Desanto LW: Laryngocele, laryngeal mucocele, large saccules and laryngeal saccular cysts: A developmental spectrum. Laryngoscope 84:1291, 1974.
62. Hollinger LD, Barnes DR, Smid LJ, Hollinger PH: Laryngoceles and saccular cysts. Ann Otol Rhinol Laryngol 87:675, 1978.
63. Johnstone JH: External laryngocele. Surgery 34:307, 1953.
64. Mattel SF, Persky M: Infiltrating lipoma of the sternocleidomastoid muscle. Laryngoscope 93:205, 1983.
65. Micheau C, Luboinski B, Lamchi P, Cachin Y: Relationship between laryngoceles and laryngeal carcinoma. Laryngoscope 88:680, 1978.
66. Soule EH: Proliferative (nodular) fasciitis. Arch Pathol 73:437, 1962.
67. Stout AP: Pseudosarcomatous fasciitis in children. Cancer 14:1216, 1961.
68. Thawley SE, Bone RC: Laryngopyocele. Laryngoscope 83:362, 1973.
69. Virchow R: Die Krankhafter Geschwulste. Berlin, A. Herschwald, 1863, pp 35–40.
70. Yarington CT, Frazer JP: An approach to the internal laryngocele and other submucosal lesions of the larynx. Ann Otol Rhinol Laryngol 75:956, 1966.

CAROTID BODY TUMORS

71. Dent TL, Thompson NW, Fry WJ: Carotid body tumors. Surgery 80:365, 1976.

72. Farr HW: Carotid body tumors: A 40-year study. CA *30*:260, 1980.
73. Grufferman S, Gillman NW, Pasternick LR, et al: Familial carotid body tumors: A case report and epidemiologic review. Cancer *46*:2116, 1980.
74. Irons GB, Wheland LH, Brown WO: Paragangliomas of the neck: Clinical and pathological analysis of 16 cases. Surg Clin North Am *57*:575, 1977.
75. Javid H, Dye WS, Hunter JA, et al: Surgical management of carotid body tumor. Arch Surg *95*:771, 1967.
76. Krupsky WC, Effeney DJ, Ehrenfeld WK, Stoney RJ: Cervical chemodectoma—Technical considerations and management options. Am J Surg *144*:215, 1982.
77. Lees CD, Levine HL, Bevin EG, Tucker HN: Tumors of the carotid body: Experience with 41 operative cases. Am J Surg *142*:362, 1981.
78. Matthews FS: Surgery of the neck. *In* Johnson AB (ed): Operative Therapeutics. Vol. III. New York, Appleton-Century-Crofts, 1950, p 315.
79. Maydl L, cited by Burn JJ: Carotid body and allied tumors. Am J Surg *95*:371, 1958.
80. Riegner K, cited by Lahey FH, Warren KW: A long-term appraisal of carotid body tumors with remarks on their removal. Surg Gynecol Obstet *92*:481, 1951.
81. Shamblin WR, Remine WH, Shepps SG, Harrison EG: Carotid body tumor: Clinical pathologic analysis of 90 cases. Am J Surg *122*:732, 1971.
82. VanAspren H, Debourfrs J, Klepshaw JL, Vinck M: Diagnosis, treatment and operative complications of carotid body tumors. Br J Surg *68*:433, 1981.
83. VanHower, L, cited by Dickenson AM, Traverse CA: Carotid body tumors: Review of the literature with report of two cases. Am J Surg *69*:9, 1945.

BENIGN TUMORS OF THE PARAPHARYNGEAL SPACE

84. Baker DC, Conley J: Treatment of massive deep lobe parotid tumors. Am J Surg *138*:572, 1979.
85. Bass RM: Approaches to the diagnosis and treatment of tumors of the parapharyngeal space. Head Neck Surg *4*:281, 1982.
86. Brown DE: Infections of the deep fascial spaces of the head and neck. Rochester, Minnesota, American Academy of Ophthalmology and Otolaryngology, 1978.
87. Coller FA, Yglesis L: Infections of the lip and face. Surg Gynecol Obstet *60*:277, 1935.
88. Gaughrangrl H: The lateral pharyngeal cleft. Ann Otol Rhinol Laryngol *68*:1082, 1959.
89. Grodinski M, Holyoke EA: The fascia and fascial spaces of the head, neck and adjacent regions. Am J Anat *63*:367, 1938.
90. Heeneman H, Gilbert JJ, Rood SR: The Parapharyngeal Space: Anatomy and Pathologic Conditions with Emphasis on Neurogenous Tumors. Rochester, Minnesota, American Academy of Ophthalmology and Otolaryngology, 1980.
91. Langinbruner DJ, Dijoni S: Pharyngomaxillary space abscess with carotid artery erosion. Arch Otolaryngol *94*:447, 1971.
92. Patey DH, Thackray AC: The pathological anatomy and treatment of parotid tumors with retropharyngeal extension (dumbbell tumors). Br J Surg *44*:352, 1956.
93. Rebuzzi DD, Johnson JT: Diagnosis and Management of Deep Space Neck Infections. Edition 2. Rochester, Minnesota, American Academy of Ophthalmology and Otolaryngology, 1978.
94. Som PM, Biller HF, Lawson W: Tumors of the parapharyngeal space: Preoperative evaluation, diagnosis and surgical approaches. Ann Otol Rhinol Laryngol Suppl *90*:3, 1981.
95. Work WP: Parapharyngeal space and salivary gland neoplasms. Otolaryngol Clin North Am *10*:421, 1977.

CHAPTER 56

Controversies in Management of Cancer of the Neck

Sharon L. Collins, M.D.

To avoid error in the diagnosis and treatment of the disease one must substitute factual data for opinions, frequently inaccurate, founded on inadequately controlled clinical impressions.

Preston, 1954

No primary cancer in the head and neck can be treated without concomitant attention directed to regional metastases, and there are many questions pertaining to the correct management of this aspect of disease. This chapter will attempt to define these controversial topics and to apply concepts from recent advances in tumor biology in order to redirect thinking in relation to therapeutic and research strategies for head and neck cancer patients. It is suggested that this chapter be read from start to finish in the order presented so that the reader will have an appropriate data base to understand reinterpretations of the traditional controversies as they emerge.

To provide a historical perspective, a review of the development of surgery for cancer of the neck is presented initially. The second major section presents work from the fields of experimental and clinical cancer research which relates to the tumor-host interaction: the role of regional lymph nodes, the process of metastasis, and the multifaceted influences of cancer treatment modalities. Discussion then proceeds to the major controversies in the management of squamous cell cancer in the neck, including a critique of the literature, the rationale and methods for elective treatment, treatment of advanced neck disease, methods of neck node biopsy, and the issue of combination therapy. Management of the neck with non-squamous cell tumors (salivary gland cancer, thyroid tumors, and malignant melanoma) is then reviewed. A concluding section proposes relevant directions for future research and relates the issues presented to the broader context of surgical oncology.

HISTORICAL DEVELOPMENT OF SURGERY FOR CANCER IN THE NECK

In the early 1800s, there was little reference to the treatment of head and neck cancer once it had spread to the "cervical glands," and it was felt that once the tumor had involved the submaxillary gland, complete removal of the disease was impossible. In 1847, Warren described an operation for removal of metastatic lymph nodes from the upper neck. Butlin, in 1900, advised the removal of cervical lymphatics through the Kocher incision and suggested routine elective excision of these tissues in the treatment of tongue cancer. It was George Crile, Sr., however, who first described a systematic operative procedure for the removal of cervical lymphatics and lymph nodes based on anatomic principles in 1906.[43] His initial report on 132 operations pioneered the mechanistic approach to head and neck cancer, in which curability was related to the magnitude of the surgical resection following principles established by Halsted for breast cancer.[95] As we shall see, the rationale for this approach can be challenged, based on a better understanding of the natural history of cancer and new biologic information. At the time, however, surgical treatment was consistent with pathologic findings and the current conception of cancer spread.

The permeation theory of metastasis was introduced by Handley in 1907 based on autopsy studies of patients who had died of breast cancer and melanoma.[97] He concluded that lymphatic metastases originated by continuous permeation of the lymphatics radiating away from the primary tumor site. Patients studied generally had far-advanced disease, and intervening vessels frequently were completely plugged by infiltrating disease. The permeation concept of lymphatic metastases was the basis for the development of incontinuity (en bloc) dissection of nodes with primary cancers for melanoma, breast cancer, and head and neck cancer.

Von Recklinghausen noticed that metastases could be found in the lymph "glands" without tumor in the intervening lymphatics, and the embolic spread of metastases is now generally accepted. Handley's concept of permeation still fits several clinical situations in head and neck cancer, such as massive recurrent cancer with obstruction of the normal lymphatic pathways leading to retrograde spread and tumors in certain sites such as large floor-of-mouth tumors with direct extension to the submandibular area.

In Crile's 1906 paper,[43] he lamented that despite significant advances in surgery for other types of cancer, treatment of cancer in the head and neck had not received comparable attention, nor had it kept abreast of progress made in other fields, and he complained that the operative treatment was hampered by tradition and conventionality—complaints still valid even 80 years later. He felt that an incomplete operation disseminated and stimulated growth of tumor. Dissection en bloc was indicated regardless of whether the glands were palpable, because palpable glands could be inflammatory, and nonpalpable glands could contain carcinoma. When there were no palpable glands, only the immediate lymphatic drainage area was excised, whereas radical dissection was performed for palpable metastases. He also felt it was important to strictly avoid handling cancer tissue as long as the lymphatic channels were intact in order to avoid further dissemination of the tumor.

Crile's procedure was formidable in the early 1900s because of the risk of infection and hemorrhage, and it was generally recommended that the neck operation should be delayed after excision of the primary tumor to decrease the risk of medastinitis. Crile decreased aspiration problems by using a nasopharyngeal tube that ended opposite the epiglottis and was stabilized with pharyngeal packing. Because blood transfusions were not available (Landsteiner discovered the first three blood group substances in the early 1900s, and the Rh factor was not discovered until the 1940s), Crile minimized troublesome venous hemorrhage by placing the patient in a semisitting position and using the rubber pneumatic suit to maintain cerebral blood flow. It is interesting that, as an early step in his neck dissection, the common carotid artery was temporarily clamped to control arterial bleeding. He also administered atropine preoperatively not only to decrease bronchial secretions but also to prevent "inhibitory collapse from direct reflex inhibition through the Vagus."

In reporting his results, Crile noted that a perusal of the literature had convinced him that one could obtain the safest conclusions only from his own experience because it was often impossible to get precise knowledge of the planned purpose and descriptions from the work of other surgeons. Crile's attitude was held by almost all senior surgeons who treated their patients based on their own personal experience and gradually modified techniques as technology improved.

Crile's experience led him to conclude that recurrent malignant tumors that had transgressed the lymphatics and invaded the deeper planes of the neck were inoperable. He felt that radical dissection of the neck was four times more effective than less radical neck operations. He did perform bilateral radical neck dissection (RND) once, and would also do resections on the neck and mouth "at the same seance" when indicated. He noted that although cancers in different sites of the head and neck are not equally curable, once the lymphatics of the neck were involved, the surgical problem and the risks were independent of the location of the primary lesion. According to Crile, because the head and neck was an exposed area, cancer there should be recognizable early, and every case should at some time be curable by complete excision. Because the cervical lymphatics were accessible and the cancer rarely penetrated the lymphatic collar of the neck, localized growth persisted for some time, and by applying comprehensive block dissections, the outcome of cancer of the head and neck should be better than for almost any other portion of the body. In maintaining that the cervical lymphatics were an effective long-term barrier against the spread of disease, he cited 4500 autopsy cases studied by a Dr. Hitchings, showing that in less than 1 per cent were secondary cancer foci located in distant organs and tissues. When Hayes Martin attempted to check on this source in 1940, Hitchings had died, and there was no way to confirm the data.

The Crile and Halsted school of thought completely dominated cancer surgery from the last decade of the nineteenth century until the present time and was consistent with prevailing knowledge of the nature of cancer spread as then understood:

1. A growing tumor first remains localized at its site of origin and then spreads to the regional lymph nodes (RLNs) and finally systemically in an orderly, predictable manner.

2. Tumor cells permeate and traverse lymphatics by direct extension.

3. Regional lymph nodes provide an effective barrier to the passage of tumor cells, leading to prolonged local retention.

4. The blood stream is of little significance as a route of metastasis for carcinomas.

5. A tumor is autonomous from its host.

It is interesting that in the discussion of Crile's 1906 paper, basic questions that have been debated for the succeeding 80 years were introduced. Surgeons were doing unilateral or bilateral, partial or radical neck dissections electively, and various types of modified neck dissections preserving the sternocleidomastoid muscle and internal jugular vein were reported. Apparently, some surgeons felt that removing neck "glands" was prophylactic in that spread of the tumor could be prevented because metastases would then have no place to lodge and grow.

By 1923, a symposium on carcinoma of the jaws, tongue, and lips* provided a forum for presentation of additional material accrued during the intervening years. By that time, it was possible to perform complete bilateral neck dissections separated by several weeks without untoward complications. The major cause of death after head and neck cancer operations was pneumonia resulting from inhalation of blood or secretions, as tracheotomies were not routinely performed. Light general or local anesthesia was used so that the conscious patient could cough. Deep ether or chloroform anesthesia was not favored because of the danger of postoperative vomiting and fatal aspiration. It was considered very important to avoid hemorrhage because bleeding necessitated sponging of the cancer surface, which allowed cells to adhere to the sponges and be resown upon a "fresh and fertile field." It was stated that the resultant new growth might kill the patient much earlier than the primary lesion would have. Cancer tissue should not be cut across or handled.

By 1923, Crile had performed 224 operations for carcinoma of the cheek, lip, tongue, mouth, and jaws with only six operative deaths. He still noted that excision of the lymphatic glands not only did not lead to cures but usually was followed by greater dissemination and more rapid cancer growth. After the operation, a single treatment with deep x-rays or radium was employed.

At the same symposium, other surgeons were cited who felt that as long as the lymphatics were nature's barriers, they should not be removed unless they were involved with cancer. Neck dissections were still gen-

---

*Surg Gynecol Obstet 36:159, 1923.

erally performed separately from the treatment of the primary tumor, which was often treated with radium implants or cautery. Bilateral suprahyoid dissections were advocated with completion of a block dissection on the involved side if disease was demonstrated—this was the origin of the concept that a suprahyoid neck dissection was an adequate biopsy technique. It was noted that cancer had not been found in the lymphatic vessels between the primary lesion and the involved nodes, thus confirming the view that, at least in the head and neck, lymph node metastasis was an embolic process rather than a direct growth of malignant cells along lymph channels. By that time, neck dissection was usually performed discontinuously from excision of the primary tumor.

In the discussion that followed these papers, certain aspects of the natural history of head and neck cancer were enumerated. It was noted that the primary lesion was not always easy to find and that immense carcinomatous masses in the neck might be the first sign of disease, whereas some patients with large primary tumors did not develop neck metastases during the course of their disease. Similar observations were made by Martin and Morfit.[152] For instance, in 1944, they asked:

why do certain primary malignant tumors behave so much like normal tissues in that they respond to growth-control influences and remain microscopic in size, yet nevertheless possess an uninhibited capacity to metastasize? Furthermore, once having metastasized, why do the same growth-control factors likewise not inhibit the rapid and bulky growth of the metastases? In these cases, one must assume that there are differences in the biologic conditions at the primary and secondary sites of growth and that in these cases, at least, the growth control function is not necessarily systemic, but local and possibly neurotropic.

One physician (Blair) noted that some of the larger tumors were "fenced around by and composed largely of inflammatory tissue that long retards gland infection, while some of the small shallow ulcers that look like abrasions of the mucosa are often the most deadly" and that "cancer is best handled as one would treat a skunk—let it alone or kill it quick; only grief can come from irritating it." Such comments indicate knowledge of the biologic heterogeneity of head and neck tumors by the cancer surgeons of the 1920s.

Another physician (Quick) noted that because of his improved results of treatment of the primary tumor with radium implants, his management of cervical nodes was becoming increasingly conservative. He noted that cervical lymphatics performed a "conservative" function, which was much more than that of a filter, in that microscopic evidence of encapsulation of tumor cells by new connective tissue and destruction by active lymphatic infiltration could be seen in some specimens. In addition, rapid recurrences with increased rate of growth were typically seen once the natural factors of immunity were interfered with, as by surgery. When nodes became palpable, a unilateral block dissection was performed and filtered radium was inserted in rubber tubing in the wound. This was noted to improve the results with respect to early recurrence. In the cases in which gross residual disease was left in the neck, implantation was performed. In addition, preliminary external radiation was used prior to any operation in all cases in which neck disease was palpa-

ble. Dr. Mueller of Philadelphia recommended radium implantation at the time of block dissection of the neck, at well known areas of frequent recurrence. The radium "seeds" that were used were enclosed in glass tubes 1 to 2 mm in diameter, containing from 1 to 5 mC of "radium emanation."

In the 1930s and 1940s, general surgeon Hayes Martin and his associates at Memorial Hospital in New York standardized the technique of radical neck dissection (RND) and reported on 1450 cases of neck dissection for head and neck cancers performed between 1928 and 1950.[151] As did Crile and Halsted, Martin felt that the lymph node constituted a protective barrier that, for a time, could confine metastatic growth to an area accessible to treatment by surgery or radiation, and that once beyond this barrier, cancer of the head and neck was to all intents hopelessly advanced. The degree to which metastasis could be prevented or controlled was the main factor that determined the patient's prognosis. In general, Martin was a "one operation fits all" surgeon. He developed the "commando" procedure (composite, jaw-neck resection) and favored incontinuity resection of the primary tumor and neck disease, radical as opposed to modified neck dissection (MND) and therapeutic rather than elective neck dissection (END). Martin's indications for neck dissection included definitive evidence that cancer was present in the cervical lymphatics, control of the primary lesion or a plan to remove it at the same time of the neck dissection, a reasonable chance of complete removal of the cervical metastatic cancer, and no clinical or x-ray evidence of distant metastasis (DM). He noted that the term "inoperable" meant different things to different surgeons, and that operability frequently depended on the experience, skill, and attitude of the individual surgeon. He also performed neck dissection in selected cases with evidence of metastasis below the clavicle for palliation of the pain and other disabling symptoms of metastatic cervical cancer, although he preferred radiation therapy (RT) in those cases in which the primary lesion was inoperable.

Martin discussed the issue of elective neck dissection at length. He took exception to the term "prophylactic" neck dissection because the term implied prevention rather than cure of metastatic cancer and because the only means of preventing metastases was to eradicate the primary tumor before spread could occur. The term prophylactic did not include cases in which neck dissection was performed because the neck was entered during excision of the primary tumor. He calculated that only 6 per cent of his 237 patients with lip cancer and 20 per cent of 120 patients with tongue cancer would have benefited from a prophylactic neck dissection—presumably these were patients who died of uncontrolled neck disease. In order to assess the attitudes of clinicians in the community concerning prophylactic neck dissection for cancer of the lip and tongue, he sent a questionnaire to 75 doctors; among 58 respondents, only 16 of 23 who favored prophylactic neck dissection were willing to specify a number representing the chance of benefiting the patient, which would justify prophylactic operation (choices were 1 in 5 to 1 in 25). The greatest number of respondents stated that they considered a 1 in 10 chance of benefit sufficient to employ prophylactic neck dissection. One surgeon stated that he would insist upon neck dissection for himself for even the smallest lip cancer. This is an interesting consideration, which every physician should think about to test his or her level of commitment to a given treatment. Many who favored prophylactic neck dissection admitted that their feelings were based on the fact that they could not provide adequate follow-up in their private practices or clinics. Martin did not consider this an acceptable indication for the procedure, with the possible exception of cases of indigent and illiterate patients who could not be depended upon to cooperate in any follow-up plan.

Obviously, it remains difficult to determine cases in which a 1-in-10 incidence of occult disease is present in the neck, and the degree of increased survival pursuant to treating such occult diseases is even more difficult to determine. Some respondents stated that they resisted any statistical basis for drawing conclusions on this question. Others preferred to individualize each case by evaluating all factors such as age, general condition, size and position of the lesion, and histologic grade to arrive at a conclusion. Others would make a decision for or against prophylactic neck dissection on the specific size in millimeters of the primary lesion. In short, many of the respondents resisted any attempt to establish the practical value of the procedure on a statistical basis, preferring to individualize each case, thus "placing the decision into the arbitrary realm subject of day-to-day variation, based on the physicians' most recent experience." (Elective neck irradiation was not an option at that time—state-of-the-art radiation therapy was administered through small portals to the neck because cancer-lethal doses over the entire neck could not be tolerated by the patient.)

Martin's somewhat derisive response to this attitude was that "even though some members of the medical profession should actually possess such occult powers to select treatment methods in individual cases without reference to or regard for statistical evidence, nonetheless, such skills are limited in their usefulness and could hardly be taught to others." One suspects that such a questionnaire today would elicit a similar variety of responses because although many statistics have accumulated in the literature since that time, almost none of the basic questions can be definitively answered from the existing data on a scientific basis.

Hayes Martin was a major pioneer in head and neck cancer surgery, and his opinion strongly influenced not only his successors at Memorial Hospital but many other surgeons. He did not condone partial neck dissection because the lymphatics along the internal jugular vein were in close association with the walls of the vein itself, and it was unlikely that any procedure short of excision of the vein could completely remove the lymph vessels and nodes in this region. Similarly, preservation of the spinal accessory nerve was unequivocally condemned. He felt that the shoulder deficit was relatively insignificant because the action was taken over in part by the major and minor rhomboids and the levator scapulae muscles. His major objection to preserving the 11th cranial nerve routinely was that in its upper portion, it ran directly through a mass of fatty, areolar, and lymphatic tissue in which were embedded the subdigastric nodes. In agreement with Crile, Martin noted that when the surgeon was faced with the necessity of excising the common or internal carotid artery in cases

of metastatic cervical cancer, there would almost inevitably be associated technical factors that precluded the successful use of a graft to restore circulatory continuity. Although reluctant to perform such heroic surgery in aged patients with limited life expectancy, the Memorial Hospital surgeons tended to risk the immediate high mortality rate in the younger age group because the long-range chance of survival was more worthwhile.

Martin did not favor elective whole-field postoperative radiation therapy, and he felt that clinicians who recommended such treatment to the entire operative field believed erroneously that a moderate dose (about one "skin erythema dose") exercised a "restraining effect" in an area of "lymphatic block," so that any remaining metastatic emboli could not progress further. He did favor occasional radiation therapy with curative intent for local recurrences after surgery, and localized postoperative radiation therapy (RT) was also considered acceptable if it was not possible to remove metastatic disease in the vicinity of the carotid artery completely.

Radiation therapy usually consisted of a course of fractionated orthovoltage radiation with supplementary gold radon "seeds" implanted into the nodes. Martin felt that the efficacy of the cervical lymphatics in blocking the further spread of head and neck cancer should encourage aggressive attempts at regional control unless there was evidence of distant metastases (DMs). In support of this principle, he cited "repeated" 5-year (or longer) neck control with radical neck dissection when the histologic examination showed multiple positive nodes, even at low levels in the neck, proving that although there was extensive disease throughout the neck, metastatic emboli had not permeated the main lymphatic ducts to produce generalized metastasis. When cancer recurred following neck dissection, either in the operative field or elsewhere, the incidence of spread below the clavicle was fairly high—23 per cent—in autopsies on 240 cases of patients with head and neck cancer at Memorial Hospital (in the 1950s).

The mortality rate associated with neck dissection in Martin's hands was 1 to 2 per cent, compared with the early figures approaching 10 per cent before the days of antibiotics, transfusion, and airway control. His data (prior to TNM staging) supported therapeutic over elective neck dissection: the 5-year cure rate with neck dissection was about 33 per cent if metastasis was present on admission, whereas if metastasis developed subsequently, the cure rate was slightly higher—36 per cent. It is not possible to state accurately the value of neck dissection in controlling metastatic cervical disease from these early reports because the neck disease was not adequately quantified and the recurrence of tumor at the primary site was not always eliminated. These problems have continued to plague assessment of therapeutic neck control in many subsequent articles.

In 1954, a book on neck dissection was published with the stated attempt of disseminating information on the indications and technique of the operation more fully to the medical community.[26] These authors felt that the "wait and see" method had little to recommend it and presented serious practical disadvantages. Cases were cited in which patients initially without palpable nodes had developed large necrotic metastases 1 month later. Intuitively, these authors stated that if the surgeon waits until metastases are large enough to be palpable, some further dispersion will probably have occurred and the cure rate will be substantially less than if neck dissection had been done earlier. They also decried the philosophy of some head and neck surgeons who felt that neck dissection should never be done until the local lesion had been cured, for operable neck masses could become inoperable while awaiting complete regression of the local lesion from radiation or healing after operation. They also noted that on their service, when bilateral neck metastases were present, a RND was usually done on the more involved side, combined with a dissection on the opposite side sparing the internal jugular vein.

From this discussion, we can see that most, if not all, of the current concepts, practices, and debates in head and neck cancer surgery were in place in the 1920s—combination surgery and radiation therapy, elective versus therapeutic neck dissection, modified neck dissection, elective neck irradiation, pre- versus postoperative RT, effect on the immune response of lymph node removal, use of radium implants for residual neck disease, etc. Although technologic advances in surgery and RT have occurred, little of a truly revolutionary nature has since transpired in the treatment or conceptualization of head and neck cancer to alter this traditional armamentarium.

RELEVANT TUMOR BIOLOGY

Role of Regional Lymph Nodes in Tumor-Host Interactions

As we have seen, controversy over the decision to perform elective neck dissection has existed since neck dissections were first performed. In general, END has historically been considered an operation with *prophylactic* potential—the ability to prevent cancer dissemination. As we shall argue later, its true merit may, in fact, lie in its utility as a *biopsy* procedure that allows the identification of occult metastatic spread to the neck. In the context of a prophylactic maneuver, the need for and timing of END have been and still are controversial because the putative role of the regional lymph node (RLN) as a barrier to cancer spread and as a possible site of effective antitumor immune response is conjectural. Many experiments over the years have attempted to elucidate the role of the RLN as a particularly hostile or favorable site for tumor growth. Some experiments indicate that, once established in the lymphatic system, tumor growth is difficult or impossible to arrest, but others seem to show that lymph nodes (LNs) are the site of effective antitumor reactions. Some of the information in this section is abstracted from *Lymphatic System Metastasis*,[265] to which the reader is referred for in-depth discussion.

Lymphatic Anatomy

Because tumors have no primary lymphatics, cancer cells presumably gain access to the lymphatic system at the invasive tumor periphery through clefts between lymphatic endothelial cells. Lymphatic vessels are continuously contracting; actin-like filaments are observed in lymphatic endothelial cells. The afferent lymphatics join a marginal sinus in the cortex of individual LNs. When cells lodge in LNs, proliferation first occurs peripherally and later involves the medulla. From there, anastomosing channels penetrate the body of the node to form hilar efferent channels into which the marginal sinuses drain directly. The efferent channels from a group of nodes form lymphatic trunks that in turn form the three terminal collecting trunks—thoracic, subclavian, and right lymphatic ducts. The ducts drain into the venous system at the junctions of the internal jugular and subclavian veins. According to the traditional view, cancer cells in the lymphatic system can gain access to the blood stream only through these terminal collecting trunks at their junctions with major blood vessels.

Lymphaticovenous Communications

Many other lymphaticovenous (LV) communications exist, however. This is understandable because embryologically, lymphatics originate from buds of venous endothelium. Substances of varying sizes have been demonstrated to pass from lymphatics to veins within LNs, including red blood cells, tumor cells, and bacteria. Cells that enter lymphatics are transported to LNs in the afferent vessels and are deposited in peripheral subcapsular sinuses of the node, but subsequent processes are variable, based on the existence of LV anastomoses. Cancer cells may permanently lodge in the LNs, may traverse nodes taking egress by efferent lymphatics or through LV communications within nodes to become hematogenously disseminated, or may completely bypass LNs to enter the blood vascular system.[75, 76] Primary hematogenous spread may occur when cells gain access to small blood vessels in the tumor stroma; such vessels develop from existing host vessels, presumably as a response to tumor angiogenesis factor.[213] Blood-borne tumor cells may also traverse interstitial spaces, invade the lymphatics, and then disseminate via lymphatics.

Thus, in addition to the classical route from the afferent channels through the medulla to the efferent channels, cells may bypass the medulla by means of the marginal sinus or may enter the blood stream in the node. Additionally, LNs may be completely bypassed through collateral channels, although this route is enhanced by local obstruction to lymphatic flow caused by metastases or reactive LN hyperplasia, including sinus histiocytosis. Tumor cells can bypass the nearest regional nodes and proceed to more remote LNs. This phenomenon of "skip metastasis" is seen not infrequently in head and neck cancer patients. There is apparently no orderly progression down lymphatic chains and thence into the blood vascular system when lymphatic depots are saturated.

The many opportunities for lymphaticovenous, venous-lymphatic, and interlymphatic communication prevent any rigid discrimination between hematogenous and lymphogenous metastasis anatomically. This two-way intercommunication may well account for confused patterns of metastasis involving the two circulatory systems and argues against metastasis being confined to one or the other, except perhaps in early, subclinical cancer. The many routes for communication

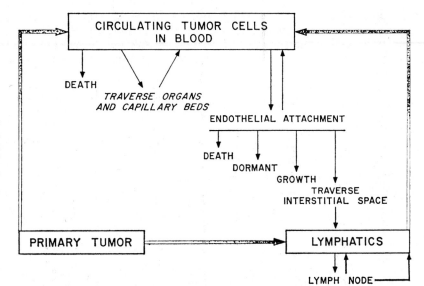

Figure 56–1. A unifying concept of tumor cell dissemination. (From Fisher B, Fisher ER: Significance of the interrelationship of the lymph and blood vascular systems in tumor cell dissemination. Prog Clin Cancer 4:84, 1970.)

between the two circulatory systems are diagrammed in Figures 56–1 and 56–2.

Although such LV communications exist, whether or not they are quantitatively significant under normal physiologic conditions is unknown. It is generally thought that these channels are probably relatively dormant until called into action by imbalance in intra-

vascular pressure precipitated by mechanical obstruction. LV shunts have been reported in lymphatic obstruction and inflammatory states and by lymphographic studies at autopsy. Obstruction is not mandatory, however, for such shunts have been noted in patients with a patent lymphatic system.[237] Reversal of lymph flow can be easily produced; retrograde flow of

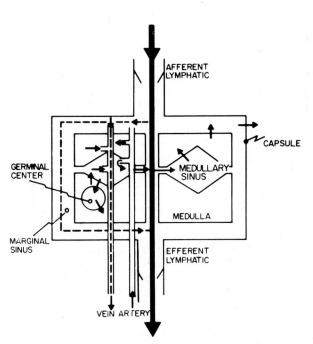

The possible flow patterns of cancer cells through lymph nodes. In addition to the classical route from the afferent channels through the medulla to the efferent channels, cells may bypass the medulla by means of the marginal sinus and also be carried in the blood stream to and from lymph nodes. Additional pathways are indicated by small arrows.

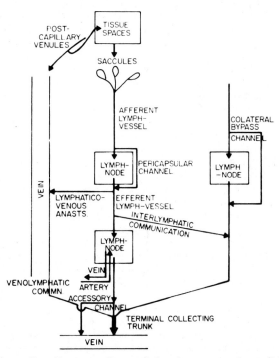

The possible traffic patterns of cancer cells from tissue spaces, or intermediate ports of entry, to the venous system by way of a terminal collecting trunk. Lymph nodes may be completely bypassed through collateral channels, or partially bypassed through the pericapsular channel. There are many opportunities for lymphaticovenous, venolymphatic, and interlymphatic communication.

Figure 56–2. Communication route between circulatory systems. (From Weiss L: The pathophysiology of metastasis within the lymphatic system. *In* Weiss L, et al (eds.): Lymphatic System Metastasis. Boston, G. K. Hall Medical Publishers, 1980, p. 2.)

lymph is enhanced, and "filtering" efficiency of LNs is decreased by inflammation, fibrosis from radiation, and tumor growth within them. Tumor emboli are able to disseminate through existing or opened anastomoses or in newly formed collateral channels.

Lymphatic Metastasis: The Filter-Barrier Concept

Whereas in some animal models LNs apparently serve as temporary filters for cancer cells, this original filter-barrier concept of lymphatic metastasis is not as compelling now as previously. One study showed that, experimentally, tumor cells easily passed through LNs even when they were filled with metastatic tumor.[146] In another experiment, a rabbit model was used to study the role of cervical LNs as a barrier to the spread of cancer.[6] Rabbits injected intravenously with V-2 carcinoma cells invariably died of pulmonary metastases, whereas intralymphatic injection of tumor cells was not always fatal, and the RLNs were thought capable of containing tumor for a variable period of time. In animals who had had a previous unilateral neck dissection, those receiving intravenous tumor cells all died within 28 to 35 days, whereas those receiving intralymphatic injections did not routinely die of multiple lung metastases. Tumor arrest within a LN occurred in less than 50 per cent of animals, and the ability to contain tumor within the node decreased with time. The fact that animals who had had neck dissection did almost as well as those with an intact cervical lymphatic system could be taken as evidence against any efficient and effective barrier system provided by the RLNs. The fact that RND did not significantly reduce the variable barrier effect was attributed by the authors, however, to the assumption of such activity by small regenerated lymphatic vessels and nodes in the dissected side of the neck or by the intact nodes in the contralateral side of the neck.

After neck dissection it is more likely that persisting RLN function is subserved by LNs not removed during operation, and regeneration of small lymphatic follicles probably occurs only in young animals. Rouvière[205] states that LNs do not regenerate postoperatively in human adults.

The filter-barrier hypothesis proposes that RLNs serve as mechanical and biologic filters in which phagocytosis assists the more mechanical phase of particulate trapping. By analogy with phagocytosis of particulate material such as India ink, first used to demonstrate the function of LNs, cells were also assumed to be susceptible to the same trapping mechanisms. Most studies deal only with the mechanical aspect of lymphatic barrier function, and the relationship between this and the biologic role of the RLN is not elucidated.

In various studies it has been shown that cancer cells can traverse nodes that themselves remain free of tumor, implying that the node is an ineffective barrier. Fisher and Fisher reported that nodes were able to trap 90 per cent of infused red blood cells and 40 per cent of V-2 carcinoma cells. The nodes did not become saturated.[75] Other studies have found that the greater the number of cells injected, the greater the passage through the node. Intermediate studies have shown that nodes are potential barriers to infused tumor cells for only a

limited time—approximately 3 weeks. Thereafter, the tumor cells are no longer effectively retained.[63, 176, 273] In one study,[108] as the primary tumor increased in size, the number of cells in the nodes remained constant. The authors concluded that the nodes had a reasonably constant holding capacity and that above such a threshold, all other tumor cells passed on into efferent channels and the general circulation.

In most experimental animal models used to investigate the filter function of the RLN, normal nodes have been subjected to an influx of a large number of tumor cells—a situation that may not be at all analogous to the requirements of the RLN in the early stages of clinical cancer spread in humans. Additionally, studies that inject particulate material or cells can create high pressures and artifacts in nodal function.

Spread of Carcinomas versus Sarcomas

What about the traditional teaching that carcinomas spread by the lymphatics and mesodermal tumors spread via the blood stream? Although it may appear clinically that *detectable* metastases are limited to one or the other system, at best this applies to comparatively early cancer. In fact, based on the anatomy discussed previously, metastases to *both* circulatory systems are *probably occurring simultaneously*, and the apparent separation may relate to the fact that it is easier to identify growing metastases in superficial, clinically palpable LNs than it is to detect similar growth in deep viscera when such metastases have arrived there via the blood stream.

An early step in the metastatic process is the detachment of cancer cells or clusters of cells from their parent tumors; clusters have better chances of survival than single cells. Single cancer cells tend to enter the blood or lymphatic systems equally, whereas cell clumps are more restricted to entering blood vessels than the smaller lymphatic channels. Because of intimacy with their own blood supply, sarcomas have a better chance than carcinomas of gaining early access to blood channels, and with their comparatively lower thrombogenic activity, they have less chance of being held up by intravascular thrombosis than carcinoma cells. Sarcomas also preferentially separate as multicellular units rather than as single cells. This would promote their survival in the blood stream and would tend to hinder their access to lymphatic systems. Conversely, the greater tendency of carcinomas to release single cells would favor early direct lymphatic spread. Such mechanical considerations may provide the explanation of the often observed tendency of carcinomas to metastasize to RLNs at a comparatively early stage of their development, whereas sarcomas at a similar stage are usually considered to spread more often by the hematogenous route, although hematogenous and lymphogenous metastases are not distinct processes.

Role of the Regional Lymph Node in the Immune Response to Tumors: Breast Cancer

Having established that the RLNs are not simple mechanical barriers that prevent dissemination of tumor cells, we are still left with the question of their functional role in initiating immune responses (ImR) that may be detrimental to cancer growth. George Crile, Jr., was among the first to offer evidence in support of the theory that the RLNs are vital in the containment of cancer. In animal experiments,[45] he showed that in mice bearing tumor in one hindfoot, removal or irradiation of the popliteal nodes between the fourth and tenth days after implantation resulted not only in decreased resistance to tumor reimplantation but also in an increased susceptibility to pulmonary metastases. Removal of the nodes after the tenth day had no demonstrable effect. Similarly, in another system, removal of RLNs shortly after a primary graft of tumor led to increased metastasis, whereas removal of nodes when the tumor was clinically detectable (approximately 10^{10} cells) had no discernible influence.[186]

The widely accepted implication of such experiments in the aggregate is that the RLNs are important in the host defense against early cancer growth, during which time they help potentiate systemic immunity, but that RLNs are defunct when the tumor burden increases. The relevance of such observations to an autologous, spontaneous human tumor system is uncertain. They certainly cannot necessarily be used to support retention or removal of LNs in patients, who by definition always have a clinically detectable tumor. Crile's experiments were criticized by Hammond and Rolley[96] because of the use of homologous tumors without demonstrable immunogenicity (with nonimmunogenic tumors the function of RLNs could not be explained on an immunologic basis) and because of failure to provide histologic evidence of tumor metastases or reimplantation. Using data from their own animal models, these authors showed that the presence or absence of RLNs had no discernable effect upon the ability to mount a primary response to inoculated immunogenic tumor or on the development of metastases or local wound recurrences, and the time of tumor removal was more important in achieving tumor control than the status of the RLNs.

Crile, Jr. believed that removal of uninvolved RLNs was detrimental to the ability of the host to control tumor growth and dissemination, and he stressed the importance of preserving the RLNs to improve cancer control unless these nodes were invaded by tumor. He studied immunologic reactivity of lymphocytes in the RLNs of breast cancer patients with a variety of in vitro tests. It was shown that regional lymphocytes reacted, provided that there was no nodal tumor involvement. In addition, the nodal lymphocytes showed more interaction with tumor cells than peripheral blood lymphocytes from the same patient.[44–47, 55]

On the basis of his experiments, Crile, Jr. challenged the classic concept of en bloc resection of primary breast cancer with its regional lymphatics and advocated subtotal mastectomy with preservation of the RLNs. Clinical studies at the Cleveland Clinic demonstrated a significantly increased 5-year survival rate when the nodes were left in situ in early breast cancer patients when compared with survival of patients undergoing radical mastectomies. Such results seemed to confirm Crile's hypothesis. With longer follow-up, the concept that axillary LNs exert an antitumor effect in early breast cancer has been criticized because the results of simple mastectomy in which the nodes are left intact are not better than those following radical mastectomy in which they are removed. This conflicting data can be explained

by the fact that it is not possible to tell whether or not the LNs contain cancer unless they are removed. Some patients undergoing simple mastectomy do harbor cancer in their LNs, whereas others do not—the latter group is expected to have a better prognosis. On the other hand, negative clinical observations of this type do not give information on any retarding effects of RLNs on cancer up to the time of surgical intervention. Similar considerations are relevant to the continuing controversy over END for head and neck cancers.

More recently, cell-surface markers have been used to detect a decrease in antibody-dependent cellular cytotoxicity in RLNs of breast cancer patients, and it was concluded that the data argued against a major tumor defense mechanism located in the draining LNs of breast cancer patients at the time of clinical diagnosis.[104] Reiss and associates[196] used a reproducible blast assay to study the role of the RLN in breast cancer and to compare nodal and systemic reactivity. Preliminary results indicated that with a very small tumor mass, immune activity existed in the RLNs when none was seen peripherally. As the tumor burden increased, the nodes began to exhibit suppression, and the peripheral lymphocytes became stimulated. Finally, with a large tumor mass, suppression was seen peripherally as well, suggesting that no major immunologic defense barrier was being breached when a LN dissection was performed in patients with a small tumor burden. Interestingly, the nodes farthest from the tumor were more stimulated than those closer to the tumor. There seemed to be an increasing involvement of systemic immunity and progressive suppression of the local immune response as the tumor burden increased.

Role of the Regional Lymph Node in the Immune Response to Tumors: Head and Neck Cancer

Schuller[214] has recently presented similar work concerning the immunologic capability of lymphocytes from cervical LNs. He attempted to characterize the regional immunologic defense provided by cervical LNs in head and neck cancer patients. An incredibly efficient in vitro clonogenic stem cell assay was used to examine tumor-lymphocyte interactions for each of 104 patients. Because the number of tumor colonies resulting from the tumor-lymphocyte mixtures differed significantly from the colony counts when tumor was grown alone, it was concluded that some type of interaction was definitely occurring between extracted RLN lymphocytes and single-cell tumor suspensions. The numbers of patients showing a reduction *or* increase in the colony counts were comparable—in other words, tumor growth was enhanced as often as it was suppressed. Interestingly, there was no difference between lymphocytes arising from any node group in the neck, showing that lymphocytes from nodes close to the primary tumor had comparable immunoreactive capabilities to lymphocytes from more distant RLNs.

The group of patients studied appeared to be unusually immunocompetent, and a number of the usual tests of systemic immune competence yielded normal results. A comparison between regional and systemic immunoreactivity showed that the helper:suppressor T-cell ratios in the nodes were generally higher than those in the serum. Unfortunately, inadequate length of follow-up did not allow correlation of this data with the patient's survival status at the time of this report.

Statistical analysis showed no difference in the neck-nodal immunoreactivity between previously untreated patients and those with recurrent disease or between patients currently free of disease when compared with those with disease. The lack of difference in results related to the patient's tumor-bearing status was taken to indicate that the regional neck nodes are capable of mounting an ImR regardless of the patient's tumor status—even in the presence of recurrent carcinoma.

The general conclusion was that dynamic interaction does occur when tumor emboli encounter lymphocytes within the RLNs of head and neck cancer patients. This study raises a number of questions with respect to experimental design, and some of the results conflict with similar studies using different tumor systems; but the author is reasonably careful not to extrapolate beyond the data, and the study certainly represents a step in the right direction with respect to obtaining scientifically based information that eventually may help to guide treatment policies for head and neck cancer patients.

Role of the Regional Lymph Node in the Immune Response to Tumors: Promoter or Inhibitor?

With any in vitro model it is not possible to assess the relevance of results to the in vivo situation, which is influenced by other intact tumor-host influences. For example, some of the lymphocytes extracted from LNs might have been "passing through," and their presence in the assay could influence the results of the test, whereas in vivo their relevance to the tumor-host interaction is unknown. Also, conclusions reached about immune reactivity vary with the assay used, and there is still little standardization. It is likely that many experimental tumor metastasis models are irrelevant artifacts of in vivo human tumor growth, and normal laboratory animals may not be appropriate for the study of the complexities of the malignant process. Human tumors appear to more closely approximate weakly immunogenic animal tumors rather than the highly antigenic tumors that are capable of eliciting true transplantation rejection and are more commonly used in experimental tumor studies.

Current majority opinion seems to feel that although the RLN could be important for the initiation of immunity, the effect probably depends on the antigenicity of the tumor under study. The RLNs seem relatively more important in the initiation of systemic immunity to weakly antigenic tumors than to strongly antigenic tumors. It is also felt that the properties of the tumor cells *per se*, rather than the filtration capacity of the LNs, may determine whether neoplastic cells are trapped. Unfortunately, it is currently impossible by any diagnostic means to detect the conversion from the N0 to the occult N+ node.

To date, the role of the RLN has not been fully defined, and conflicting experimental and clinical studies perpetuate controversies. Is the RLN, by virtue of its location, important in conferring antitumor immunity, and if so, does the tumor maintain any immunologic stimulation in the host by the time it becomes clinically detectable?

One side of the argument maintains that RLNs are not simple mechanical barriers that prevent dissemination of tumor cells but rather are organs essential to the initiation of immune responses. An intact lymphatic system constitutes the afferent limb that is necessary before a demonstrable immune response is initiated. The LNs provide the appropriate environment for development of immunologically reactive cells in the host. Effector cells then migrate through the blood stream to needed sites to express host defense. On the other hand, Wilson and Billingham[269] have demonstrated that the ImR is not exclusively generated in the regional nodes. With removal of RLNs, new pathways involve distant LNs that would not otherwise have taken part in the reaction, and the surgical removal of local nodes does not significantly reduce the primary ImR. Recirculating small lymphocytes spread activity from regional to distant nodes and are as effective in transferring immunity as the RLNs per se. Thus, the lymphocytic response is a systemic one and is not strictly limited to the LNs that drain the tumor site.

Although some evidence suggests that significant tumor cell destruction is possible in RLNs, other data from different model systems indicates that the LN does not significantly impair or retard tumor dissemination. For example, it has been shown that the dose of immunogenic tumor cells needed for successful growth in the rodent LN is lower than the dose required for "take" in the rodent footpad, suggesting some degree of immunologic privilege for tumor growth in the fertile soil of the RLN. The occurrence of large nodal metastases with very small or undetectable primary tumors (seen in about 10 per cent of head and neck cancer patients) also suggests that the RLN may be an ideal environment for cancer cell proliferation rather than destruction.

Current work on the reactivity of RLNs to human cancers is incomplete. There have been relatively few studies on the immunologic reactivity of RLNs of cancer patients to their own tumors. Some work shows that tumor-draining LNs may contain lymphocytes that are cytotoxic to cancer cells, as detected by in vitro chromium-51 cytotoxicity tests,[260] or the nodes may be anergic with respect to inhibiting tumor cell growth.[172, 260] It is imprudent at present to make any general or sweeping statements without reference to specific cancers and their hosts. Part of the difficulty in using human material to elucidate the biologic behavior of cancer cells is that small, clinically detectable, presumably early cancers may be late lesions from a biologic viewpoint in terms of host response. Although animal and in vitro models are subject to several major criticisms, exclusive use of human data provides limited insights into the basic mechanisms involved in the extremely complex process of metastasis.

Pertinent Tumor Immunology

Although the function of lymphoid tissue in the cellular and humoral defense against infection is well appreciated, its role against tumor cells is a matter of controversy. The early experimental and clinical work on the pros and cons of elective node dissection evolved during the late 1960s and 1970s when evidence in favor of "immunologic surveillance" was being accumulated. Work in the past decade has shown that the concept of host regulation of neoplasia is extremely complex and that the original immune surveillance hypothesis is simplistic, based on current understanding. A tremendous information explosion concerning the ImR has shown that many cells and cell-free factors are involved in a complex regulatory mechanism subject to positive and negative feedback modulation akin to that of the endocrine system.

The capability to clone T-cells can now provide pure populations of individual cell types that can be studied for lymphokine production and function. Similarly, the ability to produce in vitro large quantities of pure antibodies of restricted specificity (monoclonal) through techniques of cell hybridization (initially reported in 1975 by Kohler and Milstein[131] and acknowledged this year with the Nobel Prize) has proved of great practical and theoretic use to basic as well as to applied clinical research.[17, 32]

Cancer cell survival or death in the RLN is unlikely to be an all-or-none phenomenon. Destruction of tumor cells probably can occur in LNs, but only when the tumor burden is low. The mechanism of this destruction is not certain but may involve cells with immunologic reactivity. There are several candidates. T-lymphocytes account for about 85 per cent of circulating lymphocytes (lcs) and are the predominant lymphocyte population within a node. Several T-cell subpopulations have been defined: "helper" T-cells potentiate antibody production by B-cells, and "suppressor" T-cells can suppress B-cell antibody production. A current area of active investigation is the role of the host suppressor T-cells in antitumor regulation.[25, 170] A patient's peripheral blood may simultaneously contain cytotoxic and suppressor T-cells, and suppressor cells have the potential to decrease the cytotoxic reactions of other lymphoid populations and thus the potential to enhance tumor growth. Prostaglandins also act as suppressor factors pharmacologically and have been shown to be produced by both host and tumor cells.[23] Efforts to abrogate suppressor T-cell function form a major thrust in current basic tumor research.

Lymphocytes also have the ability to secrete a variety of immunoreactive substances called lymphokines, including the interleukins. Macrophages are also involved. The fact that a large number of nonspecific compounds can activate macrophages has led to the clinical use of nonspecific immunostimulants, such as bacillus Calmette Guérin (BCG), as adjuvants to conventional therapy.

There is evidence that after exposure of a RLN to an antigenic tumor, T-lymphocytes are specifically sensitized and probably activate macrophages through lymphokines. Recirculation of long-lived T-cells can bring distant LNs into the ImR. Evidence for the tumoricidal role of LN macrophages comes from studies showing favorable prognoses in breast cancer patients with sinus histiocytosis and the "starry sky" pattern in Burkitt's lymphoma in which phagocytic macrophages contain remnants of destroyed cancer cells and which has been associated with regression of LN metastases.[201] Eccles and Alexander[61] have stressed the inverse relationship between the percentage of macrophages infiltrating a tumor bed and the incidence of metastases. Decreased

activation of macrophages has also been correlated with an increase in metastasis.[19]

"Natural killer" (NK) cells, a type of nonadherent cell that is nonspecifically active against tumor cells without prior exposure to them, possibly have great importance in LN defense against tumor. It is currently not known whether NK cells are an important component of tumor rejection because normal NK activity has been found in many cancer patients with early disease, and other paradoxes remain to be resolved. Characterization of NK cell identity and in vivo activity is undergoing intensive investigation.[179]

In any event, immunologic activity of several types of LN cells to autochthonous tumors has been demonstrated by various means and is being increasingly addressed in head and neck cancer publications. It may be more relevant to study tissue-bound or intratumoral cells than their peripheral blood counterparts in an attempt to learn how these cells function in the area of the tumor, which may be completely different from the periphery. The mere morphologic finding of a particular cell type in a LN does not indicate what it is doing there, however. For example, with infected head and neck tumors, events in the RLNs are difficult to relate to specific antitumor activity as opposed to an inflammatory reaction to the contaminating organisms. Responses in the RLNs of cancer patients may well be an index of the host's general reaction to a tumor rather than a specific local record of the interactions of LN cells with cancer cells. It is currently almost impossible to discriminate between local and general events in humans, as it is not known which parameters of the ImR are relevant with respect to in vivo function. The response of LN cells to cancer may also change over time and vary based on location with respect to the tumor.

Experiments of Fisher and Fisher[76] using mouse mammary carcinoma and fibrosarcomas showed that local LNs could exhibit antitumor activity in vivo and in vitro, whereas distant uninvolved LNs did not. As the disease progressed and the animals became moribund, nodal antitumor activity was lost diffusely. The concept emerged that metastases in these animals resulted when the cytotoxic capability of their RLNs decreased. Nodal metastases may be less able than primary tumors to enhance an ImR by way of other nodes regional to them because of deficiencies in the efferent arm of the ImR. These depleted or deficient nodes could then become fertile soil for metastatic growth.

The transition from the reactive to the ineffectual LN is not easily explained; however, several possibilities exist which are not mutually exclusive. Acute-phase proteins from the host (mainly sialoglycoproteins) are known to be nonspecifically immunosuppressive by binding to and masking the reactive sites on lymphocytes and macrophages. Immunosuppressive polypeptides liberated directly from the tumor have been described. Specific blocking factors, generally tumor-associated antigens and tumor antigen-host antibody complexes, have been shown to block the reactivity of cytotoxic lymphoid cells in vitro and could do so directly in the node. Blocking factors could also exert a systemic effect by eliciting specific suppressor T-cells. Surface antigens shed from cancer cells that reach RLNs might enhance immunogenesis or shed antigen-antibody complexes could induce immunologic tolerance. The same antigen given under different conditions may produce humoral or cellular immunity.

"Lymph node paralysis,"[103] in which immunocompetent cells are trapped within tumor-draining LNs, is an example of a "sanctuary" site in which tumor cells can escape complement- and antibody-mediated lysis and effector cells. Antigen released by early tumors may attract specifically reactive cells to draining LNs, and although a proportion of these may circulate in the peripheral blood, continued local exposure to high tumor antigen doses can result in saturation of specifically reactive cell receptors and tolerance in the local ImR of the cells remaining in the node. The existence of LN paralysis can render LNs that are not directly involved with metastatic tumor functionally incompetent, although more distant nodes could respond normally to tumor antigens.

RLN "paralysis" was described by Currie and Alexander[49] with rat sarcomas and appears to have depended on an intense local release of soluble tumor antigens and could be due to either pre-emption of binding sites, elicitation of systemic suppressors, or both.

It is difficult to extrapolate answers from experimental models of metastasis in which the sudden subcutaneous injection of a large number of tumor cells could overwhelm host defense mechanisms. In the human situation, metastasis is known to occur by embolization of single tumor cells or small cell clumps. Progressive slow release of antigen could lead to immunologic tolerance in the RLNs during the processes of tumor cell attachment and circulatory arrest. Small tumor emboli could be more vulnerable to host defenses than larger (experimentally induced) tumor masses.

Significance of Cancer in the Regional Lymph Node

The fate of tumor cells in RLNs is probably variable. Small numbers of retained cancer cells can indeed give rise to tumors within LNs; however, this is not an invariable result. Hewitt and Blake[108] studied a nonimmunogenic squamous cell carcinoma of mice and found that spontaneous nodal metastases rarely occurred, although the regional nodes contained viable tumor cells detected by bioassay. The presence of cancer cells in LNs does not mean that they represent functionally implanted metastases. At the time of node dissection and histologic fixation, some visible cancer cells may be artificially arrested; in vivo this might have continued into the efferent lymph, where they would be subject to further rigors in completing the metastatic process successfully. The presence of a cancer cell in a node does not elucidate its functional status. Such a cell might undergo mitosis to become an overt metastasis, it might remain dormant for an indefinite period, or it could undergo degeneration. A clinically and histologically positive LN unambiguously indicates that tumor cells reached the node and grew there. A LN may be negative, however, because cancer cells never reached it or because they entered the node but were not retained or were destroyed. It is also well known that the more carefully metastases in LNs are sought in surgical specimens, the more often they will be found. Evidence from animal studies shows that tumor cells not detected histologically in LNs were found by bioassay.[208]

Lack of knowledge concerning the significance of occult cancer in LNs causes continuing controversy in the treatment of solid tumor systems, and therefore, the therapeutic or prophylactic significance of elective treatment to the neck is impossible to decide at present. Currently, occult disease can be detected only in a removed LN dissection specimen. Once removed, such occult disease is obviously not available to evolve further in vivo. Hence, its ultimate significance is impossible to define directly. The problem here is our current inability to detect and follow subclinical LN involvement by tumor in a noninvasive way.

Clinical Significance of Occult Nodal Cancer

The prophylactic advantage offered by elective node treatment is based on the assumption that LNs not only are ineffective barriers to tumor cells but also act as a source of further cancer dissemination. Considerable controversy has surrounded whether or not LN metastases can themselves act as generalizing sites that significantly contribute to a higher incidence of distant metastases (DMs). The same types of invasive histologic features that are seen at the periphery of primary tumors are also seen at the periphery of metastatic deposits. Several types of animal experiments, including those on parabiotic systems,[110, 130] have indicated that metastases can indeed serve as a source for further dissemination. Fidler's work also shows that metastatic lesions do have the ability to metastasize.[67] This question cannot be definitively answered in humans because it is not possible to rule out distant dormant cells (which originate from the primary tumor) as a metastatic tumor source. These cells could be reactivated and could metastasize via the blood or lymph.

The metastatic spread of head and neck tumors was analyzed by Viadana[251] in terms of this so-called "cascade" phenomenon, using data from 371 autopsy cases. The statistical significance of the association of metastases at two sites in each patient was evaluated in terms of the Chi square test applied to contingency tables. The test was run again on contingency tables with and without metastases at a third site to determine whether metastases at the third site affected the occurrence of metastases at the other two. The results indicated that the cervical LNs and lungs indeed act as generalizing sites for head and neck cancers and can thus play an important role in systemic dissemination. Of course, there are problems in reaching such a conclusion from an autopsy study because it is not known whether or not occult metastatic deposits would have become clinically significant during the patient's lifetime. Also, Viadana's statistics have been critically evaluated[39] and were found to not prove the point. Alternate conclusions can explain the findings as well as those proposed. Therefore, although it has been shown unequivocally in experimental systems that metastases can metastasize, whether or not this phenomenon is *clinically* significant from positive LNs, in the face of simultaneous hematogenous spread, is not answered by statistical analysis of autopsy studies.

Breast Cancer As a Model for Head and Neck Carcinoma

Because answers to these basic questions are not forthcoming from the head and neck cancer literature, other solid tumor systems that metastasize to LNs were reviewed in search of analogies that might prove illuminating to the controversial issues concerning the clinical relevance of the RLN. A series of consecutive studies on breast cancer provides an example of rational application of scientific information derived from the laboratory applied to a clinical cancer situation to test new hypotheses. Using information derived from experiments started in the late 1950s on animal models of metastasis, Bernard (a surgeon) and Edwin (a pathologist) Fisher and their coworkers developed several theories of metastasis which differed from those that guided the cancer surgeons of the late 1800s and early 1900s in performing radical en bloc resections of primary tumors with their draining lymphatics.

Halsted's Influence

By way of background, during the late 1800s Halsted embarked on the task of perfecting an extensive surgical approach to breast cancer aimed at decreasing an inordinately high incidence of local recurrence that was observed by the surgeons of his era. This procedure was based on the assumption that breast cancer metastasized only by contiguous spread and through the lymphatics—he did not appreciate the capacity of cancer to spread via the blood stream. He carried breast cancer operations to what now seems like ridiculous extremes—with resection of the humoral head and iliac wing—in an attempt to remove every cancer cell. His operative procedure was developed largely from experience with patients who had advanced bulky tumors, which was then the most common form of first presentation.

Halsted succeeded in achieving his desired hygienic effect accompanied by a previously unequaled control of local recurrence and late regional recurrences. The trend to attempt to improve cancer cure rates by developing progressively more radical operations resulted in the ultraradical cancer operations of the 1940s and 1950s, which extended cancer surgery to its anatomic limits. Unfortunately, with few exceptions, these more radical procedures did not significantly increase cure rates, and the cure of common neoplasms treated surgically has not changed much during the past 30 to 40 years, although patients with solid tumors who are "cured" generally have had surgery as part of their treatment program. It eventually became apparent that the Halsted radical mastectomy did not enhance survival in patients presenting with a small tumor—these patients are currently in the majority.

Nevertheless, the surgical community was so strongly influenced by Halsted that it was to take nearly half a century for investigators to re-evaluate the validity of his surgical strategy. Treatments had their basis in medical tradition rather than in testing through clinical trials until 1952. A similar scientific basis for clinical trials has been delayed for an additional 30 years for head and neck cancer, and the recent trend toward acceptance of this strategy has been introduced not by surgeons but by the participation of chemotherapists in multimodality treatment protocols for advanced head and neck cancer patients.

Clinical Breast Cancer Trials

Table 56–1 contrasts the traditional concepts of metastasis with the "alternate hypothesis" of the Fishers. They sought a clinical system that would allow testing of the alternate hypothesis, and early breast cancer appeared to meet the necessary criteria. After 10 years of planning, a consecutive series of well-designed, scientifically based, randomized prospective clinical trials were initiated and have yielded much valuable information on the significance of the RLN and tumor biology; this data can serve as a model for answering similar questions in head and neck and other solid tumors. The results recently have been summarized.[73, 78]

In the first trial, started in the early 1970s under the auspices of the National Surgical Adjuvant Breast Project (NSABP), patients with early breast cancer without clinical evidence of regional lymphadenopathy were randomized to receive radical mastectomy (RM), total (simple) mastectomy (TM), or total mastectomy plus

TABLE 56–1. Two Divergent Hypotheses of Tumor Biology

Halstedian	Alternative
Tumors spread in an orderly defined manner based upon mechanical consideration	There is no orderly pattern of tumor cell dissemination.
Tumor cells traverse lymphatics to lymph nodes by direct extension supporting en bloc dissection	Tumor cells traverse lymphatics by embolization challenging the merit of en bloc dissection.
The positive lymph node is an indicator of tumor spread and is the instigator of distant disease	The positive lymph node is an indicator of a host-tumor relationship which permits development of metastases rather than being the instigator of distant disease.
Regional lymph nodes (RLNs) are barriers to the passage of tumor cells	Regional lymph nodes are ineffective as barriers to tumor cell spread.
RLNs are of anatomic importance	RLNs are of biologic importance.
The blood stream is of little significance as a route of tumor dissemination	The blood stream is of considerable importance in tumor dissemination.
A tumor is autonomous of its host	Complex host-tumor interrelationships affect every facet of the disease.
Operable breast cancer is a local-regional disease.	Operable breast cancer is a systemic disease.
The extent and nuances of operation are the dominant factors influencing patient outcome	Variations in local-regional therapy are unlikely to substantially affect survival.

Source: Modified from Fisher B et al: The contribution of recent NSABP clinical trials of primary breast cancer therapy to an understanding of tumor biology—An overview of findings. Cancer 46:1009, 1980.

postoperative local-regional radiation (TM + RT). At 5 years, the incidence of distant disease in the three groups (those who had nodes removed, irradiated, or untreated) was similar. The time from operation to the detection of distant disease in each circumstance was not appreciably different. Overall survival of the three clinically node-negative groups did not differ significantly in frequency or in time from operation to death, indicating that the presence or absence of distant disease more closely correlated with patient survival than did the initial treatment failure site. (It is mandatory that the incidence of any distant disease following local-regional failure be included as an end point of patient response to therapy.)

In the clinically node-positive patients, there was no significant difference between those receiving RM and those with TM + RT with respect to total treatment failure, local-regional or distant treatment failure, or survival. Whereas the combination of surgery and radiation apparently reduced local recurrence, tumor-free survival was not appreciably affected. Although some patients who had TM alone required subsequent axillary dissection for delayed nodal appearance, these patients fared no worse than those in whom the axilla was treated initially.

The similarities in distant disease and survival rates and the relatively small increase in local-regional disease following TM compared to that following RM in node-negative patients were remarkable, considering that 40 per cent of the RM patients were found to have histologically positive nodes in the removed axillary contents. Because the treatment groups were equivalent with respect to all parameters available for comparison owing to the prospective randomized format, it was expected that approximately 40 per cent of women subjected to TM alone also had positive nodes that were untreated. Based on Halstedian concepts, such retained positive nodes could serve as a source of further tumor dissemination, resulting in an increase in distant treatment failure, and yet patients who underwent TM alone had about the same incidence of distant disease and survival! Survival and recurrence in more than 2000 patients were independent of the number of axillary nodes removed. (General clinical practice currently includes routine axillary dissection mainly to serve as a basis for selecting patients for adjuvant treatment.)

Findings from a later NSABP protocol and a similar large trial undertaken at the Tumor Institute of Milan[73] showed that in pathologically node-positive patients who had had RM and then received one, two, or three chemotherapeutic agents there was a significant increase in the disease-free interval over that observed in patients receiving no chemotherapy. This was the first evidence of the ability of adjuvant systemic treatment to change the natural history of a solid tumor in humans.

The Regional Lymph Node As an Indicator, not Instigator, of Metastatic Cancer

Thus, from the work of the Fishers and the NSABP we see a different significance attached to the RLN as an *indicator* of the ability of the primary tumor to metastasize rather than as an *instigator* of distant metastases per se. Although one cannot exclude a contribution to distant metastases from a regional lymph node source, the NSABP trial results indicate that this phenomenon may not be *clinically* significant.

According to the alternate hypothesis, a poor prognosis is associated with positive LNs not because the LNs themselves act as generalizing sites or because disease in them kills the patient but rather because RLN involvement indicates a host condition that permits development of metastases in general, not only in the RLNs but in the viscera as well. The quantitative amount of LN involvement is regarded as an indirect index of the severity of the disease in disseminated sites (systemic tumor burden), although the most important prognostic feature is the presence or absence of cancer in LNs. Except for indicating possibly a longer time before recurrence, one or a few positive nodes in this context are as ominous as many.

If one accepts this rationale, then removal of LNs serves as a *biopsy staging procedure* to ascertain the presence or absence of metastases and, by extension, the risk of visceral involvement, which defines high-risk patients who might benefit from systemic adjuvant therapy. Regional lymphadenectomy is *not* a prophylactic measure that prevents disease dissemination and cures the patient, for cancer cells continuously disseminate via *both* the lymphatic system and the blood stream, and spread has probably already occurred. One Fisher analogy is that local therapy aimed at LNs alone will no more effectively control DMs than removal of the speedometer of a car will reduce its speed.

Because a large proportion of women operated upon for breast cancer develop metastatic disease regardless of the extent of surgery, it is apparent that the disease is often systemic at the time of surgery. In these cases, surgical therapy has limited effect on survival, although its utility in local palliation and hygienic control of disease should not be underestimated. These results have led to the growing opinion that tumor-free survival depends upon the biology of the tumor present at operation and not upon the extent of operation. The innate virulence of the neoplasm balanced against whatever defense reactions are excited in the host constitute a biologic complex that determines the natural history of the process in the individual cancer patient.[145]

Although surgical treatment of clinically positive nodes remains unchallenged, there is now reason to believe that excision of occult nodal metastases does not contribute to cure. By analogy, elective neck dissection for head and neck cancer patients, based on the presumed presence in some of occult disease in the neck, would not be expected to be a useful therapeutic maneuver in decreasing metastatic capability. This surgical conservatism is not meant to suggest that wide resection of primary tumors is no longer important, for ceasing to attempt to obtain negative margins would invite local recurrence. Adequate local-regional treatment is essential in head and neck cancer, which tends to be locally aggressive, and the reader should not construe this discussion to favor "lumpectomy" for primary head and neck cancers.

The NSABP findings help explain why patients with positive LNs have at least a 50 per cent decreased chance of survival compared with those with uninvolved LNs. These explanations may well apply generally to solid tumor systems that exhibit lymphatic metastasis regardless of the histologic tumor type, but they need to be confirmed in each system independently to encompass the possibly unique features of tumors of different sites and histologic type. With respect to head and neck squamous cell carcinoma (SCC), the explanation for this dismal prognosis has historically been attributed to deaths related to the presence of disease in the neck per se, resulting in such events as carotid hemorrhage. Uncontrolled disease in the neck generally accompanies uncontrolled local disease and occurs as an isolated phenomenon more rarely. Especially in recent years, with better local-regional disease control, this cause of death has greatly decreased, and patients are living longer, exhibiting a new cause of death (or possibly unmasking the natural history of successfully treated local-regional disease)—the development of DMs. Thus, it may be more correct to view head and neck SCC as a systemic disease rather than as the local-regional process that has traditionally been used to support the efficacy of Halstedian surgical oncologic principles.

Solid Malignancy As a Systemic Disease: Implications Relevant to Elective Lymphadenectomy

It is being recognized that systemic dissemination can occur early in many cancers, and the systemic aspects of neoplastic growth are currently in central focus—a full circle return to the time of Galen, when cancer was regarded as a surgically incurable systemic disease. Nevertheless, there undoubtedly is variation among different tumor systems, and it is probably an incorrect overreaction to regard all cancer as a systemic disease from the inception of the primary tumor. Many surgeons resist this aspect of the "alternate hypothesis" because they have personal experience with having "cured" patients who had regional nodal involvement, and they have seen death from systemic disease in patients without LN involvement. The question they ask is, "If cancer is a systemic disease, how can anyone ever be cured?" That people are apparently cured of advanced cancer is not an indictment of the alternate hypothesis, but merely a reflection of the protean nature of tumor biology in the individual patient. A patient may die of unrelated causes apparently free of cancer and thereby achieve a "personal cure," whereas if he or she had lived longer, the natural history of the systemic nature of the cancer might have manifested itself. Alternatively, diminishing tumor burden with surgery may allow host defenses to "mop up after the surgeon's knife."[166]

Leaving clinically nonpalpable nodes, which may harbor metastases that could serve as a source of further dissemination, will continue to bother traditionally trained oncologic surgeons, who feel that unless the nodes are removed there is no way of precluding this possibility (although the NSABP data just presented suggests that "cascade" metastasis formation is not a clinically significant process). The concept that surgical cure requires removal of the last tumor cell persists, despite much evidence to the contrary—surgical traditions die hard.

An example of different conceptual frameworks concerning cancer treatment has been provided by Kardinal and Yarbro.[129] One aspect seems particularly relevant. In the Renaissance, the seven liberal arts were divided into two groups: the trivium (grammar, rhetoric, logic) and the quadrivium (arithmetic, geometry, astronomy, and acoustical proportions) representing the four quantitative methods of calculation and analysis. The trivium propagated the analytic methodology of Aristotle and Galen (rationalism), whereas the quadrivium represented the new empirical approach of Copernicus and Galileo. A simulated debate between a "trivialist" (T) and "quadrivialist" (Q) in a modern-day tumor conference follows:

Q: What is the operation of choice in this patient?
T: Radical mastectomy.
Q: But aren't survival data just as good with a less extensive operation?
T: To cure cancer, one must remove all cancer cells. To do this requires a radical operation; otherwise, lymph nodes with cancer cells may remain in the patient's body.
Q: But it does not alter survival!
T: But it is the only chance to remove all the cancer cells!

Such a debate is difficult to resolve because the conceptual frameworks of the discussants are different. The quadrivialist focuses on the measured results of various treatment alternatives. The trivialist supports the specific treatment approach because of faith in a particular conceptual framework. In order to resolve the conflict, the trivialist's mind must be open to data acquired by the scientific method.

The "trivialist" view of RLN significance is defensible only if a cancer initially spreads *only* via the lymphatics to the RLNs and is retained in them for a period of time before dissemination occurs. In such cases, complete removal of the primary lesion and the regional nodes during this phase of the disease should be curative. Even if LNs can serve as disseminating sites, they are unlikely to be the only routes of dissemination because, as we have seen, considerable scientific and anatomic data contradict the exclusivity of this mechanism of cancer spread. Hence, although it is conceivable that their removal might decrease dissemination, it is unlikely that such a procedure would eliminate all possible sources of cancer spread. If, as the alternate hypothesis suggests, tumor growth in LNs simply indicates the ability of the primary tumor to metastasize, *local therapy will not significantly affect survival,* because distant spread via the blood stream will not be addressed by local-regional therapy. This dilemma is well recognized by surgeons who accept the futility of extensive LN dissections as curative procedures in patients with cancers that have also spread to distant sites, but this is a difficult concept for Halstedian surgeons to accept as applicable to early disease.

The "quadrivialist" approach, exemplified by the NSABP trials, is more rational and scientific and asks, "Even though there is cancer in the RLNs, what effect does this have on survival?" The NSABP trial results contradict traditional Halstedian principles because presumably some of the study patients harbored occult disease in their LNs, yet their survival was not shortened by failure to treat such regional disease. Distant metastatic disease proved to be the limiting factor to survival regardless of local-regional treatment.

In the final analysis, the role of the RLN in neoplasia

is important but will remain controversial. The concept of the importance of retaining the regional nodes that are free of metastatic cells to maintain a high level of systemic tumor immunity may well be simplistic, as we have seen. The initiation of systemic tumor immunity by the RLN, if it occurs, probably depends on the antigenicity of the individual tumor and other poorly defined tumor-host interactions. Majority opinion currently seems to favor the fact that if tumor cells have reached the RLNs and a host defense has been initiated, by the time a tumor becomes clinically apparent, elective treatment of the RLNs probably will not interfere with tumor control. It is not necessary to explain the failure or success of metastasis of tumors by a single mechanism such as a defect in the RLNs. Rather, since the metastatic chain of events is only as strong as its weakest link, a deficiency in completing any stage in the complex process could bring about its failure.

Before the issues brought up in this section can be definitively resolved, the mechanisms involved in tumor-host interactions, metastasis, and the effects of various treatment modalities on them must be further investigated in the basic science laboratory and via well-controlled clinical trials that are designed to test a particular *hypothesis* and will thereby yield useful information, regardless of the outcome of the study. The current status of these areas is summarized in the following discussion.

Metastasis

Since better regional control has been achieved with combinations of conventional therapy, head and neck cancer patients are now surviving longer, only to succumb to DMs and to multiple primary tumors, and these two problems now appear to be limiting factors in the ultimate cure of these patients. A review of current understanding of basic tumor biology and metastasis will provide a perspective for interpreting the problems of head and neck cancer patients who are susceptible to both lymphatic and visceral metastases in the neck and distantly. Spread of cancer to neck nodes is not an isolated phenomenon and should be viewed within the broader context of metastasis in general. Additional information can be found in several excellent reviews of the subject.[68, 69, 242, 264, 265]

Metastasis is becoming the nemesis of treatments that otherwise can successfully eradicate the primary tumor. Metastasis is a very complicated phenomenon involving many different interactions between tumor and host, and it is influenced by humoral, cellular, endocrine, nutritional, metabolic,[59] and chronobiologic[114] factors that currently are largely undefined. Complex factors including tumor growth rate, degree of differentiation, the presence or absence of barriers to spread, blood supply, tumor-host immunologic interaction, and cancer treatment modalities have an impact upon the tumor-host relationship in ways that are also poorly understood currently.

Tumor Heterogeneity

The original concept of a tumor population as the monoclonal expansion of identical cells frozen in a particular state of differentiation is no longer valid. The UICC (International Union against Cancer) classification lists 273 types of cancer worldwide, and it is now known that cells populating a primary neoplasm, as well as those in various metastases within an individual, are not uniform but are biologically diverse and *heterogeneous*. Tumor heterogeneity exists with respect to a number of biologic characteristics, including morphologic features, cell-cycle–dependent phenomena, immunogenicity, tumorigenicity, sensitivity to treatment modalities, ploidy, cell-surface receptors, enzyme markers, hormone receptors, growth rate, metabolic characteristics, pigment production, and metastatic potential. Clonal subpopulations within individual cancers have been detected. As conventional treatment combinations are achieving better regional control, metastases resistant to conventional therapeutics are emerging as the most formidable obstacles to the cure of cancer patients.[69]

Intratumor heterogeneity is a dynamic phenomenon with a more or less continual emergence of new variant subpopulations that may differ in many characteristics and can also interact with each other to influence growth, metastasis, and sensitivity to treatment. Tumor cells apparently tend to stabilize their relative proportions and impose an equilibrium on the conglomerate population. Removal of a major clone by some treatment modality can permit the other subpopulations to proliferate unchecked and become dominant. The diversified resurgent population is likely to be resistant to the treatment modality that removed the dominant clone initially. In addition, there may be intrinsically resistant cells, and the mechanisms of their resistance may differ from those for acquired resistance.

In the past, metastatic potential generally has been correlated with features of the primary tumor such as size, site, and differentiation. Many metastasis researchers now believe that the successful establishment of metastases represents the selective emergence of pre-existing subpopulations of cells that are endowed with special properties that allow them to survive to complete the arduous and highly selective process of metastasis, which contains a number of potentially fatal steps. Using radiolabeled tumor cells, Fidler[67] observed that by 24 hours after entering the circulation, less than 1 per cent of injected cells were still viable and less than 0.1 per cent of the cells survived to produce metastases. There is also evidence that the selection process is not random. This is fortunate because a random process cannot be manipulated therapeutically, whereas a selective process can be altered once the mechanisms that regulate it are discovered. Recent experiments have shown that whereas clones with widely differing metastatic potential can be isolated from primary tumors, cloned sublines isolated from metastases exhibit a more uniform metastatic potential, suggesting that metastases are populated by a more homogeneous cell population than are primary tumors.

Tumor-Host-Treatment Interactions

Metastases proliferating in different organs can exhibit different responses to a given treatment regimen. Host factors such as neovascularization, availability of growth factors, and inflammatory responses can all influence the interactions of metastatic cells with therapeutic agents. Logistic factors may prevent adequate drug delivery to some sequestered sites. It is also not uncommon to clinically observe the regression of some metastases in one organ, whereas others in the same patient grow progressively, either with or without treatment.

Differences in the response of primary and metastatic lesions to therapeutic agents have been documented in clinical practice. The classic example of treatment selection pressure is chemotherapeutic drugs. Even if representative drug sensitivities could be determined using an in vitro system, it is still possible that in vivo modulation of the tumor-host relationship might have occurred, changing the dominant clone by the time the correct drug combination was decided, thereby rendering it ineffective in clinical use. Radiation treatment can also serve as a selective agent, and this can be different from selection provided by hyperthermia treatments.[200] There is some indirect evidence that surgery can also provide a similar selective pressure, although of the three treatment modalities, presumably it would be the least selective because the tumor mass is removed in toto. The effects of surgery can alter the tumor-host equilibrium, however, by temporarily depressing the ImR and by eliminating the suppressor effect of the primary tumor on metastases, sometimes resulting in "metastatic explosions."

Tumor growth, whether primary or metastatic, is unpredictable. Patients can present with metastatic disease from a small or even undetectable primary tumor, whereas other patients have huge primary tumors that show no evidence of metastasis during the patient's lifetime. Different and even opposite effects may be seen among tumor types or among individuals with the same type of tumor. Some patients survive well in symbiosis with multiple primary tumors over several years, whereas others succumb quickly to small, potentially curable cancers.

Despite the fact that a large primary tumor generally has a small growth fraction, micrometastases may grow rapidly, presumably because of their more favorable environment. Such relationships are relevant to certain types of therapy. It is well known, for example, that chemotherapeutic agents preferentially affect rapidly growing cell populations and hence should have relatively increased activity on micrometastatic disease. That this is not always seen clinically is another reflection of the complexity of tumor-host interactions.

Mechanisms of Metastasis

Metastasis involves the release of cells from the primary tumor, dissemination to distant sites, arrest in the microcirculation of organs, extravasation and infiltration into the stroma of those organs, and survival and growth as new tumor colonies. To establish metastases, tumor cells must complete all the steps, and interruption of the sequence at any stage can prevent the production of clinical metastases. The outcome of the process depends on host factors and tumor cell properties. Although we know much about the clinical manifestations of the metastatic process, little is yet understood about the biochemical and cellular events that determine the ultimate outcome.

It has been estimated that up to 10 per cent of tumor cells undergoing division may be shed into the circula-

tion. Even in grossly necrotic tumor areas, clonogenic cells that can produce tumors can be found. Indeed, there is some evidence that cells metastasizing under hypoxic conditions show increased survival capability. Most cells released into the blood stream are eliminated rapidly. It appears intuitively logical that the greater the number of cells released by the primary tumor, the greater the probability that some cells will successfully complete all the steps and form metastases. We know that most patients have symptomatic cancers at the time of diagnosis; thus, presumably the phase of entry into the circulation has been reached by the time of presentation, and the cancer may not be susceptible to clinical intervention.

Little is known about the mechanisms responsible for invasion of local tissues. Primary growth rate is inconsistent—many highly invasive tumors have very slow growth rates. Mechanical pressure and individual cell motility are probably important in invasion. Tissue-destructive enzymes may also function in tumor invasion, although the importance of different enzymes may vary among tumor systems or among anatomic sites within the same system. There is apparently a strong correlation between the ability of tumor cells to produce spontaneous metastases and possession of high levels of type IV collagenase. There is evidence that metastatic tumor cells exhibit a preferential attachment to type IV collagen substrates (the major structural protein of basement membranes), and circulating cells tend to degrade basement membranes to a much greater degree than cells from the primary tumor. Head and neck SCCs possess relevant degradative enzymes such as type IV collagenase and proteases.[115]

Conventional histologic assessment has proved relatively unhelpful with respect to defining individual tumor invasiveness, although new ultrastructural and immunohistochemical methods may aid in this regard. A major new direction is to define biochemical correlates of invasive potential at the primary site.[164]

Although the circulation can be a hostile environment for circulating cancer cells (blood more so than lymph), the events occurring after tumor cell arrest may be more important in tumor cell destruction. Some studies using radiolabeled tumor cells indicate that nearly all cells released into the circulation reach the favored target organ, but after initial entrapment, most cells die and only a few develop into successful metastases.

Establishment of Distant Metastases

There is a tendency for primary tumors of a particular histologic type to metastasize and grow in specific distant organs. Two hypotheses have been proposed to explain this nonrandom pattern of tumor spread. Ewing suggested that metastases were influenced purely by mechanical considerations such as anatomic and hemodynamic factors. Paget proposed the "seed and soil" hypothesis, which suggests that sites of secondary tumor growth are determined by both host and tumor factors. Certainly, the vascularity of organs may contribute to the frequency with which metastatic deposits are formed in them. For example, the lung may be a common site of metastatic development simply because it is the first capillary bed encountered by tumor cells entering the venous circulation. Host control of metastatic patterns, however, has been dramatically demonstrated using organ grafts maintained in ectopic sites. Grafts of various tissues have been implanted in the flanks of syngeneic mice that were subsequently inoculated with tumor suspensions. Tumors developed only in those grafts derived from the organs that normally supported tumor growth in the intact animal. Selective entrapment and arrest of circulating tumor cells are probably also determined by the specificity of cell-cell recognition, the control of which resides at the cell surface, and modification of many tumor cell properties can alter tumor dissemination patterns.

In addition to lytic enzymes, other substances may also function in preferential location of distant metastases. There is some evidence that the secretion of prostaglandins by head and neck SCCs is a factor that promotes preferential metastasis to bone.[33] Necrotic cell products released from the primary tumor may also have a "feeder" effect, increasing the take of viable cells released. For example, it has been shown that the dose of cells required for the successful subcutaneous implantation of a tumor is greatly reduced by adding lethally irradiated tumor cells to viable tumor cell suspensions.[107, 198] This phenomenon has obvious clinical implications with respect to using radiation therapeutically, and especially electively.

Interactions between Primary and Metastatic Tumor Deposits

Implications for surgical and other cytoreductive therapy are found in earlier reports indicating that primary tumors apparently have an inhibitory effect on the growth of DMs. In 1913, Tyzzer showed that partially removing the primary tumor in a mouse did not increase the incidence of metastasis but did increase the growth rate of metastatic tumors.[247] He postulated that increased nutrition was available to the metastases after removal of the primary tumor—the so-called "athreptic immunity theory." He also found that if a primary tumor was completely removed prior to reaching a critical size, all metastases could be prevented. This "premetastatic period" could be greatly shortened by the massage of the primary tumor—of relevance in "no-touch" surgical and biopsy techniques. In 1958, Schatten, using a mouse model concluded that a primary tumor inhibited the growth of its distant metastases upon reaching a critical size.[210] Control mice with intact primary tumors showed a significantly lower number and size of metastases than did animals whose tumors had been amputated. It was postulated that the stress of operation (amputation) lowered the animal's resistance to growth of disseminated cells, allowing more of the cells already lodged in the lungs to grow. In better designed experiments, however, control and experimental animals were sacrificed and assayed for metastases at the same time after manipulation. The tumor-bearing animals developed metastases more frequently and exhibited more tumors per mouse than did the corresponding animals undergoing amputation. Metastases that developed in the amputated group grew significantly larger than in comparable tumor-bearing animals. Amputation brought about a cessation of tumor cell shedding and thus prevented further metastasis.

A considerable body of experimental evidence indicates the existence of a regulatory mechanism monitoring total tumor mass throughout an organism. Sudden removal of a primary tumor's metastasis-inhibiting influence could explain the "disease explosion" sometimes seen after surgical excision of primary tumors. DeWys[57] demonstrated a nearly synchronous slowing of the growth rate of a primary tumor and its spontaneous metastases after the primary tumor reached a critical size. Amputation of the primary tumor renewed proliferation of lung metastases. In some nonimmunogenic model systems with well-vascularized metastases (thereby excluding poor oxygenation and nutrition as reasons for growth retardation) the existence of a "tumor-related systemic growth-retarding factor" has been hypothesized. It has also been shown experimentally that in addition to surgical removal, irradiation of a primary tumor can also be followed by growth of larger metastases than those that occur when the primary tumor is untreated.

Nearly all tumors studied have demonstrated an exponential slowing of tumor growth rate with increasing tumor mass. Released soluble factors may serve as mitotic inhibitors with a systemic effect, and this could explain an inhibitory influence of the primary tumor on metastases. Polyamines that have growth-regulating effects and are products of tumor necrosis are possible candidates in this regard.

The phenomenon of "concomitant immunity" may also be relevant here—experimental systems show that animals with a large primary tumor mass are protected from artificial intravenously induced metastases in some cases.[90] Concomitant immunity is dependent upon the presence of a large primary tumor, for it rapidly declines following removal of the primary lesion. The successful escape of metastatic disease from the control of concomitant immunity may relate to the ability of established bulky primary tumors to successfully mask their surface antigens, whereas metastatic cells may be more likely to expose tumor-specific surface antigens. In addition, some metastases have been shown to be antigenically dissimilar from the primary tumor and may thereby escape "immune surveillance" by the host. Metastasis has also been correlated with the amount of tumor-specific transplantation antigen—tumors shedding large amounts of the antigen tend to metastasize, whereas nonshedding tumors do not. In tumors that shed antigen rapidly, little antigen remains on the tumor cell membrane, so they tend to act as weakly antigenic tumors. The large amounts of antigen released can "paralyze" the ImR, allowing the growth of metastases. Thus, the rate of antigen shedding may be a factor in determining both immunogenicity of the primary tumor and its ability to metastasize or, as originally proposed by Old and coworkers, "sneak through" host defenses without recognition as foreign until the tumor load is too great for the host to counteract.

A more recent interpretation of "sneaking through" conceptualizes not a failure of immunologic recognition, but rather an interaction between tumor cells and immunologically competent lymphocytes that results in a shutdown of the cytotoxic response.[190, 191] Presumably, low doses of tumor cells stimulate a weak immunogenic response that actually promotes tumor growth, or weak tumor antigens might preferentially activate suppressor cells that restrict the antitumor ImR and thereby enhance tumor progression.[170] Thus, the response of the immune system to tumors may well be of a dual nature—during the initial stages of neoplasia, or in cases in which tumors are weakly antigenic, the response may be stimulatory, whereas the ImR to strongly antigenic tumors may inhibit cancer growth. If some human tumors are spontaneous and weakly immunogenic, then the stimulation of the T-lymphocyte system as a mode of immunotherapy could be fraught with danger.

Dormant Tumor Cells and Trauma

The role of trauma is particularly interesting in the development of metastases. Tumor cells can selectively stick to areas of raw collagen created by periodic endothelial cell contractions or trauma. In addition, when the capillary barrier is disrupted by acute injury (which may be provided by a treatment modality such as surgery or radiation), metastases can reach organs that otherwise never become the sites of metastasis in control animals. Trauma can also activate dormant tumor cells.

The phenomenon of metastatic tumor growth appearing many years after apparently effective and permanent control of the primary tumor implies that dormant tumor cells have persisted for long periods of time in symbiosis with the host. Such tumor cells must have originated from tumors prior to their removal and lain dormant until triggered by unknown mechanisms. Pulmonary metastases in rats have been activated, leading to macroscopic disease when the hosts were immunosuppressed by whole-body irradiation or thoracic duct drainage, suggesting immunologically mediated restraint of dormant tumor cells.[61] Estrogen stimulation of dormant tumor cells has also been achieved.[267]

Trauma has been implicated in the reactivation of dormant tumor cells since the early 1900s when Lubarsch[143] showed that implantation of splinters in the livers of mice resulted in secondary localization of tumor at that site. In an experimental liver tumor,[74] growth-stimulating factors from post-traumatic regenerating liver were thought to be relevant. There have also been reports of the development of metastases after a long latent interval in the area of bruises, intramuscular injections, distant skin graft donor sites, and dinitrochlorobenzene (DNCB) inoculations[37] as well as in distant surgical scars unrelated to fresh surgical wounds. One patient with "cured" carcinoma of the larynx without evidence of DMs, who concomitant with radiation therapy underwent application of a Spica cast, subsequently developed metastases in the areas traumatized. At autopsy the patient did not have any local-regional tumor—this was presumably an instance of reactivation of dormant tumor cells by trauma.[37]

Significant data has accumulated to indicate that tissue injury and inflammation activate enhanced localization, implantation, and growth of circulating cancer cells at the site of the inflammatory response—"inflammatory oncotaxis."[54, 223] Clinically this rarely occurs, possibly because the simultaneous occurrence of inflammation and circulating tumor cells is unusual or because the tumor cells, once localized to the site of inflammation, are unable to establish themselves and grow. Ischemic damage and mechanical tissue trauma have been shown experimentally to attract cancer cells to local sites.[102]

In one trauma metastasis experiment of the Fishers,[74] labeled tumor cells were injected into rats after injury to one extremity by a clean surgical excision, turpentine injection, or crushing; there was significantly greater accumulation of tumor cells in the injured extremity than in the normal control animals, and the number of cells localized increased directly with the degree of inflammatory response to the trauma. Tumor recurrence after long disease-free intervals implies either growth of dormant cells pre-existing at the points of trauma or an active attraction of dormant cells to these points from distant sources. Bernard Fisher has suggested that some local recurrences may actually represent this latter mechanism—homing of distant cancer cells to surgically traumatized areas—rather than regrowth of cells spilled or implanted in the wound during surgery.

It should be noted that surgery is not the only trauma-inducing mechanism; other cytoreductive treatments such as radiotherapy and chemotherapy can also provide a traumatic influence and may, in fact, alter the tumor-host interaction by providing longer exposure to tumor necrosis products than surgery, which presumably eliminates the tumor bulk in a few hours.

In contrast to studies showing increased number of tumor cells localizing at areas of inflammation, several studies show improved survival and fewer DMs in patients with postoperative wound or systemic infections.[184, 209] Infection has been interpreted to nonspecifically potentiate host immune mechanisms with consequent inhibition of tumor dissemination. These papers were retrospective, however, and attributed significance to one parameter when many others were uncontrolled. Such results are reminiscent of the work of Coley[38] in which a "toxin" extracted from heat-killed streptococci and *Serratia* was shown to be effective in causing the remission or cure of inoperable sarcomas, implicating bacterial wound infection in cancer regression. Nonspecific immunotherapy with bacterial products such as BCG and C-parvum as immunopotentiators evolved from such work. Immunotherapy and wound infection may not boost antitumor immunity per se but may encourage a more rapid recovery from a therapeutically induced immunosuppression.

The Challenge of Clinical Oncology

Thus, many aspects of the immune response are currently conjectural. In addition, components of the ImR are variably susceptible to different treatment modalities (see following discussion). When one adds a primary tumor to this complex mechanism it is understandable that widely varying results are obtained in experiments with different model systems and methods. Although there are a multitude of potential tumor defense mechanisms in the intact host, the tumor itself has a number of systems at its disposal to counteract immune recognition and destruction. Once a neoplasm begins to grow, it starts to interfere with host mechanisms to facilitate its own growth. It is now apparent that the means by which tumors avoid host destruction are extremely complicated and intertwined with the host immunoregulatory apparatus. Tumor cells can insidiously interact with the host's regulatory network to induce both specific and general unresponsiveness. A recent review summarizes these "escape" mechanisms[181] and is recommended to the reader to allow appreciation of the magnitude of the task faced by those who hope to intervene in the tumor-host relationship. The relative importance of various escape mechanisms also probably varies among tumors, patients, and clinical stages in a continually modulated spectrum, adding further complexity.

It is now apparent that the process by which tumor cells escape immunologic and nonimmunologic controls is not due to the simple failure of the host to recognize weak tumor antigens, as postulated in the theory of immunosurveillance. Rather, successful evasion by neoplastic cells involves dynamic interaction with the host regulatory capabilities, which can sometimes be subverted for the tumor's own use. Neoplastic cell populations are continuously differentiating in vivo and are capable of sending and receiving regulatory signals between themselves and nonmalignant immunocompetent cells.

Such tumor-host interactions have obvious implications for clinical therapy. Some alterations in the tumor-host equilibrium which have been attributed to various treatment modalities are summarized in the next section. Most studies are uncontrolled, however, and it is difficult to attribute changes to therapy rather than to tumor-host factors. Also, the metastatic process is a continuum from the growth of the primary tumor to an established metastasis, and it is rarely possible to determine just when or where a treatment modality is operative.

Treatment Modalities—Double-Edged Swords

The "big three" cancer treatment modalities are currently surgery, radiation therapy (RT), and chemotherapy, and widespread enthusiasm exists for their combined use against solid tumors in the 1980s. Although no one would suggest holding these effective treatments in reserve, the surgical oncologist must nevertheless be aware that each of them has a "down side."

As usual, disagreement exists on the precise nature of the detrimental effects of each treatment modality because a variety of parameters have been used as indicators of the tumor-host interaction, leading to difficulties in interpretation and comparison of data. Many of the measurements may be irrelevant to the in vivo tumor-host situation. It appears that both the common in vitro lymphocyte transformation assays and the in vivo skin tests measure immune competence only in a general way and may not reflect specific antitumor defenses.

There is little uniformity in administration and interpretation of tests, and without uniformity, data are not comparable and conclusions can be contradictory. Pleas for uniformity in application and interpretation of immunologic tests and the doubtful relevance of measures of nonspecific immune reactivity are receiving more attention in the recent cancer literature, including head and neck publications.[11, 18, 197] It is necessary to develop simple, reproducible, reliable tests of tumor-host parameters which are relevant to the in vivo situation, standardized among institutions, to assay specific and nonspecific antitumor effects that may exist—this is a large task.

Because alcoholics, smokers, and malnourished pa-tients show significantly decreased immune reactivity compared with normal control subjects, reduced reactivity seen in head and neck cancer patients, who typically have these associated conditions, may not be connected with tumor disease at all. Thus, there is a need for more appropriate controls—data from healthy control subjects may not be relevant.

Treatment modalities can influence the tumor-host equilibrium in unpredictable ways. With these caveats in mind, a brief review follows on the effects of various treatments on the ImR and other presumably relevant tumor-host parameters.

Surgery

Certainly, surgery has the ability to mechanically alter the local-regional tumor environment. It has been shown that lymphatics can re-establish continuity if the cut edges are in proximity, but when the gap is considerable, union is the result of development of collateral channels—usually within 2 to 3 weeks.[237] The ability to regenerate varies with the consistency of the connective tissue through which the lymphatics must grow. Dense connective tissue, such as surgical scar, can account for the difficulty with which lymphatics bypass long incisions. Lymphatic regeneration has also been noted to be slower after external irradiation, possibly owing to associated fibrosis or to an effect on dividing endothelial cells. Such mechanical effects have the ability to alter lymphatic metastatic spread. Two studies on rabbits undergoing neck dissection[6, 72] demonstrated diversion of lymph flow to the contralateral side of the neck after ipsilateral neck dissection. This could account for the appearance of delayed contralateral nodes in the presence of recurrent tumor at the primary site.

Surgical scarring can also trap spilled tumor cells, although retention of such cells at the local site does not inevitably lead to local recurrence (see biopsy discussion). Common sense dictates gentle handling of cancerous tissues, however, to decrease exposure of surgical wounds to free cancer cells and thus minimize the potential for growth. Many experimental models have shown that forceful manipulation of the primary tumor increases metastases, although clinical evidence for a detrimental effect is equivocal.

The phenomenon of "metastatic explosion" after resection of primary tumors has variously been attributed to mechanical dissemination of tumor cells at the time of operation or to release of an inhibitory influence of the primary tumor on metastases[130, 144] by tumor removal or related to the immunosuppressive effects of a major surgical procedure. Experimental studies suggest that operative stress promotes tumor "take" and increases metastatic rate, resulting in shortened survival in animals.[101, 112, 243] It is difficult to separate the immunologic effects of removal of tumor from those of operation, however.

Several recent reviews have documented the immunosuppressive effects of surgery and general anesthesia; both appear to induce a profound but transient depression in lymphocyte function[224] in patients undergoing elective noncancer surgery. Most investigators have implicated stress-induced adrenocortical release associated with the trauma of surgery and anesthesia. Other evidence suggests that surgical stress alone is probably the only significant factor because operation in adrenalectomized animals has been shown to promote tumor growth[227] and depression of T-lymphocyte function in rats following thermal and mechanical injury occurs even in the absence of adrenal function.[167]

The release of nonspecific inhibitory substances secondary to tissue trauma, activation of suppressor T-cells, and altered macrophage function have also been suggested to explain the immunosuppressive effect seen following surgery and anesthesia, but such ideas are speculative at this point. Studies in cancer patients are few and results are equivocal—some demonstrate an increase in postoperative lymphocyte function, others a decrease.[204] The duration of immunosuppression also depends on the site of the operation, blood transfusion, length of operating time, and tumor histologic features.

Because of the possible facilitation of dissemination, implantation, and propagation of tumor cells during a period of suppressed cellular immunity related to anesthesia and operation, means are being investigated to maintain and augment cellular immune competence in cancer patients during and after surgical intervention—presumably at a time when such agents would be of most use—when the tumor burden is lowest. Preliminary indications that such manipulations may be helpful appear in several recent papers.[144, 243] Because biologic response modifiers (see following section) have varying effects, depending upon the stage and type of cancer as well as their route of administration, dosage, and many other factors, caution against premature and uncontrolled use of such agents certainly pertains here.

Chemotherapy

Antineoplastic drug therapy is immunosuppressive in nature. Each agent suppresses the ImR in a slightly different manner. The suppressor effects of single chemotherapeutic agents are usually short-lived, with complete or nearly complete recovery of immune parameters within several days after cessation of therapy, and an overshoot phenomenon is occasionally observed. In addition, both chemotherapy and RT have proved carcinogenic effects—an increased risk of secondary neoplasia, particularly acute lymphocytic leukemia, is well documented.[133] Because the cancer patient must survive the index primary tumor in order to be susceptible to this delayed risk, the benefits of adjuvant chemotherapy in delaying recurrence may outweigh potential hazards in the short term, at least.

Chemotherapy is presumably effective against systemic micrometastases. In rodent systems, small deposits tend to have relatively high growth fractions and short doubling times and are therefore more susceptible to chemotherapeutic intervention. The growth of human micrometastases is thought to be substantially slower than that of volume-equivalent tumor in rodents, however, and compelling evidence of a comparable benefit for human solid tumors is currently lacking. The effectiveness of chemotherapeutic agents against micrometastases can only be inferred by alterations in the rate of clinically apparent distant metastases, for occult micrometastases cannot be detected.

Concern that chemotherapy may, in fact, *increase* metastatic rate is exemplified by a recent study,[228] in which the incidence of DMs after multimodality therapy

(anterior chemotherapy, RT, surgery) in inoperable patients with stage IV head and neck SCC (T4 and/or N3) was significantly greater than in patients treated with standard combined therapy (RT followed by surgery if operation became possible)—40 per cent versus 12.5 per cent. In comparison with average incidences of DMs of 6 to 13 per cent following RT alone and of about 15 per cent following similar multimodality treatments, the 40 per cent incidence of observed DMs appeared high, and the authors expressed concern that some alteration in the tumor-host interaction occurred after multimodality therapy, which resulted in an increased incidence of metastases. It was suggested that multimodality therapies might prove a double-edged sword; while causing significant regional regression, they might promote frequent, early DMs.

Radiation Therapy

Whereas the head and neck surgeon tends to think of the detrimental effects of RT in terms of local morbidity (woody induration, mucositis, xerostomia, potential for radionecrosis), RT also has systemic effects. Awareness of these is relevant to the issue of employing elective neck irradiation (which currently enjoys widespread use) in already immunocompromised head and neck cancer patients.

The pertinent literature is vast and conflicting, as usual, because many different animal models have been used as well as different radiation amounts, portals, and fractionation schemes. Methods of assessing the ImR have also varied considerably, and observed changes also depend on the interval after therapy when the assessment is performed.

SYSTEMIC EFFECTS OF RADIOTHERAPY

The literature on the effects of ionizing radiation on the ImR has recently been reviewed.[2, 10] With the exception of atom bomb survivor studies, almost all the data concerns RT administered for malignancy, and little is known about the effects of radiation on the normal human immune system. Irradiation suppresses both the humoral and cellular arms of the ImR, and recovery depends on the regeneration of a functional cell population from surviving lymphocyte precursors. It was originally thought that depression of cell-mediated immunity occurred primarily in patients when their thymus was included in the treatment portals, but it is presently felt that cell-mediated immunity is depressed secondary to the treatment of large volumes of blood in transit through the irradiated field, and this defect tends to persist for long periods of time after therapeutic radiation, even in clinically "cured" patients. The evidence for a long life span for lymphocytes involved in cell-mediated immunity leads to the speculation that therapeutic radiation may have a permanently deleterious effect on lymphocytes or their progenitors as they circulate through the treatment portals.

A number of papers have addressed the compromised ImR following irradiation in head and neck cancer patients.[117, 174, 233, 261] These studies all show various types of immune depression, depending upon the parameter measured, length of time after treatment, and dose received. One typical study[244] showed prolonged depression of cellular immunity in cured laryngopharyngeal cancer patients treated with RT. A relatively small number of patients that had radiation as part of their treatment and were subsequently cured (mean follow-up time, 9 years) had significantly impaired cellular immune parameters when compared to normal subjects and patients treated by surgery alone. This demonstrated that the effect of local radiation could be systemic and prolonged. The studies that show persistent depression of immunity in cured cancer patients help eliminate the criticism that persistence or appearance of reduced immune competence is due to residual tumor burden rather than to the treatment modality.

Lymphoid tissue and circulating small lymphocytes are extremely radiosensitive, and doses as low as 25 rad may produce a detectable decrease in the peripheral lymphocyte count.[48] B-lymphocytes are quite radiosensitive and probably undergo interphase as well as mitotic death following radiation. Within the functional categories of T-lymphocyte subpopulations, there is a change from extreme radiosensitivity of precursor cells to relative radioresistance of effector cells. Suppressor T-cells are thought to be particularly radiosensitive (more so than helper T-cells) and may be the only T-cell subset to undergo interphase death. Red blood cells, granulocytes, platelets, plasma cells, and mature macrophages are relatively radioresistant. Electron spin resonance studies suggest that irradiation may alter the fluidity of the plasma membrane of lymphocytes, and this could affect a variety of immune interactions.

EFFECTS OF RADIOTHERAPY ON THE LYMPHATIC SYSTEM

Irradiation is associated with changes in LNs and lymphatics, but results from different series vary. Animal studies on the alteration of barrier function of LNs following RT yield varying results, depending on the agent used to challenge the barrier. Because radiation produces nodal and perinodal fibrosis, altered filtration capacity results.

In general, within a few days of radiation, hyperemia and decreasing numbers of lymphocytes are noted, and LN hyalinization and thickening of the walls of blood vessels are also observed. Several weeks later, there is evidence of regeneration with a few germinal centers and many mitoses in the cortical areas of LNs, and repopulation of irradiated nodes, presumably by circulating lymphocyte precursors, has been observed. Thus, the acknowledged effect of radiation as a lympholytic and immunosuppressive agent may be counterbalanced by re-entry of lymphocytes from the circulating pool. It is difficult to imagine, however, that a normal functional complement of immune cells can traffic through fibrotic LNs and vessels, especially when their own functional capabilities may have been compromised by previous circulation through the radiation portals.

In irradiated cervical LNs in the dog[266] it was found that major obstruction and rerouting of lymph flow contralaterally occurred secondary to damage to lymphatic channels from local infection with subsequent scarring and fibrosis, although lymph flow was minimally distorted by radiation per se.

Although numerous patients have undergone LN dissection after irradiation, few reports describe the changes following this therapy.[111] Burge[27] reported the histologic changes in the cervical LNs of 38 RND specimens in comparison with nonirradiated controls. Doses over 4000 rad led to hyalinization and proliferation of fibrous tissue. In many nodes, no residual lymphoid follicles could be found and few mitotic figures were present.

Before becoming a famous skull-base surgeon, Ugo Fisch studied the pathophysiology of cervical lymphatics. He evaluated the barrier function of LNs in 22 RND specimens from patients that had had preoperative RT of 2000 to 7000 rad.[71] He concluded that at doses over 6000 rad, the mechanical barrier function of the LN (as assessed by passage of avian erythrocytes) was reduced. Injection and perfusion methods used in this study could have induced significant artifacts, however.

A histologic and lymphographic study of neck dissection specimens from ten patients who had received previous RT[70] showed that visualized LNs were only a few millimeters in diameter, and fibrotic changes occurred in the connective tissue and fat as well as thickening of the capsule of LNs and the wall of lymph vessels. One year following RND, no formation of collaterals was seen, but a network of tortuous subcutaneous and dermal lymphatic channels was visualized in some cases. This finding might account for the increased incidence of subdermal metastases after treatment that redirects lymph flow; this tends to occur more frequently in patients after surgical and radiation treatment than when primary tumor first presents, even with massive cervical disease. In "normal" cervical lymphatics, no filling of the dermal and subcutaneous lymphatics was seen and strict directional flow was present. After neck radiation, the caliber and number of lymph vessels and the size and number of cervical LNs were markedly decreased. The changes seen lymphographically were confirmed histologically. Fisch's conclusion was that a complete block to cervical lymph flow was observed only following RND, with partial obstruction following radiation.

It has been speculated that contralateral nodes and lymphatics can take over the immune functions normally served by the ipsilateral treated lymphatics and nodes. In cases of bilateral neck treatment, this compensatory mechanism could also be damaged.

INFLUENCE OF RADIATION ON TUMOR GROWTH

Whether or not radiation affects the incidence of DMs is controversial, and experiments have provided evidence on both sides of the issue since Primm's report in 1929 in which pulmonary metastases were increased in tumor-bearing animals who received local irradiation over those who did not. More recently, an animal study showed that extensive-field radiation (but not limited-field RT) could facilitate growth of tumors in unirradiated parts of the animal, although radiation was an effective therapeutic agent against tumor growth in the radiated field.[248] The controversy over whether observed increases in DMs are due to local effects or generalized immunologic damage is summarized by Vaage.[248]

Some of the clinical data from the NSABP has been interpreted to indicate that conventional postoperative RT may increase the risk of DMs in selected patients with breast cancer because although the incidence of tumor recurrence in the radiated field was reduced, DMs were detected earlier in the radiated patients.

In one study of DMs in patients with upper aerodigestive tract (UADT) tumors, patients whose primary lesion was treated by RT or surgery alone had essentially the same incidence of DMs. Patients receiving postoperative radiation, however, had twice the incidence of those receiving preoperative radiation. However, the sequence of modalities was not randomized, and the patients receiving postoperative RT tended to be selected for more advanced disease, with evidence of connective tissue disease in the neck or multiple levels of node involvement, and it is well known that advanced N stage greatly influences increased DMs.

In addition to the acknowledged carcinogenic potential of RT, other miscellaneous effects of radiation may have a bearing on the tumor-host interaction. There is some evidence that radiation does not destroy the immunogenicity of tumors but rather may enhance it. X-ray may also alter carcinoma cell coats in a way that promotes phagocytosis by macrophages. Some studies have shown that after irradiation, phagocytic activation of macrophages is markedly stimulated.[259] It was suggested that the damage to tumor cell membranes enhances accessability to macrophages. An electron microscopic study of injured, abnormally permeable lymphatics[34] showed opening of intercellular junctions. Endothelial swelling and increased permeability after radiation may cause circulating tumor emboli to localize at sites of such lymphatic damage preferentially, and this could influence local recurrence or distant metastases.

It is interesting that in the early days of tissue culture, adding radiated cells to the culture enhanced the growth of tumor cells that otherwise would not "take," presumably by acting as nutritive feeder cells.[193] The effects of cell-free tumor necrosis products resulting from radiation-induced tumorolysis in vivo on the tumor-host interaction are largely unknown.

In conclusion, the complexity of cancer treatment becomes more obvious as components of the immune response and tumor-host interaction are identified and dissected and their responses to different modes of therapy are assessed. A rational approach to multimodality therapy must take all these effects into consideration. For example, radiation following chemotherapy might be advantageous, as immune suppression seems to be rapidly reversed after cessation of chemotherapy. However, the potential for altering the ability of immunocytes to repair radiation damage exists, and the duration of this potential effect is unknown. Conversely, chemotherapy following radiation would have antineoplastic drugs interacting with an immune system already compromised by radiation damage. Also, prior immunosuppression by radiation may alter the antitumor efficacy of some drugs. Radiation damage to tissue on a local or regional basis may alter the biodistribution of both antitumor drugs and immunocompetent cells. This effect may work to the benefit or detriment of tumor control and emphasizes the need to study multimodality therapy in a controlled clinical setting.[149]

Biologic Response Modifiers

As we have alluded to in a previous section, the dual potential of tumor-host interactions to enhance or suppress tumor growth (a dynamic and changing equilibrium) poses problems for the interventionist who approaches the tumor-host system with a therapeutic modality. An important new concept is the *biologic therapy of cancer*, which may well become the fourth major modality of cancer treatment (immunotherapy is a subset), and a large number of agents that can affect the tumor-host interaction are being defined (Table 56–2) and are known as *biologic response modifiers* (BRMs). These agents have the potential to modify either the host or the tumor with the goal of altering the tumor-

TABLE 56–2. Biologicals and Biologic Response Modifiers

Immunomodulator and Immunostimulating Agents	
Alkyl lysophospholipids (ALP)	Lentinan
Azimexon	Levan
Bacillus Calmette-Guerin (BCG)	Muramyldipeptide (MDP)
Bestatin	Malic anhydride-divinyl ether (MVE-2)
Brucella abortus	Mixed bacterial vaccines
Corynebacterium parvum	N-137
Cimetidine	*Nocardia rubra* cell wall skeleton (CWS)
Sodium diethyldithiocarbamate (DTC)	Picibanil (OK 432)
Endotoxin	Prostaglandin inhibitors (aspirin, indomethacin)
Glucan	Thiobendazole
"Immune" RNAs	Tilorones
Therafectin	Tuftsin
Krestin	

Interferons and Interferon Inducers	
Interferons (α, β, and γ)	*Brucella abortus*
Poly 1C-LC	Viruses
Tilorones	

Thymosins	
Thymosin α-1	Other thymic factors
Thymosin fraction 5	

Lymphokines and Cytokines	
Antigrowth factors	Migration inhibitory factor (MIF)
Chalones	Maturation factors
Colony-stimulating factor (CSF)	T-cell growth factor (TCGF) (interleukin 2, IL-2)
Growth factors (transforming growth factor, TSF)	Interleukin 3 (IL-3)
Lymphoctye activation factor (LAF) (interleukin 1, IL-1)	T-cell replacing factor (TRF)
Lymphotoxin	Thymocyte mitogenic factor (TMF)
Macrophage activation factor (MAF)	Transfer factor
Macrophage chemotactic factor	B-cell growth factor (BCGF) Tumor necrosis factor (TNF)

Monoclonal Antibodies	
Monoclonal antibodies to growth-promoting factors	Anti-T-suppressor cell
Anti-T-cell	Antitumor antibody (including antibody fragments and conjugates with drugs, toxins, and isotypes)

Antigens	
Tumor-associated antigens	Vaccines

Effector Cells	
Macrophages	T-cell clones
Natural "killer" (NK) cells	T-helper cells

Miscellaneous Approaches	
Allogeneic immunization	Plasmapheresis and ex vivo treatments (activation columns and immunoabsorbents)
Bone marrow transplantation and reconstitution	Virus infection of cells (oncolysates)

Source: Oldham RK: Biologicals and biological response modifiers: Fourth modality of cancer treatment. Cancer Treat Rep *68*:221, 1984.

host interaction to favor the host and produce toxic effects against the tumor, resulting in therapeutic benefit. The important concept is that these agents are *modulatory* (stimulatory *or* suppressive), and the end result depends on the endogenous tumor-host relationship, which is currently difficult to characterize.

In general, the immune system must be normalized before it can be stimulated. Restoration of immunodeficient states can be achieved if the deficit is due to hyperactive immune mechanisms, such as increased suppressor activity. If, however, the resting state of the immune system is normal, a detrimental immunosuppressive effect may result from immunologic intervention. Awareness of this concept is crucial for the appropriate application of biologically active agents, a large number of which are becoming available for clinical trials.[106, 179] Note that indomethacin, a prostaglandin synthetase inhibitor, is a BRM. As such, the conflicting results with its use in advanced head and neck cancer patients[109, 182] are understandable, as the tumor-host situation in each test patient was probably different.

The ultimate clinical utility of BRMs must be defined carefully by ongoing preclinical and clinical studies. The availability of purified cytokine molecules and expanded, specifically cytotoxic lymphocyte populations has the potential to circumvent several steps classically required for immunotherapy—the stimulation with exogenous agents of activity in the patients themselves. Thus, effective biologic therapy of cancer is possible even in the presence of severe deficiencies in the host, and it may be possible to selectively use certain mechanisms rather than inducing the broad cascade seen after stimulation of the host.

Before some of these new leads can be followed up, a greater understanding of the regulation of immune responses and the tumor-host interaction is needed. Despite an almost irrepressible tendency to interdigitate biologic cancer therapy into current clinical trials, throwing BRMs haphazardly into the therapeutic armamentarium is probably premature at this point, and doing so is likely to lead to confusion, especially in the field of head and neck cancer, where few basic questions are answered. Biologic intervention can remove important stabilizing influences in the tumor-host equilibrium, and such alterations could result in the demise of the host sooner than if no intervention had been undertaken. Nevertheless, with the current feeling among many investigators that drugs may not provide the magic bullet needed to improve survival for solid tumor patients, rational study of BRMs may now be timely.

THE HEAD AND NECK CANCER CONTROVERSIES

Squamous Cell Carcinoma

Many of the traditional controversies revolve around elective treatment of the N0 neck:

1. What is the significance of occult neck metastases?
2. What features of the primary tumor are useful in estimating the incidence of occult neck metastases?
3. When should elective neck treatment be carried out, and what is the rationale?

4. Is functional neck dissection (FND) an oncologically effective operation?
5. What is the value of elective neck irradiation (ENI)?
6. Is END as effective as ENI?
7. Is patient survival compromised if neck dissection is done therapeutically, when disease becomes evident, rather than electively?

At the opposite end of the spectrum, controversies also revolve around appropriate treatment of the N3 neck, particularly with advanced or recurrent disease. Appropriate timing and methods for biopsy of neck disease have also generated controversy. More recently, the value of combined therapy in certain situations has been championed and questioned:

1. What is the value of radical neck dissection (RND) as a single modality?
2. What prognostic factors of neck disease accurately define patients at high risk for neck recurrence or distant spread?
3. What is the value of surgery plus radiation?
4. When should postoperative radiotherapy be added to therapeutic or elective neck dissection?
5. What is the role of multimodality treatment, including chemotherapy, for advanced neck disease?

Controversy also surrounds appropriate management of the neck with nonsquamous tumors of the head and neck: malignant melanoma, salivary gland cancer, and thyroid cancer. We shall discuss each of these topics, selecting the most valid data from the abundant literature on each, and we shall attempt to relate it to the tumor biology concepts presented previously.

First, however, it is necessary to comment on the head and neck cancer literature as a whole as background to help the reader interpret the data to be presented.

A Critical Assessment of the Literature

It is interesting and disappointing that after decades of treatment for thousands of head and neck cancer patients, it is virtually impossible to answer any basic oncology questions in a definitive and scientific manner from the publications in the literature. Therefore, "pendulum swings" of opinion concerning treatment occur about every 5 years, and controversies persist. Although most of the controversies discussed in this chapter originated before 1910, they are still debated in the 1980s. Historically, treatment of head and neck cancer patients has been dictated at major referral centers by pre-eminent head and neck surgeons, who treated their patients based on their personal experience. It is likely that patients treated in this manner, in fact, received the best available treatment. However, as a result, the number of prospective randomized studies in the head and neck cancer literature (until recently) can almost be counted on the fingers of one hand, and the less experienced surgeon has few absolute guidelines to follow.

Analysis even of a closely followed population treated at one facility only partially compensates for the major defect inherent in all retrospective studies—bias. Interpretation of retrospective nonrandomized clinical studies of cancer is clouded by difficulties in comparing the various types of treatment that originate from different criteria for selecting patients for a particular therapy.

The heterogeneous criteria for selecting patients makes it difficult to be certain that any differences or similarities relate to the therapies themselves. In a nonrandomized study, the patient's treatment is determined by many factors involving the patient, tumor, and physician. The site, stage, and anaplasticity of primary and metastatic tumors vary, and individual tumors that are identical in these factors still behave differently owing to poorly defined tumor-host interactions. The socioeconomic status, medical condition, and desires of the patient also enter into the decision making. Diagnostic and treatment expertise varies among institutions and treatment personnel, including the surgeon, radiotherapist, pathologist, ancillary care personnel, and those administering adjuvant therapy. Combination treatments are administered in varying sequences, and when radiotherapy is included, doses vary. Surgeons differ in their aggressive approach and have different criteria for operability. Physician bias based on beliefs concerning optimal therapy cannot be eliminated without randomization and strict study criteria.

The typical retrospective series in the head and neck cancer literature has been accumulated over several decades and contains many patients. Upon reading the materials and methods section, however, one quickly finds that many patients are eliminated for various reasons. This results in a small group of patients in each stratum considered. Although a regulation codified by the U.S. Food and Drug Administration states that, in a disease with high and predictable mortality rate, results of a treatment procedure may be compared quantitatively with prior historical experience based on the natural history of the disease, historical control groups are generally not held in high regard because comparison is inevitably between current and archaic modalities.

Retrospective studies also suffer from the need to retrieve information from charts; the usefulness of such information varies greatly with the level of interest on the part of those collecting it. Acceptable data can be generated only if similar documentation is present for all cases under study. In a retrospective chart review, data tend to be incomplete, inaccurate, misinterpreted, and even fabricated. Incorporation of this type of data automatically biases the statistics and invalidates the majority of such studies.

Treatment end points in the reporting of data also vary. The number of patients in individual tumor or treatment categories is often too small for statistical consideration, and relatively few papers attempt any statistical analysis. In those that do, terms such as "trends" and "approaches statistical significance" are not uncommon. Survival is the usual end point reported by head and neck surgeons, whereas radiotherapists tend to report disease control in the treated volume. The latter is more relevant in assessing the effects of treatment modalities such as surgery and RT, which are directed against local-regional disease. The argument that local-regional control is irrelevant if the patient ultimately succumbs to cancer is not particularly valid for head and neck cancer patients, in whom the lack of local control can cause extreme morbidity. It is probably less troublesome to die of intercurrent disease, unrelated events, or distant metastases than from uncontrolled local-regional head and neck cancer. Survival rates are also reported in various ways (such as determinant or absolute), and this further obscures causes of death; and end points other than survival, such as the first site of failure, are also reported. Studies that report different end points are not strictly comparable.

Some authors also compare their results with retrospective series from other institutions, a practice that is particularly meaningless because expertise varies among institutions. Staging systems also vary in different parts of the world—UICC in Europe versus AJC in North America. Additionally, some institutions such as The M. D. Anderson Hospital have used their own methods of staging (neck) for many years. Based on these and other factors, it is not legitimate to compare the results of series from different institutions, and errors are compounded when statistics from various series are averaged, especially in retrospective.

To some degree, prospective randomized controlled therapeutic trials cancel out large numbers of variables and allow reasonable comparison of therapies administered to comparable patient groups. Inaccuracies in data gathering are also minimized when the format is carefully planned and needed information is anticipated and deliberately recorded. This is not to say that every question requires a prospective randomized study to answer it. Such studies require a large number of patients, and some basic efficacy studies such as phase I chemotherapy trials do not require this format. Generally, more advanced comparison of a new method with a standard treatment does, however.

Some authors maintain that because patients at a given institution are taken in rotation by the staff physicians, this incorporates an element of randomization into the treatment policies. This assumes that individual surgeons are always consistent and that they treat patients according to criteria that do not evolve or change with additional experience.

Because few prospective randomized reports compare different therapies in the head and neck cancer literature, confusion still exists regarding optimal management. At best, one can get only indications, hints, and trends from this literature. Nevertheless, certain treatment methods have been accepted as "state of the art," despite the lack of compelling evidence in their favor, based on heavy circumstantial data.

Gilbert and Kagan[86] undertook a review of the head and neck squamous cell carcinoma literature in search of statistics with universal relevance. They found that many reports neglected to describe the extent of tumors, the selection of cases, or treatment policies in such a manner as to be readily defined. Most often, survival rates were given without a detailed report of how failure occurred. Staging systems were not identical. They found that the lack of pertinent statistical data was epidemic in this literature. They felt that articles giving survival rates on the basis of treatment with little concern for anatomic site of failure or proper staging had to be rejected, and that additional pertinent data were needed before scientific conclusions could be drawn. They concluded that most head and neck cancer patients were treated on the basis of scientific assumption and opinion, because the clinician was guided by personal experience, which was based on a select group of patients and the clinician's training. It is evident that many nebulous factors enter into head and neck cancer patient treatment when similar methods yield different results. As DeSanto[56] points out, it is desirable to differentiate what we *know* to be true from what we *believe* or would like to be true, as we study the literature. In the case of head and neck cancer, we *know* very little, and the problem of sorting out valid data will become even more complex as multimodality therapy with various adjuvant treatments becomes the rule.

With respect to the specific situation of treatment of cancer in the neck, the value of a particular therapy cannot be assessed unless only previously untreated patients are reported, and only if the primary tumor remains controlled. Uncontrolled primary tumor can seed the neck after treatment, thereby contributing to a higher incidence of recurrence than would be found if the primary tumor were under control and making it impossible to evaluate the efficacy of the previous treatment to the neck per se. Only rarely is sufficient data reported to indicate how many patients die *of* cancer in the neck rather than *with* cancer in the neck—the former category of deaths are potentially preventable by elective neck treatment. Another factor is the notorious inaccuracy of clinical examination of the neck when compared to the true pathologic state of disease found on histologic examination. The inaccuracy rate in most series varies from 30 to as high as 60 per cent. Hence, treatment results of pathologically confirmed neck disease are necessary rather than analysis of response of clinically palpable neck disease (which may not have contained tumor pathologically) to treatment. The recognized staging error in clinically evaluated necks makes direct comparisons between clinically and pathologically staged studies difficult or impossible.

In addition, the method of histologic examination of the neck dissection specimen is important. It has been shown that the more closely a neck specimen is examined, the higher the incidence of disease found in the nodes—30 to 40 per cent in the analogous situation for breast cancer. In lymphadenectomy specimens the nodes should be dissected while the tissue is in a fresh state because more nodes are found than when the specimen is preserved in formalin and the nodes are dissected after it has hardened. Random sections (usually only one or two) from a lymph node do not show small occult tumor deposits as well as serial sections do; however, the serial sections are prohibitively time-consuming, and for breast cancer, it has been found that the additional information has not been particularly useful prognostically. A method of neck node examination that constitutes a happy medium is proposed by Wilkinson and Hause.[268]

Elective Treatment of the Neck: Perspectives

The basic question that propagates the controversies concerning elective treatment of the neck is, "What is the significance of occult disease in cervical nodes?" Can occult nodal cancer deposits serve as instigators of distant metastases (DMs) by seeding different sites in a "cascade" phenomenon, or do they merely serve as indicators of the ability of the individual's tumor to metastasize? The breast cancer data discussed earlier may also apply to head and neck cancer, for both systems are solid carcinomas that metastasize to regional nodes, but the lack of controlled scientific data in the head and neck cancer literature precludes confirmation of such an analogy at this time. Some data is suggestive of similar processes, as we shall see.

THE TRADITIONAL ARGUMENTS

Proponents of elective treatment of the neck maintain that such treatment serves a prophylactic function—it has the ability to prevent some cancer-related deaths. Proponents maintain that untreated occult neck disease can shed tumor into the lymphatic or vascular systems and produce DMs while the lymph node (LN) is slowly growing to clinically detectable proportions (that is, metastases metastasize). If DMs arise *only* when LNs are involved, removing the LNs early would be important to do immediately upon diagnosis if metastases can metastasize, and if the lymphatic route is the exclusive channel. Only DMs seeded from developing nodal disease can be prevented by elective neck treatment. Patients who would benefit from elective neck treatment are those in whom metastatic nodes later develop and are not salvageable when the primary tumor remains controlled when a "watchful waiting" policy is used, or those who died of DMs with local-regional tumor control, assuming that the DMs were caused by the neck metastases.

By the same token, patients who would not have benefited from elective neck treatment include those who never develop metastatic nodes at any time, those in whom metastatic nodes later developed and were successfully treated, those in whom the primary tumor was not controlled who developed nodes later, those who died as a result of the elective neck operation, and those who developed lethal contralateral nodes. It is interesting that patients who develop DMs *only* have also been placed in the category of patients who would not have benefited. If DMs can arise as a result of nonlymphatic dissemination, as is likely, then it may be true that treatment of the neck will not affect failure at distant sites.

The traditional arguments pro and con generally relate to END as the treatment modality. We shall later discuss ENI as a method of accomplishing the same end. The arguments for and against elective neck dissection are summarized in Table 56–3.

A prerequisite for evaluation of any treatment effect is a baseline provided by the natural history of the untreated disease. Almost no papers specifically deal with this issue in the head and neck cancer literature. One by DuVal and Healy[60] includes only 10 cases, which were too advanced to be treated even palliatively. Naturally, such a baseline cannot ethically be obtained today, and most experienced head and neck oncologists would probably agree that the inevitable outcome of untreated aggressive head and neck SCC is a disagreeable death within 2 years related to uncontrolled local-regional disease.

A major impediment to evaluating the utility of treatments is the lack of definition of the true cause(s) of failure in treatment of this disease. What proportion of deaths are directly attributable to cervical metastases per se, and thereby potentially preventable by elective neck treatment? (This assumption ignores the systemic nature of metastasis.) If patients die *with* or *of* neck disease, then elective neck treatment might have been palliative, at least, if the primary tumor remained controlled. Because results are usually reported in terms of

TABLE 56–3. Traditional Arguments for and against Elective Neck Dissection

Con	Pro
RLN helpful in tumor defense—ND removes barrier to cancer spread and has deleterious immunologic effect	RLN not helpful in tumor defense
Significance of micrometastases unknown and cure rate not lower with watchful waiting for N0→N+ conversion	False negative findings on clinical examination are common; significant number of patients have occult disease and all occult nodes will become clinically significant
Careful clinical follow-up detects earliest conversion of N0→N+	Even with monthly follow-up some patients will develop inoperable neck disease with watchful waiting
Morbidity and mortality of surgery	Morbidity and mortality are negligible with surgery, especially with functional ND
ENI is as effective as END in control of occult neck disease with less morbidity	END is as effective as ENI in control of occult neck disease; RT can be held in reserve for future disease
	Do END when: enter neck during primary surgery, in patients with short, fat, difficult to examine necks and when poor follow-up anticipated

Additional Considerations

1. Elective neck treatment is prophylactic only in patients who develop inoperable neck disease with watchful waiting. Otherwise, survival is not improved because local-regional treatment does not affect distant cancer spread.
2. It is impossible to compare END and ENI efficacy because the status of neck disease is unknown when ENI is used.
3. END can serve as a biopsy, which is an indicator of the concomitant risk of systemic disease, because neck and distant metastases are manifestations of the same process—the ability of a tumor to metastasize in an individual host.
4. ENI has the potential to produce systemic morbidity based on its effect on the immune system—morbidity is not limited to the local-regional factors usually cited.

Key: RLN = Regional lymph nodes; ND = neck dissection; ENI = elective neck irradiation; RT = radiation therapy; END = elective neck dissection.

---

overall survival without tabulating causes of death and sites of failure, this question is almost impossible to answer from the existing literature.[86, 138, 150, 240]

CHANGING PATTERNS OF FAILURE

The Halstedian head and neck surgeon traditionally maintains that the risk of neck operation is justified in a selected group of patients—those with a high yield of occult positive nodes—because the earlier these nodes are found and treated, the better the result. This raises the perennial question of whether the "better result" seen in such patients is related to the neck dissection, or whether it merely reflects the natural history of disease in that individual. Patients undergoing END without positive nodes in the specimen constitute a subgroup that favorably influences the overall result compiled on all patients undergoing END.

Whereas Halstedian concepts of surgical oncology have been questioned in breast cancer, head and neck cancer has for many years been considered a prototype solid tumor system that proves their utility—that is, local-regional disease can be cured with local-regional treatments (surgery and radiation), and DMs are not a significant problem. This conclusion is now in question. For decades, the results of ineffective local-regional disease control were seen—progression of disease killed the host within a relatively short period of time. More recently, as technologic advances have allowed better combinations of standard therapy, less local-regional disease recurs and patients are living longer, only to die more frequently of DMs or second primary tumors. Overall, survival has not changed.

In a recent commentary, Goepfert[88] notes that SCC of the upper aerodigestive tract (UADT) is a heterogeneous group of entities with different biologic behaviors. At M. D. Anderson Hospital, autopsy reports for 1955 to 1965 were compared with the decade beginning in 1973. There was an increase in DMs as the cause of death (17 to 32 per cent), deaths from uncontrolled tumors above the clavicle dropped (30 to 15 per cent), there was a marked reduction of fatal treatment complications (25 to 10 per cent), the cause of death from unrelated nonmalignant diseases increased (15 to 28 per cent), and the incidence of second malignancies as the cause of death remained at 14 per cent.

PREDICTORS OF OCCULT NODAL METASTASES

Much effort has been expended in defining the incidence of occult disease in the neck, either by demonstrated pathologic examination of END specimens or as inferred from the conversion rate of clinically N0 to N+ necks after successful treatment of the primary tumor. Because there is currently no way to identify occult disease in cervical nodes other than by removing and examining them, various features of the primary tumor (site, size, differentiation) have been correlated with the incidence of occult disease in the neck with the objective of decreasing the number of needless and risky surgeries.

Most studies look at only one feature; thus, a large number of biases are not controlled, and as many papers can be found refuting as supporting the significance of any particular prognostic parameter. Lindberg's widely quoted paper,[137] which correlated the location of the primary tumor with the frequency of cervical metastases, is a clinical study of palpable nodes. Because of significant error in clinical neck evaluation and lack of pathologic correlation, the accuracy of the associations can be questioned. Pathologic staging tends to be higher than clinical staging, although false positive nodes occur, especially with floor of mouth cancers.

In 1976, Shear and associates[222] evaluated the primary site, size, and histologic differentiation in 898 cases in which cervical metastases were histologically confirmed. A logistic multiple regression analysis defined several site, size, and differentiation "clusters" that were associated with progressively increased risk of cervical metastases. If, for a given tumor, the site, size, or differentiation cluster was known, then it was possible to estimate the probability of metastasis. In this series, the indication for neck dissection was not stated; however, it was mentioned that many clinically positive nodes appeared when the primary tumor recurred, so the primary site was not always controlled in this series.

Because the literature does not show strict correlation of neck metastasis rate with any of the primary tumor factors studied to date, workers are investigating additional features of the primary tumor that might correlate better with the propensity to metastasize, such as invasive morphologic features at the periphery.[272] Eventually, biochemical correlates of primary tumor metastatic ability may be available and assessible from a biopsy specimen.

WHEN TO TREAT?

It is next necessary for the surgeon to decide what is the acceptable incidence of occult neck metastases to justify operation. This was a more serious consideration in the past when such procedures were more dangerous; now with the availability of various modified neck dissections (MND), the question of surgical morbidity is essentially moot (if one believes that such conservation neck dissections are oncologically safe). The acceptable incidence of occult disease that warrants elective neck treatment varies, depending upon the opinion of the "treatment manager." Some say that an occult metastatic rate exceeding 15 to 20 per cent would warrant elective neck treatment.[135] The incidence of occult neck disease ranges from 15 to 50 per cent, so virtually all sites and stages of epidermoid.cancer of the mouth and throat, except lip and T1 glottic tumors, would qualify for elective neck treatment on this basis. Others[178] have suggested that a 5 to 10 per cent increase in survival (which is almost impossible to determine from the literature) is sufficient to warrant elective neck treatment.

In the final analysis, percentages from series are not applicable to individual patients. The patient either will have or will not have cervical metastases—an all-or-none phenomenon—a 0 or 100 per cent incidence in the individual. Therefore, the information that 30 per cent of patients with invasive T2 floor of mouth cancers have occult neck metastases is not easily applied to the individual case.

SIGNIFICANCE OF OCCULT NODAL METASTASES

Next, what is the natural history of occult neck disease—does it *always* become clinically significant? It is possible to compile data showing that the incidence of pathologically positive nodes in END specimens (about 30 per cent average) corresponds quite closely to the N0 to N+ conversion rate without neck treatment (about 25 per cent average)—this can be interpreted to indicate that occult disease in the neck has a rather inexorable potential to manifest as clinically apparent cervical metastases[156, 160] (see Table 56–4). Not all data shows this equivalence, however. In one series, the conversion rate in surgical determinate cases with the primary tumor controlled was 8 per cent for T1 lesions, 10 per cent for T2, and 2 per cent for T3—considerably less than expected based on the presumed incidence of occult disease in the neck.[66] In a series from M. D. Anderson Hospital, only 2 to 2.5 per cent of the patients with cancer of the oral cavity whose primary lesion was

TABLE 56–4. Incidence of Lymph Node Metastasis by Primary Site in Head and Neck Squamous Cell Carcinomas

Primary Site	N+ at Presentation	N0 Clinically, N+ Pathologically	N0→N+ with No Neck Treatment
Floor of mouth	30%–59%	40%–50%	20%–35%
Gingiva	18%–52%	19%	17%
Hard palate	13%–24%		22%
Buccal mucosa	9%–31%		16%
Oral tongue	34%–65%	25%–54%	38%–52%
Nasopharynx	86%–90%		19%–50%
Anterior tonsillar pillar/retromolar trigone	39%–56%		10%–15%
Soft palate/uvula	37%–56%		16%–25%
Tonsillar fossa	58%–76%		22%
Base of the tongue	50%–83%	22%	
Pharyngeal walls	50%–71%	66%	
Supraglottic larynx	31%–54%	16–26%	33%
Hypopharynx	52%–72%	38%	

*T1N0 patients only.
†Patients received preoperative irradiation.
Source: Modified from Mendenhall WM, Million RR, Cassisi NJ: Elective neck irradiation in squamous cell carcinoma of the head and neck. Head Neck Surg 3:15, 1980.

controlled were judged to have been able to benefit from complete elective neck treatment. This series did, however, include a number of patients who had upper neck irradiation included with treatment to the primary site, and it is therefore not strictly comparable to the surgery-only series.[118]

Remember, too, that averaged data compiled from aggregate studies on different patient populations and from different institutions is invalid. Also, it appears that recurrence of the primary tumor is the most common cause of conversion of a clinically N0 to N+ neck, and therefore, disease control at the primary site is mandatory when N0 to N+ conversion rates are compared to the incidence of occult disease in END specimens.

The "alternate hypothesis," as applied to cervical metastatic cancer, would regard cervical and distant metastases as manifestations of the same biologic process—the overall ability of the tumor to metastasize in a particular host. If cancerous cervical nodes serve as indicators of concomitant DMs, then END as a diagnostic biopsy procedure—not prophylactic—would almost never be unnecessary, except for lesions with a very low metastatic rate (T1 glottic, lip) or in patients who develop contralateral neck disease only, because proper histologic examination of the neck dissection specimen would tell whether cervical metastases were present or absent. Delayed contralateral neck disease usually occurs after treatment (surgery or RT) that alters lymphatic drainage pathways in the neck and sometimes in the presence of recurrent primary disease. Delayed contralateral neck disease occurs rarely in untreated necks with the primary tumor controlled. By using END in this context, a population at high risk to develop DMs would be identified and adjuvant therapy could be instituted (in a controlled trial setting) at a time more likely to be successful than later when distant disease manifests clinically and is more quantitatively significant. This strategy would become more useful in routine clinical practice when efficacious adjuvant treatments become available, but it can be useful now in the phase of identifying useful agents.

If cervical metastases are not predictors of distant disease, however, then END would not have this potential usefulness. Is histologically proven neck disease a predictor for DMs? Once again, the literature makes it difficult to answer this question unequivocally, because DMs as causes of death are seldom listed accurately. Also, distant disease tends to occur at the same time as recurrent regional disease, thus making it difficult to determine its source as activation of dormant cells from the original tumor or from the recurrence. (Does the frequent synchronicity of local-regional recurrence and distant disease result from systemic depression in the host when all cancer control mechanisms have broken down, thus representing another aspect of the natural history of terminal disease?) Therefore, correlation of DM incidence with parameters of the initial tumor stage can only be made when DMs arise with regional disease controlled. Additionally, there is sometimes difficulty in deciding whether tumor that appears in the lung represents DMs or a second primary lesion. How the DMs are defined is also relevant—whether on a clinical or autopsy basis. In series which have looked for DMs at autopsy, they are found in as many as 50 to 60 per cent of patients with head and neck SCC, whereas the clinical detection of metastatic foci occurs in 10 to 30 per cent of cases.[1, 4, 15, 28, 53, 113, 161, 177, 184, 192, 251] It is probably more relevant to report the incidence of DMs in living patients because it is not known whether those found at autopsy would have become clinically significant.

NODAL METASTASES AS PREDICTORS OF DISTANT DISEASE

Although certain features of the primary tumor have been correlated with the incidence of DMs, the amount of disease in the neck at presentation is the feature most constantly predictive of DMs (Table 56–5). Nodal involvement presumably reflects the aggressive biologic nature of the primary lesion.[1, 15, 24, 86, 161] Lindberg[138] recently reported on 3616 patients treated from 1960 to 1974 and their sites of first failure, based on *clinical* staging. Distant metastases were the first recurrence (with local-regional tumor control) in 7.2 per cent of patients. In Merino's series,[161] 8 per cent of all patients and 23 per cent of patients with N2–3 lesions who had disease controlled above the clavicle developed DMs, implying that subclinical metastases must have occurred before or during the initial treatment. The incidence of DMs associated with advanced (N2–3) N stage was four times that associated with early N stage (N0–1)—24 per cent versus 6 per cent. In Berger and Fletcher's series[15] DMs were present in 11 per cent of early N stage cases and in 47 per cent of advanced N stage cases, the difference between these two categories of nodal disease being statistically significant. There was no relationship between the subsequent development of DMs and the location of initial nodal disease.

A second conclusion from the literature is that the incidence of DMs doubles in patients who develop a recurrence above the clavicle[118, 161, 175] (Table 56–6).

For the hypothesis that N stage is an accurate prognosticator for DMs to be acceptable, it is also necessary for patients with N0 necks to develop DMs infrequently or never. A perusal of the literature indicates that, indeed, patients staged N0 at the outset of their disease can develop DMs, but in only 3 to 5 per cent of cases.[113, 118, 138, 161, 184] There is almost no data to allow one to determine pathologically whether or not N0 patients go on to develop DMs. In one study[4] in which pathologic neck status was correlated with the incidence of DMs, there was no statistically significant difference in local recurrence, DMs, or survival in patients with positive or negative occult nodes at END. Although lacking statistical significance, it is interesting that there were no DMs in 16 patients with pathologically negative nodes, whereas there were six in 39 patients with pathologically positive nodes.

In clinically staged series, the occurrence of DMs in patients with N0 necks does not negate the correlation

TABLE 56–5. Risk of Distant Metastases by Stage

Stage	Risk	T Stage	Risk	N Stage	Risk
I	2.0%	T1	5.2%	N0	4.9%
II	5.7%	T2	9.6%	N1	11.8%
III	8.5%	T3	12.7%	N2	21.8%
IV	19.5%	T4	16.1%	N3	27.1%

TABLE 56–6. Risk of Distant Metastases Related to Initial Neck Control with Primary Lesion Controlled

| Primary Site | Clinical N Stage | Neck Controlled without Treatment (N0) or with Initial Treatment (N+) | | Neck Converted To + or Not Controlled by Initial Treatment | |
		Number of Patients	Distant Metasases	Number of Patients	Distant Metasases
Oral cavity	N0	387	3%	94	11%
Oral cavity, oropharynx	N1–2	134	12%	46	24%
Oral cavity, oropharynx	N3	20	5%	45	31%

Source: Modified from Million RR: The natural history of squamous cell carcinoma. *In* Million RR, Cassisi NJ (eds): Management of Head and Neck Cancer: A Multidisciplinary Approach. Philadelphia, J.B. Lippincott, 1984, p 29.

between neck status and the propensity to form DMs; because of the clinical error in examination of necks, some of the patients could have had microscopically positive neck nodes. Distant metastases arising in the context of a pathologically N0 neck could arise from occult neck disease not detected pathologically (if metastases metastasize), by hematogenous spread, by seeding from an unrecognized recurrent tumor or unknown second primary cancer, or from reactivation of dormant tumor cells that arose from the original tumor. In one series, N0 patients who remain without a recurrence above the clavicle had an incidence of DMs of 3 per cent versus 11 per cent in patients initially N0 who developed a recurrence above the clavicle.[118] Because the literature supports a rather compelling correlation between the presence of neck disease and the likelihood of developing DMs, it seems that an END "biopsy" would be a useful prognosticator for distant spread.

NODAL CHARACTERISTICS AS DETERMINANTS OF PROGNOSIS

Attempts have been made to define specific features of LN metastases that indicate a poor prognosis in patients—usually related to the propensity for recurrence in the neck after treatment. Factors such as the site, size, and number of positive nodes in the neck, as well as presence of nodes at multiple levels and extracapsular extension have been looked at, usually as individual parameters. In various series, each of these has been shown to be either significant or not and definite conclusions cannot be drawn from retrospective series that do not control for other sources of bias. For example, in one series the influence of smoking, alcohol intake, and weight loss during therapy were found to be important prognosticators of survival and regional recurrence—equivalent to tumor site and LN metastases.[35]

A more reliable way of assessing the individual or aggregate importance of single parameters is to use a multivariate stepwise discriminant analysis, although the utility of this approach is still limited when data is derived from retrospective studies because other sources of bias have not been eliminated or controlled.

Widespread *beliefs* concerning cervical LN prognostic parameters are that the prognosis is very poor with nodes in the lower jugular and posterior triangle areas, or with bilateral or contralateral disease. Prognostic significance has often been attributed to certain morphologic LN patterns, with lymphocyte predominance being associated with a better prognosis than unstimulated or lymphocyte-depletion patterns, presumably as a reflection of the host's ability to mount an effective antitumor immune response.[16] Sinus histiocytosis, in which macrophages proliferate in the LN sinuses, has also been considered favorable. Functional correlates of various patterns have not been characterized. Problems in attributing significance to this type of LN prognostic parameter include studying LNs from patients who have undergone radiation, which alters the lymphocyte population of nodes, and sampling bias (the cellular pattern can vary within and between RLNs). Attributing the course of cancer in a patient solely to localized interactions within a node ignores the many other clinical parameters, including treatment, which influence prognosis. Responses of RLNs to a cancer may well be an index of the host's general reaction to tumor, rather than a specific local record of the interactions of LN cells with cancer cells. Many head and neck cancers are ulcerated and contaminated, and regional node lymphocyte patterns may represent inflammatory responses rather than reactions to tumor cell antigens. Proliferative states such as sinus histiocytosis can mechanically block cancer cell traffic through the node, and the absence of local node metastases may be explicable in terms of such a bypass instead of arrest and destruction of cancer cells within the node.

In a multiple regression analysis of 23 tumor, node, and patient variables, Kraus and Panje[132] found that lower jugular node involvement and histopathologic results greater than clinical staging were significantly correlated with decreased survival. The most relevant combination of factors that predicted decreased survival were mid- and lower jugular node involvement and positive histopathologic findings. These were all stage IV patients with a "giant" cervical LN (greater than 4 cm). Of 94 patients there were 15 long-term survivors and a determinate 5-year or greater survival of 20 per cent. The mean survival time was 10 years for survivors, showing that not all patients with cervical metastases are doomed to die of cancer. Thirteen of the 15 survivors had only one positive node, however. Although nodal masses larger than 3 cm often represent a conglomerate of nodes, in this study many of the "giant" cervical nodes were single. The authors speculated that such nodes might be the site of some immune or inflammatory response to cancer indicative of a favorable tumor-host interaction.

Schuller and associates[217] performed discriminant analysis on 12 characteristics of metastatic LNs (number, percent positive, size, anatomic position) and attempted to correlate them with survival. Although involvement of the posterior triangle and noncontiguous or multiple sites were associated with a worse prognosis, whether considered individually or collectively, there was no parameter that was accurate enough to be of use to the clinician in prognostication. No mention was made of whether or not primary tumors were controlled in the survival analysis. The conclusion was that the most important information relating LN status to prognosis was whether or not tumor was present or absent in the cervical nodes, and that attributing added significance to individual features of metastatic nodes was not warranted.

SIGNIFICANCE OF MACROSCOPIC VERSUS MICROSCOPIC NODAL DISEASE

Is "microscopic" neck cancer more favorable than "macroscopic" neck disease, or are both associated with a similar prognosis? The relative significance of micro- versus macrometastases is not scientifically addressed in the head and neck cancer literature. Tulenko[246] showed 5-year cures ranging from 76 per cent in patients with histologically and clinically negative nodes to 11 per cent in those with histologically and clinically positive nodes. Histologically negative palpable nodes were associated with 79 per cent survival, and histologically positive nonpalpable nodes with a 29 per cent survival. Micrometastases were therefore about three times more curable than macrometastases.

In a retrospective study on 64 epidermoid carcinomas of the mouth and pharynx treated between 1960 and 1964[66] one third of 60 surgically determinate patients with occult positive nodes treated by END were cured, as contrasted with a 25 per cent cure rate for patients with clinically positive nodes—the difference is not statistically significant.

The relative significance of macro- versus micrometastatic LN disease is also controversial in the breast cancer literature. Some studies have shown that micrometastases (maximum diameter 2 mm) in axillary nodes, in the absence of macrometastases, are associated with an excellent prognosis and that patients with occult metastases have treatment success equivalent to that of patients with pathologically negative nodes. In some of these cases, however, the "positive" foci were characterized as tumor emboli lying free within the peripheral sinuses of the nodes, and they may not have represented true implanted metastases.[79, 116, 188]

The common practice of cutting LNs at only one or two levels will result in small nodal foci of cancer being missed. Several studies have shown that when LNs are serially sectioned, additional tumor deposits are found in 20 to 40 per cent of cancer cases, although it is generally accepted that routine sampling may be adequate for purposes of treatment planning. Cutting nodes into four nearly equal segments with proper orientation of the slices so that different surfaces are examined significantly improves the success of identifying small nodal lesions without drastically increasing the amount of work involved.[268]

EXTRACAPSULAR SPREAD

Although we have just indicated that attributing prognostic significance to any individual LN parameter other than the presence or absence of metastasis is unwarranted, general belief regards extracapsular spread (ECS) as a particularly bad prognosticator. It is intuitively understandable that spread of tumor beyond the LN capsule could result in a high incidence of neck recurrence. There are no prospective or multiple regression studies relating survival to ECS, however; and its significance as an individual parameter should be viewed with caution.

In a recent study Johnson and associates[124] retrospectively examined specimens from 516 patients with SCC treated by RND between 1973 and 1981. Recurrence rates, site of recurrence, disease-free interval, and 2-year survival were assessed for three neck conditions: pathologically negative necks and pathologically positive necks with or without ECS. Sixty per cent of patients with neck disease less than 3 cm in dimension had ECS. Histologically verified ECS was associated with a significantly poorer prognosis compared with patients without this finding. Although 90 per cent of patients with ECS got postoperative RT, the overall survival rate was only 35 per cent—two thirds died with regional disease and one third with DMs. Patients with ECS were at increased risk to develop local recurrence and DMs and had a shorter time to recurrence. Extracapsular spread decreased survival approximately 50 per cent over patients with tumor confined within LNs.

In an earlier report of this data,[125] the incidence of failure in the neck (with or without DMs) was 37 per cent, 30 per cent, and 50 per cent, respectively, for patients with no histologic neck disease, patients who had neck disease without ECS, and patients who had neck disease with ECS. The incidence of patients developing DMs alone was 50 per cent, 50 per cent, and 30 per cent for the same groups. A 50 per cent incidence of DMs in pathologically N0 patients (10 of 19) is quite surprising and does not fit with the hypothesis that the presence or absence of neck disease is a strong predictor for DMs. It does suggest, however, that biologically "early" head and neck SCC (that is, cancer not metastatic to RLNs), as clinically perceived, can be a systemic disease by virtue of hematogenous spread.

Noone and associates[173] found that if tumor was limited to the nodes, 70 per cent of patients survived 5 years, whereas if the node capsule was invaded, 48 per cent did. If there was ECS, 5-year survival was 27 per cent. Sessions[220] noted that invasion of neck soft tissue by tumor decreased treatment success by a ratio of 5:1. Snow and associates[230] found ECS in 23 per cent of nodes less than 1 cm, in 53 per cent of nodes 2 to 3 cm, and in 74 per cent of nodes greater than 3 cm. Addition of RT after RND did improve the results in patients with ECS. Zoller and associates[274] reviewed a group of patients treated by surgery alone. None of the survivors had ECS, but 36 per cent of those who died did. Of the patients who underwent RT, ECS was present in 20 per cent of the survivors and in 39 per cent of those who died.

The biologic significance of ECS is currently unclear—does it represent increased tumor burden or increased tumor aggressiveness? Johnson and associates[125] speculated that ECS may represent a more aggressive tumor and may indicate depressed host immunosurveillance with failure to contain tumor spread. Intuitively, not all ECS should have the same prognosis—node rupture in occult positive nodes may not have the same significance as nodal rupture in large, "fixed" neck masses (N3). In the former instance, neck dissection should be able to remove the disease with an adequate margin. Also, ECS is generally spoken of as an "all-or-none" phenomenon. Clearly, not all nodes in a specimen show ECS. Is ECS as significant if it occurs in only one node as if it occurs in 20? Probably ECS should now be studied in a more rigorous manner with respect to quality and quantity, and it must be correlated with patient prognosis and treatment in a prospective manner before the true significance of this finding can be assessed. Already, many surgeons are sensitized to the finding of "ECS" (although few articles describe what they mean by this and different pathologists probably have different definitions) and now conscientiously add postoperative RT to the treatment plan of any patient found to have as little as one positive node with ECS in an END specimen. This is probably not warranted on the basis of the existing literature, although the urge to use "big gun" treatment is now strongly founded on an intuitively appealing mass of suggestive evidence.

In one breast cancer series[147] extension through axillary node capsules worsened the prognosis only for those patients with fewer than three involved nodes. Rupture of the LN capsule has also been strongly associated with the presence of tumor emboli in lymphatic vessels in some cases, so associated findings may also be relevant.[171]

PERTINENT DATA FROM THE HEAD AND NECK LITERATURE

In one of the few well-constructed retrospective series that addresses many of the preceding considerations, Ogura and associates[178] evaluated the neck recurrence and survival rates of 348 patients with pharyngeal and laryngeal cancers based on whether their neck dissection specimens contained pathologically negative nodes, occult positive nodes, or palpable positive nodes. Almost half of the patients had received planned low-dose preoperative radiation but previous analysis of this group indicated that the incidence of neck recurrence was not influenced by such treatment. Patient treatment was considered homogeneous because all cases were managed by the senior author. Recurrence of tumor at the primary site was eliminated. Patients who were lost to follow-up or dead within 3 years of any cause were considered failures with respect to survival rate determination, thereby obscuring the cancer-related causes of death.

The data were analyzed by a mathematical model that made the (questionable) assumptions that an occult node would in time become palpable and that deaths due to causes other than neck recurrence were independent of the degree of node involvement (as we have seen, DMs seem significantly related to N stage). In general, for tumors in different primary locations, the incidence of neck recurrence was zero or negligible for patients with negative nodes and occult positive nodes and was only significant for patients with palpable positive nodes. Although some of the occult positive nodes undoubtedly had ECS, neck recurrence was not a problem. The survival rates of patients with occult positive nodes were generally intermediate between those with negative nodes and palpable positive nodes, although exceptions did occur. Because the causes of death were not specified, it is not possible to interpret intermediate death rates in patients with occult positive

nodes as evidence in favor of a more dismal prognosis, even with histologically positive occult neck disease. For some sites, the survival rate was not significantly different when comparing the occult node group with the palpable node group; however, for other sites the survival rate was significantly greater with occult nodes versus palpable nodes. In the latter situation, the positive influence on survival was attributed to neck dissection—this is the traditional interpretation of elective neck dissection as being prophylactic.

The causes of death were not mentioned, but because the primary tumor was controlled in all cases and the neck recurrence rate was usually the same in patients with occult positive and negative nodes, the change in survival was apparently not related to uncontrolled neck disease. When nodes were palpable, however, there was generally a significantly increased neck recurrence rate and concomitant decreased survival, presumably attributable to recurrent disease in the neck.

Based on the mathematical model, it was calculated that "elective" neck dissection (neck dissection was performed for both palpable and nonpalpable nodes) improved the survival rate 4 per cent for patients with supraglottic cancers and 11 per cent for patients with pyriform sinus cancers. It was suggested that ability to increase the survival rate 5 to 10 per cent was sufficient to justify END, as the mortality rate was less than 1 per cent for patients undergoing the procedure.

Data from a recent paper relate to many of the considerations discussed previously.[255] Failure at distant sites following multimodality treatment for stages III and IV head and neck SCC was examined. Twenty of 114 patients developed DMs as the first site of failure—all within 2 years of treatment of the primary tumor. The T stage did not relate to the subsequent incidence of DMs, but the N stage did, as found in other series previously. Patients presenting with palpable neck nodes had a higher incidence of DMs than those who presented with clinically negative necks (25 per cent versus 4 per cent). The most significant prognosticator for DMs was the pathologic extent of nodal metastases found at neck dissection. Patients with positive nodes at multiple levels had significantly greater likelihood of developing subsequent DMs than did those whose metastases were confined to one level or who had negative nodes (35 per cent versus 5 per cent). In this study, patients with N1 disease were grouped with those having negative nodes, thereby obscuring the data related to patients with negative nodes alone. The incidence of DMs was also uninfluenced by previous chemotherapy, age or sex of the patient, site of the primary tumor, or histologic grade of the primary tumor. The overall incidence of DMs in this series (20 per cent) was similar to that reported previously from the same institution.[66] However, in that series, DMs were the initial cause of failure in only 4 per cent of the patients, and failure in the head and neck area dominated. In this series, however, patients who failed did so primarily at distant sites (56 per cent), reflecting achievement of better local-regional control.

Although interpretation should be cautious, based on the retrospective nature of the series, it seemed that the addition of postoperative RT to surgery did not appreciably alter the incidence of DMs, but it did decrease the incidence of antecedent failure above the clavicle, so much so that failure at distant sites had become prominent as the primary cause of disease and death. This offset the improvement in survival which had been hoped for by combining surgery and RT. Patients considered at high risk for the development of DMs were those who had metastases to cervical nodes at multiple levels (one in three of these patients could be expected to develop DMs within 2 years), and it was suggested that such patients be enrolled in prospective studies to evaluate the efficacy of adjuvant therapy directed against systemic micrometastases. However, two of three patients would not develop DMs, and it was suggested that research to define more detailed pathologic and perhaps kinetic cancer parameters should be undertaken to help identify patients at high risk for failure at distant sites.

It is well accepted that 5-year survival is reduced by at least half when positive cervical nodes are present in a patient with head and neck SCC. But why? The material in this section has mentioned several possible mechanisms. One article that reviewed the literature stated that the biologic significance of the clinically positive neck (initially or later in the course of disease) reflected the aggressiveness of the primary tumor and its propensity to recur after either surgery or RT.[86] I would add that it also reflects the aggressiveness of the primary tumor with respect to its ability to metastasize not only to the neck but to distant sites. It is difficult to conclude from the head and neck cancer literature how many patients die *of* versus *with* neck disease, as opposed to failure at other sites. Patients dying *of* neck disease typically experience some dramatic event, such as hemorrhage from the carotid artery, in order to be so designated. One gets the feeling that many more patients die *with* rather than *of* neck disease. With more effective local-regional disease control, the dismal prognostic significance of neck disease may now relate more to the fact that it represents generalized metastatic tumor potential rather than to the fact that patients die from disease in their necks per se.

Several controversies relating to appropriate treatment of the N0 neck concern the choice of modality— surgery or RT. It is important to realize that *surgery* and *radiation therapy* are effective against local-regional disease, not systemic disease. Reporting survival as the treatment end point incorporates several causes of death that are not amenable to control by local-regional therapy per se—DMs, multiple primary tumors, and intercurrent disease. A more appropriate end point for evaluating the efficacy of local-regional treatment is control of disease in the treated volume, as radiotherapists tend to report. Laments concerning the lack of increased survival in head and neck SCC patients despite more effective combinations of surgery and RT miss this essential point.

The assessment of efficacy of single or combination treatment modalities with respect to control of neck disease requires that the method of treatment is standardized, that positive nodes are verified histologically, and that tumor control at the primary site is maintained. If we were to restrict our discussion to papers that satisfy these criteria and use appropriate statistical analysis, nothing would remain to be said at this point. Therefore, we will discuss the papers that have adequately dealt with one or more of these aspects.

Elective Neck Dissection

It is safe to say that RND is the procedure of choice for palpable metastatic SCC in the neck. Before discussing conservation neck dissection, we must evaluate the ability of RND as a single treatment modality to control neck disease. To avoid the contamination of results by combination modalities, one must resort to the older literature. Problems in interpretation arise because in earlier decades neck staging was not standardized and treatment efficacy is expected to vary with the amount of disease in the neck, which is hard to quantify. Also in the older reports, primary disease control was seldom accomplished. Therefore, recurrence in the neck following radical dissection could be attributed to either development of residual disease in the neck or from seeding from uncontrolled primary tumor. The latter seems to have been more prevalent until recently. Therefore, much of the data that putatively reflects the lack of efficacy of RND to control neck disease actually reflects the inability of initial neck treatment to control recurrent disease originating from primary tumor. Lack of primary control has become less of a problem in recent years, and we may even see an additional benefit from the recent availability of reliable flaps, which have allowed surgeons the freedom to excise primary tumors with wider margins now that large defects can be readily reconstructed.

EFFICACY OF RADICAL NECK DISSECTION

Recurrence rates of tumor in the neck from 10 to 70 per cent have been reported following RND. Two of the most widely quoted articles report rates of 26 and 36 per cent, respectively.[13, 239] In the first article,[13] primary tumor recurrence also occurred in 30 per cent of the patients (were these the same patients who developed neck recurrence?). In Strong's article[239] a neck recurrence rate of 71 per cent was found when pathologically positive nodes were present at multiple levels. In this series also, the primary tumor was uncontrolled in about 25 per cent of patients.

In the few papers that report neck control rate with primary tumor also controlled, neck recurrences range from 11 per cent for N1 disease and 19 per cent for N2 disease[212] to 25 to 30 per cent.[82] In a recent paper, DeSanto and associates[56] reported on a series of head and neck cancer patients who underwent neck dissection; 75 per cent were treated with primary surgery alone. The recurrence rate in dissected necks at 2 years was 7.5 per cent, 20.2 per cent, and 37.4 per cent for N0, N1, and N2 necks. Because failure was defined as the first sign of recurrence in the neck and because most neck recurrences were noted before primary recurrence was found, it was stated that the rate of neck recurrence was probably not influenced by uncontrolled primary disease, but this variable was not strictly eliminated.

These results seem to indicate the intuitively logical conclusion that the efficacy of RND decreases as the amount of disease increases in the neck and as it spreads from containment in the LN into adjacent soft tissue. Radical neck dissection is by no means an ineffective treatment modality, however; one must realize that the lack of control attributed to RND has in large part historically related to lack of control of tumor at the primary site.

MODIFIED NECK DISSECTIONS

With respect to less than radical neck dissections, the standard for comparison is the work of Bocca's group in Italy, who since the 1960s have been using routine elective functional neck dissection (FND), which removes the LN-bearing contents of the neck but preserves the sternocleidomastoid muscle (SCM), internal jugular vein (IJV), and spinal accessory nerve (SAN). Their rationale for performing routine END is that they did not know which tumors would metastasize and which would not. Thus, they view END in the traditional *prophylactic* context.

As we have seen, head and neck cancer surgeons have been using various types of modified neck dissection (MND) since the 1920s. Conservation neck dissection has come continually under fire during the last 25 years because it deviates from Halstedian or "Crilean" principles, which dictate that RND is necessary for the best removal of all cancer in the neck. Disapproval of conservation operations was expressed by Conley, a pre-eminent authority in the field, in 1975. As recently as 1976[156] the operation was described as "a form of surgical brinkmanship in that microscopically involved nodes had been seen hard against, and involving the adventitia of the internal jugular vein; it becomes clear that cancer in a functional neck dissection specimen is not a faithfully gift-wrapped entity." Conservation larynx cancer operations met with similar resistance initially—change evokes resistance.

Bocca maintains that the extent of a radical approach should be conceived against the cancer and not against the neck, and has always affirmed that his modified procedure is as oncologically radical as any traditional neck dissection, provided that some technical details are respected, that the nodes are still mobile, and that the dissection consists of removing the aponeurotic sheaths with the areolar tissues which they surround.[20] When so performed, FND offers oncologic safety comparable to RND while avoiding unnecessary mutilation. In response to the criticism that the preservation of the internal jugular vein and sternocleidomastoid muscle compromises oncologic safety because they cross lymphatic pathways, Bocca has pointed out that the spinal accessory nerve, thoracic duct, vagus nerve, cervical sympathetic chain, and hypoglossal nerve also cross aponeurotic spaces in an irregular fashion because their development is unrelated to the branchial apparatus, but yet these structures are preserved routinely in RND (except for the spinal accessory nerve).

Preservation of the spinal accessory nerve as a modification of RND had not generated similar controversy until our attention was redirected by Schuller and associates[215] to a fact noted by Hayes Martin in the 1940s: the spinal accessory chain includes a portion in the subdigastric area where metastatic nodes frequently occur, and preservation of this nerve in modified or FND requires cutting through and sectioning lymphatic channels connecting these LNs in the superior portion of the neck (as does preservation of the hypoglossal nerve). Schuller's report challenges the conclusion that the spinal accessory nerve can be preserved. Because studies do not mention the location of neck recurrences following various types of MND, it is difficult to know whether or not saving the spinal accessory nerve or

other structures with or without the use of postoperative RT in fact results in recurrences in the area of preserved structures.

If the surgeon can rationalize saving the spinal accessory nerve, then preservation of the internal jugular vein and sternocleidomastoid muscle in selected cases should not cause additional theoretical difficulties. In Bocca's words, "obstacles to the acceptance of the new technique are twofold; first, a theoretical objection deriving from the authority of traditional teaching, and second, a technical objection deriving from the necessity of acquiring new surgical habits. Both of these obstacles can be easily overcome if one is armed with good will, openmindedness, and constructive criticism."[20]

Certainly, FND is more time-consuming than RND, as are all operations that preserve structures rather than radically remove them, and the "occasional" head and neck surgeon is advised to remain with RND or, at most, spinal accessory nerve preservation as a standard operation. That the operation is oncologically sound in Bocca's hands does not mean that the same is true when it is performed by other surgeons who vary in expertise and ability. Considerable experience and commitment to removal of all the lymph-bearing tissue in the neck are required. Bocca's group—presumably technical experts in this operation—honestly list a number of iatrogenic complications, including injury to the internal jugular vein and section of the thoracic duct, spinal accessory nerve, phrenic nerve, sympathetic chain, and hypoglossal nerve. There is no question that it is possible to remove virtually as much LN-bearing tissue as with a RND with practice (Fig. 56–3); however, in some hands a "functional neck dissection" is little more than a disturbance of the local lymphatic drainage in the neck, with removal of a few lymph nodes.

RESULTS WITH FUNCTIONAL NECK DISSECTION

Amputating the SCM from the mastoid tip (as well as removing some tail of parotid tissue and the posterior digastric muscle) allows more complete cleansing of the LN-bearing tissue in the high jugular area. This is undoubtedly beneficial in controlling recurrent tumor at the base of skull, although this has not been documented in the literature.

In order to assess the ability of FND to control disease in the neck, the recurrence rate in the neck should be examined in cases with histologically positive nodes with the primary tumor controlled and in patients who have had a complete rather than partial (anterior, supraomohyoid) FND and no additional treatment such as pre- or postoperative RT. The location of recurrence sites in relation to preserved structures should be noted, along with the amount of disease in the neck and whether or not ECS is present. In one Italian series, albeit retrospective,[163] a group of patients with laryngeal cancer who underwent FND were compared with another selected group of patients matched as closely as possible for primary and neck tumor stage who underwent RND by the same group of surgeons previously. Although selection bias was inherent because the control group had RND, the incidence of histologic metastases was similar in both groups, but extranodal spread occurred more frequently in the group undergoing RND. No patients received pre- or postoperative RT. It

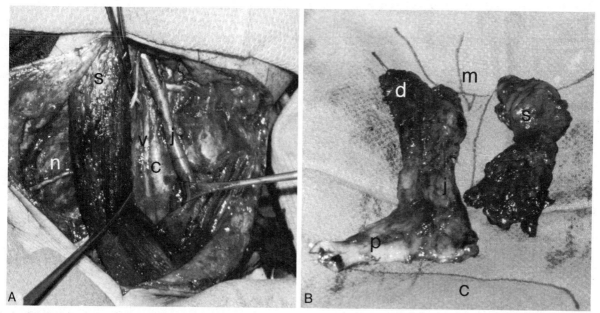

Figure 56–3. Functional neck dissection. (A) Retained structures: sternocleidomastoid muscle (s); internal jugular vein (j); vagus nerve (v); carotid artery (c); and spinal accessory nerve (n). (B) Removed lymph node–bearing tissue, separated to show relation to carotid sheath and surrounding anatomic structures. Identified areas are the angle of mandible (m), clavicle (c), submandibular gland (s), jugular chain (j), posterior triangle (p), and subdigastric area (d).

was not stated whether or not the primary tumor was controlled, nor was the location of recurrence mentioned, and it was not stated how recurrent tumors were treated and what the salvage rate was.

In the presence of histologically positive nodes, recurrences appeared in 9.4 per cent of the RND patients and in 4.5 per cent of those who had FND. With no capsular rupture, the recurrence rate was 8.3 per cent after RND and 5.3 per cent after FND. When capsular rupture was present, recurrence occurred in 12.5 per cent (one of eight cases) after RND and in no patients after FND (three cases). The series did eliminate a few patients who were planned to undergo FND but who were converted to MND or RND intraoperatively when significant ECS was noted. Overall, recurrence was definitely higher in cases with confirmed metastases (7.4 per cent versus 0.8 per cent) but was not strongly affected by the presence of capsular rupture (7 per cent without rupture, 9 per cent with rupture). Thus, based on this report, the presence of ECS does not seem to be inevitably followed by neck recurrence, even without postoperative RT.

The conclusion was that FND was as effective as RND for cervical metastatic spread from cancer of the larynx when performed en bloc with partial or total laryngectomy (a Halstedian principle) provided that the LN metastases were not greater than 3.5 cm. It was noted that the incidence of extranodal spread increased significantly when the size of the node went from 2.5 to 3 cm. Therefore, for larger nodes it was felt that the appropriate operation should be MND (spinal accessory nerve saved) or RND. FND is considered by Bocca inappropriate for "fixed" nodes that become mobile after RT or for recurrence of neck metastases after previous therapy.

In another report from the Italian surgeons the effi-

cacy of FND and RND was considered equivalent, based on evaluation of 476 operations performed from 1972 to 1978.[29] This article also provides the best description and illustration of the technique of FND in a step-by-step manner. The total number of local recurrences during 3-year follow-up was 3.5 per cent. However, this is not a reflection of the efficacy of the surgical procedure per se, because the majority of histologically positive patients received postoperative RT. Some also received preoperative RT.

Bocca has recently reported his series of cases done from 1961 to 1971.[21] This is a retrospective study comparing neck recurrence rate in a series of 1200 FNDs with that after classic RND in 414 patients, performed at the same institution by some of the same surgeons during the period of 1948 to 1960. Each operation was performed in both elective and therapeutic contexts. The data is clouded by not having eliminated recurrence at the primary site. (Recurrences at the primary site and in the neck were included, and recurrences at the primary site alone were excluded.)

The results are shown in Table 56–7. Because the

TABLE 56–7. Incidence of Neck Recurrence Based on Type and Context of Neck Dissection

Context	Type of Neck Dissection	Incidence of Recurrence
Elective	Functional	2.4%
	Radical	6.6%
Therapeutic	Functional (stages N1 and N2)	30.0%
	Radical (stages N1 and N2)	44.0%
	Radical (stage N3), lack of neck or primary control	85.0%

series was retrospective, there were more N3 cases and bilateral neck dissections performed in the later than in the earlier years (80 per cent versus 40 per cent). The 5-year cure rate with FND used in either an elective or therapeutic context in 775 patients was a respectable 92 per cent. This is a difficult statistic to evaluate, however, because there is no mention of additional postoperative treatment or salvage therapy. The neck recurrence rate after elective FND did not differ between the histologically negative and positive cases. This interesting finding probably represents reseeding of the neck from recurrent tumor at the primary site. An unspecified number of patients did have earlier RT. It is unclear in most of the Italian papers how and when postoperative RT is added. Unless the articles are read closely, the impression is that these are reports on the efficacy of surgery alone.

In a number of other studies advocating conservation neck procedures, RT is used in a planned combined approach to nodal disease, although this is not always made clear. Thus, some of the comparisons in the literature are actually between a surgical procedure alone versus a combined therapy program. At M.D. Anderson Hospital, for example, MND has been combined with planned postoperative RT as a treatment policy since about 1970 for palpable but not far advanced neck disease, with the express intent of investigating the efficacy of the combination for the control of cervical metastases.[119] The addition of RT can cause xerostomia because it is impossible to irradiate the upper jugular areas without including some mucosa of the mouth, throat, and salivary glands. Some authors point out that the morbidity resulting from combined treatment may be more significant than the rehabilitatable shoulder syndrome resulting from RND.[219] As we have described earlier, RT may also have important systemic effects that can affect the tumor-host equilibrium adversely.

Based on personal experience with Bocca's FND technique and the appeal of his oncologic rationale, I have little difficulty accepting the procedure as a useful one, even for palpable LNs, when removing them in this manner does not require peeling the nodes from the retained structures. This chapter is proposing that END can provide useful information about tumor-host biology in individual patients with clinically N0 necks, and the ability to perform a neck dissection biopsy procedure with preservation of important structures is obviously a useful corollary to this approach. I agree with Bocca that surgeons who unconditionally reject the utility of this technique are probably reacting to "theoretical objections deriving from the authority of traditional teaching." It would be interesting to know if such surgeons maintain the courage of their convictions by never performing an operation preserving the internal jugular vein on one side when bilateral neck dissection is required. In practice, many surgeons have been doing this for a long time, even in the presence of palpable disease, as an expedient. As with any conservation procedure, unless the techniques and indications are followed, the results will be inferior.

Partial Neck Dissections

The standard Bocca FND removes the entire lymphoid-bearing contents of the neck, including the pos-

terior triangle, although sometimes the submandibular gland is left in situ. Various modifications of this have evolved.

The rationale for performing a *suprahyoid* neck dissection contralaterally as a biopsy procedure and then completing a RND if positive nodes are found has been shown to be oncologically inadequate, for "skip" metastases have been reported in 20 to 60 per cent of neck dissection specimens.[82, 158] Vandenbrouck and associates[249] found positive low jugular nodes when the upper neck nodes were free of tumor in 20 per cent of neck dissections. Such discontinuous spread is not uncommon and it is impossible to predict the absence of growths in the lower neck by sampling the upper neck. Therefore, suprahyoid neck dissection should not be considered an adequate biopsy procedure, but it does have utility in obtaining a margin around primary tumors such as large floor of mouth or lip cancers. For the same reason, partial upper neck radiation is in general disrepute because patients so treated tend to develop recurrences in the neck outside the treatment port.

Supraomohyoid neck dissection has also enjoyed some popularity. In this procedure the sternocleidomastoid muscle, internal jugular vein, spinal accessory nerve, and contents of the posterior triangle inferiorly are left in situ, and the anterolateral neck contents are removed. This is considered an oncologically sound operation, for nodes seldom occur in the retained lymphatic tissue. In one paper the value of a contralateral supraomohyoid neck dissection (SOND) was evaluated.[165] One hundred seventy-seven patients with T1–4 tumors of the oral cavity, pharynx, and larynx underwent ipsilateral RND and contralateral elective SOND. Fifty-six patients had received preoperative RT of unspecified amounts; however, they had a 3 per cent incidence of pathologically positive contralateral nodes, and this was not significantly different from the 2.7 per cent incidence in patients without preoperative RT. There was also no significant difference in the incidence of pathologically positive nodes between patients with midline tumors and those with tumors that approached the midline (3 per cent versus 2.6 per cent). Although the overall recurrence rate was not alluded to in the paper, it was noted that in three patients with both clinically and pathologically negative nodes, recurrent contralateral neck disease developed. It was not mentioned whether or not the primary tumor was controlled in these patients. Based on the low incidence of contralateral occult disease and the fact that the procedure was not necessarily effective in preventing future disease, the authors concluded that contralateral SOND for treatment of primary malignancies in the sites included was not of significant prophylactic value electively.

The findings in this paper have some significance if treatment strategy were to swing toward doing more ENDs because some lesions would seem to require operations on both sides, and unless "double-teamed," bilateral FNDs would be very time-consuming. Based on the results of Morgan's paper and some evidence that neck dissection is just as effective when done therapeutically for palpable nodes as when done electively, it seems that bilateral neck dissections would, in fact, not be necessary very often. The usefulness of END as a biopsy procedure would be best realized by performing the operation on the ipsilateral side where the yield of occult positive nodes is likely to be the greatest.

Elective Neck Irradiation

As we have seen, the criteria for when to do an END are not agreed upon and, once decided upon, the type of operation to be done is almost equally controversial. Therefore, the massive circumstantial evidence in the literature that elective neck irradiation (ENI) is equally effective in this context to END has been welcomed by many surgeons as a panacea. It is widely believed that external radiation to the clinically uninvolved neck in doses of 4500 to 5000 rad will control occult metastases in 90 to 95 per cent of cases.[83] This conclusion is based on comparison of the observed rate of conversion of N0 to N+ necks after ENI and the expected rate of appearance of nodes based on the 20 to 40 per cent incidence of occult disease in the neck. We have discussed the significance of occult disease previously—such studies make the assumption that all occult LN cancer deposits will become clinically significant, and this is not supported by valid data such as the NSABP trials.

For example, Million[162] has indicated that the *average* probability of an initially clinically negative neck becoming positive is 35 per cent in patients with head and neck SCC in various sites, in whom the primary tumor is controlled by surgery alone. With the addition of ENI to the neck, however, less than 5 per cent of patients develop LN metastases. Berger and associates[14] reported that only 1.7 per cent of 469 patients developed new nodal disease after control of the primary tumor with irradiation that included the entire cervical lymph chains bilaterally. Of 185 patients treated with partial neck irradiation, 10.2 per cent developed recurrent nodal disease in marginal or unirradiated areas.

These reports must be read carefully; some compare the rate of neck recurrence in patients treated with RT in whom the primary tumor was controlled with patients undergoing RND in whom the primary tumor was not always controlled. A higher incidence of neck recurrence in the latter group is expected and cannot be attributed to failure of the neck dissection as a treatment modality. Additionally, some of the classic papers that have been used to support ENI have also had very small patient numbers. For example, Million[162] reported that eight of 23 TX N0 patients with SCC of the oral cavity had recurrence in the neck (with primary tumor controlled) when no elective neck irradiation was given, whereas none of nine TX N0 patients who received ENI had recurrence in the neck.

Elective Neck Dissection versus Elective Neck Irradiation

Comparisons between ENI and END usually cite approximately equivalent neck recurrence rates for each modality when the primary tumor is controlled—11 to 14 per cent for END and 3 to 10 per cent for ENI. A 3 to 10 per cent incidence of neck recurrence following ENI seems considerably better than the expected 20 to 40 per cent incidence. However, we have seen from some surgical series[66] that the incidence of conversion may be considerably below the expectation based on the incidence of occult disease. DeSanto and associates[56] concluded from a review of the literature that ENI results in no fewer neck recurrences than his estimated 7.5 per cent rate in the pathologically negative neck following END. Therefore, pro and con arguments involve ancillary issues. DeSanto and associates[56] state, "the prophylactic radiation or surgery issue ends where it has always ended—not at which treatment is the most beneficial, but which is the most harmful and the choice is left to the treatment manager."

Proponents of ENI counter the objection of surgeons that RT has its own associated morbidity by noting that such a morbidity rate is "very low," usually referring to local soft-tissue changes, which are indeed minimal with the dose employed in ENI. Again, however, even limited-field radiation does have potentially unfavorable systemic ramifications. This type of potential morbidity is generally not considered and has not been quantitated.

Surgeons can now argue that the morbidity of conservation END is also very low in competent hands. Whereas the doses used for ENI cause little xerostomia, loss of taste, or soft-tissue changes according to radiotherapists, some surgeons and patients consider these problems significant. With multiple primary tumors continuing to provide ongoing disease in these patients, holding RT in reserve to treat later disease is a plan deserving serious consideration. Of course, if RT helps significantly in decreasing morbidity and mortality from the index primary tumor, it should be used; inadequately treated patients may not survive to develop multiple primary tumors. Additional primary tumors can arise in radiated areas of head and neck mucosa.

Certainly, occult disease is present in the necks of patients with head and neck SCC and can develop if untreated. But does ENI actually decrease the likelihood of this occurrence? Why isn't all occult neck disease controlled with ENI? In the final analysis, *it is impossible to know the value of ENI because one does not know whether or not there was cancer in the nodes that were treated.* For the same reason, it is impossible to assess the relative efficacy of ENI versus END. To emphasize this point, if it is not known whether the nodes treated contained cancer when ENI is the treatment modality, it is possible that none of the nodes contained cancer and that the treatment actually *caused* the neck recurrences! This interpretation may seem far-fetched, and in fact, based on the incidence of occult disease in the neck, it is unlikely that *no* patients would have developed cancer if watched. However, we know from our discussion of tumor biology that the significance of micrometastatic disease in LNs is not known, and RT could select particularly malignant cell subpopulations and thereby change the natural history of occult disease in the neck to the detriment of the host. Alternatively, occult neck disease that becomes clinically evident may have the innate potential to do so, and ENI did nothing to prevent this biologic predeterminism. These two effects cannot be ruled out just because the data have been interpreted to show that ENI decreases the incidence of neck disease. Thus, the arguments that ENI provides an effective and less offensive means than END of controlling occult metastases, although supported by suggestive figures, do not stand up to scientific scrutiny.

Both ENI and END are viewed as *prophylactic* treatments, and the controversy has ignored the possible biologic significance of occult disease in the neck as a marker of the ability of the individual tumor to metastasize, thereby providing a strong prognostic indicator of the concomitant presence of distant disease and the need for adjuvant systemic treatment. Currently, only a neck dissection will provide the requisite specimen, and therefore, the argument tips heavily in favor of END. Ipsilateral END would always be useful in this context except in patients who have only contralateral neck disease. If it becomes possible to detect occult disease in nodes by some noninvasive technique, then the issue may tip back in favor of ENI, if such disease proves to be detrimental.

Elective lymphadenectomy is the only currently available method of identifying occult micrometastatic tumor in lymph nodes. A noninvasive diagnostic method that would identify occult tumor deposits would be a major breakthrough and would revolutionize the approach to diagnosing solid cancers that spread through the lymphatics. Whereas cervical lymphangiograms have been used for depicting lymphatic anatomy in vivo, they are much less valuable for detecting metastatic tumor. Blocks to the flow of dye can result from reticular hyperplasia in lymph nodes, lymphatic hyperplasia, metastatic tumor, or any combination of these, thus rendering the study of little value in detecting metastatic disease. Although CT scanning increases diagnostic accuracy (from 60 to 80 per cent in one series[84]), there are still false negative and false positive results, and CT scanning is not specific or sensitive enough to supersede clinical judgment in the management of cancer in the neck. At its current limits of detection, CT will not allow detection of small tumor deposits in lymph nodes or distinguish the large hyperplastic node from a tumor-containing node reliably.

The possibility that diagnostic imaging techniques may soon be able to detect occult disease is indicated by a recent animal study[263] in which subcutaneously injected monoclonal antibodies localized in tumor in regional lymph nodes in a guinea pig hepatocellular carcinoma model. The method requires that the lymphatic vessels be patent, and it therefore may not be useful in areas blocked by tumor in lymph nodes or in previously radiated or operated necks. Such approaches hold promise for providing the required diagnostic sophistication to detect occult cancer in lymph nodes and may ultimately be useful therapeutically if antibodies can be conjugated to toxic substances for use in adjuvant therapy against occult lymph node metastases.

The increasingly widespread acceptance of ENI as "state of the art" treatment for the N0 neck (and some now recommend elective neck treatment for cancers in all sites in the head and neck except for the nose, sinus, lip, and true vocal cord regardless of T stage) does not leave much motivation for the establishment of a randomized prospective study to address this issue, although such a need is occasionally acknowledged in the literature. Many people would probably consider such a scientific assessment a giant step backward. When it is realized that the effectiveness of neither method of treatment is truly known, the necessity for a trial reappears. Such a study would need more than two "arms." Simply comparing radiation versus dissection in equivalent groups of patients would not answer the question, because in those who received ENI it would still not be known whether or not their necks contained cancer. The appropriate study would have to be organized along the lines of the NSABP breast cancer trials, evaluating groups of patients whose necks are treated by surgery alone, RT alone, and the combination of surgery and RT as well as patients who are observed closely without neck treatment. Many stratification criteria would need to be worked out, and the type of neck dissection would have to be standardized.

Elective versus Therapeutic Neck Dissection

There is currently no statistically significant evidence in the head and neck cancer literature to indicate any detriment to patient survival by delaying neck treatment until nodes become clinically evident in patients who present with N0 necks. Several retrospective series have reached this conclusion.[135, 168, 236, 245] These studies have generally evaluated survival as it relates to the method of treatment rather than to the amount of disease in the neck.

Mustard and Rosen[168] speculated that the lower survival rate found for patients who converted in 1 year as opposed to those who remained N0 for longer than 1 year might indicate a more favorable tumor-host relationship in those who recurred later, because they had been able to control their tumor for a longer period of time by one means or another.

One randomized prospective trial in the literature addresses this issue.[249] The authors explained the need for such a trial: all the reports advocating either routine elective or delayed therapeutic neck dissection were based on comparisons from different hospitals and different treatment protocols, and they used historical comparisons from the same or different hospitals; it was impossible to compare such groups, and the results were of little value. Between 1966 and 1973, 75 patients were accrued with T1–3 N0 SCC of the oral cavity. Half of them underwent elective RND within 2 months of treatment of the primary tumor by interstitial implantation. The other patients who were treated similarly at the primary site underwent therapeutic RND when nodes became clinically palpable. The proportions of patients with different T stages were not the same in the two treatment groups. The percentage of patients in each group with histologically positive or negative nodes was the same; however, patients undergoing therapeutic neck dissection had twice the incidence of ECS. Patients with histologically positive neck nodes received postoperative RT.

Based on careful 5-year follow-up, no difference in survival was noted between the two groups. The survival similarity persisted when histologic node parameters such as ECS were assessed. In the delayed treatment group, local tumor condition or the patient's general condition precluded operation when nodes became palpable in only two patients. According to the alternate hypothesis, this is the only risk when adopting a wait-and-see policy for N0 disease—that patients who have developed contraindications to surgery or in whom disease has become inoperable will die as a result of cancer in the neck, whereas this might have been prevented by elective treatment.

These findings support the contention that elective treatment of the neck is not prophylactic—it does not prevent cancer-related deaths or increase survival. Once again, we see that survival is an inappropriate endpoint for evaluating the efficacy of a regional treatment modality. The tendency to attribute survival results to the method of treatment is probably a major misinterpretation. The survival difference may well be related to the pathologic condition of the nodes or intrinsic tumor biology and is not affected by the operation performed.

Treatment of Massive Neck Disease

The designation of massive neck disease is used in preference to the N3 neck because the N3 category describes diverse degrees of neck disease, such as bilateral or contralateral N1 disease and massive unilateral or bilateral disease. One questions whether these different categories are biologically equivalent and should be included in the same stage. Management of massive neck disease is controversial because it is difficult, and results with standard treatment combinations tend to be poor.

MANAGEMENT OF BILATERAL NECK DISEASE

In patients with bilaterally palpable nodes many surgeons perform RND on the most involved side and MND preserving the internal jugular vein on the other, and they use postoperative RT as an adjunct. In a series from M.D. Anderson Hospital[8] there were 66 patients in whom histologically positive nodes were confirmed bilaterally, and 50 determinate patients of whom 42 survived for 3 years. Postoperative RT was part of the treatment program in 13 per cent of the total group. Eight patients failed locally, regionally, or both. Twenty-two of the survivors had RND on one side and MND on the other, and received postoperative RT. Twenty of the survivors had bilateral MNDs, with only three receiving postoperative RT (two of the survivors had thyroid carcinoma, but the others had SCC). The conclusion was that patients with nodal metastases to both sides of the neck should fare as well as those with unilateral involvement if the nodal status is comparable and if they receive adequate treatment to each side of the neck. The main cause of treatment failure was attributed not to the multiplicity or bilaterality of neck nodes, but rather to the presence of cancer outside the nodes that involved other structures of the neck. Almost all recurrences occurred initially at the primary site, however, and the incidence of treatment failure in the neck without failure at the primary site was negligible.

In patients who present with simultaneous bilateral neck disease, operations on both sides of the neck are advisable, because delay may allow growth of the neck disease to the point that the second side becomes inoperable. When MND on one side would require leaving gross disease in the neck, it is better to perform bilateral RNDs. When this is done, a thorough understanding of the possible complications and relevant physiology is essential to adequately care for the patient. An excellent review is provided by McQuarrie and associates.[157]

MANAGEMENT OF "INOPERABLE" NECK DISEASE

Although the criterion of "fixation" has been eliminated from neck staging (AJC) because of its subjective nature, several papers have been published on the role of surgery in this situation. In various series, the incidence of "fixed" nodes is 6 to 7 per cent. The highest incidence, about 35 per cent, is found in patients with unknown primary tumors—an example of unpredictable tumor biology. Batsakis states that most neck metastases from unknown primary tumors are single, unilateral, and fixed.[12] The term "fixed" includes attachment to different structures, and the results included a heterogeneous group of patients; because other factors had not been controlled, the data are not worth reporting in detail.

Santos and associates[207] reported on a selected group of 12 patients from a group of 51 with fixed nodes— these were probably patients on whom sufficient data could be accumulated retrospectively. Several of them received high-dose preoperative RT, and in six of them the nodes became smaller and mobile. The two patients who survived more than 5 years were those without viable tumor in the neck dissection specimens, presumably sterilized by the preoperative RT. In the other 10 patients, histologically positive nodes were present in the specimen, and surgery did not control the disease; all but two died of disease or had clinical evidence of disease within 13 months of surgery. None of the six patients whose nodes disappeared or became smaller and mobile developed neck recurrence; however, five of six patients with fixed nodes at surgery developed recurrent disease in the neck. The majority of patients died of local recurrence or DMs. The authors concluded that surgery played little or no substantial role in improving survival in patients with head and neck SCC with fixed nodes. Addressing the ability of the local-regional treatments to control local-regional disease would have been more to the point.

Stell and Green[236] found in their personal series a 12 per cent cure rate at 5 years in patients with a fixed node in the neck treated with surgery. They felt that surgery was advisable for nodes fixed to the mandible, skin, or external carotid artery, that it was doubtful whether resection or replacement of the internal or common carotid artery was justifiable, and that fixation to the brachial plexus and cervical spine should remain as absolute contraindications to surgery.

A more recent report by Stell and associates[235] concerning patients with fixed cervical nodes (7 per cent of 2000 patients with SCC of the head and neck) showed that RT did not significantly prolong survival but that surgery did. In another paper[234] that reported on patients with bilateral fixed cervical nodes (classified N4 by the author), the conclusion was that "it is doubtful that this group (N4) should be treated at all." Only 25 per cent of the N4 group received treatment, however, and none of the newer forms of combination therapy were employed.

An opposing view is reported from M.D. Anderson Hospital.[139] The addition of RT to RND in patients with multiple, bilateral, or fixed cervical nodes from head and neck primary cancers improved local cancer control by 50 per cent. Note that the end point here was cancer control in the treated area, not survival.

Everyone agrees that treatment of patients with fixed nodes is extremely challenging; however, new modes of aggressive therapy with the addition of "up front" chemotherapy to radiation and surgery may salvage some of these unfortunate patients. Whether or not such combinations can convert "inoperable" to "operable" neck disease remains to be seen and should be assessed in appropriately designed studies. Although early reports seemed to show that neck disease was not as susceptible to shrinkage with anterior chemotherapy as was the primary tumor, additional reports more often show equivalent responses at both sites.[270]

MANAGEMENT OF THE CAROTID ARTERY AND RESIDUAL NECK DISEASE

The issue of whether or not to resect a carotid artery involved with tumor will probably continue to remain a matter of individual choice. In general, few surgeons ever resect the carotid, although a few resect it in selected situations. Most surgeons are probably more aggressive with younger patients. Carotid artery resection is poorly tolerated in patients over 65 years of age. Relative indications to operate on massive neck disease include patients who are symptomatic with Stokes-Adams attacks due to the mass effect in the neck or palliation for the unpleasant side effects of uncontrolled disease in the neck. This is usually an exercise in futility if there is not reasonable expectation of being able to remove the gross disease.

Loré and Boulos recently summarized their experience with 10 patients and listed the various tests available to assess the adequacy of collateral brain blood flow and those which predict the likelihood of major neurologic sequelae.[141] Carotid arteriography with cross-compression is relatively useless as a prognosticator of neurologic sequelae, as are most of the other tests currently available. Tests that measure actual carotid pressure are the most useful and include intraoperative distal stump pressure or oculoplethysmography, which is a noninvasive measure of the pressure in the internal carotid artery. Useful information can also be obtained by clamping the artery intraoperatively with EEG leads in place. If slow waves develop, the patient is at risk to develop major neurovascular complications.[92] Opinion differs as to the utility of this technique, which is expensive and requires interpretation.

Whether or not the carotid artery should be reconstructed (with saphenous vein preferentially) also remains controversial. If preoperative or intraoperative tests show that the patient should tolerate ligation well, it is unnecessary and probably inadvisable to reconstruct, because the revascularized segment can rupture and hemorrhage if recurrent disease develops. If salivary fistula is likely to result from the operation or if disease cannot be well cleared from the neck, revascularization should not be attempted, especially in heavily irradiated patients. Recurrent disease frequently occupies the base of the skull, and it may not be possible to perform an anastomosis distally. If the patient shows no EEG slow waves, if no fistula is likely, and if the disease can be completely removed, the carotid can be revascularized or, occasionally, preserved.

Because noninvasive tests are so inaccurate, some surgeons proceed in high-risk patients to perform a superficial temporal artery to middle cerebral artery bypass as a separate neurosurgical procedure before the major operation. This is a viable option only in certain skull base cases in which the internal but not the common or external carotid will need to be sacrificed.

What is the appropriate treatment for disease left in the neck after neck dissection? This issue is seldom addressed in the literature, and retrospective chart reviews cannot be considered accurate because of the reticence to dictate such a finding into the operative report. Carotid "peels" usually leave gross or microscopic disease in the neck. One gets the feeling from the literature that RND with postoperative RT is inadequate in handling this situation, and that recurrences are frequent.

Two institutions have reported using ^{125}I implants as an adjunct to surgery in this context. In one series[153] 18 of 48 patients were treated for cure with an actuarial survival of 50 per cent. Local-regional control was achieved in 58 per cent, and during follow-up no patient recurred in the implanted volume. Seventeen patients with a comparable disease state were treated with curative intent previously without implants and were analyzed retrospectively for comparison; their actuarial survival was 18 per cent with overall local-regional control in 21 per cent. The statistically significant difference between the two groups was attributed to the addition of the ^{125}I implants, which were either individually placed or inserted into absorbable Vicryl suture carriers. In 17 patients who received implants for local recurrence, local control was achieved in 50 per cent, but the 2 to 2½ year survival was only 17 per cent. Overall, the complication rate was 11 per cent, and the authors felt that the improved survival, high local control, and minimal complication rate made the intraoperative implantation of ^{125}I seeds useful for treatment of microscopic residual disease, although implanting in residual macroscopic disease was useless.

In the other series,[254] 124 patients with advanced head and neck cancer were treated for palliation with radioactive permanent ^{125}I implants. Complete regression occurred in 71 per cent (21 per cent later recurred), and partial regression occurred in 18 per cent (55 per cent later recurred). The incidence of serious complications was 5.5 per cent. Overall, in 64 per cent of cases the implanted lesions remained controlled until the patient's death, which usually was due to progression of cancer elsewhere in the body. The authors concluded that such implants offered useful palliation to patients with recurrent head and neck cancer without local toxicity even after full-course external radiotherapy. The technology is currently being investigated as a planned adjunct to external RT and chemotherapy in the initial management of patients with locally advanced head and neck cancers.

Other surgeons are investigating the use of high-dose intraoperative external beam RT to treat microscopic residual disease in the neck.[89] This logistically difficult treatment adjunct is also useless for macroscopic residual disease. Both of these methods need longer follow-up to assess patient benefit, long-term toxicities, and recurrence rates.

Neck Node Biopsy—When and How?

Based on the writings of Hayes Martin from Memorial Hospital in the 1940s and 1950s, it became a widely accepted dogma among head and neck surgeons that removal of an enlarged lymph node for diagnostic purposes was a disservice to patients who had cervical cancer. According to Martin, "incisional biopsy for the removal of a portion or of the whole of the cervical tumor should never be made until other methods have been unsuccessful. One of the most reprehensible surgical practices is the immediate incision or excision of a cervical mass for diagnosis without any preliminary investigation for a possible primary growth. There can be no better example of ill-advised and needless surgery."[152]

IS INITIAL OPEN NECK BIOPSY HARMFUL?

In 1978, McGuirt and McCabe[155] presented data that putatively brought Martin's dictum from the realm of personal experience to that of proven fact in a paper that has been widely quoted since. The complications of wound necrosis, local cervical recurrence, and distant metastasis were compared in 714 patients who had undergone RND, 64 of whom had a cervical node biopsy before diagnosis and definitive treatment. As a subgroup, 40 of the 64 patients were matched with an equal number of patients who had no biopsy with respect to age, sex, histologic diagnosis, site, stage of the lesion, and treatment protocol. The major conclusion was that in patients who allegedly differed only by the variable of a biopsy before treatment or not, there were "trends" toward higher complication rates (wound necrosis and regional recurrence) and a statistically significant difference in the incidence of distant metastases for previously biopsied patients. In the overall group, there were no statistically significant differences between patients in whom no biopsy was done and the group that had a biopsy at the time of definitive treatment. The histologic types of cancer were not specified in the paper.

This paper can be criticized on several counts. Although it is stated that the patient groups differed only in whether or not they had a biopsy prior to diagnosis and definitive treatment, the reader is left to accept the author's word for this because there is no mention of pathologic findings. Were all the biopsied neck nodes pathologically positive? Why did some patients have a neck biopsy and others no biopsy? Presumably, the nonbiopsied patients had the diagnosis made from a biopsy of a primary lesion, or they had no palpable neck nodes to biopsy. Patients in the latter category would be in a relatively favorable prognostic category, because the incidence of distant metastases strongly correlates with positive neck nodes. In the overall group, the indications for RND were not stated and there is no mention of pathologic findings; one cannot assume that all of these patients had positive nodes in the specimen.

Conclusions from the overall comparison group are subject to the criticisms of any retrospective study, but analysis of the subgroup of computer-matched patients is more relevant. The authors acknowledged that in this subgroup, differences in wound necrosis and regional recurrence between biopsied and nonbiopsied patients were not statistically significant. This tends to negate their speculation that any surgical disruption of lymphatic drainage or manipulation of a metastatic tumor is apt to worsen the chances for a clean surgical excision

and a cure unless that disruption is done at the time of the definitive resection. The conclusion from the matched subgroup that a difference in distant metastatic rate was statistically significant seems quite compelling until one realizes that the patients were matched for overall TNM stage and this obscures the status of the neck disease, which is the most relevant prognostic factor with respect to predicting the likelihood of distant metastases. For example, stage 4 patients can range from T4 N0 to T1 N3B. Therefore, advanced stages can include patients with very different amounts of neck disease and inherently different likelihoods of forming distant metastases. In short, the paper provides insufficient data to decide whether or not the conclusions are truly valid—that is, such conclusions are explainable on a basis not related to the neck biopsy per se. The outcome may be attributable to the presence or absence and amount of neck disease, rather than to the fact that it was biopsied. There is also no mention of the time interval between biopsy and definitive treatment, and this factor can also affect prognosis.

It should be mentioned that a dissenting view[194] emerged from a Roswell Park study in which there was no detriment to patient survival if definitive treatment followed the biopsy without significant delay. In this study, the previous biopsy of a neck node did not adversely affect the incidence of either neck recurrence or survival when appropriate surgery was performed. There is no mention of whether or not the primary tumor was controlled in patients with neck recurrence, however; and the results were compared with a historical control group from another institution (Memorial Hospital), so the study is scientifically invalid.

If one reads Martin's original paper, it is apparent from the cases presented and the discussion that the major reason for his caveat to avoid early biopsy was his experience with patients who presented to his referral center after having experienced considerable delay or absence of complete diagnosis. According to Martin, "The most frequent and tragic errors in diagnosis occur when the physician considers first such remote possibilities as tuberculosis, syphilis, or inflammatory hyperplasia, and persists in these beliefs for periods of weeks or months until the malignant growth extends locally and systemically to become incurable." Apparently, many of the referring physicians failed to recognize the probably cancerous nature of cervical masses in the adult, and treated them as benign for extended periods of time without recourse to histologic diagnosis. They also failed to recognize the probable metastatic character of histologically proved malignant cervical tumors, interpreting them as primary neck cancers, and therefore failed to examine other head and neck sites for silent or obvious primary lesions. As well, there was failure to appreciate that in cases with negative findings on initial examination of head and neck sites, serial follow-up by experienced examiners was necessary. Although transgressions and delays in diagnosis and treatment still occur, knowledge of the significance of cancer in the neck is more widespread than 40 years ago. It was mainly for these reasons that Martin advocated holding incisional biopsy in reserve as a last resort, never to be used as an initial diagnostic procedure in cases of cervical tumors. He usually employed fine needle aspiration biopsy for such diagnoses.

Martin's warning was apparently later generalized to

include the corollaries that biopsy causes cervical scarring that will complicate neck dissection, and that local node excision may lead to local and possibly general spread of the disease. These theories led to the development of "no touch" techniques for solid tumor surgery. The former objection does not generally prove a serious problem for experienced head and neck surgeons. Is there support for the latter? Is it really necessary to do the excisional biopsy only at the time of the definitive procedure?

Several early animal studies seem to show a hazard from manipulation and biopsy with respect to metastases. In one study of three different mouse systems, there was a small but significant increase in pulmonary metastases in mice that had had open biopsy before the primary cancer was amputated; in another, an increase in metastasis was found after palpation of the tumor and also after both open biopsy and fine needle biopsy.[199, 247] In a recent study[64] five syngeneic mouse systems were used to study the influence of fine needle aspiration biopsy, incisional biopsy, and excisional biopsy on tumor-related death rates. The experiments did not reveal any difference in death rates between the test groups and the control group or among the three biopsy methods. Tumor cell seeding and tumor outgrowth by way of the aspiration needle tract could be made to occur under extreme test conditions. Previous work on needle tract seeding from fine- and large-bore needle biopsies is reviewed in this article.

SIGNIFICANCE OF CANCER CELLS IN OPERATIVE WOUNDS

Many studies that have looked for cancer cells in operative wounds and wound drainage systems have found viable cells in the area; however, almost none of these studies has been able to correlate this finding with the later development of increased local or metastatic disease.[3, 80, 98, 229] A possibly analogous situation is the apparently low rate of establishment of lung tumors in patients who have had endoscopy for upper aerodigestive tract (UADT) cancers. Surely in these cases tumor cells are shed not only with manipulation but during normal physiologic events, yet no studies have shown this to be detrimental with respect to later development of pulmonary tumors.

These findings can be interpreted in the light of current knowledge of tumor biology. We know that establishment of metastasis is a multistaged process requiring successful completion of each step, and local recurrence or distant metastasis is not a foregone conclusion simply based on tumor cell contamination of a surgical wound. The trauma necessary to remove a tumor from the operative area, whether during a biopsy procedure or definitive resection, along with the necessary transection of lymphatic and blood vessels, will inevitably allow exposure of tumor emboli to the operative wound and circulation. Efforts at "no touch" cancer surgery have not proved significantly beneficial in the long run. Nevertheless, it is intuitively correct to try to decrease manipulations, such as cutting into cancer and gross spillage of tumor cells, and to keep the area clean by changing contaminated instruments and surgical attire. For the same reasons, excisional versus incisional biopsy is preferable whenever possible. Also, with respect to tumor biology, manipulation of tumor should be avoided as much as possible, because this can lead to increased shedding of tumor-associated antigens, which can theoretically compromise the host immune response.

Thus, other considerations are relevant to the method and timing of biopsy than those which simplistically assume that spilling cancer cells will automatically lead to development of local recurrence and metastases. It is probably unlikely that a tumor will disseminate lethal metastases only during the interval between biopsy and definitive surgery, based on our current thought that many solid tumors are systemic diseases from relatively early in their course.

Combination Therapy

One of the major controversies today concerns the utility and role of planned combined surgery and RT (now generally administered postoperatively) for head and neck SCC. The aggregate conclusion is that whereas the combination of surgery and RT appears to improve local-regional disease control, concomitant increases in survival have never been observed, and from this apparent discrepancy, vigorous controversy has arisen. Much of the controversy disappears when one stops to analyze what surgery and RT can reasonably be expected to do. Both of these treatment modalities are aimed at local-regional disease and can therefore be expected to affect only local-regional control rates, not overall survival. From 30 to 40 per cent of head and neck SCC patients die of causes unrelated to local-regional disease, such as DMs, multiple primary tumors, and intercurrent disease. As local-regional treatments, surgery and RT would not be expected to be effective against these additional factors, which influence survival. Survival is the wrong end point to use when assessing the utility of these treatments. Thus, the general finding that survival has not improved, although local-regional control has, is not an indictment of the efficacy of surgery and RT.

Surgeons and radiotherapists are generally arrayed at opposite ends of this controversy. DeSanto—a surgeon—argues that to see only a shift in the site of recurrence (to DMs) with combination treatment but no change in survivorship shows that it is not in the patients' best interest to treat them in two different ways for the same disease and find that the only benefit derived is a change in the cause of death.[56] He remains skeptical that the solution to the problem is to use more or different sequences of conventional treatment, and he doubts that more treatment is necessarily better. At the opposite end of the spectrum, M.D. Anderson Hospital radiotherapist Fletcher[82] argues that evaluation of the efficacy of combined treatment should not be made solely on survival rates, because patients dying of uncontrolled head and neck cancer have a very poor quality of life—worse than those dying of DMs.

Most of the studies indicating the benefit of combination therapy have originated from M.D. Anderson and Memorial-Sloan Kettering Hospitals. Several reports from M.D. Anderson, in which the primary tumor remained controlled, have led to the general conclusion that combining the two modalities produces local-regional disease control in twice as many patients as single modality therapy. They feel that the absolute 5-

year survival does not reflect this improvement because as local-regional control increases, more patients live longer but die before 5 years from DMs and other causes.

It is probably safe to conclude that by allowing better local-regional control the use of combined surgery and RT has unmasked the previously hidden natural history of head and neck SCC—the development of DMs and multiple primary tumors as additional causes of death. Despite the current emphasis on the changing patterns of mortality in head and neck SCC, with emphasis now being placed on these additional factors, one should not lose sight of the fact that this disease is locally aggressive and that failure of local-regional control is probably still the major cause of disease and death in these patients in the United States. If the pendulum swings back toward single modality treatment (surgery alone), we may be taking a giant step backward and again see uncontrolled local-regional disease re-emerge as the devastating problem it had been in the past.

EFFICACY OF COMBINATION THERAPY FOR NECK DISEASE

Combined therapy is often used for more advanced neck disease.[119–121, 139, 175, 212] For example, in one group of patients compiled between 1954 and 1968[121] the neck recurrence rate after surgery alone was 14 per cent for N1, 26 per cent for N2, and 34 per cent for N3. Corresponding recurrence rates after combination therapy were 2, 11, and 25 per cent. The benefit of combination therapy becomes more obvious as the amount of disease increases in the neck—for N2–3 disease, rather than for N1 disease. For N1 disease, it was found that RT controlled all but 8.5 per cent, that recurrences followed RND in 10.5 per cent, and there were no recurrences after combined treatment. For N2a and N2b disease, 21.5 per cent failures followed RT alone, 18.5 per cent followed RND alone, and none were found with combined treatment.[120] Lindberg and Jesse[139] stated that the size of the LN was important; they felt that combined therapy resulted in a decreased recurrence rate over surgery alone only for nodes greater than 3 cm in dimension.

There are two randomized prospective studies in the literature comparing surgery with surgery plus RT in relation to neck control. In the first,[239] patients were treated with surgery alone including RND and were compared with those who got similar surgery following 2000 rad preoperatively. Combined treatment significantly lowered the incidence of cervical recurrence, especially in patients with advanced metastatic cancer involving cervical nodes at more than one level (the control and study groups had comparable amounts of histologically positive nodes). Neck recurrences occurred in 36 per cent of operated patients with positive nodes at one level and in 71 per cent with positive nodes at multiple levels. Corresponding figures for the combined treatment group were 28 and 37 per cent. Recurrence at the primary site was not eliminated in this series, however, and occurred in 25 per cent of operated patients and 17 per cent of combined therapy patients. The author stated that excluding patients with local and regional recurrence did not significantly alter the differences in cervical recurrence rates—29 per cent in operated versus 18 per cent in combined therapy

patients. Three-year survival was about 50 per cent in both groups; patients fared better in the dissected neck but died of uncontrolled disease elsewhere.

The second randomized prospective study[231] compared three treatments for patients with SCC in the oral cavity and oropharynx—preoperative RT plus surgery, surgery plus postoperative RT, and radical RT alone. Combination therapy controlled 50 per cent of the patients. Forty-three per cent had local-regional failure only, 26 per cent had DMs only, and 24 per cent had all three. In patients dying with detectable carcinoma, 37 per cent had local-regional persistence only, 28 per cent had only DMs, and 26 per cent had all three. There was no statistically significant difference in the development of DMs in patients who received pre- versus postoperative RT, and there were no statistically significant differences between the three groups with respect to survival or disease-free interval. One of the major conclusions was that the incidence of DMs was high in spite of combined therapy and that improvement in survival, and perhaps local control, required employment of some additional modality such as long-term maintenance chemotherapy following surgery and RT.

Data from Memorial Hospital lead to the same conclusions. Vikram and associates[253] examined recurrence at various sites in 105 patients followed for at least 18 months with stage III and IV SCC of the head and neck, treated with surgery and postoperative RT. One third of the patients had "close" or involved margins, and 82 per cent had pathologically positive nodes. Postoperative RT doses varied from 4500 to 6000 rad. Overall, 30 per cent of patients developed recurrence or metastases, whereas of 93 determinate cases, 80 per cent remained free of cancer in the head and neck. In the total group, local-regional failure occurred in 18 per cent, and distant metastatic failure in 11.5 per cent. The frequency of local recurrences and DMs increased as the stage of neck disease increased (11.5 per cent for N0, 11 and 7 per cent for N1, 27 and 21 per cent for N2, and 20 and 13.5 per cent for N3). Overall, 9.5 per cent of patients recurred at the primary site, and 8.5 per cent recurred in the neck. (Were these the same patients?)

It was determined that the timing of postoperative RT was critical. When it was delivered 6 weeks or less after surgery, only 5.6 per cent of patients had local-regional recurrence, but 31 per cent recurred locally or regionally if therapy was delayed. This trend was seen regardless of the pathologic status of the nodes.

The authors concluded that local-regional control had been considerably increased when compared with a historical series from the same institution. The series used for comparison was compiled between 1960 and 1964,[66] when the incidence of patients relapsing in the head and neck region within the first 18 months was 50 to 75 per cent. When this series was compiled, however, patients presented with more advanced disease, surgical and RT techniques were relatively archaic compared with current methods, and local-regional recurrence was consequently more frequent. Changes in treatment techniques over the intervening years and in the patient population are important variables that may make this comparison group inappropriate.

Postoperative RT was given for unsatisfactory surgical margins, neck metastases at multiple levels, and pathologically positive nodes. Thus, these patients constituted a presumably high-risk group for local-regional recurrence, and the results do look impressive on the surface, but one must remember that the validity of the historical control group is questionable.

In a comparable paper that also looked at the effectiveness of postoperative RT,[241] 26 per cent of patients had a local recurrence and 6.5 per cent had cervical recurrence. The authors felt that there may be a difference in the ability of RT to control microscopic disease at the primary site and in the neck; however, this is speculative because treatment of subclinical neck disease includes some patients without pathologically positive disease.

Everyone agrees that "no surgeon should be deluded by the siren song of postoperative radiation into doing less than an adequate surgical procedure in the hopes that most disease left behind can be satisfactorily eradicated by the radiotherapist."[7]

INDICATIONS FOR COMBINING THERAPY FOR CONTROL OF NECK DISEASE

The indications for using postoperative RT for neck disease vary. Ballantyne[7] uses it when there is microscopic disease at the margins, when there are multiple positive nodes at multiple levels, and for extensive perineural lymphatic spread and soft-tissue metastasis outside the regional nodes. The M.D. Anderson Hospital group recommends postoperative RT if the surgical specimen contains disease—5000 rad to the entire neck and an additional boost to parts of the neck extensively dissected, because tumor cells in scar tissue may be hypoxic. The indications are very strong if a node is over 3 cm, if connective tissue is invaded, or if multiple nodes are positive. Even when only one small node is positive in the RND specimen, postoperative RT is usually given. Recall again that the M.D. Anderson group generally uses modified neck dissection in combination with radiation postoperatively.

Another group[51] gives postoperative RT to patients with major LN involvement of more than three positive nodes or capsular invasion. As we have seen, Johnson and associates[126] consider even such combination treatment inadequate for specimens showing ECS and recommend systemic adjuvant treatment. In the reports of Snow and associates[230] and Zoller and associates[274] RT in combination with surgery selectively benefited only patients with ECS. Other authors feel that the addition of RT to all histologically positive necks significantly decreases recurrence rates.[239]

DeSanto and coworkers[56] compared patients who received postoperative RT in a miscellaneous manner (less than 4000 rad or outside planned time limits) without known recurrence, with patients getting surgery alone or planned combined therapy. The neck recurrence rate in the miscellaneous group was no different from that for the group with stage II disease undergoing surgery alone, or for the group receiving planned combined therapy. Thus, it was suggested that the addition of RT to neck dissection for pathologically positive necks is a random event with no significant influence at all on recurrence rates in the neck.

NECK RECURRENCE FOLLOWING COMBINATION THERAPY

In a more recent paper[258] failure in the neck following combination treatment was further assessed. Ninety-four of 106 patients were N+ pathologically. The failure rate in the neck after surgery plus postoperative RT appeared to be independent of the clinical or pathologic extent of disease in the neck (presence or absence of ECS, involvement of single or multiple levels), histologic differentiation of the primary tumor, or previous chemotherapy (four patients). Overall, 11 patients developed neck recurrences—three of 54 patients with N0 and N1 necks and eight of 60 patients with N2 necks. The difference was not statistically significant. The failure rate in pathologically positive necks was 10.6 per cent. Involvement of the soft tissues of the neck resulted in recurrence in four of 33 patients compared with recurrence in seven of 61 who did not have ECS—this difference is not statistically significant. Upon finding that the failure rate in the neck after surgery and RT was independent of the pathologic state of disease in the neck, one wonders what the actual effect of RT is on different aspects of neck disease.

The number of patients developing recurrence was compared to the total of 106 patients who underwent RND. A more appropriate comparison would have been with the 94 patients who were proved to have carcinoma in the neck histologically. The state of primary tumor control is not clarified and the comparison was with a historical control group in which recurrence in the dissected neck occurred in 36.5 per cent of cases with carcinoma at one level and in 71 per cent when metastases were present at more than one level; the primary tumor was not controlled in about 20 per cent of the patients in the comparison series.

Patterns of cancer recurrence in postoperatively irradiated necks were studied at another institution.[148] Of 92 patients treated with combined therapy, 54 were pathologically N+. Overall, five patients with histologically positive nodes had recurrences when the primary tumor was controlled. Of the five isolated cervical recurrences, one was within the radiated field and four were outside the treatment portal in posterior cervical nodes. When the primary tumor was controlled, five of 18 patients with ECS recurred in the neck, whereas none of 36 without ECS recurred in the neck alone. Therefore, postoperative RT presumably controlled 13 of 18 patients at high risk for neck recurrence. It is interesting that three of 38 patients with no metastatic nodes recurred in the neck with the primary controlled. Of the 20 patients who died with malignancy, DMs developed in 10 without local-regional recurrence, although this was not analyzed according to the patient's initial N stage. There was a significantly better recurrence-free survival at 3 years for patients with zero or one metastatic node as compared to those with two or more positive nodes—69 and 54 per cent versus 37 and 30 per cent. The difference in overall survival rates was not statistically significant, however. Tumor recurrence and decreased survival were associated with two or more metastatic nodes at the time of surgery and with ECS. Postoperative RT was considered useful in decreasing ipsilateral cervical tumor recurrence only in those patients with more than two metastatic nodes. In all patients, contralateral neck recurrence was eliminated. The studies from M.D. Anderson Hospital have also shown a considerable decrease in delayed neck disease in electively irradiated contralateral necks. (Was disease present in them?)

Bartelink and associates[9] reported on the value of

postoperative RT as an adjuvant to RND in 405 patients who underwent RND from 1960 to 1975 at the Netherlands Cancer Institute. Of these, 140 patients were treated with RT either pre- or postoperatively. Indications for postoperative RT were macro- or microscopically positive margins, extranodal spread, and tumor emboli in lymphatic vessels. Therefore, this group had several presumably unfavorable prognostic factors not present in the group treated by surgery alone. The postoperative RT techniques until 1973 used orthovoltage and partial neck irradiation. Later the entire field was treated. In 70 patients the N stage was unknown, in 28 patients the T stage was unknown, and in 12 patients the number of metastases and ECS were unknown—all were typical defects in a retrospective study. A neck recurrence occurred in 38 of the 140 patients. There was no apparent difference between those receiving pre- and postoperative RT with respect to recurrence rate or survival, nor was there a relationship between the radiation dose and recurrence rate. Recurrence rate in the neck in the postoperatively irradiated patients did not differ significantly from the group having surgery alone, presumably owing to selection of patients with prognostically unfavorable signs to receive the adjuvant RT.

Comparison was then made between the postoperatively irradiated group and the 188 patients treated with surgery alone who had histologically proven LN metastases. In the group of patients with combination treatment, a lower (but not statistically significant) recurrence rate was observed. Results of combination treatment were better for patients with ECS without fixation of the nodes. Postoperative RT did not decrease the recurrence rate in 24 patients with ECS *and* fixation of nodes, giving evidence that not all "ECS" has the same significance or response to treatment. The survival rate in the combined group as a whole did not differ from the patients treated with surgery alone, but the subgroup of patients with ECS treated with combined therapy had a favorable survival rate compared with patients treated with surgery alone. Patients with recurrence at the primary site were included, however, making it almost impossible to evaluate the effects of treatment on neck control per se. The recommendation was to deliver postoperative RT to patients with prognostically bad histologic characteristics—ECS, tumor emboli in lymphatic vessels, and multiple metastatic nodes.

In Mantravadi's series,[148] postoperative RT was used to treat 43 head and neck cancer patients for micro- or macroscopic tumor at the surgical margins and 29 patients with tumor-free margins to categorize the effectiveness of postoperative RT in controlling positive margins. Most of the patients had stage III or IV tumors. In the series of 72 patients, 21 per cent had node metastases at one level, and 45 per cent had involvement at multiple levels. The status of tumor in the neck was defined as R0 (negative tumor margins), R1 (microscopically positive tumor margins), and R2 (macroscopically positive tumor margins). Tumor control was achieved in 71 per cent of R0 patients, in 73 per cent of R1 patients, and in 46 per cent of R2 patients at 3 years. (Tumor recurred at the primary site in 40 per cent of patients with positive margins versus 27 per cent of those with tumor-free margins at the primary site.) Of patients who were radiated within 6 weeks of operation,

local failure occurred in 16 per cent of R0 patients. Twenty-two per cent of patients with tumor extension into the neck soft tissue developed a recurrence in the neck after RT. Of the 10 patients with incompletely resected metastatic nodes, 50 per cent developed neck recurrence. All four patients who were radiated later than 6 weeks after surgery developed recurrent disease, although the resection margins were free of tumor. Fifty-eight per cent of R0, 78 per cent of R1, and 42 per cent of R2 patients survived 3 years. The claim for this study is for improved prognosis in patients with advanced head and neck cancer using combination surgery and postoperative RT over that achieved with surgery or RT alone, based on comparison with survival rates from another institution in patients with inadequate margins who underwent only surgical treatment (31 per cent 5-year survival).[140] The 3-year actuarial survival in this series was 64 per cent for all patients and 71 per cent for those with inadequate margins, and the authors recommend using a 5000-rad dose in patients with adequate tumor margins and with limited LN involvement within 6 weeks postoperatively. When a delay is unavoidable, 6500 rad was recommended even if tumor-free margins were achieved. The recommendation was to use postoperative RT in all head and neck cancer patients with inadequate surgical margins and for those with high-risk factors (nodes at multiple levels, ECS). In the final analysis, one must question the value of postoperative RT when the four patients with adequate margins who were radiated more than 6 weeks after surgery died with tumor. This suggests that some pathologically negative tumor margins are not biologically negative and that RT may not have too much influence on intrinsic tumor behavior.

COMBINATION THERAPY—ONCOLOGIC CONSIDERATIONS

There is also concern that the combination of surgery with radiation may in fact increase the incidence of certain causes of death such as DMs. For example, Schuller and associates[216] speculate that "it is conceivable that a combined therapy program that includes irradiation as the initial treatment may well not represent a strong enough attack on the tumor and subsequently permits microscopic seeding of tumor cells that go on to develop into distant metastases." Of course, such seeding may occur from solid tumors before they become clinically evident also.

As we have seen, tumor heterogeneity can include radiosensitivity with cell subpopulations being more or less radioresistant, probably on a basis other than mere anatomic location within the hypoxic tumor core. Preoperative RT may in some way select cells with a survival advantage—those that can escape and form DMs. Lindberg and associates found no difference in local recurrence or DMs when 5000 rad were given preoperatively versus 6000 rad given postoperatively. In a later report from M.D. Anderson Hospital[161] patients treated with preoperative RT had a significantly lower incidence of DMs than those treated with postoperative RT (10 per cent versus 20 per cent). The distribution of cases by TNM stage was similar. The incidence of DMs was higher in all postoperative groups but the difference was statistically significant only in patients with $T3–4_2$ $N2–3$ lesions. The higher incidence of DMs could not be explained by local recurrence rates above the clavicle;

the postoperative group had a lower incidence of local recurrence than the preoperative group (25 per cent versus 37 per cent). Because treatment was not randomized and because the general treatment policy was to give postoperative RT to patients with connective tissue disease or multiple levels of node involvement in the neck, there was a tendency to select the most advanced patients into the group receiving postoperative RT—such patients would be expected to have a higher endogenous incidence of DMs.

The issue of second malignant neoplasms (SMN) is also relevant to the use of combination therapy. In a recent series[257] of 114 patients who were successfully treated with combination therapy for advanced head and neck cancer between 1975 and 1980, 14 per cent developed SMNs, primarily in the lung and esophagus. Whereas local-regional and distant recurrences manifested generally within 2 years, SMNs continued to appear at a steady rate of about 6 per cent per year for at least the first 4 years. In patients who survived without relapse for 2 years, SMNs became more of a cause for concern than local-regional relapse or DMs. This incidence was similar to the 17 per cent incidence reported by Farr and Arthur.[66] In that and other earlier series[271] a common site for SMNs in patients with head and neck neoplasms was within the local area—the mouth, larynx, and pharynx. In Vikram's series,[257] SMNs in these locations were conspicuously absent, and this was interpreted to be a reflection of the prophylactic value of wide-field RT in preventing field cancerization.[226] It was acknowledged that efforts at improving survival in head and neck cancer patients in the future must incorporate strategies for the prevention, early detection, and treatment of SMNs, especially those arising in the esophagus and lung. It was suggested that elective radiation of the esophagus might decrease the subsequent incidence of esophageal cancer in these patients.

The opposite side of this issue is presented in several other papers that attribute poor survival with SMNs to the lack of available treatment modalities, especially RT, which have been used up in the treatment of the index primary tumor.[87] Obviously, a patient must survive the first cancer to develop a second one; hence, successful initial treatment is vital. However, the addition of RT in this context is not insignificant in view of SMNs as a major emerging limitation to long-term survival. If RT can reasonably be held in reserve for treatment of SMNs, survival might increase. One must also remember that ionizing radiation is an established carcinogenic agent,[134, 206, 211] but in the therapeutic context the risk:benefit ratio is strongly in favor of its use. In patients with "condemned mucosa" conservative surgery and careful observation may provide as good results as radical combination therapy.

COMBINATION THERAPY—AN UNANSWERED QUESTION

The assumption that combined surgery and RT is better than either alone for advanced head and neck cancer is now deeply engrained, based on heavy circumstantial evidence. This is an example of doggedly adhering to what we believe to be true rather than acknowledging that the answer is not known. A number of articles indicate that the issue is not resolved,[56, 218]

and most of these identify the lack of survival advantage with combination therapy as the major bone of contention. A number of series in the literature indicate that surgical therapy alone achieves survival equivalent to combined therapy,[30, 91, 183, 216] and some show that survivorship of patients on combined therapy programs is poorer than that for patients treated with surgery alone, even when treatment groups were compared by stage of lesion.[216] DeSanto and associates[56] are skeptical of the benefits of combined therapy claimed by articles that start with large numbers of patients and eliminate all but a few for analysis as a basis for conclusions. He cites Jesse and Lindberg,[122] who started with 1039 cases and drew conclusions based on analysis of 85 cases. A similar study from Memorial Hospital started with 150 cases and ended up with 22 for analysis. DeSanto, however, acknowledges case elimination in his own series—of 881 patients who underwent neck dissection, only 129 had properly defined and sequenced combined therapy. As we have repeatedly indicated, however, lack of survival advantage is not an indictment of combination therapy because one expects these local-regional treatments only to be able to improve local-regional disease control. To expect an increase in survival is to ignore the contamination of survival as an end point by factors such as DMs and intercurrent disease, which are not amenable to control local-regional treatment modalities.

The issue actually is whether we need a controlled study to prove that surgery plus RT is more effective in control of local-regional disease than either modality alone. This question is not frivolous because RT has systemic effects on host immunity, is potentially carcinogenic, and might prove more useful as a reserve treatment for SMNs. Cost-effectiveness is also of increasing concern. These considerations must be weighed against the fairly unequivocal evidence that it is the combination of surgery and RT that has accomplished our current unprecedented level of local-regional disease control. There is considerable evidence from both retrospective and prospective trials in breast cancer to conclude that local-regional treatment using surgery in combination with radiation does significantly improve the local disease control rate.

These are difficult issues to decide. A proposed Radiation Therapy Oncology Group (RTOG) study to compare conservation neck dissection and RT versus RND alone failed because the type of MND to be used could not be agreed upon. Inability to decide such technical details makes the prospect of deciding the larger issues (which studies to undertake) seem somewhat dismal.

Non–Squamous Cell Tumors

Management of the neck with "unusual" primary tumors is not well standardized. Recent developments in immunohistochemical staining of pathologic specimens can help identify the origin of "undifferentiated" neck metastases that can be hard to pinpoint with conventional light microscopy.[52, 65]

Management of lymphoma and rhabdomyosarcoma in the neck is not discussed here because it is relatively noncontroversial from a surgical viewpoint. Non–squamous cell tumors to be discussed include salivary gland and thyroid cancers and malignant melanoma. There are no controlled studies on these topics, but an attempt has been made to present the majority or expert opinion.

Salivary Gland Neoplasms

Patients with carcinoma of the salivary glands are at relatively low risk to develop cervical metastases. As a group, salivary gland cancers metastasize distantly via hematogenous routes more frequently than to the RLNs, and the incidence of cervical metastases present initially for all parotid cancers is about 13 per cent. The metastatic patterns of salivary gland tumors of various histologic types are shown in Tables 56–8 and 56–9. It is generally agreed that only high-grade mucoepidermoid and SCC have any significant propensity for neck metastasis. Adenoid cystic carcinoma apparently has the lowest incidence of neck metastases, which result more often by contiguous spread than by lymphatic embolism. This should be considered in treatment planning, and an END may be reasonable, depending on the location of the primary tumor and its proximity to the nerves that extend into the neck.

Based on a modified AJC staging system for parotid cancers,[123] stage I tumors have about a 1 per cent incidence of neck metastasis, in stage II it is 14 per cent, and in stage III it is 67 per cent. Fu and coworkers[85] found that stage I tumors had a 13 per cent incidence of neck metastasis, stage II had 13 per cent, and stage III had 33 per cent. Naturally, the histologic distribution of tumors in each series affects the reported metastatic rates. The presence of facial nerve paralysis has also been associated with a high likelihood of LN metastasis—77 per cent[62] and 66 per cent.[41] T3 parotid cancers and those associated with facial paralysis have a high association with regional node metastases.

The incidence of occult neck disease is presented in Table 56–10.[123] In Spiro's study[232] the incidence of occult

TABLE 56–8. Salivary Gland Carcinomas: Metastatic Patterns

Investigators	Number of Cases	Metastasis to Lymph Nodes (%)	Distant Metastasis (%)
Adenoid Cystic Carcinoma			
Spiro et al	242	15	42.9†
Conley and Dingman	134	16	34.0
Zielke-Temme and Wannenmacher	82	—	30.0
Eby et al	54	15	24.0
Blanck et al	35*	20	34.0
Grahne et al	21	24	43.0
Carcinoma Ex Pleomorphic Adenoma			
Spiro et al	150	25	32.0
Eneroth et al	21	24	24.0
Mucoepidermoid Carcinoma (all grades)			
Spiro et al	367 (all patients)	29	—
	342 (with follow-up)	—	15.0
	254*	28	—
Jakobsson et al	63*	8	6.5

*Parotid only.
†70% assumed.
Source: Modified from Batsakis JG: Metastatic patterns of salivary gland neoplasms. Ann Otol Rhinol Laryngol 91:465, 1982.

TABLE 56–9. Rates of Lymph Node Metastasis among Patients with Parotid Carcinoma

Histologic Type of Carcinoma	Number with Metastasis/ Total (%)
Mucoepidermoid (high-grade)	62/140 (44%)
Acinous cell	8/60 (13%)
Adenoid cystic	3/58 (5%)
Adenocarcinoma	37/144 (26%)
Arising from mixed tumor	24/117 (21%)
Squamous cell	24/65 (37%)
Undifferentiated	15/64 (23%)

Source: Johns ME: Parotid cancer: A rational basis for treatment. Head Neck Surg 3:132, 1980.

cervical nodes was 16 per cent or less for all parotid cancers except for SCC, which had a 44 per cent incidence.

When neck node metastases are palpable, RND is generally advised; the location of cervical metastases from parotid primary tumors rarely allows preservation of the spinal accessory nerve. Following surgery, RT is indicated.

In cases without palpable lymphadenopathy but with a high-grade primary tumor, such as mucoepidermoid, adenoid cystic, and squamous cell carcinoma, treatment generally consists of combined surgery and postoperative RT with the neck included, as well as the particular lymphatic drainage of the gland (such as facial nodes for parotid primary tumors). In the elective situation, failure in the neck without local recurrence is uncommon. Intraoperative treatment planning can be modified when the first echelon LNs (parotid and subdigastric) are exposed during parotidectomy. Any suspicious nodal tissue can be removed at that time to determine the need for neck dissection. If postoperative RT is to be used as an adjunct to surgery, this in itself may control any occult disease. There is no information to suggest that the neck is best treated with elective RND. Johns treats the neck as follows: during parotidectomy the upper jugular and postglandular (submandibular) nodes are inspected, and suspicious nodes are either biopsied or included in the parotid dissection.[123] The decision to use further surgery or adjunctive RT is based on the pathologic report.

Combined therapy for high-grade nonsquamous lesions has been employed for a relatively short time, but it seems to be effective in treating the neck electively. "Prophylactic" neck dissection may be indicated, but only for high-grade malignant tumors. Indications for postoperative radiation include (1) high-grade cancers,

TABLE 56–10. Rates of Occult Lymph Node Metastasis among Patients with Parotid Carcinoma*

Histologic Type of Carcinoma	Number with Metastasis/ Total (%)
Mucoepidermoid (high-grade)	10/64 (16%)
Malignant mixed	0/48 (0%)
Acinous cell	2/31 (6%)
Adenocarcinoma	2/23 (9%)
Adenoid cystic	0/19 (0%)
Squamous cell	4/10 (40%)

Source: Johns ME: Parotid cancer: A rational basis for treatment. Head Neck Surg 3:132, 1980.

TABLE 56–11. Principles of Treatment for Parotid Carcinoma

Treatment Group	Tumor Type	Treatment
Group I	T1 and T2 low-grade Mucoepidermoid low-grade Acinous cell	Superficial or total parotidectomy Preservation of facial nerve No neck dissection unless palpable nodes No irradiation
Group II	T1 and T2 high-grade High-grade T1 and T2 Adenocarcinoma Malignant mixed Undifferentiated Squamous cell (facial nerve not involved)	Total parotidectomy with resection of 1st echelon lymph nodes Resection of part of facial nerve adjacent to or involved by tumor No neck dissection unless palpable nodes Postoperative irradiation
Group III	T3 without extraparotid extension Any recurrent malignant tumors not in group IV	Radical parotidectomy (sacrifice of facial nerve with immediate reconstruction) Neck dissection Postoperative irradiation
Group IV	T4 with extraparotid extension	Radical parotidectomy with resection of skin, mandible, muscles, mastoid tip, as indicated Sacrifice of facial nerve with immediate reconstruction Neck dissection Postoperative irradiation

Source: Modified from Johns ME: Parotid cancer: A rational basis for treatment. Head Neck Surg 3:132, 1980.

(2) recurrent cancers, (3) deep lobe cancers, (4) gross or microscopic residual disease, (5) tumor adjacent to the facial nerve, (6) regional node metastases, (7) invasion of muscle, bone, skin, or nerves or extraparotid extension, and (8) T3 parotid cancer.[123] The treatment principles advocated by Johns are summarized in Table 56–11.

The foregoing considerations apply to previously untreated cancers. Recurrent disease requires more aggressive management, and neck dissection is advisable when radiation has been used previously.

Thyroid Cancer

Each histologic type of thyroid cancer has its own natural history. For papillary carcinoma, 40 to 50 per cent of patients (higher in children) have gross evidence of RLN metastases at operation. The incidence of occult disease in cervical nodes is also high—50 to 60 per cent for differentiated thyroid carcinomas (DTC), papillary and follicular. That cervical disease generally has an indolent course is inferred from data showing that patients who do not undergo elective LN dissection have a lower incidence of reported failure in the neck than would be expected from the incidence of subclinical metastasis (assuming no additional systemic treatment was given). The same is true for failure in the contralateral thyroid lobe following less than total thyroidectomy, despite the well-known multifocal nature of the primary disease.

The involved nodes from papillary cancer tend to remain free and mobile without extension of tumor through the capsule. Physiologic problems relating to uncontrolled local-regional disease is the usual cause of death in the majority of patients who die of papillary carcinoma, but following conservative operations, only 10 to 20 per cent of patients have to undergo reoperation for recurrent nodal or primary disease. The salvage rate is high unless the soft tissues of the neck are involved by recurrent cancer. Multiple operations are sometimes necessary.

Follicular carcinomas, like papillary lesions, tend to grow slowly and LN metastases are seldom seen except in the presence of extensive capsular invasion of the gland, recurrent tumor, or extraglandular extension. Survival relates to the degree of histologic invasiveness, and patients with invasive lesions tend to do poorly, with frequent local and distant failure and eventual death from cancer.

Medullary carcinoma is bilateral in almost all familial cases, and it may be unilateral or bilateral in sporadic cases. At presentation, 25 per cent of patients have palpable LNs; 50 to 75 per cent of all patients have positive LNs at operation. Involvement of mediastinal nodes is also common. With this entity, survival correlates best with nodal status and is decreased by 50 per cent in patients with positive nodes. In a Mayo Clinic series,[36] clinically apparent tumor recurrences following resection with curative attempt in 128 patients were noted in almost two thirds of the patients with positive nodes versus about 10 per cent in those with negative nodes. The majority of recurrences were local or regional (neck and mediastinum). Persistently elevated plasma calcitonin levels also indicate probable residual disease in the absence of clinically apparent cancer.

Anaplastic carcinomas are very aggressive, and local, regional, and distant failures are all common. Neck nodes are usually involved, although sometimes the primary tumor is so extensive that regional node status is difficult to assess. In contrast to the mobile nodes associated with differentiated lesions, those associated with anaplastic carcinoma are often "fixed." Cured patients (rare) have disease confined to the gland and regional nodes without extension into the soft tissues of the neck.

The biologic significance of cervical metastasis from DTCs is not entirely clear. Some authors feel that nodal disease can be a serious factor in survival, and others suggest that positive nodes might have a paradoxically favorable influence on the outcome. The general consensus of opinion is that survival for DTC appears unaffected by nodal involvement or the extent of its treatment. Elective LN dissections are not routinely performed for DTC. If positive nodes are noted at surgery, they are usually adequately dissected, using a MND that preserves the internal jugular vein, sternocleidomastoid muscle, and spinal accessory nerve. RND is rarely necessary and is used only in patients whose tumor extends through the nodal capsule. Because the majority of positive nodes occur in the mid- and lower jugular areas, some surgeons leave the submandibular gland intact if END is performed. Although the prognosis in patients with cervical nodes does not apparently depend on the extent of the surgery performed, node "plucking," which was commonly performed in earlier years, is currently discouraged in favor of a more complete MND. The surgeon must judge the need for a very careful and complete node dissection against the possibility of damaging the parathyroid blood supply.

Some surgeons are more aggressive. At the time of thyroid surgery, regardless of whether or not there are positive lateral nodes in the jugular chain, Loré[142] removes the paratracheal, tracheoesophageal, and pretracheal nodes. These nodes are sent for frozen section, and if they are positive, an ipsilateral MND is performed, preserving the sternocleidomastoid muscle and spinal accessory nerve. Loré removes the submandibular triangle contents and the internal jugular vein. If a bilateral neck dissection is indicated, the contralateral internal jugular vein is preserved.

At M.D. Anderson Hospital, if a diagnosis of cancer is not definite on frozen section, the head and neck surgeons proceed with a subtotal thyroidectomy and compartmental LN dissection, considered as the best approach to avoid re-exploration of the area, should the diagnosis of cancer be confirmed. All the LN-containing tissue of the thyroid compartment and the upper mediastinum above and below the level of the recurrent laryngeal nerve (RLN) is swept medially in continuity with the specimen.[93]

Recently, Rosen and Maitland[202] have advocated routine node sampling of the ipsilateral lower jugular chain in thyroid cancer cases to dictate the need for formal MND. This additional procedure increased their yield of detecting metastatic thyroid cancer from 15 to 42 per cent. Four of 12 positive nodal samples showed addi-

tional tumor in the neck when MND was completed. Although the authors concede the usually successful outcome for DTC regardless of neck treatment, they are uncomfortable about leaving residual disease in the neck, based on the known high incidence of occult spread to the nodes, and they advocate complete cancer clearance of occult disease to "prevent the emergence of future malignant disease in at least some patients."

Rosen and Maitland's article[202] cites the opinions of other surgeons regarding the biologic implications of occult metastatic neck disease from DTC. According to Cady, neck metastases are found more frequently in the younger age group and can serve as a source of failure, but without an apparent adverse influence on survival, whereas neck metastases are more life-threatening in older patients. Similarly, Mazzaferri and Young noted that the cancer recurrence rate was twice as high in patients initially observed to have cervical node metastasis (and even five times greater in patients over 40 years of age), but survival did not appear to be adversely affected. In one series, almost 70 per cent of a selected group of patients with papillary carcinoma who underwent END demonstrated neck disease, but in none of them did neck recurrence or death due to cancer develop.[5] Because those who die of papillary thyroid cancer usually have uncontrolled local growth that might have been prevented if the source had been removed early in the disease, END may actually be "prophylactic" in this context.

Some of the literature suggests the possibility that lymphatic involvement triggers some favorable response, such as an immune reaction, to account for the lack of adverse effect on survival of nodal involvement. Cervical LN involvement in papillary carcinoma is generally associated with an indolent clinical course. Such ideas are speculative; relevant studies seldom control for the multiple factors that can influence prognosis, such as treatment and other variables that specifically relate to thyroid cancer. The literature addressing the biologic significance of cervical nodes is usually based on cases in which positive nodes have been identified and treated and thereby incorporate treatment bias— the discovery of nodes at surgery may have been an alarming sign to the clinician, prompting more extensive treatment that otherwise might have been delayed or not instituted.

In one of the few publications dealing with pulmonary metastasis from DTC,[154] 58 patients were studied to determine the therapeutic program most capable of preventing the occurrence of such DMs. Because the cause of death could not be established for most of the patients studied, the objective of the paper was not fulfilled, but certain associations are interesting.

A correlation was found between cervical LN involvement (33 per cent in a series of 831 cases of DTC) and the occurrence of pulmonary metastases (PMs), which occurred in 11 per cent of patients with cervical LN involvement and in 5 per cent of patients without such involvement. An inverse correlation applied to other sites of DMs—the rate of bone metastasis was 4 per cent in patients with cervical nodes and 12 per cent in patients without. Cervical node involvement was found to have no adverse prognostic influence; the overall mortality was 17 per cent with node involvement and

18 per cent without. Mortality rate was 60 per cent in patients with PMs and cervical metastasis and 75 per cent in patients with PMs without cervical metastasis.

It was felt that mediastinal LN involvement, which is associated with a poor prognosis, represented secondary metastases from the PMs instead of being direct invasion from involved cervical nodes, because there was no correlation between the cervical and mediastinal LN involvement, the main histologic patterns were different at both sites, and mediastinal nodes occurred rarely as isolated lesions. Although removal of at least the upper mediastinal nodes may be easy at operation, the utility of this maneuver as a routine was questioned because surgical removal of mediastinal nodes did not influence the evolution of pulmonary lesions. Surgery was recommended, however, as a palliative procedure for complications arising from compression of the upper aerodigestive tract.

Medullary carcinoma patients generally undergo total thyroidectomy and bilateral neck dissection because of the high incidence of occult metastases. For medullary carcinoma, which has a propensity for early invasion of the soft tissues outside of the cervical lymphatics, RND is generally recommended. When bilateral procedures are undertaken, preservation of the spinal accessory nerve and internal jugular vein can be considered on the less involved side, which is usually the one without the primary tumor.[124] Lesser procedures have been advocated by other authors for patients without apparent LN metastases at operation. Parsons and Pfaff[185] dissect the central LNs between the carotid sheaths from the level of the hyoid bone to the innominate artery in the superior mediastinum. If there is obvious lymphadenopathy or if frozen section reveals positive LNs, RND(s) will be performed in preference to conservation neck surgery.

At M.D. Anderson Hospital patients with medullary carcinoma undergo MND that includes excision of the paratracheal, parapharyngeal, and periesophageal LNs.[93] When there is clinical evidence of metastasis from medullary carcinoma, classic bilateral RND should be performed; conservation of a single jugular vein may be possible if the cervical metastases are limited to one side or the involved nodes are clearly away from the jugular vein. Postoperative RT should be given because most of the failures occur in the neck and mediastinum and medullary carcinomas do not concentrate radioiodine or suppress with thyroid hormone.

Although the outcome of treatment of DTC is usually successful, the experienced clinician invariably encounters cases in which thyroid cancer follows a more aggressive and lethal course, demonstrating the spectrum of biologic activity within a given histologic type. Even though papillary cancer of the thyroid is traditionally a slowly metastasizing tumor with a good prognosis, cases have been reported of clinically occult carcinoma that presented with large metastases and caused death.[238]

Traditionally, the morphologic features of primary or metastatic lesions are used as prognosticators. A current trend is to biochemically phenotype individual tumors as markers for aggressiveness. For example, in a recent study[158] on a variety of medullary thyroid carcinomas, of which some were early and localized and others were late and diffuse, the distribution of carcinoembryonic antigen (CEA) and calcitonin was studied. Results indicated that retention of CEA (a marker for early epithelial differentiation) and loss of calcitonin (a marker for terminal differentiation or cellular maturity) may reflect a degree of maturation block in tumor from patients with aggressive disease. Additional follow-up and clinicopathologic correlation are needed to assess the specificity of such prognosticators, but this study demonstrates the current trend to attempt to derive biochemical correlates of individual tumor aggressiveness.

Malignant Melanoma

TUMOR BIOLOGY

In contrast to the usual conception of SCC as a lethal cancer by virtue of local or regional aggressiveness, it is generally conceded that malignant melanoma (melanocarcinoma) kills by distant spread and that evaluation of the RLNs for disease is a strong prognosticator of dissemination. In Handley's original description of the pathologic development of melanotic growths in relation to their operative treatment,[97] he noted that in the later stages of "melanotic sarcoma," slowly progressive lymphatic permeation receded into insignificance, and the patients died almost universally with tumor deposits resulting from blood-borne embolism—an event that occurred rarely with carcinomas, according to the current conception of the time.

When malignant melanoma (MM) proves fatal, it is as a result of involvement of distal vital organs—brain, lung, liver, adrenals, kidneys, heart, or spinal cord. This implies vascular (or lymphatic) spread which can only have originated from the primary site before the tumor was totally excised. This does not generally occur as a result of progressive disease still confined to the primary site or RLNs except in the rare case of far-advanced, ulcerated, bleeding, infected local and regional tumor masses. Cure in MM, as in other solid cancers, can only be reliably obtained by removal of the primary lesion before it has metastasized.

Some of the literature maintains that the sequence of metastasis is from primary lesion to nodes to systemic circulation, based on the observation that nodal and distant metastases coincide in 75 per cent of patients and that in the 25 per cent of patients without RLN metastases who subsequently die of distant disease, tumor cells probably spread directly through the blood stream only. A more likely explanation is that metastases originate simultaneously from the primary site through contiguous capillary lymphatic and vascular channels, and not secondarily from the lymphatics into the blood stream. In most instances, when lymphatic metastases are present, the disease has already spread to distant sites via vascular channels, and the impression that LNs seed distant sites is artificial because superficial tumor deposits are more readily identifiable than deep visceral metastases.

Biologically, it appears that the RLNs do not prevent melanoma cells from reaching the systemic circulation: 50 to 75 per cent of patients with nodal metastases subsequently develop visceral disease and die, whereas most patients (80 to 90 per cent) without nodal metastases remain free of disease at distant sites. According to Eilber and Goodnight,[61a] the RLNs can be considered an "in vitro petri dish" rather than a filter, and metastasis to the RLNs indicates that the circulating tumor cells have the capacity to survive at a distant site. This explains why 75 per cent of patients with melanoma metastatic to the RLNs die of DMs; the malignant cells have long since disseminated by way of the lymphatics or blood stream or both. Whether equivalent conditions favoring growth are present distally as they are in the RLNs is uncertain; traversing the additional distance, tumor cells can meet many more unfavorable host influences and this may explain why some patients with LN metastases survive if the disease is effectively controlled locally.

PROGNOSTIC FACTORS

In general, in the presence of LN metastases, prognosis is poor regardless of other characteristics of the primary tumor, suggesting that the presence of disease in the RLNs is the most significant indicator of prognosis. Many prognostic variables are associated with overall survival for MM, including age, sex, site of the primary tumor, ulceration, depth of invasion, blood vessel and lymphatic invasion, the number of histologically positive nodes, node palpability, pathologic stage, extent of surgical treatment, and the presence or absence of involved RLNs. Few series match patients for these prognostic variables in the same way, if at all, and the patient population varies among series. Series that have undertaken multifactorial analysis of a number of variables yield somewhat more information than series which do not (summarized by Kaiser and Ostfeld[127]), but they are still limited by the variation in patient population.

Patients with histologically proven RLN metastases survive 5 years in 20 to 50 per cent of cases, and histologic demonstration of nodal metastases predicts eventual dissemination in 50 to 75 per cent of cases. Conversely, the absence of such involvement predicts the subsequent absence of DMs in 85 per cent of patients and 5-year survival. Therefore, lymphadenectomy as a staging procedure appears to be extremely accurate. When all patients are evaluated regardless of prognostic variables, the overall 5-year survival of clinical stage I patients (local disease only) is 70 to 80 per cent, and for stage II patients (regional metastases) it is 40 per cent. Stage III is systemic disease.

Patients with superficially invasive MM (Clark's level 2 or maximum depth less than 0.75 mm) in whom the primary tumor is surgically removed have a very high cure rate and very little potential for the development of metastasis. The risk of nodal spread becomes clinically significant once the melanoma penetrates deeper than 0.76 mm into the dermis, and there is a regular association between RLN involvement and lesions more than 1.7 mm in depth. The potential for metastatic spread seems most directly related to the vertical growth or depth of invasion of the primary tumor: Clark level 2, less than 10 per cent; level 3, 40 to 52 per cent; level 5, 58 to 75 per cent.

The incidence of microscopic LN metastases is 5 to 75 per cent, with a mean value of 20 per cent. Although there is variation among series, the mean percentage of patients with micrometastases is 5 per cent for Clark level 2 disease, 14 per cent for level 3, 33 per cent for level 4, and 49 per cent for level 5.

With respect to Breslow measurements, lesions less than 0.76 mm in thickness rarely have micrometastases in the RLNs; for lesions 0.76 to 1.5 mm the incidence is 14 per cent; for those 1.5 to 4 mm it is 30 per cent; and it is 50 per cent with lesions thicker than 4 mm.

A recent 22-author paper maintains that microscopic satellites are more highly associated with RLN metastases than is primary melanoma thickness.[99] Multivariate analysis performed on 20 clinical and histologic variables from 327 clinical stage I melanoma patients who had elective regional node dissection showed that primary tumor thickness, microscopic satellites, and the interval between diagnosis and elective node dissection were the variables that most highly predicted clinically occult regional node metastases ($p = 10^{-15}$). The probability of finding occult nodal metastases from melanomas less than 0.75 mm in thickness was zero; for lesions 0.76 to 1.5 mm it was 4 per cent; for those 1.51 to 3 mm it was 14 per cent; and for those more than 3 mm it was 39.5 per cent.

TREATMENT CONTROVERSIES: HEAD AND NECK SITES

As with other head and neck cancers, it is generally agreed that patients with palpable lymphadenopathy should undergo a therapeutic regional node dissection. Clinical examination is considerably more accurate for MM than for SCC; for MM, 95 per cent of palpable nodes contain tumor histologically. Based on the natural history of this disease, therapeutic lymphadenectomy is a palliative procedure. Positive nodes may become locally disabling, and they should be removed for anticipated palliation if there is no contraindication to the operation. Nodal removal will, however, not enhance the patient's chance for survival if metastases are present in distal vital organs.

By this point, it should be no surprise to the reader that controversy continues concerning the role of elective node dissection for MM. Almost every surgeon has opinions as to when such procedures should be applied, but a scientific, clinically controlled basis for decision making is lacking. Depending upon the studies selected for review, an argument can be made either for or against elective treatment of the neck for head and neck MM, primarily based on reports of survival. Favorable reports show that patients who undergo END have better survival rates than those who don't, but these reports seldom mention the site of failure or cause of death and frequently do not relate the outcome to whether nodes were histologically positive or negative. Obviously, patients who do not harbor cancer in their neck nodes will have a better outcome than those who do, even though both groups had END. The outcome in either case may have occurred in spite of, not because of, the treatment modality.

Elective node dissection for head and neck MM has been strongly endorsed in the literature, especially for thicker lesions, primarily based on the work of Conley and Pack.[42a] The increased survival rate in Conley's series for individuals who underwent local excision plus END, over those who underwent local excision alone (76.5 per cent versus 62 per cent), was for many years the rationale for performing END for head and neck

MM, even though the selection of these patients was not random and many variables were present. In 18 per cent of Conley's 200 patients, lymphatics and cervical nodes were bypassed and systemic disease was observed. When LNs were palpable, the 5-year cure rate was 15 per cent, and the rate was 25 per cent when occult metastatic disease was present—probably an insignificant difference in a retrospective series.

A recent update of this series[42] retrospectively reviewed all cases of MM of the head and neck treated at the Pack Foundation between 1935 and 1972 and showed some of the deficits in a retrospective analysis of such patients. Classification according to Clark's level could be defined for only 289 of 660 cases; 80 per cent were levels 3 to 5. Local disease was present in 56 per cent of patients, regional disease in 33 per cent, and disseminated disease in 11 per cent. The 5-year or greater absolute survival for all cases with positive nodes (that lent themselves to analysis) was 12.6 per cent (190 cases). Survival for cases with END was 55 per cent versus 38.5 per cent without END. The pathologic status of the removed nodes was not mentioned, however, and causes of death were not specified. In the 86 patients who underwent END, 30 per cent developed DMs, and in 158 patients who had therapeutic neck dissection, 70 per cent developed DMs.

Roses and associates[203] reported on selective surgical management of cutaneous melanoma of the head and neck. Of 52 patients who had RND performed for invasive melanoma with more than 5-year follow-up, 29 had histologically negative nodes (two died of systemic melanoma) and 22 had histologically positive nodes (21 died of systemic melanoma). No patient developed local recurrence independent of systemic spread. Four patients developed local recurrence synchronously with systemic metastases. All four had clinical and histologic confirmation of nodal metastasis. No patient with micrometastases alone developed local recurrence. In all patients with histologically positive regional nodes, the nodal group immediately adjacent to the primary excision site was involved, but there was no "skipping" of metastasis to more distant nodal groups. The 5-year survival rate was only 8 per cent when regional nodes were histologically positive. Measures of Breslow's thickness were not performed in this study, however, and it is possible that a disproportionate number of patients had biologically aggressive or thick lesions. This study showed that regional node dissection failed to control the dissemination of MM of the head and neck. The authors recommended that in the absence of clinically involved nodes, sampling of immediate adjacent nodes be performed. If no metastases were demonstrated, there was no need for a conventional node dissection. If metastases were found, formal node dissection should be completed, despite the low survival figures, in an attempt to provide local control and freedom from disfiguring recurrence.

In an analysis of 100 patients with invasive primary or locally recurrent head and neck MM treated by a single surgeon between 1970 and 1978,[180] patients who had END with negative findings or only one or two positive nodes had similar 5-year survival rates—significantly better than patients with three or more positive nodes at the time of surgery. Relapse in both the group having wide excision only and the node dissection

group was most often associated with DMs. Patients who had a relapse after nodal dissection invariably presented with systemic disease, and such recurrence portended death. Again it was found that "skip" involvement of nodes did not occur; if proximal nodes were negative, distal nodes were also negative. The recommendation for lesions 0.76 to 1.5 mm and within a few centimeters of node-bearing areas was to selectively dissect nodes, removing only those nodes in the nearest group. If positive nodes were encountered, node dissection was extended to include all regional nodes (MND or RND). For lesions thicker than 1.5 mm, neck dissection was carried out except for midline or near-midline lesions. The 5-year survival rate was 56 per cent when only one or two nodes were positive, but more extensive nodal involvement was associated with a grim prognosis. This paper indicates (as do some others on SCC and breast cancer) that the prognosis of patients with minimal micrometastatic nodal disease is not significantly worse than those without demonstrable disease, although papers that show equivalent outcomes with macro- and microstatic nodal disease are also in the literature (see following discussion). Once again, the true significance of occult disease is not known. Involvement of only a few nodes may represent a low systemic tumor burden that can be controlled by host defense mechanisms.

RELEVANT DATA IN THE LITERATURE—ELECTIVE LYMPHADENECTOMY

Because of the wide variation in 5-year survival rates in published series based on differing patient populations with diverse prognostic factors, the relative merits of END cannot be resolved by retrospective analysis. One retrospective series, which attempted to evaluate comparable patient populations, reported on a selected group of patients from Australia.[50] Four groups of 15 patients were retrospectively selected from a large group of new patients registered between 1963 and 1968 and were matched for sex, age, tumor site, and depth of invasion. All patients had apparently normal nodes at first examination and underwent similar primary treatment—excision with or without skin graft. One group had elective node dissection with negative nodes microscopically. The second had elective node dissection with positive nodes microscopically. Patients in the third group were observed, and metastases never developed. In the fourth group, patients were observed, and metastases developed in the regional nodes, some of which were inoperable. The survival of patients was assessed at 5 years, although there were not enough cases for statistical evaluation. Patients who had a positive elective node dissection had a cumulative 5-year survival of 35 per cent, compared with 44 per cent in the observed group who later underwent therapeutic node dissection. Thus, survival following removal of occult positive nodes was *worse* than waiting and removing the nodes when they became clinically involved. No advantage was seen for elective node dissection over observation with later lymphadenectomy as indicated. Patients who had elective node dissection with negative nodes had a 5-year survival rate that was similar to those who were observed and never developed metastases (76 per cent). Patients who had elective node dissection with positive disease had a 5-year survival rate similar to those presenting with clinically positive nodes; the prognosis was similar if nodal disease was present, whether occult or palpable.

There are no prospective randomized studies evaluating END for patients with MM of the head and neck, but two series have evaluated elective regional node dissection in patients with MM at other sites.[225,250] Neither trial showed a statistical benefit for patients undergoing immediate elective node dissection versus delayed node dissection when nodes became palpable in patients with clinical stage I MM. Although both series have been criticized, the data is prospective, well documented, carefully obtained, and probably meaningful. It appears at present that "prophylactic" lymphadenectomy offers little therapeutic benefit. Such a procedure can, however, provide prognostic information, and currently the main indication for regional lymphadenectomy in patients with high-risk primary lesions and clinically uninvolved regional nodes aims at identifying patients at risk for recurrence. Such patients can be placed in adjuvant treatment protocols to evaluate experimental therapy in either delaying metastatic development or improving survival.

TREATMENT OF THE NECK: ADDITIONAL RECOMMENDATIONS

When the primary lesion directly overlies a LN area and when primary drainage is to a single node-bearing region, elective node dissection may be considered to avoid a later palliative operation in a previously operated field. In cases in which lymphatic drainage is ambiguous (to two or more nodal regions), such a procedure is not indicated.

There is currently no specific indication for regional lymphadenectomy in continuity with the primary excision.[221] When the primary tumor is located in proximity to positive RLNs it may be convenient to include the intervening skin to fascial soft parts. Doing a RND in continuity for head and neck MM includes the platysma muscle with the skin as a precaution against "in transit" metastases and latent satellitosis. Although some authors have recommended delaying elective LN operations for several weeks after excision of the primary tumor to allow time for any "in transit" tumor cells to reach the nodes, this view is purely speculative, and the optimal time to perform a neck dissection is at the time of excision of the primary tumor.

If the nodes are clinically involved, complete removal (RND) is indicated. For elective operations, partial neck dissections are acceptable because microscopic metastases are found only in the nodes closest to the tumor. A superficial parotidectomy should be added for preauricular, malar, and temporal lesions.[94] Clinically obvious superficial parotid metastases are excised with a margin that includes the posterior belly of the digastric muscle and a deep lobe parotidectomy. Posterior neck dissection is performed for lesions in the posterior parietal, mastoid, and occipital areas.[81] Roses and associates[203] have described a number of modifications of the standard RND for MM in various sites of the head and neck.

Malignant melanoma is a capricious disease with protean manifestations.[187] Its unpredictability is manifested when even radical surgery fails to control stage I disease and when patients who present with advanced disease remain alive after treatment of recurrent local-regional disease, with multiple primary tumors, and sometimes with DMs. Nonresectable melanomas have remained symptomless in situ without treatment for a period of years, probably related to the patient's intrinsic resistance and the biologic aggressiveness of the individual tumor, and some spontaneous cures have been reported. Therefore, when recurrent melanoma appears as a safely resectable lesion, an operative procedure should be performed regardless of the anticipated prognosis, since clinical disease-free intervals of many years can result in some instances. The vast majority of MMs that are going to recur do so within the first 2 to 3 years, and careful long-term follow-up is mandatory.

Adjunctive chemoimmunotherapy is not indicated as primary treatment and should be used only in controlled study situations. In such adjuvant trials, clinical staging is inadequate, and elective regional node dissection is necessary to provide accurate staging and to remove residual metastases, which may have a significant bearing on results.

MUCOSAL MELANOMA

Nodal disease from head and neck *mucosal melanoma* is present in 10 to 23 per cent of patients at presentation. Subsequent development of nodal metastases in the absence of primary tumor recurrence or disseminated disease is uncommon, occurring in less than 5 per cent. Hence, regional node metastasis in most series is not a significant management problem, and in very few patients do LN metastases per se contribute to death. Elective node dissection is not generally recommended because survival figures are extremely poor. There is continued attrition from DMs more than 5 years following treatment, and there is little evidence that this disease can be cured.[100]

CONCLUSION

In 1982, important future directions for research in head and neck oncology were identified as follows:[262]

1. Determining the crucial biologic factors which cause the cancer cell to differ from normal cells and factors which control the tumor-host interaction

2. Continued study of etiologic factors such as viruses, smoking, and alcohol and application to prevention programs

3. Development of effective measures to assist smokers to quit their habit and establishment of patient education programs about the health consequences of smoking

4. Continued evaluation of the effects of various treatment modalities (heat, cold, chemotherapeutic drugs, irradiation, surgery) used individually and in combination

5. Use of multi-institutional cooperative studies to accumulate a sufficient number of patients to answer these important questions.

More retrospective clinical cancer series are not needed.

It has been suggested in this chapter that cervical metastases from head and neck cancers are associated with a poor prognosis not because neck disease is an immediate cause of patient death but because cervical metastases are biologic markers of the general ability of the individual's tumor to metastasize—an accepted precept in breast cancer and malignant melanoma. As better local-regional control is achieved, more patients are living longer to develop distant metastases. It may therefore be useful to conceptualize head and neck cancer as a *systemic disease*. That more effective local-regional treatment modalities have not resulted in a corresponding increase in patient *survival* is unfortunate but understandable on this basis—surgery and radiation therapy cannot combat the systemic nature of the process, although the combination is apparently useful in decreasing local-regional recurrence.

Data were also presented to show that tumor cells spread via both hematogenous and lymphogenous routes simultaneously, and although it has been shown experimentally that metastases can metastasize, the dual nature of cancer cell dissemination seems to preclude routine *clinical* cancer cures by elective regional node dissection. If spread occurred only from involved lymph nodes, then, presumably, removing occult disease with elective lymphadenectomy would decrease the incidence of distant metastases and thus would have a *prophylactic* function. However, this does not appear to be the situation in adequately studied human solid tumor systems (breast cancer). Equivalent survival results, when node dissection is done electively or in a delayed therapeutic context, support the lack of prophylactic utility of elective lymphadenectomy.

If one accepts these arguments, as well as the apparently valid fact that cervical metastases are reliable prognosticators of distant spread, then elective node dissection does have utility as a *diagnostic biopsy procedure*, offering a means of assessing the metastasizing ability of individual tumors and identifying patients who might benefit from systemic adjuvant treatment. Although some might consider routine elective neck dissection for this purpose futile in the absence of effective adjuvant modalities, studies could still be designed to determine the significance of the regional lymph node and the efficacy of various treatment modalities along the lines of the NSABP breast cancer trials. In fact, such studies are mandatory, for although compelling analogies can be drawn between head and neck and breast cancer, individual solid tumor systems must be independently investigated.

Studies are now needed to elucidate basic tumor biology aspects of head and neck cancer, and many are under way. Ethically designed human studies and animal models that closely approximate the human SCC situation should be investigated using tests designed to measure functionally relevant parameters that approximate the in vivo tumor-host interaction. Defining the nature of tumor heterogeneity constitutes one of the major challenges to the experimental oncologist.

Ongoing attempts to identify the effects of adjuvant therapies should be employed only within the context of well-designed clinical trials. The tendency for clinical trials to be instituted is increasing. Large numbers of cooperative groups and individual institutions are now interacting, but to generate valid data, considerable organization and standardization is required. The randomized prospective clinical trial is an important mechanism for clinical problem solving, and according to Bernard Fisher[73] all treatments must be related to bio-logic considerations; otherwise the basis for therapy is relegated to the realm of speculation and personal experience. He points out that if clinical trials are designed to test the relative merits of a standard treatment with those of a new treatment, this is unlikely to be a productive undertaking, for if the second treatment does not prove better than the first (which is the case more often than not), the trial is considered a failure and has made no contribution to knowledge. The aim of a trial should be to test the validity of a biologic principle or a hypothesis resulting from basic and clinical investigations. If so designed, the results of such a trial are apt to be important and will provide information that strengthens, modifies, or discredits the original scientific considerations leading to the trial—the hypothesis. Such considerations are especially relevant to head and neck cancer trials in which the number of available patients is relatively small. Deciding relevant questions to be answered (hypotheses to test) might most efficiently be re-evaluated at a national planning level before the subjects are further dispersed into regional programs. Certainly, scientific trials would be useful in defining the risks and benefits associated with various combinations of treatment that have been accepted as standard therapy on an empirical basis, especially before adding additional treatments from the category of biologic response modifiers.

According to Fisher[73] cancer therapists are methodologically oriented and are concerned with the nuances of their particular resource rather than with concepts or scientific considerations that relate to their effort. Surgeons might ask how much of a regional node dissection is necessary, rather than what might be the biologic basis for doing the operation, for example. At the 1984 International Conference on Head and Neck Cancer, Harrison mentioned that although surgeons are intelligent, ambitious and enterprising, they show a significant need to achieve, control, resist change, and persist methodically and conventionally in a task.[99a] In this era, however, it is the responsibility of surgeons not only to modify their decisions based upon new information but also to participate in its acquisition. The trained surgical oncologist should be able to perceive areas of investigation that affect patient care but are less discernible to nonclinical specialists. Ideally, a surgical oncologist has a current understanding of tumor biology and the capability of selecting from the "oncologic concept pool" that which can be used in clinical investigations or applied to formulation of better therapeutic strategies directed toward the patient. An oncologist should also develop the ability to generate new information via laboratory and clinical research to add to the information pool. It is desirable that a subset of head and neck cancer surgeons expand beyond their methodologic orientations so that they become scientists who can introduce a different perspective into the study of cancer. When one compares the operating rooms of today with those of Halsted's time (Fig. 56–4) and then realizes that his principles of surgical oncology are still considered dogma by many cancer surgeons, the need for updating our conceptual framework becomes obvious.

It is now, as it was then, as it may ever be, conceptions from the past blind us to facts which almost slap us in the face.

W.A. Halsted, 1908

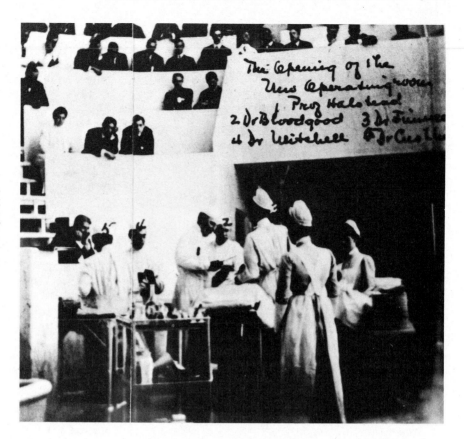

Figure 56—4. This photograph shows operating room technology during Halsted's era. Isn't it time to update our surgical oncology concepts, too? (From the Naldecon Gallery of Medical History.)

REFERENCES

1. Abramson AL, et al: Distant metastasis from carcinoma of the larynx. Laryngoscope 81:1503, 1971.
2. Anderson RE, Warner NL: Ionizing radiation and immune response. Adv Immunol 24:215, 1976.
3. Arons MS, et al: Significance of cancer cells in operative wounds. Cancer 14:1041, 1961.
4. Arons MS, Smith RR: Distant metastasis and local recurrence in head and neck cancer. Ann Surg 154:235, 1961.
5. Attie J, et al: Elective neck dissection and papillary carcinoma of the thyroid. Am J Surg 122:464, 1971.
6. Baker RR, et al: Role of the cervical lymph nodes as a barrier to metastatic tumor. Am J Surg 118:654, 1969.
7. Ballantyne AJ: Current controversy in the management of cancer of the tongue and floor of mouth. In Kagan AR, Miles JW (eds): Head and Neck Oncology. Controversy in Cancer Treatment Series. Boston, GK Hall, 1981.
8. Ballantyne AJ, Jackson GL: Synchronous bilateral neck dissection. Am J Surg 144:452, 1982.
9. Bartelink H, et al: The use of postoperative radiation therapy as an adjuvant to radical neck dissection. Cancer 52:1008, 1983.
10. Baskies AM, et al: Radiation therapy: Its effects on immune reactivity. Progr Clin Cancer 8:215, 1982.
11. Bates SE, et al: Immunologic skin testing and interpretation. A plea for uniformity. Cancer 43:2306, 1979.
12. Batsakis JG: The pathology of head and neck tumors: X. The occult primary and metastasis to the head and neck. Head Neck Surg 3:409, 1981.
13. Beahrs OH, Barber KW: The value of radical dissection of structures in the neck in management of carcinomas of the lip, mouth and larynx. Arch Surg 85:49, 1962.
14. Berger DS, et al: Elective irradiation of the neck lymphatics for squamous cell carcinoma of the nasopharynx and oropharynx. AJR 111:66, 1971.
15. Berger DS, Fletcher GH: Distant metastasis following local control of squamous cell carcinoma of the nasopharynx, tonsillar fossa and base of tongue. Radiology 100:141, 1971.
16. Berlinger NT, et al: Immunologic assessment of regional lymph node histology in relation to survival in head and neck carcinoma. Cancer 27:697, 1976.
17. Bernstein ID, et al: Monoclonal antibodies: Prospects for cancer treatment. In Mihich E (ed): Immunological Approaches to Cancer Therapeutics. New York, John Wiley & Sons, 1982.
18. Bier J, et al: The doubtful relevance of nonspecific immune reactivity in patients with squamous cell carcinoma of the head and neck region. Cancer 52:1165, 1983.
19. Birbeck MSC, Carter RL: Observations on the ultrastructure of two hamster lymphomas with particular reference to infiltrating macrophages. Int J Cancer 9:249, 1972.
20. Bocca E: Conservative neck dissection. Laryngoscope 85:1511, 1975.
21. Bocca E, et al: Functional neck dissection: An evaluation and review of 843 cases. Laryngoscope 94:942, 1984.
22. Bocca E, et al: Occult metastases in cancer of the larynx and their relevance to clinical and histological aspects of the primary tumor: A 4 year multicentric research. Laryngoscope 94:1086, 1984.
23. Bockman RS: Prostaglandins in cancer: A review. Cancer Invest 1:485, 1983.
24. Braund RR, Martin HE: Distant metastasis in cancer of the upper respiratory and alimentary tracts. Surg Gynecol Obstet 73:63, 1941.
25. Broder S, Waldmann TA: The suppressor-cell network in cancer. N Engl J Med 299:1281, 1978.
26. Brown JB, McDowell F: Neck Dissection. Springfield, Ill, Charles C Thomas, 1954.
27. Burge AJS: The significance and management of metastatic lymph nodes in the neck. Proc Roy Soc Med 68:77, 1975.
28. Burke EM: Metastasis and squamous cell carcinoma. Am J Cancer 30:493, 1979.
29. Calearo C, Teatini G: Functional neck dissection. Anatomical grounds, surgical technique, clinical observations. Ann Otol 92:215, 1983.
30. Carpenter RJ III, et al: Cancer of the hypopharynx: Analysis of treatment and results in 162 patients. Arch Otol 102:716, 1976.
31. Carr I: The pathologist's role in interpreting metastatic lymph node disease. In Weiss L (ed): Lymphatic System Metastasis. Boston, GK Hall, 1980.
32. Carrasquillo JA, et al: Diagnosis of and therapy for solid tumors with radio-labelled antibodies and immune fragments. Cancer Treat Rep 68:317, 1984.

33. Carter RL, et al: Patterns and mechanisms of bone invasion by squamous carcinomas of the head and neck. Am J Surg 146:451, 1983.

34. Casley-Smith JR: An electron microscope study of injured and abnormally permeable lymphatics. Ann NY Acad Sci 116:803, 1964.

35. Chardot C, Dartois D: De l'importance de tares associés dans la survie ã long terme des maladies attients d'epitheliomas aero digestifs supérieures. Bull Cancer 59:87, 1972.

36. Chong GC, et al: Medullary carcinoma of the thyroid gland. Cancer 35:695, 1975.

37. Cohen HJ, Laslow J: Influence of trauma on the unusual distribution of metastasis from carcinoma of the larynx. Cancer 29:466, 1972.

38. Coley WB: Late results of the treatment of inoperable sarcoma by the mixed toxins of erysipelas and bacillus prodigiosus. Am J Med Sci 131:375, 1906.

39. Colombano SP, Reese PA: The cascade theory of metastatic spread: Are there generalizing sites? Cancer 46:2312, 1980.

40. Conley JJ: Radical neck dissection. Laryngoscope 85:1344, 1975.

41. Conley J, Hamaker RC: Prognosis of malignant tumors of the parotid gland with facial paralysis. Arch Otol 101:39, 1975.

42. Conley J, Hamaker RC: Melanoma of the head and neck. Laryngoscope 87:760, 1977.

42a. Conley JJ, Pack GT: Melanoma of the head and neck. Surg Gynecol Obstet 116:15, 1963.

43. Crile G: Excision of cancer of the head and neck. JAMA 47:180, 1906.

44. Crile G Jr: Rationale of simple mastectomy without radiation for clinical stage I cancer of the breast. Surg Gynecol Obstet 120:975, 1965.

45. Crile G Jr: Results of simple mastectomy without irradiation in the treatment of stage I cancer of the breast. Ann Surg 168:330, 1968.

46. Crile G Jr: The effect on metastasis of removing or irradiating regional nodes of mice. Surg Gynecol Obstet 126:1283, 1969.

47. Crile G Jr: Possible role of uninvolved regional nodes in preventing metastasis from breast cancer. Cancer 24:1283, 1969.

48. Cronkite ET, et al: Lymphocyte repopulation and restoration of cell mediated immunity following radiation; whole-body and localized irradiation. Proceedings of the Conference on interaction of radiation and host immune defense mechanisms in malignancy. New York, Brookhaven National Laboratory, 1974.

49. Currie GA, Alexander P: Spontaneous shedding of tumor-specific transplantation antigens by viable sarcoma cells: Its possible role in facilitating metastatic spread. Cancer 29:72, 1974.

50. Davis NC: The regional lymph nodes in malignant melanoma: Is routine excision indicated? Progr Clin Cancer 6:183, 1975.

51. Decroix Y, Ghossein MA: Experience of the Curie Institute in treatment of cancer of the mobile tongue. II. Management of the neck nodes. Cancer 47:503, 1981.

52. DeLellis RA, et al: Immunoperoxidase techniques in diagnostic pathology. Am J Clin Pathol 71:483, 1979.

53. Dennington ML, et al: Distant metastasis in head and neck epidermoid carcinoma. Laryngoscope 90:196, 1980.

54. Der Hagopian RP, et al: Inflammatory oncotaxis. JAMA 240:374, 1978.

55. Deodhar S, et al: Study of the tumor cell—lymphocyte interaction in patients with breast cancer. Cancer 29:2321, 1972.

56. DeSanto LW, et al: Neck dissection: Is it worthwhile? Laryngoscope 92:502, 1982.

57. DeWys WD: Studies correlating the growth rate of a tumor and its metastasis in providing evidence for tumor-related systemic growth—retarding factors. Cancer Res 32:374, 1972.

58. Donegan JO, et al: The role of suprahyoid neck dissection in the management of cancer of the tongue and floor of mouth. Head Neck Surg 4:209, 1982.

59. Dowd PS, Heatley RV: The influence of undernutrition on immunity. Clin Sci 66:241, 1984.

60. Duval MK, Healy MJ: The natural history and effects of treatment of cancer of the tongue. Cancer 9:1842, 1956.

61. Eccles S, Alexander P: Macrophage content of tumors in relation to metastatic spread and host immune reaction. Nature 250:667, 1974.

61a. Eilber FR, Goodnight JE: Malignant melanoma: Biologic implications of regional lymph node metastases. In Weiss L (ed): Lymphatic System Metastasis. Boston, G. K. Hall, 1980.

62. Eneroth CM: Facial nerve paralysis: A criterion of malignancy in parotid tumors. Arch Otol 95:300, 1972.

63. Engeset A: Barrier function of lymph glands. Lancet 1:324, 1962.

64. Eriksson O, et al: Effects of fine needle aspiration and other biopsy procedures on tumor dissemination in mice. Cancer 54:73, 1984.

65. Falini B, Taylor CR: New developments in immunoperoxidase techniques and their application. Arch Pathol Lab Med 107:105, 1983.

66. Farr HW, Arthur K: Epidermoid carcinoma of the mouth and pharynx, 1960 to 1964. Elective radical neck dissection. Clin Bull 1:130, 1971.

67. Fidler IJ: Metastasis: Quantitative analysis of distribution and fate of tumor cell emboli labeled with ^{125}I 5-iododeoxyuridine. J Natl Cancer Inst 45:773, 1970.

68. Fidler IJ, et al: The biology of cancer invasion and metastasis. Adv Can Res 28:149, 1978.

69. Fidler IJ: Recent concepts of cancer metastasis and their implications for therapy. Cancer Treat Rep 68:193, 1984.

70. Fisch UP: Cervical lymph flow in man following radiation and surgery. Trans Am Acad Ophthalmol Otol 69:846, 1965.

71. Fisch UP: The barrier function of the lymph nodes in the neck of the human. Prog Clin Ca 4:97, 1970.

72. Fisch UP, Sigel ME: Cervical lymphatic system as visualized by lymphography. Ann Otol 73:869, 1964.

73. Fisher B: Cancer surgery: A commentary. Cancer Treat Rep 68:31, 1984.

74. Fisher B, Fisher ER: Experimental evidence in support of dormant tumor cells. Science 130:918, 1959.

75. Fisher B, Fisher ER: Barrier function of lymph nodes to tumor cells and erythrocytes: I. Normal nodes. Cancer 20:1907, 1967.

76. Fisher B, Fisher ER: Barrier function of lymph nodes to tumor cells and erythrocytes. II. Effect of x-ray, inflammation, sensitization and tumor growth. Cancer 20:1914, 1967.

77. Fisher B, Fisher ER: Metastasis revisited. In Weiss L (ed): Fundamental Aspects of Metastasis. Amsterdam, North-Holland Publishing Co., 1976.

78. Fisher B, et al: The contribution of recent NSABP clinical trials of primary breast cancer therapy to understanding of tumor biology—an overview of findings. Cancer 46:1009, 1980.

79. Fisher ER, et al: Detection and significance of occult axillary node metastasis in patients with invasive breast cancer. Cancer 42:2025, 1978.

80. Fisher JC, et al: Significance of cancer cells in operative wounds. Am J Surg 114:514, 1967.

81. Fisher SR, et al: Application of posterior neck dissection in treating malignant melanoma of the posterior scalp. Laryngoscope 93:760, 1983.

82. Fletcher GH: The role of irradiation in management of squamous cell carcinomas of the mouth and throat. Head Neck Surg 1:441, 1979.

83. Fletcher GH: Subclinical disease. Cancer 53:1274, 1984.

84. Friedman M, et al: Metastatic neck disease—evaluation by computed tomography. Arch Otol 110:443, 1984.

85. Fu K, et al: Carcinoma of the major and minor salivary glands. Cancer 40:2882, 1977.

86. Gilbert H, Kagan AR: Recurrence patterns in squamous cell carcinoma of the oral cavity, pharynx, and larynx. J Surg Oncol 6:357, 1974.

87. Gluckman JL, Crissman JD: Survival rates in 548 patients with multiple neoplasms of the upper aerodigestive tract. Laryngoscope 93:71, 1982.

88. Goepfert H: Are we making any progress? Arch Otol 110:562, 1984.

89. Goldson AL: Past, present and prospects of intraoperative radiotherapy (IOR). Semin Oncol 8:59, 1981.

90. Gorelik E: Concomitant tumor immunity and the resistance to a second tumor challenge. Adv Can Res 39:71, 1983.

91. Grandi C, et al: Surgery vs. combined therapies for cancer of the anterior floor of mouth. Head Neck Surg 6:653, 1983.

92. Grenby BL: Intraoperative monitoring of sensory evoked potentials. Anesthesiology 58:72, 1983.

93. Guillamondegui OM, Goepfert H: Thyroid cancer. In Gates G (ed): Current Therapy in Otolaryngology—Head and Neck Surgery, 1984 to 1985. St. Louis, C. V. Mosby Co., 1984, p 270.

94. Gussack GS: Cutaneous melanoma of the head and neck—a review of 399 cases. Arch Otol 109:803, 1983.

95. Halsted WS: The results of radical operations for the cure of carcinoma of the breast. Ann Surg 46:1, 1907.

96. Hammond W, Rolley R: Retained regional lymph nodes: Effects on metastasis and recurrence after tumor removal. Cancer 25:358, 1970.

97. Handley WS: The pathology of melanotic growth in relation to their operative treatment. Lancet 1:927, 1907.

98. Harris AH, Smith RR: Operative wound seeding with tumor cells: Its role in recurrences of head and neck cancer. Ann Surg 151:330, 1960.

99. Harris TJ, et al: "Microscopic satellites" are more highly associated

with regional lymph node metastasis than is primary melanoma thickness. Cancer 53:2183, 1984.

99a. Harrison DFN: International Conference on Head and Neck Cancer, July 1984. St. Louis, C. V. Mosby Co., 1985.

100. Harwood AR: Melanoma of the head and neck. In Million RR, Cassisi NJ (eds): Management of Head and Neck Cancer. A Multidisciplinary Approach. Philadelphia, J. B. Lippincott Co., 1984.

101. Hattori T, et al: Experimental studies on operative stress in surgery for cancer. J Jap Surg Soc 80:1385, 1979.

102. Hattori T, et al: Enhancing effect of thoracotomy on tumor growth in rats with special reference to duration and timing of operation. Gann 71:280, 1980.

103. Hawrylko E: Mechanisms by which tumors escape immune destruction. In Waters H (ed): The Handbook of Cancer Immunology. Vol 2. New York, Garland STPM Press, 1978, pp 1–53.

104. Heidenreich W, et al: Immunological characterization of mononuclear cells in peripheral blood and regional lymph nodes of breast cancer patients. Cancer 43:1308, 1979.

105. Herberman RB, Holden HT: Natural cell-mediated immunity. Adv Can Res 27:305, 1978.

106. Hersh E: Perspectives for immunologic and biologic therapeutic intervention. In Mihich E (ed): Immunological Approaches to Cancer Therapeutics. New York, John Wiley & Sons, 1982.

107. Hewitt HB, et al: The effect of lethally irradiated cells on transplantability of murine tumors. Br J Cancer 28:123, 1973.

108. Hewitt HB, Blake ER: Further studies of the relationship between lymphatic dissemination and lymph nodal metastasis in non-immunogenic murine tumors. Br J Cancer 35:415, 1977.

109. Hirsh B, et al: Immunostimulation of patients with head and neck cancer. Arch Otol 109:298, 1983.

110. Hoover HC, Ketcham AS: Metastasis of metastases. Am J Surg 130:405, 1975.

111. Hora JS: Pre-operative radiation therapy as an adjunctive measure to radical neck dissection: A histopathologic study. Laryngoscope 79:1921, 1969.

112. Howard RJ, Simmons RL: Acquired immunologic deficiences after trauma and surgical procedures. Surg Gynecol Obstet 39:771, 1974.

113. Hoye RC, et al: A clinicopathological study of epidermoid carcinoma of the head and neck. Cancer 15:741, 1962.

114. Hrushesky WJM: The clinical application of chronobiology to oncology. Am J Anat 168:519, 1983.

115. Huang CC, et al: Collagenase and protease activities in head and neck tumors. Otolaryngol Head Neck Surg 88:749, 1980.

116. Huvos AG, et al: significance of axillary macrometastasis and micrometastasis in mammary cancer. Ann Surg 173:44, 1971.

117. Jenkins VK, et al: Radiation therapy in head and neck cancer—role of lymphocyte response and clinical stage. Arch Otol 106:414, 1980.

118. Jesse RH, et al: Cancer of the oral cavity. Is elective neck dissection beneficial? Am J Surg 120:505, 1970.

119. Jesse RH, et al: Radical or modified neck dissection: A therapeutic dilemma. Am J Surg 136:516, 1978.

120. Jesse RH, et al: Neck nodes. In Fletcher GH (ed): Textbook of Radiotherapy. 3rd ed. Philadelphia, Lea & Febiger, 1980, p 249.

121. Jesse RH, Fletcher GH: Treatment of the neck in patients with squamous cell carcinoma of the head and neck. Cancer 39:869, 1977.

122. Jesse RH, Lindberg RD: The efficacy of combining radiation therapy with a surgical procedure in patients with cervical metastasis from squamous cancer of the oropharynx and hypopharynx. Cancer 35:1163, 1975.

123. Johns ME: Parotid cancer: A rational basis for treatment. Head Neck Surg 3:132, 1980.

124. Johnson JT: Cervical metastasis. In Gates G (ed): Current Therapy in Otolaryngology. Head and Neck Surgery, 1984–1985. St. Louis, C. V. Mosby Co., 1984, p 238.

125. Johnson JT, et al: The extracapsular spread of tumors in cervical node metastasis. Arch Otol 107:725, 1981.

126. Johnson JT, et al: Cervical metastasis: Incidence and implications of extracapsular carcinoma. Abstract No. 86, International Conference on Head and Neck Cancer, Baltimore, July 1984. In press, 1985.

127. Kaiser CW, Ostfeld D: Therapeutic considerations in the management of melanoma. J Surg Oncol 20:31, 1982.

128. Kamo I, Friedman H: Immunosuppression and the role of suppressive factors in cancer. Adv Can Res 25:271, 1977.

129. Kardinal CG, Yarbro JW: A conceptual history of cancer. Semin Oncol 6:396, 1979.

130. Ketcham AS, et al: The development of spontaneous metastasis after the removal of a "primary" tumor. II. Standardization of protocol in 5 animal tumors. Cancer 14:875, 1971.

131. Kohler G, Milstein C: Continuous cultures of fused cells secreting antibody of pre-defined specificity. Nature 256:495, 1975.

132. Kraus EM, Panje WR: Factors influencing survival in head and neck patients with "giant" cervical lymph node metastasis. Otolaryngol Head Neck Surg 90:296, 1982.

133. Kyle RA: Second malignancies associated with chemotherapeutic agents. Semin Oncol 9:131, 1982.

134. Lawson S, Som M: Second primary cancer after irradiation of larynx cancer. Ann Otol 84:771, 1975.

135. Lee JG, Krause CJ: Radical neck dissection: Elective, therapeutic and secondary. Arch Otol 101:656, 1975.

136. Levy MH, Wheelock ES: The role of macrophages in defense against neoplastic disease. Adv Cancer Res 20:131, 1974.

137. Lindberg RD: Distribution of cervical lymph node metastasis from squamous cell carcinoma of the upper respiratory and digestive tracts. Cancer 29:1446, 1972.

138. Lindberg RD: Sites of first failure in head and neck cancer. Cancer Treat Symp 2:21, 1983.

139. Lindberg RD, Jesse RH: Treatment of cervical lymph node metastasis from primary lesions of the oropharynx, supraglottic larynx and hypopharynx. AJR 102:132, 1968.

140. Looser KG, et al: The significance of "positive" margins in surgically resected epidermoid carcinomas. Head Neck Surg 1:107, 1978.

141. Loré JM, Boulos J: Resection and reconstruction of the carotid artery in metastatic squamous cell carcinoma. Am J Surg 142:437, 1981.

142. Loré JM: Cancer of the thyroid. In Gates G (ed): Current Therapy in Otolaryngology—Head and Neck Surgery, 1982–1983. St. Louis, C. V. Mosby Co., 1982, p. 243.

143. Lubarsch EE: Gewaechse Med Klin 8:1651, 1912.

144. Lundy J, et al: Immune impairment in metastatic tumor growth—the needs for an immunorestorative drug as an adjunct to surgery. Cancer 43:945, 1979.

145. MacDonald I: Biologic predeterminism in human cancer. Surg Gynecol Obstet 90:443, 1951.

146. Madden RE, Gyure L: Trans lymph nodal passage of tumor cells. Oncology 22:281, 1968.

147. Mambo MC, Gallagher S: Cancer of the breast—the prognostic significance of extranodal extension of axillary disease. Cancer 39:2280, 1977.

148. Mantravadi RVP, et al: Patterns of cancer recurrence in the postoperatively irradiated neck. Arch Otol 109:753, 1983.

149. Markoe AM: The effects of combined radiation therapy and chemotherapy on the immune response. Prog Exp Tumor Res 25:219, 1980.

150. Marcial VA, et al: Patterns of failure after treatment for cancer of the upper respiratory and digestive tracts: A RTOG report. Cancer Treat Symp 2:33, 1983.

151. Martin HE, et al: Neck dissection. Cancer 4:441, 1961.

152. Martin H, Morfit H: Cervical lymph node metastasis as the first symptom of cancer. Surg Gynecol Obstet 78:133, 1944.

153. Martinez A, et al: ^{125}I implants as an adjuvant to surgery and external beam radiotherapy in the management of locally advanced head and neck cancer. Cancer 51:973, 1983.

154. Massin J-P, et al: Pulmonary metastasis in differentiated thyroid cancer. Cancer 53:982, 1984.

155. McGuirt WF, McCabe BF: Significance of node biopsy before definitive treatment of cervical metastatic carcinoma. Laryngoscope 88:594, 1978.

156. McKelvie P: Metastatic lymph nodes in the head and neck. Proc Soc Med 69:409, 1976.

157. McQuarrie DG, et al: A physiologic approach to the problems of simultaneous bilateral neck dissection. Am J Surg 134:455, 1977.

158. Mendelsohn G, et al: Relationship of tissue CEA and calcitonin to tumor virulence in medullary thyroid carcinoma. Cancer 54:657, 1984.

159. Mendelson BC, et al: Cancer of the oral cavity. Surg Clin North Am 53:585, 1977,

160. Mendenhall WM, et al: Elective neck irradiation in squamous cell carcinoma of the head and neck. Head Neck Surg 3:15, 1980.

161. Merino OR, et al: An analysis of distant metastasis from squamous cell carcinoma of the upper respiratory and digestive tracts. Cancer 40:145, 1977.

162. Million RR: Elective neck and irradiation for Tx N0 squamous carcinoma of the oral tongue and floor of mouth. Cancer 34:149, 1974.

163. Mollinari R, et al: Retrospective comparison of conservative and radical neck dissection for larynx cancer. Ann Otol 89:578, 1980.

164. Montanden D, et al: Cancer invasiveness: Immunofluorescence and ultra-structural methods of assessment. Plast Reconstr Surg 69:365, 1982.

165. Morgan RF, et al: Value of contralateral supraomohyoid neck dissection. Am J Surg 146:439, 1983.

166. Morton EL: Changing concepts of cancer surgery: Surgery as immunotherapy. Am J Surg 135:367, 1978.

167. Munster AM, et al: Ability of splenic lymphocytes from injured rats to induce a graft-vs-host reaction. Transplantation 14:106, 1972.

168. Mustard R, Rosen I: Cervical lymph node involvement in oral cancer. AJR 90:978, 1963.

169. Nahum AM, et al: The case for elective prophylactic neck dissection. Laryngoscope 87:588, 1977.

170. Naor D: Supressor cells: Permitters and promoters of malignancy? Adv Cancer Res 29:45, 1979.

171. Nime FA, et al: Prognostic significance of tumor emboli in intramammary lymphatics in patients with mammary carcinoma. Am J Surg Pathol 1:25, 1977.

172. Nind A, et al: Lymphocyte anergy in patients with carcinoma. Br J Cancer 28:108, 1973.

173. Noone RB, et al: Lymph node metastasis in oral cancer (a correlation of histopathology with survival). Plast Reconstr Surg 53:158, 1974.

174. Nordman E, Toivanen A: Effects of irradiation on the immune function in patients with mammary, pulmonary or head and neck carcinoma. Acta Radiol Oncol 17:3, 1978.

175. Northrop M, et al: Evolution of neck disease with primary squamous cell carcinoma of the oral tongue, floor of mouth and palatine arch, and clinically positive nodes neither fixed nor bilateral. Cancer 29:23, 1972.

176. O'Brien PH, et al: Effect of irradiation on tumor-infused lymph nodes. Radiology 94:407, 1970.

177. O'Brien PH, et al: Distant metastases and epidermoid cell carcinoma of the head and neck. Cancer 27:304, 1971.

178. Ogura JH, et al: Elective neck dissection for pharyngeal and laryngeal cancers—an evaluation. Ann Otol 80:646, 1971.

178a. Old LJ, et al: Antigenic properties of chemically induced tumors. Ann NY Acad Sci 101:80, 1961.

179. Oldham RK: Biologicals and biological response modifiers: Fourth modality of cancer treatment. Cancer Treat Rep 68:221, 1984.

180. Olson RM, et al: Regional lymph node management and outcome in 100 patients with head and neck melanoma. Am J Surg 142:470, 1981.

181. Ozer H: Tumor immunity and escape mechanisms in humans. In Mihich E (ed): Immunological Approaches to Cancer Therapeutics. New York, John Wiley & Sons, 1982, p 39.

182. Panje WR: Regression of head and neck carcinoma with a prostaglandin-synthesis inhibitor. Arch Otol 107:658, 1981.

183. Panje WR, et al: Epidermoid carcinoma of the floor of mouth: Surgical therapy versus combination therapy versus radiation therapy. Otolaryngol Head Neck Surg 88:714, 1980.

184. Papac RJ: Distant metastases from head and neck cancer. Cancer 53:342, 1984.

185. Parsons JT, Pfaff WW: Carcinoma of the thyroid. In Million RR, Cassisi NJ (eds): Management of Head and Neck Cancer. A Multidisciplinary Approach. Philadelphia, J. B. Lippincott Co., 1984, p 579.

186. Pendergrast WJ, et al: Regional lymphadenectomy and tumor immunity. Surg Gynecol Obstet 142:385, 1976.

187. Perzik SL: Treatment of melanoma. In Kagan and Miles (eds): Head and Neck Oncology. Controversies in Cancer Treatment Series. Boston, G. K. Hall, 1981.

188. Pickren, JW. Significance of occult metastases. A study of breast cancer. Cancer 14:1266, 1961.

189. Polk HC, Linn BS: Selective regional lymphadenectomy for melanoma: A mathematical aid to clinical judgment. Ann Surg 174:402, 1971.

190. Prehn RT: Tumor progression and homeostasis. Adv Cancer Res 23:203, 1976.

191. Prehn RT, Lappé MA: An immunostimulation theory of tumor development. Transplant Rev 7:26, 1971.

192. Probert JC, et al: Patterns of spread of distant metastases in head and neck cancer. Cancer 33:127, 1974.

193. Puck TT, Marcus PI: A rapid method for viable cell titration and clone production with HeLa cells in tissue culture: The use of X-irradiated cells to supply conditioning factors. Proc Natl Acad Sci USA 41:432, 1955.

194. Razack M, et al: Influence of initial neck node biopsy on the incidence of recurrence in the neck and survival in patients who subsequently undergo curative resectional surgery. J Surg Oncol 9:347, 1977.

195. Reed GF, Miller WA: Elective neck dissection—1970. Laryngoscope 80:1292, 1970.

196. Reiss CK, et al: The role of the regional lymph node in breast cancer: A comparison between nodal and systemic reactivity. J Surg Oncol 22:249, 1983.

197. Renk CM, et al: Comparison of the techniques used for monitoring humoral immunity in cancer patients. J Surg Oncol 19:155, 1982.

198. Révész L: Effect of tumor cells killed by X-rays upon the growth of admixed viable cells. Nature 178:1391, 1956.

199. Riggins RS, Ketcham AS: Effect of incisional biopsy on the development of experimental tumor metastasis. J Surg Res 5:200, 1965.

200. Rofstad EK, Brustad T: Differential responses to radiation and hyperthermy of cloned cell lines derived from a single human melanoma xenograft. Int J Radiat Oncol Biol Phys 10:857, 1984.

201. Roos E, Dingemans KP: Mechanisms of metastasis. Biochim Biophys Acta 560:135, 1979.

202. Rosen EB, Maitland A: Changing the operative strategy for thyroid cancer by node sampling. Am J Surg 146:504, 1983.

203. Roses DF, et al: Selective surgical management of cutaneous melanoma of the head and neck. Ann Surg 192:629, 1980.

204. Roth JA, et al: Effects of operation on immune response in cancer patients: Sequential evaluation of in vitro lymphocyte function. Surgery 79:46, 1976.

205. Rouvière M: Anatomy of the Human Lymphatic System. Ann Arbor, Mich., Edwards Bros., Inc., 1938.

206. Sakamoto A, et al: History of cervical radiation and incidence carcinoma of the pharynx, larynx and thyroid. Cancer 44:718, 1979.

207. Santos VB, et al: Role of surgery in head and neck cancer with fixed nodes. Arch Otol 101:645, 1975.

208. Sato H: Cancer metastasis and ascites tumor. NCI Monograph 16:141, 1964.

209. Schantz ST, et al: Improved survival associated with postoperative wound infection in larynx cancer: An analysis of its therapeutic implications. Otolaryngol Head Neck Surg 88:412, 1980.

210. Schatten WE: An experimental study of postoperative tumor metastases: I. Growth of pulmonary metastases following total removal of primary leg tumor. Cancer 11:455, 1958.

211. Schindel J, Castoriano IM: Late appearing (radiation induced) carcinoma. Arch Otol 95:205, 1972.

212. Schneider JJ, et al: Control by irradiation alone of nonfixed clinically positive lymph nodes from squamous cell carcinoma of the oral cavity, oropharynx, supraglottic larynx and hypopharynx. Am J Roentgenol 123:42, 1975.

213. Schor AM, Schor SL: Tumor angiogenesis. J Pathol 141:385, 1983.

214. Schuller DE: An assessment of neck node immunoreactivity in head and neck cancer. Laryngoscope 94(Suppl 35), 1984.

215. Schuller DE, et al: Spinal accessory lymph nodes: A prospective study of metastatic involvement. Laryngoscope 88:439, 1978.

216. Schuller DE, et al: Symposium: Adjuvant cancer therapy of head and neck tumors: Increased survival with surgery alone versus combination therapy. Laryngoscope 89:582, 1979.

217. Schuller DE, et al: The prognostic significance of metastatic cervical lymph nodes. Laryngoscope 90:557, 1980.

218. Schuller DE, et al: Conservative neck dissection—radical approach? Arch Otol 107:642, 1981.

219. Schuller DE, et al: Analysis of disability resulting from treatment including radical neck dissection or modified neck dissection. Head Neck Surg 6:551, 1983.

220. Sessions DG: Surgical pathology of cancer of the larynx and hypopharynx. Laryngoscope 86:814, 1976.

221. Shah JP, Goldsmith HS: Incontinuity versus discontinuous lymph node dissection for malignant melanoma. Cancer 26:610, 1970.

222. Shear M, et al: The prediction of lymph node metastasis from oral squamous cell carcinoma. Cancer 37:1901, 1976.

223. Shine T, Wallack MK: Inflammatory oncotaxis after testing the skin of the cancer patient. Cancer 47:1325, 1981.

224. Shochat SJ, et al: Evaluation of cellular immunity and adrenocortical activity in surgical patients. J Surg Res 26:332, 1979.

225. Sim FH, et al: A prospective randomized study of the efficacy of routine elective lymphadenectomy in management of malignant melanoma—preliminary results. Cancer 41:948, 1978.

226. Slaughter DP, et al: Field cancerization in oral stratified epithelium. Cancer 6:963, 1956.

227. Slawikowski GJM: Tumor development in adrenalectomized rats given inoculations of aged tumor cells after surgical stress. Cancer Res 20:316, 1960.

228. Slotman GJ, et al: The incidence of metastasis after multimodality therapy for cancer of the head and neck. Cancer 54:2009, 1984.

229. Smith RR, Hilberg AW: Cancer cell seeding of operative wounds. J Natl Cancer Inst 16:645, 1955.

230. Snow GB, et al: Prognostic factors of neck node metastsis. Clin Otol 7:185, 1982.

231. Snow JB, et al: Randomized preoperative and postoperative radia-

tion therapy for patients with carcinoma of the head and neck: Preliminary report. Laryngoscope 90:930, 1980.

232. Spiro RH, et al: Cancer of the parotid gland: A clinical-pathologic study of 288 primary cases. Am J Surg 130:452, 1975.
233. Stefani S, Kerman RH: Lymphocyte response to PHA before and after radiation therapy in patients with carcinomas of the head and neck. J Laryngol Otol 91:605, 1977.
234. Stell PM: Fixed bilateral cervical nodes. J Laryngol Otol 96:851, 1983.
235. Stell PM, et al: The fixed cervical lymph node. Cancer 53:336, 1984.
236. Stell PM, Green JR: Management of metastases to the lymph glands of the neck. Proc R Soc Med 69:411, 1976.
237. Sterns EE: Current concepts of lymphatic transport. Surg Gynecol Obstet 138:773, 1974.
238. Strate SM, et al: Occult papillary carcinoma of the thyroid with distant metastases. Cancer 54:1093, 1984.
239. Strong E: Preoperative radiation and radical neck dissection. Surg Clin North Am 49:271, 1969.
240. Strong EW: Sites of treatment failure in head and neck cancer. Cancer Treat Symp 2:5, 1983.
241. Suen JY, et al: Evaluation of the effectiveness of postoperative radiation therapy for the control of local disease. Am J Surg 140:577, 1980.
242. Sugarbaker E: Cancer metastasis: A product of tumor-host interaction. Curr Probl Cancer 3:1–59, 1979.
243. Tanemura H, et al: Influences of operative stress on cell mediated immunity and on tumor metastasis and their prevention by nonspecific immunotherapy: Experimental studies in rats. J Surg Oncol 21:189, 1982.
244. Tarpley JL, et al: Prolonged depression of cellular immunity in cured laryngopharyngeal cancer patients treated with radiation therapy. Cancer 35:638, 1975.
245. Terz JJ, Farr HW: Carcinoma of the tonsillar fossa. Surg Gynecol Obstet 3:581, 1967.
246. Tulenko J, et al: Cancer of the tongue. Comments on surgical treatment. Am J Surg 112:562, 1966.
247. Tyzzer EE: Factors in the production and growth of metastases. J Med Res 28:309, 1913.
248. Vaage J, et al: Radiation-induced changes in established tumor immunity. Cancer Res 34:129, 1974.
249. Vandenbrouck C, et al: Elective versus therapeutic radical neck dissection in epidermoid carcinoma of the oral cavity—results of a randomized clinical trial. Cancer 46:386, 1980.
250. Veronesi U, et al: Inefficacy of immediate node dissection in Stage I melanoma of the limbs. N Engl J Med 297:627, 1977.
251. Viadana E: The metastatic spread of "head and neck" tumors in man—an autopsy study of 371 cases. Z Krebsforsch 83:293, 1975.
252. Vikram B: The importance of the time interval between surgery and postoperative radiation therapy in the combined management of head and neck cancer. Int J Radiat Oncol Biol Phys 5:1837, 1979.
253. Vikram B, et al: Elective postoperative radiation therapy in Stage III and IV epidermoid carcinoma of the head and neck. Am J Surg 146:580, 1980.

254. Vikram B, et al: I^{125} implants in head and neck cancer. Cancer 51:1310, 1983.
255. Vikram B, et al: Failure at distant sites following multimodality treatment for advanced head and neck cancer. Head Neck Surg 56:730, 1984a.
256. Vikram B, et al: Failure at the primary site following multimodality treatment in advanced head and neck cancer. Head Neck Surg 6:720, 1984b.
257. Vikram B, et al: Second malignant neoplasms in patients successfully treated with multimodality treatment for advanced head and neck cancer. Head Neck Surg 6:734, 1984c.
258. Vikram B, et al: Failure in the neck following multimodality treatment for advanced head and neck cancer. Head Neck Surg 6:724, 1984d.
259. Vorbrodt A, et al: The effects of x-rays on some cytochemical properties of macrophages and carcinoma cell surfaces. Acta Histochem 44:29, 1972.
260. Vose VM: Human tumour-lymphocyte interactions in vitro. V. Comparison of the reactivity of tumour-infiltrating blood and lymph node lymphocytes with autologous tumour cells. Int J Can 20:895, 1977.
261. Wara WM, et al: Immunosuppression following radiation therapy for carcinoma of the nasopharynx. AJR 123:482, 1975.
262. Ward PH, et al: Important unanswered research questions. Ann Otol Rhinol Laryngol (Suppl) 100:11, 1982.
263. Weinstein JN, et al: Monoclonal antitumor antibodies in the lymphatics. Cancer Treat Rep 68:257, 1984.
264. Weiss L: A pathobiologic overview of metastasis. Semin Oncol 4:5, 1977.
265. Weiss L, Gilbert HY, Ballon SC (eds): Lymphatic System Metastasis. Boston, G. K. Hall, 1980.
266. Welsh LW, et al: Effects of irradiation on cervical lymph nodes. Ann Otol 88:502, 1979.
267. Wheelock ES, et al: The tumor dormant state. Adv Cancer Res 34:107, 1981.
268. Wilkinson EJ, Hause L: Probability in lymph node sectioning. Cancer 33:1269, 1974.
269. Wilson DB, Billingham RE: Lymphocytes and transplantation immunity. Adv Immunol 7:189, 1967.
270. Wolf GT, et al: Predictive factors for tumor response to preoperative chemotherapy in patients with head and neck squamous cell carcinoma. Cancer 54:2869, 1984.
271. Wynder EL, et al: A study of the etiological factors in cancer of the mouth. Cancer 10:1300, 1957.
272. Yamamoto E: Mode of invasion and lymph node metastasis in squamous cell carcinoma of the oral cavity. Head Neck Surg 6:938, 1984.
273. Zeidman I, Buss JM: Experimental studies on the spread of cancer in the lymphatic system. I. Effectiveness of the lymph node as a barrier to the passage of embolic tumor cells. Cancer Res 14:403, 1954.
274. Zoller M, et al: Guidelines for prognosis in head and neck cancer with nodal metastasis. Laryngoscope 88:135, 1978.

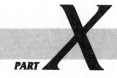

PART **X**

Dental and Jaw Tumors

CHAPTER 57

Odontogenic Cysts and Tumors

CLINICAL EVALUATION AND PATHOLOGY

R. Keith McDaniel, B.A., D.D.S., M.S.

Tooth development is a complex process involving tissues derived from ectoderm, neuroectoderm, and mesoderm. It is an ongoing phenomenon, involving multiple sites and occurring over a long duration of time—beginning 6 to 7 weeks in utero and reaching completion in early adulthood. The various stages in normal odontogenesis are dependent upon proper epithelial-mesenchymal relationships, morphogenesis, fibrillogenesis, and mineralization.[29]

Considering the complexity, multiplicity of sites, and duration of the odontogenic process, it is not surprising that a multitude of aberrations may occur in the forms of hamartomas, cysts, or neoplasms. Although relatively few of the odontogenic cysts or tumors have a recurrent or aggressive behavior, it is extremely important to distinguish them from the innocuous ones.

By correlating the clinical, radiographic, and histopathologic features of a specific odontogenic lesion, the clinician—after referring to previous studies and current classifications—should be able to reach a definitive diagnosis, estimate the behavior of the lesion, and effect proper treatment.

CLASSIFICATION

Although Scultet described cystic tumors of the jaws as "tumeurs liquides des machoires" as early as 1654[1] and odontogenic cysts were described by Fauchard (1746) and John Hunter (1780),[21] it was much later when the first categorization of odontogenic tumors was proposed. Broca, after coining the term *odontoma* in 1866, proposed the first classification of odontogenic tumors in 1868.[1] Some years later, Malassez (in 1884 and 1885) demonstrated that the radicular cyst originated from epithelial rests in the periodontal ligament; he also proposed a classification of odontogenic cysts and tumors based upon a common origin from odontogenic epithelial rests.[1, 11, 12] Subsequently, Bland-Sutton proposed the subdivision of *odontomes* into five categories: (1) aberrations of the *enamel organ*, (2) aberrations of the *follicle*, (3) aberrations of the *papilla*, (4) aberrations of the *whole tooth germ*, and (5) *anomalous odontomes*.[4]

In 1946, Thoma and Goldman proposed a classification of odontogenic tumors based upon the germ-cell layer of origin.[30] This classification—later modified by

the American Academy of Oral Pathology[18]—separated odontogenic cysts from odontogenic tumors and subdivided the tumors into three categories: *ectodermal, mesodermal,* and *mixed.*

A more functional classification was suggested by Pindborg and Clausen in 1958,[13] later modified by Gorlin, Chaudhry, and Pindborg,[8] which divided odontogenic tumors into two main groups: *epithelial* and *mesodermal.* The epithelial tumors were further subdivided into (1) epithelial tumors without inductive changes in the connective tissue and (2) epithelial tumors with inductive changes in the connective tissue.

In 1971, a classification of odontogenic tumors and cysts was published by the World Health Organization.[14] More recently, Reichart and Ries proposed a systematic classification of odontogenic tumors which is based upon the histogenetic, organogenetic, and embryologic aspects of tooth development. This classification not only considers the inductive principle which unites odontogenic epithelium and mesenchyme but also distinguishes the cellular derivatives of ectomesenchyme from those of mesenchyme.[16]

REVIEW OF TOOTH DEVELOPMENT

In the mammalian embryo, three definitive germ layers (ectoderm, endoderm, and mesoderm) form during the first 3 weeks of development. Subsequently, the endodermal layer gives origin to the digestive tract and the mesodermal layer gives rise to connective tissue (including cartilage and bone), smooth and striated muscle, blood, blood vessels, and the urogenital system. The ectodermal layer differentiates into the nervous system, the epidermis of skin and its appendages, most of the epithelium of the oral cavity, and the epithelium of the ear, nose, and eye. A neural tube forms from neural folds (neuroectoderm) at the cephalad end of the embryo and eventually develops into the brain and spinal cord. Neural crest cells along the neural tube migrate and give rise to sensory ganglia, sympathetic neurons, Schwann cells, melanocytes, meninges, cartilage of the branchial arches, and embryonic connective tissue of the facial area and oral cavity (*ectomesenchyme*).[29]

After 37 days of development, horseshoe-shaped bands of thickened epithelium (the *dental lamina*) develop in each jaw and form a series of bud-like ingrowths into the underlying ectomesenchyme. In each developing tooth bud, the dental lamina divides to form the enamel organ—a cap-like structure that is composed of inner and outer enamel epithelium separated by the stellate reticulum. The condensed ectomesenchyme beneath the enamel organ is known as the *dental papilla* and forms the dentin and pulp of the tooth (Fig. 57–1). Ectomesenchyme that surrounds the dental papilla and enamel organ is called the *dental follicle*[29] (Fig. 57–1).

Following the "inductive" effect of the inner enamel epithelium on the dental papilla, *odontoblasts* develop from undifferentiated ectomesenchymal cells and begin to form dentin. After the initial deposition of dentin, cells of the inner enamel epithelium differentiate into *ameloblasts* and begin to secrete enamel—the ectodermal tissue covering of the tooth crown. It has been determined, through experimental studies, that the ectomesenchyme rather than the epithelium is the determinant for tooth development and also determines the shape of the tooth.[29]

The root of the tooth, composed of dentin, is formed by odontoblasts, which develop following the formation of Hertwig's root sheath—a double layer of epithelial cells arising in the *cervical loop.* When the outer layer of dentin matrix starts to calcify, the cells of Hertwig's root sheath form a double-layered and fenestrated network

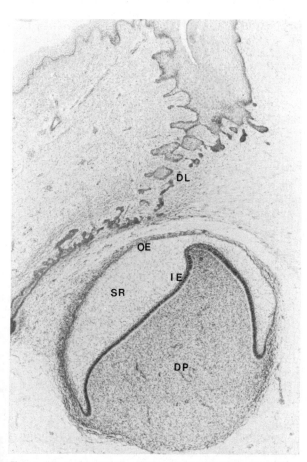

Figure 57–1. Developing tooth. DL = Dental lamina; SR = stellate reticulum; OE = outer enamel epithelium; IE = inner enamel epithelium; DP = dental papilla. (×40)

of epithelial cells around the tooth, within the periodontal ligament. The epithelial network ultimately disintegrates and fragments, leaving discrete epithelial remnants. These clusters of epithelial cells are known as the *rests of Malassez* and, unless stimulated to proliferate by changes in their environment (for example, inflammation), they appear to be functionless.[24, 28, 29] At about the same time, ectomesenchymal cells of the dental follicle differentiate into *cementoblasts*, which in turn secrete a layer of cementum on the root surface.[24]

Another epithelial component of the developing enamel organ that disintegrates, leaving remnants, is the dental lamina. These epithelial rests, which are found in dental follicles and gingival tissues, are known as *dental lamina rests* and the *rests of Serres.* Although many dental lamina rests keratinize and are eventually discharged during childhood, some of them persist in adult tissues. Stout and coworkers studied 67 human fetuses (7 to 32 weeks of age) and found that most of the dental laminae are fragmented after 10 to 12 weeks of development. Histologic studies, by the same investigators, of gingival material from 266 adults showed a 34 per cent incidence of epithelial rests in the gingiva.[27] Histologically, most of the dental lamina rests observed by Bhaskar appeared "basaloid," and others appeared "squamoid" or contained "clear cells."[3] Stanley and his colleagues observed epithelial hyperplasia and squamous metaplasia in dental lamina remnants within dental follicles, apparently related to inflammation and age.[25] Other factors to be considered as possible stimuli of epithelial proliferation are systemic disease, mechanical trauma, and an increase in local blood supply.[2] Dental lamina rests are known to give rise to epithelial hamartomas,[2, 19] various types of cysts,[3, 6] and ameloblastomas.[26]

Baden and associates recognized and reported three instances of *odontogenic gingival epithelial hamartoma*—an entity they considered to be a "transitional stage between a developmental anomaly and a true odontogenic tumor."[2] Clinically, the three cases presented as asymptomatic nodules on the gingiva of adults (55, 59, and 65 years of age). The nodules, which were in the canine-premolar regions, ranged in size from 2.5 mm to "pea-sized." Microscopically, the lesions were characterized by nests, cords, and clusters of odontogenic epithelium in a myxoid or dense fibrous stroma. Some epithelial cords resembled the proliferative stage of the dental lamina, and others were arranged in "ameloblastic-like" follicles.[2] Another case occurring in the incisor region of a 40-year-old female was reported by Sciubba and Zola.[19]

Another interesting, but uncommon, histologic feature of the dental lamina is the presence of melanocytes. Lawson and associates[10] studied the dental laminae and tooth buds in 17 human fetuses and found melanocytes in nine (three of 11 Caucasians and six of six blacks). These observations of neuroectodermal-derived melanocytes in the dental primordia provide evidence that neural crest cells are involved in odontogenesis and give an explanation for the presence of melanin in certain epithelial odontogenic lesions.[10, 23] In addition to being found in the calcifying odontogenic cyst, melanin has been noted in odontogenic keratocysts, a gingival cyst,[9] ameloblastomas,[23] and an epithelial odontogenic tumor in a black patient.[17] Soames[23] studied the ultrastructural features of melanocytes in a pigmented cal-cifying odontogenic cyst and observed two forms:

1. Cells containing small numbers of premelanosomes with few fully melanized melanosomes.

2. Cells with large numbers of premelanosomes and fully melanized melanosomes.

ODONTOGENIC CYSTS

Since the late 19th century when the early categorizations of jaw cysts were attempted, numerous classifications have been published. The classification presented here in Table 57–1 represents a slight modification of that published by Shear in 1983.[21] Discussion will be limited to those cysts of odontogenic origin.

Developmental Odontogenic Cysts

Gingival Cysts of Infants

Gingival cysts of infants are also known as dental lamina cysts, Epstein's pearls, and Bohn's nodules. These small, multiple, keratin-filled cysts, first described by Epstein in 1880,[32] are commonly found on the palate and alveolar ridges of young infants. The cysts that are located on the midpalatine raphe are thought to arise from epithelial islands that are entrapped during fusion of the palatal folds and nasal processes, and those occurring on the alveolar ridges represent keratinized remnants of the dental lamina.[21, 37] In a study of 55 human fetuses 8 to 22 weeks of age, Moreillon and Schroeder[35] observed that dental lamina–derived microkeratocysts develop and increase in number (up to 190 cysts per fetus) between 12 and 22 weeks of development. The midpalatal cysts, however, reach a peak number (less that 20 cysts per fetus) by week 14 and do not become more numerous with time. Fromm[33] designated cysts located on the midpalatine raphe as "Epstein's pearls," cysts on the crest of the alveolar ridges as "dental lamina cysts," and cysts on the buccal and lingual aspects of the alveolar ridges as "Bohn's nodules."

Clinical Features. Gingival cysts of infants appear as raised white or pink nodules that range from 1 to 5 mm in diameter. They may be solitary, but are often multiple. The cysts are not found on the soft palate[35] and rarely occur in children over the age of 3 months. Cataldo and Berkman[31] examined 209 infants 1 to 5 weeks of age and found the median palatal raphe to be the most common site (65.1 per cent), followed by the maxillary alveolar mucosa (36.5 per cent) and mandibular alveolar mucosa (9.9 per cent).

Incidence. Monteleone and McLellan[34] observed the cysts in the midpalatine raphe of 79 per cent of black infants and 85 per cent of Caucasian infants. Fromm[33] found gingival cysts in 75.9 per cent of 1367 infants. Cataldo and Berkman[31] reported an 80 per cent incidence on the palatal or alveolar mucosa of 209 newborn infants. Stout and associates[37] observed epithelial remnants or gingival cysts in 68 per cent of 109 infants, but found only one true cyst in 266 adults.

Histopathology. The cyst is lined by thin (two to four cells in thickness) keratinizing epithelium that exhibits a parakeratotic surface. The cyst cavity, in most cases, is filled with keratin. The epithelial lining lacks the columnar basal layer and "corrugated" appearance that are commonly seen in the odontogenic keratocyst. Stages of development may be observed, ranging from squamous metaplasia of dental lamina remnants to keratin pearl formation.

Behavior. The vast majority of dental lamina cysts are discharged shortly after birth and therefore require no treatment. Following discharge of the keratin, the cyst wall fuses with the oral epithelium.[35]

Gingival Cysts of Adults

This developmental lesion may be defined as an epithelium-lined cyst that occurs in the gingival soft tissue and may cause superficial bone erosion but does not arise within bone. Various theories of origin have been proposed:

1. Odontogenic epithelial rests.

2. Traumatic implantation of surface epithelium.

3. Cystic degeneration of deep projections of surface epithelium.

4. Reduced enamel epithelium.

Most authorities favor origin from dental lamina rests.[50, 53] Wysocki and associates, noting clinical and histomorphologic similarities in the gingival cyst of the adult and the lateral periodontal cyst, proposed a common histogenesis.[53]

Frequency. Browne[43] studied 540 cysts and found a 0.2 per cent incidence of gingival cysts. Buchner and Hansen[44] retrieved 33 gingival cysts from 21,503 surgical specimens—an incidence of only 0.15 per cent. Shear reported that 0.3 per cent of 1345 cysts represented gingival cysts.[21]

Clinical Features. Gingival cysts are more common in the mandible, 77 per cent of them occurring there (33 of 43 reported cases). The most common location is the

TABLE 57–1. Cysts of the Jaws

Epithelial Cysts
I. Odontogenic
  A. Developmental
    1. Gingival cyst of infants (dental lamina cyst, Epstein's pearls, Bohn's nodules)
    2. Gingival cyst of adults
    3. Lateral periodontal cyst
    4. Dentigerous (follicular) cyst
    5. Odontogenic keratocyst: nevoid basal cell carcinoma syndrome
    6. Calcifying odontogenic cyst
  B. Inflammatory
    1. Radicular cyst
    2. Residual cyst
    3. Inflammatory lateral periodontal cyst
    4. Paradental cyst
II. Nonodontogenic (fissural)
  A. Nasopalatine duct (incisive canal) cyst
  B. Median palatine and median mandibular cysts
  C. Nasolabial (nasoalveolar) cyst

Nonepithelial cysts
I. Traumatic bone cyst (simple, unicameral, solitary, hemorrhagic bone cyst)
II. Aneurysmal bone cyst

Source: Modified after Shear M: Cysts of the Oral Regions, 2nd ed. Boston, Wright-PSG, 1983, p. 3.

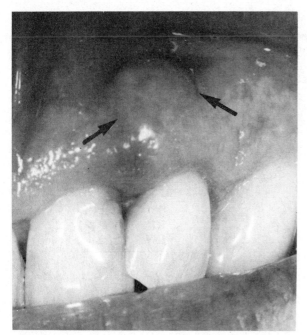

Figure 57–2. Gingival cyst of the adult. The cyst presented as a fluctuant painless swelling on the maxillary gingiva of a 56-year-old female.

cuspid–first premolar region, nearly always on the buccal or facial surface.[39, 44, 48, 53]

The majority of the cysts occur in patients who are between 40 and 59 years of age. In a study of 33 gingival cysts, Buchner and Hansen noted that 21 occurred in the fifth or sixth decades.[44] The mean age of 10 patients in the study of Wysocki and associates was 50.7 years.[53] The age of reported cases ranges from 7 years to 77 years.[39, 44, 48, 53] Of 59 cases in the literature, 35 (59 per cent) were in females and 24 (41 per cent) were in males.

The lesions appear as painless, circumscribed swellings on the gingiva and are white, red, or blue-gray. They are usually less than 1 cm in diameter (range of 0.1 cm to 1.5 cm)[44] and, when palpated, are soft and fluctuant (Fig. 57–2). The differential diagnosis often includes lipoma, mucocele, and pigmented nevi. Pressure resorption of underlying bone may result in a saucerization of the cortical surface, but this may or may not be evident radiographically as a slight radiolucency.[44]

Histopathology. Most of the gingival cysts of the adult are lined by thin nonkeratinized squamous epithelium without rete peg formation, which ranges from one to three cells in thickness. Some cysts appear to be devoid of contents, and others contain amorphous eosinophilic material. Clear cells and localized thickenings (plaques) in the epithelial lining have been described. Two uncommon variants in the adult cysts are (1) a keratinized stratified squamous epithelial lining with keratin in the lumen, similar to the dental lamina cyst of infants, and (2) a thin stratified squamous epithelial lining with a parakeratotic corrugated surface, similar to the odontogenic keratocyst.[44, 49] A gingival cyst with melanocytes in the epithelial lining was reported by Grand and Marwah in 1964.[46]

Behavior. The gingival cyst of adults tends to grow very slowly and does not have a tendency to recur.

Lateral Periodontal Cyst

The developmental type of lateral periodontal cyst is characterized by (1) its location, which is lateral to the tooth root and above the root apex of canine or premolar teeth; (2) its small size, shape, and radiographic appearance; and (3) its histomorphologic and clinical features, which exclude an inflammatory origin. Although it has been proposed that the cyst develops from reduced enamel epithelium or the rests of Malassez,[50, 51] Wysocki and associates[53] favor an origin from dental lamina rests. Those investigators further suggest that the lateral periodontal cyst and the gingival cyst of the adult represent intraosseous and extraosseous manifestations of the same lesion.[53]

Incidence. Browne, in a study of 540 cysts, found 15 lateral periodontal cysts (2.8 per cent).[43] An incidence of 1.5 per cent was reported by Shear (20 of 1345 cysts).[49] Owing to the fact that some published studies of lateral periodontal cysts included gingival cysts, it is difficult to accurately determine the number of lateral periodontal cysts reported in the literature. Also, some reports included inflammatory lateral cysts as well as the developmental type. It is estimated that more than 100 instances of lateral periodontal cysts have been published.

The lesion occurs about twice as often in males as in females (49 of 69 cases).[43, 49, 53]

Clinical Features. Most commonly, the lateral periodontal cyst occurs in the mandible. Of 98 cases in the literature, 73 (74 per cent) were located there.[45, 47, 49, 51, 53] In a study of 39 cases by Wysocki and associates, 26 were located in the incisor-cuspid-premolar area of the mandible and 13 occurred in the lateral incisor region of the maxilla.

Signs and Symptoms. Lateral periodontal cysts are usually asymptomatic and are first noticed on routine dental radiographs. The associated teeth are vital and should not be extracted.

Radiographic Features. The characteristic radiographic appearance is that of a round or ovoid radiolucency, with sharply defined margins, and usually less than 1 cm in diameter. The cysts are located in a lateral position to the tooth root, between the apex of the root and the cervical portion of the tooth (Fig. 57–3A).

Histopathology. Similar to the gingival cyst of the adult, the lateral periodontal cyst is nearly always lined by thin (one to four cells in thickness) nonkeratinizing squamous epithelium. Occasionally, the lining epithelium is composed of cuboidal or short columnar cells.[53] Wysocki and associates noted the presence of glycogen-rich clear cells, which resembled dental lamina cells, in the epithelial lining and fibrous wall.[53] Occasional focal collections of chronic inflammatory cells may be found in the fibrous wall, but in most cases, they are not present. Uncommon variations include:

1. Epithelial thickenings (plaques) in the lining.
2. The presence of mucous cells.[43]
3. A lining composed of thin keratinized squamous epithelium with a palisaded columnar basal layer and a corrugated surface—features of the odontogenic keratocyst (if the microscopic criteria of an odontogenic keratocyst are fulfilled, it should be treated accordingly).
4. A multilocular (botryoid) configuration.

The *botryoid odontogenic cyst* was recognized by Weathers and Waldron in a report of two cases.[52] One cyst

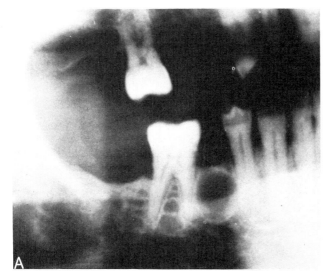

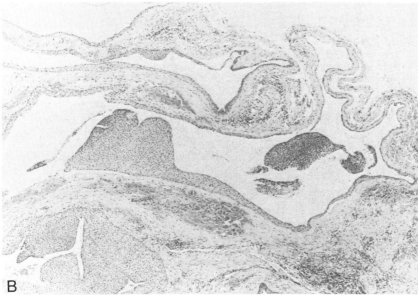

Figure 57–3. Botryoid odontogenic cyst. (*A*) A well-circumscribed radiolucency located between the roots of the mandibular left first premolar and first molar teeth. (B) Multilocular cyst lined by thin squamous epithelium with bulbous plaques. (×40) (Courtesy of Dr. Michael Patton.)

occurred in a 51-year-old female, and the other was found in an 85-year-old male. Both were located within the mandible in the cuspid-premolar region and were thought to arise from odontogenic epithelial rests. The gross appearance of the largest lesion was described as resembling a "bunch of grapes," hence the term "botryoid." Microscopically, the cysts were divided into multiple compartments, each lined by thin, nonkeratinizing squamous epithelium, which exhibited focal "buds" of clear cells (Fig. 57–3B). Since 1973, there have been numerous observations and some reports of multilocular or botryoid cysts. In a review of 39 lateral periodontal cysts, Wysocki and associates found three examples that were polycystic.[53] One of the five cases reported by Standish and Shafer had the microscopic features of a multilocular cyst, with microcysts in the fibrous wall.[51] It is probable that the botryoid cyst is a variant of the lateral periodontal cyst.

Behavior. The lateral periodontal cyst does not have a tendency to recur.

Dentigerous (Follicular) Cyst

The dentigerous cyst is defined as a developmental cyst that encompasses the crown of an unerupted tooth. It develops after the crown of the tooth has completely formed and fluid accumulates between the reduced enamel epithelium (which lines the dental follicle) and the enamel. Unless secondarily infected, most of the cysts are symptomless and are first detected on radiographs. When the patient is aware of an abnormality, it is frequently described as a swelling or asymmetry that has developed slowly.

Incidence. The dentigerous cyst is one of the most common odontogenic cysts, second in frequency to the radicular cyst. Of 8850 jaw cysts reported in the literature, 1592 (18 per cent) were dentigerous cysts.[54, 55, 58, 62] According to calculations by Mourshed, about 3 per cent of the patients with one or more unerupted teeth will have a dentigerous cyst.[61]

Clinical Features. The cysts are most frequently detected in the second, third, and fourth decades of life.

In a study of 206 dentigerous cysts by Shear, 63.6 per cent (131) occurred in that age group.[62] The median age of 81 patients with this type of cyst was 36.6 years.[55]

In a survey of 176 cases by Mourshed, 61.3 per cent occurred in males and 38.7 per cent occurred in females.[61] Browne also noted a predilection in males: 70 per cent of 81 cases.[55] In a larger series of 218 instances of dentigerous cysts by Shear, 62 per cent were found in males and 38 per cent were in females.[62]

The third molar region of the mandible and the canine region of the maxilla are the two most common sites for a dentigerous cyst to develop, followed by the mandibular premolar and maxillary third molar areas. Shear reviewed 184 cases and found that 66 per cent of the cysts were located in the mandible and 34 per cent were in the maxilla; 69 per cent of those in the mandible were associated with third molar teeth, and 58 per cent of the maxillary cysts were associated with canine teeth.[62] In Mourshed's series of 128 dentigerous cysts, 74 per cent occurred in the mandible, and 69 per cent of them involved the third molar area.[61] Browne also found dentigerous cysts to be more common in the mandible than in the maxilla: 54 per cent (42 of 78) were found in the mandible, and 46 per cent (36 of 78) were found in the maxilla.[55]

Radiographic Features. The usual radiographic appearance is that of a unilocular radiolucency, with a well-defined sclerotic margin, which encircles the coronal portion of an erupted tooth (Fig. 57–4A). There is great variation in the size of dentigerous cysts, ranging from less than 2 cm to more than 10 cm in its greatest dimension. The largest cysts, usually located in the body and ramus of the mandible, may cause considerable expansion of bone cortices and give the appearance of multilocular radiolucencies. Displacement of associated teeth and severe root resorption of adjacent teeth may occur as sequelae of an enlarging dentigerous cyst. Struthers and Shear noted a greater tendency for root resorption by dentigerous cysts (55 per cent) when compared with radicular cysts (18 per cent) and primordial cysts (0 per cent).[64]

Histopathology. The dentigerous cyst is lined by stratified squamous epithelium, which usually is nonkeratinizing and ranges from three to 12 cells in thickness. Rete pegs are usually absent (Fig. 57–4B). Variations observed and reported by Browne included:

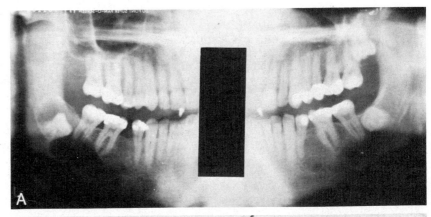

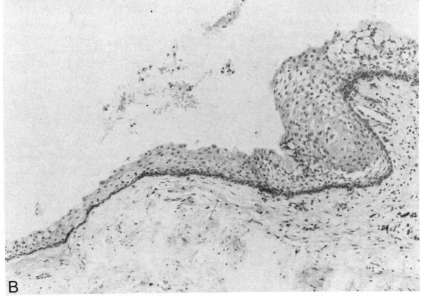

Figure 57–4. Dentigerous cyst. (A) A large radiolucency associated with the crown of the embedded third molar tooth in a 49-year-old male. (B) The cyst is lined by nonkeratinizing stratified squamous epithelium with focal collections of mucous cells. (×100) (Courtesy of Dr. J. L. McClendon.)

1. Mucous cells in 42 per cent of 81 dentigerous cysts.
2. Keratin in 2.5 per cent.
3. Mineralized bodies in 7.4 per cent.
4. Hyaline bodies in 1.2 per cent.[55]

The fibrous wall, composed of loose or collagenous fibrous connective tissue, often contains nests or strands of odontogenic epithelium. An inflammatory infiltrate—which varies in severity—is frequently observed. Occasionally, focal deposits of cholesterol and foreign body giant cells are present.

Behavior. The vast majority of dentigerous cysts have no tendency to recur. However, the capability of the lining epithelium to undergo metaplasia and form mucous cells or keratin, as previously stated, creates a potential site for neoplastic transformation. Eversole and associates, in a review of central epidermoid carcinomas and central mucoepidermoid carcinomas, noted a significant association with odontogenic cysts.[59] Seventy-five per cent of 32 instances of central epidermoid carcinoma were associated with an odontogenic cyst, and 48 per cent of 27 instances of central mucoepidermoid carcinoma were associated with a cyst or impacted tooth.[59] Browne described two examples of malignant change in longstanding dental cysts and provided evidence of a preceding keratin metaplasia of the cyst lining.[56]

Odontogenic Keratocyst

The term *odontogenic keratocyst* was first used by Philipsen to describe certain jaw cysts that exhibited keratinization of their epithelial linings.[77] Shear recognized the keratinizing odontogenic cyst as a separate entity and used the term *primordial cyst*.[80] In 1963, Pindborg and Hansen published a paper entitled "Clinical and Roentgenologic Aspects of Odontogenic Keratocysts," which was the compilation of a study of 30 cases. Significantly, there was a 62 per cent recurrence rate in 16 of the cases.[78]

For the past two decades, numerous reports and studies of odontogenic keratocysts have appeared in the literature. It is now generally accepted that the odontogenic keratocyst (1) is a distinct entity with characteristic microscopic features, (2) has a much higher recurrence rate when compared with other odontogenic cysts, and (3) may be associated with the multiple nevoid basal cell carcinoma syndrome.

Authorities are at variance, however, on the synonymous use of the terms "odontogenic keratocyst" and "primordial cyst." In the opinion of some authors, "primordial cyst" is to be preferred owing to the origin of the cyst from primordial odontogenic epithelium and the nonspecificity of "keratocyst." Others, however, reserve "primordial cyst" for a cyst that arises from a breakdown of the stellate reticulum in the enamel organ before mineralization occurs. In other words, a cyst forms in place of a tooth. Using the latter definition for primordial cyst, Brannon, in his extensive study of 312 keratocysts, found that only 44.4 per cent of the primordial cysts fulfilled the microscopic criteria of the odontogenic keratocyst.[66] Odontogenic keratocysts are thought to develop from two sources: (1) the dental lamina or its epithelial remnants[67, 81] and (2) basal cell hamartia of the overlying oral mucosa.[81, 83]

Incidence. Data from 15 series reviewed by Shear,[81] showing the frequency of odontogenic keratocysts (when compared with other types of odontogenic and jaw cysts), indicated that the mean frequency of odontogenic keratocysts was 9.2 per cent and the range of frequency was 3.2 to 21.8 per cent.

Clinical Features. Odontogenic keratocysts may be detected at any age; there are reported cases in the first and ninth decades of life. Data from three series totaling 446 cases[66, 68, 80] reveal a greater frequency in the second, third, and fourth decades (54.2 per cent, or 243 of 446 cases). In Hodgkinson's study[74] of 79 cases, the mean age was 41.8 years. Ahlfors and associates reported the mean age of 255 patients with odontogenic keratocysts to be 41 years.[65]

There is a male predilection, which ranges from 1.44:1 to 2:1.[65, 66, 68, 74]

Invariably, the mandible is affected more frequently than the maxilla. Brannon noted a 65 per cent incidence in the mandible, Payne found 65.5 per cent, Hodgkinson 72 per cent, Shear 75 per cent, Ahlfors 75 per cent, and Browne 83 per cent.[65, 66, 68, 74, 76, 81] In the mandible, 70 to 78 per cent[61, 68] of the cysts occur in the posterior region. In the maxilla, the posterior region is also affected most often, but to a lesser degree: 35 to 52.5 per cent.[66, 74] In eight instances studied by Brannon, the cysts were quite extensive, crossing the midline.[66]

Multiple cysts occur in one of every 14 patients (7 per cent) with an odontogenic keratocyst.[65, 66, 81] One third to one half of those patients with multiple cysts have the nevoid basal cell carcinoma syndrome.[65, 66, 81]

Radiographic Features (Fig. 57–5A). The majority of the cysts appear radiographically as unilocular radiolucencies with well-defined sclerotic borders. Brannon interpreted 32 of 52 cases as unilocular and 17 as bilocular or multilocular.[66] Hodgkinson and associates, in a review of 79 cases, reported 54 per cent as unilocular and 46 per cent as loculated. Those investigators noted that locular or multilocular lesions usually occurred in the mandible and were seldom observed in the maxilla.[74] The size of the cysts varied from 1 to 9 cm, with a mean diameter of 3.3 cm.[74] Large cysts may result in buccal and lingual expansion, and perforation of the cortical plate has been reported.[81] Wright and associates reported four examples of odontogenic keratocysts that appeared radiographically as periapical lesions.[85]

Signs and Symptoms. One half (50.3 per cent) of the 312 patients in Brannon's series were symptomatic; swelling and drainage were the most common findings, followed by pain, paresthesia, and trismus.[66] A detectable swelling was apparent in 85 per cent of the 79 patients studied by Hodgkinson and associates; in these patients pain was a symptom in 24 per cent, and oral drainage was a complaint in 15 per cent.[74]

Histopathology. The characteristic histopathologic features of the odontogenic keratocyst (Fig. 57–5B) are as follows:

1. A thin, epithelial lining, devoid of rete pegs, composed of keratinizing stratified squamous epithelium, which ranges from three to six cells in thickness.

2. A parakeratotic surface in 80 per cent[81] to 97 per cent[65] of the cases.

3. An orthokeratotic surface in 3 per cent[65] to 10 per cent[66] of the cases.

4. A well-defined basal layer composed of palisaded basophilic columnar cells, cuboidal cells, or both.[66]

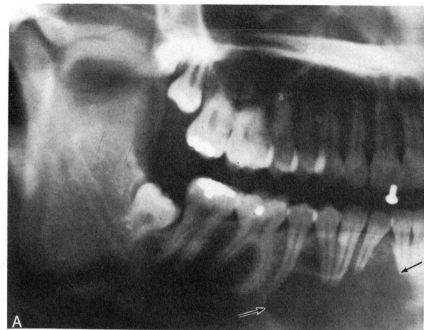

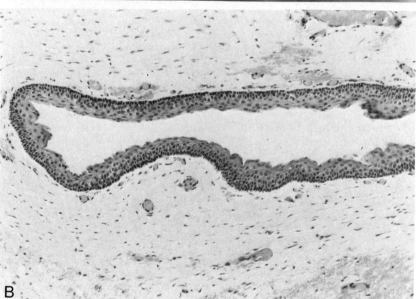

Figure 57–5. Odontogenic keratocyst. (A) Large multilocular cyst in the mandible of a 16-year-old female with the nevoid basal cell carcinoma syndrome. (Courtesy of Dr. J. L. McClendon.) (B) In a typical odontogenic keratocyst, the lining shows parakeratosis, corrugation of the surface, and a prominent basal cell layer. (×100)

5. A suprabasilar split in 36 per cent[66] to 53 per cent[65] of the cases.

  6. Budding of the basal layer.

  7. Satellite cysts in the fibrous wall.

  8. Epithelial rests in the wall.

  9. Dystrophic calcifications.

  10. Inflammation and cholesterol clefts.

  11. Epithelial dysplasia.

Features 6 through 11 are considered more variable.[65, 66]

Behavior. The review of 21 separate reports on the recurrence rate of odontogenic keratocysts revealed a range of recurrence from 5 to 62.5 per cent.[65, 66, 67, 69, 81] The most recent studies by Ahlfors and associates,[65] Forssell,[72] and Vedtofte and Praetorius[84] found recurrence rates of 27, 40, and 51 per cent, respectively.

Wright, after finding only one recurrence in 24 orthokeratinized odontogenic keratocysts, suggested that cysts with an orthokeratinized lining are less likely to recur than those with parakeratinized linings.[86] This was substantiated in a recent report by Ahlfors and coworkers.[65] They found that all recurrent, multiple, or syndrome-associated cysts were parakeratinized; all the orthokeratinized cysts were single, and none recurred.[65]

Nevoid Basal Cell Carcinoma Syndrome. First described as a syndrome by Gorlin and Goltz,[73] the *nevoid basal cell carcinoma syndrome* is also known as the *Gorlin-Goltz syndrome* and the *basal cell nevus syndrome*. It is characterized by the following:

1. Basal cell carcinomas of the skin, often at an early age.

2. Multiple odontogenic keratocysts of the jaws.

3. Bifid ribs and other skeletal anomalies.

4. Frontal and parietal bossing of the skull.

5. Broad nasal root.

6. Calcification of the falx cerebri.

7. Palmar or plantar pits.

8. Autosomal dominant inheritance with marked penetrance and variable expressivity.

Odontogenic keratocysts have been observed in 65 per cent[75] to 77 per cent[82] of the patients with this syndrome, and they occur at a relatively early age.[75] The cysts have been detected in patients as young as 6 years old, although they are most often recognized during adolescence or early adulthood.[68, 75] Multiplicity of cysts is common, and they may appear radiographically as unilocular or multilocular radiolucencies. The most common sites are the premolar and first molar regions of the mandible and the second molar region of the maxilla.[73]

Syndrome-associated keratocysts are considered to have a much higher recurrence rate than single keratocysts. In an analysis of 13 cases of nevoid basal cell carcinoma syndrome by Donatsky and associates, 85 per cent of the patients with the syndrome showed recurrences of the odontogenic keratocysts within 2 years.[71]

Microscopically, there are no basic differences between single cysts, multiple cysts, or syndrome-associated cysts.[68] There are, however, certain microscopic features that are more frequently observed in syndrome-associated cysts when compared with single recurrent cysts:[65]

1. A lining that is exclusively parakeratinized (in both forms).

2. Budding of basal layer (50 vs. 14 per cent).

3. Epithelial islands in cyst wall (50 vs. 15 per cent).

4. Satellite cysts in cyst wall (50 vs. 2 per cent).

5. Mural proliferation (42 vs. 2 per cent).

6. Suprabasilar split (92 vs. 77 per cent).

Multiple odontogenic keratocysts have also been reported in association with Marfan's syndrome and Noonan's syndrome.[70]

Calcifying Odontogenic Cyst

The calcifying odontogenic cyst (Gorlin cyst, keratinizing and calcifying epithelial odontogenic cyst) was first recognized as a distinct entity by Gorlin and associates in a report of 15 cases.[91] It is characterized by a variable epithelial lining that has a distinct columnar basal layer and masses of ghost cells undergoing keratinization and calcification (Fig. 57–6)—features that resemble the cutaneous calcifying epithelioma of Malherbe. Most of the cysts occur in an intraosseous location, but some are entirely extraosseous. It is not uncommon for them to be associated with unerupted teeth or complex odontomas.[88, 93] Prior to 1962, one case was reported as a variant of cholesteatoma, and several were described as atypical variants of ameloblastoma.[91]

Owing to its varied nature with some features of an odontogenic tumor, the lesion has been classified both as a cyst and as a neoplasm.[90, 95] Praetorious and associates described three variants of the calcifying odontogenic cyst:

1. A unilocular cyst with moderate proliferations of epithelium and sparse amounts of dysplastic dentin.

2. A unilocular cyst that produces compound or complex odontomas.

3. A unilocular cyst with extensive ameloblastoma-like proliferations of epithelium.[96]

Incidence. The calcifying odontogenic cyst is not common; Altini and Farman found eight cases in 411 odontogenic tumors and developmental cysts (less than 2 per cent).[88] More than 130 cases have been published in the world literature since Gorlin's initial contribution.[80, 90, 92, 94, 96]

Clinical Features. Freedman and associates, in a review of 70 cases, found the age range to be 7 years to

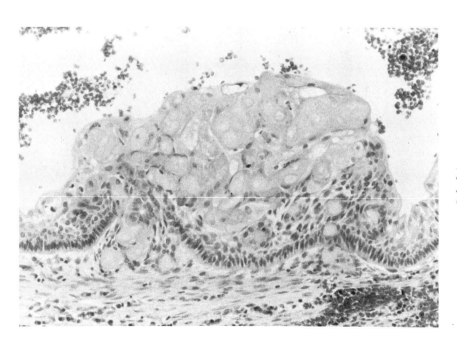

Figure 57–6. Calcifying odontogenic cyst. Note the columnar basal layer and the eosinophilic "ghost" cells. (×200)

82 years, with a mean age of 38.4 years; almost one half of the patients, however, were younger than 31 years of age.[90] Altini and Farman noted a peak incidence in the second decade.[88] Nagao and colleagues reported 23 cases and an age range of 9 to 71 years, with a mean age of 21 years and a peak incidence in the second decade.[94]

Distribution between the sexes is nearly equal; of 93 cases, 44 (47 per cent) were male and 49 (53 per cent) were female.[90, 94]

Nearly as many calcifying odontogenic cysts occur in the mandible as in the maxilla; 43.5 per cent of 92 lesions were in the mandible, and 56.5 per cent involved the maxilla.[90, 94] More than three out of four are intraosseous and are located anterior to the first molar teeth.[90]

Radiographic Features. Radiographically, the intraosseous lesions usually appear as unilocular radiolucencies with well-demarcated borders. The size of the cyst may range from 1 to 8 cm, with an average diameter of 3 cm. Some examples may appear multilocular or show irregular radiopacities, but others may have an ill-defined periphery. Cortical expansion, resorption of adjacent tooth roots and association with unerupted teeth have been reported in some cases.[90, 99] Three of ten intraosseous cysts reported by McGowan and Browne were in the periapical region of associated teeth and, therefore, simulated radicular cysts.[92] Extraosseous lesions may cause a saucerization of adjacent cortical bone.[96]

Histopathology. Out of a total of 82 lesions reviewed by Freedman and associates and McGowan and Browne, 72 were cystic and ten were solid.[90, 92] The cystic lesions are lined by squamous epithelium six to eight cells in thickness, with a prominent basal layer of columnar cells and a loose-appearing middle layer that resembles stellate reticulum. The cells toward the lumen exhibit keratinization and karyolysis, resulting in the ghost cell appearance. Multinucleated foreign body giant cells may be observed in association with masses of keratin. Dystrophic mineralization occurs in some of the ghost cells.[98] Varying amounts of dentinoid (dysplastic dentin) have been described.[96] Melanin pigmentation within the epithelial cells has been reported in more than seven cases.[90, 91, 97, 100]

Signs and Symptoms. A painless, slow-growing swelling is the most common complaint in both the intraosseous and extraosseous lesions. Fifty per cent of the 70 cases reviewed by Freedman and associates complained of a swelling, but only one third of them had pain associated with the enlargement.[90]

Behavior. Calcifying odontogenic cysts usually do not recur, although occasional instances have been reported.[91, 92]

Inflammatory Odontogenic Cysts

Radicular Cyst

The radicular cyst (apical periodontal cyst) may be defined as an inflammatory odontogenic cyst, usually located at the apex of the root of a nonvital erupted tooth; the cyst arises from the rests of Malassez in the periodontal ligament. In rare instances, it may be found lateral to the root rather than apical. Like other types of inflammatory cysts, the radicular cyst does not recur if it is adequately curetted.

Incidence. The radicular cyst is the most common odontogenic cyst. In Shear's review of 1345 jaw cysts, 55 per cent (740) of them were radicular or residual cysts.[113] Browne and Ahlfors reported higher frequencies of 74.3 per cent (402 of 540 cysts)[103] and 70.7 per cent (4182 of 5914 jaw cysts).[101]

Clinical Features. Although radicular cysts may occur in any decade of life, few cases are seen in the first, eighth, and ninth decades. Most of the cysts are diagnosed during the second, third, and fourth decades, and the greatest number occur in the second decade.[102, 113]

There is a male preponderance. In Browne's study of 380 cysts, 60 per cent (225) were found in males and 40 per cent (153) were found in females.[103] Shear reported that 58 per cent of 664 cysts affected males and 42 per cent affected females.[113]

Although radicular cysts may develop in any of the tooth-bearing areas of either jaw, the highest frequency is in the anterior maxillary region. The combined series of Bhaskar and of LaLonde and Luebke reflected an 82 per cent incidence in the maxilla (997 of 1218 cysts),[102, 107] and Shear reported that 60 per cent of 789 cysts occurred in the maxilla.[113] The anterior region of the maxilla was affected in 42 per cent of the patients in LaLonde and Luebke's study and in 37 per cent of Shear's cases.[107, 113]

Radiographic Features. Radiographically, the radicular cyst appears as a round or ovoid radiolucency, with sharply defined sclerotic borders, which is in continuity with the root apex of the involved tooth (Fig. 57–7A). Because the radicular cyst is the end result of an inflammatory sequence (pulpitis → apical periodontitis → periapical granuloma → epitheliated periapical granuloma → radicular cyst), it is difficult to differentiate radiographically between radicular cysts and periapical granulomas. Various studies indicate that 53 to 67 per cent of periapical radiolucencies with diameters larger than 1 cm are radicular cysts.[106, 109, 110]

Signs and Symptoms. Although pain and discomfort may be experienced during the preceding stages of pulpitis or apical periodontitis, radicular cysts often are asymptomatic. Many of them are not detected until pulp vitality tests indicate a nonvital tooth and subsequent radiographs are taken. Symptoms consisting of pain and swelling may be present when the cyst is infected. In rare cases, a sinus tract may extend from the periapical lesion, through bone, to the oral mucosal surface (parulis) or the skin surface.

Histopathology. The radicular cyst is lined by nonkeratinizing stratified squamous epithelium, which usually ranges between six and 15 cells in thickness. Frequently, the epithelial lining appears hyperplastic and edematous. Invariably, there is a dense infiltrate of plasma cells and lymphocytes in the fibrous wall, and polymorphonuclear leukocytes may be present within the epithelium and connective tissue (Fig. 57–7B). Features that are more variable include (1) mucous cells in the lining,[103] (2) hyaline bodies of Rushton in the epithelium, and (3) cholesterol with associated lipid-laden macrophages in the fibrous wall. Hyaline bodies (Rushton bodies) are straight, curved, laminated, or hairpin-shaped structures, about 1 mm in length, that have an eosinophilic glassy appearance (Fig. 57–7C).[112] Rushton considered them to be of odontogenic origin, resembling

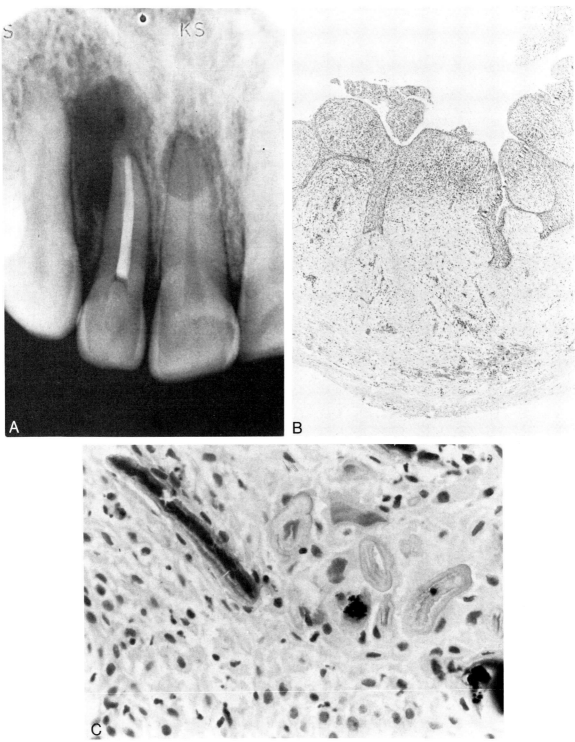

Figure 57–7. Radicular cyst. (*A*) The cyst appears as a well-defined radiolucency at the apex of an endodontically treated maxillary left lateral incisor. (Courtesy of Dr. Alan Selbst.) (*B*) The photomicrograph shows the hyperplastic epithelial lining and a prominent inflammatory component which are characteristic of the radicular cyst. (×40) (*C*) Hyaline (Rushton) bodies in the epithelial layer of a radicular cyst. (×400)

the keratinized layer of the epithelial attachment of a tooth. Subsequently, some investigators suggested a hematogenous origin for the bodies, but others favored an epithelial cell origin.[113] Yamaguchi, after completing extensive histologic, histochemical, and ultrastructural studies of hyaline bodies, could not confirm a keratinous nature and considered them to be particular products formed by odontogenic epithelium.[115]

Residual Cyst

As defined by Weine, "A residual cyst is any type of odontogenic cyst that persists in the bone after the tooth with which it was associated has been removed."[114] In Bhaskar's review of 2308 periapical lesions, only 84 (3.7 per cent) were classified as residual cysts.[102] Craig, in a review of 1051 odontogenic cysts, found 223 residual cysts (21.2 per cent).[104]

Although many residual cysts develop following the extraction of a tooth with a radicular cyst, others may arise from epithelial remnants in a periapical granuloma, and still others occur after the removal of an impacted tooth with a dentigerous cyst. Radiographically, the cyst appears as a well-circumscribed radiolucency in the edentulous area formerly occupied by the offending tooth. Occasionally, a residual cyst may be in close association with the root of a remaining tooth, mimicking a radicular cyst and resulting in unnecessary endodontic treatment.[114] The microscopic features of the residual cyst are very similar to those of the radicular cyst.

Inflammatory Lateral Periodontal Cyst

Occasionally, an inflammatory cyst of odontogenic origin arises in a lateral, rather than apical, relationship to the roots of anterior or posterior teeth. When the cyst is associated with pulpitis or a nonvital tooth, it should be designated as a lateral radicular cyst. If, however, the cyst develops from activation of the rests of Malassez by inflammation in a periodontal pocket, the term "inflammatory lateral periodontal cyst" would seem most appropriate. Microscopically, both cysts appear quite similar, exhibiting a nonkeratinizing squamous epithelial lining and a dense infiltrate of chronic inflammatory cells in the fibrous wall.

Paradental Cyst

First defined as a specific type of inflammatory odontogenic cyst by Craig, the paradental cyst arises in relation to partially erupted mandibular third molar teeth that have been affected by pericoronitis.[104] In his study of 49 such lesions, Craig observed a consistent location near the buccal bifurcation of the third molar tooth (Fig. 57–8A), often associated with an enamel projection from the bifurcation. The cysts usually occurred in the third decade, were more common in males than in females (5:1), and made up 4.7 per cent (49) of 1051 odontogenic cysts.[104] Some of the paradental cysts were apparent on radiographs as well-defined or superimposed radiolucencies; others, however, were not suspected prior to the removal of the associated tooth.[104] Microscopically, the cysts are lined by hyperplastic,

nonkeratinizing stratified squamous epithelium (Fig. 57–8B) and exhibit occasional hyaline bodies or calcifications. The fibrous wall invariably contains a dense infiltrate of acute and chronic inflammatory cells, and this may be accompanied by focal deposits of cholesterol, hemosiderin, or dystrophic calcifications. The cyst is of uncertain pathogenesis, but it probably arises from reduced enamel epithelium[104] or from the rests of Malassez.[113]

ODONTOGENIC TUMORS

Odontogenic tumors, ranging from hamartomatous processes to neoplastic proliferations, are extremely variable in their rate of development, radiographic appearance, histopathology, and behavior. Although many histologic variants have been recognized, it is often difficult to determine the precise nature of such lesions. As Minderjahn has aptly stated,

A lack of knowledge of etiology, extraordinary rarity, polymorphism in their nature and lack of agreement on a commonly accepted nomenclature and classification put nearly insurmountable difficulties in the way of every experiment to gather and analyze the clinical behavior of the different forms of these tumors.[136]

Pindborg and Clausen proposed a classification of odontogenic tumors based on embryologic principles, that is, the embryonal inductive influence that the cells of one tissue exert upon the cells of another tissue.[139] This classification was slightly modified by Gorlin[128] (Table 57–2). Recently, Reichart and Ries introduced a systematic classification based on the histogenetic, organogenetic, and embryologic aspects of tooth development[141, 142] (Table 57–3). In this discussion of the clinical and pathologic features of odontogenic tumors, both classifications will be employed.

TABLE 57–2. Classification of Odontogenic Tumors

Epithelial Odontogenic Tumors
Minimal inductive change in connective tissue:
 1. Ameloblastoma
 2. Adenomatoid odontogenic tumor
 3. Calcifying epithelial odontogenic tumor
Marked inductive change in connective tissue:
 1. Ameloblastic fibroma
 2. Ameloblastic fibrosarcoma
 3. Odontoma
  a. Ameloblastic odontoma
  b. Ameloblastic dentinosarcoma
  c. Complex odontoma
  d. Compound odontoma

Mesodermal Odontogenic Tumors
 1. Myxoma
 2. Odontogenic fibroma
 3. Cementoma
  a. Periapical cemental dysplasia
  b. Benign cementoblastoma
  c. Cementifying fibroma
  d. Familial multiple (gigantiform) cementomas

Source: Based on classification of Pindborg and Clausen[139]; modified by Gorlin RJ, *In* Gorlin RJ, Goldman HM (eds): Thoma's Oral Pathology. 6th ed. St. Louis, The C. V. Mosby Co., 1970.[128]

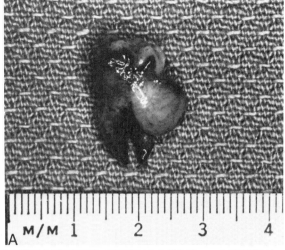

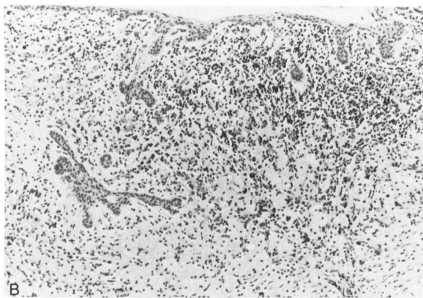

Figure 57–8. Paradental cyst. (*A*) Typical location in the bifurcation of a mandibular third molar tooth. (*B*) Microscopic appearance of the cyst lining. (×100) (Courtesy of Dr. J. L. McClendon.)

Ameloblastic Tumors

Ameloblastic tumors are epithelial tumors with minimal inductive change in the connective tissue. They include the ameloblastoma, adenomatoid odontogenic tumor, calcifying epithelial odontogenic tumor, and squamous odontogenic tumor.

Ameloblastoma

One of the most significant odontogenic tumors in terms of behavior and frequency, the ameloblastoma (adamantinoma, adamantoblastoma, basiloma, epithelioma ameloblastoides) was first recognized by Cusack in 1827[120] and was later described by Falksson.[124] The term *adamantinoma* was introduced to denote the tumor by Malassez in 1885. Ivy and Churchill, favoring terminology that did not imply a calcifying neoplasm, suggested the name ameloblastoma.[133] Ameloblastomas are generally considered to originate from one of several structures[128]:

1. Remnants of the dental lamina or remnants of Hertwig's sheath.
2. The enamel organ.
3. The epithelium of odontogenic cysts, particularly the dentigerous cyst.
4. Basal cells of the surface epithelium.

Incidence. In a review of 706 odontogenic tumors by Regezi and associates, ameloblastomas composed 11 per cent (78 of 706 tumors). The overall incidence was 0.14 per cent (78 of 54,534 biopsies).[140]

Clinical Features. Most ameloblastomas are diagnosed in the third, fourth, or fifth decades of life; 62.5 per cent of 1152 instances in the literature occurred in patients 20 to 49 years of age.[135, 140, 146, 148] Very few of the tumors have been detected during the first decade of life. In a review of 1036 cases by Small and Waldron, the mean age of the ameloblastoma patient, at the time of diagnosis, was 38.9 years.[148] Cases have been reported in the newborn and in the elderly (birth to 84 years of age).[118]

Distribution of the tumors between the sexes is

TABLE 57–3. Reichart and Ries Classification of Odontogenic Tumors*

	Ameloblastic	Ectomesenchymal	Mesenchymal	Neuroectodermal (in strict sense)
Ameloblastic	Ameloblastoma Adenomatoid odontogenic tumor Calcifying epithelial odontogenic tumor Squamous odontogenic tumor			
Ectomesenchymal	Ameloblastic fibroma Ameloblastic fibroodontoma Complex odontoma Compound odontoma	Cementoblastoma Odontogenic myxoma Odontogenic fibroma Dentinoma		
Mesenchymal	"Adamantino" hemangioma	Periapical cemental dysplasia Gigantiform cementoma Cementifying fibroma	Fibroma Lipoma Hemangioma	
Neuroectodermal (in strict sense)	Ameloblastoma with neurinoma	"Central pacinian neurofibroma"	Neurofibroma	Melanotic and neuroectodermal tumor of infancy

*Based on histogenesis.
Source: Adapted from Reichart PA, Ries P: Considerations on the classification of odontogenic tumors. Int J Oral Surg *12*:323, 1983. Copyright Munksgaard International Publishers Ltd., Copenhagen, Denmark.

nearly equal; 50.4 per cent (644) of 1277 cases occurred in males, and 49.6 per cent (633) were in females.[135, 140, 146, 148]

Ameloblastomas occur about four times as often in the mandible as in the maxilla. Of 1207 reported instances, 80.8 per cent (975) were located in the mandible and 19.2 per cent (232) were in the maxilla.[135, 140, 146, 148] In both jaws, the posterior region is most commonly affected (69.8 per cent of 336 cases[140, 148]) (Table 57–4). In a study of 24 *maxillary* ameloblastomas by Tsaknis and Nelson, 80 per cent were posterior in location and the mean age was 45.6 years. Significantly, 12 of the 24 cases involved the maxillary antrum, and eight of 16 cases recurred.[150]

Signs and Symptoms. Typically, early symptoms are absent and the tumors are seldom diagnosed in the early stages of development.[148] A slow-growing, painless swelling is the most common complaint of patients with advanced tumors. Melisch and coworkers noted that 75 per cent of patients complained of a swelling, but only 33 per cent complained of pain. Other manifestations,

TABLE 57–4. Localized Sites of Ameloblastoma

Site	Frequency
Mandible	81%
Posterior region	56.7%
Premolar region	16.2%
Anterior region	8.1%
Maxilla	19%
Posterior region	14.6%
Premolar region	2.5%
Anterior region	1.9%

which are less common, include mobile teeth, ill-fitting dentures, malocclusion, ulcerations, draining sinuses, and nasal obstruction.[135]

The size of ameloblastomas may range from small, asymptomatic lesions measuring less than 1 cm up to disfiguring tumor masses measuring as large as 16 cm.[150] The mean size of the tumors reviewed by Tsaknis and Nelson was 4.2 cm[150]; Sehdev and associates reported the mean size of mandibular lesions as 4.7 cm, and those in the maxilla measured 5 cm.[146]

Radiographic Features. The ameloblastoma appears radiographically as a radiolucency, with no calcified or radiopaque components. At one end of the radiographic spectrum, the tumors may appear unilocular, with or without association with a tooth. At the other end of the spectrum, the radiographic appearance is that of an expansile, multilocular radiolucency with distinct compartmentalization. The unilocular lesion that surrounds the crown of a tooth is indistinguishable from a dentigerous cyst. The differential diagnosis of a multilocular radiolucency should include cherubism, giant cell granuloma, odontogenic myxoma, aneurysmal bone cyst, and odontogenic keratocyst.

Histopathology. Microscopically, the ameloblastoma is composed of nests, strands, and cords of ameloblastic epithelium, all separated by relatively small amounts of fibrous connective tissue stroma. There are two predominant patterns, *follicular* and *plexiform*. In the *follicular* type (Fig. 57–9A), the epithelial islands contain central portions that are composed of a loose network resembling the stellate reticulum of the enamel organ. The epithelium at the periphery is composed of tall columnar cells, with polarized nuclei, and these cells resemble the cells of the inner enamel epithelium. In the *plexiform*

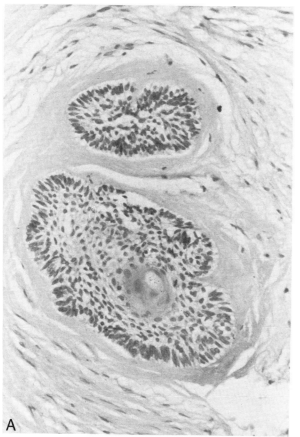

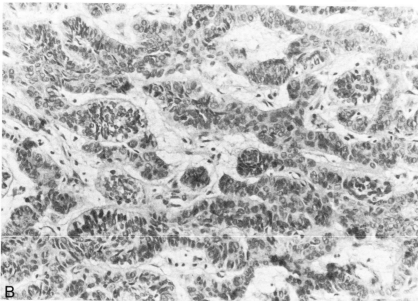

Figure 57–9. Ameloblastoma. (*A*) Follicular pattern with early squamous metaplasia. (*B*) Plexiform pattern resembling the dental lamina. (×200) (*C*) Ameloblastoma with extensive granular cell component. (×100) (*D*) A segment of cystic ameloblastoma that may be misinterpreted as an odontogenic cyst. (*E*) Islands of ameloblastoma adjacent to cystic areas.

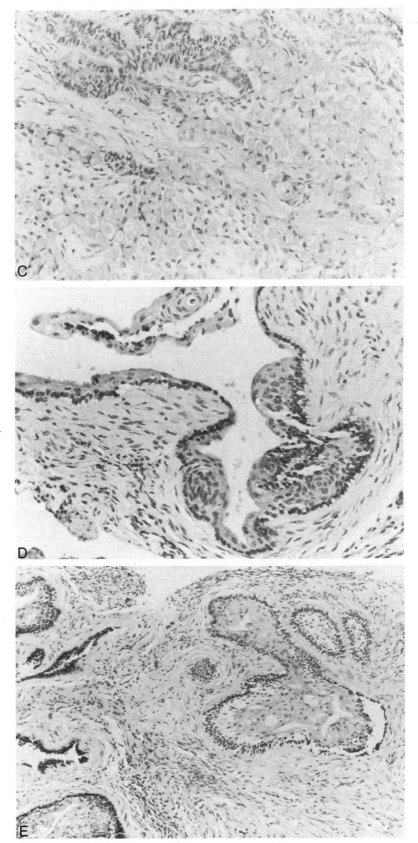

Figure 57–9 Continued.

type (Fig. 57–9B), the epithelium is arranged in anastomosing strands and cords, which resemble the dental lamina. The epithelial cells are closely apposed and, morphologically, appear basaloid or cuboidal. The stellate reticulum is not well defined in plexiform tumors.

Of the two types, the follicular pattern is more common,[128, 148] although both variations have been observed in the same tumor. One third of the maxillary ameloblastomas studied by Tsaknis and Nelson were plexiform, one sixth were follicular, and one half exhibited both patterns.[150]

Cystic degeneration may occur in the central stellate area of the follicles[128, 130, 132] and also in the stroma,[128, 132] resulting in a cystic ameloblastoma. It is most likely to occur in tumors that are predominantly follicular in pattern.[130] Happonen and Newland, in a study of 12 cystic ameloblastomas by light and electron microscopy, observed areas of squamous metaplasia in the stellate reticulum. It was noted consistently that these acanthomatous changes preceded the development of squamous-lined cystic areas, and microcyst formation occurred only in areas of squamous metaplasia. As the cystic lumina increased in size, some areas of the squamous lining became compressed and flattened, resembling the lining of a dentigerous cyst (Fig. 57–9D).[130]

When squamous metaplasia of the stellate reticulum-like areas is extensive and forms islands of keratinizing squamous epithelium, the tumor is often referred to as *acanthomatous ameloblastoma* (Fig. 57–9E). Calcification of metaplastic epithelium in ameloblastomas has been reported.[128]

The preceding acanthomatous and cystic changes are observed quite frequently in cystic ameloblastomas, and care should be taken to avoid misinterpreting them. If the biopsy specimen is too superficial or not representative, the acanthomatous changes may be misdiagnosed as a squamous cell carcinoma; and the cystic lining, if compressed, may be misdiagnosed as a dentigerous cyst.

There are other histopathologic variations in ameloblastoma, including the following:

1. An abundance of granular cells[131, 135] (Fig. 57–9C) (granular cell ameloblastoma).
2. Numerous blood vessels in the stroma[128, 147] (ameloblastic hemangioma).
3. The presence of neuromatous elements[128, 147] (ameloblastic neuroma).
4. The presence of mucin-producing epithelial cells[145] (mucin-producing ameloblastoma).

In the recent classification of odontogenic tumors by Reichart and Ries, the granular cell ameloblastoma and ameloblastic neuroma are classified as *ameloblastic-neuroectodermal* tumors, and the ameloblastic hemangioma is categorized as an *ameloblastic-mesenchymal* tumor.[142]

Behavior. The conventional ameloblastoma has a capacity for continued growth and a tendency to infiltrate between bony trabeculae. The recurrence rate for ameloblastomas treated by enucleation or curettage is reported to be 55 to 90 per cent.[127, 146]

UNICYSTIC AMELOBLASTOMA (Figs. 57–10A and 57–10B)

The development of ameloblastoma in the wall of an odontogenic cyst has long been recognized, and many cases have been reported.[144] Robinson and Martinez reported 20 instances of unilocular cystic lesions, each of which clinically and radiographically mimicked a dentigerous or primordial cyst but microscopically had the features of an ameloblastoma. The lesions exclusively involved the posterior regions of the mandible, and 14 of the 20 patients were younger than 30 years of age. The treatment for all the lesions had been enucleation, and follow-up data (2 to 14 years) revealed a recurrence rate of 25 to 33 per cent. The young age of the patients and relatively low rate of recurrence, when compared with conventional ameloblastomas, prompted those investigators to propose the term *unicystic ameloblastoma* and to recommend simple enucleation as the preferred treatment.[144] Gardner and Corio reported 38 similar cases, all located in the mandible, in patients ranging from 8 to 35 years of age. They found only four recurrences in 34 cases.[126, 127] Eversole and coworkers studied 31 unicystic ameloblastomas that affected patients 14 to 68 years of age (average 26.9 years). The lesions appeared radiographically as pericoronal, interradicular, or periapical radiolucencies, and all were located in the mandible. With the exception of one case, all had been treated by curettage or enucleation. The overall recurrence rate was 18 per cent (follow-up periods ranged from less than 2 to 25 years).[123]

PERIPHERAL AMELOBLASTOMA

The *peripheral ameloblastoma* is a term used to describe a neoplasm, with microscopic features of ameloblastoma, which arises in the soft tissue overlying a tooth-bearing region of the jaws.[151] At least 30 cases of this uncommon odontogenic tumor have been published, including some cases that were diagnosed as basal cell carcinoma.[116, 119, 125, 137, 138] In a review of 27 cases by Moskow and Baden, 65 per cent of the lesions were located in the mandible, and 35 per cent were in the maxilla. The most common sites were the lingual gingiva of the mandible and the soft-tissue tuberosity area of the maxilla. Origin from the basal cell layer of the epithelium was described in two thirds of the cases; the remaining one third arose from dental lamina rests. One neoplasm developed from the wall of a soft-tissue cyst. The age of patients ranged from 20 to 93 years, with a mean age of 51 years. Microscopically, most of the tumors were diagnosed as acanthomatous types of ameloblastoma. Recurrences were uncommon, reportedly 20 per cent or less.[137]

Adenomatoid Odontogenic Tumor (Fig. 57–11A)

More than 150 cases have been reported since Stafne first recognized the adenomatoid odontogenic tumor as a distinct entity.[157, 165] For many years it was considered to be a variant of ameloblastoma and was named accordingly: adamantinoma, adenoameloblastoma, and ameloblastic adenomatoid tumor.[157] In 1969, Philipsen and Birn proposed the term *adenomatoid odontogenic tumor*, which is generally accepted today.[160] The precise origin of the tumor is unknown, but several sites have been suggested:

1. Outer enamel epithelium.[155]
2. Inner enamel epithelium.[164]
3. Enamel organ.[158, 162, 163]

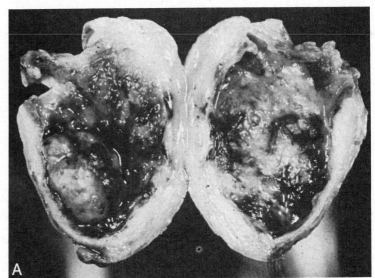

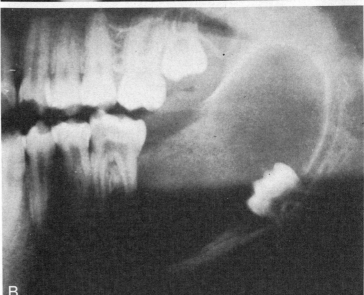

Figure 57–10. Unicystic ameloblastoma. (*A*) Bisected gross specimen. (From Gardner DG, Corio RL: Plexiform unicystic ameloblastoma. Cancer *53*:1730, 1984.) (*B*) Unicystic ameloblastoma in the mandible of a 17-year-old male. The radiographic appearance is identical to that of a dentigerous cyst. (Courtesy of Dr. Michael Fesler.)

4. Enamel epithelium.[167]

5. Basal cell layer of the epithelium.[169]

Some authors consider the lesion to be a hamartomatous proliferation of odontogenic tissue[153, 156, 164] but others regard it as a neoplasm.[168]

Incidence. Three per cent (22) of the 706 odontogenic tumors reviewed by Regezi and associates were adenomatoid odontogenic tumors.[161]

Clinical Features. The tumor characteristically affects a young age group. Courtney and Kerr, following a study of 20 cases, reported that 80 per cent occurred between the ages of 10 and 20 years; one patient was 5 years old, and the oldest patient was 37 years of age.[156] Giansanti and coworkers reviewed 105 instances of adenomatoid odontogenic tumors, 74 (70.4 per cent) of which affected patients between 10 and 19 years of age. The mean age was 17.8 years, with an age range of 5 to 53 years.[157]

Females develop the tumor almost twice as often as males; 65.4 per cent (89) of 136 cases in the literature occurred in females, and 34.6 per cent affected males.[153, 156, 157, 167]

Adenomatoid odontogenic tumors are more common in the maxilla than the mandible and usually involve the anterior region. A review of data representing 141 cases indicates that 66 per cent of the tumors were located in the maxilla and 34 per cent were in the mandible. In both the maxilla and mandible, 76 per cent of the lesions occurred in the anterior region.[153, 156, 157, 167]

Seventy-four per cent of the cases reviewed by Giansanti and his colleagues were associated with impacted permanent teeth.[157] Bedrick and coworkers described an unusual adenomatoid odontogenic tumor, which consisted of two lobes, one lobe within the bone of the maxilla and the other partially in bone and soft tissue.[154] At least seven extraosseous lesions have been re-

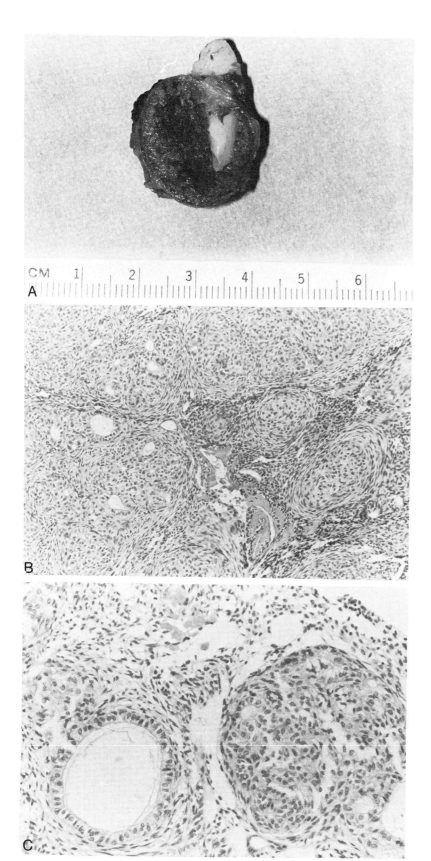

Figure 57–11. Adenomatoid odontogenic tumor. (A) Bisected gross specimen of a tumor associated with an unerupted tooth in the mandible of a 15-year-old male. (B) Whorled nests of epithelial cells in duct-like configurations. (×100) (C) Note the amorphous eosinophilic material and the columnar cells lining the duct-like structures. (×200)

ported.[156, 157] Six were located in the maxilla, some of them presenting in the central incisor area as labial gingival swellings.

Signs and Symptoms. The most common symptom is that of a painless swelling.[156, 157] About two of three cases reviewed by Giansanti and associates exhibited intraoral swelling, and approximately one of five showed extraoral swelling.[157] Pain and tooth mobility were less frequently encountered.

Radiographic Features. Typically, the adenomatoid odontogenic tumor appears radiographically as a unilocular radiolucency around the crown of an impacted tooth, resembling a dentigerous cyst. In some cases, calcifications may be detectable, appearing as radiopaque "flecks" or dense radiopacities. The margins are usually well defined and sclerotic.[156, 157] Occasionally, the lesions are associated with roots of teeth and are situated in periapical or interradicular relationships.[157] The vast majority of the tumors measure between 1.5 and 3.0 cm,[157] but large lesions up to 12 cm have been reported.[168]

Histopathology. Characteristically, there is a thick-walled cystic structure with a prominent intraluminal proliferation of odontogenic epithelium. The epithelial proliferation is composed of cuboidal or columnar cells in duct-like rosettes or solid configurations (Fig. 57–11B). The duct-like structures are lined by a single layer of cuboidal or columnar epithelium with nuclei that are polarized away from the lumina. Ultrastructurally, the duct-lining cells are similar to preameloblasts[10] and may be distinguished from the smaller, spindle-shaped cells, which comprise the interstitial areas; Smith and associates classified them as type I and type II cells.[163] Eosinophilic amorphous material is present consistently in the lumina of the duct-like structures and between the cells lining them (type I cells) (Fig. 57–11C). Histochemically and ultrastructurally, the eosinophilic material is considered to be epithelial basement membrane material[156, 167] or enamel matrix.[159]

Calcifications in several forms may be observed: (1) irregular dystrophic bodies, (2) laminated or ring-like calcifications, and (3) large globular masses.[153] Yamamoto and coworkers, in an ultrastructural study of intraluminal calcifications in an adenomatoid odontogenic tumor, observed features that closely resembled the relationship between enamel and reduced enamel epithelium in normal odontogenesis. Electron diffraction of the calcifications showed an apatite pattern, also resembling enamel.[170]

Behavior. Giansanti and coworkers found no recurrences in 33 cases that were followed from 1 to 10 years.[157] Courtney and Kerr were able to follow ten cases for periods from 1 to 7 years and did not find a single recurrence.[156]

Calcifying Epithelial Odontogenic Tumor

The calcifying epithelial odontogenic tumor (CEOT, Pindborg tumor), a distinctive and relatively rare neoplasm, was first recognized as a separate entity by Pindborg in 1955.[184] Earlier, the tumor had been described by Thoma and Goldman as "adenoid adamantoblastoma,"[189] by Ivy as "unusual ameloblastoma,"[182] and by Stoopack as "cystic odontoma."[188]

The tumor is thought to arise from the epithelial elements of the enamel organ, but the specific site of origin is controversial. The stratum intermedium was considered to be the originating site by Gon,[181] whereas Chaudhry favored the reduced enamel epithelium[177] and Mori and Makino singled out the inner enamel epithelium.[183]

Incidence. Compared with other types of odontogenic tumors, the calcifying epithelial odontogenic tumor is uncommon. Regezi and colleagues, in a review of 706 odontogenic tumors, found only six cases of calcifying epithelial odontogenic tumors (less than 1 per cent).[186] In 1976, Franklin and Pindborg reviewed and analyzed 113 cases from the world literature. They calculated that approximately 1 per cent of all odontogenic tumors (including odontomas) are calcifying epithelial odontogenic tumors.[179] Since 1976, at least 27 additional cases have been published.[172, 174, 175, 186, 187, 191] Ai-Ru and associates calculated the frequency of occurrence to be 1.8 per cent (4 of 221 odontogenic tumors).[172]

Clinical Features. In the 113 cases reviewed by Franklin and Pindborg, the ages of patients ranged from 8 to 92 years, with a mean age of 31.4 years.[179] The average age of nine cases described by Ai-Ru and associates was 34.2 years (range of 20 to 64 years).[172] Regezi and associates reported a higher average age of 41 years (range of 29 to 62 years) in six patients.[186]

The distribution of the calcifying epithelial odontogenic tumor is nearly the same in males as in females. Of 112 cases reviewed by Franklin and Pindborg, 49 per cent (55) occurred in males and 51 per cent (57) occurred in females.[179] Ai-Ru and associates reported nine of the tumors; females were affected in seven cases, and males were involved in two cases.[172] Regezi and associates reported an equal sex distribution in six cases.[186]

Two thirds of the tumors occur in the mandible (89 of 132 reported cases), and one third are found in the maxilla.[172, 174, 175, 179, 186, 187, 191] There is a marked predilection for the molar region in both jaws. One of every two cases is associated with an unerupted or embedded tooth.[179] Baunsgaard and associates described a calcifying epithelial odontogenic tumor in the maxillary antrum that encroached upon the nasal cavity, producing nasal symptoms.[175]

At least ten instances of *peripheral calcifying epithelial odontogenic tumor* in extraosseous locations have been described,[171, 172, 179, 183, 190] usually presenting as gingival swellings in the anterior mandible. Two of the reported cases had features of the clear cell variant of calcifying epithelial odontogenic tumor,[171, 190] whereas the other cases presented a more typical microscopic appearance. Two sites of origin have been suggested: (1) dental lamina remnants and (2) the basal layer of the gingival epithelium.[172]

Signs and Symptoms. The most common presenting complaint is that of a painless, slow-growing mass. Rarely, the patient may complain of pain, nasal stuffiness, headaches, epistaxis, or proptosis.[179] In some cases, there are no symptoms.

Radiographic Features. Depending upon the stages of development, calcifying epithelial odontogenic tumors may present variable radiographic appearances. Some lesions are well-defined radiolucencies (Fig. 57–12A), whereas others are primarily radiopaque. Intermediate stages occur, and the radiopaque component ranges from small flecks to large irregular calcified areas.

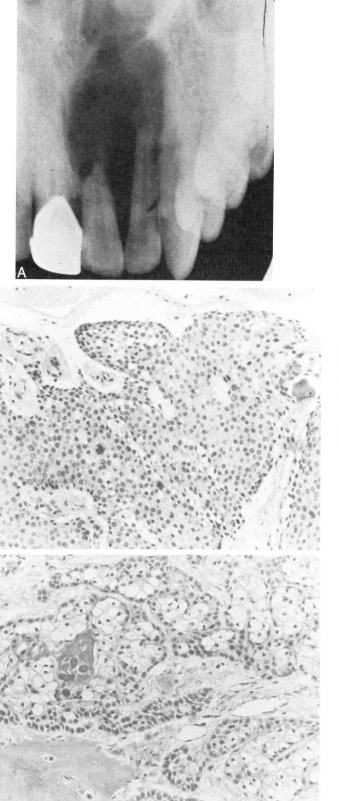

Figure 57–12. Calcifying odontogenic tumor (CEOT). (*A*) This tumor in the anterior maxilla of a 26-year-old female has resulted in external root resorption. Radiographically and microscopically, this tumor was less calcified than most. (Courtesy of Dr. Anne Schmitt.) (*B*) Typical tumor consisting of sheets of polyhedral epithelial cells with focal calcifications. (×200) (*C*) Clear cell variant. (×200)

The most common radiographic finding is that of a unilocular radiolucency, frequently associated with an embedded tooth, which may be interpreted as a dentigerous cyst. Large lesions may appear multilocular, and some may have poorly defined borders.

Histopathology. Calcifying epithelial odontogenic tumors have a characteristic microscopic appearance: sheets or islands of polyhedral epithelial cells with prominent cell borders, intercellular bridges, and occasional ring-like calcifications (Liesegang rings) (Fig. 57–12B).

Eosinophilic homogeneous substance is present in the fibrous stroma and cytoplasm of the tumor cells and has been variously reported as amyloid,[178] keratin,[176] basal lamina,[173] and enamel matrix.[176, 181] The eosinophilic substance stains positively with amyloid stains (Congo red and thioflavin T) and therefore has been interpreted as a form of amyloid. Ultrastructural study of the material was conducted by El-Labban and colleagues, who described two types of structures: (1) sheets of fine filaments measuring 10 to 12 nm in diameter and (2) aggregates of lamina densa fragments, probably secreted by tumor epithelium. They concluded that the fine filamentous material is a form of amyloid that represents a degradation product of lamina densa.[178] Following a histochemical study, Gon suggested that the amyloid-like material might represent an attempt at matrix formation prior to calcification.[181] Mori and associates demonstrated histochemical similarities between the homogeneous substance and enamel matrix.[183] Yamaguchi and associates, noting an absence of basal lamina between the tumor cells and the homogeneous substance, suggested that the homogeneous substance is originally formed by tumor cells and subsequently is transported to the stroma.[191]

Considerable variation in the epithelial component has been reported. Multinucleated cells, pleomorphic cells, giant cells, and bizarre nuclear forms have been observed, sometimes arranged in cribriform or adenoid patterns.[171] Atypical tumors that are composed of strands of epithelial cells and globules of eosinophilic homogeneous material but lack calcifications were reported by Regezi and associates[186] and Smith and associates.[187]

Infrequently, the epithelial cells have a vacuolated cytoplasm and appear as "clear cells" (Fig. 57–12C). Anderson and associates considered the clear cells to represent a degenerative process.[173] Yamaguchi and associates noting a similarity between the glycogen-rich clear cells and epithelial cells of the enamel organ, considered the clear cells to be a feature of cytodifferentiation rather than degeneration.[191]

Behavior. The calcifying epithelial odontogenic tumor is considered to have a rate of recurrence which is much lower than that of the ameloblastoma. In the large series reviewed by Franklin and Pindborg, 14 per cent of the patients had a recurrence.[179]

Squamous Odontogenic Tumor

Since the first six cases were described by Pullon and his colleagues in 1975,[200] 11 acceptable cases of this uncommon odontogenic tumor have been reported.[192–198] Prior to its designation as *squamous odontogenic tumor* by Pullon and associates, the tumor had been variously referred to as "epithelial odontogenic tumor," "benign epithelial odontogenic tumor," "acanthomatous ameloblastoma," or "acanthomatous ameloblastic fibroma."[200]

The epithelial origin of the squamous odontogenic tumor and its apparent tendency to arise in the periodontal ligament suggest that the tumor arises from the rests of Malassez. Most authors have held this view,[194–196, 198–201] although some have also considered the surface mucosa[200] and the rests of Serres[192] as possible sites of origin.

By definition, the tumor is a discrete mass of fibrous connective tissue with a prominent squamous epithelial component; it is not a cystic structure with a proliferation of epithelium in the wall. Some cases reported in the literature represent the latter.[194–196, 198]

Clinical Features. In the 17 acceptable cases, the age of the patients ranged from 11 to 67 years. Cataldo and coworkers calculated the average age of 18 patients to be 36.3 years, with 66 per cent of lesions occurring in people younger than 32.[193] There was a slight female predilection: 57 per cent (12 of 21 cases) occurred in females.

Cataldo and associates noted a nearly equal distribution of cases between the maxilla and mandible. Ten cases occurred in the maxilla, and 10 occurred in the mandible, with both jaws involved in three cases. The incisor-canine area was the most common site in the maxilla, and the premolar region of the mandible was most often affected.[193]

Signs and Symptoms. The squamous odontogenic tumor may be symptomless and diagnosed fortuitously from a radiograph. The most common sign or symptom in 16 cases reviewed by Goldblatt and associates was tooth mobility (eight of 16 cases), and in one third of the cases, tooth mobility was the only sign or symptom. Pain and tenderness following percussion of the associated teeth were also observed. A "vise-like" pressure sensation was experienced by one patient.[193, 196]

Radiographic Features. The usual radiographic appearance of the squamous odontogenic tumor is that of a well-defined semicircular radiolucency that involves the alveolus and surrounds the roots of teeth. Some lesions, particularly when multiple, may exhibit radiographic features that resemble adult or juvenile periodontitis.[199, 200] Root resorption was described in one case.[192] In the maxilla, the tumors do not appear well defined and are more likely to perforate the facial or palatal alveolar plates of bone, extending into adjacent soft tissue.[196, 197, 199, 200]

Histopathology. Characteristically, the tumor is composed of multiple, irregularly shaped islands of benign-appearing squamous epithelium scattered randomly in a mature fibrous stroma. The epithelial islands assume variable shapes, from round to comma-shaped to irregular. The periphery of the epithelial islands appears well defined and is composed of flattened or cuboidal cells that lack any resemblance to the palisaded columnar cells of the ameloblastoma. Keratinization and focal areas of cystic degeneration have been observed in the central portions of the islands. Intraepithelial eosinophilic masses and laminated calcified structures have been described.[194, 197, 199, 200]

Microscopically, it may be difficult to distinguish between the squamous odontogenic tumor and similar-appearing epithelial proliferations in the wall of a cyst.

Wright reported instances of squamous epithelial proliferations in the walls of four dentigerous cysts and one lateral radicular cyst that were histomorphologically identical to the squamous odontogenic tumor.[203] None of the cases showed any tendency to develop into solid tumors, and none recurred.

Behavior. As a result of the limited number of reported cases and, in most instances, an inadequate follow-up period, the long-term behavior of this tumor is difficult to determine at this time. The majority of cases have been managed by conservative surgical procedure and have not recurred.[193, 196]

Ameloblastic and Ectomesenchymal Tumors

Ameloblastic and ectomesenchymal tumors are epithelial tumors with marked inductive change in connective tissue. The following tumors will be discussed:

1. Ameloblastic fibroma.
2. Ameloblastic fibro-odontoma and odontoameloblastoma.
3. Odontomas, complex and compound.
4. Odontogenic fibroma.

Ameloblastic Fibroma

Once considered to be an immature stage of odontoma known as "soft mixed odontoma,"[204] the ameloblastic fibroma is now thought to represent a specific neoplastic entity.[205, 207, 218] Although it bears a superficial microscopic resemblance to ameloblastoma, the ameloblastic fibroma is an entirely different lesion that occurs at a younger age and, most important, behaves in a less aggressive fashion.

The pathogenesis of the tumor is thought to result from a proliferation of ameloblasts that subsequently induce a formation of ectomesenchyme. The loose reticular appearance of the ectomesenchymal stroma resembles that of the embryonic dental papilla.

Incidence. Approximately 60 ameloblastic fibromas have been reported in the medical literature.[205, 206, 210–217,]

[219] Regezi and associates reported that the ameloblastic fibroma composed 2 per cent (15) of 706 odontogenic tumors.[214]

Clinical Features. The ameloblastic fibroma occurs between the ages of 6 months and 42 years, the average age at the time of discovery being 14.6 years.[218] Significantly, four of every 10 cases occur in children younger than 10 years of age, and three of every four cases occur before the age of 19.[218, 219]

The sex distribution is nearly equal. In Slootweg's review of 55 cases, 29 occurred in males, and 26 occurred in females.[218]

There is a marked tendency for ameloblastic fibroma to affect the mandible. Eighty-three per cent (46 of 55 cases) were located in the mandible, and only 17 per cent were maxillary.[218] The vast majority of the tumors in both jaws develop in the posterior regions.[218, 219]

Signs and Symptoms. A painless swelling was the most common presenting sign in nearly 60 per cent of the cases reviewed by Trodahl.[219] Pain, tenderness, and drainage were less common presenting signs or symptoms.[219] Disturbance of tooth eruption has been a prominent clinical feature cited in some previous reports, occurring in up to one third of the cases.[213, 219]

Radiographic Features. The tumors appear radiographically as sharply defined radiolucencies, often with sclerotic borders, which vary from 1 cm to 8.5 cm in diameter.[219] Most of the lesions appear multilocular (3:1), whereas lesions of small size appear unilocular.[219] Expansion of the cortex is often observed, but perforation of the cortex is rare.[221] Three of every four tumors are associated with unerupted teeth.[219]

Histopathology. The ameloblastic fibroma is characterized by the presence of scattered strands, cords, rosettes, or islands of odontogenic epithelial cells in an immature cellular stroma that resembles the dental papilla (Fig. 57–13). The epithelium may be cuboidal and double-layered, resembling the dental lamina, or may be columnar and palisaded with a stellate reticulum, resembling the ameloblastoma. The loose, primitive appearance of the stroma differs markedly from the

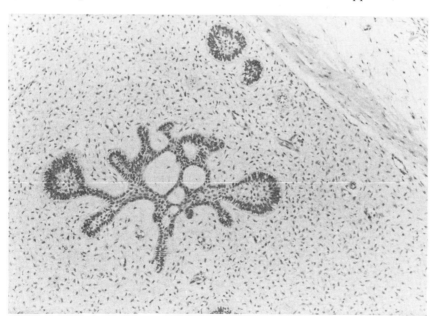

Figure 57–13. Ameloblastic fibroma. Islands of odontogenic epithelium in a stroma that resembles dental pulp tissue. (× 100)

mature fibrous connective tissue stroma seen in the ameloblastoma. There is little pleomorphism or variability in the stromal cells. Mitoses are rare. In some instances, an amorphous, eosinophilic hyaline-like material surrounds the epithelium.[220] The periphery of the tumor is well circumscribed or encapsulated. A case of cystic ameloblastic fibroma with melanin pigment in the epithelial component was reported by Edwards and Goubran.[206]

Behavior. Generally, recurrence of the tumor is considered unlikely if the initial treatment is adequate. There are, however, several reports of recurrent ameloblastic fibromas.[205, 211, 217] Although Trodahl reported a 43.5 per cent rate of recurrence (ten of 23 cases), Zallen and coworkers calculated the cumulative rate of recurrence for the tumor to be 18.3 per cent.[219, 221]

Ameloblastic Fibro-odontoma and Odontoameloblastoma

Hooker is credited with separating these two entities as *ameloblastic fibro-odontoma* and the rare *odontoameloblastoma*.[228, 233] As currently defined, the *ameloblastic fibro-odontoma* contains elements of ameloblastic fibroma combined with features of an odontoma (enamel and dentin) (Fig. 57–14B).[234] In a review of 77 cases, Tsagaris reported a median age of 13 years, with three of every four cases occurring in patients younger than 20 years. Only one recurrence was found in 29 cases, and inadequate surgical removal was considered to be a causative factor in it.[238] Miller and colleagues reported no recurrences in seven cases, with follow-up periods ranging from 3 months to 12 years.[233] The majority of reported cases

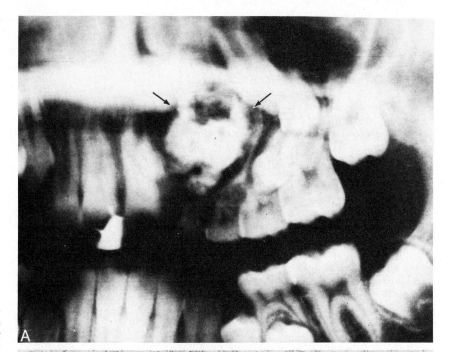

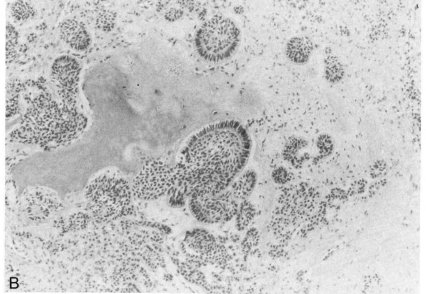

Figure 57–14. Ameloblastic fibro-odontoma. (*A*) Large tumor in the maxilla of a 9-year-old male. (Courtesy of Dr. Mario Luna.) (*B*) Photomicrograph illustrating the soft tissue component of an ameloblastic fibro-odontoma. (×100)

have occurred in the posterior mandible or the anterior maxilla.[233, 237] Slootweg regards the ameloblastic fibroodontoma to be an immature complex odontoma.[237]

Contrary to the nonrecurrent nature of the previous entity, the *odontoameloblastoma* is a locally aggressive, recurrent tumor that is thought to have a rate of recurrence similar to the conventional ameloblastoma.[232] Microscopically, it is composed of enamel and dentin in a mature fibrous stroma with an epithelial component that is identical to ameloblastoma.[234] Radiographically, the odontoameloblastoma and ameloblastic fibro-odontoma usually appear as well-defined radiolucencies with variable irregular radiopacities (Fig. 57–14*A*).

Complex and Compound Odontomas

Although odontomas are usually classified as odontogenic "tumors," they are more accurately defined as malformations or hamartomas. Four subcategories are recognized: complex odontoma, compound odontoma, ameloblastic fibro-odontoma, and odontoameloblastoma. The *complex odontoma*, as defined by the World Health Organization, is a malformation in which all the dental tissues are represented, with the individual tissues being well formed but occurring in a more or less disorderly pattern. The *compound odontoma* is defined as a malformation in which all the dental tissues are represented in a more orderly pattern than in the complex odontoma, so that the lesion consists of many tooth-like structures. Of all the odontogenic hamartomas and tumors, the compound odontoma achieves the highest degree of differentiation.

Incidence. Thirty per cent of the 706 odontogenic tumors reviewed by Regezi and associates were complex odontomas.[243] In a study of 149 odontomas by Budnick, 76 (51 per cent) were the complex type and 73 (49 per cent) were compound.[239]

Clinical Features. Most of the odontomas are detected between the ages of 10 and 30 years. The average age at detection is calculated to be 14.8 years for the complex odontoma and 20.3 years for the compound type.[239]

Reviews of the literature by various investigators have resulted in conflicting conclusions. One author indicated a nearly equal sex distribution,[247] another reported a slight male predominance,[239] and yet another found a marked predilection in males (2:1).[244]

Complex odontomas are more common in the mandible (56 per cent), usually in the posterior region. Compound odontomas show a marked predilection for the maxilla (78 per cent), usually in the anterior region.[244] Odontomas have been reported in unusual sites: McClatchey and associates described a complex odontoma in the retrotympanic area of a young child;[240] Mendelsohn and coworkers reported a giant complex odontoma in the maxillary antrum of a 9-year-old male.[241]

Signs and Symptoms. A swelling or expansion of the buccal plate was the most common sign or symptom. Pain occurs in about 50 per cent of the cases, and absence of a corresponding tooth is observed in 75 per cent. Eighteen per cent of the lesions are discovered fortuitously.[247]

Radiographic Features. Odontomas appear radiographically as irregular radiopaque masses surrounded by a narrow radiolucent band (Fig. 57–15*A*). The complex odontoma presents as a solid radiopacity, whereas the compound type contains multiple tooth-like structures. The differential diagnosis includes condensing osteitis, cementifying fibroma, and benign cementoblastoma.

Histopathology. Microscopically, there is a mixture of enamel, enamel matrix, dentin, pulp tissue, and cementum, which may be arranged in an orderly or haphazard fashion (Fig. 57–15*B*).

Behavior. Odontomas do not recur after simple enucleation. Displacement of tooth buds and resorption of unerupted teeth may occur.

Odontogenic Fibroma

The odontogenic fibroma is an uncommon and poorly understood entity. It is defined as a central odontogenic tumor, of probable ectomesenchymal-epithelial derivation, which is composed of a moderately cellular fibrous connective tissue stroma with variable strands or nests of inactive odontogenic epithelium. Two types have been defined by Gardner: the simple type and the World Health Organization (WHO) type.[251] The *simple* type is composed of scattered rests of odontogenic epithelium in a delicate or dense collagenous stroma (Fig. 57–16). The *WHO* type exhibits numerous strands of odontogenic epithelium and calcifications in the stroma resembling dysplastic dentin or cementum.[249, 251] Care should be taken to avoid misdiagnosing a hyperplastic dental follicle as an odontogenic fibroma. At least 15 odontogenic fibromas have been described in the literature, but very few have been subclassified.[248, 249, 252, 253]

Clinical Features. In a review of 11 cases by Dahl and coworkers, the age distribution ranged from 11 to 80 years, with a mean age of 34 years and a median age of 23 years. Six of the tumors occurred in males, and five were found in females.[248]

Of 15 cases in the literature, 12 (80 per cent) were located in the mandible, and four were in the maxilla.[248, 249, 252–255]

Signs and Symptoms. The tumors are reported to have a slow, persistent growth that results in asymptomatic cortical expansion.[255]

Radiographic Features. Radiographically, the odontogenic fibroma appears as a multiloculated radiolucency that may be associated with unerupted or displaced teeth.[248, 255]

Behavior. Of the 15 cases in the literature, there has been only one recurrence.[252]

Ectomesenchymal (Mesodermal) Tumors

Myxoma

The myxoma (odontogenic myxoma, myxofibroma) is a locally aggressive tumor with no metastatic potential; it arises from primitive mesenchyme, probably derived from the dental apparatus. The precise origin of the tumor has been controversial, generating numerous histochemical and ultrastructural studies.[259, 262–266, 271] Most of the ultrastructural investigations have described the proliferating cell as fibroblast-like but with sufficient differences to warrant the specific designation of *myxoblast*. The majority of the cells appear to be metabolically active and secretory, producing the abundant quantities

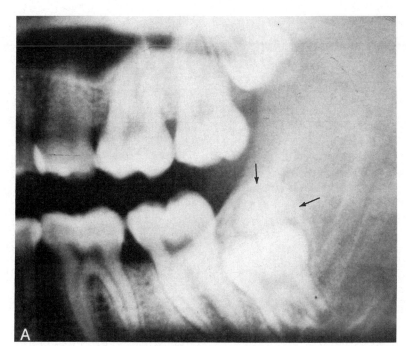

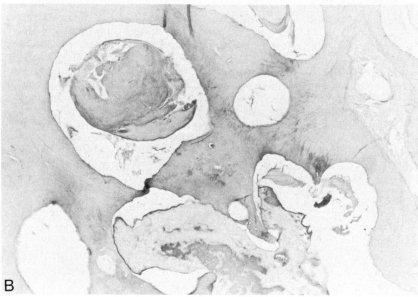

Figure 57–15. Complex odontoma. (*A*) Radiopaque mass overlying the crown of an unerupted third molar tooth. (Courtesy of Dr. Terence Furman.) (*B*) Admixture of the dental hard tissues. (×100)

of mucoid matrix.[259, 262, 266, 272] The electron microscopic features of epithelial islands in the tumor were studied by Harrison[264] and by Hendler and associates.[266] Both concluded that the epithelial cells contained well-developed cellular organelles and were therefore metabolically active, differing from inactive epithelial inclusions such as the rests of Malassez.[264, 266] Yura and coworkers described a myxoma that, by virtue of prominent epithelial cell rests and close association with an embedded third molar, strongly suggested an odontogenic origin.[273]

Incidence. The myxoma is relatively uncommon. Three per cent of 706 odontogenic tumors reviewed by Regezi and associates were myxomas.[270] More than 125 cases have been reported in the medical literature.

Clinical Features. Although about 60 per cent of myxomas arise within the second and third decades,[260] the tumor has affected individuals between the ages of 8 years and 70 years of age. The calculated mean age in four separate studies is as follows: 26.5 years (White and associates, nine cases); 30 years (Zimmerman and Dahlin, 26 cases); 32.7 years (Kangur and associates, 18 cases); and 34 years (Gundlach and Schulz, nine cases).[262, 267, 272, 274]

The tumor is slightly more common in the mandible (60 of 106 cases) than the maxilla (46 of 106 cases).[256–258, 260, 262, 267, 271, 273] The posterior regions are most often affected in both jaws.[260–262, 271] Rarely, the tumor may involve the mandibular condyle and condylar neck.[264, 271]

Signs and Symptoms. The main symptom is a slow, progressive swelling and bony expansion.[262, 266] Mobile

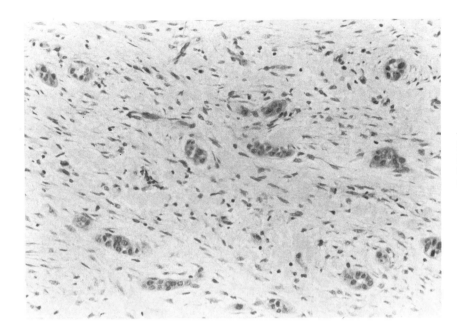

Figure 57–16. Central odontogenic fibroma (simple type). Small nests and cords of odontogenic epithelium in a collagenous stroma. (×200)

teeth, malposed teeth, and unerupted teeth are often a direct consequence of tumor enlargement. Facial asymmetry may be quite prominent. Pain or paresthesia rarely occurs.

Radiographic Features. The radiographic appearance of the myxoma is that of a unilocular or multilocular radiolucency with indistinct borders. Delicate septa in rectangular, square, or triangular shapes may impart a "honeycombed" appearance. The bone cortex may appear thin or perforated. In the maxilla, the maxillary sinus may be involved by tumor. An embedded tooth, missing tooth, or encompassed tooth bud may be associated with the tumor.[264]

Histopathology. Microscopically, the myxoma has a stroma composed of homogeneous ground substance that appears slightly basophilic. Scattered throughout the mucoid ground substance are stellate-shaped cells with branching cytoplasmic processes (Fig. 57–17). Thin bundles of collagen are variable features, and mitotic figures are very rarely seen. Occasionally, strands of inactive odontogenic epithelium are observed.

Behavior. The rate of recurrence in the literature ranges from 10 per cent[258] to 33 per cent.[256] Killey and Kay emphasized the aggressive behavior of the myxoma in a report of four cases, three of which caused extensive bone destruction and recurred several times.[268]

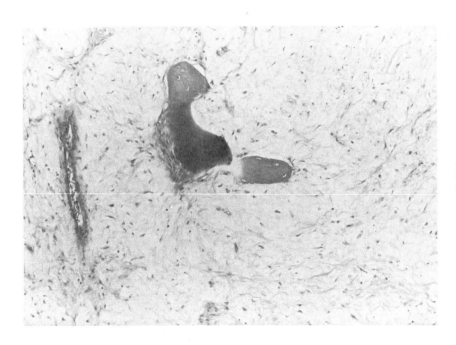

Figure 57–17. Odontogenic myxoma. Note the trabecula of bone which is surrounded by tumor. (×100)

Benign Cementoblastoma

The benign cementoblastoma (true cementoma) is defined by the World Health Organization as "a neoplasm characterized by the formation of sheets of cementum-like tissue, which may contain a very large number of reversal lines and be unmineralized at the periphery of the mass or in the more active growth areas."[287] It is solely ectomesenchymal in origin, developing without inductive phenomena, and is considered to be the only true neoplasm of cemental origin.[276, 280, 287]

Norberg, in a dissertation on odontomes, is credited with the first description of this benign tumor of cementum.[286] Since then, at least 57 instances have been reported.[280, 282, 285, 289] The lesion is characterized as a well-circumscribed radiopaque mass attached to the root of an erupted permanent tooth (Fig. 57–18A).[278]

Incidence. The benign cementoblastoma is a rare odontogenic neoplasm, composing less than 1 per cent of the 706 tumors reviewed by Regezi and associates.[288]

Clinical Features. Of 31 instances reviewed by Farman and coworkers, the youngest patient was 10 years old and the oldest was 72 years of age. The average age at detection of the tumor was 25.5 years. Fifty per cent of the tumors were detected in patients between 10 and 20 years of age.[282]

Cementoblastomas show a slight predilection for males. Of 45 cases studied by Farman and associates, 25 (55.6 per cent) occurred in males, and 20 (44.4 per cent) were in females.[282] An example of the tumor in an 8-year-old female was reported by Esguep and others.[280]

Three of every four lesions are located in the mandible. Thirty-eight of 50 cases (76 per cent) in Farman's review were mandibular, and almost half of them were associated with the mandibular first molar. Of the cases that did not involve the first molar, nearly all of them

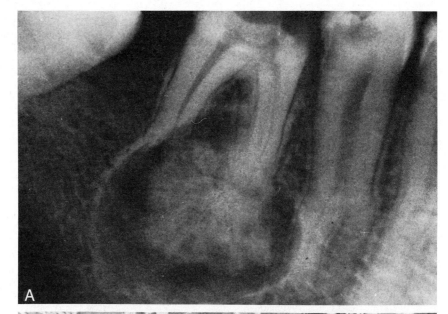

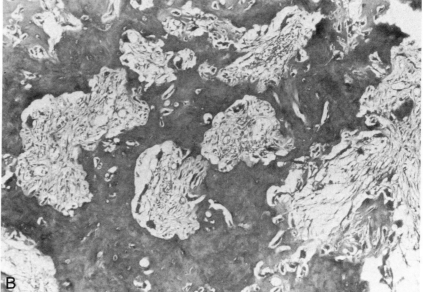

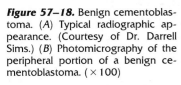

Figure 57–18. Benign cementoblastoma. (*A*) Typical radiographic appearance. (Courtesy of Dr. Darrell Sims.) (*B*) Photomicrography of the peripheral portion of a benign cementoblastoma. (×100)

were associated with premolars, second molars, or third molars; none of the reported cases developed around incisor teeth.[282] All the tumors in the mandible were attached to single teeth, whereas some maxillary lesions were fused to two or more teeth.[275, 278, 282] Involvement of the maxillary sinus has been described in at least two instances.[275, 278]

Signs and Symptoms. Expansion of the jaws, swelling, or facial asymmetry is the most common clinical feature, reported in about two thirds of the cases.[275, 278] Pain, usually of low intensity, is a significant symptom in 50 per cent of the reported cases.[275, 278]

Radiographic Features. The typical cementoblastoma appears radiographically as a well-circumscribed, round radiopaque mass—with a radiolucent periphery—which is fused to a single or multiple roots of a tooth. The affected roots usually appear partially resorbed. The differential diagnosis should include condensing osteitis, odontoma, cementifying fibroma, and benign osteoblastoma.

Histopathology. Microscopically, the tumor consists of a central mass of mineralized cementum, with numerous reversal lines, which is fused to the tooth root. At the periphery, there are variable quantities of cellular fibrous stroma and unmineralized trabeculae of cementum, which are bordered by numerous, large hyperchromatic cementoblasts (Fig. 57–18B). Occasional multinucleated "clast" cells may be observed. The microscopic differential diagnosis should include osteoid osteoma, benign osteoblastoma, and osteosarcoma.

Behavior. The cementoblastoma is considered to be benign with an unlimited growth potential, but little tendency to recur.[277, 279, 282] The rate of growth has been estimated to be approximately 0.5 cm per year.[276, 289]

Ectomesenchymal and Mesenchymal (Mesodermal) Tumors

Along with the ectomesenchymally derived cementoblastoma, the following lesions are included in the broad category of "cementomas":

1. Periapical cemental dysplasia.
2. Cementifying fibroma.
3. Gigantiform cementoma.

They are considered to be of periodontal membrane origin[292] and are composed of an ectomesenchymal cell component (cementum) and a mesenchymal component (fibrous tissue).

Periapical Cemental Dysplasia

According to Regezi and associates, periapical cemental dysplasia (cementoma, periapical fibrous dysplasia, periapical osteofibrosis) accounts for 8 per cent of the odontogenic tumors.[296] It is an innocuous, small lesion that develops at the root apex of a *vital* tooth. Three stages have been described:

1. The initial or osteolytic stage (radiolucent), during which there is a hyperplasia of cementoblasts and fibrous tissue in the periodontal membrane, resulting in periapical bone resorption.
2. The calcifying or cementoblastic stage (mixed radiolucent-radiopaque), during which spicules of cementoid and cementum are deposited in the fibrous stroma.

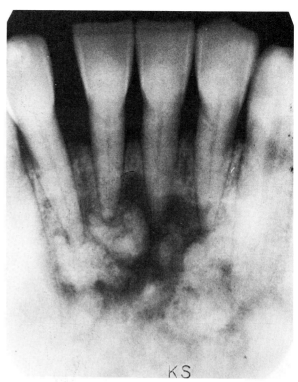

Figure 57–19. Periapical cemental dysplasia, mature stage. (Courtesy of Dr. Paul Stimson.)

3. The mature stage (radiopaque with a thin radiolucent band), which represents calcification into a localized solidified mass (Fig. 57–19).[292]

The lesions usually occur in females (14:1 female to male ratio) who are between the ages of 25 and 45 years.[304] More than 90 per cent of the lesions involve the mandible and are most often associated with the incisor or canine teeth. About seven of every ten patients are black. Most of the lesions are small, usually less than 1 cm in diameter, and are multiple in 70 per cent of the patients.[304] There is an absence of symptoms, there is no local expansion of bone, and all associated teeth are vital.

The radiographic appearance of periapical cemental dysplasia varies from a well-defined radiolucency of the initial lesion to the radiopaque mass of the mature lesion. Depending upon the stage of development, the microscopic features are also varied. The early stage appears as a cellular fibrous stroma without a mineralized component; the intermediate stage contains variable numbers of rounded cementicles and cementoid material; and the mature stage contains larger cementicles, which coalesce to form masses of cementum. Periapical cemental dysplasia is a self-limiting lesion that requires no treatment.

Cementifying Fibroma

Composing about 2 per cent of the odontogenic tumors,[296] the cementifying fibroma (cemento-ossifying fibroma) presents as a solitary, well-circumscribed radiolucent-radiopaque lesion that usually occurs in the premolar-molar region of the mandible. In a study of

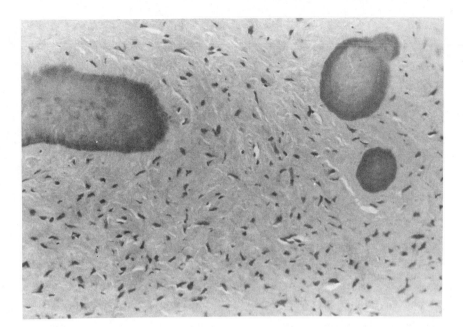

Figure 57–20. Central cementifying fibroma. (×200)

43 cases by Waldron and Giansanti, more than half of the tumors occurred in patients between the ages of 20 and 40 years, with a range of 15 to 70 years. Eighty-four per cent of the lesions affected females, and 86 per cent were located in the mandible.[301] Radiographically, the cementifying fibroma is well delineated and may appear as a radiolucency or a dense radiopacity, depending upon the amount of cementum within the lesion. The size of the lesion ranges from 1 to 7 cm, with the majority of tumors (85 per cent) measuring less than 4 cm in diameter.[301] Microscopically, the lesion consists of a cellular fibrous stroma containing scattered droplets of acellular cementum or rounded and fused basophilic masses of cementum-like tissue (Fig. 57–20). The cementifying fibroma rarely recurs following conservative enucleation.

Gigantiform Cementoma

The gigantiform cementoma is defined as a rare cementoid lesion that is characterized by progressive expansile growth in multiple jaw quadrants, resulting in marked facial deformity. A microscopic picture of variously sized, cementum-like calcific masses in a moderately dense fibrous stroma has been described.

From nosologic and pathogenetic standpoints, the gigantiform cementoma is controversial, and its designation as a separate diagnostic entity is questionable. Several instances—some with apparent familial association—have been reported since Agazzi and Belloni's original cases in 1953.[290, 291, 295, 300, 303] Other cases in the literature with similar clinical, radiographic, and histopathologic features have been described by different terms, such as florid osseous dysplasia, chronic sclerosing osteomyelitis, multiple enostosis, and sclerotic cemental masses.[295]

Another entity with a hereditable tendency and a superficial resemblance to gigantiform cementoma is autosomal dominant cemental dysplasia, which was defined by Sedano and coworkers.[297]

Melanotic Neuroectodermal Tumor of Infancy

Melanotic neuroectodermal tumor of infancy (melanotic ameloblastoma, melanotic progonoma, retinal anlage tumor) is a rare, distinctive neoplasm containing melanin; it primarily affects the maxilla of infants during the first year of life (Fig. 57–21). In the literature, several theories of histogenesis have been proposed for the tumor: (1) it represents a melanocarcinoma derived from enclaved epithelial rests; (2) it is odontogenic in origin; or (3) it is neuroectodermal in origin.[305]

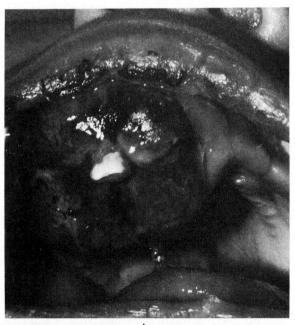

Figure 57–21. Melanotic neuroectodermal tumor of infancy in the anterior maxilla of a 3-month-old female infant. (Courtesy of Dr. Paul Edwards.)

As a result of studies by Borello and Gorlin,[305] Koudstaal and associates,[310] and Nikai and associates,[313] there is now general agreement that the tumor is derived from the neural crest. It is classified with the odontogenic tumors only in an extended sense, based upon the common origin of tumor melanocytes and dental lamina melanocytes from the neural crest.

Incidence. Approximately 65 instances of this rare tumor have been reported in the medical literature.[305–308, 310–316] A review of 53 cases was published by Borello and Gorlin in 1966.[305]

Clinical Features. The tumor most often affects infants younger than 6 months of age. The age of affected infants in the study by Borello and Gorlin ranged from 3 weeks of age to 12 months, with a mean age of 4.1 months. The sex distribution was nearly equal: 26 of 49 cases occurred in males, and 23 cases were in females.[305]

Seventy-nine per cent (44 of 56 cases) were located in the maxilla, usually in the anterior region. Sites other than the anterior maxilla include the anterior mandible, anterior fontanel, temporal bone, frontal area, brain, cerebellum, mediastinum, epididymis, and shoulder.[305–316]

Radiographic Features. Radiographically, the melanotic neuroectodermal tumor of infancy appears as a radiolucency with indistinct borders. In its typical location in the anterior maxilla, the tumor frequently results in destruction of the anterior alveolar process and displacement of partially formed deciduous teeth. The usual size of the tumor varies between 0.5 cm and several centimeters.

Histopathology. Microscopically, the tumor is composed of a prominent fibrous connective tissue stroma that contains numerous alveolar spaces lined by large, melanin-containing cuboidal cells. The spaces contain small hyperchromatic nonpigmented cells, which may exhibit a delicate fibrillar cytoplasm, and on occasion are present in sufficient numbers to completely fill the spaces. Less common microscopic features include the presence of odontogenic epithelium[305] and focal areas of osteogenesis.[316]

Behavior. The melanotic neuroectodermal tumor of infancy is considered a benign neoplasm with a recurrence rate of 15 per cent.[307, 315] Nagase and coworkers reviewed 17 instances of recurrent melanotic neuroectodermal tumors, 12 of which were described as "rapidly growing."[312] A malignant melanotic neuroectodermal tumor with multiple metastases occurring in a stillborn infant was reported by Stowens and Lin in 1974.[315] A second malignant case reported by Dehner and associates was initially diagnosed in the maxilla of a 4-month-old boy and subsequently metastasized, resulting in the death of the patient almost 3 years later.[307] The initial tumor was composed of melanin-containing cells and small dark cells, whereas the metastatic tumor at autopsy was solely composed of small, dark neuroblastoma-like cells.[307]

Malignant Odontogenic Tumors

Odontogenic Carcinomas

When malignant epithelial neoplasms arising from the odontogenic apparatus occur, albeit rarely, they are difficult to diagnose and classify. Some of the reported cases have developed as a result of malignant transformation of a conventional ameloblastoma and retain the histopathologic features of ameloblastoma in the primary tumor and metastatic lesions. Such tumors have been called *malignant ameloblastomas*.

In others, however, the tumor arises from an ameloblastoma but appears poorly differentiated—the so-called *ameloblastic carcinoma*. A third type, the *primary intraosseous carcinoma* (primary intra-alveolar epidermoid carcinoma), is indistinguishable from keratinizing or nonkeratinizing squamous cell carcinoma of oral mucosal origin and is often diagnosed by exclusion.[320, 327–329] In addition, Browne and Gough[318] reported two cases of squamous cell carcinoma that developed as a result of malignant change in the lining of longstanding odontogenic cysts. Elzay[320] proposed a classification of odontogenic carcinomas:

Type 1: Arising ex odontogenic cyst
Type 2: Arising ex ameloblastoma
    a. Well-differentiated (malignant ameloblastoma)
    b. Poorly differentiated (ameloblastic carcinoma)
Type 3: Arising de novo
    a. Nonkeratinizing
    b. Keratinizing

Type 2A: Malignant Ameloblastoma. In a review of the literature by Slootweg and Müller, 20 cases were collected—11 in females and nine in males. The age of patients ranged from 6 to 54 years, with a mean age of 31.3 years. The tumors were almost exclusively located in the mandible (18 of 20 cases). Metastatic involvement was reported in the lung (16 instances), lymph nodes (four instances), spleen, kidney, liver, ilium, ribs, and vertebrae. Eleven of 16 patients died 9 months to 9 years after metastatic disease was noted.[329]

Type 2B: Ameloblastic Carcinoma. Slootweg and Müller also made a compilation of data on reported cases of less differentiated and anaplastic ameloblastic tumors. Twenty-five cases were described, 15 in males and ten in females. The age of patients ranged from 4 years to 75 years, with a mean age of 33.2 years. Eighty per cent of the tumors (20 of 25 cases) were located in the mandible. Sites of metastases included the lungs, lymph nodes, chest wall, liver, peritoneum, brain, intestine, skull, and vertebrae. Seven of nine patients with less differentiated or dedifferentiated tumors died 1 month to 2 years after metastases were first noted. Six of seven patients with anaplastic tumors (without verification of metastases) died 1 year to 45 years after the initial diagnosis of the tumor.[329]

Type 3: Primary Intraosseous Carcinoma. Twelve documented cases of primary intraosseous carcinoma, excluding tumors developing in cysts, were reviewed by Elzay.[320] There was a 3:1 predilection for males, and all but one of the cases were located in the mandible. The age of patients ranged from 4 years to 75 years, with an average age of 45.2 years. Microscopically, the tumors were nonkeratinizing in 58 per cent of the cases, exhibited peripheral palisading in 58 per cent of the cases, and showed a plexiform or alveolar pattern in 67 per cent of the cases. The prognosis is poor, with a 2-year survival rate of only 40 per cent.[320]

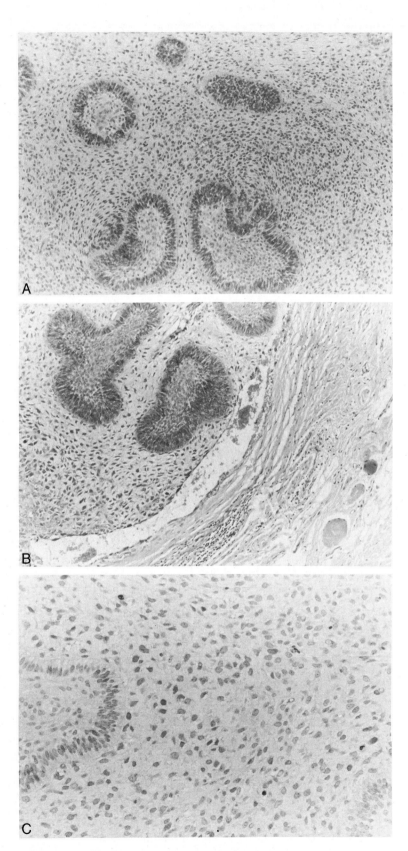

Figure 57–22. Recurrent ameloblastic fibrosarcoma in a 35-year-male. This tumor is the third recurrence during a 14-year period. (*A*) Islands of ameloblastic epithelium in a cellular, sarcomatous stroma. (*B*) Infiltration of the neoplasm into soft tissue. (×100) (*C*) Note the pleomorphism of the stromal cells and numerous mitoses. (Courtesy of Dr. Jose Lomba).

Ameloblastic Fibrosarcoma

As defined by Pindborg and colleagues, the ameloblastic fibrosarcoma is a "neoplasm with a similar structure to the ameloblastic fibroma but in which the mesodermal component shows the features of a sarcoma."[325] A mineralized component consisting of dentin or enamel may also be present.

Incidence. The rarity of the neoplasm is evidenced by the paucity of reported cases. Approximately 30 instances have been described.[317, 319, 321, 323, 328] Leider and coworkers presented the largest series in which they reviewed 11 cases from the literature and added six of their own.[323]

Clinical Features. The average age of the 17 patients in Leider's study was 31 years, with an age range of 13 years to 78 years.[323] When compared with the mean age of patients with the benign counterpart, that is, ameloblastic fibroma, the average ameloblastic fibrosarcoma patient is about 15 to 18 years older.

The distribution between the sexes is about equal, with 11 of 21 cases occurring in females, and 10 occurring in males.[317, 319, 321, 323]

Ameloblastic fibrosarcomas are more common in the mandible than in the maxilla. Seventeen of 24 reported cases were located in the mandible, and seven were in the maxilla. In both mandible and maxilla, the tumors most often occurred in the posterior regions.[317, 319, 321, 323, 328]

Signs and Symptoms. The most common clinical manifestations observed in affected patients were pain and swelling.[323] The swelling is often preceded by pain, a feature that helps to differentiate the ameloblastic fibrosarcoma from other odontogenic tumors.[328] Less frequently, paresthesia of the lower lip, bleeding, and ulceration were reported.[323]

Radiographic Features. Radiographically, the tumors are characterized by diffuse, poorly defined radiolucencies that often exhibit gross expansion and thinning of the cortices. The lesion may appear multilocular and may resemble the ameloblastoma or ameloblastic fibroma, but the peripheral margins are indistinct, irregular, or ragged. Root resorption is a common feature. Progressive, recurrent tumors will result in a marked degree of facial asymmetry or disfigurement.

Histopathology. Microscopically, the tumor differs from its benign counterpart by exhibiting a sarcomatous fibrous stroma (Fig. 57–22A). The cellularity of the stroma, the interlacing pattern of spindle cells, and the presence of numerous mitoses are key features (Fig. 57–22C). The odontogenic epithelial component does not show malignant features. Dysplastic dentin is occasionally observed in association with the odontogenic epithelial islands.[323, 328]

Behavior. The majority of ameloblastic fibrosarcomas are clinically characterized by multiple recurrences over several years (Fig. 57–22A–C).[323, 328] There are a few reports of tumors that metastasized,[319, 321, 328] but the tendency to metastasize appears to be much lower than that of the odontogenic carcinomas.[328] There are several documented cases of ameloblastic fibrosarcomas that developed in pre-existing benign counterparts (ameloblastic fibroma or ameloblastic fibro-odontoma).[317, 319, 321, 328] The histopathologic study of some of the tumors indicated that the epithelial component of the tumor diminishes, and even disappears, as malignant transformation progresses.[323, 325, 328]

REFERENCES

GENERAL REVIEW

1. Baden E: Terminology of the ameloblastoma: History and current usage. J Oral Surg 23:40, 1965.
2. Baden E, Moskow BS, Moskow R: Odontogenic gingival epithelial hamartoma. J Oral Surg 26:702, 1968.
3. Bhaskar SN: Gingival cyst and the keratinizing ameloblastoma. Oral Surgery–Oral Pathology Conference No. 13, Walter Reed Army Medical Center. Oral Surg 19:796, 1965.
4. Bland-Sutton JB: Odontomes. Trans Odont Soc G Brit 20:32, 1888.
5. Broca P: Recherches sur un nouveau groupe de tumeurs designe sous le nom d'odontomes. Gaz Hebd Med Chir 5:19, 1868.
6. Browne RM: The pathogenesis of odontogenic cysts: A review. J Oral Pathol 4:31, 1975.
7. Eversole LR, Tomich CE, Cherrick HM: Histogenesis of odontogenic tumors. Oral Surg 32:569, 1971.
8. Gorlin RJ, Chaudhry AP, Pindborg JJ: Odontogenic tumors: Classification, histopathology, and clinical behavior in man and domesticated animals. Cancer 14:73, 1961.
9. Grand NG, Marwah AS: Pigmented gingival cyst. Oral Surg 17:635, 1964.
10. Lawson W, Abaci IF, Zak FG: Studies on melanocytes. V. The presence of melanocytes in the human dental primordium: An explanation for pigmented lesions of the jaws. Oral Surg 42:375, 1976.
11. Malassez L: Note sur la pathogénie des kystes dentaires dits periostiques. J Conn Med Prat (Paris) 7:98, 1884.
12. Malassez L: Sur la pathogénie des kystes folliculaires des machoires. Comptes Rend Soc Biol (Paris) 2:639, 1885.
13. Pindborg JJ, Clausen F: Classification of odontogenic tumors. Acta Odont Scand 16:293, 1958.
14. Pindborg JJ, Kramer IRH, Torloni H: Histological Typing of Odontogenic Tumors, Jaw Cysts, and Allied Lesions. Geneva, World Health Organization, 1971, pp. 15–23.
15. Reichart PA, Ries P: Zur Bedeutung der neuralleistenzellen in der histogenese und klassifikation der odontogenen tumoren. Dtsch Z Mund-Kiefer-Gesichts-Chir 3:23, 1979.
16. Reichart PA, Ries P: Considerations on the classification of odontogenic tumours. Int J Oral Surg 12:323, 1983.
17. Richardson JF, Balogh K, Merk F, Booth D: Pigmented odontogenic tumor of jawbone. Cancer 34:1244, 1974.
18. Robinson HBG (ed): Oral Pathology. Proceedings of the Fifth Annual Meeting of American Academy of Oral Pathology, 1951. Oral Surg 5:177, 1952.
19. Sciubba JJ, Zola MB: Odontogenic epithelial hamartoma. Oral Surg 45:261, 1978.
20. Shear M: The unity of tumours of odontogenic epithelium. Br J Oral Surg 2:212, 1965.
21. Shear M: Cysts of the Oral Regions, 2nd ed. Boston, Wright-PSG, 1983, p 3.
22. Slootweg PJ, Rademakers LHPM: Immature complex odontoma: A light and electron microscopic study with reference to eosinophilic material and epithelio-mesenchymal interaction. J Oral Pathol 12:103, 1983.
23. Soames JV: A pigmented calcifying odontogenic cyst. Oral Surg 53:395, 1982.
24. Spouge JD: A new look at the rests of Malassez. J Periodontol 51:437, 1980.
25. Stanley HR Jr, Krogh HW, Pannkuk E: Age changes in the epithelial components of follicles (dental sacs) associated with impacted third molars. Oral Surg 19:128, 1965.
26. Stoelinga PJW: Studies on the dental lamina as related to its role in the etiology of cysts and tumors. J Oral Pathol 5:65, 1976.
27. Stout FW, Lunin M, Calonius PEB: A study of epithelial remnants in the maxilla. Abstracts of the 46th General Meeting of The International Association for Dental Research, March 1968, San Francisco, Cal. Abstracts 419, 420, 421:142, 1968.
28. Ten Cate AR: The epithelial cell rests of Malassez and the genesis of the dental cyst. Oral Surg 34:956, 1972.
29. Ten Cate AR: Oral Histology. St. Louis, The C. V. Mosby Co., 1980.
30. Thoma KH, Goldman HM: Odontogenic tumors: Classification based on observations of epithelial, mesenchymal, and mixed varieties. Am J Pathol 22:433, 1946.

GINGIVAL CYST OF INFANTS

31. Cataldo E, Berkman MD: Cysts of the oral mucosa in newborns. Am J Dis Child 116:44, 1968.
32. Epstein A: Uber Eithelperlen in der mundhohle neugeborener Kinder. Ztschr Heilk 1:59, 1880.

33. Fromm A: Epstein's pearls, Bohn's nodules, and inclusion cysts of the oral cavity. J Dent Child 34:275, 1967.
34. Monteleone L, McLellan MS: Epstein's pearls (Bohn's nodules) of the palate. J Oral Surg 22:301, 1964.
35. Moreillon MC, Schroeder HE: Numerical frequency of epithelial abnormalities, particularly microkeratocysts, in the developing human oral mucosa. Oral Surg 53:44, 1982.
36. Shear M: Cysts of the Oral Regions. 2nd ed. Boston, Wright-PSG, 1983, pp 35–39.
37. Stout FW, Lunin M, Calonius PEB: A study of epithelial remnants in the maxilla. Abstracts of the 46th General Meeting of the International Association for Dental Research, March 1968, San Francisco, Cal. Abstracts 419, 420, 421:142, 1968.
38. Wysocki GP, Brannon RB, Gardner DG, Sapp P: Histogenesis of the lateral periodontal cyst and the gingival cyst of the adult. Oral Surg 50:327, 1980.

GINGIVAL CYST OF THE ADULT AND LATERAL PERIODONTAL CYST

39. Alexander WN, Griffith JG: Gingival cysts: Report of two cases. J Oral Surg 24:339, 1966.
40. Baker RD, D'Onofrio ED, Corio RL, et al: Squamous cell carcinoma arising in a lateral periodontal cyst. Oral Surg 47:495, 1979.
41. Bhaskar SN, Laskin DM: Gingival cysts: Report of three cases. Oral Surg 8:803, 1955.
42. Bhaskar SN: Gingival cyst and keratinizing ameloblastoma. Oral Surgery–Oral Pathology Conference No. 13, Walter Reed Army Medical Center. Oral Surg 19:796, 1965.
43. Browne RM: Metaplasia and degeneration in odontogenic cysts in man. J Oral Pathol 1:145, 1972.
44. Buchner A, Hansen LS: The histomorphologic spectrum of the gingival cyst in the adult. Oral Surg 48:532, 1979.
45. Fantasia JE: Lateral periodontal cyst. Oral Surg 48:237, 1979.
46. Grand NG, Marwah AS: Pigmented gingival cyst. Oral Surg 17:635, 1964.
47. Moscow BS, Siegel K, Zegarelli EV, et al: Gingival and lateral periodontal cysts. J Periodontol 41:249, 1970.
48. Reeve CM, Levy BP: Gingival cysts: A review of the literature and a report of four cases. Periodontics 6:115, 1968.
49. Shear M: Cysts of the Oral Regions. 2nd ed. Boston, Wright-PSG, 1983, pp 40–55.
50. Shear M, Pindborg JJ: Microscopic features of the lateral periodontal cyst. Scand J Dent Res 83:103, 1975.
51. Standish SM, Shafer WG: The lateral periodontal cyst. J Periodontol 29:27, 1958.
52. Weathers DR, Waldron CA: Unusual multilocular cysts of the jaws (botryoid odontogenic cysts). Oral Surg 36:235, 1973.
53. Wysocki GP, Brannon RB, Gardner DG, and Sapp P: Histogenesis of the lateral periodontal cyst and the gingival cyst of the adult. Oral Surg 50:327, 1980.

DENTIGEROUS (FOLLICULAR) CYST

54. Ahlfors E, Larsson A, Sjögren S: The odontogenic keratocyst: A benign cystic tumor? J Oral Maxillofac Surg 42:10, 1984.
55. Browne RM: Metaplasia and degeneration in odontogenic cysts in man. J Oral Pathol 1:145, 1972.
56. Browne RM, Gough NG: Malignant change in the epithelium lining odontogenic cysts. Cancer 29:1199, 1972.
57. Cahill DR, Marks SC Jr: Tooth eruption: Evidence for the central role of the dental follicle. J Oral Pathol 9:189, 1980.
58. Craig GT: The paradental cyst: A specific inflammatory odontogenic cyst. Br Dent J 141:9, 1976.
59. Eversole LR, Sabes WR, Rovin S: Aggressive growth and neoplastic potential of odontogenic cysts. Cancer 35:270, 1975.
60. Harris M, Goldhaber P: The production of a bone resorbing factor by dental cysts in vitro. Br J Oral Surg 10:334, 1973.
61. Mourshed F: A roentgenographic study of dentigerous cysts. Oral Surg 18:47 (Part 1), 54 (Part 2), and 466 (Part 3), 1964.
62. Shear M: Cysts of the Oral Regions. 2nd ed. Boston, Wright-PSG, 1983, pp 56–75.
63. Stanley HR, Diehl DL: Ameloblastoma potential of follicular cysts. Oral Surg 20:260, 1965.
64. Struthers PJ, Shear M: Root resorption produced by the enlargement of ameloblastomas and cysts of the jaws. Int J Oral Surg 5:128, 1976.

ODONTOGENIC KERATOCYST

65. Ahlfors E, Larrson A, Sjögren S: The odontogenic keratocyst: A benign cystic tumor? J Oral Maxillofac Surg 42:10, 1984.

66. Brannon RB: The odontogenic keratocyst. Part I. Oral Surg 42:54, 1976.
67. Brannon RB: The odontogenic keratocyst. Part II. Oral Surg 43:233, 1977.
68. Browne RM: The odontogenic keratocyst: Histological features and their correlation with clinical behavior. Br Dent J 131:249, 1971.
69. Chuong R, Donoff RB, Guralnick W: The odontogenic keratocyst. J Oral Maxillofac Surg 40:797, 1982.
70. Connor JM, Price Evans DA, Goose DH: Multiple odontogenic keratocysts in a case of Noonan syndrome. Br J Oral Surg 20:213, 1982.
71. Donatsky O, Hjorting-Hansen E, Philipsen HP, Fejerskov O: Clinical, radiologic, and histopathologic aspects of 13 cases of nevoid basal cell carcinoma syndrome. Int J Oral Surg 5:19, 1976.
72. Forssell K: The primordial cyst: A clinical and radiographic study. Proc Finn Dent Soc 76:129, 1980.
73. Gorlin RJ, Goltz RW: Multiple nevoid basal cell epithelium, jaw cysts, and bifid rib: A syndrome. N Engl J Med 269:908, 1960.
74. Hodgkinson DJ, Woods JE, Dahlin DC, Tolman DE: Keratocysts of the jaw. Cancer 41:803, 1978.
75. Howell JB, Byrd DL, McClendon JL, Anderson DE: Identification and treatment of jaw cysts in the nevoid basal cell carcinoma syndrome. J Oral Surg 25:129, 1967.
76. Payne TF: An analysis of the clinical and histopathologic parameters of the odontogenic keratocyst. Oral Surg 33:538, 1972.
77. Philipsen HP: On "keratocysts" in the jaws. Tandlaegebladet 60:963, 1956.
78. Pindborg JJ, Hansen J: Studies on odontogenic cyst epithelium: II. Clinical and roentgenologic aspects of odontogenic keratocysts. Acta Pathol Microbiol Scand 58:283, 1963.
79. Rud J, Pindborg JJ: Odontogenic keratocysts: A follow-up study of 21 cases. J Oral Surg 27:323, 1969.
80. Shear M: Primordial cysts. J Dent Assoc S Afr 15:211, 1960.
81. Shear M: Cysts of the Oral Region. 2nd ed. Boston, Wright-PSG, 1983, pp 4–34.
82. Southwick GJ, Schwartz RA: The basal cell nevus syndrome: Disasters occurring among a series of 36 patients. Cancer 44:2294, 1979.
83. Stoelinga PJW, Peters JH: A note on the origins of keratocysts of the jaws. Int J Oral Surg 2:37, 1973.
84. Vedtofte P, Praetorius F: Recurrence of the odontogenic keratocysts in relation to clinical and histological features: A 20 year follow-up study of 72 patients. Int J Oral Surg 8:412, 1979.
85. Wright BA, Wysocki GP, Larder TC: Odontogenic keratocysts presenting as periapical disease. Oral Surg 56:425, 1983.
86. Wright J: The odontogenic keratocyst: Orthokeratinized variant. Oral Surg 51:609, 1981.

CALCIFYING ODONTOGENIC CYST

87. Abrams AM, Howell FV: The calcifying odontogenic cyst: Report of four cases. Oral Surg 25:594, 1968.
88. Altini M, Farman AG: The calcifying odontogenic cyst: Eight new cases and a review of the literature. Oral Surg 40:751, 1975.
89. Fejerskov O, Krogh J: The calcifying ghost cell odontogenic tumor—or the calcifying odontogenic cyst. J Oral Pathol 1:273, 1972.
90. Freedman PD, Lumerman H, Gee JK: Calcifying odontogenic cyst. Oral Surg 40:93, 1975.
91. Gorlin RJ, Pindborg JJ, Clausen FP, Vickers RA: The calcifying odontogenic cyst—a possible analogue of the cutaneous calcifying epithelioma of Malherbe. Oral Surg 15:1235, 1962.
92. McGowan RH, Browne RM: The calcifying odontogenic cyst: A problem of preoperative diagnosis. Br J Oral Surg 20:203, 1982.
93. Nagao T, Nakajima T, Fukushima M, Ishiki T: Calcifying odontogenic cyst with complex odontoma. J Oral Maxillofac Surg 40:810, 1982.
94. Nagao T, Nakajima T, Fukushima M, Ishiki T: Calcifying odontogenic cyst: A survey of 23 cases in the Japanese literature. J Maxillofac Surg 11:174, 1983.
95. Pindborg JJ, Kramer IRH, Torloni H: Histological Typing of Odontogenic Tumors, Jaw Cysts, and Allied Lesions. Geneva, World Health Organization, 1971.
96. Praetorius F, Hjørting-Hansen E, Gorlin RJ, Vickers RA: Calcifying odontogenic cyst: Range, variations and neoplastic potential. Acta Odontol Scand 39:227, 1981.
97. Saito I, Suzuki T, Yamamura J, et al: Calcifying odontogenic cyst: Case reports, variations, and tumorous potential. J Nihon Univ Sch Dent 24:69, 1982.
98. Sapp JP, Gardner DG: An ultrastructural study of the calcifications in calcifying odontogenic cysts and odontomas. Oral Surg 44:754, 1977.
99. Shear M: Cysts of the Oral Regions. 2nd ed. Boston, Wright-PSG, 1983, pp 79–86.

100. Soames JV: Pigmented calcifying odontogenic cyst. Oral Surg 53:395, 1982.

RADICULAR CYST

101. Ahlfors E, Larsson A, Sjögren S: The odontogenic keratocyst: A benign cystic tumor? J Oral Maxillofac Surg 42:10, 1984.
102. Bhaskar SN: Oral Surgery–Oral Pathology Conference No. 17, Walter Reed Army Medical Center. Periapical lesions. Oral Surg 21:657, 1966.
103. Browne RM: Metaplasia and degeneration in odontogenic cysts in man. J Oral Pathol 1:145, 1972.
104. Craig GT: The paradental cyst. Br Dent J 141:9, 1976.
105. Grossman LI, Rossman SR: Correlation of clinical diagnosis and histopathologic findings in 101 pulpless teeth with areas of rarefaction. J Dent Res 34:692, 1955 (abstract).
106. LaLonde ER: A new rationale for the management of periapical granulomas and cysts: An evaluation of histopathological and radiographic findings. J Am Dent Assoc 80:1056, 1970.
107. LaLonde ER, Luebke RG: The frequency and distribution of periapical cysts and granulomas. Oral Surg 25:861, 1968.
108. Main DMG: Epithelial jaw cysts: A clinicopathological reappraisal. Br J Oral Surg 8:114, 1970.
109. Morse DR, Patnik JW, Schacterle GR: Electrophoretic differentiation of radicular cysts and granulomas. Oral Surg 35:249, 1973.
110. Mortensen H, Winther JE, Birn H: Periapical granulomas and cysts: An investigation of 1,600 cases. Scand J Dent Res 78:241, 1970.
111. Natkin E, Oswald RJ, Carnes LI: The relationship of lesion size to diagnosis, incidence, and treatment of periapical cysts and granulomas. Oral Surg 57:82, 1984.
112. Rushton MA: Hyaline bodies in the epithelium of dental cysts. Proc R Soc Med 48:407, 1955.
113. Shear M: Cysts of the Oral Regions, 2nd ed. Boston, Wright-PSG, 1983, pp 114–141.
114. Weine FS, Silverglade LB: Residual cysts masquerading as periapical lesions—three case reports. J Am Dent Assoc 106:833, 1983.
115. Yamaguchi A: Hyaline bodies of odontogenic cysts: Histological, histochemical and electron microscopic studies. J Oral Pathol 9:221, 1980.

CLASSIFICATION OF ODONTOGENIC TUMORS AND AMELOBLASTOMA

116. Anneroth G, Johansson B: Peripheral ameloblastoma: A case report (personal communication).
117. Baden E: Terminology of the ameloblastoma: History and current usage. J Oral Surg 23:40, 1965.
118. Baden E: Odontogenic tumors. Pathol Annu 6:475, 1971.
119. Birkholz H, Sills AH, Reid RA: Peripheral ameloblastoma. J Am Dent Assoc 97:658, 1978.
120. Cusack JW: Report of the amputations of portions of the lower jaw. Dublin Hosp Rec 4:1, 1827.
121. Donath K: Odontogene kiefertumoren: Klassifikation, pathogenese, and haufigkeit. Dtsch Med Wschr 102:1291, 1977.
122. Eversole LR, Tomich CE, Cherrick HM: Histogenesis of odontogenic tumors. Oral Surg 32:569, 1971.
123. Eversole LR, Leider AS, Strub D: Radiographic characteristics of cystogenic ameloblastoma. Oral Surg 57:572, 1984.
124. Falksson R: Zur kenntnis der kieferzysten. Virchow's Arch (Pathol Anat) 76:504, 1879.
125. Gardner DG: Peripheral ameloblastoma. Cancer 39:1625, 1977.
126. Gardner DG: Plexiform unicystic ameloblastoma: A diagnostic problem in dentigerous cysts. Cancer 47:1358, 1981.
127. Gardner DG, Corio RL: The relationship of plexiform unicystic ameloblastoma to conventional ameloblastoma. Oral Surg 56:54, 1983.
128. Gorlin RJ: Odontogenic tumors. In Gorlin RJ, Goldman HM (eds): Thoma's Oral Pathology. 6th ed. St Louis, The C. V. Mosby Co., 1970.
129. Gorlin RJ, Meskin LH, Brodey R: Odontogenic tumors in man and animals: Pathologic classifications and clinical behavior—a review. Ann NY Acad Sci 108:722, 1963.
130. Happonen R-P, Newland JR: Cyst formation in ameloblastoma: A histopathologic and electron microscopic study. Proc Finn Dent Soc 78:224, 1982.
131. Hartman KS: Granular cell ameloblastoma. Oral Surg 38:241, 1974.
132. Lucas RB, Thackray AC: Cystic formation in adamantinoma. Br Dent J 93:62, 1952.
133. Ivy RH, Churchill HR: The need of a standardized surgical and pathological classification of the tumors and anomalies of dental origin. Am Assoc Dent Sch Trans 7:240, 1930.

134. Malassez L: Sur le rôle des débris épithéliaux paradentaires. Arch Physiol Norm Pathol 5:309 and 6:379, 1885.
135. Mehlisch DR, Dahlin DC, Masson JK: Ameloblastoma: A clinicopathologic report. J Oral Surg 30:9, 1972.
136. Minderjahn A: Incidence and clinical differentiation of odontogenic tumors. J Maxillofac Surg 7:142, 1979.
137. Moskow BS, Baden E: The peripheral ameloblastoma of the gingiva: Case report and literature review. J Periodontol 53:736, 1982.
138. Patriklou A, Papanicolaou S, Stylogianni E, Sotiriadou S: Peripheral ameloblastoma: Case report and review of the literature. Int J Oral Surg 12:51, 1983.
139. Pindborg JJ, Clausen F: Classification of odontogenic tumors; suggestion. Acta Odont Scand 16:293, 1958.
140. Regezi JA, Kerr DA, Courtney RM: Odontogenic tumors: Analysis of 706 cases. J Oral Surg 36:771, 1978.
141. Reichart P, Ries R: Zur bedeutung der neuralleistenzellen in der histogenese und klassifikation der odontogenen tumoren. Dtsch Z Mund-Kiefer-Gesichts-Chir 3:23, 1979.
142. Reichart PA, Ries P: Considerations on the classification of odontogenic tumors. Int J Oral Surg 12:323, 1983.
143. Robinson HBG: Ameloblastoma: A survey of three hundred and seventy-nine cases from the literature. Arch Pathol (Chicago) 23:831, 1937.
144. Robinson L, Martinez MG: Unicystic ameloblastoma. Cancer 40:2278, 1975.
145. Sapp JP, Milder D: Mucin-producing ameloblastoma: Light microscopic, ultrastructural and histochemical features (abstract). Presented at the Annual Meeting of the American Academy of Oral Pathology, Boston, Mass., May 1984.
146. Sehdev MK, Havos AG, Strong EW, et al: Ameloblastoma of maxilla and mandible. Cancer 33:324, 1974.
147. Shear M: Unity of tumours of odontogenic epithelium. Br J Oral Surg 2:212, 1965.
148. Small IA, Waldron CA: Ameloblastomas of the jaws. Oral Surg 8:281, 1955.
149. Spouge JD: Odontogenic tumors: A unitarian concept. Oral Surg 24:392, 1967.
150. Tsaknis PJ, Nelson JF: The maxillary ameloblastoma: An analysis of 24 cases. J Oral Surg 38:336, 1980.
151. Wesley RK, Borninski ER, Mintz S: Peripheral ameloblastoma: Report of case and review of the literature. J Oral Surg 35:670, 1977.
152. Yokobayashi Y, Yokobayashi T, Nakajima T, et al: Marsupialization as a possible diagnostic aid in cystic ameloblastoma: Case report. J Maxillofac Surg 11:137, 1983.

ADENOMATOID ODONTOGENIC TUMOR

153. Abrams AM, Melrose RJ, Howell FV: Adenoameloblastoma: A clinical pathologic study of ten new cases. Cancer 22:175, 1968.
154. Bedrick AE, Solomon MP, Ferber I: The adenomatoid odontogenic tumor: An unusual clinical presentation. Oral Surg 48:143, 1979.
155. Bhaskar SN: Adenoameloblastoma: Its histogenesis and report of 15 new cases. J Oral Surg 22:213, 1964.
156. Courtney RM, Kerr DA: The odontogenic adenomatoid tumor: A comprehensive study of twenty new cases. Oral Surg 39:424, 1975.
157. Giansanti JS, Someren A, Waldron CA: Odontogenic adenomatoid tumor (adenoameloblastoma): Survey of 111 cases. Oral Surg 30:69, 1970.
158. Lucas RB: A tumor of enamel organ epithelium. Oral Surg 10:652, 1957.
159. Mori M, Makino M, Imai K: The histochemical nature of homogeneous amorphous materials in odontogenic epithelial tumors. J Oral Surg 38:96, 1980.
160. Philipsen HP, Birn H: The adenomatoid odontogenic tumor; ameloblastic adenomatoid tumor; or adenoameloblastoma. Acta Pathol Microbiol Scand 75:375, 1969.
161. Regezi JA, Kerr DA, Courtney RM: Odontogenic tumors: Analysis of 706 cases. J Oral Surg 36:771, 1978.
162. Schlosnagle DC, Someren A: The ultrastructure of the adenomatoid odontogenic tumor. Oral Surg 52:154, 1981.
163. Smith RRL, Olson JL, Hutchins GM, et al: Adenomatoid odontogenic tumor: Ultrastructural demonstration of two cell types and amyloid. Cancer 43:505, 1979.
164. Spouge JD: The adenoameloblastomes. Oral Surg 23:470, 1967.
165. Stafne EC: Epithelial tumors associated with developmental cysts of the maxilla: Report of 3 cases. Oral Surg 1:887, 1948.
166. Subbuswamy SG, Shamia RI: Oral and maxillofacial tumours in northern Nigeria: An analysis over five years. Int J Oral Surg 10:255, 1981.
167. Takaki M: Adenomatoid ameloblastoma: An analysis of 9 cases by

histopathological and electron microscopic study. Bull Tokyo Med Dent Univ 14:487, 1967.
168. Tsaknis PJ, Carpenter WM, Shade NL: Odontogenic adenomatoid tumor: Report of case and review of the literature. J Oral Surg 35:146, 1977.
169. Yazdi I, Nowparast B: Extraosseous adenomatoid odontogenic tumor with special reference to the probability of the basal-cell layer of oral epithelium as a potential source of origin. Oral Surg 37:249, 1974.
170. Yamamoto H, Kozawa Y, Hirai G, et al: Adenomatoid odontogenic tumor: Light and electron microscopic study. Int J Oral Surg 10:272, 1981.

CALCIFYING EPITHELIAL ODONTOGENIC TUMOR

171. Abrams AM, Howell FV: Calcifying epithelial odontogenic tumors: Report of four cases. JADA 74:1231, 1967.
172. Ai-Ru L, Zhen L, Jian S: Calcifying epithelial odontogenic tumors: A clinicopathologic study of nine cases. J Oral Pathol 11:399, 1982.
173. Anderson HC, Kim B, Minkowitz S: Calcifying epithelial odontogenic tumor of Pindborg: An electron microscopic study. Cancer 24:585, 1969.
174. Aufdermaur M: Pindborg tumor. Cancer Res Clin Oncol 101:227, 1981.
175. Baunsgaard P, Lontoff E, Sorensen M: Calcifying epithelial odontogenic tumor (Pindborg tumor): An unusual case. Laryngoscope 93:635, 1983.
176. Chaudhry AP, Holte NO, Vickers RA: Calcifying epithelial odontogenic tumor: Report of a case. Oral Surg 15:843, 1962.
177. Chaudhry AP, Hanks CT, Leifer C, Gergiulo EA: Calcifying epithelial odontogenic tumor: A histochemical and ultrastructural study. Cancer 30:519, 1972.
178. El-Labban NG, Lee KW, Kramer IRH, Harris M: The nature of the amyloid-like material in a calcifying epithelial odontogenic tumor: An ultrastructural study. J Oral Pathol 12:366, 1983.
179. Franklin CD, Pindborg JJ: The calcifying epithelial odontogenic tumor: A review and analysis of 113 cases. Oral Surg 42:753, 1976.
180. Gardner DG, Michaels L, Liepa E: Calcifying epithelial odontogenic tumor: An amyloid-producing neoplasm. Oral Surg 26:812, 1968.
181. Gon F: The calcifying epithelial odontogenic tumor: Report of a case and a study of its histogenesis. Br J Cancer 19:39, 1965.
182. Ivy RH: Unusual case of ameloblastoma of mandible: Resection followed by restoration of continuity by iliac bone graft. Oral Surg 1:1074, 1948.
183. Mori M, Makino M: Calcifying epithelial odontogenic tumor: Histochemical properties of homogeneous acellular substances in the tumor. J Oral Surg 35:631, 1977.
184. Pindborg JJ: Calcifying epithelial odontogenic tumor. Acta Pathol Microbiol Scand Suppl 111:71, 1955 (abstract).
185. Pindborg JJ: A calcifying epithelial odontogenic tumor. Cancer 11:838, 1958.
186. Regezi JA, Kerr DA, Courtney RM: Odontogenic tumors: Analysis of 706 cases. J Oral Surg 36:771, 1978.
187. Smith RA, Hansen LS, DeDecker D: Atypical calcifying epithelial odontogenic tumor of the maxilla. J Am Dent Assoc 100:706, 1980.
188. Stoopack JC: Cystic odontoma of the mandible. Oral Surg 10:807, 1957.
189. Thoma KH, Goldman HM: Odontogenic tumors: Classification based on observations of epithelial, mesenchymal, and mixed varieties. Am J Pathol 22:433, 1946.
190. Wertheimer FW, Zielinski RJ, Wesley RK: Extraosseous calcifying epithelial odontogenic tumor (Pindborg tumor). Int J Oral Surg 6:266, 1977.
191. Yamaguchi A, Kokubu JM, Takagi M, Ishikawa G: Calcifying epithelial odontogenic tumor: Histochemical and electron microscopic observations on a case. Bull Tokyo Med Dent Univ 27:129, 1980.

SQUAMOUS ODONTOGENIC TUMOR

192. Carr RF, Carlton DM Jr, Marks RB: Squamous odontogenic tumor: Report of case. J Oral Surg 39:297, 1981.
193. Cataldo E, Less WC, Giunta JL: Squamous odontogenic tumor: A lesion of the periodontium. J Periodontol 54:731, 1983.
194. Doyle JL, Grodjesk JE, Dolinsky HB, Rafel SS: Squamous odontogenic tumor: Report of three cases. J Oral Surg 35:994, 1977.
195. Fay JT, Banner J, Rothouse L, et al: Squamous odontogenic tumors arising in odontogenic cysts. J Oral Med 36:35, 1981.
196. Goldblatt LI, Brannon RB, Ellis GL: Squamous odontogenic tumor: Report of five cases and review of the literature. Oral Surg 54:187, 1982.

197. Hopper TL, Sadeghi EM, Pricco DF: Squamous odontogenic tumor: Report of a case with multiple lesions. Oral Surg 50:404, 1980.
198. Leventon GS, Happonen R-P, Newland JR: Squamous odontogenic tumor: Report of two cases and review of the literature. Am J Surg Pathol 5:671, 1981.
199. McNeill J, Price HM, Stoker NG: Squamous odontogenic tumor: Report of case with long-term history. J Oral Surg 38:466, 1980.
200. Pullon PA, Shafer WG, Elzay RP, et al: Squamous odontogenic tumor: Report of six cases of a previously undescribed lesion. Oral Surg 40:616, 1975.
201. Swan RH, McDaniel RK: Squamous odontogenic proliferation with probable origin from the rests of Malassez (early squamous odontogenic tumor?). J Periodontol 54:493, 1983.
202. Van der Waal I, deRijcke BM, Van der Kwast WAM: Possible squamous odontogenic tumor: Report of case. J Oral Surg 38:460, 1980.
203. Wright JM: Squamous odontogenic tumorlike proliferations in odontogenic cysts. Oral Surg 47:354, 1979.

AMELOBLASTIC FIBROMA

204. Cahn LR, Blum T: Ameloblastic odontoma: Case report critically analyzed. J Oral Surg 10:169, 1952.
205. Carr RF, Halperin V, Wood C, et al: Recurrent ameloblastic fibroma. Oral Surg 29:85, 1970.
206. Edwards MB, Goubran GF: Cystic, melanotic ameloblastic fibroma with granulomatous inflammation. Oral Surg 49:333, 1980.
207. Gardner DG: The mixed odontogenic tumors. Oral Surg 57:395, 1984.
208. Gardner GD, Smith FA, Weinberg S: Ameloblastic fibroma, a benign tumor treatable by curettage. J Canad Dent Assoc 35:306, 1969.
209. Gorlin RJ, Meskin LH, Brodey R: Odontogenic tumors in man and animals: Pathological classification and clinical behavior. A review. Ann NY Acad Sci 108:722, 1963.
210. Gupta DS, Gupta MK, Wadkar MA, Soni PH: Ameloblastic fibroma or ameloblastic fibrosarcoma: A case report. J Indian Dent Assoc 54:445, 1982.
211. Huebsch RF, Stephenson TD: Recurrent ameloblastic fibroma in a 3-year old boy. Oral Surg 9:707, 1956.
212. Lysell L, Sund G: Ameloblastic fibroma: Report of two cases. Br J Oral Surg 16:78, 1978.
213. Nilsen R, Magnusson BC: Ameloblastic fibroma. Int J Oral Surg 8:370, 1979.
214. Regezi JA, Kerr DA, Courtney RM: Odontogenic tumors: Analysis of 706 cases. J Oral Surg 36:771, 1978.
215. Sawyer DR, Nwoku AL, Mosadomi A: Recurrent ameloblastic fibroma: Report of two cases. Oral Surg 53:19, 1982.
216. Sedano HO: Ameloblastic fibroma: Report of two cases. Oral Surg 17:475, 1964.
217. Shafer WG: Ameloblastic fibroma. Oral Surg 13:317, 1955.
218. Slootweg PJ: An analysis of the interrelationship of the mixed odontogenic tumors—ameloblastic fibroma, ameloblastic fibro-odontoma, and the odontomas. Oral Surg 51:266, 1981.
219. Trodahl JN: Ameloblastic fibroma: A survey of cases from the Armed Forces Institute of Pathology. Oral Surg 33:547, 1972.
220. van Wyk CW, van der Uyver PC: Ameloblastic fibroma with dentinoid formation/immature dentinoma: A microscopic and ultrastructural study of the epithelial-connective tissue interface. J Oral Pathol 12:37, 1983.
221. Zallen RD, Preskar MH, McClary SA: Ameloblastic fibroma. J Oral Maxillofac Surg 40:513, 1982.

AMELOBLASTIC FIBRO-ODONTOMA AND ODONTOAMELOBLASTOMA

222. Anneroth G, Modeer T, Twetman S: Ameloblastic fibro-odontoma in the maxillae: A case report. Int J Oral Surg 11:130, 1982.
223. Bernhoft L, Bang G, Gilhous-Moe O: Ameloblastic fibro-odontoma. J Oral Surg 8:241, 1979.
224. Frissell CT, Shafer WG: Ameloblastic odontoma: Report of case. Oral Surg 6:1129, 1953.
225. Daley TD, Lovas GL: Ameloblastic fibro-odontoma: Report of a case. J Can Dent Assoc 48:467, 1982.
226. Gardner DG: The mixed odontogenic tumors. Oral Surg 57:395, 1984.
227. Hanna PJ, Regezi JA, Hayward JR: Ameloblastic fibro-odontoma: Report of a case with light and electron microscopic observations. J Oral Surg 34:820, 1976.
228. Hooker SP: Ameloblastic odontoma: An analysis of twenty-six cases. Oral Surg 24:375, 1967 (abstract).

229. Hutt PH: Ameloblastic fibro-odontoma: Report of a case with documented four-year follow-up. J Oral Maxillofac Surg 40:1, 1982.
230. Jacobsohn PH, Quinn JH: Ameloblastic odontomas. Oral Surg 26:829, 1968.
231. Josephsen K, Larsson A, Fejerskov O: Ultrastructural features of the epithelial-mesenchymal interface in an ameloblastic fibro-odontoma. Scand J Dent Res 88:79, 1980.
232. LaBriola J, Steiner M, Bernstein ML, et al: Odontoameloblastoma. J Oral Surg 38:139, 1980.
233. Miller AS, Lopez CF, Pullon PA, Elzay RP: Ameloblastic fibro-odontoma: Report of seven cases. Oral Surg 41:354, 1976.
234. Monteil RA, Knoche JF: Etude de l'évolution du terme odontome depuis sa création jusqu'au concept anatomo-pathologique actuel. Actual Odontostomatol 130:583, 1980.
235. Pindborg JJ, Kramer IR, Torloni H: International Histological Classification of Tumors, No. 5. Histological Typing of Odontogenic Tumors, Jaw Cysts, and Allied Lesions. Geneva, World Health Organization, 1971.
236. Sanders DW, Kolodny SC, Jacoby JK: Ameloblastic fibro-odontoma: Report of case. J Oral Surg 32:281, 1974.
237. Slootweg PJ: Epithelio-mesenchymal morphology in ameloblastic fibro-odontoma: A light and electron microscopic study. J Oral Pathol 9:29, 1980.
238. Tsagaris GT: A Review of the Ameloblastic Fibro-odontoma. M.S. Thesis, George Washington University, Washington, D.C., 1972.

COMPLEX AND COMPOUND ODONTOMAS

239. Budnick SD: Compound and complex odontomas. Oral Surg 42:501, 1976.
240. McClatchey KD, Hakimi M, Batsakis JG: Retrotympanic odontoma. Am J Surg Pathol 5:401, 1981.
241. Mendelsohn DB, Hertzanu Y, Glass RBJ, et al: Giant complex odontoma of the maxillary antrum. S Afr Med J 63:704, 1983.
242. Monteil RA, Knoche J-F: Etude de l'évolution du terme odontome depuis sa création jusqu'au concept anatomo-pathologique actuel. Actual Odontostomatol 132:583, 1980.
243. Regezi JA, Kerr DA, Courtney RM: Odontogenic tumors: Analysis of 706 cases. J Oral Surg 36:771, 1978.
244. Slootweg PJ: An analysis of the interrelationship of the mixed odontogenic tumors—ameloblastic fibroma, ameloblastic fibro-odontoma, and the odontomas. Oral Surg 51:266, 1981.
245. Slootweg PJ, Rademakers LHPM: Immature complex odontoma: A light and electron microscopic study with reference to eosinophilic material and epithelio-mesenchymal interaction. J Oral Pathol 12:103, 1983.
246. Sprawson E: Odontomes. Br Dent J 62:177, 1937.
247. Stasinopoulos M: Mixed calcified odontogenic tumors. Br J Oral Surg 8:93, 1970.

ODONTOGENIC FIBROMA

248. Dahl E, Wolfson SH, Haugen JC: Central odontogenic fibroma. Review of literature and report of cases. J Oral Surg 39:120, 1981.
249. Dunlap CL, Barker BF: Central odontogenic fibroma of the WHO type. Oral Surg 57:390, 1984.
250. Freedman PD, Cardo VA, Kerpel SM, Lumerman H: Desmoplastic fibroma (fibromatosis) of the jawbones: Report of a case and review of the literature. Oral Surg 46:386, 1978.
251. Gardner DG: The central odontogenic fibroma: An attempt at clarification. Oral Surg 50:425, 1980.
252. Heimdal A, Isacsson G, Nilsson L: Recurrent central odontogenic fibroma. Oral Surg 50:140, 1980.
253. Schofield IDF: Central odontogenic fibroma: Report of case. J Oral Surg 39:218, 1981.
254. Slootweg PJ, Muller H: Central fibroma of the jaw, odontogenic or desmoplastic: A report of five cases with reference to differential diagnosis. Oral Surg 56:61, 1983.
255. Wesley RK, Wysocki GP, Mintz SM: The central odontogenic fibroma. Clinical and morphologic studies. Oral Surg 40:235, 1975.

ODONTOGENIC MYXOMA

256. Barros RE, Dominguez FV, Cabrini RL: Myxoma of the jaws. Oral Surg 27:225, 1969.
257. Gandra YR, de Abreu EM, di Hipolito O Jr, et al: Central myxoma of the mandible in a child: Report of case. J Oral Surg 39:769, 1981.
258. Ghosh BC, Huvos AG, Gerold FP, Miller TR: Myxoma of the jaw bones. Cancer 31:237, 1973.
259. Goldblatt LI: Ultrastructural study of an odontogenic myxoma. Oral Surg 42:206, 1976.

260. Gorlin RJ, Chaudhry AP, Pindborg JJ: Odontogenic tumors: Classification, histopathology, and clinical behavior in man and domesticated animals. Cancer 14:73, 1961.
261. Gorlin RJ, Goldman HM (eds): Thoma's Oral Pathology. 6th ed. St. Louis, The C.V. Mosby Co., 1970.
262. Gundlach KKH, Schulz A: Odontogenic myxoma—clinical concept and morphological studies. J Oral Pathol 6:343, 1977.
263. Harbert F, Gerry RG, Dimmette RM: Myxoma of the maxilla. Oral Surg 2:1414, 1949.
264. Harrison JD: Odontogenic myxoma: Ultrastructural and histochemical studies. J Clin Pathol 26:570, 1973.
265. Hasleton PS, Simpson W, Craig RDP: Myxoma of the mandible—a fibroblastic tumor. Oral Surg 46:396, 1978.
266. Hendler BH, Abaza NA, Quinn P: Odontogenic myxoma: Surgical management and an ultrastructural study. Oral Surg 47:203, 1979.
267. Kangur TT, Dahlin DC, Turlington G: Myxomatous tumors of the jaws. J Oral Surg 33:523, 1975.
268. Killey HC, Kay LW: Fibromyxomata of the jaws. Br J Oral Surg 2:124, 1965.
269. LeDoussal V, Mahe E, Hebert H: Les fibromyxomes odontogènes: Etude histologique, histochimique et ultrastructurale d'un cas avec revue de la littérature. Arch Anat Cytol Pathol 29:325, 1981.
270. Regezi JA, Kerr DA, Courtney RM: Odontogenic tumors: Analysis of 706 cases. J Oral Surg 36:771, 1978.
271. Stewart SS, Baum SM, Arlen M, Elevezabal A: Myxoma of the lower jaw. Oral Surg 36:800, 1973.
272. White DK, Chen S-Y, Mohnac AM, Miller AS: Odontogenic myxoma: A clinical and ultrastructural study. Oral Surg 39:901, 1975.
273. Yura Y, Yoshida H, Yanagawa T, et al: An odontogenic myxofibroma related to an embedded third molar of the mandible: Report of a case. Int J Oral Surg 11:265, 1982.
274. Zimmerman DC, Dahlin DC: Myxomatous tumors of the jaws. Oral Surg 11:1069, 1958.

BENIGN CEMENTOBLASTOMA

275. Abrams AM, Kirby JW, Melrose RJ: Cementoblastoma: A clinical-pathologic study of seven new cases. Oral Surg 38:394, 1974.
276. Anneroth G, Isacsson G, Sigurdsson A: Benign cementoblastoma (true cementoma). Oral Surg 40:141, 1975.
277. Cherrick HM, King OH, Lucatorto FM, Suggs DM: Benign cementoblastomas: Clinicopathologic evaluation. Oral Surg 37:54, 1974.
278. Corio RL, Crawford BE, Schaberg SJ: Benign cementoblastoma. Oral Surg 41:524, 1976.
279. Curran JB, Collins AP: Benign (true) cementoblastoma of the mandible. Oral Surg 35:168, 1973.
280. Esguep A, Belvederessi M, Alfaro C: Benign cementoblastoma: Report of an atypical case. J Oral Med 38:99, 1983.
281. Eversole LR, Sabes WR, Dauchess VG: Benign cementoblastoma. Oral Surg 36:824, 1973.
282. Farman AG, Kohler WW, Nortje CJ, Van Wyk CW: Cementoblastoma: Report of case. J Oral Surg 37:198, 1979.
283. Hamner JE III, Scofield HH, Cornyn J: Benign fibro-osseous jaw lesions of periodontal membrane origin. Cancer 22:861, 1968.
284. Langdon JD: The benign cementoblastoma—just how benign? Br J Oral Surg 13:239, 1976.
285. Monks FT, Bradley JC, Turner EP: Central osteoblastoma or cementoblastoma? A case report and 12 year review. Br J Oral Surg 19:29, 1981.
286. Norberg O: Zur kenntis der dysonto genetischen geschwulste der kieferknochen. Vischr Zahnheilk 46:321, 1930.
287. Pindborg JJ, Kramer IRH, Torloni H: Classification of Odontogenic Tumors. Geneva, World Health Organization, 1971.
288. Regezi JA, Kerr DA, Courtney RM: Odontogenic tumors: Analysis of 706 cases. J Oral Surg 36:771, 1978.
289. Vindenes H, Nilsen R, Gilhuus-Moe O: Benign cementoblastoma. Int J Oral Surg 8:318, 1979.

CEMENTAL LESIONS (EXCLUDING CEMENTOBLASTOMA)

290. Agazzi C, Belloni L: Gli odontomi duri dei mascelari. Arch Ital Otol (Supp. 16) 64:5, 1953.
291. Cannon JS, Keller EE, Dahlin DC: Gigantiform cementoma: Report of two cases (mother and son). J Oral Surg 38:65, 1980.
292. Hamner JE III, Scofield HH, Cornyn J: Benign fibro-osseous jaw lesions of periodontal membrane origin. Cancer 22:861, 1968.
293. Krausen AS, Pullon PA, Gulmen S, et al: Cementomas—aggressive or innocuous neoplasms? Arch Otolaryngol 103:349, 1977.
294. Pindborg JJ, Kramer IRH, Torloni H: Histological typing of odontogenic tumors, jaw cysts and allied lesions. International Classi-

fication of Tumors, No. 5, Geneva, World Health Organization, 1971.

295. Punniamoorthy A: Gigantiform cementoma: Review of the literature and a case report. Br J Oral Surg 18:221, 1980.

296. Regezi JA, Kerr DA, Courtney RM: Odontogenic tumors: Analysis of 706 cases. J Oral Surg 36:771, 1978.

297. Sedano HO, Kuba R, Gorlin RJ: Autosomal dominant cemental dysplasia. Oral Surg 54:642, 1982.

298. Sugimura M, Okunaga T, Yoneda T, et al: Cementifying fibroma of the maxilla—report of a case. Int J Oral Surg 10:298, 1981.

299. Sweet RM, Bryarly RC, Kornblut AD, Corio RL: Recurrent cementifying fibroma of the jaws. Laryngoscope 91:1137, 1981.

300. Van der Waal I, Van der Kwast WAM: A case of gigantiform cementoma. Int J Oral Surg 3:440, 1974.

301. Waldron CA, Giansanti JS: Benign fibro-osseous lesions of the jaws: A clinical-radiologic-histologic review of sixty-five cases. II. Benign fibro-osseous lesions of periodontal ligament origin. Oral Surg 35:340, 1973.

302. Waldron CA, Giansanti JS, Browand BC: Sclerotic cemental masses of the jaws (so-called chronic sclerosing osteomyelitis, sclerosing osteitis, multiple enostosis, and gigantiform cementoma). Oral Surg 39:590, 1975.

303. Winer HJ, Goepp RA, Olsen RE: Gigantiform cementoma resembling Paget's disease: Report of a case. J Oral Surg 30:517, 1972.

304. Zegarelli EV, Kutscher AH, Napoli N, et al: The cementoma—a study of 230 patients with 435 cementomas. Oral Surg 17:219, 1964.

MELANOTIC NEUROECTODERMAL TUMOR OF INFANCY

305. Borello ED, Gorlin RJ: Melanotic neuroectodermal tumor of infancy—a neoplasm of neural crest origin. Report of a case associated with high urinary excretion of vanilmandelic acid. Cancer 19:196, 1966.

306. Brekke JH, Gorlin RJ: Melanotic neuroectodermal tumor of infancy. J Oral Surg 33:858, 1975.

307. Dehner LP, Sibley RK, Sauk JJ Jr, et al: Malignant melanotic neuroectodermal tumor of infancy: A clinical, pathologic, ultrastructural, and tissue culture study. Cancer 43:1389, 1979.

308. Dooling EC, Chi JG, Gilles FH: Melanotic neuroectodermal tumor of infancy: Its histological similarities to fetal pineal gland. Cancer 39:1535, 1977.

309. Kerr DA, Pullon PA: A study of the pigmented tumors of jaws of infants (melanotic ameloblastoma, retinal anlage tumor, progonoma). Oral Surg 18:759, 1964.

310. Koudstaal J, Oldhoff J, Panders AK, Hardonk MJ: Melanotic neuroectodermal tumor of infancy. Cancer 22:151, 1968.

311. Lindahl F: Malignant melanotic progonoma: One case. Acta Pathol Microbiol Scand (Sect. A) 78:532, 1970.

312. Nagase M, Ueda K, Fukushima M, Nakajima T: Recurrent melanotic neuroectodermal tumour of infancy: Case report and survey of 16 cases. J Maxillofac Surg 11:131, 1983.

313. Nikai H, Ijuhin N, Yamasaki A, et al: Ultrastructural evidence for neural crest origin of the melanotic neuroectodermal tumor of infancy. J Oral Pathol 6:221, 1977.

314. Stokke T: Pigmented jaw tumor in an infant: A melanocytoma. Acta Odont Scand 26:657, 1968.

315. Stowens D, Lin T-H: Melanotic progonoma of the brain. Hum Pathol 5:105, 1974.

316. Williams AO: Melanotic ameloblastoma ("progonoma") of infancy showing osteogenesis. J Pathol Bact 93:545, 1967.

MALIGNANT ODONTOGENIC TUMORS

317. Adekeye EO, Edwards MB, Goubran GF: Ameloblastic fibrosarcoma. Oral Surg 46:254, 1978.

318. Browne RM, Gough NG: Malignant change in the epithelium lining odontogenic cysts. Cancer 29:1199, 1972.

319. Chomette G, Auriol M, Guilbert F, et al: Ameloblastic fibrosarcoma: A clinical and anatomopathological study of three cases. Histoenzymological and ultrastructural data. Arch Anat Cytol Pathol 30:172, 1982.

320. Elzay RP: Primary intraosseous carcinoma of the jaws: Review and update of odontogenic carcinomas. Oral Surg 54:299, 1982.

321. Howell RM, Burkes EJ Jr: Malignant transformation of ameloblastic fibro-odontoma to ameloblastic fibrosarcoma. Oral Surg 43:391, 1977.

322. Kalmar JR, Weathers DR: Primary intraosseous squamous cell carcinoma of the jaws: A report of four cases and review of the literature with 5-year survival data (abstract). Presented at the Annual Meeting of the American Academy of Oral Pathology, Boston, Mass., May 1984.

323. Leider AS, Nelson JF, Trodahl JN: Ameloblastic fibrosarcoma of the jaws. Oral Surg 33:559, 1972.

324. Melrose RJ, Abrams AM, Mills BG: Florid osseous dysplasia. Oral Surg 41:62, 1976.

325. Pindborg JJ, Kramer IRH, Torloni H: Histological Typing of Odontogenic Tumors, Jaw Cysts, and Allied Lesions. Geneva, World Health Organization, 1971.

326. Reichart PA, Zobl H: Transformation of ameloblastic fibroma to fibrosarcoma: Report of a case. Int J Oral Surg 7:503, 1978.

327. Shear M: Primary intra-alveolar epidermoid carcinoma of the jaw. J Pathol Biol 97:645, 1969.

328. Shear M, Altini M: Malignant odontogenic tumors. J Dent Assoc South Afr 37:547, 1982.

329. Slootweg PJ, Müller H: Malignant ameloblastoma or ameloblastic carcinoma. Oral Surg 57:168, 1984.

MANAGEMENT OF ODONTOGENIC CYSTS AND TUMORS

Edward Ellis III, D.D.S., M.S. • Raymond J. Fonseca, D.M.D.

Before the management of the odontogenic tumors is presented, cysts of the jaws and their management will be discussed briefly. Although cysts are tumors only in the broadest sense of the word, the principles in their management are very useful for the more benign odontogenic tumors. Also, they are more common in clinical practice than are the odontogenic tumors.

Oral tumors may be classified as *odontogenic* or *non-odontogenic*. "Odontogenic" signifies a tumor composed of cells whose primary purpose is (or was) to form teeth or tooth-related structures. Aberrations from the normal pattern of odontogenesis may occur at any stage in tooth development and give rise to odontogenic tumors. These tumors may, in their development, produce teeth or tooth-like structures. They are unique to the jaws, and most of these lesions are intraosseous. All of them display distinctive histologic anatomy and variable clinical expression. However, the odontogenic tumors are benign, with few exceptions, and therefore do not require radical surgery for cure. In fact, many are treated with enucleation or curettage.

In odontogenic tumors treated with partial removal

of the jaw, immediate reconstruction has been the rule. As the reconstructive efforts constitute a vital aspect of the therapeutic regimen, this topic will be explored along with the discussion of the curative extirpative surgery.

CYSTS OF THE JAWS

A cyst is defined generally as an epithelium-lined sac filled with fluid or soft material. The prevalence of cysts in the jaws can be related to the abundant epithelium that gets into bone through the process of tooth formation and along lines where the surfaces of embryologic jaw processes fuse. We therefore may divide cysts of the jaws into two types: those arising from odontogenic epithelium (odontogenic cysts) and those from oral epithelium that is trapped between fusing processes during embryogenesis (fissural cysts) (Table 57–5).

The stimulus that causes resting epithelial cells to proliferate into the surrounding connective tissue has not been determined. Inflammation seems to play a major role in those arising in granulomas from infected dental pulps.

There is a tendency for residual fragments of cyst membrane to produce recurrent cysts. This necessitates complete excision of the epithelial lining of the cyst at the time of operation. Some cysts (for example, keratocysts) behave more aggressively in both destructive characteristics and recurrence rates. Cysts have been known to destroy large portions of the jaws and to push teeth into the most remote areas of the jaws (mandibular condyle, mandibular angle, and coronoid process). Enlargement of cysts is caused by a gradual expansion, and most are discovered on routine dental radiography. Cysts are asymptomatic unless they are secondarily infected. The overlying mucosa is normal in color and consistency; there are no sensory deficits from encroachment on nerves. Palpation with firm pressure may indent the surface of an expanded jaw with characteristic rebound resiliency.

The radiographic appearance of cysts is characteristic and exhibits a distinct, dense periphery of reactive bone (condensing osteitis) with a radiolucent center. Most cysts are unilocular in nature; however, multilocularity is often seen in some dentigerous cysts and cystic ameloblastomas. Cysts do not usually cause resorption of the roots of teeth, but when seen, one should be suspicious of neoplasm. The epithelial lining of cysts may, on rare occasions, undergo ameloblastic or malignant changes. Therefore all must be submitted for pathologic examination.[6]

Fissural Cysts

A number of different types of fissural (or inclusion) cysts of bone occur in the jaws and are assumed to be caused by proliferation of epithelium trapped along lines of fusion of embryologic processes. These are true epithelium-lined cysts and may be classified as follows:
1. Nasopalatine duct cyst.
2. Median maxillary cyst.
3. Globulomaxillary cyst.
4. Median mandibular cyst (Table 57–5).

These cysts are associated with vital teeth unless affected by other forms of disease. Preservation of the teeth must therefore be assured. Those occurring in the maxilla may be lined by respiratory or squamous epithelium.

Nasopalatine Duct Cyst (Incisive Canal Cyst). This is the most common of the fissural cysts and must be differentiated from the normal nasopalatine canal. They can grow to a large size and are removed by a palatal approach to avoid disrupting the blood supply to the dental pulps of the anterior teeth (Figs. 57–23 and 57–24).

TABLE 57–5. Epithelial Cysts of the Jaws

Fissural
  Nasopalatine duct (incisive canal)
  Median maxillary (midpalatine)
  Globulomaxillary
  Median mandibular

Odontogenic
  Periodontal
    Apical
    Lateral
    Residual
  Dentigerous
  Odontogenic keratocyst
    Nevoid basal cell carcinoma syndrome
  Keratinizing and calcifying odontogenic cyst

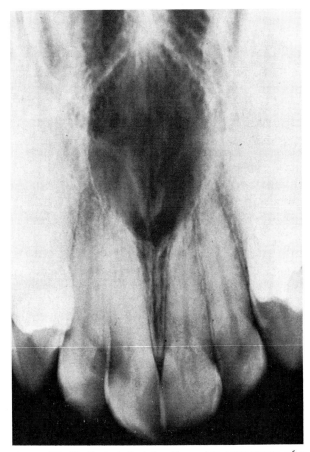

Figure 57–23. Typical dental radiographic appearance of a nasopalatine duct cyst. These teeth are vital.

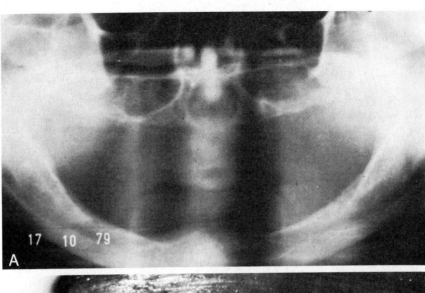

Figure 57–24. Nasopalatine duct cyst. (*A*) Panoramic radiographic appearance of a large nasopalatine duct cyst in an edentulous patient. (*B*) Cyst being enucleated at surgery via a palatal approach. (*C*) Cyst and aspirated fluid after removal.

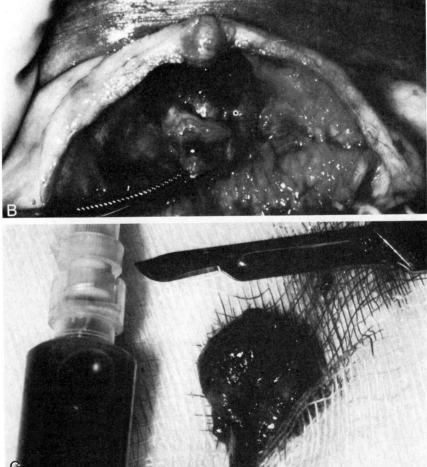

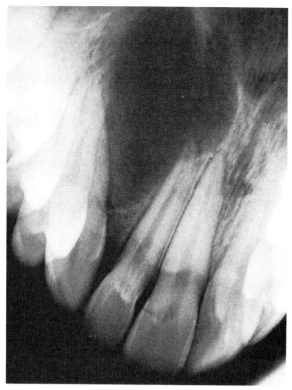

Figure 57–25. Typical dental radiographic appearance of a globulomaxillary cyst. Note divergence of roots of teeth.

Median Maxillary (Palatal) Cyst. This cyst is formed by epithelium trapped in the suture between the two lateral palatal shelves and may involve the nose and maxillary sinus. They are rarely symmetric in location and may appear to be located more to one side of the palatal midline than the other.

Globulomaxillary Cyst. This cyst is formed from epithelial remnants between the medial nasal and maxillary processes. The location is characteristic and occurs between the incisor and cuspid tooth. It frequently causes divergence of their roots and is often pear-shaped (Fig. 57–25).

Median Mandibular Cyst. This is an extremely rare cyst and may result from epithelium entrapped within a cleft in the mandibular symphysis.

Odontogenic Cysts

The odontogenic cysts are derived from proliferation of the epithelium associated with the developing dental apparatus. Several types of cysts may occur, depending chiefly upon the stage of odontogenesis during which they originate, and various investigators have attempted to devise a classification and system of nomenclature of the lesions. Controversy exists in classification, however. One which is simple, yet helpful, is presented in Table 57–5.

Periapical (Radicular) Cyst. These cysts are the most common of all cystic lesions of the jaws and result from inflammation or necrosis of the dental pulp (Fig. 57–26). Pulp vitality tests will help in making a diagnosis. A vital tooth rules out the possibility of an associated radicular cyst. Endodontic treatment of the tooth is followed by a period of observation, for it is impossible to differentiate between a cyst and periapical granuloma on a radiograph. If the radiolucency remains static or enlarges, a cyst should be suspected and periapical surgical excision of the lesion should be undertaken. Alternatively, extraction with enucleation via the tooth socket can be readily accomplished when the cyst is small. When large, a mucoperiosteal flap may be reflected, and access to the cyst is obtained through the labial plate of bone. This leaves the alveolar crest intact to ensure adequate bone height following healing.

Lateral Periodontal Cyst. This is an uncommon cyst that is usually small and appears between the roots of the mandibular bicuspid teeth[46] (Fig. 57–27). This cyst is associated with vital teeth and may result from proliferation of epithelial rests within the periodontal ligament. When possible, it is treated by surgical excision without damage to the adjacent tooth roots.

Residual Cyst. This cyst is a radicular cyst that has been overlooked after extraction of the causative tooth (Fig. 57–28). It either remains static or enlarges and is treated by enucleation.

Dentigerous Cyst (Follicular Cyst). The dentigerous cyst originates through alteration of the reduced enamel epithelium after the crown of the tooth has been completely formed. Fluid accumulates between the reduced enamel epithelium and the tooth crown. Therefore, it is always associated with the crown of a tooth, most commonly the impacted mandibular third molar.[11, 42]

The dentigerous cyst is capable of becoming an aggressive lesion with expansion of bone, facial asymmetry, and extreme displacement of teeth (Fig. 57–29). It is more often unilocular than multilocular. The possibility of ameloblastic or malignant change should be considered in any cyst, particularly dentigerous cysts that show multilocularity. It is imperative that thorough histologic examination of the specimen be undertaken to detect these changes.

Odontogenic Keratocyst (Primordial Cyst). A primordial cyst is one that arises from the enamel organ prior to formation of the calcified tissues and thus is found in place of a tooth. However, it may occur with a full complement of teeth and in this case probably represents degeneration of a supernumerary tooth. All primordial cysts have been found to histologically represent keratocysts; thus, great controversy and confusion have been focused on the difference between the odontogenic keratocyst and primordial cyst.[20, 40] However, a keratocyst is one with distinctive histologic characteristics that many feel can be associated with dentigerous, lateral periodontal, and residual cysts as well as "primordial" cysts.[16] Others contend that an odontogenic keratocyst found in conjunction with an impacted tooth or the apex of a root is a collision phenomenon.[47]

Radiographically, these cysts may produce multilocularity and great invasion of the jaw, and surprisingly, in many cases, expansion is not marked. They sometimes appear so destructive that an odontogenic tumor is suspected (Fig. 57–30).

The controversy surrounding the odontogenic keratocyst stems from their aggressive clinical behavior and their markedly increased rate of recurrence.[16] Reported recurrence rates have been between 20 and 60 per cent.[42] Reasons for locally aggressive behavior are based upon the increased mitotic activities and increased cellularity

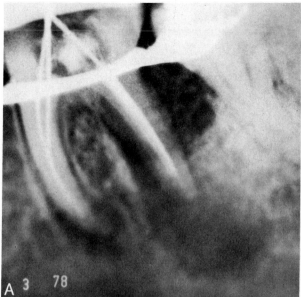

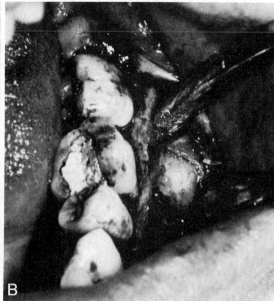

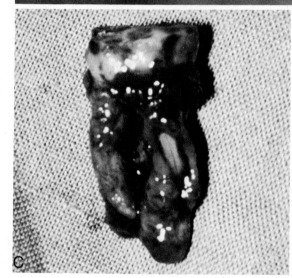

Figure 57–26. Radicular cyst attached to a tooth that previously had undergone root-canal therapy. (*A*) Dental radiographic appearance. (*B*) Cyst wall exposed at time of extraction. (*C*) Extracted tooth with cyst attached to root.

Figure 57–27. Typical dental radiographic appearance of lateral periodontal cyst. These teeth are vital.

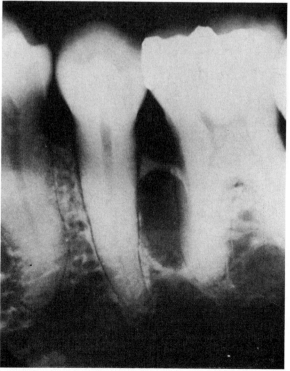

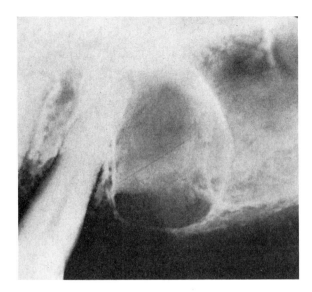

Figure 57–28. Typical dental radiographic appearance of a residual cyst in the maxilla.

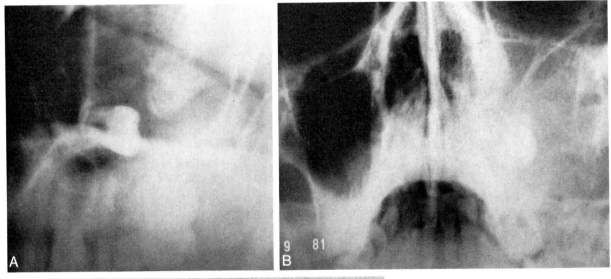

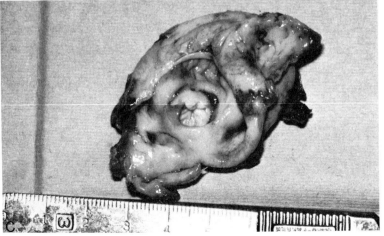

Figure 57–29. Dentigerous cyst causing extreme displacement of the maxillary third molar tooth. (*A*) Lateral radiographic view (note clouding of the sinus). (*B*) Waters view. (*C*) Specimen after enucleation. Note the relationship of the tooth crown to the lumen of the cyst.

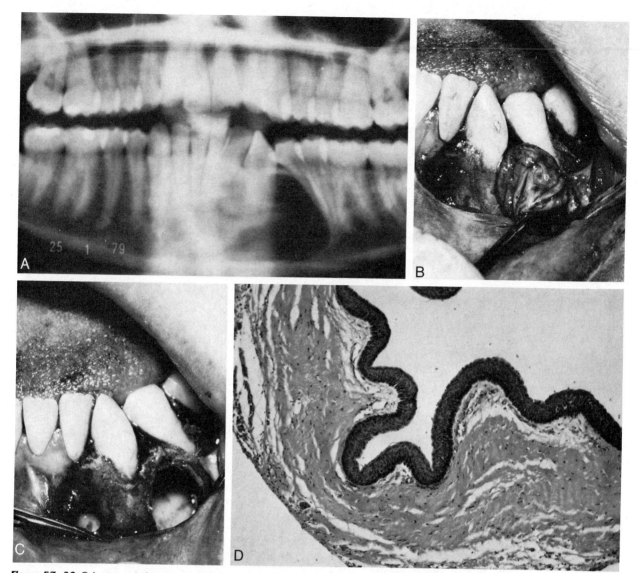

Figure 57–30. Odontogenic keratocyst in a 16-year-old female. (A) Radiographic appearance demonstrating displacement of teeth and considerable destruction of the mandible. These teeth are vital. (B) Cyst being enucleated. (C) Defect in mandible following enucleation. (D) Typical histologic appearance of odontogenic keratocyst.

of the odontogenic keratocyst's epithelium.[33, 49, 53] Daughter or satellite cysts, found in the periphery of the main cystic lesion, may be incompletely removed, contributing to the increased rate of recurrence. The cystic lining is usually very thin and readily fragments, making thorough enucleation difficult.

Because little has been written comparing treatment modalities for the odontogenic keratocyst, present treatment has been based largely on the surgeon's past experience. From our experience, when an odontogenic keratocyst is clinically suspected, the minimal treatment should be a careful enucleation with an aggressive curettage of the bony cavity. Should a recurrence develop, treatment must then be predicated on several factors: if the area is accessible, another attempt at enucleation could be undertaken; if inaccessible, bony resection with 1-cm margins should be considered.

Whatever the treatment, the patient must be followed closely for recurrence because odontogenic keratocysts have recurred years following treatment.

Stoelinga[47] contends that recurrences result from invasion of the bone from epithelium in soft tissues. Support for this is offered by recurrences within bone grafts placed following resections. He has noted a constant fusion of the cystic wall with the oral mucosa in at least one area of the cyst. It is usually along the anterior border of the ascending mandibular ramus where no bone is present. Histologic sections of this area demonstrate an abundance of epithelial cells and strands of cells. Many of the cells are cystic or in the process of becoming so.

Stoelinga feels that excision of soft tissue within the bony perforation, including the overlying oral mucosa, should be done in order to cure the lesion. Cauterizing select areas that are inaccessible with Carnoy's solution is then performed. In his hands, a 5 to 6 per cent recurrence rate was obtained using this method.

Nevoid Basal Cell Carcinoma Syndrome. This genetic syndrome is transmitted as an autosomal dominant characteristic with a high rate of penetrance.[5, 24] These patients demonstrate multiple keratocysts of the jaws. Other abnormalities include nevoid basal cell carcinomas, skeletal deformities of vertebra and ribs, palmar skin pits, and ectopic calcification of soft tissues. The keratocysts in these patients appear earlier and are characterized by multiplicity, bilaterality, and continued development.[35] This is an important surgical point because continued formation of new cysts may occur for years and can make it difficult to distinguish recurrence from new cyst formation. In any event, these patients require lifelong monitoring of their cutaneous lesions and jaw cysts.

Keratinizing and Calcifying Odontogenic Cyst. This cyst is a unique lesion because it possesses some features of a cyst but also has many characteristics of a solid neoplasm. Most of these cysts occur centrally within bone and in the mandible. Radiographically, they may appear as cysts, but they may contain variable amounts of calcified radiopaque material, ranging from tiny flecks to large masses. These lesions may obtain large dimensions, involving much of the jaw. Treatment is similar to that of the odontogenic keratocyst.

Surgical Treatment of Jaw Cysts

Cysts of the jaws are treated in one of three basic methods:

1. Enucleation.
2. Partch marsupialization.
3. A staged combination of the two procedures.

Enucleation is the treatment of choice whenever possible; however, several factors may mitigate against this procedure. Proximity of the cyst to vital and important structures can mean unnecessary sacrifice of tissue if enucleation is carried out on some large cysts of the jaws. Therefore, a preliminary Partch operation may permit the repair of bone to re-establish new bone for protection of the maxillary sinus, nasal cavity, and inferior alveolar canal. It can also conserve the nerve and blood supply to involved teeth.[27] The Partch operation may also be useful in cysts that have weakened the involved jaw to the point at which pathologic fracture might occur if enucleation were attempted (Fig. 57–31A).

The initial Partch procedure must provide an opening large enough to obtain a representative specimen of the cyst wall for biopsy and histologic diagnosis (Fig. 57–31B). The opening must be large enough to permit complete inspection of the inner aspect of the cystic wall in order to rule out abnormal thickenings that may represent neoplastic transformation of the epithelial lining. The margins of the oral epithelium are sutured to the cystic wall, and the surgically created window must be kept patent. The patient is given an irrigating syringe and instructed in its use so that daily irrigations can be performed to prevent infection (Fig. 57–31C). Antibiotics are prescribed for 1 week.

Following a Partch operation, initial healing is rapid, but the size of the cavity may not decrease appreciably past a certain point. The objectives of the Partch procedure have been accomplished at this time, and a secondary enucleation may be undertaken without injury to adjacent structures (Fig. 57–31D to F). This reduces the morbidity and accelerates complete healing to obliterate the defect. Another advantage, which we have noticed in using the Partch operation, is the development of a thickened cystic lining, which makes the secondary enucleation an easier procedure.

Enucleation of cysts should be done with care in an attempt to remove the cyst in one piece without fragmentation. This reduces the chances of recurrence by increasing the chance of total removal. Those cysts that surround tooth roots, or that are in inaccessible areas of the jaws, require aggressive curettage to remove fragments of cyst lining that could not be removed with the bulk of the cyst wall. Should obvious devitalization of teeth occur during a cystectomy, endodontic treatment of the teeth should be undertaken. This helps to prevent odontogenic infection of the cystic cavity from the necrotic dental pulp.

Following enucleation, a water-tight primary closure should be accomplished. There is no advantage to packing open large cystic cavities. If the primary closure should break down, the bony cavity needs to be packed open. We see no advantage to begin packing and be committed to packing changes from the onset. Several surgeons advocate bone grafting large cystic cavities. This may be done with autogenous or allogeneic bone. However, the end result is the same, and there appears to be no advantage unless there is the chance of postoperative pathologic fracture. In this case, packing with autogenous or allogeneic bone will increase the rate of consolidation of the bony defect. This would increase strength in a shorter period of time.

Another indication for grafting would be cysts that have destroyed normal bone contours, such as alveolar ridges, where reconstruction is necessary for future prosthetic considerations. In either of these cases, however, one must weigh the advantages of grafting a cystic cavity that will fill with host bone over a slower period of time against the morbidity of harvesting bone and the potential for graft loss due to infection. This latter consideration is important when dealing with transoral placement of bone grafts in areas where primary closure may be difficult. Jaws that have been expanded by cysts will slowly remodel to a more normal contour with time. Radiographic evidence of bony fill will take 6 to 12 months.

ODONTOGENIC TUMORS

Basic Surgical Procedures

The therapeutic goal of any extirpative surgical procedure is to remove the entire lesion, leaving no neoplastic cells that could proliferate and cause a recurrence of the lesion. The methods used to achieve this goal vary tremendously and depend on the nature of the lesion. Excision of an oral carcinoma necessitates an aggressive approach that must sacrifice adjacent structures in an attempt to thoroughly remove the lesion. Using this approach on an odontoma would be a tragedy. It therefore becomes imperative to histologically

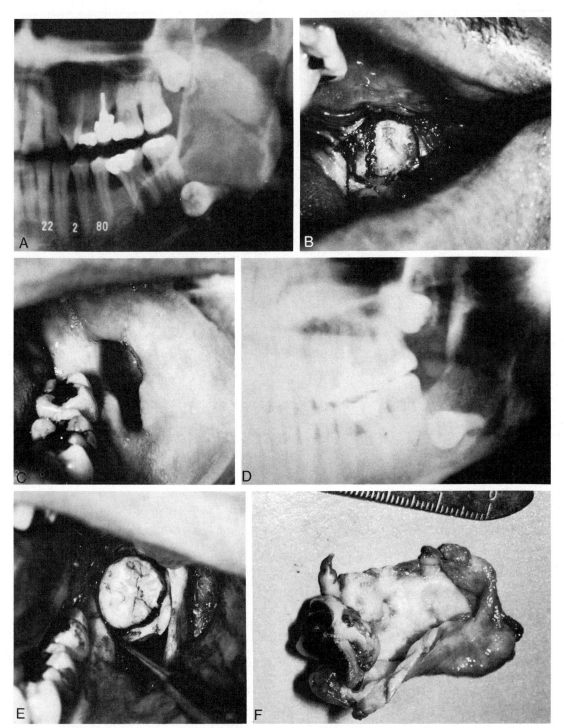

Figure 57–31. Large destructive dentigerous cyst that has compromised the strength of the mandible and has displaced the third molar tooth to the inferior border of the mandible. (*A*) Radiographic appearance showing extent of lesion. Note extension into the coronoid and condylar processes of the mandible. (*B*) Cyst wall exposed after removal of overlying cortical plate in anterior ramus. The exposed cyst wall was excised and submitted for histologic examination. (*C*) Appearance of window created into cyst to allow daily irrigations and to decompress cyst after 3 weeks. (*D*) Radiographic appearance of cyst after 9 months. Note the amount of bone that has been regenerated. (*E*) Cyst being enucleated with involved third molar tooth. (*F*) Specimen after enucleation. Note the thickness of the wall of the cyst.

identify the lesion with biopsy. Other factors that must be evaluated prior to extirpative surgery are the anatomic location of the lesion, its confinement to bone, the duration of the lesion, and the possible methods for reconstruction following surgery.

Aggressiveness of the Lesion

Surgical therapy of odontogenic tumors ranges from enucleation or curettage to composite resection. Histologic diagnosis positively identifies and therefore directs the treatment of the lesion. Owing to the wide range of behavior of odontogenic tumors, the prognosis is related more to the histologic diagnosis than to any other single factor.

Location of the Lesion

Anatomic Location. The location of an odontogenic tumor within the jaws may severely complicate the surgical excision and therefore jeopardize the prognosis. A very benign tumor in an inaccessible area, such as the mandibular condyle, presents an obvious problem surgically and from the standpoint of the functional rehabilitation of the patient. Conversely, a more aggressive tumor in an easily reachable and resectable area, such as the anterior mandible, offers a better prognosis.

Another important consideration with the more aggressive odontogenic tumors is whether they are within the mandible or the maxilla. Maxillary ameloblastomas, for example, exhibit much more aggressive behavior than their mandibular counterpart. Further, the adjacent maxillary sinuses and nasopharynx allow the tumor to grow asymptomatically to large sizes with symptoms occurring late.

The proximity of the very benign tumors to adjacent neurovascular structures and teeth is an important consideration because preservation of these structures should be attempted. Frequently, the apices of adjacent tooth roots are completely uncovered during a surgical procedure, stripping the dental pulps of their blood supply. These teeth should undergo endodontic treatment to prevent an odontogenic infection, which may complicate healing and jeopardize the success of bone grafts placed in an adjacent area.

The amount of involvement within a particular site, such as the body of the mandible, has bearing on the type of surgical procedure necessary to obtain a cure with the more aggressive lesions. When possible, the inferior border of the mandible is left to maintain continuity. This can be accomplished by marginal resection of the involved area. When the tumor extends through the entire thickness of the involved jaw, a partial resection then becomes mandatory (Fig. 57–32).

Intraosseous versus Extraosseous Location. An odontogenic tumor confined to the interior of the jaw, without perforation of the cortical plates, offers a better prognosis than those that have invaded surrounding soft tissues. In the latter case, the soft tissue in the area of the perforation should be locally excised. A supra-periosteal excision of the involved jaw should be undertaken in those cases in which the cortical plate has been reduced to the point of being eggshell thin without obvious perforation.

Duration of the Lesion

Several of the odontogenic tumors exhibit slow growth and may become static in their size. The odontomas, for example, may be discovered in the second decade of life, and their size may remain unchanged for many years. The slower growing lesions seem to follow a more benign course, and treatment should be individually tailored to each case.

Functional Rehabilitation of the Patient

After the primary objective of eradicating an odontogenic tumor has been achieved, the most important consideration is the residual defects resulting from the extirpative surgery. Best results are attained when reconstructive procedures and principles are considered preoperatively. Methods of grafting, fixation principles, soft-tissue deficits, dental rehabilitation, and patient preparation must be thoroughly evaluated and adequately handled preoperatively.

When reconstructing defects in the mandible, specific treatment goals or objectives should be established. One should tailor reconstructive surgery in an attempt to satisfy these goals. The first and foremost objective should be restoration of mandibular continuity. This not only allows bilateral harmonious function of the masticatory apparatus but restores symmetry to the face for optimal esthetic results. A second treatment objective is the restoration of alveolar bone height. Prosthetic rehabilitation depends on an adequate alveolar bony base, and this should be provided at the time of reconstructive surgery, if possible. An extension of these objectives is to restore adequate bulk to the mandible to prevent pathologic fracture during function and to provide symmetry. Examples of reconstructing residual defects will be presented in discussions of several specific odontogenic tumors.

Treatment of Specific Odontogenic Tumors

A discussion of the surgical management of specific odontogenic tumors is made easier by the fact that many odontogenic tumors behave, and therefore are treated, in a similar fashion. The three main modalities of surgical excision of odontogenic tumors are (1) enucleation, or curettage, (2) marginal or partial resection, and (3) composite resection.

Conservative Treatment. The very benign odontogenic tumors behave more as hamartomas than true neoplasms and are therefore treated conservatively. Odontomas, for example, may be treated as cysts by using simple enucleation, with little chance of recurrence. Other odontogenic tumors that may be treated with enucleation or curettage are the ameloblastic fibroma, the ameloblastic fibro-odontoma, the keratinizing and calcifying odontogenic cyst, the adenomatoid odontogenic tumor, the cementoblastoma, and the central cementifying (ossifying) fibroma.

More Aggressive Treatment. The next group of odontogenic tumors behave more aggressively and require wide margins of uninvolved tissue to adequately excise the lesions. The most frequently encountered tumor in this group is the *ameloblastoma.* Other odontogenic tu-

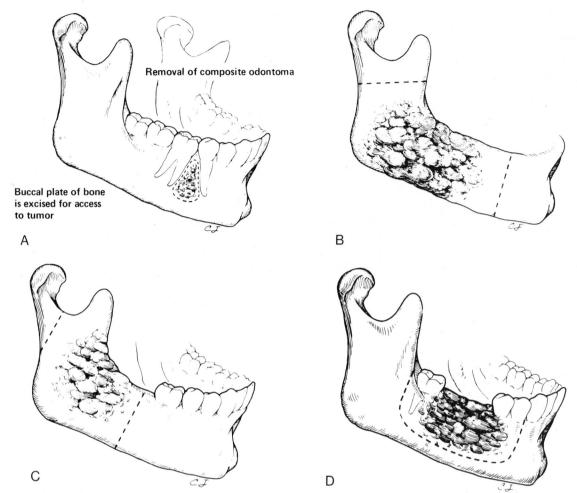

Figure 57–32. Techniques for removing odontogenic tumors. (A) Simple enucleation or curettage via removal of buccal plate of bone. (B) Partial resection of the mandibular body and ramus, leaving this condylar and coronoid processes intact for future reconstruction. (C) Partial resection of the mandibular body and ramus, leaving the condylar process intact for future reconstruction. (D) Marginal resection leaving the inferior border of the mandible intact.

mors treated similarly are the odontogenic (fibro-) myxoma, the calcifying epithelial odontogenic tumor (Pindborg), the squamous odontogenic tumor, and the ameloblastic odontoma.

Radical Treatment. Malignant varieties include primary introsseous carcinoma, malignant ameloblastic carcinoma, and the ameloblastic fibrosarcoma. Management of these tumors requires more radical intervention, with consideration of radiation and chemotherapy, in addition to surgery.

Benign Odontogenic Tumors

Odontoma. Odontomas are the most frequently encountered odontogenic tumor, and although they may be detected at any age, they develop at the time normal odontogenic structures are differentiating. Treatment for odontomas, whether of the compound or complex variety, should be similar to that for an impacted supernumerary tooth. Because cystic or ameloblastomatous change can occur, as well as continued growth

with distortion and destruction of normal tissues, excision is mandatory. Early removal is usually indicated to prevent interference with subsequent tooth eruption (Fig. 57–33). Surgical removal of these benign tumors is always conservative. They can be approached as an impacted tooth with removal of the overlying bone and enucleation of the calcified masses and their surrounding soft tissues. Multiple sectioning of the calcified masses is frequently necessary to enable removal without excessively enlarging the osseous opening and to prevent fracture of the involved jaw (Fig. 57–34). A thin layer of connective tissue or epithelial lining is usually present, affording a cleavage plane for simple enucleation. Because the growth potential of odontomas is usually limited and because they are easily removed, recurrence is extremely uncommon. The ameloblastic odontoma and ameloblastic fibro-odontoma bear great resemblance to the common odontoma; therefore, submission of these lesions for pathologic examination is mandatory.[42]

Ameloblastic Fibroma. The ameloblastic fibroma is a

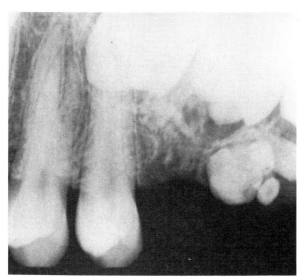

Figure 57–33. Typical radiographic appearance of an odontoma in the maxilla. Note the impedance to eruption of the permanent teeth.

true mixed odontogenic tumor that occurs in younger patients than does the ameloblastoma. An accurate diagnosis is mandatory because it is frequently mistaken for an ameloblastoma. Treatment of this lesion is not similar to that for an ameloblastoma. This benign expansile lesion does not actively infiltrate bone, from which it readily separates. Surgical treatment consists of enucleation of the lesion and curettage of the underlying bony crypt. Sacrifice of teeth or tooth buds within the lesion is frequently necessary because the posterior mandible is the site where the majority of these lesions occur.

Differentiation between the ameloblastic fibroma and ameloblastic fibrosarcoma may be histologically difficult in certain cases. Malignant change of the fibrous stroma may be apparent only in certain areas of the tumor and can be missed on incisional biopsy. Further, it is now widely conceded that although most ameloblastic fibromas are adequately treated with conservative methods, in some instances rapid recurrence after adequate excision has been noted. Therefore, the clinical behavior of well-differentiated ameloblastic sarcoma overlaps that of aggressive ameloblastic fibromas. This has led some to question the conservative treatment of ameloblastic fibromas, recommending conservative resection rather than enucleation or curettage.[3] Given the rarity of the more aggressive ameloblastic fibromas and the ameloblastic fibrosarcoma, we do not recommend resection for the ameloblastic fibroma. However, should recurrence occur with rapidity following adequate treatment, resection of the recurrent tumor should be considered. Additionally, thorough histologic examination of the entire lesion is mandatory, for malignant change may occur in only one area of the lesion.

Ameloblastic Fibro-odontoma. The ameloblastic fibro-odontoma is a tumor that may be a more mature form of the ameloblastic fibroma, in which histodifferentiation has progressed to the point of manufacture of dentin and enamel. It is a distinctive odontogenic tumor that must be clearly separated from the ameloblastic

odontoma because of the marked difference in clinical behavior of the two. The ameloblastic fibro-odontoma occurs in a similar age group and location as does the ameloblastic fibroma. They have the same limited growth potential (although some have attained considerable size). They are usually well circumscribed and usually are associated with an impacted tooth. Within the radiolucent area, solitary or multiple radiopacities may be identified on radiographs. During surgery, this tumor will appear to have a connective tissue capsule and is easily enucleated. The surgical bed should undergo curettage.

Should ameloblastic proliferation extend to a surgical margin, we would not recommend additional surgery. Instead, we would follow the patient with periodic clinical and radiographic examinations for evidence of recurrence. In our experience, a recurrence is extremely rare, and additional surgery for this tumor has not been necessary.

Adenomatoid Odontogenic Tumor. The adenomatoid odontogenic tumor is an uncommon epithelial odontogenic tumor which was formerly known as the adeno-ameloblastoma or ameloblastic adenomatoid tumor. These latter designations are unfortunate in that they imply ameloblastoma behavior characteristics that this tumor does not clinically exhibit.[9, 23, 37] These lesions behave as a cyst with expansive, not invasive, growth. Therefore, distinction between it and an ameloblastoma is imperative. Clinically, these lesions are usually asymptomatic, but there may be localized painless swelling. Two thirds are discovered in the second decade of life, two thirds occur in the maxilla, two thirds are seen in females, and two thirds are associated with an impacted tooth, two thirds of which are canines.[42] Most of them are located in the anterior part of the jaws in contrast to the ameloblastoma. Radiographically, the lesion appears as a well-demarcated radiolucent lesion that may be associated with the crown of an unerupted tooth (Fig. 57–35). This lesion mimics a dentigerous cyst when found in this manner. However, there may be flecks of opacification within the lesion.[10] Enucleation is curative. If associated with an impacted tooth, it should be removed with the lesion. Recurrences have not been reported, even after incomplete removal.[1]

Cementoblastoma. The cementoblastoma is a benign tumor of cementoblasts, which form a solid calcified tumor that is attached to the surface of a tooth root, usually a mandibular bicuspid or molar. This lesion may continue to enlarge slowly, expanding the cortical plates of the affected jaw. The tooth is vital unless affected by some other disease process. Care must be taken to differentiate this lesion from hypercementosis or chronic focal sclerosing osteomyelitis (condensing osteitis), both of which may superficially resemble it. Its radiographic appearance is characterized by a spherical expansile opaque mass that is attached to the tooth root with a radiolucent periodontal membrane space separating it from adjacent bone (Fig. 57–36). Treatment consists of surgical removal of the lesion and can be accomplished in one of two ways: surgical extraction of the tooth with the associated lesion can be undertaken with care to avoid fracture of the involved jaw, or a more conservative modality would be to first treat the tooth endodontically and then to perform periapical surgical removal of the lesion and a portion of the involved root.

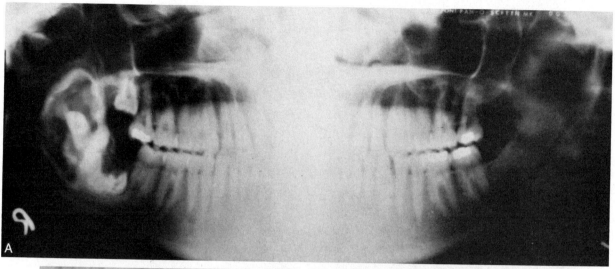

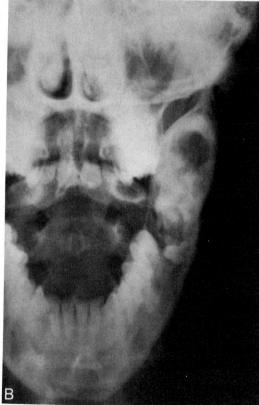

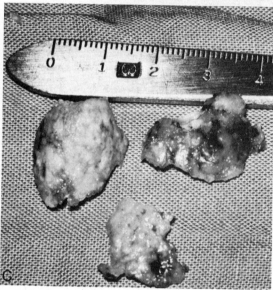

Figure 57–34. Large odontoma in the mandibular ramus. (*A*) Panoramic view. (*B*) Frontal view demonstrating mediolateral expansion of ramus. (*C*) Specimen after removal. The tumor was multiply sectioned to prevent fracture of the mandible during surgery.

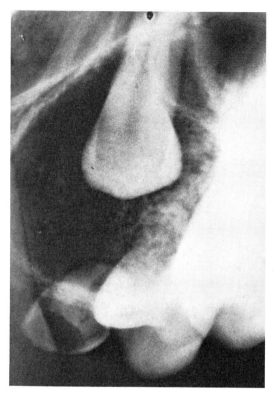

Figure 57–35. Radiographic appearance of an adenomatoid odontogenic tumor in the maxilla. Note its association with an impacted canine tooth and flecks of opacity within the radiolucent center.

Cementifying Fibroma (Cemento-ossifying Fibroma). This lesion may not represent a true odontogenic neoplasm. It is probably a variant of the ossifying fibroma, which was discussed in the preceding chapter.

Ameloblastoma. The ameloblastoma is a rare epithelial neoplasm that most commonly is found within the

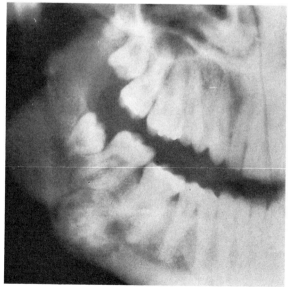

Figure 57–36. Radiographic appearance of a cementoblastoma.

bony structure of the jaws. With the exception of the odontoma, it is the most common odontogenic neoplasm.[39] The majority of ameloblastomas are located in the mandibular third molar area, although rare, soft-tissue ameloblastomas have been reported. A number of important factors must be considered in planning the treatment of an ameloblastoma. These factors include the patient's health, age, functional and esthetic concerns, and the type, size, and location of the lesion. For instance, elderly, debilitated patients may not be candidates for radical resection of their neoplasm because the functional compromise of the surgical and postsurgical period may be more deleterious than the disease itself.

It is essential to distinguish between the three clinical types of ameloblastoma—the intraosseous solid or multicystic lesion, the well-circumscribed unicystic type, and the rare peripheral (extraosseous) ameloblastoma—because they require different forms of treatment.[19]

Ameloblastomas may invade the intertrabecular spaces of cancellous bone but do not invade compact bone, although they may erode it. Small lesions in the body of the mandible are often treated by a marginal resection of the mandible, leaving the inferior border of the mandible intact. This form of therapy will leave the mandible continuous, enhancing postsurgical function and esthetics.

Ameloblastomas in the posterior part of the maxilla should be treated more extensively than similar lesions in the mandible because the tumor may spread to the pterygopalatine fossa, temporal fossa, or base of the skull. Such tumor extensions are not easily resectable.[50]

The occurrence of the unicystic ameloblastoma has been studied in 20 patients presenting with unilocular cystic lesions with clinical, radiographic, and gross features that were similar to those of non-neoplastic cysts.[41] The majority of these lesions mimicked a dentigerous cyst. The rate of recurrence for this group of lesions, as determined by long-term follow-up, was distinctly lower than that for multilocular ameloblastomas. This indicates that the unicystic ameloblastoma is a much less aggressive variety of neoplasm. Enucleation with good follow-up examination is probably sufficient for tumors that have proliferated into the cystic lumen. More extensive surgery is indicated for those involving the periphery of the fibrous connective tissue wall of the lesion.

Various modes of therapy have been advocated for treating intraosseous ameloblastomas, including curettage with and without cryotherapy,[15] radiotherapy,[25] and marginal or radical resection.[29, 32, 43] In one review of the treatment of 245 cases of ameloblastoma,[7] the lowest incidence of recurrence (4.5 per cent) occurred in 89 patients treated by radical jaw resection. The recurrence rate for conservative surgery (120 patients) was 59 per cent, and for radiotherapy (36 patients) it was 42 per cent. It was noted that 25 per cent of the patients treated with radiotherapy died of postradiation sarcoma rather than their primary disease. Although the use of a combination of local curettage and cryotherapy has been reported to offer the advantage of treating a broad area of bone without destruction of the basic structural matrix of this tissue,[34] the more conventional approach to erradication of this tumor is segmental or radical resection.

As previously stated, a marginal resection of the mandible is indicated when a tumor-free margin of bone can be preserved at the inferior border (see Fig. 57–32B). This affords the patient a minimal decrease in masticatory and functional limitation. The procedure can be accomplished by using an intraoral incision. The teeth immediately involved with the ameloblastoma should be removed with the tumor, and a primary closure of the soft tissues is obtained (Fig. 57–37).

If the tumor is large, recurrent, or in the ramus or angle of the mandible, a partial hemimandibulectomy (resection) is indicated. If there has been no perforation of the cortical plates, this can be accomplished via an intraoral route. Where perforation of the cortical plates has occurred, a supraperiosteal dissection of the involved mandible is undertaken via an intraoral or extraoral route. The involved teeth and bone are removed with at least a 1-cm margin of uninvolved bone on the proximal and distal ends of the lesion. If the tumor is in the mandibular ramus, the posterior border and condylar process of the ramus should be saved, if at all possible, to aid in immediate or delayed reconstructive efforts (Fig. 57–38).

The reconstruction of the defect caused by resection of the mandible can be immediate or delayed. Some feel that the presence of a simultaneous intraoral-extraoral defect, in addition to the high recurrence of the ameloblastoma, contraindicate an immediate reconstruction of the mandible. Instead, a space-maintaining device is placed at the time of resection, and a secondary reconstruction is performed weeks to months later.[2, 31] When delayed reconstruction is opted for, consideration should be given to maintain the residual mandibular fragments in their normal anatomic relationship with intermaxillary fixation, external pin fixation, Kirshner wire fixation, splints, or a combination of these modalities. This prevents cicatricial and muscular deformation and displacement of the segments and simplifies secondary reconstructive efforts (Figs. 57–39 to 57–41).

Our clinical results and the work of others[2] have shown that immediate reconstruction is a viable option and has the advantages of one surgical procedure and an early return to function with a minimal compromise in facial esthetics. A major disadvantage would be a recurrence within the grafted bone, but this is very rare.[12] Another possible disadvantage is the loss of the graft from infection. The risk of infection may be higher when placing a graft transorally or in an extraoral wound that had oral contamination during the extirpative surgery.

Considering that the recurrence rate is substantial in these tumors, prudent planning and meticulous surgery are mandatory prior to attempting reconstruction in order to minimize risk of failure due to recurrence. Three choices for immediate reconstruction are possible. One is to perform the entire surgical procedure intraorally, first removing the tumor and then grafting the defect. Another method is to perform the tumor removal by a combined intraoral-extraoral route. A water-tight oral closure is obtained, followed immediately by grafting the defect through the extraoral incision. The third method is useful when the tumor has not caused destruction of the alveolar crest bone, and when no extension of the tumor into oral soft tissues has occurred. In this case, extraction of the involved teeth is

performed followed by a waiting period of 6 to 8 weeks for healing of the gingival tissues. The tumor is then removed, and the defect is grafted through an extraoral incision, taking care to avoid perforation of the oral soft tissues. This latter procedure is the only type of immediate reconstruction in which oral contamination can be avoided.

We have had good success with two types of grafting systems. The first involves the use of an split autogenous ilium graft with cancellous autogenous bone placed around the graft (Figs. 57–38 and 57–42). The second technique utilizes an allogeneic freeze-dried portion of a mandible, iliac crest, or split ribs, which act as a strut or biologic scaffold, wired to the proximal and distal portions of the residual mandible. Fresh autogenous cancellous bone obtained from the ilium is then compressed into this allogeneic tray (Fig. 57–43). Intermaxillary fixation or external pin fixation is used concomitantly for several weeks to immobilize the fragments. In many instances, a secondary vestibuloplasty procedure is indicated if prosthetic function is to be restored.

Mural Ameloblastoma. Ameloblastomas arising in the wall of cysts occasionally occur, representing approximately 5 to 6 per cent of all ameloblastomas.[45] The dentigerous cyst is implicated in over 80 per cent of these lesions.[45, 49] Toller,[49] in a review of a number of surveys, has estimated that the frequency of recurrence following conservative treatment by enucleation of *solid* ameloblastomas is more than 50 per cent. Shteyer and coworkers[45] found a recurrence rate of less than 10 per cent following enucleation of *mural* ameloblastomas.

In view of these statistics, we recommend enucleation for mural ameloblastomas with periodic clinical and radiographic follow-up examinations. Should recurrence be found, treatment is then based on whether the recurrence represents a cystic lesion or a solid tumor. If another cyst is apparent, a repeat enucleation should be undertaken. If multilocularity, invasion of soft tissues, or evidence of solid tumor becomes apparent, marginal or partial jaw resection should be accomplished, and the lesion should be treated as an ameloblastoma.

Ameloblastic Odontoma. This has the clinical characteristics and behavior of the ameloblastoma and should be managed similarly. The presence of calcific structures does not imply a more benign nature in this tumor.

Calcifying Epithelial Odontogenic Tumor (Pindborg Tumor). This tumor is extremely rare and bears little microscopic similarity to the typical ameloblastoma. The tumor behaves similarly to an ameloblastoma and is locally invasive with tendencies for recurrence. The treatment for this lesion is similar to that described for an ameloblastoma (Fig. 57–44).

Odontogenic Myxoma (Odontogenic Myxofibroma). This is a benign, slow-growing lesion that is locally aggressive. It occurs most frequently in the posterior region of the mandible and will recur if initial therapy is too conservative. Owing to the loose gelatinous nature of this lesion, it is difficult to remove it completely. Therefore, the prognosis is good, but recurrence rates high. Small lesions are best treated by vigorous curettage followed by electrical or chemical cauterization, cryotherapy, or mechanical fulguration with an acrylic bur (Fig. 57–45). Large lesions are best treated by partial

Text continued on page 1504

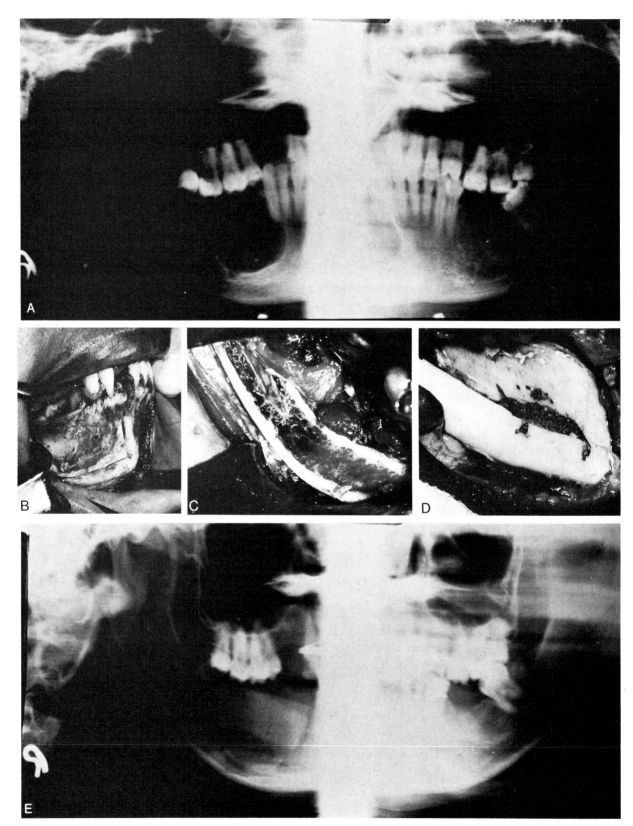

Figure 57–37. Ameloblastoma of the mandibular body treated by marginal mandibular resection and immediate reconstruction with autogenous corticocancellous graft. (*A*) Unilocular tumor in right body of the mandible. (*B*) Intraoral resection of tumor, leaving the inferior border of the mandible intact. (*C*) Defect following removal of the tumor. Note intact inferior border of the mandible. (*D*) Autogenous corticocancellous ilium graft placed through extraoral incision once the intraoral incision had been sutured. Graft secured to residual mandible with heavy resorbable suture. (*E*) Immediate postoperative panoramic radiograph showing the graft in place, adequately restoring alveolar height for future prosthetic rehabilitation.

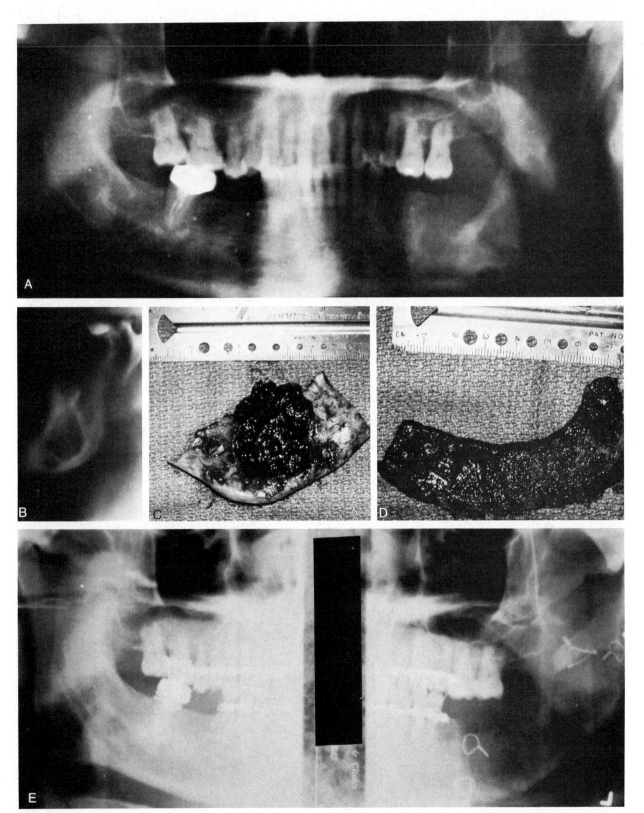

Figure 57–38. Ameloblastoma of the mandibular ramus treated by partial mandibular resection and immediate reconstruction with autogenous corticocancellous graft. (*A*) Panoramic radiograph showing a questionable radiolucency in the left mandibular ramus. (*B*) Tomograms demonstrating the extent of the lesion. (*C*) Resected specimen showing remnants of muscle tissue where a supraperiosteal dissection was carried out. (*D*) Autogenous corticocancellous ilium graft prior to placement in defect. (*E*) One year postoperative panoramic radiograph showing result.

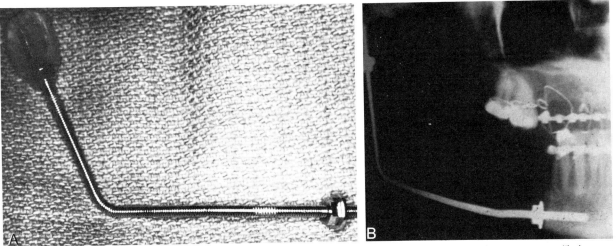

Figure 57–39. Threaded pins are used to replace missing parts of the mandible. (A) Pin fashioned to replace the mandibular ramus (including condyle) and a portion of the mandibular body. (B) Radiograph of pin in place.

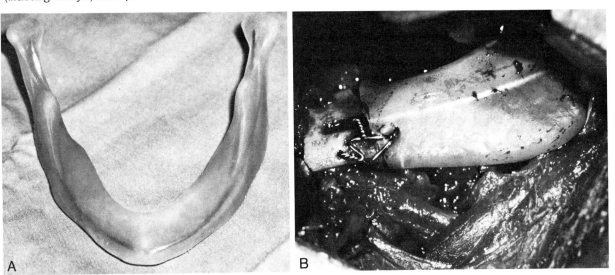

Figure 57–40. Space-maintaining device used for delayed reconstruction of a mandibular defect. (A) An acrylic mandible that can be used in part or in toto. (B) A portion of the acrylic mandible used to maintain the position of the hard and soft tissues following partial resection of a mandibular tumor. This is removed at the time of the reconstructive procedure.

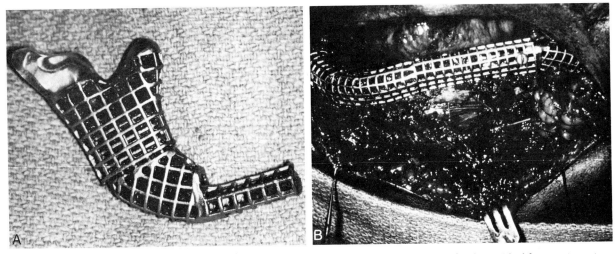

Figure 57–41. Alloy crib used to restore mandibular defect. These cribs serve as fixation devices for the residual fragments, as trays to carry particulate bone grafts, and as prosthetic replacement for parts of mandible such as the mandibular condyle. (A) Alloy framework used to replace the mandibular ramus, including the mandibular condyle. Note that the framework is packed with particulate bone graft. (B) Mandibular body and symphysis.

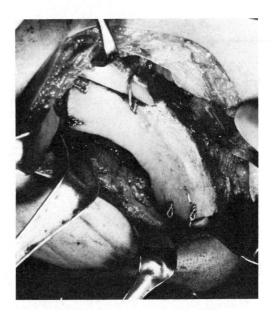

Figure 57–42. Grafted defect following removal of a tumor in the mandibular ramus. Note the posterior aspect of the ramus has been preserved to serve as a "handle" to secure the bone graft to the mandibular condyle.

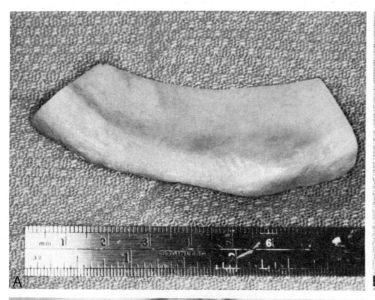

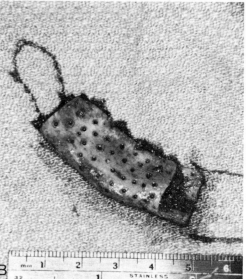

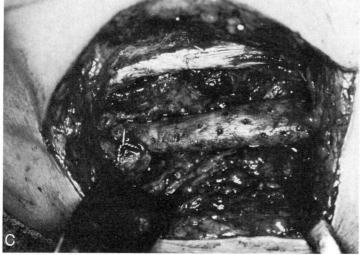

Figure 57–43. Allogeneic ilium graft used to restore mandibular continuity defect. (A) Graft prior to modification. (B) Graft has been hollowed out, and several holes have been drilled through the cortices. The center of the allogeneic graft has been packed with fresh autogenous cancellous particles. (C) The graft is wired in place.

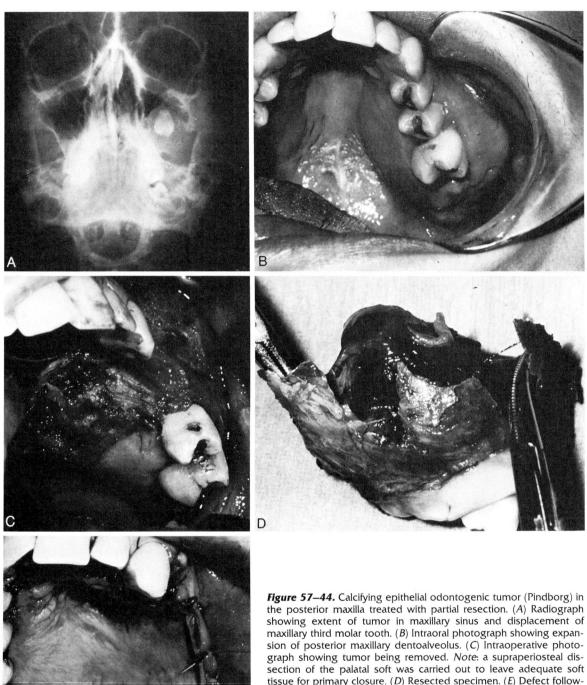

Figure 57–44. Calcifying epithelial odontogenic tumor (Pindborg) in the posterior maxilla treated with partial resection. (*A*) Radiograph showing extent of tumor in maxillary sinus and displacement of maxillary third molar tooth. (*B*) Intraoral photograph showing expansion of posterior maxillary dentoalveolus. (*C*) Intraoperative photograph showing tumor being removed. *Note:* a supraperiosteal dissection of the palatal soft was carried out to leave adequate soft tissue for primary closure. (*D*) Resected specimen. (*E*) Defect following primary closure.

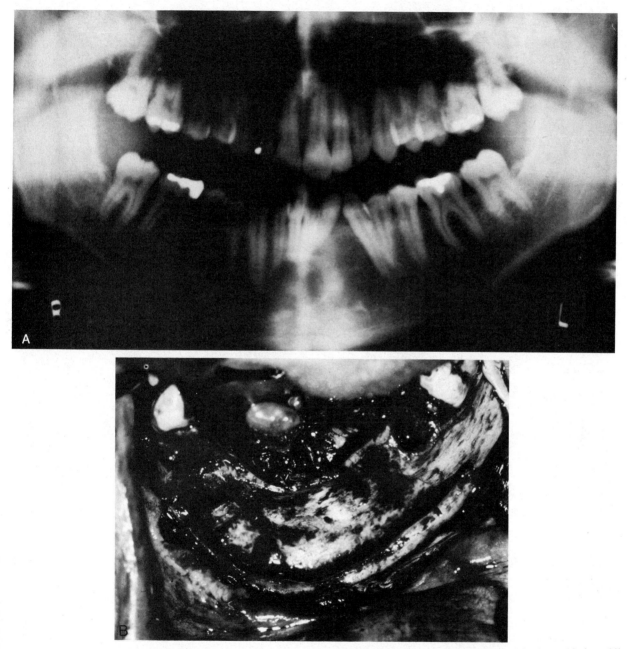

Figure 57–45. Myxoma in the mandibular symphysis treated conservatively with curettage and saucerization with bur. (*A*) Preoperative panoramic radiograph showing multilocular radiolucency. (*B*) Intraoperative photograph demonstrating defect following marginal mandibular resection, curettage, and saucerization. Note intact lingual plate of mandible. This defect was not grafted.

Illustration continued on following page

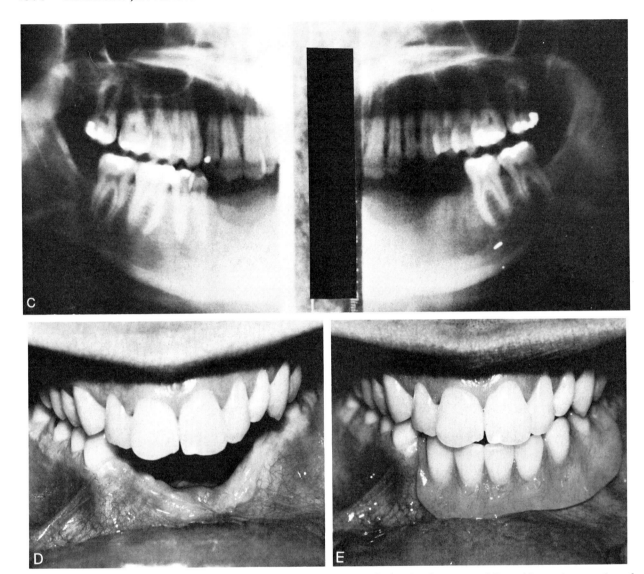

Figure 57–45 Continued. (C) One year postoperative panoramic radiograph showing bony remodeling with good restoration of alveolar height. (D) Intraoral photograph 1 year postoperatively, demonstrating resultant defect. (E) Prosthetic replacement of sacrificed dentition.

jaw resection with immediate reconstruction (Figs. 57–46 and 57–47). A detailed description of this procedure is presented for the treatment of the ameloblastoma.

Squamous Odontogenic Tumor. Surgical management of this uncommon and controversial lesion is probably best handled by an initial conservative attempt at eradication using curettage or enucleation. Because most of these lesions occur within the dentoalveolus, the removal of involved teeth is usually indicated. When perforation of the buccal and lingual plates of bone are found with involvement of soft tissues, more extensive and aggressive surgery is indicated.

Although conservative excision and extraction of the involved teeth has been adequate treatment in most cases,[8, 13, 17, 38, 51] en bloc resection[13] or hemimaxillectomy[28] has been necessary to eradicate the disease in some

cases because of its extent and involvement of adjacent structures, such as buccal, palatal, or lingual soft tissues, maxillary sinus, nasal floor, and nasal spine.[21]

It is important that this lesion not be mistaken for an acanthomatous ameloblastoma, for which treatment is more radical.

Malignant Odontogenic Tumors

Primary Intraosseous Carcinoma. This tumor is a squamous cell carcinoma arising within the jaw, having no initial connection with the oral mucosa. It presumably develops from residual odontogenic epithelium within the jaws.[36] In an excellent review by Elzay,[14] in which nine cases were treated by surgical excision or resection, at least one recurrence occurred in six cases. Multiple recurrences were reported in several instances.

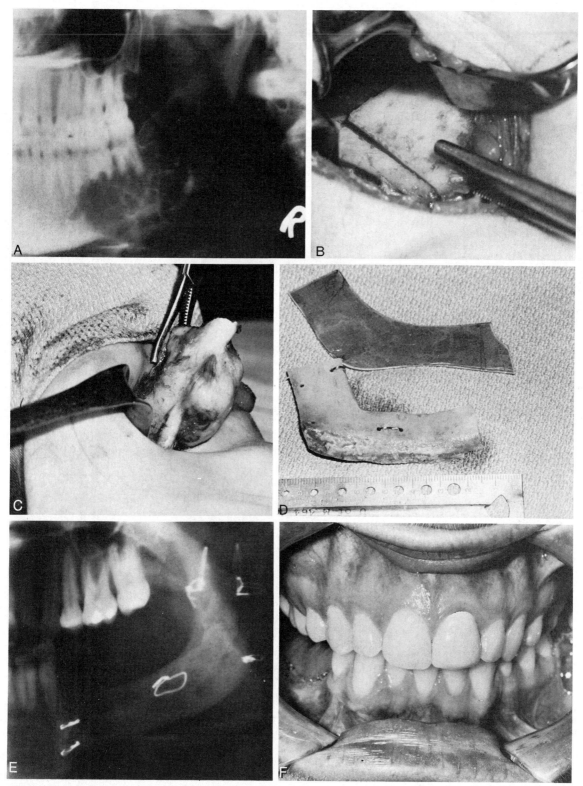

Figure 57–46. Myxoma of the posterior mandibular body and ramus treated with partial resection and immediate reconstruction with autogenous corticocancellous graft. (*A*) Multilocular radiolucency in the right mandibular ramus. (*B*) Inverted "L" osteotomy of the mandibular ramus demonstrated at the time of surgery. This operation left the mandibular condylar and coronoid processes intact along with the posterior border of the ramus. (*C*) Intraoral removal of the tumor along with involved teeth. The intraoral incisions were then closed primarily and immediate reconstruction was performed extraorally. (*D*) Surgical template fabricated preoperatively using radiographs to determine proper graft size during harvesting. (*E*) One year postoperative radiograph showing good mandibular structure and alveolar bone height. (*F*) Occlusion 1 year postoperatively.

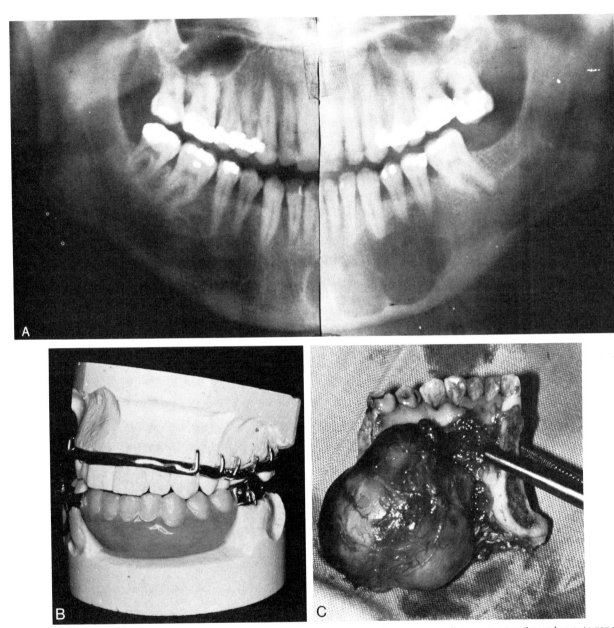

Figure 57–47. Myxoma of the mandibular symphysis treated with partial resection and immediate reconstruction using autogenous corticocancellous graft. (*A*) Multilocular radiographic appearance of lesion. (*B*) Custom arch bar and prosthetic fixation device fabricated prior to surgery. (*C*) Specimen following removal. Note lingual expansion.

Illustration continued on opposite page

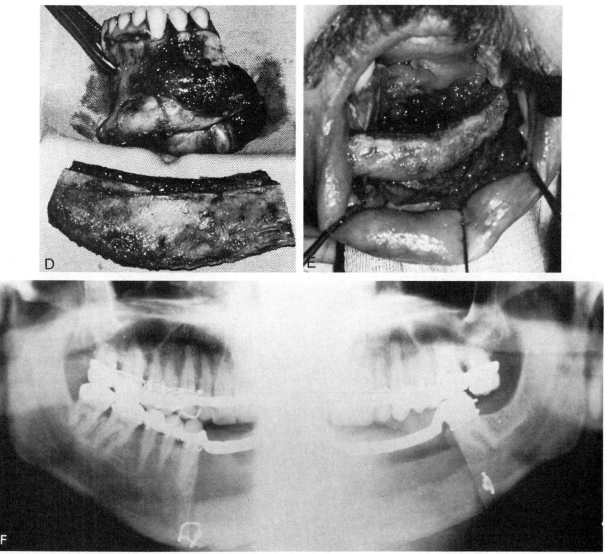

Figure 57–47 *Continued.* (*D*) Specimen used to size the autogenous corticocancellous ilium graft. (*E*) Graft secured into place using transoral approach. (*F*) Postoperative panoramic radiograph showing graft and fixation devices in place.

Following recurrence, radiation or chemotherapy was utilized. Six of the nine patients treated received radiation treatment subsequent to surgery. Three of them were alive after 2 years. Three patients received chemotherapy in addition to radiation treatment, and one was alive after 2 years. Eight of the patients had clinical or histologic evidence of metastasis to cervical lymph nodes, and three out of four patients were alive after 2 years and were reported to have lymph node involvement. As demonstrated by Elzay's review, the prognosis is extremely poor. Shear[44] reported a 5-year survival rate of 30 to 40 per cent.

Treatment of the involved jaw is similar to epidermoid carcinoma of the oral cavity which has invaded the bone. Treatment should consist of surgical resection, and ipsilateral neck dissection is necessary if there is clinical evidence of nodal involvement. Radiation or chemotherapy may be utilized in conjunction with surgery to effect an improved prognosis.

Malignant Ameloblastoma. This is an extremely rare lesion. Three commonly discussed modes of metastasis are via hematogenous spread, lymphatic spread, and the unusual mechanism of aspiration of tumor cells. The treatment of malignant ameloblastoma is by either radiotherapy or chemotherapy.

Ameloblastic Fibrosarcoma. The ameloblastic fibrosarcoma or ameloblastic sarcoma is a rare tumor that rarely metastasizes.[30] However, fatal cases usually have been associated with uncontrollable local infiltration. This is in contrast to the typical fibrosarcoma of the head and neck that metastasized in 25 per cent of a series of 40 cases reported by Swain and co-workers.[48] Inadequate surgical intervention and biopsy appear to be associated with rapid growth in some reported cases.[22, 51] Therefore, treatment of these lesions as a low-grade fibrosarcoma, with radical resection, is appropriate as the first mode of therapy. The limited information available at present suggests that chemotherapy should be reserved for intractable cases.[22, 30] Radiation therapy has not been found to be an effective mode of treatment.[26, 30]

An allied lesion, the ameloblastic odontosarcoma, is much rarer than the ameloblastic fibrosarcoma. It differs in that dysplastic enamel and dentin are formed within the tumor. Treatment should be similar to the ameloblastic fibrosarcoma.[4]

The authors would like to thank Dr. James R. Hayward, Professor and former Chairman, Department of Oral and Maxillofacial Surgery, The University of Michigan, for his contributions to this chapter.

REFERENCES

1. Abrams AM, Melrose RJ, Howell FV: Adenoameloblastoma: A clinical pathologic study of ten new cases. Cancer 22:175, 1968.
2. Adekeye EO: Reconstruction of mandibular defects by autogenous bone grafts. A review of 37 cases. J Oral Surg 36:125, 1978.
3. Adekeye EO, Edwards MB, Goubran GF: Ameloblastic fibrosarcoma: Report of a case in a Nigerian. Oral Surg 46:254, 1978.
4. Altini M, Smith I: Ameloblastic dentinosarcoma: A case report. Int J Oral Surg 5:142, 1976.
5. Anderson DE, McClendon JL, Howell JB: Genetics and skin tumors with special reference to basal cell nevi. In Clinical Conference on Cancer, M.D. Anderson Hospital and Tumor Institute, 1962; Tumors of the Skin: Chicago, Year Book Medical Publishers, 1964.
6. Angelopoulos AF, Tilson HB, Stewart FW, Jaques WE: Malignant transformation of the epithelial lining of the odontogenic cysts. Oral Surg 22:415, 1966.
7. Becker R, Pertl A: Zur therapie des ameloblastoms. Dtsch Zahn-Mund-Kieferheilk 49:423, 1967.
8. Carr RF, Carlton DM, Jr, Marks RB: Squamous odontogenic tumor: Report of case. J Oral Surg 39:297, 1981.
9. Cina MT, Dahlin DC, Gores RJ: Ameloblastic adenomatoid tumors: A report of four new cases. Am J Clin Pathol 39:59, 1963.
10. Courtney RM, Kerr DA: The odontogenic adenomatoid tumor. Oral Surg 39:424, 1975.
11. Dachi SF, Howell FV: A survey of 3,874 routine full-mouth radiographs. II. A study of impacted teeth. Oral Surg 14:1165, 1961.
12. Dolan EA, Angelillo JC, Georgiade NG: Recurrent ameloblastoma in autogenous rib graft. Report of case. Oral Surg 51:357, 1981.
13. Doyle JL, Grodjesk JE, Dolinsky HB, Rafel SS: Squamous odontogenic tumor: Review of three cases. J Oral Surg 35:994, 1977.
14. Elzay RP: Primary intraosseous carcinoma of the jaws: Review and update of odontogenic carcinomas. Oral Surg 54:299, 1982.
15. Emmings FG, Gage AA, Koepf SW: Combined currettage and cryotherapy for recurrent ameloblastomas of the mandible. Report of case. J Oral Surg 29:41, 1971.
16. Eversole LR, Sabes WR, Rovin S: Aggressive growth and neoplastic potential of odontogenic cysts with special reference to central epidermoid and mucoepidermoid carcinomas. Cancer 35:270, 1975.
17. Fay JF, Banner J, Rothouse L, et al: Squamous odontogenic tumor arising in odontogenic cysts. J Oral Med 26:35, 1981.
18. Frankel KA, Smith JD, Frankel LS: Soft tissue ameloblastoma in a 92 year-old woman. Arch Otolaryngol 103:499, 1977.
19. Gardner DG, Pecak AM: The treatment of ameloblastoma based on pathological and anatomic principles. Cancer 46:2514, 1980.
20. Gardner DG, Sapp JP, Wysocki GP: Epithelial cysts of the jaws. Bull Int Acad Pathol 17:6, 1976.
21. Goldblatt LI, Brannon RB, Ellis GL: Squamous odontogenic tumor: Review of five cases and review of the literature. Oral Surg 54:187, 1982.
22. Goldstein G, Parker FP, Hugh GSF: Ameloblastic sarcoma. Pathogenesis and treatment with chemotherapy. Cancer 37:1673, 1976.
23. Gorlin RJ: Odontogenic tumors. In Gorlin RJ, Goldman HM (eds): Thoma's Oral Pathology. 6th Ed. St. Louis, The C.V. Mosby Co., 1970.
24. Gorlin RJ, Yunis JJ, Tuna N: Multiple nevoid basal cell carcinoma, odontogenic keratocysts and skeletal anomalies: A syndrome. Acta Derm-Venereol (Stockh) 43:39, 1963.
25. Hair JAG: Radiosensitive adamantinoma. Br Med J 1:105, 1963.
26. Hatzifotiadis D, Economou A: Ameloblastic sarcoma in the maxilla: A case report. J Maxillofac Surg 1:62, 1973.
27. Hayward JR: Cysts of bone and soft tissue lesions. In Hayward JR (ed): Oral Surgery. Springfield, Charles C Thomas, 1976.
28. Hopper TL, Sadeghi EM, Pricco DF: Squamous odontogenic tumor: Review of case with multiple lesions. Oral Surg 50:404, 1980.
29. Horrman PJ, Baden EO, Rankow RM, Potter GD: The fate of uncontrolled ameloblastoma. Oral Surg 26:419, 1968.
30. Howell RM, Burkes EJ Jr: Malignant transformation of ameloblastic fibro-odontoma to ameloblastic fibrosarcoma. Oral Surg 43:391, 1977.
31. Kluft O, Van Dop F: Mandibular ameloblastoma (resection with primary reconstruction)—A case report with concise review of the literature. Arch Chir Neerl 28:289, 1976.
32. Lucas RB, Thrackray AC: The histology of adamantinoma. Br J Cancer 5:289, 1951.
33. Main DMG: Epithelial jaw cysts: A clinicopathological reappraisal. Br J Oral Surg 8:114, 1970.
34. Marciani RD, Trodahl JH, Suckiel, MJ, Dubick MN: Cryotherapy in the treatment of ameloblastoma of the mandible: Report of cases. J Oral Surg 35:289, 1977.
35. McClatchey KD: Odontogenic lesions—tumors and cysts. In Batsakis JG (ed): Tumors of the Head and Neck—Clinical and Pathological Considerations. 2nd ed. Baltimore, Williams & Wilkins Co., 1979.
36. Pindborg JJ, Kramer IRH, Torloni H: Histologic Typing of Odontogenic Tumours, Jaw Cysts and Allied Lesions. Geneva, World Health Organization, 1972, pp 35–36.
37. Philipsen HP, Birn H: The adenomatoid odontogenic tumor: Ameloblastic adenomatoid tumor or adenoameloblastoma. Acta Pathol Microbiol Scand 75:375, 1969.
38. Pullon PA, Schafer WG, Elzay RP, et al: Squamous odontogenic tumor. Review of six cases of a previously undescribed lesion. Oral Surg 40:616, 1975.

39. Regezi JA, Kerr DA, Courtney RM: Odontogenic tumors: Analysis of 706 cases. J Oral Surg 36:771, 1978.
40. Robinson HBG: Primordial cyst *vs.* keratocyst. Oral Surg 40:362, 1975.
41. Robinson L, Martinez MG: Unicystic ameloblastoma: A prognostically distinct entity. Cancer 40:2278, 1977.
42. Shafer WG, Hine MK, Levy BM: A Textbook of Oral Pathology. 3rd ed. Philadelphia, W. B. Saunders Co., 1974.
43. Shatkin S Hofmeister FS: Ameloblastoma: A rational approach to therapy. Oral Surg 20:421, 1965.
44. Shear M: Primary intra-alveolar epidermoid carcinoma of the jaw. J Pathol 97:645, 1969.
45. Shteyer A, Lustmann J, Lewin-Epstein J: The mural ameloblastoma: A review of the literature. J Oral Surg 36:866, 1978.
46. Standish SM, Shafer WG: The lateral periodontal cyst. J Periodont 29:27, 1958.
47. Stoelinga J: Personal communication from a lecture presented at The University of Michigan School of Dentistry, May 1983.
48. Swain RE, Sessions DG, Ogura JH: Fibrosarcoma of the head and neck: A clinical analysis of forty cases. Ann Otol 83:439, 1974.
49. Toller PA: Autoradiography of explants from odontogenic cysts. Br Dent J 131:57, 1971.
50. Tsaknis PJ, Nelson JF: The maxillary ameloblastoma: An analysis of 24 cases. J Oral Surg 38:336, 1980.
51. Villa BG: Ameloblastic sarcoma in the mandible. Report of case. Oral Surg 8:123, 1955.
52. Wright JM Jr: Squamous odontogenic tumorlike proliferation in odontogenic cysts. Oral Surg 47:354, 1979.
53. Wysocki GP, Sapp JP: Scanning and transmission electron microscopy of odontogenic keratocysts. Oral Surg 40:494, 1975.

CHAPTER 58

Non-odontogenic Tumors

CLINICAL EVALUATION AND PATHOLOGY

Robert O. Greer, Jr., D.D.S., Sc.D. • **Michael D. Rohrer, D.D.S., M.S.**
Stephen Kent Young, D.D.S., M.S.

The jaws are relatively uncommon anatomic sites for primary skeletal neoplasms. Osteosarcoma, for example, is recognized as the most common primary malignancy of bone, accounting for greater than 20 per cent of all primary osseous malignancies[5, 6]; however, it is a rare neoplasm in the head and neck (jaws, facial bones, and skull). The first part of this chapter will deal specifically with the unique aspects of nonodontogenic tumors of bone with a special emphasis on clinicopathologic features, epidemiology, and diagnostic findings.

BENIGN BONE-FORMING TUMORS

Osteoma

Osteomas have been classically described as slowly but progressively growing central, peripheral, or subperiosteal osteogenic tumors containing mature cancellous or compact bone. Osteomas are relatively uncommon in the jaws, facial bones, and skull.

The pathogenesis of this neoplasm is unclear, although an ivory osteoma was demonstrated on the right side of an Egyptian skull of Roman vintage,[8] and multiple composite osteomas have been found coincident with other tumorous conditions. Quite frequently, the terms osteoma and exostosis are used interchangeably, but these lesions are not identical. *Exostoses* are exceedingly common in the jaw bones and have been documented in over 30 per cent of the population in the United States. They are not true neoplasms; rather they are bony excrescences that represent osseous anatomic variation rather than true disease.

The actual occurrence of osteoma in the jaws, facial bones, and skull is so often misinterpreted that Dahlin[5] did not include this tumor in his statistical review of 6221 bone tumors, stating that a clear line of distinction between obviously dysplastic lesions of bone and completely benign "true" osteomas is not possible. Childrey reported 15 osteomas among 3510 asymptomatic patients based on paranasal sinus radiographs.[3] The Finnish and West German literature indicates that the incidence of osteomas varies from 0.1 to 1 per cent of all patients examined in large otolaryngology clinics.[7]

Most osteomas are identified in young adults, and the male-female ratio is generally reported to show greater than a 2 to 1 male predominance.[7]

The etiology of the osteoma is unknown. Some authorities have suggested that the lesion is caused by trauma or infection.[5] Other researchers suggest that osteoma is a form of osseous hamartoma.[6] Hallberg and Bagley suggested that osteomas of the paranasal sinuses arise from the junctional region of membranous and endochondral bone in that area.[7]

Although there has been some attempt at classification and staging of osteomas on the basis of histologic findings, there are no definitive staging mechanisms.

Clinical Findings

The most common clinical presentation of osteoma is that of a well-circumscribed protuberance of bone or a central dense medullary mass. The vast majority of osteomas in the jaws and facial bones are very slow growing and produce few symptoms unless they become large enough to produce facial asymmetry. Occasionally, patients with large osteomas of the orbit may present with ophthamologic complaints including exophthalmos, blindness, or even pneumoencephalos. Exceedingly large osteomas of the mandible have been reported to cause unusual visual defects and problems with balance and stability, supposedly related to their close proximity to the carotid sinus and internal carotid artery.[10] Osteomas are most frequently identified in the mandible. Lesions of the maxillary sinus are not common, and osteomas only rarely occur in the sphenoid sinus.[8] Salinger[13] quoted Malan,[11] who, from a total of 458 cases in the paranasal sinuses, found 41 cases of osteoma in the maxillary sinus. Lautenbach[9] reported 36 cases equally distributed in the maxilla and the mandible and documented a 3:1 female-to-male ratio; however, Hallberg[7] has reported a ratio greater than 2:1 of male predominance. A rare form of osteoma, *osseous choristoma*, has been reported by Cutright[4] in the oral soft tissues, generally beneath ill-fitting dentures. This "tumor" is actually a form of osseous metaplasia and not a true osteoma.

Radiographically, subperiosteal osteomas appear as dense radiopaque masses, whereas endosteal lesions appear as well-circumscribed sclerotic masses. Tumor progression cannot be related to the degree of osteosclerosis identified on the radiograph.

Pathology

Osteomas are classically described as having three relatively distinct histologic patterns. The *trabecular osteoma (spongy osteoma)* is composed of osseous trabeculae arranged in a lamellar fashion and often rimmed by active osteoblasts. A peripheral cortical bony margin is usually identified, and abundant fatty and fibrofatty marrow may surround the trabecular component. Destruction of adjacent bone is rarely if ever present. This lesion is often considered to be identical to the so-called osteocartilaginous exostosis of long bones. The *compact osteoma (ivory osteoma)* is usually composed of dense masses of lamellar bone with little evidence of marrow spaces (Fig. 58–1). This lesion has very little evidence of osteoblastic activity; connective tissue is sparse, and there is usually no attempt at haversian system formation. Batsakis[1] has described a third variant, *osteoma durum,* which has a histologic pattern that lies between that of the compact osteoma and trabecular osteoma.

Differential Diagnosis

Gardner's syndrome is a rare inherited disease characterized by epidermoid and sebaceous cysts of the skin, multiple skin fibromas, multifocal impacted and supernumerary teeth, multiple osteomas, and intestinal polyposis. The presence of multiple osteomas should arouse the suspicion of an associated Gardner's syndrome when such lesions are found distributed throughout the bones of the jaws and face. The polyps in Gardner's syndrome, largely confined to the colon, show a tendency toward malignant transformation, often stated to be as great as 40 per cent.[14]

Osteoma can also mimic osteoblastoma and osteoid osteoma. These lesions, however, show more cellularity, and both are frequently associated with considerable jaw pain. Both neoplasms also have a rapid growth potential, unlike the slow-growing true osteoma. The clinician may often find it difficult to distinguish osteoma from a true *solid odontoma.* The latter lesion contains odontogenic remnants and tooth structure elements along with osteodentin. These features are not present in an osteoma.

Treatment and Prognosis

The treatment of choice for osteoma is complete surgical excision, and the lesions rarely, if ever, recur following complete removal. Brunner and Spiesman,[2] however, have reported secondary intercranial complications following removal of osteomas from the paranasal sinuses.

Ossifying Fibroma

Ossifying fibroma is a gradually expanding, well-circumscribed fibro-osseous lesion of bone that perhaps has more synonyms than any other jaw lesion. The lesion has been variously referred to in the literature as osteofibroma, fibro-osteoma, cemento-ossifying fibroma, cementifying fibroma, juvenile active ossifying fibroma, and benign sclerotic fibro-osseous lesion of periodontal ligament origin. The term ossifying fibroma was first popularized in the British literature, although Menzel[27] first made reference to a so-called osteofibroma of bone in 1872. The lesion gained its current nosology from Montgomery[28] in 1927.

Ossifying fibroma is almost certainly a lesion that arises from cells within the periodontal ligamant.[33] The lesions are for the most part restricted to the tooth-bearing areas of the jaws and are, in terms of histogenesis, probably best described as dysplastic lesions of membrane bone. A few investigators continue to con-

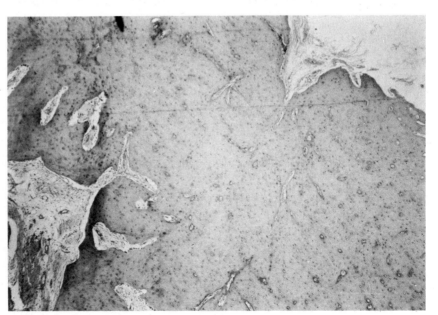

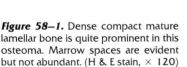
Figure 58–1. Dense compact mature lamellar bone is quite prominent in this osteoma. Marrow spaces are evident but not abundant. (H & E stain, × 120)

sider the lesions to be true neoplasms because of their ability to attain rather immense size.[16] Waldron and Giansanti,[33] who have probably reviewed and characterized fibro-osseous lesions of the jaws to a greater extent than any modern authorities, prefer to view ossifying fibroma within a spectrum of fibro-osseous lesions of periodontal ligament origin. At one end of their continuum, they group a number of reactive but nonexpansile lesions variously known as periapical cemental dysplasia, periapical cementoma, or periapical osteofibroma. They suggest that other growths with identical histomorphologic features possess the innate ability to grow progressively along lines that are consistent with a benign neoplasm; ossifying fibroma is considered to be such a lesion. Ossifying fibroma shows a rather marked predisposition for development in the mandible, and occasionally more than one lesion can be present in the jaw.[23, 25, 33] Waldron has reported a significant female predisposition,[32] although some authorities maintain that there is no sex predilection.[21, 22]

There have been a host of classification and staging criteria developed for ossifying fibroma over the past 100 years. *Fibro-osteoma* is often considered to be a unique entity distinct from ossifying fibroma. Reed and Hagy[29] suggest that the term fibro-osteoma be reserved for lesions of the maxilla and paranasal sinuses. Hamner and associates[22] suggest that the term fibro-osteoma should be reserved for gigantiform or exceedingly large fibro-osseous lesions that have the same behavior pattern as ossifying fibroma. Our own belief is that the two lesions are exactly the same entity, regardless of their size or site, and should be recognized as such. Compulsive subclassification is of little help to the clinician or surgeon who must manage such a lesion.

Ossifying fibroma can occur in any age group, but the third and fourth decades are by far the most common periods of occurrence. A so-called *juvenile active ossifying fibroma* has been reported.[31, 33] This lesion is generally suggested to be an exceedingly aggressive lesion that possesses the potential to kill the patient by local extension into vital structures. Although the term is frequently used among clinicians and pathologists

alike, there have been no well-documented series of cases reported in the literature, and many pathologists regard the tumor to be either a low-grade osteosarcoma or an active cementoblastoma. We have been able to clinically and radiographically relate this lesion to ossifying fibroma but do not consider it a useful diagnostic term because the biology of the lesion has not been well delineated.

Four distinct developmental stages of ossifying fibroma have been recognized by Billing and Ringertz.[15] These maturation stages include:

1. Osteoid fibroma, a soft, fibrous lesion and the least differentiated of all ossifying fibromas.

2. A moderately mature stage.

3. A mature or so-called osteoma stage.

4. A well-differentiated "eburnifying" fibroma that is commonly identified in the ethmoid or frontal bone.

Although these four stages have been recognized since 1946, it is difficult to establish a distinct clinical category for each stage because stages often overlap.

Clinical Findings

Most ossifying fibromas occur as asymptomatic, monostotic fibrous lesions of the jaws or bones of the face with features that are similar to fibrous dysplasia. The lesion shows a striking predisposition for the mandible. Long bone lesions are much rarer than lesions of the jaws. Waldron and Giansanti[33] report that most ossifying fibromas present as slow-growing expansile lesions of the jaw. In their review of 65 cases they found that at the time of diagnostic biopsy or surgical removal, tumor duration ranged from 6 months to 10 years, with the duration in most cases lasting less than 5 years.

The radiographic appearance of ossifying fibroma is generally quite dynamic. The tumor may present as a predominantly lytic lesion with variable amounts of radiopaque foci or as a solitary cyst-like lesion. During late stages of evolution, the lesion may become quite diffuse and homogeneous with a dense radiopaque appearance (Fig. 58-2). In most instances, regardless of

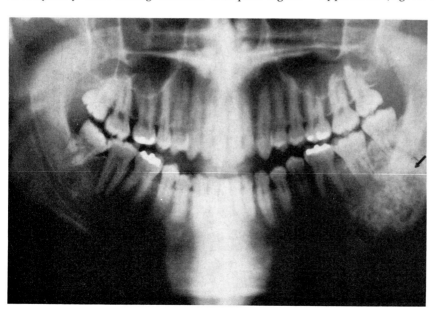

Figure 58–2. Large ossifying fibroma of the posterior mandible with coalescent radiolucent and radiopaque zones. Note that both the anterior and inferior margins of the lesion are well circumscribed.

the stage of maturation, the lesion will show radiolucent borders that are well defined and smoothly contoured. Eighty-five per cent of the lesions identified by Waldron and Giansanti[33] were less than 4 cm in size. On rare occasions ossifying fibromas blend into normal bone, causing some degree of difficulty in distinguishing them from fibrous dysplasia. Occasionally the tumor may cause gross displacement of the mandibular canal.[19] Bone scintigraphy with [99]mTc polyphosphate has seen widespread use in the diagnosis of skeletal disease; rarely, it has been used as a diagnostic aid for ossifying fibroma to reveal the full extent of the lesion, especially if it involves soft tissue.

Ossifying fibroma shows varying degrees of occurrence, depending on the population reviewed. Dehner[17] reviewed a series of 40 tumors of the mandible and maxilla recorded over a 20-year period at the Barnes Hospital and the Washington University School of Medicine. He found that 64 per cent of the tumors were fibro-osseous lesions and that half of these were ossifying fibromas. Greer and Mierau,[20] however, found only four ossifying fibromas in an extensive review of 191 tumors of the oral mucosa and jaws in children seen at the University of Colorado over an 8-year period. Regezi and associates[30] reviewed a series of 706 odontogenic tumors submitted to the department of oral pathology at the University of Michigan over a 4-year period and found cementifying fibroma to account for only 2 per cent of their cases. Khanna and Khanna[24] reviewed a series of primary tumors of the jaws in African children and noted a very high percentage of cemento-ossifying fibromas, with 28.5 per cent of 122 primary tumors of the jaws in children being diagnosed as such. Most ossifying fibromas occur in the second, third, or fourth decade of life, predominantly in close approximation to the roots and periapical areas of the teeth.

Pathology

Grossly, ossifying fibroma usually consists of multiple gritty or partially calcified pieces of hard and soft tissue.

Histologically, the tumor is composed of a similar admixture of fibrous and calcified tissue (Fig. 58–3). The supporting stroma is usually composed of interlacing fascicles of collagen, or loose proliferating fibroblasts that are stellate in character. This stroma may be richly or poorly vascularized, and endothelial cell proliferation is frequently identified. Lamellar bone may be seen distributed throughout the fibrocellular stroma, or anastomosing retiform osseous trabeculae may blend into the supporting connective tissue (Fig. 58–4). Lesional bone polarizes, showing widely spaced parallel lines of birefringence. Globular calcifications, frequently described as cementoid, may be found in the tissue sample as well. The term *cemento-ossifying fibroma* or *cementifying fibroma* has been employed when such globules are prominent. The distinction between cementoid and osteoid material is for all practical purposes of academic interest only and does not alter the biologic behavior of the tumor.

Differential Diagnosis

The most significant feature that helps distinguish ossifying fibroma from fibrous dysplasia is typically the circumscribed nature of the former. Lucas, however, has pointed out that the clinical and radiographic appearances of ossifying fibroma and fibrous dysplasia may be identical,[26] and Eversole and associates[18] suggest that the histopathologic findings of all fibro-osseous lesions is in fact a spectrum with lamellar bone, woven bone, osteoblastic rimming of osseous trabeculae, spheroid calcifications, and cementicals—features that can be found in all fibro-osseous lesions.

Waldron and Giansanti[33] reported that the stroma of fibrous dysplasia is much more fibrous than that of ossifying fibroma. These authors maintain that ossifying fibroma has an exceedingly prominent vascular stroma, unlike that of fibrous dysplasia. The common belief that cranial-facial fibrous dysplasia contains no lamellar bone and little, if any, osteoblastic rimming is rarely adhered to today. Numerous authorities have documented that lamellar bone activity with prominent osteoblastic rim-

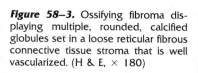

Figure 58–3. Ossifying fibroma displaying multiple, rounded, calcified globules set in a loose reticular fibrous connective tissue stroma that is well vascularized. (H & E, × 180)

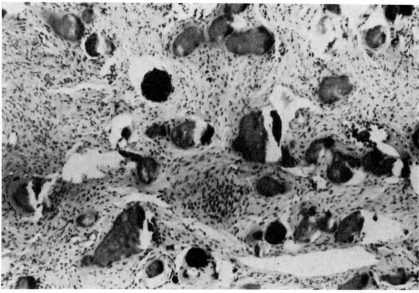

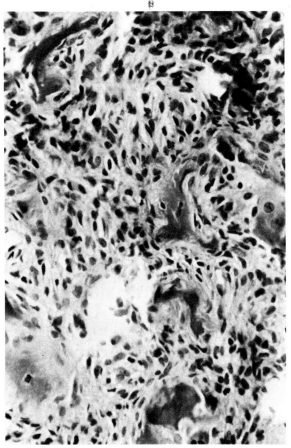

Figure 58–4. Retiform osseous trabeculae rimmed by osteoblasts are prominent in this ossifying fibroma. (H & E, × 250)

ming can be a component of both fibrous dysplasia and ossifying fibroma.[18, 33] Silver impregnation techniques may indeed outline the feathery irregular margins of fibrous dysplasia, but careful scrutiny of multiple tissue levels or serial sections of an ossifying fibroma will demonstrate that irregular feathery or twisted disoriented fibers can be found in this lesion as well.

Osteoblastoma and osteoid osteoma had been confused with ossifying fibroma in the past. These two entities are clinically unique and should not be classified as variants of ossifying fibroma. Osteoblastoma has a somewhat more limited growth potential than osteoid osteoma or ossifying fibroma, and microscopically, the osseous trabeculae of osteoblastoma are generally broader, larger, and more widely separated than in osteoid osteoma or ossifying fibroma.

Cementoblastoma may also be confused with an actively growing ossifying fibroma; however, the most dynamic feature that separates the two is the fusion of cementoblastoma to the root surfaces. Globules of cementum and layered areas of cementogenesis are typical microscopic features of cementoblastoma. These features are acutely absent in ossifying fibroma.

Treatment and Prognosis

Treatment of ossifying fibroma is most often affected by complete surgical removal using curettage, enuclea-tion, or excision. When curettage is employed, eburnation or saucerization of the bone should be completed. Small maxillary lesions may be excised via a window excision in the alveolar bone, although large lesions may require extensive surgery. Radiation therapy is contraindicated in the management of ossifying fibroma. The so-called "juvenile active ossifying fibroma" may require aggressive surgical management.

Osteoblastoma

Osteoblastoma is an exceedingly rare primary neoplasm of bone that constitutes approximately 1 per cent of all primary bone tumors.[44] Huvos[8] reported that just over 360 cases have been documented in the world literature. The tumor has been variously referred to as benign osteoblastoma, giant osteoid osteoma, osteogenic fibroma, and osteoblastic osteoid tissue-forming tumor. It is a progressively growing lesion that is frequently painful and is characterized by an absence of any reactive perifocal bone formation.[8]

The etiology of osteoblastoma is unknown. Dahlin[5] questioned whether osteoblastoma is correctly classified as a true neoplasm because it has been reported that some osteoblastomas seem to regress after incomplete surgical removal. Dahlin has also reported that histologic fields within osteoblastoma are similar to those seen in aneurysmal bone cyst. This histologic feature in association with a rather remarkable clinical similarity between the two lesions suggests that both are slightly different manifestations of a reaction to some yet unknown agent.[5] Other authors maintain that osteoblastoma represents an exuberant attempt at repair of a hematoma of bone.[47] Despite these varied etiologic proposals, osteoblastoma is most widely accepted as a true neoplasm of bone.

Clinical Findings

Osteoblastoma most often involves the long bones of the appendicular and the vertebral skeleton. These two sites account for well over 60 per cent of all lesions. The maxilla and mandible are much less frequently involved. Smith and associates[48] reviewed a series of 24 cases of osteoblastoma and found that 15 occurred in the mandible and eight occurred in the maxilla. In one case the jaw involved was not specified. Osteoblastoma occurs most often in tooth-bearing areas, with the premolar-molar region being the most common site. Occasionally, lesions may involve the coronoid process. As with its long bone and vertebral counterparts, osteoblastoma of the jaws affects males more frequently than females, with a reported ratio of 2:1.[6] Smith and associates[48] found the average age for patients with jaw osteoblastoma to be 17.2 years, with women averaging slightly older (18 years) than men (16.8 years). The overall age range was from 5 to 37 years. Greer and Berman reviewed a series of 12 osteoblastomas of the jaws and reported ages that ranged from 8 to 20 years, with a mean age of 18 years.[38] These authors reported a mandibular propensity with only two of their cases occurring in the maxilla.

Osteoblastomas produce a wide range of signs and symptoms, depending on their location and the extent of the lesion.[8] Lesions of the spinal column can cause parasthesia, muscle weakness, pain, muscle spasms, and stiffness. Those in the extremities often result in swelling, pain, and atrophy along with functional impairment. The clinical picture of osteoblastoma of the jaw also varies with the location of the lesion and is usually diagnostically nonspecific. Pain is a common symptom, and although it may occasionally be severe, it is usually tolerable.[36, 37, 40] Of 24 cases reviewed by Smith and colleagues, swelling localized to the area of the tumor was the principal symptom in 19. Among those lesions producing a noticeable swelling, 17 caused pain and two were painless. Two lesions produced pain without a noticeable swelling. These authors reported no sensory disturbances, even in cases in which the tumor was contiguous with the mandibular nerve. One lesion presented as a mass protruding through an extraction socket.[35] The only asymptomatic case reviewed was a lesion of the coronoid process of the mandible.[41]

The duration of a patient's complaints prior to diagnosis appear to be less than for extragnathic sites, with the onset of pain and other symptoms ranging from weeks to several years. All 24 osteoblastomas reviewed by Smith and associates[48] were tender to palpation, and some had erythema overlying the mucosa. The buccal and lingual cortices were generally intact but most often were expanded, and teeth ranged from unaffected to tender to percussion to quite mobile. In general, laboratory data including serum calcium, phosphorus, and phosphatase values are within normal limits.

Osteoblastoma shows a varied radiographic picture in gnathic sites. Lesions can range in size from 2 cm to 10 cm in diameter; they may contain calcifications or may be totally radiolucent with peripheral bony sclerosis (Fig. 58–5). The radiographic appearance is often complicated by the presence of a dentition. The tumor most often begins centrally, producing a rather well-circumscribed radiolucent zone. As the lesion progresses, there develops an osteolytic defect that may contain speckled mineral deposits surrounded by an expanded or eroded remnant of the cortex.[35] Dahlin has reported that occasionally the tumor can be surrounded by a thin layer of bone beneath an expanded periosteum, thereby giving an appearance similar to that of an aneurysmal bone cyst.[5] Mandibular tumors usually have a classic appearance consisting of a spherical calcified tumor surrounded by a well-defined radiolucent zone. The tumor may directly abut or totally surround the root of a tooth, causing displacement or erosion. There is usually no evidence of a surrounding area of osteosclerosis, as is characteristic of osteoid osteoma. On occasion, a sun ray pattern of osseous trabeculae may be noted, mimicking osteosarcoma, Ewing's sarcoma, or actively growing fibrous dysplasia. Martin and associates[43] reported that bone scanning may be of some value in evaluating the extent of the spread of osteoblastoma; however, their studies were done on osteoblastoma of the axial skeleton, and to date, technetium bone scanning has not been shown to be of marked diagnostic significance in the jaws. Arteriography for jaw osteoblastomas appears to be of little diagnostic value, and tomography is generally only used to determine the degree of ossification or the lateral extent of the tumor.

Pathology

Gross inspection will generally reveal the tumor to be hemorrhagic, purplish to red, often gritty and friable, or densely calcified (Fig. 58–6). The central portions of large lesions are often cystic, and rarely do lesions

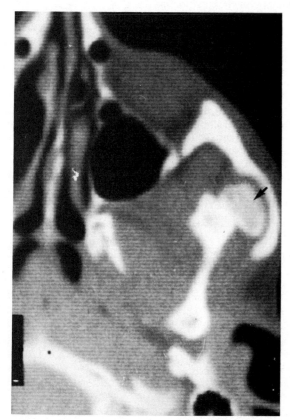

Figure 58–5. This CT scan shows well-delineated osteoblastoma of the condyle. (Courtesy of Dr. Randal James.)

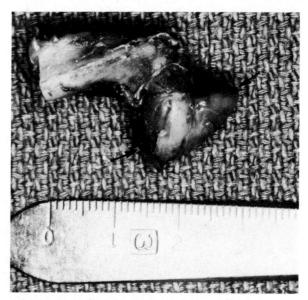

Figure 58–6. Gross surgical specimen of osteoblastoma showing expansile condylar osteoblastoma. (Courtesy of Dr. Randal James.)

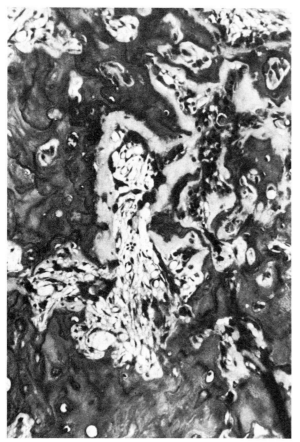

Figure 58–7. Osteoblastoma composed of a proliferation of osseous trabeculae rimmed by layered osteoblasts. Note the considerable remodeling of bone and the marked hyperchromic nuclei of osteoblasts. (H & E, × 300)

exceed 4 cm in size. Greer and Berman found that all the jaw osteoblastomas they reviewed were at least 1 cm in diameter at the time of pathologic examination. Huvos[8] reported that a constant histologic hallmark of osteoblastoma is that of cellular osteoblastic type tissue with ample intercellular osteoid material without evidence of cartilaginous cells during any stage of maturation.

Osteoblastoma of the jaws is histologically indistinguishable from its counterpart in the long bones and vertebral column. The tumor is classically composed of a highly vascularized stroma with abundant trabeculae of osteoid and immature bone in various phases of calcification. Individual trabeculae are usually rimmed by plump, often layered proliferating osteoblasts (Fig. 58–7). These osteoblasts tend to have hyperchromatic nuclei but mitotic activity is rare. Multinucleated osteoclasts are frequently seen throughout the supporting stroma. Areas of necrosis may be seen within osteoblastoma. Adjacent to these areas of necrosis, vascular channels, spindly fibroblastic tissue, and woven bone are usually prominent.

Differential Diagnosis

Owing to its cellularity, rapid growth, and potential for destruction, osteoblastoma may be confused with a host of osteogenic neoplasms (Table 58–1) clinically and microscopically. Osteosarcoma may have cartilaginous production, whereas osteoblastoma is free of such production unless there has been a pathologic fracture.[8] In addition, osteosarcoma contains areas of malignant osteoid in compact strands with little evidence of stroma and a paucity of blood vessels. Osteoblastoma, on the other hand, has an abundance of woven bone and thick osteoid with a lamellar layering of osteoblasts, a richly vascularized stroma, and a regular serrated margin around the woven bone or osteoid. There are no known reports of malignant change of osteoblastoma to osteosarcoma in the jaw bones.

The distinction between osteoblastoma and osteoid osteoma may be even more difficult. Aszodi[34a] reviewed a series of ten cases of extragnathic osteoblastoma and compared them with ten cases of extragnathic osteoid osteoma. He found that patients with osteoid osteoma possessed approximately 10 per cent more osteoid than osteoblastoma, but the number of osteoblasts in both lesions was essentially the same. Although this point of histologic variation is well conceived for extragnathic sites, it remains extremely difficult to distinguish osteoblastoma from osteoid osteoma in the jaws.

Fibrous dysplasia, especially the craniofacial variety described by Waldron and Giansanti,[33] may also be confused with osteoblastoma. The most useful means

TABLE 58–1. Differential Diagnostic Considerations for Osteoblastoma of the Jaws

Tumors	Histologic Features	Radiographic Features	Symptoms
Osteoblastoma	No cartilage production unless fracture, rich vascular stroma	Peripheral or perifocal osseous reaction minimal; lesion >2 cm	Variable pain
Osteosarcoma	Cartilage production common; sparce stroma	Variable, ranging from lucent to markedly sclerotic, poorly delineated	Variable pain
Osteoid osteoma	No cartilage production unless fracture, central nidus; stroma ranges from well vascularized to dense fibrous	Peripheral or perifocal osseous reaction marked; lesion <2 cm	Persistent pain
Fibrous dysplasia	Woven, globular or lamellar bone; stroma ranges from well vascularized to dense fibrous	Poorly defined merging border, little peripheral osseous reaction	Generally painless but expansile and occasionally tender

of differentiating between the two is by microscopic examination of the tissue. Woven bone set in a fibrous stroma is more characteristic of fibrous dysplasia. This histologic pattern is far from the predominant blastic and richly vascular histologic pattern of osteoblastoma. Some reported osteoblastomas show a strong clinical, radiographic, and histologic resemblance to cemento-blastoma.[35, 40, 42, 45] Abrams and associates[34] reported extreme difficulty in distinguishing osteoblastomas from cementoblastomas in the most active and cellular areas of the tumors; however, they found broad trabecular regions with limited cellularity to be a prominent feature that is possibly unique to cementoblastoma. Many authors conclude that the attachment of a tumor to a tooth root justifies a diagnosis of cementoblastoma; however, Larsson[42] suggests that this finding is not absolutely diagnostic because an osteoblastoma may envelope the roots of a tooth, resulting in clinical findings characteristic of cementoblastoma.

Finally, ossifying fibroma may be confused with osteoblastoma. A rich osteoblastic stroma and layering of osteoblasts are prominent features of osteoblastoma and are not common to ossifying fibroma.

Treatment and Prognosis

Treatment and follow-up data on osteoblastoma in gnathic sites are rather sparse. Of the 24 cases reviewed by Smith and colleagues,[48] follow-up ranged from 0 to 9 years. In only two of their cases were recurrences reported. Data from gnathic and extragnathic sites indicate that in nonexpanded bone, treatment by either curettage or local excision is likely to achieve success. The possibility of recurrence, however, mandates close follow-up.[48] In six of the 12 cases that were reviewed by Greer and Berman[38] and in which follow-up was reported, there had been no recurrences during periods ranging from 1 to 3 years. Some authors suggest that there is a possibility that osteoblastoma can develop malignant histologic features and pursue an aggressive course, resulting in death from the effects of local extension.[39, 46] Schajowicz and Lemos[46] believe that the term malignant osteoblastoma should be applied to these nonmetastasizing but locally aggressive tumors. No such tumors have ever been recorded in the jaws.

Osteoid Osteoma

Osteoid osteoma is a relatively slow growing, usually well-demarcated osseous lesion that classically grows to no greater than 1 cm in diameter. The lesion typically has a central nidus of bone destruction. Osteoid osteoma was first described as a distinct entity in 1935 by Jaffe,[52] who described five cases of the lesion and their specific clinicopathology. The lesion was originally thought to occur only within spongy bones, but it is now well recognized that osteoid osteoma can develop in the cortices of long bones, the jaws, and the facial skeleton. There has been rather considerable confusion regarding usage of the terms osteoblastoma and osteoid osteoma. Many authors consider that osteoid osteoma in the jaw bones is closely linked to osteoblastoma and is probably no more than a clinical and morphologic variant of the latter.[37] The principal reason for this confusion is dictated by the fact that the histologic appearance for both

lesions can be quite similar. Differentiation between the two in the jaws has been suggested primarily on the basis of size, site of involvement, and degree of reactive sclerosis.[56] Lesions larger than 1 cm in diameter have usually been termed osteoblastoma. Osteoid osteomas of the jaws were reviewed in 1968 by Greene and associates,[51] who identified six cases in the literature and added one of their own. By 1970 a total of only 12 cases had been reported in the English literature.[50]

The etiology of the osteoid osteoma has yet to be determined. There is a question as to whether or not the lesion represents a true neoplasm because it appears to have some self-limited growth potential. Recent reports have suggested a vascular origin for the lesion,[50, 57] but others[49] indicate that osteoid osteomas represent undergrown osteoblastomas.

Osteoid osteoma is most frequently identified in the cortex or the medullary bone, although it may be located in a midcortical, subperiosteal, or endosteal location. The subperiosteal form is rarest. The lesion has been recorded in nearly every bone in the skeleton and shows a special predilection for bones of the legs. Of 12 osteoid osteomas of the jaws reported by Farman,[37] seven were in the mandible and five were in the maxilla.

The sex distribution was equal among the 12 cases, and the age at diagnosis ranged from 4 to 77 years, although the vast majority of the osteoid osteomas that were reviewed occurred in young adults. This age finding is consistent with long bone findings, in which most osteoid osteomas have been reported in patients between the ages of 10 and 25. The lesion is rarely identified in patients older than 30 years of age. Although a male predilection has been noted in bones of the axial skeleton, no such predilection has been noted in the jaw bones.

Osteoid osteoma has limited growth potential and rarely exceeds 1 cm in greatest diameter. A peripheral rim of osteosclerosis is a common radiographic feature in long bones. The lesion often has been reported to be associated with pain that is relieved by aspirin. Within the medullary bone of the maxilla or mandible, the lesion is characterized radiographically by a central area of radiolucent destruction surrounded by a relatively densely sclerotic border. If the lesion involves the cortex, the adjacent cortical bone often becomes strikingly thickened by new periosteal bone formation. Most osteoid osteomas show some radiographic evidence of a central radiolucent nidus. In those lesions where the center of the nidus is composed of poorly mineralized osteoid tissue, a marked radiolucency is noted. In those lesions in which the nidus is denser and is composed of mineralized bone, a central calcified osseous nidus can be noted. A so-called annular sequestrum may be depicted in association with osteoid osteoma of the long bones and vertebral column but is a distinct rarity in the jaws. Differential diagnosis on the basis of radiographic findings is often difficult. Osteoid osteoma may be confused with Garré's osteomyelitis, osteosarcoma, or a fracture undergoing repair. If a faintly distinct and rarified peripheral periosteal reaction is noted in the mandible in association with a nonvital tooth, Garré's osteomyelitis is the preferred differential radiographic diagnosis.

Technetium bone scanning may be of value in determining the extent of an osteoid osteoma, and tomography may be helpful in determining the degree of ossification as well as the extent of the tumor. Arteriography is nondiagnostic because only reactive hyperemia in the lesional area is visualized.[55]

Pathology

The gross appearance of osteoid osteoma is variable. The central nidus may occur entirely within the cortex, or it may be located in the spongy bone. The nidus ranges in shape from oval to globular and is generally quite well demarcated from the surrounding peripheral bone. The nidus often has the consistency of granulation tissue with a gritty-meaty quality.

The classic microscopic appearance of osteoid osteoma is that of a central nidus surrounded by a peripheral limiting zone of cortical bone. Jaffe[52] postulated three evolutionary stages of nidus formation in osteoid osteoma:

1. An initial stage characterized by a proliferation of densely packed prominent osteoblasts set in a rich, highly vascularized stroma.

2. An intermediate phase rich in osteoblasts with interlacing osteoid zones.

3. A mature or compact stage in which the osteoid becomes well mineralized or calcified.

It is not always possible to identify the central osteoid nidus, and Huvos[8] has reported that in 10 to 15 per cent of the cases of osteoid osteoma microscopic confirmation of the nidus is not possible. This difficulty underlines the importance of submitting all clinically suspicious tissue that is removed from the jaw bones for thorough evaluation for a confirmatory nidus if osteoid osteoma is the suspected diagnosis.

Electron microscopic studies have shown no essential difference between the structure of the cells of osteoblastoma and osteoid osteoma. Ultrastructural findings typically show evidence of rapid peripheral bone formation surrounding a central nidus similar to light microscopic findings. Johnson and Steiner indicate that the characteristic osteoblastic resorption of bone is induced by cells that have little, if any, affinity for osteoid.[54, 58]

Differential Diagnosis

Histologically, osteoid osteoma can be distinguished from osteoblastoma if a central nidus is identifiable, although a highly vascular stroma with trabeculae rimmed by osteoblasts can be seen in both lesions. Osteoid osteoma differs from benign osteoblastoma primarily because of its broader, longer, and more widely separated osteoid trabeculae.[8] Osteoid osteoma is also considered by most authorities to be less cellular, less vascular, and much less rich in osteoblastic activity.[52, 53] Although these distinctions are quite prominently referred to in studies of bones from areas other than the facial skeleton and jaws, it is exceedingly difficult to distinguish between osteoblastoma and osteoid osteoma in the jaws. So difficult is the distinction that Farman and coworkers[37] deem it advisable to consider the two lesions a single entity.

Treatment and Prognosis

Osteoid osteoma will continue to grow in the absence of surgical intervention. Removal of the nidus of the lesion with complete curettage and eburnation or saucerization of the surrounding bone is generally considered adequate surgery and will typically effect a cure, although occasionally, resections are deemed necessary. Recurrence has been reported in long bones, but we are unaware of any recurrence of osteoid osteoma in the jaws.

MALIGNANT BONE-FORMING TUMORS

Osteosarcoma

Osteosarcoma is recognized as the most common primary malignancy of bone, accounting for greater than 20 per cent of all primary osseous malignancies; however, osteosarcoma is rarely encountered in the mandible or maxilla. Coley, in a review of 985 cases of osteosarcoma, reported that only 62 cases (6 per cent) involved the jaws.[62] Garrington,[68] in an analysis of 56 cases of osteosarcoma of the jaws, reported a 6.5 per cent incidence for osteosarcoma in all age groups. In a review of 60 tumor and tumor-like conditions of the maxilla and mandible in children recorded on the surgical pathology and autopsy services of the Barnes Hospital and Washington University School of Medicine, Dehner[17] documented 14 primary and secondary malignant tumors; among these only three osteosarcomas were accessioned. Kahnna and Kahnna, in an exhaustive review of 122 primary tumors of the maxilla and mandible, found no cases of osteosarcoma during a 17-year period.[24] Greer and Mierau[20] recorded only two instances of osteosarcoma, both in the mandible, in their review of 191 childhood tumors of the jaws seen at the University of Colorado during a 7-year period.

Although osteosarcoma of long bones has a peak incidence between the ages of 10 and 25 years, the peak age of onset in the jaws is approximately a decade later. Males are affected approximately twice as frequently as females.[66] On rare occasions, multiosseous osteosarcomas have been reported either as a metastasis from a single primary site or as a result of multicentric tumor formation.[74]

Although the peak frequency of craniofacial osteosarcoma is the second or third decade of life, it is important to note that craniofacial osteosarcoma has been reported in children and adolescents.[6] There is some indication that patients with mandibular lesions tend to be slightly younger than those with maxillary lesions, although Finkelstein[66] in a review of 24 cases from the M.D. Anderson Hospital reported that patients with mandibular lesions were approximately 10 years older than those with maxillary lesions.

A single etiology for osteosarcoma of the jaws has not been determined. It has been postulated that the lesion may be initiated by radiation, pre-existing bone disorders, or trauma. Experimental support for the concept that the tumor may be related to a disturbance of bone growth and maturation during periods of osteoblastic activity has been offered by Baserga and associates.[59] Paget's disease and fibrous dysplasia are the most common pre-existing benign lesions associated with osteosarcoma.[71] Tillman, in a review of 24 cases of Paget's disease involving the jaws, found sarcoma of all types to be a complication in three cases.[75]

Several studies have shown that osteosarcoma of long bones has an increased incidence in canines.[73] Osteosarcoma has also been produced experimentally in several species of animals using a variety of physical and chemical agents. Cottier and associates[63] have suggested that a hormonal factor may be involved in tumor histiogenesis. Osteosarcoma has been reported in patients who have received injections of Thorotrast radioactive contrast medium,[76] and injections of Moloney murine sarcoma virus has resulted in high-grade malignant osteosarcomas in rats.[65, 67]

Osteosarcoma of the craniofacial bones is not divided into subtypes on the basis of clinical staging. There are, however, four unique histologic subtypes that will be discussed in this subsection.

Juxtacortical or *parosteal* osteosarcoma, which originates on the external surface of a bone in relationship to the periosteum or to the immediate parosteal connective tissue, is exceedingly rare in the jaws. The incidence has been reported to range from 1.7 per cent to less than 1 per cent of all bone tumors, and by 1976 only 107 examples of the tumor have been reported, with three from the mandible and one from the maxilla.[72] The neoplasm occurs most often in the third decade of life.

Multiosseous osteosarcoma or multicentric osteosarcoma has also occasionally been reported in the jaws.[74] Individuals with genetically transmissible retinoblastoma have an increased incidence of femoral osteogenic sarcoma,[69] but a predisposition toward secondary osteosarcoma of the jaws has not been reported in individuals with retinoblastoma.

Clinical Findings

The most common symptom of osteosarcoma affecting the jaws and facial skeleton is the presence of a mass, lump, or swelling (Fig. 58–8).[6] Caron and associates,[60] in a review of 43 cases of osteogenic sarcoma of the facial and cranial bones, found that the most common complaint noted by patients was a painful swelling. The tumor is more common in the mandible than the maxilla, and the body of the mandible is involved more often than the symphysis, angle, or ascending ramus. Maxillary lesions may arise from any portion of that bone. However, they most often occur along the alveolar ridge. Curtis[64] has recently reported that mobility of teeth, cortical expansion, and soft-tissue swelling are features common to both maxillary and mandibular osteosarcomas. Pain and paresthesia more often accompany mandibular tumors, and nasal obstruction, discharge, and epistaxis dominate as symptoms of maxillary tumors. Many patients feel that the symptoms associated with osteosarcoma are directly of dental origin; therefore, extraction as an initial treatment modality was seen in 40 to 50 per cent of maxillary and mandibular tumors reviewed by Curtis.[64]

Caron and associates[60] have reported that serum al-

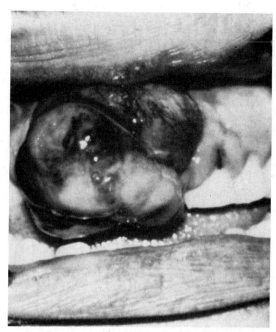

Figure 58–8. Expansile lobulated osteosarcoma of the anterior maxilla. (Courtesy of the Western Society of Oral Pathologists slide collection, Dr. Phillip Sapp and John Given.)

kaline phosphatase values may be elevated in the presence of osteosarcoma of the jaws and facial bones. In a review of 22 patients, they found elevated levels in six individuals.

Osteosarcoma of the jaws and facial skeleton shows a variable radiographic pattern. Lesions can range from totally radiolucent, poorly delineated unicentric lesions to dense radiopaque masses with a prominent "sunburst" appearance. The sunburst pattern has been shown to be nonspecific and can be encountered not only in osteosarcoma but also in osteomyelitis, Ewing's sarcoma, and benign fibro-osseous lesions, such as ossifying fibroma and fibrous dysplasia. Although osteosarcoma often does not result in alteration of maxillary or mandibular bony contours in its early phase, the lesion is quite rapidly progressive, and frequently, within a period of 6 to 8 weeks, bony contours become altered.

Roentgenographic evidence of a symmetrically widened periodontal membrane space may be a significant early finding in osteosarcoma of the jaws (Fig. 58–9). Garrington[68] initially documented the fact that insipient osteosarcoma is often first associated with destruction of the periodontal ligament. Although a widened periodontal membrane space is certainly not diagnostic of osteosarcoma, the presence of this radiographic sign, along with either a diffuse sclerotic or lytic lesion and paresthesia, should heighten the clinician's index of suspicion.

Occasionally metastatic carcinoma, especially prostatic and lung carcinoma, can mimic osteosarcoma of the mandible. These lesions are usually lytic and have poorly defined serrated margins. Multiosseous osteosarcoma should also be considered in the differential

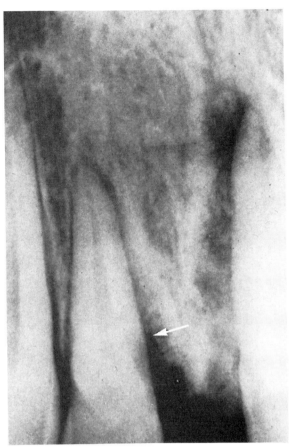

Figure 58–9. Arrow demonstrates characteristic widening of the periodontal ligament space in osteosarcoma of the maxilla. (Courtesy of the Western Society of Oral Pathologists, Dr. Phillip Sapp and John Given.)

diagnosis of multicentric poorly defined lytic lesions of the mandible or maxilla of undetermined origin.

Angiography, bone scans, and xeroradiography have all shared some acclaim as diagnostic methods for osteosarcoma in long bones. Although all three may be of some benefit in determining the operability of patients by delineating the extent of the tumor, their use in the jaws has been of little benefit. Computerized tomographic (CT) scanning may prove to be the most definitive of the new diagnostic procedures for determining anatomic limits of osteosarcomas in the jaws and craniofacial regions.

The roentgenographic appearance of *juxtacortical osteosarcoma* is often remarkably different from that of conventional medullary osteosarcoma. This special variant of osteosarcoma is likely to present as a large irregular and densely opaque ossified tumor mass adherent to and blending with the regional bony cortex.

Pathology

Osteosarcoma is classically divided into four histologic subtypes: fibroblastic, chondroblastic, osteoblastic, and telangiectatic. The vast majority of osteosarcomas in the jaws are osteoblastic. Telangiectatic osteosarcoma within the jaw bones and craniofacial skeleton is the rarest of the four subtypes. In order to render a diagnosis of osteosarcoma, one must find histologically undeniable areas of a sarcomatous stroma and direct production of tumor osteoid and bone from malignant connective tissue. Tumor stroma is characteristically composed of anaplastic spindle or oval cells with hyperchromatic nuclei, and tumor foci at the periphery of the specimen tend to be poorly mineralized (Fig. 58–10). There is general agreement among bone pathologists that osteosarcomas of the jaws display an appreciably lesser degree of anaplasia than their long bone counterparts.[5, 68] Multinucleated giant cell forms that are histologically benign may be seen in osteosarcoma; thus, benign giant cell tumors may be difficult to distinguish from osteosarcoma.

The ultrastructure of osteosarcoma has been well characterized by Williams and associates.[77] These authors have shown the most characteristic diagnostic ultrastructural feature to be the presence of dilated cisternae of rough endoplasmic reticulum and the variable presence and hydroxyapatite crystals overlying a collagenous matrix (Figs. 58–11 and 58–12). Garrington and associates reviewed a series of 56 cases of osteosarcoma microscopically and found no correlation between the histologic appearance of the tumor and the eventual prognosis.[68]

Differential Diagnosis

Chondrosarcoma may be easily confused with osteosarcoma. It is, however, a lesion of cartilaginous derivation and will not show neoplastic osteoid or bone developing directly from a sarcomatous stroma. Malignant fibrous histiocytoma may also resemble osteosarcoma histologically. Dahlin[5] has indicated that the principal features that allow its distinction from osteosarcoma are as follows:

1. Malignant giant cells with nuclei that possess a histiocytic appearance with indentation of the nuclei.
2. A storiform fibrogenic pattern.
3. Histiocytic mononuclear cells distributed focally throughout the neoplasm.
4. Considerable anaplasia with atypical mitoses and nuclear anisocytosis.

Although on rare occasions odontogenic tumors, ossifying fibroma, and osteoblastoma may produce considerable amounts of mineralized product, simulating osteosarcoma both clinically and radiographically, histologic distinction between the lesions should be relatively simple. Periosteal osteosarcoma of the jaws and facial skeleton should be distinguished from benign lesions that can display a juxtacortical position such as osteochondroma and myositis ossificans. Microscopically, these lesions demonstrate a zonal arrangement with active fibroblasts at the center and maturing bone trabeculae at the periphery. Periosteal osteosarcoma, on the other hand, has bony trabeculae that dominate the base of the lesion.

Treatment and Prognosis

The treatment for osteosarcoma in the craniofacial region remains ablative surgery, although radiation therapy and combined chemotherapeutic regimens in association with surgery have shown some success.

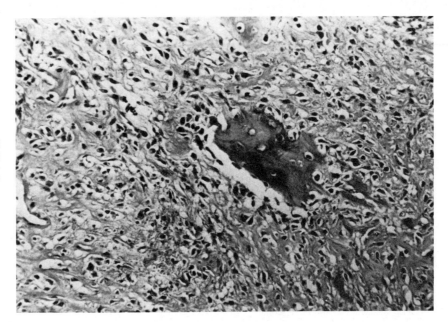

Figure 58–10. Osteosarcoma showing scattered foci of tumor osteoid arising directly from sarcomatous stroma. Calcific osteoid production is prominent throughout the neoplasm. (H & E, × 240)

Chambers and Mahoney[61] reported on the management of a series of osteosarcomas of the craniofacial bones using external beam radiation therapy with dosages as high as 16,000 rad. These authors found that the overall short-term disease free survival rate in their series of 33 patients was 76 per cent.

Osteosarcoma of the jaws and bones of the cranium and face has a better prognosis than in its long bone counterparts. Garrington and colleagues[68] reported a 35 per cent 5-year survival rate in 34 patients they followed, and Curtis and associates[64] reported that approximately 26 per cent of their patients with maxillary lesions and 35 per cent of their patients with mandibular lesions survived 5 years. Finkelstein reported a 32.3 per cent 5-year survival rate in his series of jaw osteosarcomas.[66]

Schwartz and Alpert[70] reported a 13 per cent incidence of metastasis in analyzing data concerning the metastatic potential of mandibular osteosarcoma. The majority of their metastatic lesions were identified in the lung. Upper cervical lymph node metastases occur much less frequently.

MALIGNANT CARTILAGINOUS TUMORS

Chondrosarcoma

Chondrosarcoma is a malignant neoplasm devoid of tumor osteoid with evidence of fully developed cartilaginous structures. Chondrosarcoma is an exceedingly rare primary tumor of the jaw and facial skeleton (10

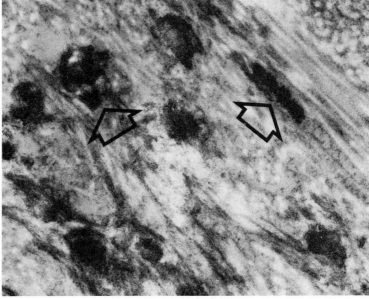

Figure 58–11. Osteosarcoma. Hydroxyapatite crystals (arrows) are being deposited on collagen fibers. (EM, × 32,500)

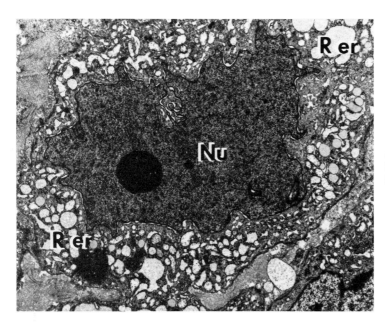

Figure 58–12. Neoplastic osteoblast typically exhibits large irregularly shaped nuclei (Nu) and a prominent rough endoplasmic reticulum (Rer). (EM, × 4800)

per cent of all chondrosarcomas), yet excluding multiple myeloma, it represents the second most common primary malignancy of bone. Dahlin, in a review of 470 chondrosarcomas, found 24 in the head and neck region.[5] Pritchard and colleagues reviewed 358 cases of chondrosarcoma of bone seen at the Mayo Clinic between 1909 and 1975, and they were able to document only 24 cases in the head and neck region.[92] The maxilla, mandible, nasal septum, sphenoid sinus, and ethmoid sinuses are the most common head and neck sites of origin for chondrosarcoma.

Chondrosarcoma can be identified as either peripheral or central, depending on its osseous location. A so-called juxtacortical or periosteal chondrosarcoma has been reported and is thought to be the equivalent of the juxtacortical osteosarcoma. It is rare in the jaws.

Chaudhry and colleagues[78] reviewed 52 chondrogenic jaw lesions and found that malignant cartilaginous neoplasms outnumbered benign ones by a ratio of 2:1. Blum[78] has suggested that chondrogenic neoplasms of the jaws be viewed with a great degree of suspicion, based on the realization that all cartilaginous jaw lesions might be at least potentially malignant. Batsakis[1] has suggested that the combination of a paucity of cases in the jaws and facial skeleton, linked with both the propensity for recurrence and subsequent aggressive behavior by an apparently benign jaw neoplasm such as a chondroma, lends some credence to the theory that lesions diagnosed as chondromas in this location are frequently in reality incipient chondrosarcomas.

The exact origin of chondrosarcoma in the jaws has not been determined. It is well known, however, that chondrosarcoma may be induced by irradiation. Fitzwater and associates[83] reviewed a series of 168 cases of radiation-induced bone sarcomas and found that 9 per cent were chondrosarcomas. Chondrosarcoma has also been reported to arise from pre-existing Paget's disease of bone,[94] and rarely, chondrosarcoma has been reported to arise in association with fibrous dysplasia[82] and the solitary bone cyst.[84]

Some authors have postulated that the predisposition of chondrosarcoma for the posterior mandible and anterior maxilla supports the concept that the lesion arises from cartilaginous remnants of the nasal capsule and Meckel's cartilage. However, Greer and associates discount this theory, emphasizing that chondrosarcoma can arise de novo from osseous tissues without the presence of cartilaginous rest.[6]

The Armed Forces Institute of Pathology had recorded 60 well-documented cases of chondrosarcoma of the jaws by 1974. The age range in their cases was from 12 to 80 years, with an average age of 32. This average age is identical with the age recorded for cases of osteosarcoma of the jaws at that institution. Among 264 patients with chondrosarcoma of all anatomic sites studied at Memorial Hospital from 1949 to 1973, an average age of 41.5 years was recorded. Males and females appear to be affected equally, although Huvos has noted a male predominance.[8]

Clinical Findings

Although rapidly expanding high-grade medullary chondrosarcomas of the long bones have been reported to cause excrutiating pain,[90] the chief clinical findings in lesions of the jaws and facial skeleton tend to be painless expansion of the cortical plates, loosening of teeth, nasal stuffiness, nasal discharge, epistaxis, and diplopia. The rare *juxtacortical chondrosarcoma* of the jaws may occur as a symptomless elevated nodule with little, if any, discomfort and only a barely visible palpable swelling. Until recently, it was uniformly accepted that the mandible was more commonly a site for chondrosarcoma than the maxilla; however, Terezhalmy and Bottomley[93] have suggested that the tumor is found with equal frequency in both arches, while Huvos notes a maxillary predilection.[8]

Chondrosarcoma of the jaws shows a variable radiographic pattern. Potdar[91] found no specific radiographic changes suggestive of a cartilaginous tumor in half of

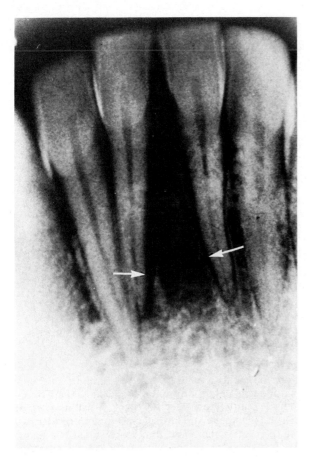

Figure 58–13. Mandibular chondrosarcoma resulting in a feathered, motheaten radiolucency with interseptal bone destruction. (Courtesy of Dr. Roy Eversole.)

the cases he reviewed. Medullary chondrosarcomas of the jaws most often demonstrate large, thick-walled areas of radiolucency with central areas of compartmentalized medullary bone destruction (Fig. 58–13). Within these areas of destruction, so-called "cotton-wool" type calcifications may be identified. Occasionally, chondrosarcoma will present with a ground-glass appearance or a sunburst radiographic appearance. Cortical destruction occurs late in the course of the disease, and periosteal bone formation is often limited. When periosteal bone formation occurs it may mimic Paget's disease of bone. Some authors have noted that a uniform widening of the periodontal membrane space, similar to that seen in osteosarcoma, can be observed with chondrosarcoma.[6] In late stage disease the primary lesion may penetrate the cortical plate and extend into adjacent soft tissues, resulting in a fuzzy soft-tissue peripheral shadow on subsequent radiographic examination.

Attempts to correlate angiography and tumor grade in long bones have shown that the more abundant the vascularity of the tumor, the more malignant the tumor tends to appear on subsequent microscopic examination. Although angiography may be useful in identifying the portion of a tumor that is most vascular, it is not possible to separate low-grade chondrosarcoma of the jaws from benign chondroma on the basis of the relative vascularity of the lesion. Features that favor a benign

cartilaginous lesion include slow growth, abundant intralesional calcification, and sclerotic peripheral lesional borders. Rapid enlargement, a paucity of intralesional calcifications, and peripheral lytic borders presume a diagnosis of chondrosarcoma.

Pathology

Central medullary chondrosarcomas are generally characterized by blue-white, often opalescent translucent lobular tissue, which on cut sections may show a mucoid character. The peripheral margin of the tumor will show abundant or sparse reactive bone, depending on the rapidity of tumor growth.

Diagnosis of chondrosarcoma on the basis of microscopic findings can be exceedingly challenging. In order to render a proper diagnosis, thorough evaluation of radiographs, clinical history, and multiple tissue samples is mandatory.

Histologic diagnostic criteria for chondrosarcoma were first established by Lichtenstein and Jaffe[88] in 1943. More recently, Evans and co-workers[81] have attempted to associate histologic grades of chondrosarcoma with the ultimate biologic behavior of the tumor. Chondrosarcoma continues to be defined as a malignant tumor composed of fully developed cartilage without tumor osteoid being directly formed from a sarcomatous stroma. Myxoid changes, calcification, and ossification may, however, be present. Lesions regarded as grade 1 by Evans and coworkers contain small, dense-staining chondrocyte nuclei and focal areas with slightly enlarged nuclei and at least a few multinucleated forms. Mineralization in the form of osseous development at the edge of the cartilaginous lobules is common. Abundant cellularity and significant numbers of enlarged nuclei and mitotic figures are rarely observed in grade 1 lesions. Grade 2 chondrosarcomas contain increased cellularity, sometimes at the periphery of tumor lobules, and nuclei that are much larger than those of grade 1 lesions (Fig. 58–14). These alterations indicative of a higher grade lesion may be focal and therefore may not be evident in inadequately sampled tissue. Grade 3 chondrosarcoma shows pronounced nuclear enlargement and prominent multinucleation. Cartilaginous lobulation is sparse, and spindle cell forms are abundant in grade 3 disease.

Grade 3 lesions have the gravest prognosis. Marcove and associates[89] reviewed a series of 152 chondrosarcomas arising in the pelvic bones and found that 56 were grade 1, 53 were grade 2, and 43 were grade 3. Although a similar large series of cranial-facial chondrosarcomas has not been reviewed, Chaudhry and associates[79] have suggested that the largest percentage of tumors identified in their review of jaw tumors were grade 1 lesions.

Differential Diagnosis

A recently identified clear cell variant of chondrosarcoma has been reported by Unni and associates.[95] The tumor affects males more often than females and shows a marked predilection for secondary centers of ossification in the epiphyses and abutting metaphyses of long bones. These lesions show an abundance of giant cells, osteoid, and large clear cells resembling chondroblasts. This variant is rarely seen in the jaws.

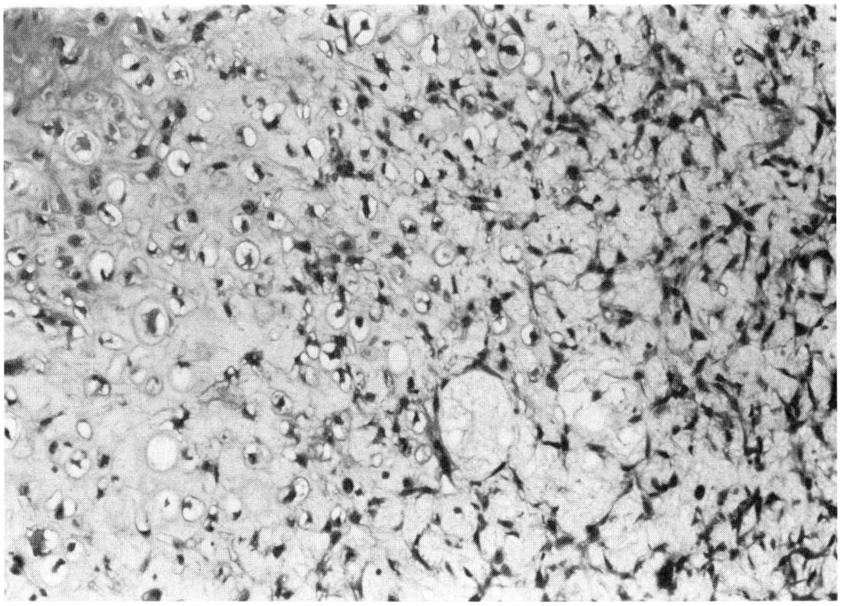

Figure 58–14. Moderately well differentiated grade 2 chondrosarcoma showing pleomorphic cartilaginous cells with atypical hyperchromatic nuclei. The cartilaginous matrix is easily identifiable. (H & E, × 180)

MESENCHYMAL CHONDROSARCOMA

Mesenchymal chondrosarcoma is an exceedingly rare malignant neoplasm that was first described by Lichtenstein in 1959.[87] Since that time, fewer than 100 cases have been reported in the literature. The neoplasm is characterized by a "bimorphic histologic pattern" consisting of sheets, clusters, and cords of highly undifferentiated small round cells that often have a slight spindling quality with an admixture of chondroid matrix that ranges from poorly differentiated to well differentiated (Fig. 58–15). The tumor may be confused with hemangiopercytoma because of its rich vascularity. However, identification of a cartilaginous substructure should substantiate a diagnosis of mesenchymal chondrosarcoma. The tumor is most commonly identified in the second and third decades of life, and this is significantly earlier than in chondrosarcoma. In a recent review of 81 cases, Joshi and associates[84a] found that 42 per cent of mesenchymal chondrosarcomas were identified in extraskeletal sites. The lesion shows a slight female predilection. Fifteen of approximately 100 reported cases have been reported in the maxilla and mandible. The tumor is radioresistant, and the management modality of choice is radical surgical excision.

BENIGN CHONDROBLASTOMA

Benign chondroblastoma is an exceptionally rare neoplasm in the jaws. It is characterized by a mixture of compact clusters of round to polyhedral cells with distinct nuclear membranes and eosinophilic cytoplasm. The chondromatous character is revealed by transition of tumor cells to areas of mature hyaline cartilage. The classic histologic feature is one of variable amounts of focal calcification between tumor cells. Calcification appears to be most prominent in areas of necrosis and chondromatous transformation. The tumor is most often identified in the epiphyses of long bones. Dahlin and Ivans[80] reported only eight chondroblastomas in the jaws, facial bones, and cranial skeleton, an incidence of less than 2 per cent. The chondroblastoma is a benign neoplasm, and cure is effected by simple curettage. Recurrence is rare and usually follows inadequate surgery.

CHONDROMYXOID FIBROMA

Chondromyxoid fibroma was initially described as a distinct tumor of bone by Jaffe and Lichtenstein in 1948.[86] Since that time, only a few cases have been reported in the jaws, facial bones, and skull.[5] The majority have been identified in the mandible. The tumor, primarily a lesion of young adults, is histologically composed of lobular, spindle-shaped, or stellate cells with a myxoid or chondroid intercellular matrix. Multinucleated giant cells are common. The tumor shows a pseudolobular growth pattern in which crowding and condensation of tumor cells at the periphery are common.

Treatment and Prognosis

Chondrosarcoma of the jaws and facial bones requires radical local surgical excision with an adequate margin of surrounding tissue. In cases of residual disease, radiation therapy has been employed, but it is not generally recommended as a primary management modality. Chemotherapy has also been employed as an adjuvant, and recently, radioactive sulfur (^{35}S) has been introduced as a management modality. The prognosis for chondrosarcoma of the jaws is grave, with 5-year survival rates approximating those of osteosarcoma.

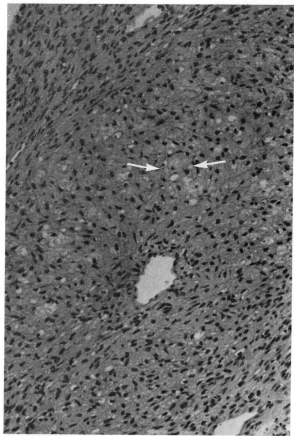

Figure 58–15. Mesenchymal chondrosarcoma composed of a richly vascular accumulation of undifferentiated round and spindle-shaped cells. Arrows identify a central area of chondroid matrix. (H & E, × 200) (From Greer RO, Mierau GW, Favara BE: Tumors of the Head and Neck in Children. New York, Praeger Publishers, 1983.)

TUMORS OF FIBROUS CONNECTIVE TISSUE ORIGIN

Desmoplastic Fibroma

Desmoplastic fibroma of extra-abdominal sites is an exceedingly rare tumor. Sugiura[105] reported that only 50 cases had been reported in the world literature by 1976. In 1978, Freedman and associates[97] reviewed the world literature concerning desmoplastic fibroma of the jaw and added one case of their own. These investigators were able to adequately document only 26 cases involving the jaws since Jaffe first reported the lesion as a separate entity from central fibrous lesions of bone in 1958.[99]

Desmoplastic fibroma is characterized by bundles of abundant collagen fibers separated by spindle-shaped fibroblasts with elongated or oval nuclei.[102] Etiologic factors responsible for desmoplastic fibromatosis are difficult to evaluate. The two most readily accepted causative factors for desmoid tumors of the anterior abdominal wall (trauma and pregnancy) cannot be invoked in extra-abdominal desmoids.[96] A hormonal eti-

ologic factor has been postulated but has not been proved.[96]

The desmoid tumor of extra-abdominal sites can affect all age groups. Masson and Soule[101] reported that the head and neck region accounted for 12 per cent of 284 desmoid tumors in all body locations in their review of these tumors in children and adults. The extra-abdominal desmoid tumor in the head and neck region is principally a lesion of young adults when soft tissue and bony sites are considered as a group. Masson and Soule[101] found a fairly uniform distribution of cases during the first five decades of life and noted that females outnumbered males three to one.

Freedman and associates,[97] in their review of desmoid tumors of the jaws, found a mean age of 15.7 years. Over 90 per cent of their cases occurred in patients during the first three decades of life. They found no sexual predisposition for the tumors.

Clinical Findings

Desmoplastic fibroma of jaw bones affects the mandible much more frequently than the maxilla. Freedman and associates[97] and Taguchi and Kaneda[106] found that approximately 70 per cent of the lesions they reviewed occurred in the molar-ramus-angle region of the mandible. The lesions grow slowly but progressively, and although most early lesions do not produce significant symptoms, the most common clinical manifestation of a lesion that has grown to a significant enough size to elicit symptoms is one of a painless swelling. The characteristic radiographic appearance of desmoplastic fibroma is a loculated, clearly defined radiolucency of bone (Fig. 58–16).[106] Freedman and associates reported that 34 per cent of the lesions they reviewed showed some degree of root resorption of the teeth in association with the lesion.[97] Slootweg and Muller[103] reported on two desmoplastic fibromas of the jaws and found that the most common presentation was that of a unilocular radiolucency with distinct margins. Jaw films of their lesions showed that the teeth appeared to be "hanging in air."

On the basis of radiographic findings, desmoplastic fibroma must be differentiated from central odontogenic fibroma of the jaw, giant cell granuloma, the radiolucent phase of fibrous dysplasia, and central osseous fibrosarcoma. Occasionally, a desmoid tumor of the jaw can produce a multilocular cystic quality, mimicking ameloblastoma, hemangioma, and aneurysmal bone cyst.

Pathology

The desmoid tumor is grossly composed of an admixture of whitish gray rubbery firm tissue that may contain areas of calcification. The histologic pattern is that of a rich proliferation of abundant collagen fibers that are woven and intertangled in layers (Fig. 58–17).[6] Cellularity is sparse. Only scattered whorles of fibroblasts with oval or fusiform nuclei can be identified distributed between collagen bundles. The center of the lesion may contain branching vascular clefts, foci of inflammatory cells, and rarely, scattered multinucleated giant cells. The periphery of the lesion is often so heavily collagen-

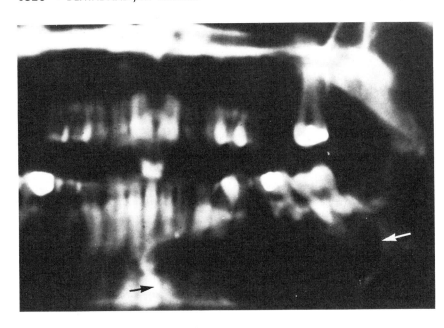

Figure 58–16. Desmoplastic fibroma of the mandible extending from ascending ramus to the midline (Courtesy of Dr. Doran Ryan; from Greer RO, Mierau GW, Favara BE: Tumors of the Head and Neck in Children. Philadelphia, Praeger Publishers, 1983.

ized that only elongated, dark-staining nuclei or metaplastic ossification or cartilaginous formation may be seen.

The lesion classically has an innocuous bland histologic appearance, and mitotic activity is rarely, if ever, present, although the presence of occasional mitosis does not mandate a diagnosis of a more aggressive neoplasm.

Differential Diagnosis

Histologic differentiation of desmoplastic fibroma from well-differentiated fibrosarcoma may be exceedingly difficult. Stout[104] reported that his attempts to find reliable methods of distinguishing between the two

diseases and detecting potential metastasizing tumors proved less than successful. Lesions with anaplastic forms and significant numbers of atypical mitoses should be classified as fibrosarcomas. Lesions with thick, wavy collagen bundles accompanied by sparsely cellular uniform fibroblasts with little or no mitotic activity are more compatible with desmoplastic fibroma. Above all, it should be noted that any suggestion that the term desmoid tumor (desmoplastic fibromatosis) and well-differentiated fibrosarcoma are interchangeable is unwarranted.

Desmoplastic fibroma should also be distinguished from central odontogenic fibroma of the jaws. Gardner postulated that all true central fibromas of the jaw should be accepted as either odontogenic fibroma or

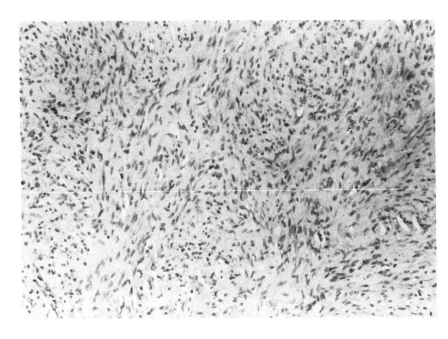

Figure 58–17. Desmoplastic fibroma of the mandible showing a rich collagenous stroma with interlacing bands and clusters of fibroblasts. (H & E, × 220)

desmoplastic fibroma.[98] He further suggested that all central jaw fibromas should be considered desmoplastic fibromas if they do not appear to arise from the odontogenic apparatus. Slootweg and Muller, however,[103] suggest that this approach harbors the danger that the concept of the well-defined desmoplasmic fibroma will become nebulous if the same diagnostic label is attached to every jaw fibroma for which an odontogenic origin cannot be proved conclusively. Huvos[8] has reported that in the case of a central fibrous lesion of the jaws, the lack of associated dental abnormalities and the abundant collagen-forming properties distinguish the desmoplastic fibroma from the more noncollagenized central odontogenic fibroma, which is often associated with unerupted teeth. A so-called periosteal desmoid tumor has been identified.[100] This lesion is histologically identical to the central osseous desmoplastic fibroma but is rarely encountered in the jaw bones.

Treatment and Prognosis

The treatment of choice for desmoplastic fibroma of the maxilla or mandible is en block surgical resection along with adjacent surrounding normal tissue. Sugiura[105] reported a recurrence of 12 of 50 cases of jaw desmoid tumors he reviewed. Masson and Soule[101] reported that 70 per cent of the patients in their Mayo Clinic series with head and neck desmoid tumors experience one or more recurrences.

Slootweg and Muller[103] reviewed two desmoplastic fibromas that were treated with enucleation and with excision and curettage, respectively. The lesion that was enucleated required no further therapy. The lesion that was treated with excision and curettage was treated 2 years after the initial surgery with re-excision and 5 years after the initial surgery with a block resection. Neither patient had evidence of disease after 15 years of follow-up. Huvos has reported that extensive curettage followed by cryosurgery holds promise as a current treatment for desmoplastic fibroma,[8] but there is little information concerning this management modality in the jaw region.

Fibrosarcoma

Fibrosarcoma is a rare neoplasm, accounting for 0.5 per cent of all malignancies and 2 to 10 per cent of all bone sarcomas.[108] The sites of origin of extragnathic fibrosarcoma in the head and neck in order of frequency are: soft tissues of the face and neck, the maxillary antrum, the paranasal sinuses, and nasopharynx.[108] When the jaws are involved, the mandible and maxilla are nearly equally represented and endosteal sites outnumber periosteal sites.[114, 115] Huvos and Higinbotham[115] reviewed a series of 130 skeletal fibrosarcomas and found that 19 occurred in the jaws, the facial skeleton, or the skull. Medullary fibrosarcoma accounted for 11 cases, and periosteal fibrosarcoma accounted for eight cases. These authors found that fibrosarcoma occurs more commonly in the mandible than the maxilla.[115] Most patients with fibrosarcoma of the jaws are 40 years or older.[108]

Fibrosarcoma in the head and neck region in children is a rather distinctive entity. The vast majority of the fibrosarcomas of infants and children are diagnosed within the first 5 years of life. Of 110 patients studied by Soule and Pritchard, 68 patients were in the first 5 years of life at the time of tumor discovery.[116]

The etiology of fibrosarcoma is unknown, although there are occasional reports of fibrosarcoma arising in burn scars or at the site of a clinically draining sinus tract or in association with fibrous dysplasia, Paget's disease, or giant cell tumor.[6] Postradiation fibrosarcoma can occur in the oral tissues, usually the tongue, following radiation therapy for carcinoma,[116] but such fibrosarcomas are exceedingly rare in the jaws. A hereditary predisposition for fibrosarcoma has been proposed but remains to this date unproved.

Clinical Findings

The principal clinical symptom of fibrosarcoma of the jaws is the presence of a mass or swelling. Pain is not a constant feature but may occur along with paresthesia, trismus, or pathologic fractures. Although there are no distinguishing routine roentgenologic features of fibrosarcoma, nearly all patients present with evidence of a radiolucent defect of variable size (Fig. 58–18). Root surfaces in the region may exhibit erosion.[118] The site of origin within the jaws remains obscure, although the periodontal ligament has been suggested as the most likely origin.

Pathology

Grossly, fibrosarcomas are composed of dense, gray-white masses of tissue that may contain cystic or myxomatous areas. Perforation of the labial or linqual cortices may produce contiguous soft-tissue masses, especially in the body and angle of the mandible.

Histologically, fibrosarcoma of bone is identical to fibrosarcoma arising in soft tissues.[111] Tumors are usually divided into well-differentiated, moderately differentiated, or undifferentiated histologic types.[117] *Well-*

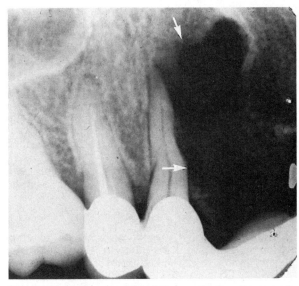

Figure 58–18. Fibrosarcoma of the maxilla showing a moth-eaten and multilocular radiolucency anterior to the premolars. (Courtesy of Dr. John F. Richardson.)

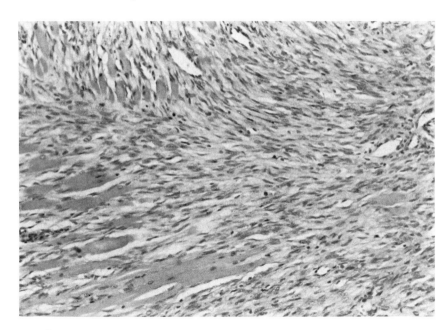

Figure 58–19. Moderately well differentiated fibrosarcoma showing infiltration of skeletal muscle adjacent to the mandible. (H & E, × 220)

differentiated neoplasms show an interwoven mixture of well-differentiated cells and fibers. Fibroblasts appear regular in size and shape, and the nuclear and cytoplasmic tintorial qualities of the cells are usually uniform. Well-developed collagen, arranged in bands and fascicles, generally surrounds tumor cells, and mitoses are rare. *Moderately differentiated* fibrosarcoma shows a characteristic herringbone distribution of cells; mitoses are sparse; and although ground substance and collagen are quite evident, they are not as dominant as in the well-differentiated counterpart (Figs. 58–19 and 58–20). Anaplastic *undifferentiated fibrosarcomas* are extremely cellular with abundant pleomorphism, mitotic figures, and tumor giant cells. Spindly fibroblasts show marked pleomorphism in most instances.

Dahl and associates[112] have described two forms of fibrosarcoma in children; a desmoplastic type and a medullary type. Desmoplastic tumors are locally aggressive and histologically similar to fibrosarcoma in adults. Medullary tumors have been reported to be less biologically aggressive.

Batsakis[108] has emphasized that no histologic feature or group of features has been successfully related to the clinical behavior or prediction of the biologic course of fibrosarcoma regardless of subtype, and although Huvos[8] reports that patients with high-grade (undifferentiated) fibrosarcomas (medullary or periosteal) of long bones may benefit from preoperative and adjuvant chemotherapy, this treatment modality has not been used enough in jaw cases to determine its effectiveness.

Differential Diagnosis

Distinction between juvenile desmoplastic fibromatosis and well-differentiated fibrosarcoma in the jaw of a child can be exceedingly difficult. The best histologic rule to follow when faced with a diagnosis of fibrosarcoma versus juvenile desmoplastic fibromatosis of childhood is to consider the parameters defined by Stout,[117] who stipulates that a diagnosis of well-differentiated

fibrosarcoma should be made only if mitotic activity is present, if there is nuclear pleomorphism, or if vascular invasion is observed.

Fibrous histiocytoma probably has been given more synonyms than any other pathologic entity in the medical literature. It may be confused with the fibrosarcoma of the jaws; however, the lack of a pinwheel or storiform arrangement of the cells in the presence of a fibrocollagenous malignancy generally negates a diagnosis of fibrous histiocytoma. Pleomorphic rhabdomyosarcoma can be an alternative light microscopic diagnosis for fibrosarcoma. Distinction between the two can often be made on the basis of electron microscopy. The large cells of pleomorphic rhabdomyosarcoma exhibit specific myofilaments and Z band material, which are absent in fibrosarcoma.

On occasion, fibrosarcoma may be difficult to distinguish from a fibroblastic osteosarcoma. Histochemical evaluation may prove helpful in that it will show no alkaline phosphatase activity by the tumor cells in fibrosarcoma, but increased alkaline phosphatase activity will be recorded with osteosarcoma.[110]

The fibroblasts of fibrosarcoma show no specific ultrastructural features; however, they have an abundance of rough endoplasmic reticulum. Activated tumor fibroblasts (myofibroblasts) often display numerous fine filaments in their peripheral cytoplasm as well as attachment plaques, foci of basal lamina–like material, pinocytotic vesicles, and occasional poorly developed cell junctions. The rare odontogenic neoplasm—ameloblastic fibrosarcoma—has a microscopic picture that is analogous to that of a benign ameloblastic fibroma with a mesodermal component that has the cytologic features of a malignant fibrosarcoma. Adekeye and associates[107] have suggested that the lesion is in fact a tumor of odontogenic origin. Some authors, including myself (R.O.G.), however, consider that in many instances the tumor actually represents a fibrosarcoma with entrapped epithelial odontogenic rests, which are in no way a functional part of the tumor but are entrapped

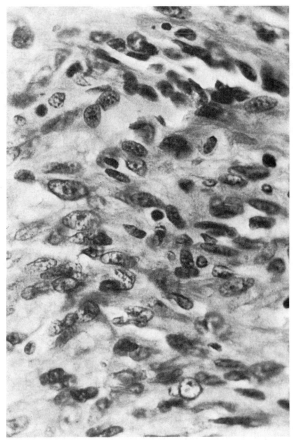

Figure 58–20. This high-power photomicrograph demonstrates the abundant growth substance generally associated with fibrosarcoma of the jaws and facial skeleton. (H & E, × 140)

fortuitously. Until a large series of these cases are reviewed longitudinally, it is probably best to identify such lesions as fibrosarcomas without appending the ameloblastic label.

Treatment and Prognosis

The treatment of choice for fibrosarcoma of the jaws is complete wide local excision with a generous border of clinically or radiographically normal tissue. The prognosis for jaw tumors appears to be somewhat better than the prognosis for other bones. Dahlin and Ivins[113] reviewed 100 cases of fibrosarcoma of bone, including 13 cases of the mandible, and found a 5-year survival rate of 28.7 per cent. Eversole and associates[114] have reported a 5-year survival rate of 27 per cent. The prognosis for periosteal lesions is much better than that for medullary lesions, with nearly a 50 per cent survival rate reported after 5 years.[108]

TUMORS OF HISTIOCYTIC AND FIBROHISTIOCYTIC ORIGIN

Malignant Fibrous Histiocytoma of Bone

In the early 1960s, the concept that neoplastic histiocytes could differentiate into fibroblasts, both morphologically and functionally, was introduced. Results of both tissue culture and ultrastructural studies supported this concept of "facultative fibrogenesis."[127, 132] Acceptance of this concept led to the reclassification of a number of soft-tissue lesions such as dermatofibrosarcoma protuberans, juvenile xanthogranuloma, sclerosing hemangioma, and nodular tenosynovitis under the term fibrous histiocytomas. In 1964, O'Brien and Stout demonstrated a malignant counterpart to the benign fibrous histiocytoma of soft tissue.[131] It was not until 1972 that Feldman and Norman described the first cases of primary malignant fibrous histiocytomas in bone.[121]

Primary malignant fibrous histiocytoma of bone was not readily accepted by pathologists. The histologic variability of these tumors and the histologic similarities to osteogenic sarcoma and fibrosarcoma delayed acceptance. Dahlin and associates even published an article in 1977 entitled "Malignant (Fibrous) Histiocytoma of Bone—Fact or Fancy?" in which they discussed this dilemma.[119]

Malignant fibrous histiocytomas of bone are rare, but they are more common than benign fibrous histiocytomas of bone.[119] The tumor occurs most commonly in the femur and tibia. In five of the largest series of primary malignant fibrous histiocytomas of bone published (126 cases), only six cases involved the maxilla or mandible.[119, 120, 124, 126, 134]

Malignant fibrous histiocytoma of bone can occur at any age, but it seems to be more common in the fourth and fifth decades. Too few cases have been reported in the jaws to evaluate age or sex predilection.

The etiology of malignant fibrous histiocytomas is unknown. However, in long bones there is a strong association between medullary bone infarcts and the subsequent development of osteosarcoma and malignant fibrous histiocytoma. These sarcomas have been noted secondary to medullary infarcts in caisson workers and in patients with sickle cell disease.[128, 129, 130] Sarcomas of bone have also been noted in previously radiated areas. Weiner and associates reported a 1-year-old girl who was irradiated for bilateral retinoblastomas and developed a malignant fibrous histiocytoma 20 years later in the maxilla.[137]

Clinical Findings

The clinical findings are those of any primary malignant neoplasm, with pain and swelling being the predominant features (Fig. 58–21).[133, 136, 137] In maxillary lesions, sinusitis and proptosis may be seen initially.[135]

Radiographic findings are nonspecific and are simply those of malignant neoplasia. The lesions reported in the jaws present as ill-defined, destructive lytic lesions. The intraosseous extent of the tumor frequently exceeds that seen on plain radiographs or tomograms. Technetium-99 polyphosphonate total body scans are helpful in delineating the intraosseous extent of the tumor. Selective biplanar angiography is extremely useful in defining the extraosseous extension of the neoplasm.[134]

Pathology

The gross appearance of malignant fibrous histiocytomas varies with the cellular composition. Lesions that are firm and white to gray usually contain large amounts

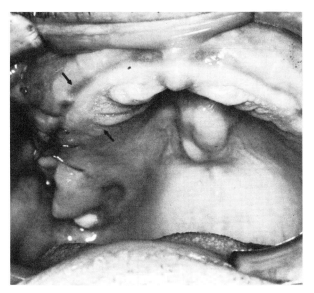

Figure 58–21. Malignant fibrous histiocytoma showing expansion of the labial and lingual posterior maxillary alveolus.

pattern about inconspicuous blood vessels. Interspersed are histiocytic cells, which may show pleomorphism. The fibroblastic cells are spindle-shaped, and the histiocytic cells have large, oval, indented nuclei and abundant cytoplasm. Normal and atypical mitotic figures may be seen in both cell types. Xanthoma cells (lipid-containing histiocytes) and siderophages (hemosiderin-containing histiocytes) may also be present. Malignant giant cells are a constant finding. In some cases, these tumor giant cells have huge, bizarre nuclei that dominate the picture. Variable numbers of inflammatory cells, predominantly lymphocytes, are seen. Metaplastic osteoid or chondroid may be present.

Electron microscopy shows at least two cell lines (histiocytic and fibroblastic) present. The fibroblastic cells have a rich, rough endoplastic reticulum, and the histiocytic cells contain numerous lysosomes and phagocytic vacuoles. Recently, small numbers of undifferentiated mesenchymal cells have been observed by electron microscopy. It has been suggested that they represent the cell of origin with differentiation along fibroblastic or histiocytic lines.[122]

Differential Diagnosis

The principal lesions considered in the differential diagnosis of malignant fibrous histiocytoma of bone are osteosarcoma and fibrosarcoma. In most cases, differentiation from osteogenic sarcoma is not difficult because of the presence of abundant, malignant osteoid deposition. However, in osteolytic osteosarcomas, malignant osteoid may be present in extremely small quantities, and differentiating it from collagen may be difficult. Dahlin reported the presence of questionable or definitive osteoid in 18 of 35 cases of malignant fibrous histiocytomas.[119] The storiform patterns and malignant giant cells can also be seen in osteosarcoma. In cases in which malignant osteoid formation or other histologic features are debatable, histochemical and ultrastructural

of collagen, and lesions that are solid pink with yellow areas are associated with a high lipid content.

The light microscopic picture of malignant fibrous histiocytomas is extremely variable, depending on the path of differentiation of the neoplastic cells, either histiocytic or fibroblastic (Fig. 58–22). Some tumors consist of sheets of histiocytes exhibiting phagocytosis, and others are predominantly fibroblastic and resemble a fibrosarcoma. This variation in appearance is responsible for the variation in names—malignant fibrous histiocytoma, malignant fibrous xanthoma, and malignant histiocytoma.

The most typical pattern is a cellular tumor composed of spindle cells arranged in a storiform or cartwheel

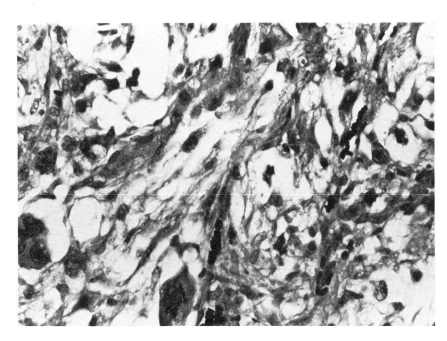

Figure 58–22. Malignant fibrous histiocytoma with fibroblastic stroma intermixed with tumor giant cells and histiocytes. (H & E, × 100)

studies may be beneficial. The presence of alkaline phosphatase in tumor cells and elevated serum alkaline phosphatase favors the diagnosis of osteosarcoma.[123, 134] Ultrastructurally, the identification of cells with histiocytic features favors malignant fibrous histiocytoma. Any tumor in which malignant osteoid can unequivocally be demonstrated should be classified as osteosarcoma.

Several histologic features help differentiate fibrosarcoma from malignant fibrous histiocytoma. Fibrosarcomas usually manifest a herringbone pattern, with mild cellular pleomorphism, rare multinucleated tumor giant cells, and no histiocytic component. However, malignant fibrous histiocytomas have a storiform pattern with marked cellular pleomorphism in the presence of multinucleated tumor giant cells. Ghandur-Mnaymneh and associates[123] observed that the amount of collagen production in fibrosarcoma varies inversely with the degree of malignancy and cellular pleomorphism. The more differentiated the tumor, the more abundant the collagen. However, in malignant fibrous histiocytoma there is no apparent relationship between the extent of collagen production and the degree of anaplasia.[123] Ultrastructurally, malignant fibrous histiocytoma shows the presence of cells with histiocytic properties that are not present in fibrosarcomas.

Treatment and Prognosis

The biologic behavior of this tumor is still not clearly established because of the limited number of cases reported and the short-term follow-up available. In 1982 Ghandur-Mnaymneh and associates reviewed the literature and found 74 cases in which there was follow-up of more than 5 years or until death. Of the 74 cases, 47 patients were dead of their disease or developed pulmonary metastases within 5 years, yielding a 5-year survival rate of 34.5 per cent.[123] This 5-year survival rate is comparable to that of deeply situated, soft-tissue, malignant fibrous histiocytomas.[125] It is lower than the rate reported by Huvos[124] of 67 per cent and by Dahlin[119] of 57.1 per cent in their series of cases.

There is no established correlation between histologic pattern and prognosis in bone lesions. The myxoid variant of malignant fibrous histiocytoma in soft tissue appears to have a more favorable prognosis.[138]

Surgery appears to be the preferred method of therapy. Too few cases are available for review in the jaws to give any indication as to the preferred mode of treatment or prognosis.

Histiocytosis X

Histiocytosis X is the designation given to three disease complexes that have varying clinical presentations but are tied together because of their similar histologic appearance. The disorders embraced under the term histiocytosis X by Lichtenstein in 1953 include (1) *eosinophilic granuloma*, (2) *Hand-Schüller-Christian syndrome*, and (3) *Letterer-Siwe syndrome*.[147] Prior to being grouped under the name histiocytosis X, these various syndromes were classified as nonlipid reticuloendothelioses. They represent a spectrum of diseases ranging from discrete isolated lesions (eosinophilic granuloma) to a rapidly disseminated form (Letterer-Siwe). However, some investigators believe the single designation of histiocytosis X is an oversimplification and that these clinical syndromes represent at least two separate entities that may have different etiologies and histologic pictures.[139, 152, 158]

The first proposed complex, which includes eosinophilic granuloma and Hand-Schüller-Christian syndrome, is represented by unifocal or multifocal eosinophilic granulomas of bone with or without extraskeletal manifestations. This is a relatively benign form that has a favorable prognosis and may display spontaneous remission. However, death may occur in the multifocal form with diffuse organ involvement. The second complex (Letterer-Siwe syndrome) is represented by a fulminant histiocytic proliferation with generalized organ involvement and an extremely poor prognosis.[152] The histologic differences between these two disease complexes will be discussed in the pathology section.

No reliable information is available on the incidence of histiocytosis X. A review of 1120 cases of histiocytosis X on file at the Armed Forces Institute of Pathology yielded 114 (10 per cent) cases with oral involvement. Those with oral involvement were classified as follows: monostotic eosinophilic granuloma, 53 per cent; polyostotic eosinophilic granuloma, 25 per cent; chronic disseminated form (Hand-Schüller-Christian syndrome), 12 per cent; and acute disseminated form (Letterer-Siwe syndrome), 10 per cent.[142]

The etiology of histiocytosis X remains obscure. Some investigators have considered the acute disseminated form to be a neoplastic process, but unifocal and multifocal eosinophilic granulomas may represent a benign reactive response to an unidentified antigen or infectious agent.[139, 148, 152, 158] Both Cline and Golde[139] and Lieberman and associates[148] believe that Letterer-Siwe disease represents a lymphomatous process, possibly histiocytic lymphoma.

The high incidence of spontaneous regression and the fact that the disease will respond to low doses of radiation and chemotherapy do not fit the pattern typical of malignant neoplasms.[151, 155] In addition, certain clinical and pathologic similarities have been observed between histiocytosis X and various immunologic disorders such as severe combined immunodeficiency disease, graft-versus-host disease, and hypersensitivity reactions. Osband and associates reported that 12 of 17 patients with histiocytosis X had circulating lymphocytes that were spontaneously cytotoxic to cultured human fibroblasts or that produced antibody to autologous erythrocytes. Also, histamine H2 surface receptors were lacking on T-lymphocytes, suggesting a suppressor-cell deficiency. Administration of calf thymus extract produced clinical remission and correction of the lymphocyte abnormalities in 10 patients.[155]

Also supporting the concept of a possible defect in the immunoregulatory mechanisms is the fact that the proliferating cell in histiocytosis X is indistinguishable from the Langerhans cell, a dendritic histiocyte.[149, 150] Langerhans cells are believed to act as tissue macrophages that interact closely with lymphocytes, play an important role in cell-mediated immunity, and may be responsible for osteoclastic activating factor and eosinophilic infiltration, which are features seen in histiocytosis X.[141]

Nesbit and associates believe there is a definite rela-

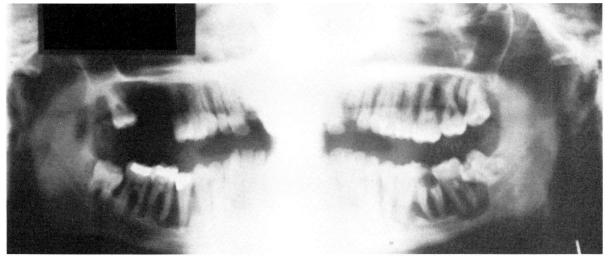

Figure 58–23. Histiocytosis X in a 19-year-old with bone loss in all four quadrants. The classic pattern of "teeth floating in air" is seen in the posterior mandibular quadrants. Severe periodontal disease must be considered in the differential diagnosis. (Courtesy of Dr. Robert Livingston.)

tionship between histiocytosis X and a defect in the thymus and the T-lymphocytes. Two postulates were offered to explain this relationship: (1) primary lymphocytic defect with secondary histiocytosis or (2) primary monocytic macrophage defect with secondary immunodeficiency.[151]

Clinical Findings

The monostotic or solitary eosinophilic granuloma occurs in children and young adults with a 2:1 male predominance.[143] Patients present with solitary osseous involvement. Polyostotic eosinophilic granuloma also occurs predominantly in the first two decades of life but exhibits mutiple bone involvement and possible extraskeletal involvement. Hand-Schüller-Christian disease, or chronic disseminated histiocytosis X, may really represent a form of multifocal eosinophilic granuloma in which the patient exhibits the classic triad of skull lesions, exophthalmos, and diabetes insipidus. In fact, this triad occurs in less than 10 per cent of those cases diagnosed as Hand-Schüller-Christian disease.[153] The acute disseminated form of histiocytosis X (Letterer-Siwe syndrome) generally occurs in infants less than 3 years of age and manifests multiple organ involvement with extraskeletal involvement predominating.

Oral involvement of both bony and soft tissue can occur in any form of the disease complex. In the series reported by Hartman, 67 per cent of the lesions were intraosseous defects, with 76 per cent involving the mandible.[142] The most common presenting symptoms are swelling and pain. Gingival lesions are frequently associated with adjacent bone involvement and are characterized by a nonspecific red swelling with ulceration, which may be mistaken for gingivitis. In children who present with loose teeth or premature loss of teeth, histiocytosis X must be considered.

Radiographically, jaw lesions primarily are unilocular, well-defined radiolucencies. When the alveolar bone adjacent to the teeth is involved, it imparts a radio-

graphic appearance of teeth "floating in air" (Fig. 58–23). Polyostotic eosinophilic granuloma, when it involves the jaws, has a radiographic appearance similar to severe periodontal disease or juvenile periodontitis. Lesions in the skull in histiocytosis X are characteristically punched-out in appearance and are often multiple (Fig. 58–24).

Work-up of the patient for multifocal involvement is essential when the diagnosis of eosinophilic granuloma is rendered. Siddiqui and associates recently reported that a radiographic skeletal survey should be the primary diagnostic test and bone scans should be obtained only when the radiographs are normal or equivocal.[157]

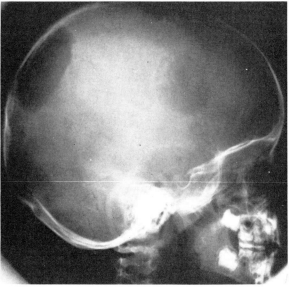

Figure 58–24. Histiocytosis X in a 2-year-old with "punched-out" lesions in the skull. (Courtesy of Dr. Robert E. Primosch.)

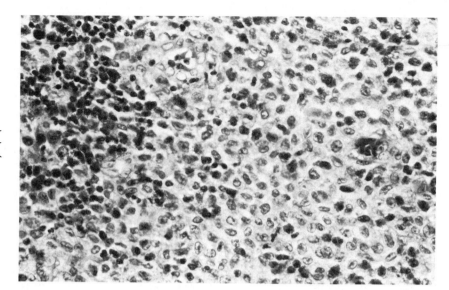

Figure 58–25. Histiocytosis X characterized by sheets of histiocytes infiltrated by scattered eosinophils. (H & E, × 100)

Pathology

The spectrum of lesions seen in histiocytosis X are characterized by a proliferation of histiocytes, usually in sheets with a variable number eosinophils, plasma cells, and lymphocytes (Fig. 58–25). The histiocytes contain an abundant eosinophilic cytoplasm, frequently containing phagocytized material. The nuclei are large, ovoid, and indented with a small nucleolus. Mitotic figures are rarely detected. Multinucleated giant cells, foam cells (lipid-containing histiocytes), and necrosis are often present. Oberman reported fewer eosinophils in lesions from patients with acute disseminated disease.[154] Foam cells said to be characteristic of Hand-Schüller-Christian disease may be found in any clinical category.[142, 148, 154]

Newton and Hamoudi published a study of histiocytosis X in childhood and observed two distinct morphologic lesions.[152] One lesion consisted of mature histiocytes with distinct cell borders with the absence of eosinophils, giant cells, necrosis, and fibrosis. Phagocytosis was scant or absent. Clinically, these patients represented Letterer-Siwe syndrome and died shortly of their illness. The second morphologic type was characterized by sheets of histiocytes with indistinct cell borders, always accompanied by eosinophils and giant cells and frequently by fibrosis and necrosis. The patients with this histologic picture followed the more benign course.[152] Some investigators have found prognostic significance in these morphologic criteria,[145] but others have failed to make any correlation.[154, 156]

Electron microscropy may be beneficial in confirming the diagnosis of histiocytosis X by detecting the presence of Langerhans or Birbeck granules within the cytoplasm of the Langerhans cells (Fig. 58–26). These rod-like or tennis racket–shaped inclusion bodies are not present

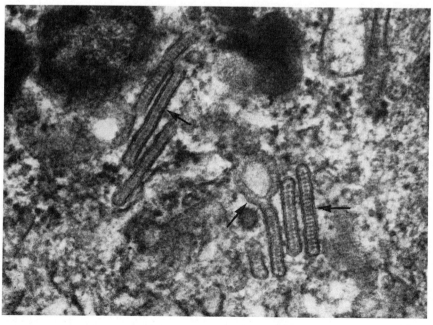

Figure 58–26. The unique ultrastructural feature of the Langerhans cell is a rod-shaped, or occasionally "racquet"-shaped, organelle (arrows) of variable length with a central striated line. (EM, × 146,000)

in normal histiocytes. Langerhans cells appear to be pathognomonic for histiocytosis X, but they are not unique to this disease and, therefore, need to be viewed in the proper context. It has been reported that Birbeck granules are not present in all cases of histiocytosis X, and their presence may be a favorable prognostic sign.[152] However, Mierau and associates do not support the preceding contention and found that these cytoplasmic inclusions are a constant feature in this group of diseases.[149]

Differential Diagnosis

Light microscopic diagnoses of these lesions are usually straightforward. The lesions may be confused with reactive histiocytic lesions, but in these cases microscopic or historical evidence of an inciting agent is usually present. However, if difficulty is encountered, ultrastructural evaluation reveals the absence of Langerhans cells in reactive histiocytic lesions. Acute disseminated histiocytosis X can be differentiated from lymphoma or malignant histiocytosis by the benign appearance of cells in histiocytosis X.

Treatment and Prognosis

The most significant factors that affect prognosis are age of onset, extent of involvement, the rapidity of disease progression, and the presence or absence of crucial organ involvement (liver, lung, and hematopoietic system).[146] Komp and associates proposed the following staging system. Patients without organ dysfunction who were over 2 years of age form the best-risk group. The intermediate-risk group was defined as consisting of those children under 2 years of age without organ dysfunction, and the poor-risk group is defined as organ dysfunction at any age.[144]

Monostotic eosinophilic granuloma usually responds to curettage or simple excision. Hartman reported a 16 per cent recurrence rate for oral solitary lesions.[142] Multifocal eosinophilic granuloma may be treated with a combination of surgery, radiation, or chemotherapy, depending on the extent of the disease. The primary mode of treatment for the acute disseminated disease form is chemotherapy.

GIANT CELL AND FIBRO-OSSEOUS LESIONS OF THE JAWS

Central Giant Cell Granuloma

Giant cell reparative granuloma of the jaws was defined in 1952 by Jaffe as a local reparative reaction, possibly to hemorrhage. Previously, these jaw lesions had been interpreted simply as giant cell tumors and were thought to be similar to the true neoplastic giant cell tumors of long bones. However, Jaffe concluded that the jaw lesions only mimic the true giant cell tumor and could be differentiated by both clinical and histologic criteria.[169]

Many investigators[160, 161, 168] support this concept, but others[159, 166, 175] believe giant cell reparative granuloma of the jaws is analogous, if not identical, to the true giant cell tumor of bone. Whether these two lesions are different, identical, or part of a spectrum of giant cell lesions, the diagnostic entity of giant cell (reparative) granuloma has been accepted. Since Jaffe's original description, the lesion is now commonly referred to as central giant cell granuloma. A more thorough discussion of the relationship of central giant cell granuloma to true giant cell tumors will be discussed under differential diagnosis.

The etiology of central giant cell granuloma is extensively debated. Intramedullary hemorrhage secondary to trauma or possibly inflammation has been proposed.[168, 169] However, a history of trauma can be elicited in only a few cases.[175] Batsakis proposed these lesions to be the result of injury imposed upon the periodontal membrane, the odontogenic mesenchyma, or the dental sac or its ancestral cells.[161] Although the exact cause of these lesions is unknown, most authors consider them to be reactive.[160, 161, 169, 175]

Central giant cell granuloma is not a common lesion. In a review by Austin of 968 benign tumors of the jaws, central giant cell granulomas accounted for only 3.5 per cent of the lesions.[160] Greer and Mierau documented a 3.6 per cent incidence in a review of 109 tumors of the oral mucosa and jaws in children.[165] Central giant cell granuloma occurs much less frequently than its peripheral soft-tissue counterpart (peripheral giant cell granuloma), to which it is histologically identical.

Central giant cell granulomas occur predominantly in children and young adults: approximately 75 per cent of the lesions occur in the first three decades of life.[160, 175] Lesions have been reported into the eighth decade of life.[159] It is more common in females.[159, 160, 175]

Central giant cell granulomas occur more frequently in the mandible. The majority of lesions, both maxillary and mandibular, occur in the anterior portion.[159, 160, 175] Waldron and Shafer reported that 21 per cent of the lesions they evaluated crossed the midline, an unusual feature for lesions of the jaws.[175]

At one time, these tumors were thought to be limited to the jaws. However, lesions of the facial skeleton (ethmoid, sphenoid, and temporal), though rare, have been reported.[163, 168] Recently, a central giant cell granuloma involving a finger was described.[162]

Clinical Findings

Pain and local swelling are the two most frequent clinical findings (Fig. 58–27A). However, many lesions may be asymptomatic and are discovered on routine examination. Austin and co-workers reported that pain occurred in 25 per cent of their cases, and one presented with paresthesia.[160]

Radiographically, central giant cell granulomas can appear as either unilocular or multilocular radiolucencies, which are fairly well delineated (Fig. 58–27B). Marked expansion and thinning of the cortical plates are frequently observed, but perforation is seldom seen.[175] Displacement of teeth and root resorption may also be observed.

Pathology

Grossly, central giant cell granuloma is composed of multiple hemorrhagic fragments of soft tissue. Histologically, the lesion is characterized by the proliferation of

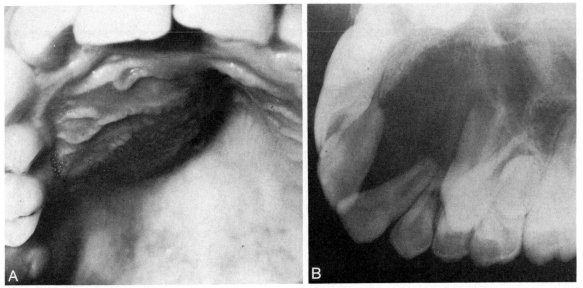

Figure 58–27. Central giant cell granuloma in a 12-year-old girl presenting with expansion of the hard palate (*A*) and a maxillary radiolucency with displacement of teeth (*B*).

young fibroblastic connective tissue, which is richly vascular. Some areas may exhibit significant collagen formation. A variable number of multinucleated giant cells are always present (Fig. 58–28). The distribution of these giant cells is usually diffuse but may vary. The giant cells can often range from very small cells with only a few nuclei to exceedingly large cells with dozens of nuclei. Multiple foci of hemorrhage are present throughout the lesion, and phagocytosis is common with hemosiderin deposition. Mitoses in stromal cells are relatively common.[175] Occasional spicules of newly formed bone or osteoid are commonly seen.

Electron microscopy is of little value in the diagnosis

of this lesion or in the differential diagnosis from true giant cell tumor or peripheral giant cell granuloma.[166, 173]

Differential Diagnosis

Lesions with histologic findings similar to those of central giant cell granuloma of the jaws include hyperparathyroidism, cherubism, aneurysmal bone cyst, and true giant cell tumor of bone.

Although rare, true neoplastic giant cell tumors of bone have been reported in the jaws.[169, 174] Several cases have been reported in association with Paget's disease of bone.[170] Therefore, if one accepts the proposition that

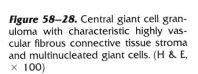

Figure 58–28. Central giant cell granuloma with characteristic highly vascular fibrous connective tissue stroma and multinucleated giant cells. (H & E, × 100)

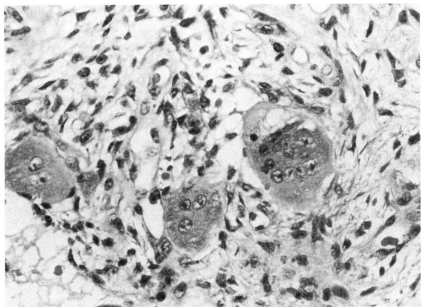

central giant cell granuloma and giant cell tumor are distinct entities, the clinician and pathologist are faced with a diagnostic dilemma in distinguishing between these two neoplastic lesions.

Batsakis[161] summarized the pertinent clinical-pathologic differences as follows:

1. True giant cell tumors are rare in bones of the skull, face, and jaws.

2. Osteoid formation or other evidence of osteogenic activity is not characteristic of true giant cell tumors, except when it is peripheral to a fracture site or injury.

3. True giant cell tumors are remarkably devoid of hemorrhage, lipid-laden histiocytes, hemosiderin, and an inflammatory cellular component.

4. Giant cell granulomas occur more frequently in the first two decades of life, but true giant cell tumors occur more commonly in the third to fourth decades.

Some authors believe that giant cells are more abundant and slightly larger in true giant cell neoplasm.[161, 168] These entities also differ in their response to treatment. Giant cell granulomas are self-limiting in their clinical behavior and usually respond to simple curettage, but giant cell tumor of bone is more aggressive and frequently recurs if incompletely excised. In 1981 the first acceptable case of malignant "true" giant cell tumor of bone was described in the jaws.[171]

Histologically, brown tumor of primary or secondary hyperparathyroidism and central giant cell granuloma are indistinguishable. Therefore, it is recommended that when the diagnosis of central giant cell granuloma is rendered, serum calcium and phosphorus levels should be acquired in order to rule out hyperparathyroidism.[174]

Cherubism is a rare autosomal dominant condition affecting the jaws of children.[167] The histopathologic appearance of cherubism is very similar, if not identical, to that of central giant cell granuloma.[160, 165] The clinical presentation is most helpful in distinguishing this entity from central giant cell granuloma. Cherubism typically appears as a bilateral, painless swelling of the jaws and is most often seen at the angle of the mandible. The age of onset is 2 to 3 years, with gradual, rapid progression seen during the first 2 to 3 years of the disease. The symmetry of the swelling is usually a striking feature. However, the disease may begin as a unilateral swelling. Radiographically, the lesions are multilocular with osseous expansion. Serum calcium and phosphorus levels are normal.

Aneurysmal bone cyst is an uncommon lesion of the jaws, but it has a similar clinical and radiographic appearance to that of central giant cell granuloma. Both lesions do exhibit a similar fibroblastic stroma containing zones of giant cells. However, histologically, aneurysmal bone cysts are dominated by cavernous blood-filled spaces, a feature not seen in central giant cell granuloma.

Treatment and Prognosis

Central giant cell granuloma is a benign condition that is usually managed by curettage or complete surgical excision and has a low recurrence rate.[159] Andersen and associates reported a 13 per cent recurrence rate.[159] However, aggressive central giant cell granulomas have been reported.[164] Malignant change has not been demonstrated except following radiation therapy.[172]

Aneurysmal Bone Cyst

The aneurysmal bone cyst is a non-neoplastic lesion of bone of unknown pathogenesis, being much more common in other parts of the body than in the jaws. This process was first discussed as a separate entity by Jaffe and Lichtenstein when they acknowledged in their major article on solitary unicameral bone cyst that a bone lesion with particular characteristics did not fit into the clinical or pathologic criteria for inclusion as that particular entity.[187] Two patients suffered what Jaffe and Lichtenstein termed an aneurysmal cyst. In 1950, Lichtenstein wrote about a group of these lesions, which he and Jaffe had studied since 1942.[188] He proposed the term, "aneurysmal bone cyst," admitting that both the terms "aneurysmal" and "cyst" were not being used in their strict meanings. The name, he said, was chosen for convenient reference because he could think of no better alternative at that time and the terms then in use, such as "hemorrhagic cyst" or "benign bone aneurysm," favored by Ewing, were inconvenient and nonspecific. More than 30 years later, after extensive investigation, the proposal of Lichtenstein still stands. No better name has surfaced, and the lesion has retained its individuality and mysterious etiology.

Although many articles have been written on the aneurysmal bone cyst since 1950, little improvement has been made on the description by Lichtenstein. The aneurysmal bone cyst is a solitary, localized, fibrous, expansile lesion that has been found in all bones but seems to favor the vertebral column and long bones. The lesion characteristically erodes through the cortex, but it is limited by a thin shell of new periosteal bone. The interior architecture of the bone is completely destroyed and replaced by cavernous, blood-filled spaces around and through which are found fibrous connective tissue septa.

The cause of the aneurysmal bone cyst is still unknown, although many theories have been proposed. Lichtenstein still adheres to the view that some persistent local alteration in hemodynamics, perhaps intraosseous arteriovenous shunts, leads to increased venous pressure.[189] Dabska and Buraczewski theorize that there is some factor that causes blood under pressure to "blow out" first smaller and then larger vessels, with the resulting increased local blood pressure destroying bone.[182] Trauma has been implicated by several authors, who suggest that the aneurysmal bone cyst may be initiated by the resulting subperiosteal hematoma.[181, 186, 192] In the jaws, aneurysmal bone cyst and central giant cell reparative granuloma are regarded as possibly different manifestations of the same process, which is an abnormal reaction to an insult to bone.[186, 193] Clough and Price suggest that the process, which may be a result of trauma, takes place in the more vascular active tissues of the immature skeleton.[181] The relationship to trauma, however, is still ambiguous.

Many investigators have found aneurysmal bone cysts in association with other benign bone lesions[178, 179, 191, 192] or even with malignant lesions.[181] These lesions included fibrous dysplasia, hemangioma, chondromyxoid fibroma, chondroblastoma, nonossifying fibroma, and others. This author (M.R.) has seen two aneurysmal bone cysts of the mandible associated with an ossifying-cementifying fibroma and a chondroblastoma. Twenty-one per cent of reported aneurysmal bone cysts of the jaws are reported to have developed in association with various bone lesions, including fibro-osseous lesions.[185] Although Tillman and associates[193] found no associated bone lesions in their study of 95 aneurysmal bone cysts from the Mayo Clinic, Biesecker and associates claimed that 32 per cent of the 66 cases in their series had an accompanying bone lesion.[178] Their hypothesis states that a primary lesion of bone initiates an osseous, arteriovenous fistula and thereby creates, via its hemodynamic forces, the secondary reactive bone lesion, which is termed an aneurysmal bone cyst.

Aneurysmal bone cysts constitute 1.5 per cent of nonodontogenic and nonepithelial cysts of the jaws and 1.9 per cent of all aneurysmal bone cysts of the skeleton.[185] In the period of time during which 95 cases of aneurysmal bone cysts were collected at the Mayo Clinic, Tillman and associates found that there occurred 177 giant cell tumors and 700 osteogenic sarcomas. Of the 95 aneurysmal bone cysts, one was in the mandible, and one in the maxilla.[193] In Biesecker's study of 66 cases, two occurred in the mandible.[178] In an analysis of 50 cases of the jaws, El Deeb and associates found that the mandible was affected in 55 per cent of the cases, and the maxilla was involved in 45 per cent.[185]

The male-to-female ratio shows a slight female predominance in aneurysmal bone cysts of the jaws, just as in other parts of the skeleton. Over two thirds of all cases, in the jaws and the rest of the skeleton, occur in patients under the age of 20 years.[178, 184, 185, 186, 193]

Clinical Findings

The aneurysmal bone cyst of the jaw is nearly always discovered because of complaints of localized swelling and occasionally a developing malocclusion. The lesions in the jaws are usually painless and are most common in the body of the mandible.[177] Although the cyst frequently erodes through the overlying cortical bone, a thin shell of new periosteal bone is always found so that there is no soft-tissue extension.

The radiographic features of aneurysmal bone cysts are not characteristic, and the differential diagnosis in the jaws includes odontogenic cysts or tumors, traumatic bone cyst, central giant cell reparative granuloma, benign fibro-osseous lesions, histiocytosis X, central hemangioma, myxoma, hyperparathyroidism, osteogenic sarcoma, Ewing's sarcoma, metastatic cancer, and cherubism.

The lesion appears radiographically as an expansile, cystic mass and is usually unilocular but may be multilocular (Fig. 58–29). As the lesion increases in size, the appearance is more likely to resemble a "soap bubble" or "honeycomb," not because of true bony septa, according to Lichtenstein, but because of spurs and ridges on the endosseous surface of the expanded shell.[188] The newly formed subperiosteal bone that is almost always present at the periphery of the lesion is not visible radiographically.[193]

The definitive diagnosis depends on the correlation of clinical, radiographic, and histologic findings. No laboratory studies are reported to be of value. However, one clinical test has been reported to help differentiate the aneurysmal bone cyst from other benign osseous cystic lesions. Chari and Reddy recorded intracystic

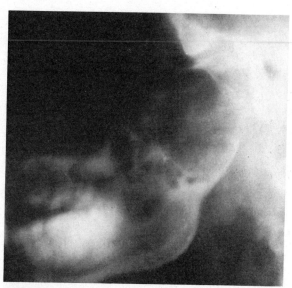

Figure 58–29. Tomogram of aneurysmal bone cyst shows large, multilocular radiolucency of the ramus and posterior body of the mandible. (Courtesy of Dr. N. Robert Markowitz.)

pressures of benign osseous cysts with a spinal manometer. Of 16 consecutive cystic lesions, 12 were noted to have a gradual rise of the column of blood in the manometer, which oscillated synchronously with the peripheral pulse rate. All of these were proved by subsequent histologic examination to be aneurysmal bone cysts.[180] Another study showed that three of six aneurysmal bone cysts subjected to manometric studies showed increased pressures as high as the arteriolar blood pressure.[178]

Pathology

The aneurysmal bone cyst completely destroys the inner architecture of the involved bone and transforms it into a tissue resembling a blood-filled sponge. When the lesion is unroofed, there is nearly always a "welling up" of blood, but no spurting. In the study of 95 cases from the Mayo Clinic, however, it was reported that a few cysts were found to contain clear fluid, presumably lesions of very long duration.[193] Ordinarily, the bulk of the lesion consists of cavernous spaces filled with unclotted blood. Some lesions contain fibrous or granular tissue, which composes a large part of the lesion.[183]

The most significant feature of the histologic findings is that the blood-filled spaces are lined not by endothelium but by compressed fibrous tissue (Fig. 58–30).[176] Throughout the fibrous tissue, there are numerous small capillaries, and frequently there are multinucleated giant cells of the osteoclast type. Lichtenstein stated that the lack of fibromuscular or elastic walls suggested that the spaces were extensively distended capillaries or venules and the lack of microscopically evident thrombosis suggested a free, if sluggish, circulation.[188] Very often, numerous hemosiderin-laden macrophages are associated with the large amount of extravasated blood. At the periphery of the lesion, new trabeculae of subperiosteal bone are very frequently encountered.[193]

Electron microscopic studies have determined that the most common cell in the aneurysmal bone cyst is the fibroblast.[176, 192] Other cells found are myofibroblasts,

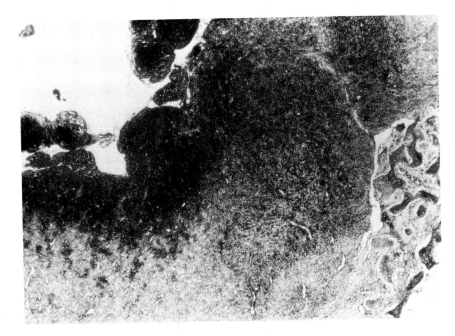

Figure 58–30. Aneurysmal bone cyst showing large, connective tissue–lined blood-filled space with newly formed, reactive bone at the periphery. (H & E, × 10)

osteoblasts, histiocytes, and primitive mesenchymal cells. There is nothing special about the multinucleated giant cells, which resemble osteoclasts. Osteoid and bone arise from metaplastic changes of the spindle cell stroma.[192]

Differential Diagnosis

Histologically, the aneurysmal bone cyst in the jaws can be confused with several other lesions. Owing to the presence of giant cells, there is always the possibility of confusion with central giant cell granuloma or a lesion of hyperparathyroidism. The delicate network of osteoid often seen could be confused with the histologic appearance of benign osteoblastoma, benign chondroblastoma, or cementoblastoma. The histologic features of the aneurysmal bone cyst and the traumatic or simple bone cyst overlap, making the distinction on this basis very difficult or impossible in some cases.[183] The presence of the variable sized, blood-filled spaces, unlined by endothelial cells, is the key to histologic recognition.

The most important histologic task is to recognize that this lesion is benign. Although the mitotic index may be rather high in some of the spindle fibroblast areas, hyperchromatism and pleomorphism are lacking. It is extremely important and sometimes difficult to distinguish aneurysmal bone cyst from telangiectatic osteosarcoma.[183, 190, 191, 192] Low-power investigation will not distinguish the cytologic subtleties of malignancy to differentiate between these lesions.

Ruiter and associates found there were significant differences in the recurrence rate, depending on mitotic activity, with increased recurrences in lesions with seven or more mitoses per high-power field.[191]

Treatment and Prognosis

The recurrence rate of aneurysmal bone cysts in the jaws of 26 per cent is similar to that in other bones.[185] Tillman and associates found a 21 per cent recurrence

rate, with recurrences being more common in patients less than 15 years of age.[193] Ruiter and associates discovered that 30.5 per cent of their 105 cases recurred.[191]

Although radiation therapy has been advocated in the past for lesions in the vertebral column presenting a great danger to the spinal cord, there appears to be no justification for irradiating a lesion in the jaws. In the series from the Mayo Clinic by Tillman and associates, osteosarcoma developed in three of 95 patients. All three had undergone radiation therapy.[193] Aho and others performed an electron microscopic study of an aneurysmal bone cyst that had been irradiated and had undergone malignant transformation. They concluded that radiotherapy of an osseous lesion may lead to sarcomatous transformation in cells capable of osteoid production and that osteosarcomas induced by irradiation have similar ultrastructural characteristics.[176]

Cherubism

Cherubism is a fairly easily recognized, although quite rare, hereditary disease affecting only the jaws. Jones, in 1933, was the first to describe the clinical entity in reporting the condition in three Jewish siblings as "familial multilocular cystic disease of the jaws."[200] It is characterized by firm, painless, usually symmetric swellings of the jaws, affecting either the mandible alone or the mandible and maxilla. The term, "cherubism," which Jones coined, refers to the severely affected cases in which the patients have involvement of the maxilla in the infraorbital ridge area, resulting in a "gaze to heaven" due to the exposure of sclera below the iris and above the lower eyelid. This feature causes the patient's expression to resemble that of the cherubs of Renaissance art.

Although sporadic cases have been reported, the disease is considered to be transmitted by an autosomal dominant gene, with nearly complete penetrance in males and between 50 to 75 per cent in females.[204, 205]

Males are therefore affected more often, and no ethnic predilection has been observed.[195]

Cherubism has long been referred to as "hereditary fibrous dysplasia," but Dahlin and others prefer to place it in the category of the more general fibro-osseous lesions.[196] Other than the facts that cherubism is a benign, self-limited disease of the jaw bones seen in children, there is no relationship to fibrous dysplasia, and that reference should cease to be used. The term cherubism has become accepted and should continue to be used in naming this disease, with the original intent, as a clinical diagnostic term.

Clinical Findings

Cherubism has a very early clinical onset, the youngest reported patient being 14 months.[199] Rapid progression of the disease may occur over the next few years, with stabilization occurring before puberty. Von Wowern has thoroughly studied all nine documented cases in Denmark and claims that girls stabilize earlier than boys, at age 10, but boys reach that stage at about age 14.[205] After puberty, a slow regression occurs, and between 20 and 30 years of age the fibrous tissue appears to be replaced by sclerotic bone, which undergoes remodeling and recontouring so that these adults show very little jaw expansion.[201] Bixler and Garner report a family in which a boy who previously appeared as a typical cherub had an essentially normal appearance by age 18 years.[194]

Facial swelling is the first abnormality noted. The mandible is most commonly affected. Involvement of the maxilla occurs less frequently, is usually less extensive, and occurs only in conjunction with mandibular disease. Origination in the maxilla most likely is in the tuberosity, the molar area corresponding to the areas of the mandible originally affected.

The dental pathologic picture is quite characteristic and, according to Von Wowern, is very uniform in all patients.[205] Teeth are affected only in areas of bone involvement. Aplasia of all third molars is noted in the jaws affected. When the mandible is involved, the second molars are also missing. In patients with maxillary involvement, second molars are either missing or malformed. Mandibular first molars are present, but with malformed roots. The pulp is normal in teeth in the involved areas. Grunebaum reports two patients, however, in whom no teeth were missing.[197] No patients have been reported to have involvement of other parts of the skeleton.

Almost all authors note enlarged submandibular lymph nodes with gradual regression. No cause for this has been discovered, and biopsy uniformly reveals lymphoid hyperplasia. Explanations of the lymphadenopathy range from an inflammatory response, due to gingival inflammation around malposed teeth, to lymph node hyperplasia, which is often seen in children.

Involvement of the maxilla can result in an alteration of the palatal vault, the palate becoming high and narrow owing to expansion of the alveolar processes.[197, 203]

A young patient who has bilateral swelling and might be suspected of having cherubism should also be investigated for fibrous dysplasia, bilateral parotid enlargement, masseteric hypertrophy, fibromatosis gingivae, and infantile cortical hyperostosis. These can be differentiated from cherubism by radiographic examination.

Radiographically, the lesions of cherubism are bilateral, multiple, multilocular, well-defined radiolucencies of the mandible and maxilla (Fig. 58–31). The cortex over the expanded area is thin and in some areas may be absent.[195] The molar and retromolar areas appear to be the sites of original involvement, with progressive growth to involve the body of the mandible and the entire anteroposterior width of the ramus. The condyles are not involved.[195, 201]

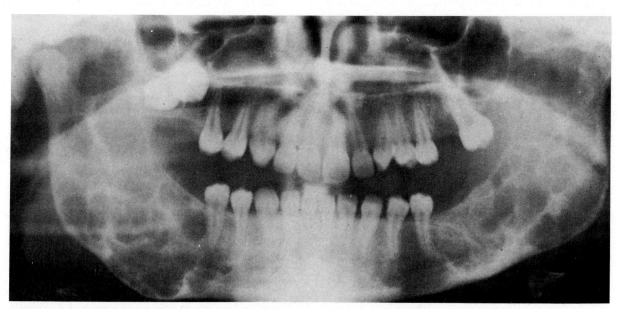

Figure 58–31. Cherubism with typical bilateral multilocular radiolucencies in the mandible. (Courtesy of Dr. Charles Dunlap.)

Differential Diagnosis

The differential diagnosis is usually a radiographic consideration and should include ameloblastoma, infantile cortical hyperostosis, histiocytosis X, hyperparathyroidism, true giant cell tumor, central giant cell granuloma, and odontogenic cysts or tumors. The major factor differentiating all these diseases from cherubism is the bilaterality of cherubism. Infantile cortical hyperostosis affects only the cortex with no loculation. Ameloblastoma is rare in young children and is unicentric. Histiocytosis X is destructive rather than expansive. Giant cell tumor occurs in older patients and is extremely rare in the jaws. Central giant cell granuloma occurs in older patients and is found in more anterior areas, premolar regions, and symphysis regions, unlike the distribution of cherubism. Hyperparathyroidism may produce cyst-like, expansile lesions in the jaws but is rare in young children and has characteristic biochemical features as well as being asymmetric.

Usually, as the disease regresses in early adulthood, the multilocular radiolucencies are replaced by bone described as being sclerotic, or having a "ground-glass" quality; however, this has not been reported uniformly.[199, 205]

Chemical laboratory studies are not helpful because values such as serum calcium and serum phosphorus are within normal limits for cherubism patients. Alkaline phosphatase may be elevated or normal.[199, 205] An elevation in a child is hard to interpret and, therefore, less than useful as a diagnostic criterion.

Pathology

Biopsy examination shows that tissue from lesions of cherubism is virtually identical in all patients and is not specific. The histologic findings cannot be differentiated from central giant cell granuloma, true giant cell tumor, or the localized bone lesions of hyperparathyroidism. Microscopic sections show numerous proliferating, spindle-shaped fibroblasts in a loose fibrillar stroma in which there are numerous thin-walled blood vessels. Multinucleated giant cells are plentiful. Several authors have noted a peculiar perivascular cuffing of collagen.[198, 199, 205] Some series have shown that bone formation is never seen in the lesions,[205] but other examples show sparse osseous trabeculae dispersed at random.[202]

Lesions of cherubism do not appear like fibrous dysplasia of bone, and confusion should not exist when the lesions are examined histologically. A correlation between radiographic, clinical, and histologic findings should establish a definite diagnosis of cherubism.

Treatment and Prognosis

The prognosis depends on the location and extent of the disease rather than on the histopathologic findings because there are virtually no histologic variations. In most patients, a slow regression occurs after puberty, with sclerosis of bone and remodeling. The prognosis is improved if only the mandible is involved rather than both jaws. Anterior as well as posterior involvement makes the situation more difficult, and maxillary involvement, owing to anatomic considerations, presents more serious treatment problems. Treatment must be determined for each patient individually, taking into account the high probability of eventual regression.

The use of radiation in any form to treat benign processes in jaw bones is highly discouraged, if not condemned, owing to the risk of transformation of the process from benign to malignant or the initiation of osteosarcoma.

Fibrous Dysplasia

Fibrous dysplasia is a pathologic condition of bone of unknown etiology with no apparent familial, hereditary, or congenital basis. Lichtenstein[219] first coined the term in 1938, and in 1942 he and Jaffe[221] separated it from other fibro-osseous lesions. The process seems to involve replacement of the spongiosa and a filling of the medullary cavity of the affected bone by a peculiar fibrous tissue that calcifies in an abnormal pattern through osseous metaplasia and increases the mass of the bone involved.[220]

Because there is no perceptible periosteal component with fibrous dysplasia, the enlargement is due to proliferation of abnormal tissue.[228] Several patterns are recognized:

1. Monostotic, involving one bone only.
2. Polyostotic, involving several bones.
3. Albright's syndrome,[207, 208] the polyostotic form associated with endocrine abnormalities (usually premature sexual development in females), abnormal pigmentation (café au lait spots), and other extraskeletal abnormalities.[221] Polyostotic fibrous dysplasia with oral pigmentation but without the other stigmata of Albright's syndrome has been reported.[209] A possible relationship of primary hyperparathyroidism and fibrous dysplasia has been suggested.[210]

A most interesting feature of the disease is that it almost always becomes quiescent after puberty, although this is not always the case, and in fact, the disease may begin in an adult.[211, 216]

The monostotic form is 30 to 40 times more common than the polyostotic, and the jaws are the most common location for the monostotic lesions.[213] Fibrous dysplasia involves the maxilla more frequently than the mandible.[212] Females are more commonly affected than males, and the process usually appears in late childhood or occasionally in early adulthood.

Many theories exist concerning the cause of fibrous dysplasia, including trauma with a nonspecific disturbance in local bone reaction,[222, 224] a congenital anomaly or development,[221] "perverted" activity of mesenchymal bone-forming cells,[220, 226] and a complex endocrine disturbance with local bone susceptibility. The most readily acceptable theory at this time is the abnormal activity of mesenchymal cells.

Clinical Findings

The most common presentation of fibrous dysplasia in the craniofacial area is a slowly progressing asymmetry of the maxilla, the mandible, or if in the skull, the occipital area. These enlargements are unilateral and are usually painless. In affected jaws, the teeth in the area of fibrous dysplasia are normal and are firmly attached in the alveolus, although they may be displaced, and erupting teeth may be impacted. Although the process is unilateral, it is very often seen crossing the midline. Ingrowth into the maxillary sinus may produce symptoms due to blockage of drainage, and growth into the orbit will cause displacement of the eyeball, with or without visual disturbances. Fibrous dysplasia in the temporal bone may obstruct the external auditory meatus.[218]

The most characteristic, although not pathognomonic, feature of fibrous dysplasia in the craniofacial region is the radiographic appearance. For any abnormality other than fracture, there may be an alteration in the calcified content of that bone of 30 to 60 per cent.[228] In fibrous dysplasia of the jaws and skull, there seems to be consistently a large osseous component.[211] The classic description is that of a "ground-glass" or "orange peel" radiopacity. This is not well circumscribed, the borders being very diffuse and not restricted to any anatomic landmarks (Fig. 58–32). Mottling or pagetoid appearances are also seen, and it is reported that 16 to 20 per cent may be cyst-like.[212, 223] No periosteal reaction is noted. Any new subperiosteal bone is most likely due to inflammation, and fibrous dysplasia does not seem to cause this in the jaws. Where teeth are involved, no particular abnormality of the lamina dura is noticed (such as loss of the lamina dura found in ground-glass changes of bone seen in jaws in hyperparathyroidism). Some cases of chronic osteomyelitis can be incorrectly diagnosed as fibrous dysplasia, and a complete review of the radiographic distinctions has been made by Johannsen.[217] Radionuclide imaging of the head of a patient with fibrous dysplasia shows increased uptake of the isotope, probably owing to the high degree of vascularity increasing the blood pool, and this might be

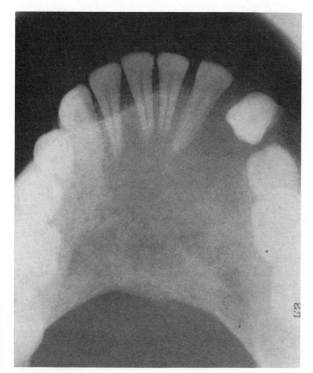

Figure 58–32. Fibrous dysplasia in a 15-year-old male showing ground-glass radiopacity, bony expansion, and tooth displacement.

confused with a variety of tumors, an arteriovenous malformation, or Paget's disease.[214]

It should be emphasized that it is utter folly to attempt to make the diagnosis of fibrous dysplasia, or for that matter of any fibro-osseous lesion of the jaws, from clinical or radiographic or histopathologic features in isolation. It is necessary to use a combination of all three.[206] Much valuable time has been wasted, especially by pathologists, in examining histologic sections for hours, looking for minute cellular variations, when the combination of clinical, radiographic, and histologic evidence will yield a definite diagnosis. No clinical laboratory tests are very helpful at this point. Serum chemistry values of calcium, phosphorus, and alkaline phosphatase are usually normal but may be increased. The alkaline phosphatase level is very often difficult to evaluate in patients of the affected age group because it is not uncommon for the levels to be normally elevated in children and adolescents.[206]

Pathology

Fibrous dysplasia of the jaws is considered a fibro-osseous lesion and thus is not classified as a neoplasm. It is more accurately considered a metabolic or developmental derangement of bone, resulting from an abnormal function of undifferentiated mesenchymal bone-forming cells.

The gross pathologic examination can be varied, but in the jaws the tissue is composed of gray to brown fibrous tissue that has enough osteoid trabeculae to give it a firm and decidedly gritty consistency. It may or may not have to be decalcified for histologic examination. Lesions arising from thin bones such as the maxilla may bulge into adjacent cavities or soft-tissue zones in a polypoid fashion.[211]

Histologically, the major feature is the proliferation of uniform fibroblasts that produce a dense collagen matrix. The fibroblastic cells may show a swirling or storiform arrangement similar to that seen in fibrous histiocytoma. However, this fibrous tissue contains trabeculae of osteoid and bone in a completely meaningless arrangement. These trabeculae have been referred to as "Chinese characters" (Fig. 58–33). Trabeculae may show prominent reversal lines similar to that seen in Paget's disease. No evidence of encapsulation is seen on the microscopic level; instead, there is a fusing and blending of abnormal and normal bone.[206] The histologic findings are essentially those of a fibro-osseous lesion and reveal nothing diagnostic for fibrous dysplasia if viewed in isolation.

The most common differential diagnosis for a lesion such as this in the jaws is ossifying fibroma or ossifying-cementifying fibroma. Uncounted hours of examination and untold pages of print have been devoted to the differentiation between ossifying fibroma and fibrous dysplasia on purely histologic grounds. Much attention has been given to woven bone. Many pathologists will not make the diagnosis of fibrous dysplasia if, by polarization, the trabeculae are not composed of immature, woven bone. Also, the early literature emphasized the contrast between trabeculae rimmed by osteoblasts and trabeculae seeming to arise directly from fusiform fibroblasts. Ossifying fibroma was supposed to contain mature, lamellar bone rather than woven

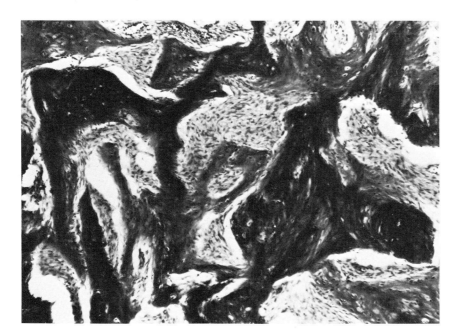

Figure 58–33. Fibrous dysplasia showing irregular, bony trabeculae in a fibrous connective tissue stroma. (H & E, × 100)

bone and was always supposed to be rimmed by osteoblasts. With the experience of a large number of cases, these distinctions are no longer considered reliable.[212, 222, 227] Fibrous dysplasia may be examined at any stage of development, and the early lesions will demonstrate woven bone in the trabeculae, but the more mature, arrested lesions will have more mature, lamellar trabeculae. Serial biopsies in a patient showed a change from woven bone to a lamellar bone with osteoblastic rimming.[212] Osteoblasts are often seen rimming trabeculae in fibrous dysplasia. Therefore, the value of the histologic examination is in confirming the benign nature of the process and the placement of the lesion into the group of fibro-osseous lesions, from which it can be extricated with a combination of clinical, radiographic, and histopathologic findings.

Treatment and Prognosis

The prognosis of fibrous dysplasia is generally very good. The deforming lesion of the jaws may recur, but usually the response to a conservative surgical approach is favorable. Mitotic figures are occasionally found in the actively proliferating lesions but have no correlation to possible malignancy.[211]

Surgical treatment should be cosmetic in nature, and no attempt should be made to remove all the process, as there is no distinct border noted radiographically or histologically. The process nearly always "burns itself out" around the age of puberty. Occasional cases of "aggressive fibrous dysplasia" are reported, but no difference in the histologic findings are noted when compared to the usual, more indolent cases.[225] With an aggressive, rapidly expanding fibrous dysplasia, histologic examination is necessary and valuable to exclude a malignant disease.

Malignant transformation does occur rarely, the incidence being less common than in Paget's disease, which is a fraction of 1 per cent.[220] It is also possible to have malignant change without prior radiation exposure. This is most often seen in the craniofacial region and long limb bones.[220] In a review of 29 cases of malignant degeneration of fibrous dysplasia, Gross and Montgomery found that 13 of the 29 patients had received prior radiation treatment for the fibrous dysplasia.[215] Radiation therapy should be avoided if practical. Any lesion of fibrous dysplasia that suddenly exhibits an accelerated growth phase or severe pain must be suspected of having undergone malignant transformation. Regional lymph node dissection is not routinely advocated, as metastasis in the instance of malignant transformation is usually by the hematogenous route, with the lung being the most usual target site.[215]

TUMORS AND TUMOR-LIKE CONDITIONS OF BLOOD VESSELS ARISING IN THE SKELETAL SYSTEM

Hemangioma of Bone

Hemangiomas of bone are rare tumors, composing only 0.7 per cent of all osseous neoplasms.[242] Watson and McCarthy reviewed 1056 cases of blood and lymph vessel tumors between the years 1931 and 1939 and found only five cases of central hemangiomas of bone.[239] The vertebral column and skull are the two most common sites. By 1975 only 53 cases of central hemangiomas of the jaws had been reported in the literature.[235] Although they are very rare, they represent a potentially lethal situation resulting from extensive hemorrhage following biopsy or tooth extraction.

The peak incidence for central hemangiomas of the jaws is in the second decade of life, with females predominating 2:1.[234] One half to two thirds of the tumors occur in the mandible, with the molar region most frequently involved.[234, 235]

The etiology of hemangiomas is uncertain. Some of the lesions may actually be tumor-like malformations or hamartomas, and others may be true neoplasms.[233] Shira and Guernsey believe that the hemangioma is a true neoplasm that is of mesenchymal origin and develops from congenital rests that differentiate by a process of endothelial proliferation into blood vessels,[237] but Shklar and Meyer support the theory that hemangiomas are developmental malformations or hamartomas.[238]

Clinical Findings

The most common clinical signs and symptoms of hemangiomas are expansion of the buccal cortex, spontaneous gingival bleeding from around the necks of teeth in the involved area, tooth mobility, and pain or numbness. Root resorption has been observed in approximately 30 per cent of the cases.[231] Severe epistaxis may be seen in lesions involving the maxilla. In large lesions in which there has been arteriovenous fistula formation, thrills or bruits may be detected. Because the majority of these lesions are slow growing and painless, 60 per cent of the patients have symptoms for more than 1 year before seeking medical attention.[234]

Hemangiomas present with a variety of radiographic appearances, many of which can mimic other lesions. Therefore, aspiration prior to surgical intervention of a radiolucent lesion of the jaws is essential.

In a very thorough review of radiographic patterns seen in vascular tumors of the jaws, Worth and Stoneman,[241] reported that most central hemangiomas of the jaws manifest a multilocular appearance, frequently described as "soap-bubble" or "honeycomb" radiolucencies (Fig. 58–34). Unfortunately, other tumors of the jaws such as ameloblastoma, myxoma, and central giant cell granulomas also exhibit this appearance.

Hemangiomas in the skull characteristically present with a "sunray" appearance in which trabeculae of bone radiate from the surface toward the periphery. This pattern has also been noted in some jaw lesions, but infrequently.[236, 241]

Radiolucent cystic lesions in which bony trabeculae radiate from the center of the lesion in a fan-like or spoke-wheel pattern is very suggestive of central hemangiomas. Occasionally, hemangiomas can appear as well-corticated, cyst-like cavities that may resemble single odontogenic cysts, emphasizing the need for needle aspiration of radiolucent jaw lesions. Arteriography is an aid in diagnosis and is essential for treatment planning.

Pathology

On gross examination, hemangiomas present as brownish red lesions. Histologically, they are classified as capillary, cavernous, and mixed hemangiomas. The classification of these lesions is academic, for there is no correlation between histologic type, clinical behavior, response to treatment, and prognosis. Cavernous hemangiomas are composed of large, thin-walled, vascular spaces engorged with blood, lined by a single layer of endothelial cells in a connective tissue stroma and interspersed between bony trabeculae. Capillary hemangiomas are composed of numerous capillary channels that have been reported in some cases to radiate outward in a sunburst pattern.[230] Some hemangiomas contain elements of both and are designated as mixed.

Weinstein and associates published a study of a case of a cavernous hemangioma in the mandible that exhibited areas of fibrosis and ossification, and they designated this lesion as a scirrhous hemangioma.[240] Choukas and associates reported a similar lesion in the maxilla under the designation of a sclerosing hemangioma.[229] These lesions probably represent the third stage (the sclerotic phase in which ossification occurs) of hemangioma development proposed by Hitzrot.[232] Stage 1 is

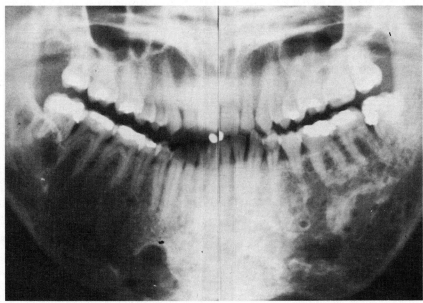

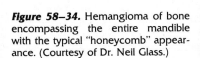

Figure 58–34. Hemangioma of bone encompassing the entire mandible with the typical "honeycomb" appearance. (Courtesy of Dr. Neil Glass.)

characterized by a richly vascular state, and the intermediate phase of the lesion features cystic areas with organized blood clot.

Electron microscopy is of little value in the diagnosis of hemangioma because of the characteristic light microscopic appearance.

Treatment and Prognosis

A number of different treatment methods and combinations have been employed in the treatment of central hemangiomas—radiation therapy, injection of sclerosing agents, surgery, and embolization—with success depending on the specific case. Factors that must be taken into consideration to determine the treatment modality of central hemangiomas are lesion location, size, and vascular supply.

Hemangioendothelial Sarcoma (Angiosarcoma) of Bone

This extremely rare, malignant vascular tumor of bone has been referred to by a variety of names—angiosarcoma, hemangiosarcoma, hemangioendothelioma, malignant hemangioendothelioma, and angioblastic sarcoma. This confusion in nomenclature results from the rarity of the tumor, the variation in biologic behavior, and a difference in behavior from soft-tissue angiosarcomas. The well-differentiated malignant endothelial tumors of bone exhibit an indolent course and have been diagnosed as hemangioendotheliomas by some investigators, and the more poorly differentiated lesions have been labeled angiosarcomas or malignant hemangioendotheliomas.[234] In addition, malignant endothelial neoplasms of bone have a less aggressive behavior than soft-tissue angiosarcomas. For these reasons, Wold and associates prefer the term hemangioendothelial sarcoma, for it clearly indicates the cell of origin and its malignant potential and distinguishes it from its soft-tissue counterpart.[253]

In the largest reported series (112 cases) of hemangioendothelial sarcomas of bone, only three occurred in the maxilla and mandible.[253] In a series of 49 cases published by Huvos in 1979, three involved the mandible.[247] Zachariades and associates reviewed the world literature in 1980 and reported a total of 46 cases of hemangioendothelial sarcoma in the oral cavity. Only 17 cases (33 per cent) were bony lesions.[255]

In the series reported by Wold, most cases occurred in the third decade of life, with an age range of 5 to 84 years.[253] The same age distribution is found in lesions of the jaws.[252, 255]

Approximately 20 to 25 per cent of the cases of hemangioendothelial sarcomas present with multifocal, osseous involvement.[247, 253] In two of the larger series, none of the multifocal cases have involved the jaws.

The etiology of hemangioendothelial sarcomas is unknown, but it has been reported developing in a chronic osteomyelitis of the tibia.[248]

Clinical Findings

Hemangioendothelial sarcomas of bone usually present with pain and swelling, but some tumors manifest as reddish, granulomatous, soft-tissue gingival lesions that clinically resemble pyogenic granulomas.[244, 251, 255]

This extraosseous presentation results from the tumor eroding through the cortex or proliferation from an extraction site.

Radiographically, these lesions are ill-defined osteolytic radiolucencies with a minimal periosteal reaction with no specific characteristics.[254] One case exhibited abnormal widening of the periodontal ligament space about the roots of the teeth in the region of the tumor, a change similar to that seen in osteogenic sarcoma.[251] Angiography is beneficial in delineating the extent of the neoplasm.[247]

Pathology

Grossly, the lesions are soft and highly vascular with irregular borders. Microscopically, they are characterized by neoplastic vascular channel formation (Fig. 58–35). The neoplastic vessels exhibit an anastomosing pattern separated by a loose connective tissue stroma. The tumors may show a variety of histologic appearances, ranging from well to poorly differentiated. The well-differentiated lesions exhibit well-formed vessels lined by plump, mildly atypical endothelial cells with few mitoses. The more anaplastic the endothelial cells appear, and the less well formed the vascular channels, the less differentiated the tumor. Papillary tufting, a common feature of soft-tissue angiosarcomas, is infrequently seen in angiosarcomas of bone.[253]

Differential Diagnosis

Well-differentiated hemangioendothelial sarcomas may be difficult to differentiate from hemangiomas of bone. In benign hemangiomas, the endothelial cells are usually flat and inconspicuous, but in well-differentiated hemangioendothelial sarcoma the cells are prominent, crowded, and hyperchromatic. Undifferentiated tumors may have "spindle cell" areas or "epithelial" areas in which differentiation from fibrosarcoma or metastatic carcinoma may be difficult.[253]

A reticulum stain is helpful in differentiating this lesion from a hemangiopericytoma, which is also very rare in bone. In hemangiopericytoma, the tumor cells (pericytes) are located outside the reticular vessel sheath, and in hemangioendothelial sarcomas they are internal to the reticular sheath.[250] Immunoperoxidase staining for factor VIII has also been reported to be helpful in diagnosing tumors of endothelial origin.[246]

Ultrastructurally, in hemangiopericytomas, the vessels are lined by a single layer of cells, which are essentially normal, but in hemangioendotheliomas the tumor cells are crowded. In addition, the neoplasms differ in spacing of tumor cells in relation to the surrounding extracellular material. In hemangioendothelioma, extracellular material is abundant, thus separating the tumor cells; in hemangiopericytomas, the material is relatively thin, segregating the cells into tightly packed masses.[245, 249]

Treatment and Prognosis

Prognosis varies with histologic grading. Patients with those tumors classified as well-differentiated or low-grade lesions have a survival rate of 95 per cent, but patients with undifferentiated or high-grade tumors have a 20 per cent survival rate.[253] Huvos reported that

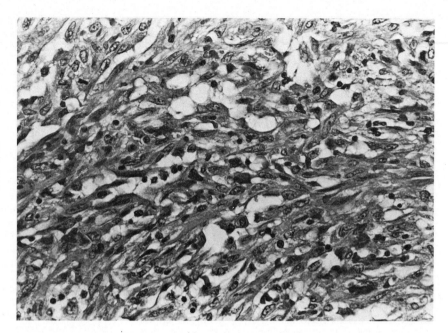

Figure 58–35. Hemangioendothelial sarcoma with poorly formed neoplastic vessels lined by atypical cells similar to those infiltrating the stroma. (H & E, × 100)

patients with multifocal lesions have a better prognosis than those with unifocal lesions.[247] Wold and associates, however, found prognosis to be based not on centricity, but rather on histologic grade.[253] Surgical excision is still the principal mode of therapy. Too few cases have been reported in the jaws to determine any variation in response to treatment and prognosis compared with other locations.

MISCELLANEOUS TUMORS

Ewing's Sarcoma

Ewing's sarcoma is an uncommon malignant tumor of bone. It accounts for only about 6 per cent of all bone tumors seen at Mayo Clinic[260] and only about 4 per cent of those seen at the Washington University School of Medicine.[284] Ewing's sarcoma is primarily a lesion of long tubular bones or innominate bones. The femur is the most common site, with 60 per cent of all cases involving the lower extremities and pelvis.[272] Involvement of the facial bones and skull is extremely rare, amounting to less than 1 per cent of all reported Ewing's sarcomas.[272] When Ewing's sarcoma does occur in the jaws, it occurs more frequently in the mandible than in the maxilla.[257] An extraskeletal form of Ewing's sarcoma has been described, but it is very rare in the head and neck region.[256, 264, 283]

Ewing's sarcoma is a disease of young people, regardless of site; 88 per cent of such tumors occur in persons between 6 and 20 years of age.[272] There is a slight male predominance, the male-female ratio being 3:2.[267, 272] Ewing's sarcoma is seldom seen in either American or African blacks.[265, 276, 287]

The histogenesis of Ewing's sarcoma has been a subject of speculation since James Ewing first described the tumor in 1921 in an article entitled "Diffuse Endothelioma of Bone.''[262] Possible cells of origin discussed since its original description are endothelial,[262, 263, 273] mesenchymal,[268] myeloblast,[270] pericyte,[279] and smooth muscle cell.[285] The controversy continues, with many investigators supporting the cell of origin as being a primitive mesenchymal cell[261] and others supporting an endothelial cell origin.[273, 280]

Clinical Findings

The most common symptoms of Ewing's sarcoma are pain[258, 259, 286] and swelling[275, 288] of the affected region. However, patients may have a more insidious onset that is characterized by slight fever, anemia, leukocytosis, and an increased sedimentation rate.[258] Additionally, patients have presented with tooth mobility or extrusion.[258, 288] Radiographic findings are nonspecific and can mimic either infectious or other neoplastic processes. In the jaws, the tumor produces an ill-defined osteolytic lesion (Fig. 58–36). In long bones, varying degrees of periosteal thickening frequently are seen, producing the classic "onion-skin" appearance.[267] Periosteal thickening is infrequently seen in jaw lesions.

Metastases to other bones and to the lungs are frequently encountered in Ewing's sarcoma. At least 25 per cent of patients with Ewing's sarcoma have evidence of metastases at the time of diagnosis or completion of treatment.[284] Therefore, full-chest tomography, bone scans, and marrow aspiration are indicated prior to initiation of therapy.[281] Several cases have been reported of Ewing's sarcoma metastasizing to the mandible.[258, 271, 286]

Pathology

Grossly, Ewing's sarcoma has a heterogeneous pattern, with white to yellow areas of viable tissue, hemorrhagic areas, and friable areas of necrosis. Ewing's sarcoma has been classically described as a neoplasm composed of sheets of uniform, small, round cells. However, the Intergroup Ewing's Sarcoma Study char-

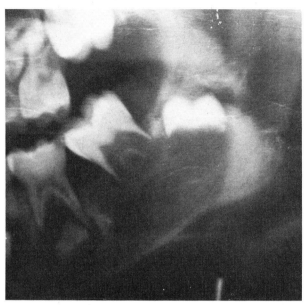

Figure 58–36. Ewing's sarcoma in a 5-year-old presented with mobility of the first permanent molar and an associated ill-defined radiolucency. (Courtesy of Drs. Jim Hix and Perry McGinnis.)

of pseudorosettes is responsible for the resemblance of Ewing's sarcoma to neuroblastoma. Nucleoli are not prominent, and mitoses are minimal. Zones of coagulation necrosis and hemorrhage are prominent. No correlation between clinical course or response to therapy and histologic variations has been reported. Extraskeletal tumors are histologically identical to those in bone.[256, 264, 283]

Much emphasis has been placed on the presence of glycogen in the cytoplasm of the tumor cells, and, ultrastructurally, at least some of the cells in Ewing's sarcoma will contain cytoplasmic glycogen.[272] However, in approximately 5 to 10 per cent of the cases, periodic acid–Schiff (PAS) staining will be negative for glycogen.[267] The presence of glycogen is helpful in distinguishing this tumor from neuroblastoma and lymphomas of bone, which are both glycogen negative. However, the absence of glycogen disclosed by light microscopy does not negate the diagnosis of Ewing's sarcoma.

Ultrastructural features seen in Ewing's sarcoma are nonspecific. In addition to the presence of cytoplasmic glycogen, intercellular connections of desmosomal type are present in 56 per cent of the cases reported by Greer and associates.[266]

Differential Diagnosis

Four malignant neoplasms must be considered in the differential diagnosis: metastatic neuroblastoma, lymphoma of bone, embryonal rhabdomyosarcoma, and small cell osteosarcoma. Although neuroblastoma is frequently metastatic to the skull, it can be distinguished from Ewing's sarcoma by an intravenous pyelogram, analysis of urine for catecholamines and vanillylmandelic acid, and negative tumor glycogen.

Non-Hodgkin's lymphomas of bone usually involve an older age group than does Ewing's sarcoma. Histologically, lymphomas are glycogen negative, and the cells have a more distinct cytoplasmic border. Reticulum

acterizes it as a dimorphic tumor with the predominant cell being a large cell (two to three times the diameter of a lymphocyte) with clear cytoplasm and indistinct boundaries.[272] These predominant, fully viable cells alternate with clusters of smaller cells, which have pyknotic, clumpy nuclei. The tumor has very little intercellular stroma, and the cells lack cohesion (Fig. 58–37). The tumor exhibits a variety of histologic patterns, the most common of which is the diffuse pattern composed of sheets of cells. Tumor cells may also cluster around blood vessels. Other patterns described are organoid, trabecular, and pseudorosette. The occasional presence

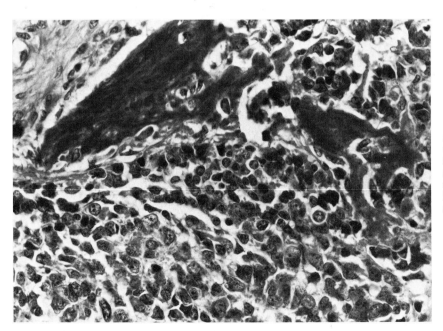

Figure 58–37. Ewing's sarcoma demonstrating the dimorphic pattern of small cells with pyknotic nuclei interspersed among sheets of large cells with indistinct borders. Spicules of bone undergoing resorption are seen at the top. (H & E, × 100)

fibers in lymphomas penetrate individual cells or cell groups, but in Ewing's sarcoma these fibers are confined to fibrous septa and vascular walls.[267] Additionally, electron microscopy and cell surface markers may be helpful in the diagnosis of lymphoma.

Embryonal rhabdomyosarcoma can frequently invade bone and present as a primary bone tumor. This is especially true in the head and neck region, where erosion of the mandible may be the initial symptom.[281] Light or electron microscopy may be beneficial in demonstrating the characteristic features of rhabdomyoblasts. The presence of malignant osteoid production is the most reliable criteria to distinguish small cell osteosarcoma from Ewing's sarcoma.

Treatment and Prognosis

Ten years ago the prognosis for Ewing's sarcoma was poor, regardless of therapy or extent of the disease. Recent reports still indicate that survival rates may be less than 20 per cent if metastatic disease or extraosseous extension is present at the time of the initial diagnosis.[266, 269, 274] However, with early, aggressive use of chemotherapy in combination with surgery or radiation therapy in patients with nonmetastatic Ewing's sarcoma, the disease-free survival rate is approximately 75 per cent.[277, 281, 282] Limited data on Ewing's sarcoma of the head and neck precludes any assessment as to the prognosis or the effectiveness of therapy in this area. However, Pomeroy and Johnson reported improved survival rates for Ewing's sarcoma involving peripheral locations (below the knee and elbow, and the mandible) when contrasted with lesions of the trunk.[278]

Primary Salivary Gland Tumors within Bone

One of the processes one must consider in a differential diagnosis of radiolucent lesions of the jaws is an intraosseous salivary gland neoplasm. A very interesting feature of these lesions is the virtual uniqueness of the type of neoplasm; rather than being a mirror of the various types of salivary gland tumors that arise in soft tissue, nearly all are central mucoepidermoid carcinomas. Central mixed tumors and central adenoid cystic carcinomas have rarely been reported.[292, 294]

The central mucoepidermoid carcinoma is a rather uncommon lesion, and few pathologists or medical centers have large series for analysis. When such a salivary gland tumor occurs in the maxilla or mandible, it resembles an osteolytic tumor of odontogenic origin or an odontogenic cyst. No clinical or radiologic method is available for diagnosis without resorting to a biopsy.

The most interesting aspect of central salivary gland tumors is the question of etiology. One does not consider salivary gland tissue to be normally found within the jaw bones. The most accepted theories of origin of these neoplasms include enclavement of embryonal salivary gland tissue,[291] ectopic salivary gland tissue,[290, 301] and mucous metaplasia of the lining of odontogenic cysts.[295, 296, 297, 299] The most telling piece of evidence is probably the histologic typing of the intraosseous salivary gland neoplasms. Rather than mimicking the distribution of salivary gland neoplasms found in major or minor glands, only a few have been found to be a type other than mucoepidermoid carcinomas. It would be reasonable to expect that if the cause of the intraosseous lesions was entrapment of embryonal salivary gland tissue, or if the cells of origin were from aberrant salivary gland tissue, the type of salivary gland neoplasms found in the jaws would approximate the distribution found in soft tissue. Therefore, the idea of these salivary gland tumors arising by mucous metaplasia within the epithelial lining of odontogenic cysts is most appealing. Mucous cells have been demonstrated in the lining of 5.5 per cent of follicular cysts (associated with impacted teeth).

Origin from the other two sources may be possible. In 1963, Bhaskar described the events that could lead to entrapment of salivary glands in the retromolar region within the mandible and presented two cases that he felt supported his thesis.[291] Another possibility frequently mentioned is origin from the so-called static bone cavity or "Stafne bone cyst." This is not a true cyst, and although it sometimes appears as a well-circumscribed radiolucency in the molar-bicuspid region of the mandible, it simply represents a depression in the bone in which rests the submandibular gland. The static bone cavity is always found below the mandibular canal. Most authors consider this very unlikely as a possible site of origin for intraosseous salivary gland neoplasms, although Browand and Waldron felt this could be a possibility because two of the tumors in their series developed below the inferior alveolar canal.[293]

The various theories of cell of origin (other than the unlikely static bone cavity) have one thing in common: the ultimate origin for these neoplasms is the oral epithelium. Entrapped embryonal salivary gland tissue, aberrant salivary gland tissue, and the dental follicle, which is the origin of the follicular (dentigerous) cyst, are all initially derived from embryonic oral epithelium. It may be far simpler to agree with Smith and associates in accepting that one cannot determine the pathogenesis of this neoplasm and simply considering the pluripotentiality of oral epithelium as the explanation for the development of intraosseous salivary gland neoplasms.[303]

In a series of 54 mucoepidermoid tumors of intraoral minor salivary glands, Melrose and associates found only one (1.8 per cent) to be intrabony.[300] Spiro and associates found less than 1 per cent of cases of mucoepidermoid carcinomas in a 30-year period at Memorial Sloan-Kettering Cancer Center to have been central in bone.[304] Grubka and associates reviewed the literature in 1983 and found only 38 cases that met the criteria for mucoepidermoid carcinomas of intraosseous origin.[297]

Several authors have developed criteria for determining the intraosseous origin of mucoepidermoid salivary gland neoplasms. Browand and Waldron have summarized these criteria as follows:

1. Presence of intact cortical plates.
2. Radiographic evidence of bone destruction.
3. Histopathologic confirmation.
4. Positive mucin staining.
5. Absence of primary salivary gland neoplasms in salivary glands or other tissues that can mimic the histologic architecture of salivary neoplasms.
6. Exclusion of an odontogenic tumor.[293]

Controversy surrounds the classification of mucoepidermoid salivary neoplasms. This includes controversy over whether the name should be mucoepidermoid "carcinoma" or "tumor." The extremes of opinion are exemplified by Batsakis,[289] who believes all are malignant and therefore should be named "carcinoma," and Melrose and associates,[300] who feel that the well-differentiated lesions behave exactly like a common mixed tumor and the neoplasms should be called "tumor" to prevent excessive therapy. Smith and associates feel the consensus favors treating even the well-differentiated mucoepidermoid neoplasms as low-grade cancers.[303] Most pathologists classify the mucoepidermoid neoplasms as "low-grade" and "high-grade," that is, low-grade malignancy and high-grade malignancy.

Clinical Findings

Intraosseous salivary gland neoplasms usually present with a rather rapid onset, producing symptoms in less than a year. A painless swelling is usually noticed, although pain may be a presenting symptom. In the largest series reported, Grubka and associates found a slight female predominance.[297] Smith and associates reported that females were affected twice as often as males.[303] The most common location is the posterior mandible near an impacted third molar or where a third molar had been extracted. Anterior locations are extremely rare, with only the fourth case being reported in the anterior of the mandible in 1983.[297] The average age of onset is the mid-fifties, and virtually no age group is exempt, the youngest patient having been reported at 1 year.

The location is in agreement with the various theories of etiology because the retromolar area is highly populated with minor salivary glands, and entrapment of embryonal or ectopic glands would be highly likely in this area. Also, the theory of development from the lining of follicular cysts is supported because the most commonly impacted tooth is the mandibular third molar, and a dental follicle exists only around the crown of a developed, but unerupted tooth.

The preoperative diagnosis of virtually all intraosseous salivary gland neoplasms is odontogenic cyst (follicular or residual) or ameloblastoma. The radiographic findings are most often a well-circumscribed unilocular or a multilocular radiolucency (Fig. 58–38).

Pathology

Gross pathologic features are not consistent. Many central salivary gland neoplasms are firm and tan to yellowish, and others show variably sized cysts containing mucus or congealed mucinous material. Microscopically, the central salivary gland neoplasms will appear the same histologically as their counterparts in major or minor salivary glands, with the exception that there is no associated normal salivary gland tissue. The histologic features of central mucoepidermoid carcinomas by which a determination of "high" or "low" grade malignancy is made are related to the relative amount of mucinous gland-like tissue and epitheloid tissue present. The more mucinous-appearing, the lower the grade; therefore, the more squamous-appearing, the higher the grade. An excellent description of the histopathologic features of salivary gland tumors is presented by Batsakis[289] and will not be reviewed here.

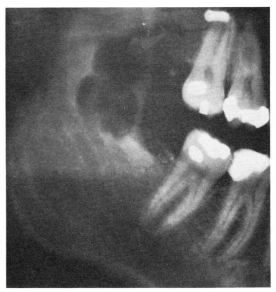

Figure 58–38. Central mucoepidermoid carcinoma in a 26-year-old showing a multilocular radiolucency in mandibular ramus. (Courtesy of Drs. Wayne Littlefield and Raymond Smith.)

Differential Diagnosis

The most significant lesions to consider in a differential diagnosis are odontogenic cysts and tumors and squamous cell carcinomas and adenocarcinomas, either primary or metastatic. The most common location of central salivary gland neoplasms, the posterior body of the mandible, is also the most common location for follicular (dentigerous) cysts and ameloblastomas. The body of the mandible is likewise the most frequent site of metastases to the head and neck area from subclavicular origins.

The most helpful ancillary study is the mucin stain, as nearly all central salivary gland neoplasms are mucoepidermoid carcinomas. However, there can be problems with interpretation of these findings, for linings of odontogenic cysts may indeed undergo mucous metaplasia and even ciliation.[298] Also, the differentiation between a high-grade mucoepidermoid carcinoma and a squamous cell carcinoma may be difficult, if not impossible. This differentiation is most likely moot, however, because the behavior will be essentially the same. If there is a question of possible metastasis to the jaws from a distant site, a thorough work-up is necessary; the prognostic implication of a metastasis is so devastating that radical or mutilating treatment is generally not offered.[302]

Treatment and Prognosis

All authors agree that the histologic grade of the majority of the central mucoepidermoid carcinomas has very little to do with prognosis; hence, the lack of agreement over whether they should all be called "carcinomas" or "tumors." Many low-grade, well-differentiated mucoepidermoid carcinomas have recurred, metastasized to regional lymph nodes, or caused death. The rare central mixed tumor or central adenoid cystic carcinoma should be treated much as their counterparts in soft tissue.

Smith and associates state that the consensus is in favor of treating well-differentiated mucoepidermoid carcinomas as low-grade cancers, that is, by wide local excision with electrocoagulation of the tumor edges; whereas the anaplastic, or high-grade mucoepidermoid carcinomas should be treated radically.[303] Many reports link proximity of tumor to surgical margins as the most important factor in local recurrence, regardless of histologic type. The Mayo Clinic series indicates that total en bloc excision of maxillary tumors should be performed whenever possible, and mandibular lesions can be treated by relatively conservative local excision.[303] In this series of nine patients, the three who died all had maxillary lesions. Central mucoepidermoid carcinomas do not readily metastasize, but they have the potential to do so; close follow-up is essential. The 5-year survival rate is excellent, and the overall prognosis is good.

Primary Lymphoma of Bone

Malignant lymphomas, as would be expected, arise in bone as well as other extranodal sites in the body. In 1939 Parker and Jackson established primary lymphoma of bone as a separate entity.[320] Because of a distinct clinical behavior, primary malignant lymphomas of bone should be separated from other lymphomas and certainly from Ewing's sarcoma. The majority of patients with lymphoma of bone will be shown to have more extensive disease after meticulous clinical and pathologic staging.[324] Although uncommon, primary lymphomas of the jaws do occur and must be recognized and appropriately treated. No attempt will be made to include a discussion of the various classifications of lymphomas now being used. A general, all-inclusive term, suggested by Dahlin[312] for discussion of bone lymphomas is "malignant lymphoma," which includes references in the literature to reticulum cell sarcoma and the various lymphocytic and lymphoblastic lymphomas. Braunstein states that Hodgkin's disease never originates in bone. Bone involvement signifies dissemination beyond the original nodal site.[307] Boston and associates claim that, although unusual, Hodgkin's disease was found in the large Mayo Clinic series of primary lymphomas of bone.[306] Burkitt's lymphoma is a distinct entity and will be discussed separately, because of its particular relationship to the jaws.

When one encounters a lymphoma producing an osseous lesion, one of three conditions may be occurring. As both Batsakis[305] and Dahlin[312] state:

1. The lesion may be considered to be primary in the involved bone.

2. Similar lesions may be found in other bones, regional or distant lymph nodes, or any other part of the body and the bone lesion in question may be considered to be either a primary or a secondary focus.

3. A lesion in bone may be found in a patient with known malignant lymphoma when the bone lesion is obviously secondary.

Minimal criteria for primary bone lymphomas include origination in a single bone with metastases limited to only regional lymph nodes, and distant metastases should follow the appearance of the primary bone lesion by at least 6 months.

Primary malignant lymphomas compose approximately 5 to 7 per cent of all malignant bone tumors.[306, 311, 312] The most common site in the jaws is the area of the maxillary antrum, although in this area it is difficult to be sure of primary bony involvement. Discounting the cases involving the maxillary antrum, the mandible is the most common jaw location and is the third most common site overall, after tubular long bones and the innominate bone.[310] Males predominate in all series, the male-female ratio being approximately 3:2. In a large series from the Mayo Clinic, the average age was 44 years, with most of the patients being in the fifth and sixth decades. Fewer than 15 per cent of the patients were less than 20 years of age; this is a great distinguishing factor from Ewing's sarcoma, in which 70 per cent of the patients were that young. In this particular series, 9 per cent of the primary bone lymphomas were located in the mandible.[306]

Staging of primary malignant lymphomas of bone is moot, for the determination that the lesion is primary is the significant factor in its treatment and prognosis.

Clinical Findings

Virtually all patients initially complain of pain at the site of the lesion. Approximately one third will have an associated mass, and in the jaws it is more common to have a palpable mass along with nerve involvement and loosening of teeth.[314, 316] Often, despite extensive local destruction, the systemic manifestations of malignant disease such as weight loss, fever, and malaise are very minimal. The average duration of symptoms before treatment is 10 to 14 months.[305, 306] A very interesting aspect of primary lymphoma of bone in comparison to other malignancies is the relative well-being of the patient.

Radiographic features are variable and have no pathognomonic characteristics.[305, 306, 314] Often, by the time of radiographic evaluation, the lesion is extensive. Commonly, they have a mottled, patchy appearance and no distinct outline. Primary lymphomas of bone very infrequently cause destruction of the cortex with soft-tissue extension (Fig. 58–39A and B). Phillips and associates have identified nine radiographic signs they feel are valuable for helping to make a prognosis for primary lymphoma of bone and they seem to be related to imminent or actual soft-tissue extension.[322]

Bone may respond to the presence of tumor by increased osteoblastic activity or so-called reactive bone formation.[319] Often small areas of calcification can be seen in these masses. One half of the lesions will most likely have reactive bone proliferation or some degree of radiopacity.[305, 306, 314] Periosteal bone formation commonly occurs in lymphoma, most frequently developing as a response to tumor that penetrates the cortex into the subperiosteal region.[319]

The diagnosis cannot be made radiographically. The most commonly suspected diseases in children are metastatic lesions, histiocytosis X, osteomyelitis, osteosarcoma, Ewing's sarcoma, and leukemia. In adults, chronic osteomyelitis, histiocytosis X, osteosarcoma, and metastasis are the more common considerations.

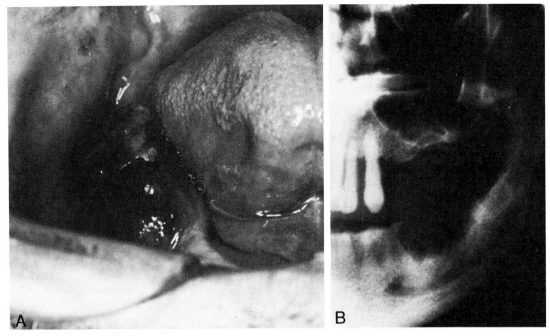

Figure 58–39. Primary lymphoma of bone presenting as a bluish, soft-tissue swelling (*A*) and a fairly well demarcated radiolucency with cortical destruction (*B*). (Courtesy of Dr. Richard M. Courtney.)

Initial evaluation for other sites of disease with nuclear bone scans, skeletal radiographic surveys, and lymphangiography is extremely important. A biopsy is necessary to establish the diagnosis.

Laboratory studies are of no use unless there is a protein abnormality indicative of multiple myeloma.

Pathology

Grossly, the malignant lymphomas of bone almost always involve some soft-tissue extension and no distinctive features, appearing similar to lymphomas in other parts of the body: soft and friable with areas of necrosis. Margins in the bone are indistinct; the boundaries are much more extensive than indicated by radiographs.

Histologically, the cell usually referred to in the past as the reticulum cell, or histiocyte, is the most common cell. This is recognized now as a misnomer, a descriptive term for large "transformed" cells of diverse origins, i.e., B- and T-lymphocytes, null cells, and the rare true "histiocytic" cell lymphoma.[317] Follicle or nodule formation is minimal or absent.[313] Exact categorization has not always been practical because of variations within individual tumors. It has been reported that histiocytic lymphoma is the most common form.

Boston and associates state that the probability of survival of the patients in their large study was not correlated to histologic appearance.[306] Essentially no further classification of morphologic and biologic variation was attempted for primary bone lymphomas until 1980, when Mahoney and Alexander divided primary "histiocytic" lymphoma in bone into two groups, depending on the presence or absence of cleavage and convolution of nuclei.[317] In 1982, Dosoretz and associates attempted to determine whether histologic features of

these lesions could serve to identify biologically distinctive subpopulations within this heterogeneous disease.[313] Using cell size, nuclear morphologic features, nucleolar prominence, pleomorphism, and staining qualities as parameters, they found that primary lymphomas of bone were easily classifiable only when grouped according to nuclear morphologic features and cell size. Size was determined in relation to a benign histiocyte, and nuclei were either noncleaved, cleaved, or hyperlobated (pleomorphic). Patients with lymphomas composed of cells with cleaved nuclei had a significantly better survival rate with no evidence of disease than those with lymphomas with noncleaved or pleomorphic nuclei, which did not differ significantly from each other. Cell size was found to be of no predictive value.[313]

Differential Diagnosis

Histologically, the differential diagnosis would include metastatic carcinoma, usually easily distinguishable, and other "round cell" tumors of bone. Myeloma is almost always easily recognized owing to the plasmacytoid cells. Evaluation of monoclonal serum proteins will help distinguish the occasional myeloma that is difficult to differentiate from lymphoma. Ewing's sarcoma is usually distinguishable by cytologic characteristics, but when this is not easy, staining tissues fixed in 80 per cent ethanol with the periodic acid–Schiff (PAS) stain for glycogen will show glycogen in cells of Ewing's sarcoma but not lymphoma.[323] Glycogen has been identified in Ewing's sarcoma cells by electron microscopy, and this may become important in distinguishing Ewing's sarcoma from malignant lymphoma. Mahoney and Alexander found glycogen in 1 per cent of the cells in primary lymphoma of bone by electron microscopy and felt the observation of glycogen in cells in isolation would not differentiate malignant lymphoma from Ewing's sarcoma. Metastatic neuroblastoma, metastatic alveolar rhabdomyosarcoma, and undifferentiated large cell carcinomas can be differentiated from primary lymphoma of bone by electron microscopy.[317] As in nodal lymphomas, Reed-Sternberg cells are necessary for the diagnosis of Hodgkin's disease.

Treatment and Prognosis

The most significant aspect of the primary lymphoma of bone is its prognosis, which is significantly better than other primary malignant tumors of bone.[305] Thirteen of 17 patients in Parker and Jackson's original series were alive 6 months to 14 years after their initial symptoms appeared.[320] Boston and associates at the Mayo Clinic found in their large study that the probability of 5-year survival with a primary lymphoma of bone is nearly twice as strong as when additional foci are found elsewhere.[306] An excellent prognosis for patients with osseous Hodgkin's disease when treated with combined-modality therapy has been documented.[318] Dosoretz feels that the large number of patients alive and free of disease at follow-up intervals of 5 years and longer indicates that primary lymphoma of bone is a local disease process in a significant number of patients at the time of presentation.[313] Cortical destruction and soft-tissue extension form a grave prognostic sign in the jaws.

Burkitt's Lymphoma

A type of malignant lymphoma with a distinct relationship to the jaws is Burkitt's lymphoma. As Burkitt himself said, "If it had been known at that time that the tumor developed from B-cell lymphocytes, the eponym would presumably not have been used."[308] In 1958, Denis Burkitt, a British surgeon serving at the university teaching hospital in Kampala, Africa, first published his findings concerning a disease affecting the jaws of African children.[309] As a surgeon, he saw an opportunity to have an article published in the prestigious *British Journal of Surgery*, but he admits now that the original article got minimal attention in the surgery journal. Burkitt's own account of the discovery and early work concerning this newly discovered disease is very interesting.[308] His study of what he calls the "geography of disease" began when he was confronted with children suffering from rapidly growing tumors of the jaw, usually in the maxilla. The children's teeth were loose, and their faces were grossly distorted. Associated with the jaw lesions were abdominal masses and, unexpectedly, paraplegia. Also, a characteristic feature was the absence of involvement of peripheral lymph nodes. It was soon realized that this was the most common tumor of the region. Early in his investigation, it became apparent that the disease was common in some areas and virtually unknown in others. Burkitt felt that if he could find geographic boundaries, clues to its cause might be found. The original survey and interviews, which defined the "lymphoma belt" and upon which all the rest of the research was based, cost $75.

Burkitt's next step was what he called a "geographic biopsy." Just as a surgeon takes a sample from the edge of a lesion to examine both diseased and normal tissue, he decided to examine the edge of the "lymphoma belt." Burkitt discovered that the tumor was limited by an altitude barrier that fell progressively as distance from the equator increased, and this was interpreted as a temperature barrier. Also, the tumor was more prevalent where the rainfall was high and less common where the rainfall was low. This climatic dependence inevitably suggested the implication of some biologic agent and vectors.

In 1961, Dr. M. A. Epstein happened to attend a lecture by Burkitt, and this began the intensive study that led to the discovery of the Epstein-Barr virus and its relationship to Burkitt's lymphoma as well as to nasopharyngeal carcinoma in the Orient and its involvement as the cause of infectious mononucleosis.

The first hypothesis to explain the geographic distribution was that this reflected a vectored virus. The Epstein-Barr (EB) virus, however, is not vectored and is equally prevalent in areas where Burkitt's lymphoma is common or rare. Some other explanation involving the virus had to be sought. The relationship to malaria was recognized, and the next hypothesis was that intense and persistent malarial infection resulted in hyperplasia of the lymphoreticular system, possibly allowing the EB virus to become oncogenic in this situation. No evidence for this was found, and the hypothesis was abandoned. The hypothesis that has survived for 15 years is that the EB virus in the presence of immunodepression might well be oncogenic.

In an excellent review of Burkitt's lymphoma, Ziegler summarizes that the cause of Burkitt's lymphoma is still obscure but includes EB virus. Besides the EB virus, genetic factors, manifest by a t(8;14q) chromosomal translocation; environmental factors, such as malaria; mediating immunoregulatory determinants; and the possible role of an RNA virus may all play a role.[326]

Burkitt's lymphoma is a neoplasm of B-lymphocytes, characterized by the presence of immunoglobulin and other B-cell markers on the cell surface. It is clear now that this is not exclusively an African disease but is truly found worldwide. However, certain clinical differences make it reasonable to distinguish the disease on geographic grounds. Burkitt's lymphoma is now usually described as either the African, or endemic, form or the nonedemic form.

Clinical Findings

The most common symptom of African Burkitt's lymphoma is a swelling of the jaws, usually the maxilla. In patients with the nonendemic form of the disease, the jaw lesions are uncommon, with abdominal involvement being prevalent.[305] Both forms are equally susceptible to chemotherapy, are clustered by time and space, are not found at high altitudes, and are related to the EB virus. However, the nonendemic form shows lower titers to the EB virus than the African form, and the EB virus genome is not detected in the tumors with as much certainty. Relapse patterns are different, with both forms showing early relapses resistant to treatment, but the nonendemic cases have not yet shown a late relapse pattern similar to the African cases.

Burkitt found that the jaw lesions, often involving all

four quadrants, were related to tumors in other sites, commonly in the kidneys, adrenal glands, and ovaries, but only extremely rarely to those in peripheral lymph nodes, bone marrow, lungs and mediastinum, liver, and spleen. Occasionally, patients have isolated tumors of the thyroid gland, distal long bones, skin, breasts, testes, and parotid glands. Retroperitoneal or extradural tumors often cause paraplegia, either by vascular compromise or direct invasion of the spinal cord.[326]

The African patients' mean age is from 7 to 9 years, and in American patients it is 11 to 12 years.[305, 326] Older patients are most often found in nonendemic cases. Nonendemic Burkitt's lymphoma patients more commonly present with intra-abdominal tumors with symptoms of intestinal obstruction or abdominal mass.

Kinetic studies of Burkitt's lymphoma have revealed that this is the fastest growing human tumor, with a cell doubling time of 24 hours.[326] This may result in extremely rapid progression of symptoms. A child may present with loose teeth and jaw lesions and then may suffer kidney failure before the diagnosis of Burkitt's lymphoma is made. Gonadal involvement is always bilateral.[305]

Diagnostic radiology is of great significance in Burkitt's lymphoma, not only in suggesting the disease before histologic confirmation but in assessing the extent of the disease. One of the first radiographic signs is the loss or break of the lamina dura around deciduous or permanent teeth. Later, larger radiolucent defects are seen, and teeth may be seen to supererupt (Fig. 58–40A, B, and C). The radiographic findings in the maxilla often include extension into the antrum. Cortical disruption usually occurs, but rarely is ulceration through the skin seen. Conventional tomograms and CT scanning are valuable in determining the extent of bone destruction and the size of the soft tissue component.[319] Intravenous pyelography should be performed to detect renal tract involvement and possibly other intra-abdominal involvement, such as retroperitoneal masses and ovarian tumors.[325]

Pathology

Histologic sections of tissue from Burkitt's lymphoma lesions of the jaw are indistinguishable between the African and nonendemic types. The tumors are composed of sheets of rather monotonous, undifferentiated lymphoreticular cells, which have little variation in the size and shape of their nuclei. Nucleoli are prominent; mitotic activity may be. Interspersed among the sheets

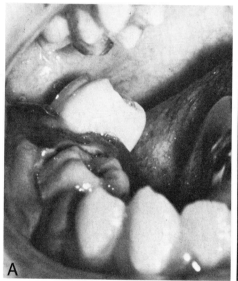

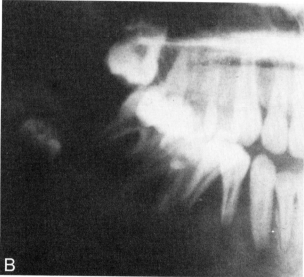

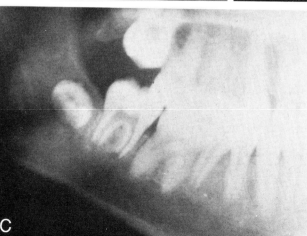

Figure 58–40. Burkitt's lymphoma in a 12-year-old male. (*A*) Posterior mandibular swelling with supereruption of the molar. (*B*) Radiograph at time of presentation showing diffuse radiolucency in posterior mandible and extrusion of the tooth. (*C*) Twenty-one days after initiation of chemotherapy, tooth is in normal position and radiopacity has returned to normal. (Courtesy of Dr. Joseph A. Regezi.)

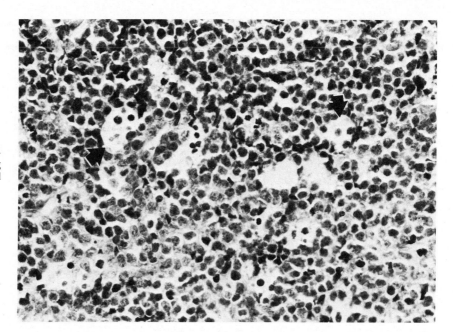

Figure 58–41. Burkitt's lymphoma exhibiting phagocyte (arrow) engulfing tumor cells rendering the typical "starry sky" pattern. (H & E, × 100)

of cells are large macrophages with clear cytoplasm, which is usually seen to contain cellular debris. According to Batsakis,[305] the cells stain positively with methyl green pyronine. This can be prevented by prior digestion with ribonuclease. Cytoplasmic lipid droplets are usually present, and some cells may stain positively with periodic acid–Schiff (PAS), demonstrating coarse cytoplasmic granules. The macrophages, which are not neoplastic, but rather are benign and reactive, provide the well-known "starry sky" pattern. The solid sheets of darkly staining, uniform, undifferentiated lymphocytic cells make up the dark "sky," and the phagocytic histiocytes constitute the "stars" (Fig. 58–41). This feature is not diagnostic of Burkitt's lymphoma, but seeing it should cause a pathologist to consider this disease high on the differential diagnosis list. Although the macrophage activity is considered a hallmark of benign hyperplasia in lymph nodes, it may be seen in adult, child, and animal lymphomas of various types.[305]

The neoplastic cells are monoclonal and have distinguishing surface markers, and some carry a chromosome 8 to 14q translocation. Katayama and associates[315] consider the ultrastructure of the tumor to be nearly diagnostic.

The differential diagnosis of jaw lesions suspected to be Burkitt's lymphoma would include other lymphoreticular neoplasms, sarcomas, neuroblastomas, benign lymphoid hyperplasia, Ewing's sarcoma, leukemic infiltrates, and undifferentiated carcinoma.

Prompt diagnosis is mandatory. Definitive treatment must be initiated within 24 to 48 hours of admission, for patients may present in emergent situations with airway, intestinal, or ureteral obstruction or renal failure as a result of the rapidly expanding tumor mass. Also, patients with large tumors are in danger of urate nephropathy due to the excessive production of uric acid from DNA catabolism.[326] Tissue biopsy with imprint preparations and well-fixed tissue sections are the methods of choice for definitive diagnosis.

Treatment and Prognosis

Prognosis is directly related to the tumor burden on initial presentation, the only other factor determining survival being age; patients below 13 years survive significantly longer than older patients.[326] Early death is attributable to rapidly growing or very large tumors that lead to fatal complications. Previously, many patients had frequent central nervous system relapses even after aggressive chemotherapy had achieved systemic remissions. Patients at highest risk for this complication are those with head and neck or paraspinal tumors or marrow involvement.

The extremely rapid proliferation of the tumor cells probably accounts for the extreme sensitivity to chemotherapeutic agents. Burkitt's lymphoma is one of the few malignant neoplasms that can be cured by drugs alone. It is also the most likely human neoplasm to be virus-induced.

REFERENCES

OSTEOMA

1. Batsakis JG: Tumors of the Head and Neck. Clinical and Pathological Considerations. 2nd ed. Baltimore, Williams & Wilkins Co., 1979, p 405.
2. Brunner H, Spiesman IG: Osteoma of the frontal and ethmoid sinuses. Ann Otol Rhinol Laryngol 57:714, 1948.
3. Childrey JH: Osteomas of the sinuses, of the frontal and sphenoid bone. Arch Otolaryngol 30:63, 1939.
4. Cutright DE: Osseous and chondromatous metaplasia caused by dentures. Oral Surg 34:625, 1972.
5. Dahlin DC: Bone Tumors. General Aspects and Data in 6,221 Cases. 3rd ed. Springfield, Charles C Thomas, 1978.
6. Greer RO, Mierau GW, Favara BF: Tumors of the Head and Neck in Children. New York, Praeger Publishers, 1983, p 125.
7. Hallberg OE, Bagley JW: Origin and treatment of osteomas of the paranasal sinuses. Arch Otolaryngol 51:750, 1950.
8. Huvos AG: Bone Tumors Diagnosis, Treatment and Prognosis. Philadelphia, W. B. Saunders Co., 1979, p 1.
9. Lautenbach E: Klinische und histologische studien an osteomen. Dtsch Zahn Mund Kieferheilkd 43:4344, 1964.

10. MacLennan WD, Brown RD: Osteomas of the mandible. Br J Oral Surg 12:219, 1974.
11. Malan E: Chirargia degli osteomi delle cauita pneumatiche perifacciali. Arch Ital Chir 48:1, 1938.
12. Mikaelian DO, Lewis WJ, Behringer WW: Primary osteoma of the sphenoid sinus. Laryngoscope 86:728, 1976.
13. Salinger S: The paranasal sinuses. Malignant tumors. Arch Otolaryngol 30:633, 1939.
14. Shiffman MA: Familial multiple polyposis associated with soft and hard tissue tumors. JAMA 182:514, 1962.

OSSIFYING FIBROMA

15. Billing L, Ringertz N: Fibro-osteoma, a pathologicoanatomical and roentgenological study. Acta Radiol 27:129, 1946.
16. Champion AHR, Maule AW, Wilkenson FC: 'Case report of an endosteal fibroma of the mandible. Br Dent J 86:3, 1946.
17. Dehner LP: Tumors of the mandible and maxilla in children. I. Clinicopathologic study of 46 histologically benign lesions. Cancer 31:364, 1973.
18. Eversole LR, Sabes WB, Rovin J: Fibrous dysplasia: A nosologic problem in diagnosis of fibro-osseous lesions of the jaws. J Oral Pathol 1:189, 1972.
19. Farman AG, Nortje CJ, Grotepass FW: Pathological conditions of the mandible. Their effect on the radiographic appearance of the inferior dental (mandibular) canal. Br J Oral Surg 15:64, 1977.
20. Greer RO, Mierau GW: Tumors of the Oral Mucosa and Jaws in Infants and Children. Denver, University of Colorado Medical Center Press, 1980.
21. Hamner JE III, Lightbody PM, Ketcham AS, et al: Cemento-ossifying fibroma of the maxilla. Oral Surg 26:579, 1968.
22. Hamner JE III, Scofield HH, Cornyn J: Benign fibro-osseous jaw lesions of periodontal ligament origin. An analysis of 249 cases. Cancer 22:861, 1968.
23. Kenneth S, Curran JB: Giant cemento-ossifying fibroma. Report of a case. J Oral Surg 30:513, 1972.
24. Khanna S, Khanna NN: Primary tumors of the jaws in children. J Oral Surg 37:800, 1979.
25. Landon JD, Rapidis AD, Patel MF: Ossifying fibroma—one disease or six? An analysis of 39 fibro-osseous lesions of the jaws. Br J Oral Surg 14:1, 1976.
26. Lucas RB: Pathology of Tumors of the Oral Tissues. 3rd ed. London, Churchill Livingstone, 1976, p 399.
27. Menzel A: Ein fall von osteofibroma des unterkiefers. Arch Klin Chir 13:212, 1972.
28. Montgomery AH: Ossifying fibromas of the jaws. Arch Surg 15:30, 1927.
29. Reed RJ, Hagy DM: Benign nonodontogenic fibro-osseous lesions of the skull. Report of two cases. Oral Surg 19:214, 1965.
30. Regezi JA, Kerr D, Courtney RM: Odontogenic tumors: Analysis of 706 cases. J Oral Surg 36:771, 1978.
31. Shafer WG, Waldron CA: Fibro-osseous lesions of the jaws. Paper delivered at the Thirteenth Annual Meeting of the American Academy of Oral Pathology, Atlanta, April 4, 1976.
32. Waldron CA: Fibro-osseous lesions of the jaws. J Oral Surg 28:58, 1970.
33. Waldron CA, Giansanti JS: Benign fibro-osseous lesions of the jaws: A clinical-radiological-histologic review of sixty-five cases. Part II. Benign fibro-osseous lesions of periodontal ligament origin. Oral Surg 35:340, 1973.

OSTEOBLASTOMA

34. Abrams AM, Kirby JW, Melrose RJ: Cementoblastoma: A clinical-pathologic study of seven new cases. Oral Surg 38:394, 1974.
34a. Aszódi K: Benign osteoblastoma: Quantitative histological distinction from osteoid osteoma. Arch Orthop Unfallchir 88:359, 1977.
35. Brady CL, Browne RM: Benign osteoblastoma of the mandible. Cancer 30:329, 1972.
36. Dahlin DC, Johnson EW Jr: Giant osteoid osteoma. J Bone Joint Surg 36:559, 1954.
37. Farman AG, Nortje CJ, Grotepass F: Periosteal benign osteoblastoma of the mandible: Report of a case and review of the literature pertaining to benign osteoblastic neoplasms of the jaws. Br J Oral Surg 14:12, 1976.
38. Greer RO, Berman DN: Osteoblastoma of the jaws. Current concepts and differential diagnosis. J Oral Surg 36:304, 1978.
39. Jackson JR, Bell MEA: Spurious "benign osteoblastoma," a case report. J Bone Joint Surg 59:397, 1977.
40. Kent JN, Castro HF, Girotti WR: Benign osteoblastoma of the maxilla: Case report and review of the literature. Oral Surg 27:209, 1969.
41. Kopp WK: Benign osteoblastoma of the coronoid process of the mandible. Report of a case. J Oral Surg 27:653, 1969.
42. Larsson A, Foroberg O, Sjögren S: Benign cementoblastoma—cementum analogue of benign osteoblastoma? J Oral Surg 36:299, 1978.
43. Martin N, Preston DF, Robinson RG: Osteoblastoma of the axial skeleton shown by skeletal scanning. Case report. J Nucl Med 17:187, 1976.
44. McLeod RA, Dahlin DC, Beabout JW: The spectrum of osteoblastoma. Am J Roentgenol 126:321, 1976.
45. Remagen W, Prein J: Benign osteoblastoma. Oral Surg 39:279, 1975.
46. Schajowicz F, Lemos C: Malignant osteoblastoma. J Bone Joint Surg 58:202, 1976.
47. Shafer WG, Hine MK, Levy BM: A Textbook of Oral Pathology. 3rd ed. Philadelphia, W. B. Saunders Co., 1974.
48. Smith RA, Hansen LS, Resnick D, Chan W: Comparison of the osteoblastoma in gnathic and extragnathic sites. Oral Surg 54:285, 1982.

OSTEOID OSTEOMA

49. Flaherty RA, Pugh DG, Dockerty MB: Osteoid osteoma. Am J Roentgenol Radium Ther Nucl Med 76:1041, 1956.
50. Golding JSR: The natural history of osteoid osteoma with a report of 20 cases. J Bone Joint Surg (Br) 36:218, 1954.
51. Greene GW Jr, Natiella JR, Sprig PN Jr: Osteoid osteoma of the jaws. Oral Surg 26:342, 1968.
52. Jaffe HL: Osteoid-osteoma. A benign osteoblastic tumor composed of osteoid and atypical bone. Arch Surg 31:709, 1935.
53. Jaffe HL, Mayer L: An osteoblastic osteoid tissue forming tumor of a metacarpal bone. Arch Surg 24:550, 1932.
54. Johnson AD: Clinical problems in osteoid-osteoma. Evidence of osteoblastic aversion to osteoid. Bull Hosp Joint Dis 23:80, 1962.
55. Marsh BW, Bonfiglio M, Brody LP, Ennecking WF: Benign osteoblastoma: Range of manifestations. J Bone Joint Surg 57:1, 1975.
56. Miller AS, Rambo HM, Bowser MW, Gross M: Benign osteoblastoma of the jaws. Report of three cases. J Oral Surg 38:694, 1980.
57. O'Hara JP, Tegtmeyer C, Sweet DE, et al: Angiography in the diagnosis of osteoid-osteoma of the head. J Bone Joint Surg (Am) 57:163, 1975.
58. Steiner GC: Ultrastructure of osteoid osteoma. Hum Pathol 7:309, 1976.

OSTEOSARCOMA

59. Baserga R, Lisco H, Cater D: The delayed effects of external gamma irradiation on the bones of rats. Am J Pathol 39:455, 1961.
60. Caron AS, Hajdu SI, Strong EW: Osteogenic sarcoma of the facial and cranial bones. A review of forty-three cases. Am J Surg 122:719, 1971.
61. Chambers RG, Mahoney WP: Osteogenic sarcoma of the mandible: Current management. Am Surg 36:463, 1970.
62. Coley B: Neoplasms of Bone. New York, Paul B. Hoeber, 1960, p 298.
63. Cottier R, Keller H, Roos B: Generalized hyperostosis interna and osteosarcoma in a total body x-ray; irradiated female Swiss albino mice with hormonally active ovarian tumors. Pathol Microbiol 27:458, 1964.
64. Curtis ML, Elmore JS, Sotereanos GC: Osteosarcoma of the jaws. Report of case with review of the literature. J Oral Surg 32:125, 1974.
65. Czitim AA, Pritzker KPH, Langer C, et al: Virus-induced osteosarcoma in rats. J Bone Joint Surg (Am) 58:303, 1976.
66. Finkelstein JB: Osteosarcoma of the jaw bones. Radiol Clin North Am 8:425, 1970.
67. Friedlander GE, Mitchell MS: A laboratory model for the study of the immunobiology of osteosarcoma. Cancer 36:1631, 1975.
68. Garrington GE, Scofield HH, Cornyn J, et al: Osteosarcoma of the jaws. Analysis of 56 cases. Cancer 26:377, 1967.
69. Jensen RD, Miller RW: Retinoblastoma—epidemiologic characteristics. N Engl J Med 285:307, 1971.
70. Schwartz DT, Alpert M: The clinical course of mandibular osteogenic sarcoma. Oral Surg 16:769, 1963.
71. Slow IH, Stein D, Friedmann EW: Osteogenic sarcoma arising in a pre-existing fibrous dysplasia. Report of a case. J Oral Surg 29:126, 1971.
72. Solomon MP, Biernacki J, Slippen M, Rosen Y: Parosteal osteogenic sarcoma of the mandible. Arch Otolaryngol 101:754, 1975.
73. Solovier Yu N, Ponomarkov VI: Clinicomorphologic analysis of spontaneous bone sarcoma in dogs. Arch Pathol 3:36, 1971.

74. Stroneck GG, Dahl EC, Fonseca RJ, Breda JA: Multiosseous osteosarcoma involving the mandible. Metastatic or multicentric? Oral Surg 52:271, 1981.
75. Tillman HH: Paget's disease of bone. Oral Surg 15:1225, 1962.
76. Tsuya A, Tanaka T, Mori T, et al: Four cases of Thorotrast injury and estimation of absorbed tissue dose in critical organs. J Radiat Res 4:126, 1963.
77. Williams AH, Schwinn CP, Parker JW: The ultrastructure of osteosarcoma. A review of twenty cases. Cancer 37:1293, 1976.

CHONDROSARCOMA

78. Blum T: Cartilage tumors of the jaws. Report of three cases. Oral Surg 72:1320, 1954.
79. Chaudhry AP, Robinovitch MR, Mitchell DF, Vickers RA: Chondrogenic tumors of the jaws. Am J Surg 102:403, 1961.
80. Dahlin DC, Ivans JC: Benign chondroblastoma. A study of 125 cases. Cancer 30:401, 1972.
81. Evans HL, Ayala A, Romsdahl NM: Prognostic factors in chondrosarcoma of bone. A clinicopathologic analysis with emphasis on histologic grading. Cancer 40:818, 1977.
82. Feintuch TA: Chondrosarcoma arising in a cartilaginous area of previously irradiated fibrous dysplasia. Cancer 31:877, 1973.
83. Fitzwater JE, Caband HE, Farr GH: Irradiation-induced chondrosarcoma. A case report. J Bone Joint Surg (Am) 58:1037, 1976.
84. Grabias S, Mankin HJ: Chondrosarcoma arising in histologically proved unicameral bone cyst. A case report. J Bone Joint Surg (Am) 56:1501, 1974.
84a. Joshi K, Abrol BM: Extraskeletal mesenchymal chondrosarcoma. Indian J Pathol Microbiol 21:261, 1978.
85. Krolls SO, Schaffer RC, O'Rear JW: Chondrosarcoma and osteosarcoma of the same patient. Oral Surg 50:146, 1980.
86. Lichtenstein L: Bone Tumors, 4th ed. St. Louis, The C. V. Mosby Co., 1972.
87. Lichtenstein L: Unusual benign and malignant chondroid tumors of bone. Cancer 12:1142, 1959.
88. Lichtenstein L, Jaffe HL: Chondrosarcoma of bone. Am J Pathol 19:553, 1943.
89. Marcove RC, Mike V, Hutter RVP, et al: Chondrosarcoma of the pelvis and upper end of the femur. An analysis of factors influencing survival time in 113 cases. J Bone Joint Surg (Am) 54:561, 1972.
90. O'Neal LW, Ackerman LV: Chondrosarcoma of bone. Cancer 5:551, 1952.
91. Potdar GG: Chondrogenic tumors of the jaws. Oral Surg 30:649, 1970.
92. Pritchard PJ: Chondrosarcoma: A clinicopathologic and statistical analysis. Cancer 45:149, 1980.
93. Terezhalmy GT, Bottomley WK: Maxillary chondrogenic sarcoma. Management of a case. Oral Surg 44:539, 1977.
94. Thompson AD, Turner-Warwick RT: Skeletal sarcomata and giant cell tumor. J Bone Joint Surg (Br) 37:266, 1955.
95. Unni KK, Dahlin DC, Beabout JW, et al: Chondrosarcoma: A clear cell variant. A report of 16 cases. J Bone Joint Surg (Am) 58:676, 1976.

DESMOPLASTIC FIBROMA

96. Das Gupta TK, Grasfield RD, O'Hara J: Extra-abdominal desmoids: A clinicopathologic study. Ann Surg 170:109, 1969.
97. Freedman P, Cardo VA, Kerpel SM, et al: Desmoplastic: Fibroma (fibromatosis) of the jaw bones. Oral Surg 46:386, 1978.
98. Gardner DG: The central odontogenic fibroma. An attempt at clarification. Oral Surg 50:425, 1980.
99. Jaffe HL: Tumors and Tumorous Conditions of Bones and Joints. Philadelphia, Lea & Febiger, 1958.
100. Kimmelstiel P, Rapp IH: Cortical defect due to periosteal desmoids. Bull Hosp Joint Dis 12:286, 1951.
101. Masson JK, Soule DH: Desmoid tumors of the head and neck. Am J Surg 12:615, 1966.
102. Schajowicz F: Tumors and tumor-like lesions of bone and joints. New York, Springer-Verlag, 1981, pp 335–339.
103. Slootweg PJ, Muller H: Central fibroma of the jaw, odontogenic or desmoplastic. A report of five cases with reference to differential diagnosis. Oral Surg 56:61, 1983.
104. Stout AP: Fibrosarcoma in infants and children. Cancer 15:1028, 1962.
105. Sugiura I: Desmoplastic fibroma. Case report and review of the literature. J Bone Joint Surg (Am) 58:126, 1976.

106. Taguchi N, Kaneda T: Desmoplastic fibroma of the mandible. Report of a case. J Oral Surg 38:441, 1980.

FIBROSARCOMA

107. Adekeye EO, Edwards MB, Goubron GF: Ameloblastic fibrosarcoma. Report of a case in Nigeria. Oral Surg 46:254, 1978.
108. Batsakis JG: Tumors of the Head and Neck. Clinical and Pathological Considerations. 2nd ed. Baltimore, Williams & Wilkins Co., 1979, pp 271–272.
109. Batsakis JG, Fox JE: Supporting tissue neoplasms of the larynx. Surg Gynecol Obstet 131:989, 1970.
110. Brozmanova E, Skrovina B: Biochemical and haematological findings in malignant bone tumour. Neoplasma 21:75, 1974.
111. Conley J, Stout AP, Healey WV: Clinicopathologic analysis of 84 patients with an original diagnosis of fibrosarcoma of the head and neck. Am J Surg 114:564, 1967.
112. Dahl I, Save S, Soderbergh J, Angerwall L: Fibrosarcoma in early infancy. Pathol Eur 8:193, 1973.
113. Dahlin DC, Ivins JC: Fibrosarcoma of bone. A study of 114 cases. Cancer 23:35, 1969.
114. Eversole LR, Schwartz WD, Sabes WR: Central and peripheral fibrogenic and neurogenic sarcoma of the oral regions. Oral Surg 36:49, 1973.
115. Huvos AG, Higinbotham NL: Primary fibrosarcoma of bone. A clinicopathologic study of 130 patients. Cancer 33:837, 1975.
116. Lucas RB: Pathology of Tumors of the Oral Tissues. 3rd ed. New York, Churchill Livingstone, 1976.
117. Stout AP: Fibrous tumors of the soft tissues. Minn Med 4:455, 1960.
118. Van Blacom CW, Mason JMK, Dahlin DC: Fibrosarcoma of the mandible. Oral Surg 32:428, 1971.

MALIGNANT FIBROUS HISTIOCYTOMA OF BONE

119. Dahlin DC, Unni KK, Matsuno T: Malignant (fibrous) histiocytoma of bone—fact or fancy? Cancer 39:1508, 1977.
120. Feldman F, Lattes R: Primary malignant fibrous histiocytoma (fibrous xanthoma) of bone. Skeletal Radiol 1:145, 1977.
121. Feldman F, Norman D: Intra- and extraosseous malignant histiocytoma (malignant fibrous xanthoma). Radiology 104:497, 1972.
122. Fu Y, Gabbiani G, Kaye GI, et al: Malignant soft tissue tumors of probable histiocytic origin (malignant fibrous histiocytomas): General considerations and electron microscopic and tissue culture studies. Cancer 35:176, 1975.
123. Ghandur-Mnaymneh L, Zych G, Mnaymneh W: Primary malignant fibrous histiocytoma of bone: Report of six cases with ultrastructural study and analysis of the literature. Cancer 49:698, 1982.
124. Huvos AG: Primary malignant fibrous histiocytoma of bone: Clinicopathologic study of 18 patients. NY State J Med 76:552, 1976.
125. Kearney MM, Soule EH, Ivins JC: Malignant fibrous histiocytoma, a retrospective study of 167 cases. Cancer 45:167, 1980.
126. McCarthy EF, Matsuno T, Dorfman HD: Malignant fibrous histiocytoma of bone: A study of 35 cases. Hum Pathol 10:57, 1979.
127. Merkow LP, Frich JC Jr, Silifkin M, et al: Ultrastructure of a fibroxanthosarcoma (malignant fibroxanthoma). Cancer 28:372, 1971.
128. Michael RH, Dorfman HD: Malignant fibrous histiocytoma associated with bone infarcts. Clin Orthop 118:180, 1976.
129. Mirra JM, Bullough PG, Marcove RC, et al: Malignant fibrous histiocytoma and osteosarcoma in association with bone infarcts. J Bone Joint Surg 56:932, 1974.
130. Mirra JM, Gold RH, Marafiote R: Malignant (fibrous) histiocytoma arising in association with bone infarct in sickle-cell disease: Coincidence of cause and effect? Cancer 39:186, 1977.
131. O'Brien JE, Stout AP: Malignant fibrous xanthomas. Cancer 17:1445, 1964.
132. Ozzello L, Stout AP, Murray MR: Cultural characteristics of malignant histiocytomas and fibrous xanthomas. Cancer 16:331, 1963.
133. Slootweg PJ, Müller H: Malignant fibrous histiocytoma of the maxilla. Oral Surg 44:560, 1977.
134. Spanier SS: Malignant fibrous histiocytoma of bone. Orthop Clin North Am 8:947, 1977.
135. Spector GJ, Ogura JH: Malignant fibrous histiocytoma of the maxilla: A report of an unusual lesion. Arch Otolaryngol 99:385, 1974.
136. Webber WB, Wienke EC: Malignant fibrous histiocytoma of the mandible: A case report. Plast Reconstr Surg 60:629, 1977.
137. Weiner M, Sedlis M, Johnston AD, et al: Adjuvant chemotherapy of malignant fibrous histiocytoma of bone. Cancer 51:25, 1983.

138. Weiss SW, Enzinger FM: Myxoid variant of malignant fibrous histiocytoma. Cancer 39:1672, 1977.

HISTIOCYTOSIS X

139. Cline MJ, Golde DW: A review and reevaluation of the histiocytic disorders. Am J Med 55:49, 1973.
140. Greer RO Jr, Mierau GW, Favara BE: Tumors of the Head and Neck in Children: Clinicopathologic Perspectives. New York, Praeger, 1983.
141. Groopman JE, Golde DW: The histiocytic disorders: A pathophysiologic analysis. Ann Intern Med 94:95, 1981.
142. Hartman KS: Histiocytosis X: A review of 114 cases with oral involvement. Oral Surg 49:38, 1980.
143. Huvos AG: Bone Tumors: Diagnosis, Treatment and Prognosis. Philadelphia, W. B. Saunders Co., 1979.
144. Komp DM, Herson J, Starling KA, et al: A staging system for histiocytosis X: A Southwest Oncology Group Study. Cancer 47:798, 1981.
145. Lahey ME: Histiocytosis X: An analysis of prognostic factors. J Pediatr 87:184, 1975.
146. Lahey ME: Prognostic factors in histiocytosis X. Am J Pediatr Hematol Oncol 3:57, 1981.
147. Lichtenstein L: Histiocytosis X. Integration of eosinophilic granuloma of bone, "Letterer-Siwe disease," and "Schüller-Christian disease" as related manifestations of a single nosologic entity. Arch Pathol 56:84, 1953.
148. Lieberman PH, Jones CR, Dargeon HWK, et al: A reappraisal of eosinophilic granuloma of bone, Hand-Schüller-Christian syndrome and Letterer-Siwe disease. Medicine 48:375, 1969.
149. Mierau GW, Favara BE, Brenman JM: Electron microscopy in histiocytosis X. Ultrastruct Pathol 3:137, 1982.
150. Murphy GF, Harrist TJ, Bhan AK, et al: Distribution of cell surface antigens in histiocytosis X cells: Quantitative immunoelectron microscropy using monoclonal antibodies. Lab Invest 48:90, 1983.
151. Nesbit ME Jr, O'Leary M, Dehner LP, et al: Histiocytosis, continued: The immune system and the histiocytosis syndromes. Am J Pediatr Hematol Oncol 3:141, 1981.
152. Newton WA Jr, Hamoudi AB: Histiocytosis: A histologic classification with clinical correlation. Perspect Pediatr Pathol 1:251, 1973.
153. Nolph MB, Luikin GA: Histiocytosis X. Otolaryngol Clin North Am 15:635, 1982.
154. Oberman HA: Idiopathic histiocytosis: A clinicopathologic study of 40 cases and review of the literature on eosinophilic granuloma of bone, Hand-Schüller-Christian disease and Letterer-Siwe disease. Pediatrics 28:307, 1961.
155. Osband ME, Lipton JM, Lavin P, et al.: Histiocytosis X: Demonstration of abnormal immunity, T-cell histamine H₂-receptor deficiency, and successful treatment with thymic extract. N Engl J Med 304:146, 1981.
156. Risdall RJ, Dehner LP, Duray P, et al: Histiocytosis X (Langerhans' cell histiocytosis): Prognostic role of histopathology. Arch Pathol Lab Med 107:59, 1983.
157. Siddiqui AR, Tashjian JH, Lazarus K, et al: Nuclear medicine studies in evaluation of skeletal lesions in children with histiocytosis X. Radiology 140:787, 1981.
158. Vogel JM, Vogel P: Idiopathic histiocytosis: A discussion of eosinophilic granuloma, the Hand-Schüller-Christian syndrome, and the Letterer-Siwe syndrome. Semin Hematol 9:349, 1972.

CENTRAL GIANT CELL GRANULOMA

159. Andersen L, Ferjerskov O, Philipsen HP: Oral giant cell granulomas: A clinical and histological study of 129 new cases. Acta Pathol Microbiol Scand (A) 81:606, 1973.
160. Austin LT Jr, Dahlin DC, Royer RQ: Giant-cell reparative granuloma and related conditions affecting the jawbones. Oral Surg 12:1285, 1959.
161. Batsakis JG: Tumors of the Head and Neck. Clinical and Pathological Considerations. 2nd ed. Baltimore, Williams & Wilkins Co., 1979.
162. Bertheussen KJ, Holck S, Schiødt T: Giant cell lesion of bone of the hand with particular emphasis on giant cell reparative granuloma. J Hand Surg 8:46, 1983.
163. Friedberg SA, Eisenstein R, Wallner LJ: Giant cell lesions involving the nasal accessory sinuses. Laryngoscope 79:763, 1969.
164. Granite EL, Aronoff AK, Gold L: Central giant cell granuloma of the mandible. Oral Surg 53:241, 1982.
165. Greer RO Jr, Mierau GW: Tumors of the Oral Mucosa and Jaws in Infants and Children. Denver, University of Colorado Medical Center Press, 1980.

166. Greer RO Jr, Mierau GW, Favara BE: Tumors of the Head and Neck in Children: Clinicopathologic Perspectives. New York, Praeger, 1983.
167. Gorlin RJ, Goldman HM: Thoma's Oral Pathology. 6th ed. St. Louis, The C. V. Mosby Co., 1970.
168. Hirschl S, Katz A: Giant cell reparative granuloma outside the jaw bone: Diagnostic criteria and review of the literature with the first case described in the temporal bone. Hum Pathol 5:171, 1974.
169. Jaffe HL: Giant-cell reparative granuloma, traumatic bone cyst, and fibrous (fibro-osseous) dysplasia of the jawbones. Oral Surg 6:159, 1953.
170. Miller AS, Elzay RP, Levy WM: Giant cell tumor of the jaws associated with Paget disease of bone: Report of two cases and review of the literature. Arch Otolaryngol 100:233, 1974.
171. Mintz GA, Abrams AM, Carlsen GD, et al: Primary malignant giant cell tumor of the mandible: Report of a case and review of the literature. Oral Surg 51:164, 1981.
172. Sabanas AO, Dahlin DC, Childs DS Jr, et al: Postradiation sarcoma of bone. Cancer 9:528, 1956.
173. Sapp JP: Ultrastructure and histogenesis of peripheral giant cell reparative granuloma of the jaws. Cancer 30:1119, 1972.
174. Smith GA, Ward PA: Giant-cell lesions of the facial skeleton. Arch Otolaryngol 104:186, 1978.
175. Waldron CA, Shafer WG: The central giant cell reparative granuloma of the jaws: An analysis of 38 cases. Am J Clin Pathol 45:437, 1966.

ANEURYSMAL BONE CYST

176. Aho HJ, Aho AJ, Einola S: Aneurysmal bone cyst, a study of ultrastructure and malignant transformation. Virchows Archiv (Pathol Anat) 395:169, 1982.
177. Batsakis JG: Tumors of the Head and Neck. Clinical and Pathological Considerations. 2nd ed. Baltimore, Williams & Wilkins Co., 1979.
178. Biesecker JL, Marcove RC, Huvos AG, Mik'e V: Aneurysmal bone cysts. A clinicopathologic study of 66 cases. Cancer 26:615, 1970.
179. Buraczewski J, Dabska M: Pathogenesis of aneurysmal bone cyst. Relationship between the aneurysmal bone cyst and fibrous dysplasia of bone. Cancer 28:597, 1971.
180. Chari PR, Reddy CRR: A clinical test to differentiate aneurysmal bone cyst from other benign osseous cystic lesions. Aust NZ J Surg 50:614, 1980.
181. Clough JR, Price CH: Aneurysmal bone cyst: Pathogenesis and long term results of treatment. Clin Orthop 97:52, 1973.
182. Dabska M, Buraczewski J: Aneurysmal bone cyst. Pathology, clinical course and radiologic appearances. Cancer 23:371, 1969.
183. Dahlin DC: Bone Tumors. General Aspects and Data on 6221 Cases. 3rd ed. Springfield, Charles C Thomas, 1978.
184. Daugherty JW, Eversole LR: Aneurysmal bone cyst of the mandible: Report of case. J Oral Surg 29:737, 1971.
185. El Deeb M, Sedano HO, Waite DE: Aneurysmal bone cyst of the jaws. Report of a case associated with fibrous dysplasia and review of the literature. Int J Oral Surg 9:301, 1980 (review).
186. Gruskin SE, Dahlin DC: Aneurysmal bone cysts of the jaws. J Oral Surg 26:523, 1968.
187. Jaffe HL, Lichtenstein L: Solitary unicameral bone cyst with emphasis on the roentgen picture, the pathologic appearance and the pathogenesis. Arch Surg 44:1004, 1942.
188. Lichtenstein L: Aneurysmal bone cyst. A pathological entity commonly mistaken for giant-cell tumor and occasionally for hemangioma and osteogenic sarcoma. Cancer 3:279, 1950.
189. Lichtenstein L: Diseases of Bone and Joints. 2nd ed. St. Louis, The C. V. Mosby Co., 1975.
190. Reed RJ, Rothenberg M: Lesions of bone that may be confused with aneurysmal bone cyst. Clin Orthop 35:150, 1964.
191. Ruiter DJ, van Rijssel TG, van der Velde EA: Aneurysmal bone cysts: A clinicopathological study of 105 cases. Cancer 39:2231, 1977.
192. Steiner GC, Kantor EB: Ultrastructure of aneurysmal bone cyst. Cancer 40:2967, 1977.
193. Tillman BP, Dahlin DC, Lipscomb PR, Stewart JR: Aneurysmal bone cyst: An analysis of ninety-five cases. Mayo Clin Proc 43:478, 1968.

CHERUBISM

194. Bixler D, Garner LD: Cherubism: A family study to delineate gene action on mandibular growth and development. Birth Defects 7:222, 1971.

195. Cornelius EA, McClendon JL: Cherubism: Hereditary fibrous dysplasia of the jaws. Am J Roentgenol 106:136, 1969.
196. Dahlin DC: Bone Tumors. General Aspects and Data on 6221 Cases. 3rd ed. Springfield, Charles C Thomas, 1978.
197. Grunebaum M: Nonfamilial cherubism: Report of two cases. J Oral Surg 31:632, 1973.
198. Hammer JC: The demonstration of perivascular collagen deposition in cherubism. Oral Surg 27:129, 1969.
199. Hamner JE, Ketcham AS: Cherubism: An analysis of treatment. Cancer 23:1133, 1969.
200. Jones WA: Familial multilocular cystic disease of the jaws. Am J Cancer 17:946, 1933.
201. Lawrence D, Nogrady MB, Cloutier AM: Cherubism: A case report. Am J Roentgenol 108:468, 1970.
202. Lichtenstein L: Diseases of Bone and Joints. 2nd ed. St. Louis, The C. V. Mosby Co., 1975.
203. Markwell BD: Cherubism: A case report. Br J Oral Surg 21:251, 1968.
204. Talley DB: Familial fibrous dysplasia of the jaws. Oral Surg 5:1012, 1952.
205. Von Wowern N: Cherubism. Int J Oral Surg 1:240, 1972.

FIBROUS DYSPLASIA

206. Adekeye EO, Edwards MB, Goubran GF: Fibro-osseous lesions of the skull, face and jaws in Kaduna, Nigeria. Br J Oral Surg 18:57, 1980.
207. Albright F: Polyostotic fibrous dysplasia: A defense of the entity. J Clin Endocrinol 7:307, 1947.
208. Albright F, Butler AM, Hampton AO, et al: Syndrome characterized by osteitis fibrosa disseminata, areas of pigmentation and endocrine dysfunction, with precocious puberty in females; report of five cases. N Engl J Med 16:727, 1937.
209. Bowerman JE: Polyostotic fibrous dysplasia with oral melanotic pigmentation. Br J Oral Surg 6:188, 1969.
210. Caudill R, Saltzman DO, Gaum S, et al: Possible relationship of primary hyperparathyroidism and fibrous dysplasia: Report of a case. J Oral Surg 35:483, 1977.
211. Dahlin DC: Bone Tumors. General Aspects and Data On 6221 Cases. 3rd ed. Springfield, Charles C Thomas, 1978.
212. Eversole LR, Sabes WR, Rovin S: Fibrous dysplasia: A nosologic problem in the diagnosis of fibro-osseous lesions of the jaws. J Oral Pathol 1:189, 1972.
213. Firat D, Stutzman L: Fibrous dysplasia of the bone. Review of twenty-four cases. Am J Med 44:421, 1968.
214. Fitzer PM: Radionuclide angiography—brain and bone imaging in craniofacial fibrous dysplasia (CFD): Case report. J Nucl Med 18:709, 1977.
215. Gross CW, Montgomery WW: Fibrous dysplasia and malignant degeneration. Arch Otolaryngol 85:97, 1967.
216. Henry A: Monostotic fibrous dysplasia. J Bone Joint Surg 51:300, 1969.
217. Johannsen A: Chronic sclerosing osteomyelitis of the mandible. Acta Radiol Diag 18:360, 1977.
218. Kinnman JEG, Hong CE, Lee EB, et al: Fibrous dysplasia of the face and skull. Pract Otorhinolaryngol 31:11, 1969.
219. Lichtenstein L: Polyostotic fibrous dysplasia. Arch Surg 36:874, 1938.
220. Lichtenstein L: Diseases of Bone and Joints. 2nd ed. St. Louis, The C. V. Mosby Co., 1975.
221. Lichtenstein L, Jaffe HL: Fibrous dysplasia of bone. Arch Pathol 33:777, 1942.
222. Marlow CD, Waite DE: Fibrous-osseous dysplasia of the jaws: Report of case. J Oral Surg 23:632, 1965.
223. Obisesan AA, Lagundoye SB, Daramola JO, et al: The radiologic features of fibrous dysplasia of the craniofacial bones. Oral Surg 44:949, 1977.
224. Schlumberger HG: Monostotic fibrous dysplasia. Milit Surg 99:504, 1946.
225. Schofield IDF: An aggressive fibrous dysplasia. Oral Surg 38:29, 1974.
226. Talbot IC, Keith DA, Lord IJ: Fibrous dysplasia of the cranio-facial bones. A clinicopathological survey of seven cases. J Laryngol Otol 88:429, 1974.
227. Williams JL, Faccini JM: Fibrous dysplastic lesions of the jaws in Nigerians. Br J Oral Surg 11:118, 1973.
228. Worth HM, Stoneman DW: Osteomyelitis, malignant disease, and fibrous dysplasia. Some radiologic similarities and differences. Dent Radiogr Photogr 50:1, 1977.

HEMANGIOMA OF BONE

229. Choukas NC, Toto PD, Valaitis J: Sclerosing cavernous hemangiomas of the maxilla. Oral Surg 16:17, 1963.
230. Gorlin RJ, Goldman HM: Thoma's Oral Pathology. 6th ed. St. Louis, The C. V. Mosby Co., 1970.
231. Hayward JR: Central cavernous hemangioma of the mandible: Report of four cases. J Oral Surg 39:526, 1981.
232. Hitzrot JM: Hemangioma cavernsum of bone. Ann Surg 65:476, 1917.
233. Huvos AG: Bone Tumors: Diagnosis, Treatment and Prognosis. Philadelphia, W. B. Saunders Co., 1979.
234. Lund BA, Dahlin DC: Hemangiomas of the mandible and maxilla. J Oral Surg 22:234, 1964.
235. Piercell MP, Waite DE, Nelson RL: Central hemangioma of the mandible: Intraoral resection and reconstruction. J Oral Surg 33:225, 1975.
236. Sherman RS, Wilner D: The roentgen diagnosis of hemangioma of bone. Am J Roentgenol Radium Ther Nucl Med 86:1146, 1961.
237. Shira RB, Guernsey LH: Central cavernous hemangioma of the mandible: Report of case. J Oral Surg 23:636, 1965.
238. Shklar G, Meyer I: Vascular tumors of the mouth and jaws. Oral Surg 19:335, 1965.
239. Watson WL, McCarthy WD: Blood and lymph vessel tumors: Report of 1,056 cases. Surg Gynecol Obstet 71:569, 1940.
240. Weinstein I, Yamanaka H, Fuchihata H: Resection and reconstruction of the mandible for removal of a central hemangioma. Oral Surg 16:2, 1963.
241. Worth HM, Stoneman DW: Radiology of vascular abnormalities in and about the jaws. Dent Radiogr Photogr 52:1, 1979.
242. Wyke BD: Primary hemangioma of the skull: A rare cranial tumor: Review of the literature and report of a case with special reference to the roentgenographic appearances. Am J Roentgenol Radium Ther Nucl Med 61:302, 1949.

HEMANGIOENDOTHELIAL SARCOMA (ANGIOSARCOMA) OF BONE

243. Batsakis JG: Tumors of the Head and Neck. Clinical and Pathological Considerations. 2nd ed. Baltimore, Williams & Wilkins Co., 1979.
244. Gandhi RK, Kinare SG, Parulkan GB, et al: Hemangiosarcoma (malignant hemangioendothelioma) of the mandible in a child. Oral Surg 22:359, 1966.
245. Greer RO Jr, Mierau GW, Favara BE: Tumors of the Head and Neck in Children: Clinicopathologic Perspectives. New York, Praeger, 1983.
246. Guarda LA, Ordonez NG, Smith JL Jr, et al: Immunoperoxidase localization of factor VIII in angiosarcomas. Arch Pathol Lab Med 106:515, 1982.
247. Huvos AG: Bone Tumors: Diagnosis, Treatment and Prognosis. Philadelphia, W. B. Saunders Co., 1979.
248. Olmi R, Rubbini L: Hemangiosarcoma developed in a chronic osteomyelitis of the tibia. Chir Organi Mov 61:765, 1975.
249. Ramsey HJ: Fine structure of hemangiopericytoma and hemangioendothelioma. Cancer 19:2005, 1966.
250. Stout AP: Hemangiopericytoma: A study of twenty-five new cases. Cancer 2:1027, 1949.
251. Toto PD, Lavieri J: Primary hemangiosarcoma of the jaw. Oral Surg 12:1459, 1959.
252. Wesley RK, Mintz SM, Wertheimer FW: Primary malignant hemangioendothelioma of the gingiva. Oral Surg 39:103, 1975.
253. Wold LE, Unni KK, Beabout JW, et al: Hemangioendothelial sarcoma of bone. Am J Surg Pathol 6:59, 1982.
254. Worth HM, Stoneman DW: Radiology of vascular abnormalities in and about the jaws. Dent Radiogr Photogr 52:1, 1979.
255. Zachariades N, Papadakou A, Koundouris J, et al: Primary hemangioendotheliosarcoma of the mandible: Review of the literature and report of case. J Oral Surg 38:288, 1980.

EWING'S SARCOMA

256. Angervall L, Enzinger FM: Extraskeletal neoplasm resembling Ewing's sarcoma. Cancer 36:240, 1975.
257. Batsakis JG: Tumors of the Head and Neck. Clinical and Pathological Considerations. 2nd ed. Baltimore, Williams & Wilkins Co., 1979.
258. Carl W, Schaaf NG, Gaeta J, et al: Ewing's sarcoma. Oral Surg 31:472, 1971.

259. Crowe WW, Harper JC: Ewing's sarcoma with primary lesion in mandible: Report of case. J Oral Surg 23:156, 1965.

260. Dahlin DC: Bone Tumors. General Aspects of Data on 6,221 Cases. 3rd ed. Springfield, Charles C Thomas, 1978.

261. Dickman PS, Liotta LA, Triche TJ: Ewing's sarcoma: Characterization in established cultures and evidence of its histogenesis. Lab Invest 47:375, 1982.

262. Ewing J: Diffuse endothelioma of bone. Proc NY Pathol Soc 24:17, 1921.

263. Ewing J: Further report on endothelial myeloma of bone. Proc NY Pathol Soc 24:93, 1924.

264. Gillespie JJ, Roth LM, Wills ER, et al: Extraskeletal Ewing's sarcoma: Histological and ultrastructural observations in three cases. Am J Surg Pathol 3:99, 1979.

265. Glass AG, Fraumeni JF Jr: Epidemiology of bone cancer in children. J Natl Cancer Inst 44:187, 1970.

266. Greer RO Jr, Mierau GW, Favara BE: Tumors of the Head and Neck in Children: Clinicopathologic Perspectives. New York, Praeger, 1983.

267. Huvos AG: Bone Tumors: Diagnosis, Treatment and Prognosis. Philadelphia, W. B. Saunders Co., 1979.

268. Jaffe HL: Tumors and Tumorous Conditions of the Bones and Joints, Philadelphia, Lea & Febiger, 1958.

269. Johnson RE, Pomeroy TC: Evaluation of therapeutic results in Ewing's sarcoma. Am J Roentgenol 123:583, 1975.

270. Kadin ME, Bensch KG: On the origin of Ewing's tumor. Cancer 27:257, 1971.

271. Kelly JR, Barr ES: Ewing's sarcoma with involvement of the head and neck. J Dent Child 43:423, 1976.

272. Kissane JM, Askin FB, Nesbit ME Jr, et al: Sarcomas of bone in childhood: Pathologic aspects. Natl Cancer Inst Monogr 56:29, 1981.

273. Llombart-Bosch A, Peydro-Olaya A, Gomar F: Ultrastructure of one Ewing's sarcoma of bone with endothelial character and a comparative review of the vessels in 27 cases of typical Ewing's sarcoma. Pathol Res Pract 167:71, 1980.

274. Mendenhall CM, Marcus RB, Enneking WF, et al: The prognostic significance of soft tissue extension in Ewing's sarcoma. Cancer 51:913, 1983.

275. Mikaelian DO, Scherr SA, Delucca LE: Primary Ewing's sarcoma of the mandibular ramus: A case report. Otolaryngol Head Neck Surg 88:211, 1980.

276. Miller RW: Etiology of childhood bone cancer: Epidemiologic observations. Recent Results Cancer Res 54:50, 1976.

277. Nesbit ME Jr, Perez CA, Tefft M, et al: Multimodal therapy for the management of primary, non-metastatic Ewing's sarcoma of bone: An intergroup study. Natl Cancer Inst Monogr 56:255, 1981.

278. Pomeroy TC, Johnson RE: Prognostic factors for survival in Ewing's sarcoma. Am J Roentgenol 123:598, 1975.

279. Povysil C, Matejovsky Z: Ultrastructure of Ewing's tumor. Virchows Arch Pathol Anat 374:303, 1977.

280. Roessner A, Voss B, Rauterberg J, et al: Biologic characterization of human bone tumors. I. Ewing's sarcoma. A comparative electron and immunofluoresence microscopic study. J Cancer Res Clin Oncol 104:171, 1982.

281. Rosen G: Current management of Ewing's sarcoma. Progr Clin Cancer 8:267, 1982.

282. Rosen G, Caparros B, Nirenberg A, et al: Ewing's sarcoma: Ten-years experience with adjuvant chemotherapy. Cancer 47:2204, 1981.

283. Soule EH, Newton W Jr, Moon TE, et al: Extraskeletal Ewing's sarcoma: A preliminary review of 26 cases encountered in the Intergroup Rhabdomyosarcoma Study. Cancer 42:259, 1978.

284. Spjut HJ, Dorfman HD, Fechner RE, et al: Tumors of Bone and Cartilage. Atlas of Tumor Pathology. 2nd Ser., Fasc. 5, Washington, D.C., Armed Forces Institute of Pathology, 1971.

285. Stern R, Wilczek J, Thorpe WP, et al: Procollagens as markers for the cell of origin of human bone tumors. Cancer Res 40:325, 1980.

286. Weir JC Jr, Amonett MR, Krolls SO: Tumorous conditions of the fibula, supraorbital area and mandible. J Oral Pathol 8:313, 1979.

287. Williams AO: Tumors of childhood in Ibadan, Nigeria. Cancer 36:370, 1975.

288. Zamur J: Ewing's sarcoma of the mandible. Mt Sinai J Med 49:352, 1982.

CENTRAL SALIVARY GLAND NEOPLASMS

289. Batsakis JG: Tumors of the Head and Neck. Clinical and Pathological Considerations. 2nd ed. Baltimore, Williams & Wilkins Co., 1979.

290. Batsakis JG, Regezi JA: The pathology of head and neck tumors: Salivary glands, part 4. Head Neck Surg 1:340, 1979.

291. Bhaskar SN: Central mucoepidermoid tumors of the mandible. Report of 2 cases. Cancer 16:721, 1963.

292. Breitenecker G, Wepner F: A pleomorphic adenoma (so-called mixed tumor) in the wall of a dentigerous cyst. Oral Surg 36:63, 1973.

293. Browand BC, Waldron CA: Central mucoepidermoid tumors of the jaws. Report of nine cases and review of the literature. Oral Surg 40:631, 1975.

294. Dhawan IK, Bhargava S, Nayak NC, et al: Central salivary gland tumors of jaws. Cancer 26:211, 1970.

295. Eversole LR, Sabes WR, Rovin S: Aggressive growth and neoplastic potential of odontogenic cysts with special reference to central epidermoid and mucoepidermoid carcinomas. Cancer 35:270, 1975.

296. Fredrickson C, Cherrick HM: Central mucoepidermoid carcinoma of the jaws. J Oral Med 33:80, 1978.

297. Grubka JM, Wesley RK, Monaco F: Primary intraosseous mucoepidermoid carcinoma of the anterior part of the mandible. J Oral Maxillofac Surg 41:389, 1983.

298. Krikos GA: Histochemical studies of mucins of odontogenic cysts exhibiting mucous metaplasia. Arch Oral Biol 11:633, 1966.

299. Marano PD, Hartman KS: Central mucoepidermoid carcinoma arising in a maxillary odontogenic cyst. J Oral Surg 32:915, 1974.

300. Melrose RJ, Abrams AM, Howell FV: Mucoepidermoid tumors of the intraoral minor salivary glands: A clinicopathologic study of 54 cases. J Oral Pathol 2:314, 1973.

301. Miller AS, Winnick M: Salivary gland inclusion in the anterior mandible. Oral Surg 31:790, 1971.

302. Rohrer MD, Colyer J: Mental nerve paresthesia: Symptom for widespread skeletal metastatic adenocarcinoma. J Oral Surg 39:442, 1981.

303. Smith RL, Dahlin DC, Waite DE: Mucoepidermoid carcinomas of the jawbones. J Oral Surg 26:387, 1968.

304. Spiro RH, Huvos AG, Berk R, et al: Mucoepidermoid carcinoma of salivary gland origin. A clinicopathologic study of 367 cases. Am J Surg 136:461, 1978.

PRIMARY LYMPHOMA OF BONE AND BURKITT'S LYMPHOMA

305. Batsakis JG: Tumors of the Head and Neck. Clinical and Pathological Considerations. 2nd ed. Baltimore, Williams & Wilkins Co., 1979.

306. Boston HC, Dahlin DC, Ivins JC, et al: Malignant lymphoma (so-called reticulum cell sarcoma) of bone. Cancer 34:1131, 1974.

307. Braunstein EM: Hodgkin's disease of bone: Radiographic correlation with the histological classification. Radiology 137:643, 1980.

308. Burkitt DP: The discovery of Burkitt's lymphoma. Cancer 51:1777, 1983.

309. Burkitt DP: A sarcoma involving the jaws in African children. Br J Surg 46:218, 1958.

310. Campbell RL, Kelly DE, Burkes EJ: Primary reticulum-cell sarcoma of the mandible. Review of the literature and report of a case. Oral Surg 39:918, 1975.

311. Coley BL, Higinbotham NL, Groesbeck HP: Primary reticulum-cell sarcoma of bone—Summary of 37 cases. Radiology 55:641, 1950.

312. Dahlin DC: Bone Tumors. General Aspects and Data on 6221 Cases. 3rd ed. Springfield, Charles C Thomas, 1978.

313. Dosoretz DE, Raymond AK, Murphy GF, et al: Primary lymphoma of bone. The relationship of morphologic diversity to clinical behavior. Cancer 50:1009, 1982.

314. Huvos AG: Bone Tumors. Diagnosis, Treatment and Prognosis. Philadelphia, W. B. Saunders Co., 1979.

315. Katayama I, Uehara H, Gleser RA, et al: The value of electron microscopy in the diagnosis of Burkitt's lymphoma. Am J Clin Pathol 61:540, 1974.

316. Kayavis JG, Papanayotou PH, Antoniadis DZ, et al: Reticulum cell sarcoma of the mandible: Report of case. J Oral Surg 38:210, 1980.

317. Mahoney JP, Alexander RW: Primary histiocytic lymphoma of bone. A light and ultrastructural study of four cases. Am J Surg Pathol 4:149, 1980.

318. Newcomer LN, Silverstein MB, Cadman EC, et al: Bone involvement in Hodgkin's disease. Cancer 49:338, 1982.

319. Parker BR, Marglin S, Castellino RA: Skeletal manifestations of leukemia, Hodgkin's disease, and non-Hodgkin's lymphoma. Semin Roentgenol 15:302, 1980.

320. Parker F Jr, Jackson H Jr: Primary reticulum cell sarcoma of bone. Surg Gynecol Obstet 68:45, 1939.

321. Peterson DE, Hovland EJ, Williams LT: Poorly differentiated nodular lymphoma associated with the mandible. J Oral Med 36:70, 1981.

322. Phillips WC, Kattapuram SV, Doseretz DE, et al: Primary lymphoma of bone: Relationship of radiographic appearance and prognosis. Radiology *144*:285, 1982.
323. Schajowicz F: Ewing's sarcoma and reticulum cell sarcoma of bone—with special reference to the histochemical demonstration of glycogen as an aid to differential diagnosis. J Bone Joint Surg (Am) *41*:349, 1959.

324. Sweet DL, Mass DP, Simon MA, et al: Histiocytic lymphoma (reticulum cell sarcoma) of bone. Current strategy for orthopaedic surgeons. J Bone Joint Surg *63*:79, 1981.
325. Whittaker LR: Burkitt's lymphoma. Clin Radiol *24*:339, 1973.
326. Ziegler JL: Burkitt's lymphoma. N Engl J Med *305*:735, 1981 (review).

SURGICAL TREATMENT OF NON-ODONTOGENIC TUMORS

Richard F. Scott, D.D.S., M.S. • Edward Ellis III, D.D.S., M.S.

A number of tumors arising from nonodontogenic origins may present in the jaws. They may be either benign or malignant, although the benign entities predominate. Metastatic tumors in the jaws have occasionally been reported; however, the discussion of their individual treatment is beyond the scope of this chapter. Those benign tumors arising from a connective tissue and producing bone will be discussed first. They include the osteoma, ossifying fibroma, osteoid osteoma, and osteoblastoma. The malignant varieties of nonodontogenic tumors are discussed later. They occur much less frequently than do the odontogenic or nonodontogenic benign tumors. Their prognosis, for the most part, has been disappointingly poor.

BENIGN BONE-FORMING TUMORS

Osteoma

Osteomas represent benign proliferations of either compact or cancellous bone. They may occur in either the maxilla or the mandible and most often present as solitary lesions except when associated with Gardner's syndrome. When these tumors arise from the inner cortical plates they are termed *central* osteomas. These tumors are most often slow-growing and asymptomatic. Observation of these lesions with periodic clinical and radiographic follow-up is an accepted therapeutic modality.

Surgical intervention should be accomplished if the lesion becomes symptomatic. Symptoms may include pain from compression of the inferior alveolar neurovascular bundle, cortical expansion, ulceration of the overlying mucosa, and interference with the dental apparatus. The latter may involve inhibition of normal eruption patterns or root resorption. Surgery should be conservative in nature and should consist essentially of enucleation. Surgery is facilitated by the fact that the majority of these lesions are well circumscribed, and a few may even be encapsulated by a thin fibrous band. They are approached intraorally. Access is gained by the development and reflection of a full-thickness mucoperiosteal flap. The flap is designed to allow for closure over solid bone. The neurovascular bundle as

well as local dental anatomy should be preserved. The wound bed is irrigated following removal of the tumor and is closed primarily. Radiographic follow-up should reveal normal bone fill. The osteoma does not recur following surgical removal.

When osteomas arise from the outer cortical plate, surgical intervention is more often indicated. This is due solely to the fact that they become symptomatic more rapidly. They may interfere with mastication and the fabrication of prosthetic appliances, and they may occasionally reach sufficient size to produce facial asymmetry. The surgical management of this form is identical to that of their central counterpart. When presenting in the posterior ramus, they may require an extraoral surgical approach (Fig. 58–42).

When multiple osteomas of the jaws are present, the clinician must consider the possible presence of Gardner's syndrome. The management of the osteomas in this syndrome is similar to that for solitary osteomas, although the management of the associated colonic polyposis obviously takes precedence.

Ossifying Fibroma

The ossifying fibroma is a benign neoplasm that bears a striking similarity both clinically and histologically to its odontogenic counterpart, the cementifying fibroma. It exhibits a predilection for the mandible in young adults.[117, 118] It is slow-growing but may eventually reach significant size and produce deformity. Consequently, it is managed with surgical excision after preliminary biopsy has confirmed its presence. The lesion will be found to be well demarcated from adjacent normal bone, and enucleation is the treatment of choice. Effort should be exerted to preserve surrounding normal anatomy such as teeth, neurovascular structures, and normal bone. An intraoral approach with primary wound closure is utilized. In cases in which the lesion has reached significant size, making postoperative mandibular fracture a possibility, the jaws should be immobilized with intermaxillary fixation during the early healing phase. Recurrence following surgical removal is not expected (Fig. 58–43).

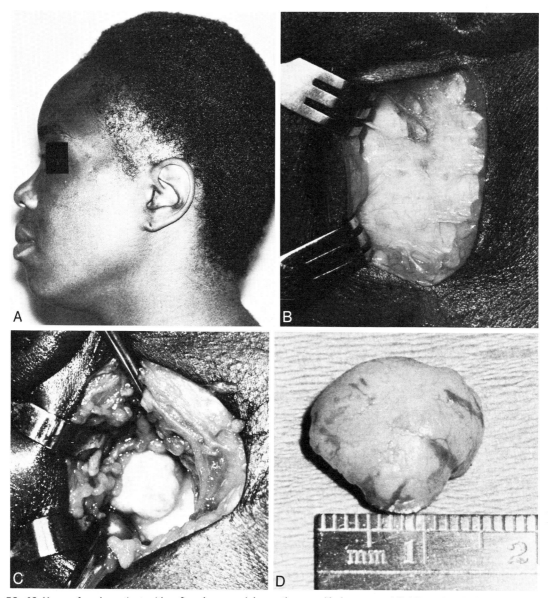

Figure 58–42. Young female patient with a firm, bony nodule on the mandibular ramus. (A) Minimal disfigurement is seen in the preauricular area. The patient had complained of increasing pain in the area for the last 6 months. (B) Post-ramal approach to the mandibular ramus. (C) Osteoma of the mandibular ramus visualized and removed with osteotome. (D) Surgical specimen.

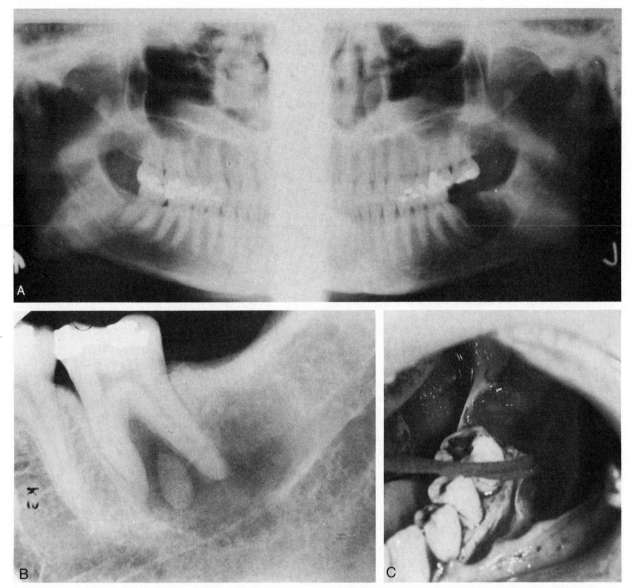

Figure 58–43. Ossifying fibroma. (*A*) Preoperative panorex of patient with a lesion of the left mandible confirmed by biopsy to be an ossifying fibroma. (*B*) Periapical radiography of the same lesion. Note the mixed radiolucent-radiopaque appearance. The encroachment on the inferior alveolar canal produced significant preoperative discomfort in this patient. (*C*) Surgical defect following removal of this lesion. Note the inferior alveolar neurovascular bundle being retracted with umbilical tape.

Osteoid Osteoma

The osteoid osteoma is an uncommon lesion of the jaws.[56, 80] Its two salient characteristics are its pathognomonic radiograhic picture and its ability to produce pain. Radiographs will show an ovoid radiolucency, usually 1 cm or less in dimension with a sclerotic border. Clinically, it produces pain that seems severe in relation to the lesion's size. The ability of osteoid osteoma to refer pain to adjacent structures should be considered in the differential diagnosis of unexplainable pain in the maxilla and mandible.[56] The nidus of these lesions may be quite vascular. The lesion is well outlined by preoperative technetium-99m bone scans. The treatment of choice is surgical excision.[10, 56, 67, 80] At the time of surgery, the margins of the lesion may be indistinguishable from surrounding normal bone. Therefore, careful preoperative planning is essential. Small amounts of normal osseous structure are generally sacrificed from around the periphery of the lesion to ensure complete removal. Recurrence is not expected.

It is important to differentiate between this lesion and that of periapical cemental dysplasia, which may, at certain stages of its development, mimic osteoid osteoma on radiographs. As Greene points out, however, the multiplicity of sites, the association with the apices of teeth, and the absence of pain would distinguish periapical cemental dysplasia from osteoid osteoma.[56]

Osteoblastoma

This lesion has also been called the giant osteoid osteoma. It shares several properties with the osteoid osteoma, especially its ability to produce pain and its vascularity. Care must be taken to differentiate the osteoblastoma from the osteosarcoma.[84, 118] This benign entity has been reported to occur in both the maxilla and the mandible.[65]

Radiographically, it will often appear as well circumscribed. Owing to its vascularity, it is well outlined by bone scans. Surgical excision via an intraoral approach is the preferred treatment, with emphasis on conservatism.[84, 118]

GIANT CELL AND FIBRO-OSSEOUS LESIONS OF THE JAWS

Central Giant Cell Granuloma

Controversy has existed in the surgical management of this lesion because it is often confused with more aggressive lesions, such as the malignant giant cell tumor.[66, 142] It may also be confused with other giant cell lesions, such as the aneurysmal bone cyst, cherubism, lesions of hyperparathyroidism, and fibrous dysplasia. In this group of lesions, perhaps more so than in any other, it is paramount that the clinician consider the total clinical history, radiographic and laboratory data, and histologic appearance before a definitive diagnosis is made. Failure to do this may result in significant mismanagement. For example, in central giant cell lesions associated with hyperparathyroidism, the surgical intervention should be directed not at the jaw lesions but at the cause of the systemic disease, usually parathyroid adenomas.

Most surgeons would agree that the treatment of choice for this lesion is aggressive curettage.[66, 118, 142] This curettage must include the bony walls of the cavity and meticulous curettage around the roots of teeth projecting into the bony cavity. Often the degree of bony destruction around these teeth will render them mobile and will necessitate the employment of dental splinting or in some instances extraction (Fig. 58–44). The wound should be irrigated thoroughly and inspected carefully for residual nests of the lesion.

It is wise to keep in mind the rich capillary vasculature of these lesions and to anticipate consistent hemorrhage in the operative site until the lesion is completely removed. In large lesions the possibility of the need for transfusion should be kept in mind (Fig. 58–45).

Upon adequate removal, the prognosis is excellent, and recurrence is rare. The expected postoperative course is that of complete bone filling of the residual defect. Endodontic therapy may be required in those teeth affected by the lesion.

It is suggested that all patients with a diagnosis of central giant cell granuloma be screened preoperatively for serum calcium and serum phosphate levels to rule out the possibility of hyperparathyroidism.

Aneurysmal Bone Cyst

These lesions most often are seen in patients under the age of 20 years, and they appear as rapidly growing, expansile, solitary lesions.[33] They may represent a variation of the central giant cell granuloma.[33] Histologically, they are found to contain numerous cavernous or sinusoidal blood-filled spaces. This accounts for the brisk and persistent oozing found upon removing these lesions. As with the central giant cell tumor, this hemorrhage will persist until the lesion is removed, and in large lesions significant blood losses may be incurred. Preoperative work-up must differentiate these lesions from central hemangiomas and arteriovenous fistulas. In general, the aneurysmal bone cyst is not under systemic pressures and bruits and thrills are not present. Preoperative needle aspiration and biopsy are essential for confirmation.

Once the diagnosis is established, the treatment of choice is surgical removal. When size and access allow, curettage is performed.[87] Cauterization of the curetted bed is often indicated. These lesions are best approached via the intraoral route. When the lesion is large and poorly situated, such as in the ramus, en bloc excision may be required. Radiation therapy is contraindicated.[33] Although recurrence has been reported in other sites, those lesions affecting the jaws usually do not recur.[33, 87]

Cherubism

The natural history of this condition dictates its management. Although it manifests itself in early childhood and may progress until puberty, this lesion tends to become static and show signs of regression in adulthood.[2] Total regression to normal contours has been observed, although changes may persist throughout life. It is best to avoid treatment in these patients and to let the process run its natural course.[2] If deformity persists in adulthood, surgical recontouring may be attempted. However, acceptable results may not be obtained with

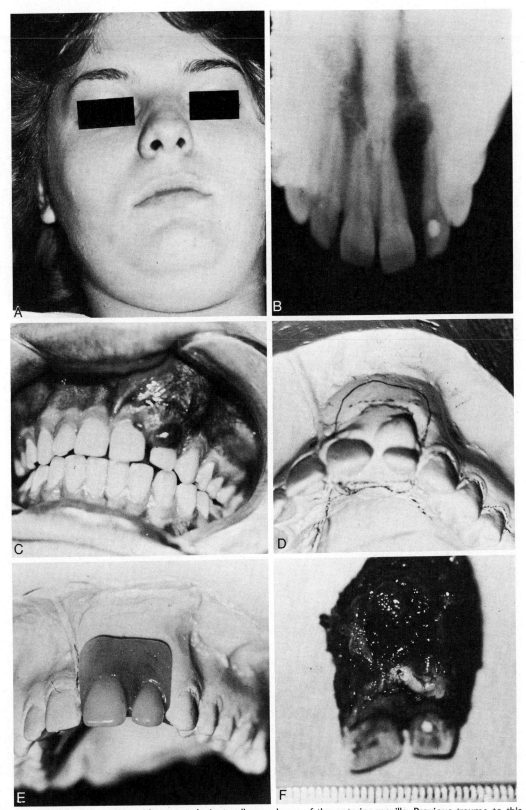

Figure 58—44. Young female patient with a central giant cell granuloma of the anterior maxilla. Previous trauma to this area had occurred. (*A*) Minimal distention is seen in the anterior left maxilla. (*B*) Occlusal radiograph showing displacement of adjacent teeth and extent of lesion. (*C*) The tumor is apparent in the anterior maxilla and exhibits cortical expansion and vestibular extension. (*D*) A dental model made from an alginate impression highlights the lesion and provides for preoperative planning and prosthetic considerations. (*E*) Temporary prosthetic appliance fabricated on the study model preoperatively and inserted at the time of surgery. (*F*) Surgical specimen showing the gritty nature of the lesion.

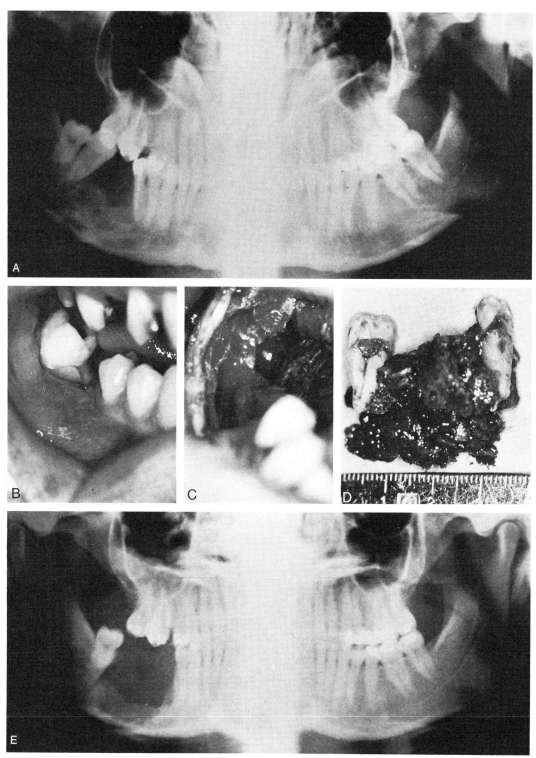

Figure 58–45. Mandibular central giant cell granuloma. (*A*) Preoperative radiograph showing bony destruction between mandibular first bicuspid and mandibular third molar. (*B*) Clinical view of lesion showing cortical expansion and loss of vestibular depth. The scar from the previous biopsy is evident. (*C*) Intraoperative view of the lesion. Note the neurovascular bundle in the inferior portion of the defect. This was preserved in this patient. (*D*) Surgical specimen. The bicuspid and molar were sacrificed because of their intimate relation to the tumor and near total loss of bone support. (*E*) Postoperative panorex showing surgical defect.

one intervention because of the nature of the intraosseous expansion and the need for symmetry. Rarely, it may be necessary to intervene during the prepubertal phase of the process.[2, 144] One example is in the child with large mandibular lesions who actively engages in contact sports (Fig. 58–46). In this instance, pathologic fracture is a risk. This patient may be treated with curettage and followed for osseous repair of the cavitation. However, it must be remembered that cure is not the intent of such a procedure. Such intervention has not been associated with accelerated growth of the lesion. Radiation therapy is contraindicated.

Fibrous Dysplasia

It should be re-emphasized that with this group of lesions it is imperative that the clinician review the entire history and presentation of the disease prior to embarking on a treatment. Much confusion has existed in the terminology and diagnosis of this lesion since the term "fibrous dysplasia" was introduced by Lichtenstein in 1938.[66] That two forms of this disease exist, a polyostotic and monostotic form, is little debated.[118] However, especially with the monostotic form, confusion has persisted as to what clinical, radiographic, and histologic criteria are required before the diagnosis of fibrous dysplasia can be made. The surgeon must work closely with the pathologist and provide the total clinical picture. Care must be taken to differentiate this lesion from the numerous osteogenic neoplasms.[86]

Once a lesion from the craniofacial anatomy has been biopsied and confirmed to be fibrous dysplasia, the clinician must rule out the possibility of other skeletal involvement. Radiographic surveys should be performed, or if available, bone scanning utilizing technetium diphosphonate should be done. These scans provide excellent diagnostic information because of the active and vascular nature of these lesions.

Once the diagnosis has been made, whether it be polyostotic or monostotic fibrous dysplasia, a commitment to long-term follow-up must be made. Numerous cases have been reported in which longstanding lesions have undergone spontaneous malignant transformation, usually to osteosarcoma.[143]

Surgical eradication of the disease is generally impractical. This is certainly true of the polyostotic form and is often the case with the monostotic form. In particular, the monostotic form of the disease is often not diagnosed until it reaches considerable size. Because its boundaries are not usually well demarcated from surrounding bone, surgical ablation would necessitate large en bloc resections, resulting in severe facial deformity. If the monostotic lesion is small, however, surgical excision with long-term follow-up is the treatment of choice. In large lesions, osseous recontouring to eliminate facial asymmetry is the preferred treatment.[50, 58, 66, 118] A transoral approach is advocated (Fig. 58–47). This should be delayed, despite patient and parent protests, until the patient has reached adulthood. This delay is predicated on the observation that these lesions appear in childhood, grow slowly during adolescence and become less active or quiescent following the onset of puberty.[76, 143] Also, it has been observed that surgery, with periosteal reflection, during the lesion's more active growth phase is a stimulus for con-

tinued growth.[38] Indeed, some surgeons advocate incisional biopsy through mucosa, periosteum, and lesional tissue without reflecting a mucoperiosteal flap.

Although periodic osseous recontouring via a transoral approach to eliminate facial deformity is advocated, it is best to retain as a general principle the wisdom of minimizing the number of times the lesion undergoes surgery.

Reports of sarcomatous change in lesions of fibrous dysplasia following radiation therapy have appeared in the literature.[143] However, fibrous dysplasia seldom jeopardizes the life of the patient, and such hazards must be kept paramount in the mind of the treating clinician.

OTHER TUMORS AND TUMOR-LIKE CONDITIONS OF THE JAWS

Hemangioma of Bone

Central hemangiomas of bone may be hamartomas rather than true neoplasms. Clinically, they may exhibit a variety of patterns, ranging from small, relatively dormant lesions to those showing progressive expansion and destruction. Histologically, they are classified as capillary, mixed, and cavernous. The latter group has the most significance to the surgeon owing to the possibility of severe blood loss and even exsanguination.[88] Reports of fatal outcomes from such lesions have appeared in the literature. Diagnosis and evaluation of the lesion has been enhanced with the use of arteriography techniques. In the pretreatment evaluation of the patient, it is essential to perform needle aspiration of the lesion. If radiographic evidence indicates a thin cortical plate, this may be accomplished by simply puncturing into the lesion with an 18-gauge needle affixed to an aspirating syringe. If the cortex is too thick for this approach, a small perforation may be made with a dental bur, followed by needle aspiration. The quantity and character of the aspirated blood should be observed. Bright red blood or a return with sufficient pressure to elevate the syringe plunger argue against further exploration such as biopsy. Preoperative arteriographic studies are required of large lesions or those with abundant hemorrhage on aspiration.

Methods of treating central hemangiomas vary. They include surgery, radiation therapy, sclerosing agents, cryotherapy, and embolization followed by surgery.[59, 70, 88] In relatively static lesions curettage is the treatment of choice. It may be necessary to perform ipsilateral external carotid ligation prior to curettage. This decision should be based on preoperative arteriograms and should be planned ahead of time. In lesions in which the rate of blood flow through the hemangioma is slow, radiation therapy or sclerosing agents (such as sodium morrhuate) injected into the lesion have proved effective.[59] In the latter case, both repeated injections over several weeks and single injections have proved effective. An intense inflammatory reaction with accompanying edema, pain, and paresthesia should be expected. These should subside within several weeks.[59]

In larger lesions with pulsatile properties or arteriovenous shunting present, conservative methods are usually inadequate. Surgical resection preceded by carotid ligation and ligation of peripheral feeders is the recommended treatment. Elective tracheotomy should

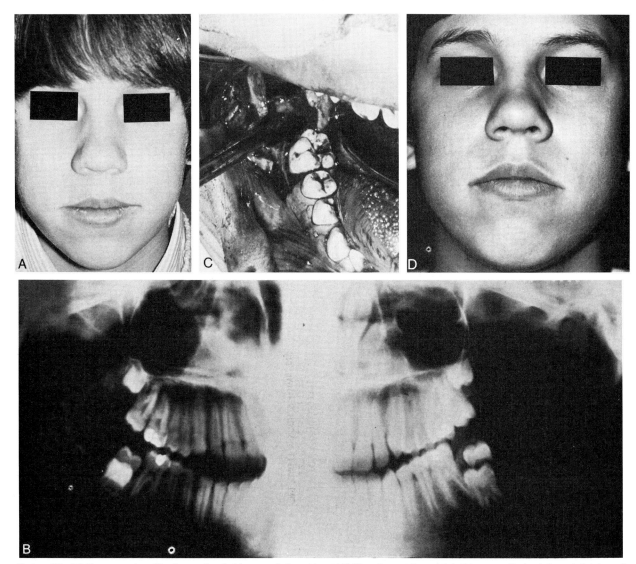

Figure 58–46. Young male with diagnosis, via biopsy, of cherubism. (*A*) The disease is restricted to mandibular left and right rami. Because of this patient's desire to participate in contact sports and the subsequent risk of pathologic fracture, surgical intervention was thought to be prudent. Note the bilateral fullness in the area of the rami. (*B*) Preoperative radiograph showing the extent of the lesions bilaterally. Note also the displacement of both right and left mandibular second and third molars. (*C*) Intraoperative photograph showing transoral approach to the lesion. Note the expansion of the cortical plates and the multilocular appearance produced by the bony septa. (*D*) One year postoperative photograph of patient. Approximately 90 per cent of the surgical defect has been filled in with new bone.

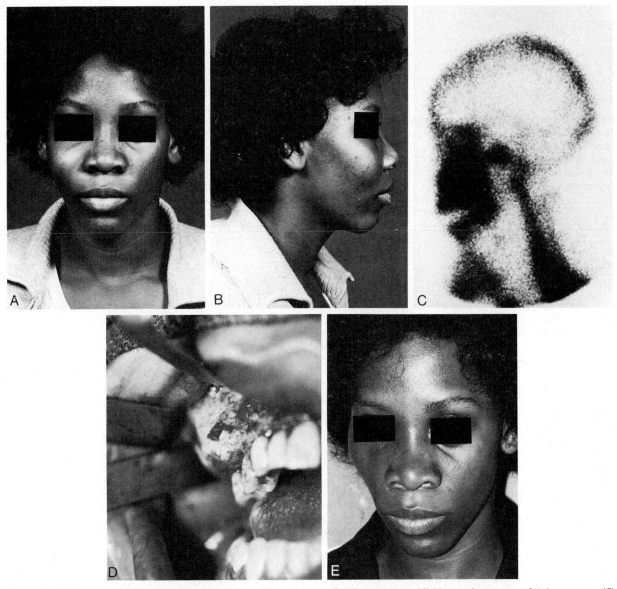

Figure 58–47. Young female patient with fibrous dysplasia producing facial asymmetry. (*A*) Note enlargement of right zygoma. (*B*) Profile view again showing enlargement of right zygoma. (*C*) Technetium bone scan showing active uptake in area of lesion. (*D*) Intraoperative view showing maxillary lesion on the lateral aspect of the posterior alveolar bone and extending up the molar strut to zygoma. The surgical objectives were to obtain debulking and recontouring only. (*E*) Six-month postoperative view of patient showing improved facial contour and improved symmetry.

be considered. Immediate reconstruction with autologous bone from the ilium is recommended.[59]

Recent refinements in embolization techniques utilizing fluoroscopy may eliminate the need for presurgical carotid ligation and may serve as an effective means of decreasing hemorrhage at the time of surgery.

In summary, the clinical and radiographic presentation of the lesion should dictate the appropriate therapy. Radical resection should be avoided in cases in which the lesion is not exhibiting progressive expansion or when more conservative management (such as sclerosing techniques) aimed at local destruction of the endothelial lining can be utilized (Fig. 58–48).

Histiocytosis X

Histiocytosis X is a disease characterized by the proliferation of mature histiocytes. It has been divided into three clinical entities as follows: (1) Letterer-Siwe disease, an acute disseminated form; (2) Hand-Schüller-Christian disease, a chronic disseminated form; and (3) eosinophilic granuloma, a localized form of the disease. It may sometimes be difficult to distinguish among the three. Treatment and prognosis vary with the presenting form.[118]

In Letterer-Siwe disease, the initial presentation usually appears during the first year of life. Its clinical course is rapid and usually fatal. Chemotherapy with cytotoxic drugs has been employed with limited success.

In Hand-Schüller-Christian disease, the initial presentation occurs somewhat later and may arise in adults. It affects a number of organs, including the liver, spleen, lymph nodes, and bone. Characteristically the patient exhibits punched-out bone lesions of the skull, diabetes insipidus, and exophthalmus. Radiation therapy and local curettage have been employed for the bone lesions. Cytotoxic drugs, such as 6-mercaptopurine, vinblastine, nitrogen mustard, and cyclophosphamide, have been used to combat other systemic involvement. The median survival is from 10 to 15 years.

The localized form of histiocytoses X, eosinophilic granuloma, is most amenable to treatment. The lesions occur in bone and are usually well circumscribed. When appearing in the jaws, they must be distinguished from periapical abscesses, periodontal disease, and odontogenic cysts. Vigorous curettage with long-term follow-up is the treatment of choice. The adjacent teeth are often sacrificed owing to the loss of alveolar support. The prognosis is good.

Desmoplastic Fibroma of the Jaws

In recent years, increasing attention has been given to a group of benign but locally aggressive intraosseous proliferations of connective tissue. Because of the growth pattern and often alarming radiologic features, they are readily mistaken for malignancies. The desmoplastic fibroma of bone is the name given to these lesions. The tumor is mainly located in long bones, but it may occur in a wide variety of bones. Most patients are in the 10- to 19-year age group.[119] The first report describing a desmoplastic fibroma occurring in the jaw bones was published in 1965.[57] Almost 30 have since been reported.[16, 18, 27, 30, 35, 44, 46, 48, 61, 62, 90, 96, 101, 106, 112, 122, 141] The vast majority have been located in the mandible.

Clinically, desmoplastic fibroma of the jawbones is a slowly expanding tumor, with swelling often being the only symptom. It is radiolucent and tends to be quite large when discovered. The radiographic appearance may easily be mistaken for a malignancy because the cortical plates may be thinned, and the radiolucent areas exhibit a honeycombed appearance. The tumors have been found to penetrate into soft tissues and muscle in more than half of the reported cases. Trismus is the result of involvement of the muscles of mastication.[57, 61]

Desmoplastic fibroma of the jaws has been treated by curettage, resection, segmental resection, and irradiation. The paucity of reported cases and the short follow-up periods make it difficult to accurately evaluate the therapeutic effectiveness of these treatment modalities. In the report by Freedman and colleagues,[48] which reviewed the treatment of 22 jaw lesions, 19 had no recurrences, with follow-up ranging from 3 months to 8 years. Twelve of these patients had been treated by excision (presumably curettage), six by resection, and one by irradiation. In only one case has recurrence been diagnosed as fibrosarcoma with metastases.[30] Given these results, it seems that thorough curettage in lesions that have not destroyed the cortical plates and have not invaded soft tissues is appropriate with adequate follow-up. If destruction of the cortical plates or invasion of adjacent tissues is noted, resection should be undertaken. Immediate reconstruction should be entertained if block resection is contemplated.

It must be concluded that diagnosis and treatment of this benign but aggressive tumor pose great problems. The importance of cooperation between pathologist and surgeon must be stressed. Re-evaluation of treatment and histologic testing must be undertaken for any fibrous lesion that does not respond favorably to conservative therapy. There is always the possibility that the histologic diagnosis may have been incorrect and a fibrosarcoma may have been overlooked.

PRIMARY MALIGNANCIES OF THE JAWS

Figure 58–49 demonstrates the surgical management of a *typical* primary malignancy of the mandible without distant metastases. Each case, however, must be individualized based upon the histologic and clinical picture upon presentation. This is not meant to indicate the method for treatment of *all* primary malignancies of the jaws.

Osteosarcoma of the Jaws

Although osteosarcoma is the most common primary malignancy of bone, it is a rare tumor. Approximately 6.5 per cent of all osteosarcomas arise in the jaws.[14, 17, 24, 91, 113, 149] The outstanding presenting symptoms are local pain and swelling, although osteosarcomas occurring within the jaws may produce less pain than those in the long bones.[51]

There is good evidence to suggest that the biologic behavior of osteogenic sarcomas of the jaws is distinctly different from osteosarcomas of long bones. The age of occurrence is at least a decade older for osteosarcomas of the jaws.[21, 51, 104] Osteosarcomas of other bones tend to rapidly metastasize to distant sites, whereas those in

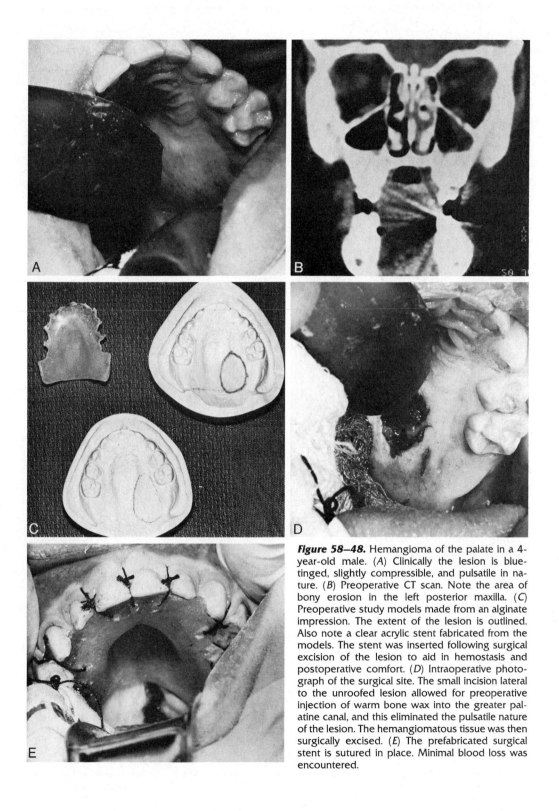

Figure 58–48. Hemangioma of the palate in a 4-year-old male. (*A*) Clinically the lesion is blue-tinged, slightly compressible, and pulsatile in nature. (*B*) Preoperative CT scan. Note the area of bony erosion in the left posterior maxilla. (*C*) Preoperative study models made from an alginate impression. The extent of the lesion is outlined. Also note a clear acrylic stent fabricated from the models. The stent was inserted following surgical excision of the lesion to aid in hemostasis and postoperative comfort. (*D*) Intraoperative photograph of the surgical site. The small incision lateral to the unroofed lesion allowed for preoperative injection of warm bone wax into the greater palatine canal, and this eliminated the pulsatile nature of the lesion. The hemangiomatous tissue was then surgically excised. (*E*) The prefabricated surgical stent is sutured in place. Minimal blood loss was encountered.

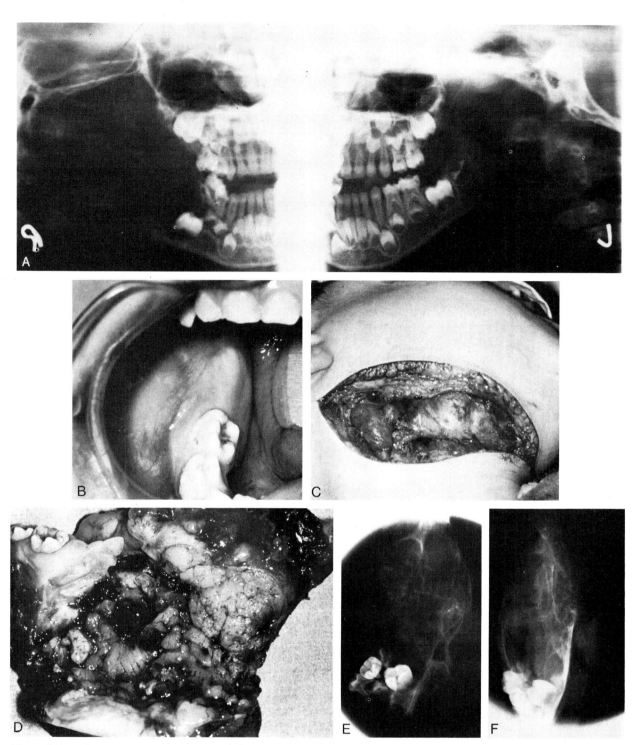

Figure 58–49. Surgical treatment of a primary malignancy of the mandibular ramus. A 4-year-old white male with an expansile lesion of his right mandibular ramus that was proved at biopsy to be Ewing's sarcoma. No metastases were discovered in the preoperative work-up. (*A*) Preoperative panoramic radiograph demonstrating a multilocular radiolucency of the right mandibular ramus and body. (*B*) Intraoral photograph showing gross enlargement of the posterior mandible. (*C*) Surgical photograph showing the enlarged mandible. (*D*) Surgical specimen which included the right hemimandible (to the canine region), the pterygoid muscles, the submandibular gland, and suprahyoid lymph nodes. (*E*) Lateral radiograph of the surgical specimen showing extent of destruction. (*F*) Occlusal radiograph of the surgical specimen showing the mediolateral expansion of the mandible. (*G*) Postoperative panoramic radiograph of patient. Although the margins were clear, the tumor was very close to the margin in one area. The patient subsequently underwent a course of radiotherapy and chemotherapy. Three and one-half years later, with no recurrences, reconstruction of his mandibular defect was undertaken. (*H*) Photograph showing incision placement inferiorly in the neck to facilitate closure. (*I*) Intraoperative photograph showing developed graft-bed. Note the distal mandibular stump and the tunnel up to the mandibular fossa where the condyle is to be placed.

Illustration continued on opposite page

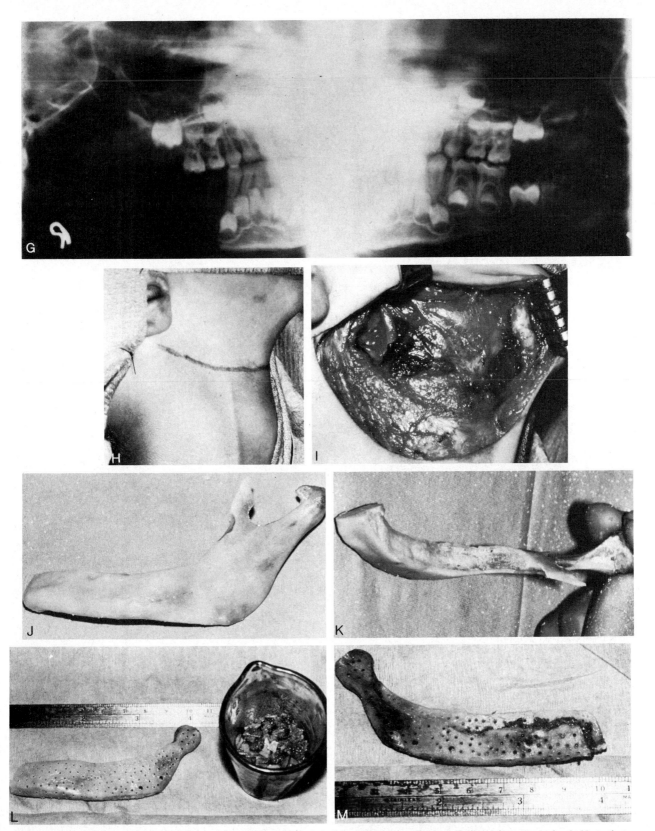

Figure 58–49 *Continued.* (*J* and *K*) Photograph of adult allogeneic freeze-dried mandible as obtained from tissue bank. Note that this hemimandible was from the opposite side as that which the patient required. (*L*) Photograph of allogeneic graft after modifications, including removal of the coronoid process, thinning the cortices, hollowing out the medullary spaces, and decreasing the size of the condyle. The autogenous corticocancellous chips in the specimen jar were obtained from the patient's ilium. (*M*) Photograph of the allogeneic crib packed with autogenous corticocancellous chips.

Illustration continued on following page

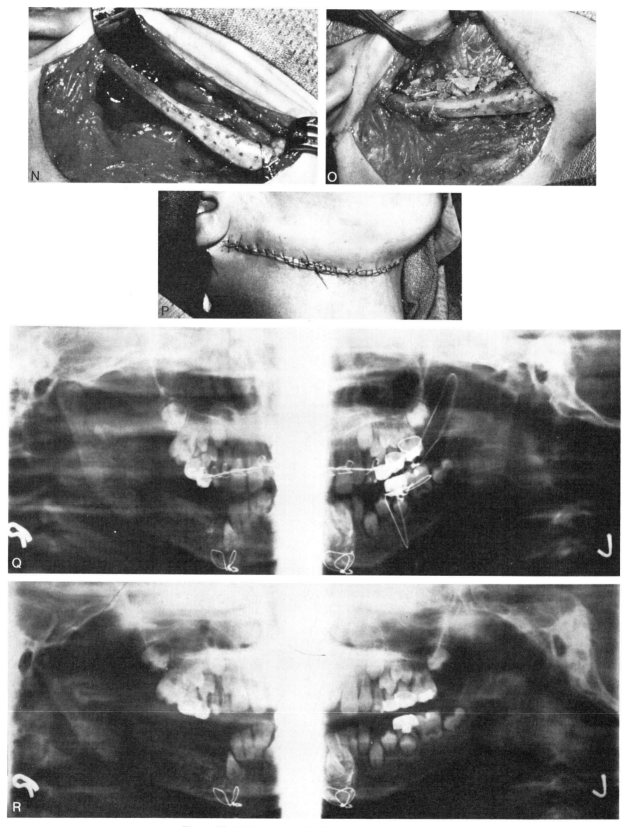

Figure 58–49 Continued. See legend on opposite page.

the jaws remain locally invasive for a long time prior to metastasizing. Radical surgical resection has been the standard treatment of osteosarcoma of the jaws and is the single most effective therapeutic measure.[51, 114] This usually involves hemimandibulectomy for mandibular tumors and maxillectomies for maxillary tumors.

Preoperative radiotherapy has been used to decrease the size of the tumors in several instances.[21, 22, 51, 104, 114] Chambers and Mahoney[22] and Russ and Jesse[114] reported better prognoses in patients who underwent preoperative radiotherapy prior to surgical resection. They both[22, 114] use intraosseous radium needles for mandibular osteosarcomas and external beam radiation if extension into soft tissues is present. The dose given to bone is 10,000 to 16,000 rad, followed immediately by resection.

Postoperative radiotherapy has also been suggested by some. Radiotherapy has been used as the only treatment in nonresectable cases, however, results have been disappointing.[21, 51] Lymph node dissections should be accomplished if nodes are palpable, as this improves survival. However, prophylactic lymph node dissection is probably not warranted, as most metastases are hematogenous.[77] Chemotherapy has been used for recurrences with little success. The combined use of ablative surgery, radiotherapy, and chemotherapy has been advanced over the past decade for the treatment of osteosarcomas of the jaws.[34]

The prognosis of patients with osteosarcoma of the jaws is relatively good, especially when compared to survival rates with osteosarcomas in general. Kragh and coworkers[77] found a 31 per cent 5-year survival rate in patients treated for osteosarcomas of the jaws and facial bones. Garrington and coworkers[51] found a 35 per cent 5-year survival rate in their series. Russ and Jesse[114] reported 50 per cent and 71 per cent 5-year survival rates for maxillary and mandibular osteosarcomas, respectively, in the patients who received definitive treatment at their institution. Recurrences are usually local; however, metastases have been reported in approximately one third to one half of cases,[21, 51] most commonly to the lung.

The juxtacortical osteosarcoma, also called parosteal osteosarcoma, is an uncommon variant. It is extremely rare in the jaws, with less than ten reported cases.[4, 13, 109] The biologic nature of these lesions tends to be less aggressive than that of the central osteosarcoma, with local recurrences and rare distant metastases. However, owing to the limited number of reports, it is difficult to thoroughly evaluate the optimal mode of therapy. Aggressive surgical resection is probably the favored treatment at this time.

Chondrosarcoma of the Jaws

Before 1930, chondrosarcomas were included with the group of osteosarcomas. In that year, Phemister[100] emphasized that sarcomas of bone consisting largely of cartilage are best designated as chondrosarcomas. In 1939, Ewing,[41] in the revised registry classification, separated the chondrosarcomas from the osteosarcomas. Since that time, there have been less than 100 cases of chondrosarcomas involving the jaws.[3, 15, 23, 60, 78, 79, 95, 103, 116, 123] Reliable data concerning this tumor have been difficult to obtain because of this paucity of reported cases. However, the pathogenesis and accepted treatment of the chondrosarcoma can be obtained from those reports available.

The clinical difficulty when dealing with cartilaginous tumors is determining whether or not they are benign or malignant. Many authorities have said that it is often difficult or impossible to distinguish histologically between benign chondromas and chondrosarcomas.[93] Although the zone between innocent tumors and overt chondrosarcomas may still be incompletely understood, it is certainly evident from clinical experience and published reports that chondrogenic neoplasms are far more often malignant than benign in their clinical or biologic course.[5, 23] Clinically, chondrosarcomas of the jaws are relatively fast-growing, invasive, and destructive. Cartilaginous tumors of the jaws have a great tendency to recur unless adequately treated. Benign lesions, following recurrence, are often found to be more cellular or to have already turned frankly malignant. Hence, all cartilaginous tumors of the jaws, benign or malignant, should be radically excised with a portion of the normal local tissues to prevent local recurrence. They cause death usually by direct extension to the base of the skull, and also through distant metastasis, chiefly to the lungs and bones.[23, 103, 108] Chondrosarcomas appear to be radioresistant, and there is no predictable effective chemotherapeutic agent.[108, 111] However, these agents have been used adjunctively with surgery or in inoperative cases for palliation.

The prognosis for patients with chondrosarcomas of the jaws is disappointingly poor. When chondrosarcomas of the jaws have been compared with those arising in long bones, a much poorer prognosis was observed in jaw tumors. The review by Chaudhry and coworkers[23] indicates that chondrosarcomas of the jaws carry a worse prognosis than osteosarcomas of the jaws. This can be attributed to a number of factors, including the high recurrence rates, the inability to detect the extent of this tumor by radiographs, aggressive local extension, and occasional metastases.

The mesenchymal chondrosarcoma, a highly characteristic chondroid neoplasm, should be treated in the same way as the chondrosarcoma of the jaws when found in this location.

Fibrosarcoma of the Jaws

Fibrosarcomas of the jaws are extremely rare neoplasms and, as such, little is known about their clinical behavior and responses to treatment. Two types of fibrosarcomas of the jaws are generally recognized: the

---

Figure 58–49 *Continued.* (*N*) Intraoperative photograph of the graft in place. Note the amount of dead space medial to the graft. (*O*) Photograph showing dead space obliteration by suturing underlying soft tissues to graft. Autogenous corticocancellous chips packed around graft prior to closure. (*P*) Photograph immediately following closure. Note improved mandibular contour. (*Q*) Immediate postoperative panoramic radiograph showing fixation techniques and graft placement. (*R*) Six-month postoperative panoramic radiograph showing graft consolidation and continued eruption of right mandibular canine tooth. The patient had no malocclusion and good functional movements.

periosteal and the endosteal. The periosteal fibrosarcoma is a soft-tissue sarcoma and has a much better prognosis than the endosteal variety.[5] The endosteal (medullary) fibrosarcoma metastasizes early via the hematogenous route and tends to recur locally, making its eradication difficult. They invade by direct extension along fascial planes with ill-defined margins to form bulky solid pseudoencapsulated masses that eventually involve adjacent bone with progressive fixation.

The treatment for either type of fibrosarcoma is wide surgical excision. These tumors are extremely radioresistant. Local recurrence is associated with inadequate resection, and these recurrences may be so bulky as to negate curative resection. Death is often due to uncontrolled local growth, with metastases infrequently causing death.

Ewing's Sarcoma of the Jaws

Ewing's sarcoma is considered a primary malignancy of bone and extraskeletal soft tissues. The jaws have the lowest rate of involvement of this tumor (1 to 10 per cent), with the long bones of the lower extremities and pelvis being most frequently affected.[31, 32, 36, 54, 103, 110, 130, 140] The mandible is more often affected than the maxilla. Patients are young, usually within the first three decades, and males are affected more often than females.

Ewing's sarcoma is a neoplasm that manifests rapid hematogenous spread. Metastases are common; estimates that 15 to 30 per cent of patients have either asymptomatic or symptomatic metastases at the time of initial diagnosis were offered by Johnson and Pomeroy.[72] If not present at initial diagnosis, metastasis within the first 6 months after diagnosis is likely.[7, 130, 135] The lungs and other bones are the sites most often affected.

In the past, Ewing's sarcoma has been one of the most lethal forms of cancer, with reported survival rates ranging from 0 to 15 per cent.[7, 31, 32, 42, 130] Recently, more encouraging results have been reported with the use of a combination of therapeutic modalities.[39, 55, 89, 99, 105, 134] Therapeutic procedures for Ewing's sarcoma have varied from local resection to amputation, radiation therapy, and chemotherapy. In the jaws, radiotherapy has been the most frequently employed treatment.[45, 104, 110] These tumors have been uniformly sensitive to radiotherapy. However, results with radiation therapy have been poor or, at best, equivocal. In the investigations of Roca and coworkers,[110] Potdar,[104] and Ferlito,[45] only three of 18 patients were alive 5 years after treatment. The combination of several treatment modalities may hold promise for eradicating this tumor. Reasonable survival rates by the combined use of chemotherapy in addition to radiotherapy has been offered by Pomeroy and Johnson,[102] among others.[68, 99] The low number of Ewing's sarcoma of the jaws and the multitude of treatment combinations preclude any meaningful assessment of therapeutic effectiveness and prognosis. However, there is hope that improved chemotherapy in conjunction with radiotherapy (and perhaps surgery) will allow better chances of survival in the future.

Malignant Fibrous Histiocytoma of the Jaws

In spite of its increased recognition as one of the more common sarcomas of deep and superficial soft tissue, malignant fibrous histiocytoma is a relatively rare tumor in the head and neck region, particularly in the oral cavity. Less than 20 have been reported in the mouth.[9, 26, 64, 71, 81, 92, 121, 125, 128, 139, 148] One per cent of fibrous histiocytomas prove malignant.[97] The malignant form of this tumor has an infiltrative and invasive characteristic, with involvement of regional lymph nodes and a tendency for distant metastasis.[97, 126] For these tumors in the head and neck, distant metastases occur in about 25 per cent of cases.[9] Most metastases have occurred in the regional lymph nodes or lungs. Once metastasis is proved, the prognosis is poor, with an average life expectancy of approximately 13 months.[69] The 5-year survival rate is around 50 per cent.

Wide surgical excision is advised for treatment of a malignant fibrous histiocytoma.[63, 75, 126, 139, 150] Most recurrences are the result of inadequate primary excision. Margins should be checked by frozen section. If adenopathy is present, lymph node dissection should be employed. Spanier and coworkers[127] reported encouraging results of radiotherapy and chemotherapy for the treatment of patients with metastasis; however, Feldman and Norman,[43] Soule and Enriquez,[126] Jones and coworkers,[73] and Hutchinson and Friedberg[63] claimed that radiotherapy was ineffective. In a case reported by Spector and Ogura,[128] the excised radiated specimen was histologically identical to the pre-irradiation biopsy specimen. The role of chemotherapy is unclear in the treatment of this lesion. Soule and Enriquez,[126] Webber and Weinke,[148] and Hutchinson and Friedberg[63] reported regression of tumor when radiotherapy and chemotherapy were employed in combination.

Primary Salivary Gland Tumors within the Jaws

Salivary gland inclusions in the mandible are no longer considered rare and have been reported with some regularity since Stafne's original description in 1942. Salivary gland inclusions have not been reported in the maxilla; however, mucous glands are found in the walls of nasopalatine duct cysts and in the nasopalatine canal.[1] As with epithelium in any location, neoplastic degeneration can occur in these inclusions, giving rise to primary intraosseous salivary gland neoplasms. Close to 100 have been reported in the literature. The majority are mucoepidermoid carcinomas and have occurred primarily in the mandible; however, both benign[120, 136, 147] and other malignant salivary gland neoplasms[37, 47, 132, 137] have also been reported.

In general, these neoplasms behave similarly to their extraosseous counterparts and, as such, should be treated accordingly. Complete surgical excision is the preferred treatment for these lesions, with radiation therapy used for recurrences or inoperable cases. Although the adenoid cystic carcinoma is generally thought to be radioresistant,[12] several investigators feel that it may temporarily arrest the tumor or decrease its size.[27, 74, 124, 129] The central mucoepidermoid carcinoma is locally aggressive but does not readily metastasize, and when it does, it usually involves the regional lymph nodes.

Non-Hodgkin's Lymphoma of the Jaws

Malignant lymphoma is a primary malignant tumor of lymphoreticular tissue, composed of histiocytic or lymphocytic derivatives in varying degrees of differentiation. It may be a homogeneous proliferation of a single cell type or a mixture of histiocytic and lymphocytic components. Rappaport[107] has classified these tumors by their cell type and histologic pattern. The histologic pattern consists of nodular or diffuse patterns within a given cell type. Any malignant lymphoma of any cellular composition may have a nodular or diffuse histologic pattern. The nodular histologic pattern carries a more favorable prognosis.[20]

Non-Hodgkin's malignant lymphoma may occur in nodal or extranodal sites, may be localized or multifocal in origin, and may spread by noncontiguous routes, possibly hematogenous. The most common site in the oral cavity is Waldeyer's ring area. Primary intraosseous malignant lymphomas do occur, but are rare. The most common form seems to be histiocytic lymphoma when found in the jaws.[40] Campbell and colleagues,[19] in reviewing the literature of histiocytic lymphoma of the mandible (reticulum cell sarcoma), noted a male predominance of 3:1. The age range of these patients was from 8 to 69 years, with a mean age of 32.2 years. Swelling was the most common symptom with histiocytic lymphoma of the mandible, followed by pain and paresthesia of the lip on the affected side. Gerry and Williams[52] reported mobility of the teeth as a symptom. The radiographic appearance of malignant lymphomas of the jaws is nonspecific, exhibiting predominant areas of osteolytic changes with less prominant areas of osteoblastic change. The lesions tend to be locally destructive and are not significantly different from other malignancies on radiographs.

Treatment for intraosseous malignant lymphomas of the jaws is similar to that for their soft-tissue counterparts in the head and neck area. Following staging (techniques vary from one institution to another), most lymphomas, with the possible exception of Burkitt's, are treated with radiotherapy (usually megavoltage).[5, 49, 83, 138, 146] These tumors are usually radiosensitive, and when treated early, the prognosis for radiocurability is good. Wang and Fleischli[145] recommended that initial therapy be in the form of radiation, with a total dose of 4500 to 5000 roentgens over a 4- to 5-week course, with a field including the regional nodes. Variant modalities of chemotherapy combined with radiation are highly recommended.[11, 83] The combined chemotherapy,* such as VEP, VEMP, MOPP, and MVPP,[82, 98] and the combined chemotherapy and radiation therapy raises the 5-year survival rate to 70 per cent instead of 50 per cent for radiotherapy only in stage I and to 60 per cent instead of 33 per cent in stage II.

The role of surgery in the treatment of intraosseous lymphomas has been disputed. Its role has become one of an adjunctive nature, debulking large lymphomas (especially the Burkitt's type) prior to radiotherapy or chemotherapy. Burkitt's lymphomas respond well to alkylating agents, and remissions in over 90 per cent of patients can be obtained. The place of radiotherapy in the management of this tumor is unclear.

---

*VEP = Vincristine, Endoxan (cyclophosphamide), prednisolone; VEMP = vincristine, Endoxan, 6-mercaptopurine, and prednisolone; MOPP = nitrogen mustard, Oncovin (vincristine), procarbazine, and prednisolone; MUPP = nitrogen mustard, vinblastine, procarbazine, and prednisolone.

REFERENCES

1. Abrams A, Howell F, Bullock W: Nasopalatine cysts. Oral Surg 16:306, 1963.
2. Anderson DE, McClendon JL, Cornelius EA: Cherubism: Hereditary fibrous dysplasia of the jaws. I. Genetic considerations. II. Pathologic considerations. Oral Surg 15:17, 1962.
3. Arlen M, Tollefsen HR, Huvos AG, Marcove RC: Chondrosarcoma of the head and neck. Am J Surg 120:456, 1970.
4. Banergee SC: Juxtacortical osteosarcoma of mandible: Review of the literature and report of a case. J Oral Surg 39:535, 1981.
5. Batsakis JG: Tumors of the Head and Neck. 2nd ed. Baltimore, Williams & Wilkins Co., 1979.
6. Bernier JL, Bhaskar SN: Aneurysmal bone cysts of the mandible. Oral Surg 11:1018, 1958.
7. Bhansali SK, Desai PB: Ewing's sarcoma: Observations on 107 cases. J Bone Joint Surg 45:541, 1963.
8. Biesecker LJ, Marcove RC, Huvos AG, Mike V: Aneurysmal bone cysts: A clinicopathologic study of 66 cases. Cancer 26:615, 1970.
9. Blitzer A, Lawson W, Biller H: Malignant fibrous histiocytoma of the head and neck. Laryngoscope 87:1479, 1977.
10. Borello ED, Sedano HO: Giant osteoid osteoma of the maxilla. Report of a case. Oral Surg 23:563, 1967.
11. Boston CH Jr, et al: Reticulum cell sarcoma of bone. Cancer 34:1131, 1974.
12. Bradley JC: A case of cylindroma of the mandible. Br J Oral Surg 5:186, 1968.
13. Bras JM, Donner R, van der Kwast WAM, et al: Juxtacortical osteogenic sarcoma of the jaws—review of the literature and report of a case. Oral Surg 50:535, 1980.
14. Brody GL, Fry LR: Osteogenic sarcoma—experience at the University of Michigan. U Mich Med Bull 29:80, 1963.
15. Buchner A, Ramon Y, Begleiter A: Chondrosarcoma of the maxilla—report of a case. J Oral Surg 37:822, 1979.
16. Bullens R, Boddaert J, Schautteet H, DeFloor E: Fibrome desmoid osseux du maxillaire inférieur. Cas exceptionnel d'un enfant de quinze mois. Rev Stomatol 76:45, 1975.
17. Cade S: Osteogenic sarcoma. J R Coll Surg Edinb 1:79, 1955.
18. Calatrava L, Donado M: Comentarios sobre los fibromas desmoplasticos. Rev Esp Estomatol 23:421, 1975.
19. Campbell RL, Kelly DE, Burkes JE Jr: Primary reticulum-cell sarcoma of the mandible. Oral Surg 39:918, 1975.
20. Carbone PJ: Non-Hodgkin's lymphoma: Recent observations on natural history and intensive treatment. Cancer 30:1511, 1972.
21. Caron AS, Hajdu SI, Strong EW: Osteogenic sarcoma of the facial and cranial bones. Am J Surg 122:719, 1971.
22. Chambers RG, Mahoney WD: Osteogenic sarcoma of the mandible: Current management. Ann Surg 36:463, 1970.
23. Chaudhry AP, Robinovitch MR, Mitchell DF, Vickers RA: Chondrogenic tumors of the jaws. Am J Surg 102:403, 1961.
24. Coventry MB, Dahlin DC: Osteogenic sarcoma. J Bone Joint Surg 39:741, 1957.
25. Cramer LM: Gardner's syndrome. J Plast Reconstr Surg 29:402, 1962.
26. Crissman JD, Henson SL: Malignant fibrous histiocytoma of the maxillary sinus. Arch Otolaryngol 104:228, 1978.
27. Cunningham CD, Smith RO, Enriquez P, Singleton GT: Desmoplastic fibroma of the mandible. A case report. Ann Otol Rhinol Laryngol 84:125, 1975.
28. Curkovic M: Osteoma of the maxillary sinuses: Report of case. Arch Otolaryngol 54:53, 1951.
29. Dabska M, Buraczewski J: Aneurysmal bone cyst: Pathology, clinical course and radiographic appearances. Cancer 23:371, 1969.
30. Dahlin DC: Bone Tumors. 2nd ed. Springfield, Charles C Thomas, 1967, pp 212–221.
31. Dahlin DC, Coventry MB, Scanlon PW: Ewing's sarcoma: A critical analysis of 165 cases. J Bone Joint Surg 43:185, 1961.
32. Dahlin DC: Bone Tumors: General Aspects and Data on 6,221 Cases. 3rd ed. Springfield, Charles C Thomas, 1978, pp 274–287.
33. Daugherty JW, Eversole LR: Aneurysmal bone cyst of the mandible: Report of case. J Oral Surg 29:737, 1971.
34. de Fries HO, Kornblut AD: Malignant disease of the osseous adnexae: Osteogenic sarcoma of the jaws. Otolaryngol Clin North Am 12:129, 1979.
35. Dehner LP: Tumors of the mandible and maxilla in children. I. Clinicopathologic study of 46 histologically benign lesions. Cancer 31:364, 1973.
36. deSantos LA, Jing BS: Radiographic findings of Ewing's sarcoma of the jaws. Br J Radiol 51:682, 1978.
37. Dhawan IK, Bhargava S, Nayak NC, Gupta RK: Central salivary gland tumors of the jaws. Cancer 26:211, 1970.

38. Dierks E, Caudill RJ, O'Leary JD: Surgical recontouring of a panfacial fibro-osseous deformity. J Oral Surg 37:682, 1979.

39. Donaldson SS: A story of continuing success—radiotherapy for Ewing's sarcoma. Int J Radiat Oncol Biol Phys 7:279, 1981.

40. Eisenbud L, Sciubba J, Mir R, Sachs SA: Oral presentations in non-Hodgkin's lymphoma: A review of thirty-one cases. Oral Surg 56:151, 1983.

41. Ewing J: Review of classification of bone tumors. Surg Gynecol Obstet 68:971, 1939.

42. Falk S, Alpert M: Five-year survival of patients with Ewing's sarcoma. Surg Gynecol Obstet 124:319, 1967.

43. Feldman F, Norman D: Intra- and extraosseous malignant histiocytoma (malignant fibrous xanthoma). Radiology 104:497, 1972.

44. Ferguson JW: Central fibroma of the jaws. Br J Oral Surg 12:205, 1974.

45. Ferlito A: Primary Ewing's sarcoma of the maxilla: A clinicopathological study of four cases. J Laryngol Otol 92:1007, 1978.

46. Fisker AB, Philipsen HP: Desmoplastic fibroma of the jaw bones. Int J Oral Surg 5:285, 1976.

47. Freedman SI, et al: Primary malignant mixed tumor of the mandible. Cancer 30:167, 1972.

48. Freedman PD, Cardo VA, Kerpel SM, Lumerman H: Desmoplastic fibroma (fibromatosis) of the jawbones. Report of a case and review of the literature. Oral Surg 46:386, 1978.

49. Fuller LM: Results of intensive regional radiation therapy in the treatment of Hodgkin's disease and the malignant lymphomas of the head and neck. Am J Roentgenol Radium Ther Nucl Med 99:340, 1967.

50. Gardner AF, Halpert L: Fibrous dysplasia of the skull with special reference to the oral regions. Dent Pract Dent Rec 13:337, 1963.

51. Garrington GE, Scofield HH, Cornyn J, Hooker SP: Osteosarcoma of the jaws—Analysis of 56 cases. Cancer 20:377, 1967.

52. Gerry RG, Williams SF: Primary reticulum-cell sarcoma of the mandible. Oral Surg 8:568, 1955.

53. Giansanti JS, Waldron CA: Peripheral giant cell granuloma: Review of 720 cases. J Oral Surg 27:787, 1969.

54. Glaubiger DL, Makuch R, Schwarz J, et al: Determination of prognostic factors and their influence on therapeutic results in patients with Ewing's sarcoma. Cancer 45:2213, 1980.

55. Graham-Pole J: Ewing's sarcoma: Treatment with high dose radiation and adjuvant chemotherapy. Med Pediatr Oncol 7:1, 1979.

56. Greene GW Jr, Natiella JR, Spring PN Jr: Osteoid osteoma of the jaws. Report of a case. Oral Surg 26:342, 1968.

57. Griffith JG, Irby WB: Desmoplastic fibroma. Report of a rare tumor of the oral structures. Oral Surg 20:269, 1965.

58. Hayward J, McLarkey D, Megguier J: Monostotic fibrous dysplasia of the maxilla. J Oral Surg 31:625, 1973.

59. Hayward JR: Central cavernous hemangioma of the mandible: Report of four cases. J Oral Surg 39:526, 1981.

60. Henderson ED, Dahlin DC: Chondrosarcoma of bone—a survey of 288 cases. J Bone Joint Surg 45:1450, 1963.

61. Hinds EC, Kent JN, Fechner RE: Desmoplastic fibroma of the mandible: Report of case. J Oral Surg 27:271, 1969.

62. Hovinga J, Ingenhoes R: A desmoplastic fibroma in the mandible. Int J Oral Surg 3:41, 1974.

63. Hutchinson JC, Friedberg SA: Fibrous histiocytoma of the head and neck: A case report. Laryngoscope 88:1950, 1978.

64. Huvos AG: Primary malignant fibrous histiocytoma of bone. NY State J Med 76:552, 1976.

65. Jaffe HL: Benign osteoblastoma. Bull Hosp Joint Dis 17:141, 1956.

66. Jaffe HL: Giant-cell reparative granuloma, traumatic bone cyst, and fibrous (fibro-osseous) dysplasia of the jaw bones. Oral Surg 6:159, 1953.

67. Jaffe HL: Osteoid-osteoma. Arch Surg 31:709, 1935.

68. Jaffe N, Traggis D, Salian S, Cassady JR: Improved outlook for Ewing's sarcoma with combination chemotherapy (vincristine, actinomycin D and cyclophosphamide) and radiation therapy. Cancer 38:1925, 1976.

69. Jahrsdoerfer RA, Sweet DE, Ritz-Hugh GS: Malignant fibrous xanthoma with metastases to the cerebellopontine angle. Arch Otolaryngol 102:117, 1976.

70. James JN: Cavernous hemangioma of the mandible. Proc R Soc Med 47:797, 1964.

71. Jee AJ, Domboski M, Milobsky SA: Malignant fibrohistiocytoma of the maxilla presenting with endodontically involved teeth. Oral Surg 45:464, 1978.

72. Johnson RE, Pomeroy TC: Evaluation of therapeutic results in Ewing's sarcoma. Am J Roentgenol 123:583, 1975.

73. Jones FE, Soule EH, Coventry MB: Fibrous xanthoma of synovium (giant-cell tumor of tendon sheath, pigmented nodular synovitis).

A study of one hundred eighteen cases. J Bone Joint Surg 51:76, 1969.

74. Kaneda T, Nobusuke M, Takeuchi M, Yamashita T: Primary central adenoid cystic carcinoma of the mandible. J Oral Maxillofac Surg 40:741, 1982.

75. Kauffman SL, Stout AP: Histiocytic tumors (fibroma, xanthoma, and histiocytoma) in children. Cancer 14:469, 1961.

76. Khosla V, Korobken M: Monostotic fibrous dysplasia of the jaw. J Oral Surg 29:507, 1971.

77. Kragh LV, Dahlin DC, Erich JB: Osteogenic sarcoma of the jaw and facial bones. Am J Surg 96:496, 1958.

78. Kragh LV, Dahlin DC, Erich JB: Cartilaginous tumors of the jaws and facial regions. Am J Surg 99:852, 1960.

79. Krolls SO, Schaffer RC, O'Rear JW: Chondrosarcoma and osteosarcoma of the jaws in the same patient. Oral Surg 50:146, 1980.

80. Kruger G (ed): Textbook of Oral and Maxillofacial Surgery. 5th ed. The C. V. Mosby Co., 1979.

81. Kyriakos M, Kempson RL: Inflammatory fibrous histiocytoma. Cancer 37:1584, 1976.

82. Larsen RR, Hill GJ, Ratzer ER: Reticulum-cell sarcoma in head and neck surgery. Am J Surg 123:338, 1972.

83. Lian S, Nagai T, Kawasaki H, et al: Reticulum-cell sarcoma of the jaws. Oral Surg 50:110, 1980.

84. Lichtenstein L: Benign osteoblastoma: A category of osteoid and bone forming tumors other than classical osteoid osteoma which may be mistaken for giant cell tumor or osteogenic sarcoma. Cancer 9:1044, 1956.

85. Lichtenstein L: Aneurysmal bone cyst. Observations on 50 cases. J Bone Joint Surg (Am) 39:873, 1957.

86. Lichtenstein L, Jaffe HL: Fibrous dysplasia of bone. Arch Pathol 33:777, 1942.

87. Lovely F: Recurrent aneurysmal bone cyst of the mandible. J Oral Maxillofac Surg 41:192, 1983.

88. Lund BA, Dahlin D: Hemangiomas of the mandible and maxilla. J Oral Surg 22:234, 1964.

89. Marcove RC, Rosen G: Radical en bloc excision of Ewing's sarcoma. Clin Orthop 153:86, 1980.

90. Marlette RH, Gerhard RC: Intraosseous "fibroma" and "fibromyxoma" of the mandible. Report of three cases. Oral Surg 25:792, 1968.

91. McKenna RJ, Schwinn CP, Soong KY, Higinbotham NL: Sarcomata of the osteogenic series. J Bone Joint Surg 48:1, 1966.

92. Merrick RE, Rhone DP, Chilis TJ: Malignant fibrous histiocytoma of the maxillary sinus. Arch Otolaryngol 106:365, 1980.

93. Miles AC: Chondrosarcoma of the maxilla. Br Dent J 88:257, 1950.

94. Miller AS, Rambo H, Bowser M, Gross M: Benign osteoblastoma of the jaws: Report of three cases. J Oral Surg 38:694, 1980.

95. Myers EM, Thawley SE: Maxillary chondrosarcoma. Arch Otolaryngol 105:116, 1979.

96. Nussbaum GB, Terry JJ, Joy ED: Desmoplastic fibroma of the mandible in a 3 year old child. J Oral Surg 34:1117, 1976.

97. O'Brien JE, Stout AP: Malignant fibrous xanthoma. Cancer 17:1445, 1964.

98. Otsuka H: Incidence of malignant lymphomas and undifferentiated carcinomas in the pharynx. Saishin-Igaku 26:937, 1971.

99. Perez CA, Tefft M, Nesbit M, et al: The role of radiation therapy in the management of nonmetastatic Ewing's sarcoma of bone. Report of the Intergroup Ewing's Sarcoma Study. Int. J Radiat Oncol Biol Phys 7:141, 1981.

100. Phemister DB: Chondrosarcoma of bone. Surg Gynecol Obstet 50:216, 1930.

101. Pindborg JJ, Hjörting-Hansen E: Atlas of Diseases of the Jaws. Copenhagen, Munksgaard, 1974.

102. Pomeroy TC, Johnson RE: Combined modality therapy of Ewing's sarcoma. Cancer 35:36, 1975.

103. Potdar GG, Srikhande SS: Chondrogenic tumors of the jaws. Oral Surg 30:649, 1970.

104. Potdar GG: Ewing's tumors of the jaws. Oral Surg 29:505, 1970.

105. Pritchard DJ: Indications for surgical treatment of localized Ewing's sarcoma of bone. Clin Orthop 153:39, 1980.

106. Rabhan WN, Rosai J: Desmoplastic fibroma. Report of ten cases and review of the literature. J Bone Joint Surg 50:487, 1968.

107. Rappaport H: Tumors of the hematopoietic system. In Atlas of Tumor Pathology. sec. 3, fasc. 8, Washington, D.C., Armed Forces Institute of Pathology, 1966.

108. Richter KJ, Freeman NS, Quick CA: Chondrosarcoma of the temporomandibular joint: Review of case. J Oral Surg 32:777, 1974.

109. Roca AN, Smith JL, Jing BS: Osteosarcoma and parosteal osteogenic sarcoma of the mandible and maxilla. Am J Clin Pathol 54:625, 1970.

110. Roca AN, Smith JL, MacComb WS, Jing BS: Ewing's sarcoma of the maxilla and mandible: Study of six cases. Oral Surg 25:194, 1965.

111. Roser SM, Nicholas TR, Hirose FM: Metastatic chondrosarcoma to the maxilla: Review of the literature and report of case. J Oral Surg 34:1012, 1976.

112. Rouchon C, Brocheriou C, Costa A, Jacob A: Fibromes desmoïdes osseux de la mandibule à propos d'un cas. Rev Stomatol 76:527, 1975.

113. Rowe NH, Hungerford RW: Osteosarcoma of the mandible. J Oral Surg 21:42, 1963.

114. Russ JE, Jesse RH: Management of osteosarcoma of the maxilla and mandible. Am J Surg 140:572, 1980.

115. Salmo NAM, Shukur ST, Abulkhail A: Bilateral aneurysmal bone cysts of the maxilla. J Oral Surg 39:137, 1981.

116. Sato K, Ueda T: Osteogenic tumors of the jaws: Chondrosarcoma of the mandible. Report of a case. Jpn J Surg 21:482, 1975.

117. Schwarz E: Ossifying fibroma of the face and skull. Am J Roentgenol Radium Ther Nucl Med 91:1012, 1964.

118. Shaffer W, Hine M, Levy B: A Textbook of Oral Pathology. 3rd ed. Philadelphia. W. B. Saunders Co., 1974.

119. Siguira I: Desmoplastic fibroma: Case report and review of the literature. J Bone Joint Surg 58:126, 1976.

120. Simpson WA: Stafne's mandibular defect containing a pleomorphic adenoma: Report of case. J Oral Surg 23:533, 1965.

121. Slootweg PJ, Muller H: Malignant fibrous histiocytoma of the maxilla. Oral Surg 44:560, 1977.

122. Slootweg PJ, Müller H: Central fibroma of the jaw, odontogenic or desmoplastic. Oral Surg 56:61, 1983.

123. Smith TS, Schaberg SJ, Pierce GL, Collins JT: Chondrosarcoma of the maxilla. J Oral Maxillofac Surg 40:803, 1982.

124. Smith LC, Lane N, Rankow RN: Cylindroma—adenoid cystic carcinoma. A report of fifty-eight cases. Am J Surg 110:519, 1965.

125. Solomon MP, Sutton AL: Malignant fibrous histiocytoma of the soft tissues of the mandible. Oral Surg 35:653, 1973.

126. Soule E, Enriques P: Atypical fibrous histiocytoma, malignant fibrous histiocytoma, malignant histiocytoma, and epithelioid sarcoma. Cancer 30:128, 1972.

127. Spanier SS, Enneking WF, Enriquez P: Primary malignant fibrous histiocytoma of bone. Cancer 36:2084, 1975.

128. Spector GJ, Ogura JH: Malignant fibrous histiocytoma of the mandible. Plast Reconstr Surg 60:629, 1977.

129. Spiro RH, Huvos AG, Strong EW: Adenoid cystic carcinoma of salivary origin—a clinicopathologic study of 242 cases. Am J Surg 128:512, 1974.

130. Spjut HJ, Dorfman HD, Fechner RE, Ackerman LV: Tumors of bone and cartilage. In Atlas of Tumor Pathology. Series 2, Fascicle 5. Washington, D.C., Armed Forces Institute of Pathology, 1971, pp 216–229.

131. Stafne EC: Bone cavities situated near the angle of the mandible. J Am Dent Assoc 29:1969, 1942.

132. Stoll HC, Marchetta FC: Tumors of salivary gland origin presenting as primary jaw tumors. Oral Surg 10:1262, 1957.

133. Tanner HC Jr, Dahlin DC, Childs DS Jr: Sarcoma complicating fibrous dysplasia. Probable role of radiation therapy. Oral Surg 14:837, 1961.

134. Tefft M: Treatment of Ewing's sarcoma with radiation therapy. Int J Radiat Oncol Biol Phys 7:277, 1981.

135. Telles NC, Rabson AS, Pomeroy TC: Ewing's sarcoma: An autopsy study. Cancer 41:2321, 1978.

136. Thoma KH, Goldman HM: Oral Pathology. 5th ed. St. Louis, The C. V. Mosby Co., 1960, pp 1323–1343.

137. Toth BB, Byrne RP, Hinds EC: Central adenocarcinoma of the mandible. Oral Surg 39:436, 1975.

138. Van Sickels JE, Plotkin RJ, Hershman DL: Histiocytic lymphoma of the mandible. J Oral Surg 38:359, 1980.

139. Van Hale HM, Handlers JP, Abrams AM, Strahs G: Malignant fibrous histiocytoma, myxoid variant metastatic to the oral cavity. Oral Surg 51:156, 1981.

140. Vohra VG: Roentgen manifestations in Ewing's sarcoma: A study of 156 cases. Cancer 20:727, 1967.

141. Wagner JE, Lorandi CS, Ebling H: Desmoplastic fibroma of bone: A case in the mandible. Oral Surg 43:108, 1977.

142. Waldron CA, Schafer WG: The central giant cell reparative granuloma of the jaws: An analysis of 38 cases. Am J Clin Pathol 45:437, 1966.

143. Waldron CA: Giant cell tumors of the jaw bones. Oral Surg 6:1055, 1953.

144. Waldron CA: Familial incidence of bilateral giant cell tumors of jaw. Oral Surg 4:198, 1951.

145. Wang CC, Fleischli DJ: Primary reticulum-cell sarcoma of bone with emphasis on radiation therapy. Cancer 22:994, 1968.

146. Wang CC: Malignant lymphoma of Waldeyer's ring. Radiol 92:1335, 1969.

147. Ward GE: Tumors of the jaws. Oral Surg 5:675, 1952.

148. Webber W, Wienke E: Malignant fibrous histiocytoma of the mandible. Plast Reconstr Surg 60:629, 1977.

149. Weinfeld MS, Dudley HR Jr: Osteogenic sarcoma. J Bone Joint Surg 44:269, 1962.

150. Weiss SW, Enzinger FM: Malignant fibrous histiocytoma: An analysis of 200 cases. Cancer 41:2250, 1978.

151. Zimmerman DC, Dahlin DC, Stafne EC: Fibrous dysplasia of the maxilla and mandible. Oral Surg 11:55, 1958.

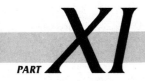

PART *XI*

Tumors of the Thyroid and Parathyroid Glands

CHAPTER 59

Clinical Evaluation of Thyroid Tumors

Robert L. Peake, M.D.

One of the most difficult problems associated with thyroid disease is the management of solitary thyroid nodules because (1) they are very common (up to 4 per cent of the population may be afflicted with nodular disease of the thyroid,[70, 71, 77, 78] (2) carcinomas of the thyroid are rare compared with benign disease (fewer than 10 per cent of nodules are carcinomas) and (3) most carcinomas of the thyroid are cured by early surgical removal.

Following the report by Cole and co-workers in 1945 that 24 per cent of solitary thyroid nodules were carcinomas at surgery,[13] debate raged through the medical literature for the next 15 to 20 years as to the true incidence of this finding: The point is often lost that prior to this time very few thyroidectomies had been performed to detect carcinomas and the incidence had been considered very low. Most subsequent reports from departments of surgery recorded an incidence of carcinoma of 10 to 40 per cent[11, 12, 15, 42, 44] and reports from internists recorded an incidence of 1 to 15 per cent.[7, 51, 69, 72, 81] The reasons for these great disparities were that surgeons tended to report only operated cases that had a pathologic diagnosis and cases were included in which carcinomas were found in the gland at sites other than the primary nodule. The most important factor for the higher incidence in the surgical series was the selection of patients for surgery according to their risk for carcinoma. On the other hand, reports from departments of medicine included patients in whom the nodule was determined to be benign by physical examination, scan, and clinical course; these nodules were not seen by the surgeons, nor was there histologic confirmation that the lesion was benign. Many studies excluded patients who had been found by physical examination to have obvious signs of cancer. Crile summarized these arguments by stating that either he could report the incidence of carcinoma in solitary nodules as 24.5 per cent or he would have to remove 6675 solitary nodules to prevent one patient from dying with thyroid carcinoma.[16] There was general agreement that the incidence of carcinoma in multinodular goiter was less than 5 per cent, but, again, histologic confirmation was often lacking.

It is now agreed that the incidence of carcinoma in nodular goiter is much less than 10 per cent because nodular goiter is very common and diagnosed thyroid carcinoma is rare (Table 59–1). As demonstrated in the table, careful autopsy studies indicate that the true incidence of carcinoma of the thyroid is probably higher but most of these lesions are occult sclerosing papillary carcinomas (less than 1.5 cm in diameter) and of little or no clinical significance. As Sampson stated: "Despite

TABLE 59–1. Incidence of Thyroid Nodules and Thyroid Carcinoma

	Per Million Population	Per Cent	Author
Clinical thyroid nodules	40,000	4	DeGroot and Stanbury, 1975[20]; Van Herle, 1982[80]; Martin, 1930[46]; Franzell and Foote, 1958[30]
New cases thyroid carcinoma	25–36/yr	0.003	DeGroot and Stanbury, 1975[19]
Death from thyroid carcinoma	3–6/yr	0.0005	DeGroot and Stanbury, 1975[19]; Silverberg, 1983[67]
Autopsy studies			
"Clinical" nodularity	60,000	4–8	Schlesinger, 1938[63]
Nodularity	300,000	20–40	Jaffe, 1930[43]; Hazard and Kauffman, 1952[37]; Mortensen et al., 1955[53]
Carcinoma			
Older studies	100–20,000	0.01–2	Schlesinger, 1938[63]; Hazard and Kauffman, 1952[37]; Mortensen, et al., 1955[53]
Omstead County, Minn.	57,000	5.7	Sampson et al., 1954[59]
Ann Arbor, Mich.	130,000	13.0	Nishigama et al., 1977[54]
Japanese	210,000	21.0	Sampson[60]

TABLE 59–2. Relative Incidence and Mortality from Thyroid Carcinoma*

Type of Carcinoma	Year 1983	New Cases (%)	Deaths	Deaths Due to Carcinoma (%)	Deaths As a Percentage of New Cases
All carcinomas	855,000	100.0	440,000	100.0	51.5
Thyroid	10,200	1.2	1,050	0.2	0.1
Lung	135,000	15.8	117,000	26.6	13.7
Breast (invasive)	114,900	13.4	37,500	8.5	4.4
Colon and rectum	126,000	14.7	58,100	13.2	6.8
Lip	4,600	0.5	175	0.04	0.02
Tongue	4,900	0.6	2,000	0.5	0.2
Other mouth conditions	9,800	1.1	2,775	0.6	0.3
Pharynx	7,800	0.9	4,200	1.0	0.5
Larynx	1,100	1.3	3,700	0.8	0.4

*Adapted from Silverberg E, Lubera JA: Ca 33:2, 1983.[67]

the relative frequency of local nodal metastasis in our series, 517 of 518 persons with an occult thyroid carcinoma reached the end of their life span without any awareness or manifestations of the presence of tumor."[61]

Because thyroid carcinoma can often be cured—or at least the patient is expected to have a very long survival if it is surgically removed (Table 59–2)—many authors have proposed surgical removal of all thyroid nodules. Others have felt that because of the slow-growing nature of well-differentiated thyroid carcinoma, patients can be observed for prolonged periods with or without thyroid hormone suppression before a decision is made for or against surgery. Again, the arguments can be vehement for either position, but most of us try to apply selection criteria with the hope that we can choose patients for surgery who have a higher risk of having thyroid carcinoma. (See "Patient Evaluation" later in this chapter.) In spite of our best efforts at this selection, only 20 to 40 per cent of patients undergoing surgery for thyroid nodules are found to have carcinoma. Fine-needle biopsy is a technique anticipated to improve this statistic, with the finding of carcinoma in 50 to 75 per cent of patients at surgery and a marked decrease in surgical removal of benign nodules.[35, 57] It is hoped that this will not be at the expense of carcinomas going undetected. (Fine-needle biopsy is discussed in detail under "Diagnostic Techniques" later in this chapter.)

ETIOLOGY, INCIDENCE, AND EPIDEMIOLOGY

The normal thyroid gland has a smooth external surface, but it may contain small foci of colloid-filled follicles or nodules. Even in "normal" thyroid glands, there are often a large number of nodules, both microscopic and macroscopic. In autopsy studies in humans, nodularity can be detected in 40 to 50 per cent of cases and appears to increase with age.[37, 43, 53] Similar changes were noted in the thyroids of aging mice, although the changes observed were in individual follicles and discrete nodularity was not commonly seen.[74] Nodularity that exceeds 1 cm in size can often be appreciated clinically. With the detection of more than one nodule, the names applied are *multinodular goiter*, *nontoxic nodular goiter*, or *adenomatous goiter* (Fig. 59–1). The inci-

dence of nodularity is two to four times more common in females than in males.

Iodine Deficiency

Because the incidence of nodular goiter has been noted to be higher in areas of the world where iodine is relatively deficient, it is tempting to speculate that a goiter is caused by periods of iodine deficiency or periods of increased requirement for thyroid hormone, i.e., during puberty, pregnancy, or other stressful episodes. The periods of relative hormone insufficiency

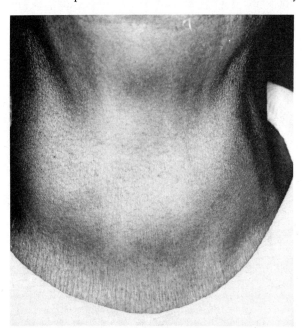

Figure 59–1. Photograph of a 58-year-old woman with a history of thyroid enlargement over 10 to 12 years. Growth had been slow but progressive. There was a strong family history for goiters, and some were proven to be Hashimoto's thyroiditis. On physical examination the thyroid was considered four to five times normal size with multiple nodular areas. Thyroid scan and antithyroid antibodies were compatible with a clinical diagnosis of Hashimoto's thyroiditis, and thyroid hormone in suppressive doses was initiated.

would lead to increased thyroid-stimulating hormone (TSH) and diffuse hyperplasia. The return of adequate iodine and normal thyroid hormone production could then lead to a decrease in thyroid gland hyperplasia, but it is not clear how this process leads to focal areas of colloid-filled modules.[26, 34, 75] Intermittent exposure to goitrogenic substances in the food or water supply could also result in a similar mechanism.[45] Other possible disorders include inherited defects in thyroid hormone synthesis[73] or autoimmune thyroid disease (Hashimoto's thyroiditis).[3] These disorders might exaggerate the hyperplasia-involution process by decreasing the ability of the gland to respond to relative iodine deficiency.

Similar lesions have been produced by alternating iodine-deficient and -sufficient diets in experimental animals.[26, 34] Prolonged and severe iodine deficiency and/or prolonged high dose goitrogen in animals leads to a very hyperplastic gland and then to adenomas that progress to tumors and have the appearance of papillary or follicular carcinoma. With even more prolonged stimulation, autonomous and anaplastic tumors can be produced with pulmonary metastases.[27, 55, 66, 90]

Thus, it is possible to build a historical and experimental case for the role of chronic iodine deficiency or goitrogen ingestion in the pathogenesis of colloid nodules and colloid multinodular goiter and even the development of thyroid neoplasia. This appears to be particularly true if the iodine insufficiency is intermittent and recurrent. Unfortunately, it is seldom possible to reconstruct these conditions in patients presenting with these problems. It is also difficult to explain the continued presence of these conditions in the United States, where the supply of iodine has been sufficient and possibly even excessive for almost 50 years.

Radiation in Childhood

The association between head and neck irradiation and thyroid carcinoma in children and young adults was first made in 1950 by Duffy and Fitzgerald.[22] Initially, radiation therapy was performed for an enlarged thymus gland and repeated respiratory infections, but more recent exposures have been for the treatment of enlarged tonsils and adenoids or for acne.[25]

In large recall studies of patients irradiated in this way, the actual incidence of carcinoma was 7 to 9 per cent, with a usual latent period before diagnosis of 10 to 20 years, and tumors were found as long as 30 years after irradiation.[25] Nodules of the thyroid or abnormalities on radionuclide scanning were found in approximately 27 per cent of patients screened. Nodules and adenomas are often multiple, the adenomas often appearing bizarre and atypical. Although the carcinomas found were usually small papillary tumors, and although death or significant metastatic disease was rare, 33 per cent of those patients sent to surgery for nodules were found to have carcinoma. More than 90 per cent of the tumors found were papillary or mixed papillary-follicular carcinomas, and 82 per cent were less than 1.5 cm in size. Forty-seven per cent of the tumors were multicentric, and this same incidence was found in sites other than the nodule for which surgery was performed. Thus, it is possible that the true incidence of carcinoma in irradiated patients may still be underestimated and more radical or near-total thyroidectomy in these indi-

viduals may be recommended for a tumor that is associated with very low mortality.[18]

External irradiation and radioactive iodine (^{131}I) have been employed both alone and in combination with long-term goitrogen to induce benign and malignant tumors of the thyroid. As previously noted, there appears to be a progression of tumors—from adenomas to invasive carcinomas initially dependent on excessive TSH to sustain their growth, to autonomous, metastasizing carcinomas.[21, 29]

Again, it is difficult to extrapolate these experimental results regarding neoplasia to the pathogenesis of clinical thyroid neoplasia except when we refer to the period following atomic explosions in Japan[59] or the Marshall Islands.[14] No increased incidence of thyroid neoplasia was noted in a screening study of children in Utah following lesser exposures to radiation.[85] It remains possible, however, that our increasing exposure to increasing industrial and medical uses of radiation will replace iodine deficiency in the continued pathogenesis of thyroid neoplasia.

CLASSIFICATION AND STAGING OF CARCINOMA OF THE THYROID

The TNM classification for carcinoma of the thyroid is shown in Table 59–3.[36] Although this classification may be useful in collecting data on carcinoma of the thyroid and in comparing thyroid cancers to other types of cancer, I do not believe that this system is useful for clinical or therapeutic decisions unless it is modified by determining the predominant tumor type. Since each of the thyroid tumors has an expected or usual clinical course and metastatic pattern, one must first make decisions on this basis and it is impossible to lump these tumors as "thyroid cancer." To omit doing this frequently leads to overaggressive and unnecessary treatment of papillary carcinoma and, potentially, to undertreatment of more aggressive tumors.

In other words, it would be foolhardy (1) to compare

TABLE 59–3. TNM Clinical Classification of Thyroid Cancer

T—Primary Tumor
  T0—No palpable tumor
  T1—Single tumor confined to the gland. No deformity
  T2—Multiple tumors or single tumor producing deformity of the gland
  T3—Tumor extending beyond the gland

N—Regional Lymph Nodes
  N0—No palpable nodes
  N1—Movable homolateral nodes
    N1a—Nodes not considered to contain growth
    N1b—Nodes considered to contain growth
  N2—Movable contralateral or bilateral nodes
    N2a—Nodes not considered to contain growth
    N2b—Nodes considered to contain growth
  N3—Fixed nodes

M—Distant Metastases
  M0—No evidence of distant metastases
  M1—Distant metastases present

TABLE 59–4. Classification of Thyroid Carcinoma According to Histologic Type

Carcinoma Type	Metastases		Surgical Treatment	^{131}I Follow-up and Treatment	Prognosis
	Local	*Distant*			
Papillary*	Very common	Rare and late	Lobectomy or near-total	Seldom useful	Excellent
Follicular*	Rare	Common	Near-total or total	Beneficial	Good
Medullary	Common	Common	Total	Not indicated	Long-term survival
Anaplastic	Common	Common	Usually not beneficial; x-ray therapy	Not beneficial	Poor

*Mixed papillary and follicular carcinomas are common tumors and follow the course of the predominant tumor type, usually papillary.

an anaplastic or a medullary carcinoma with lymph node metastases without demonstrable distant metastases (yet) to a papillary carcinoma with lymph node metastases or (2) to state that an invasive follicular carcinoma without demonstrable cervical lymph node or distant metastases has a better prognosis than a papillary carcinoma with lymph node metastases. The TNM classification can be used if it is modified and interpreted in view of the expected course for an individual tumor type.

A classification that is more useful clinically involves separating thyroid carcinomas according to their predominant histologic type and defining their clinical course, treatment, and prognosis on this basis (Table 59–4). Exceptions to the clinical course do occur, but they are so rare that one should not modify therapy on this basis. Mixed papillary and follicular carcinomas are common, but they can be expected to behave as the predominant tumor type. I will not attempt to delve into the controversies and relative benefits of different approaches to therapy (such as whether to give ^{131}I) and will leave this for complete discussions in other sections of this book. Instead, I will present my opinions regarding the preoperative, operative, and postoperative decisions one must make.

Papillary Carcinoma

Papillary carcinoma is the most common type of tumor, accounting for approximately 60 per cent of all thyroid cancers and the most common type of tumor associated with irradiation of the head and neck in childhood. This association may account for the fact that this tumor has its peak incidence in the third or fourth decade of life (Figs. 59–2 and 59–3). The tumor is also common in young persons who have not had a history of irradiation. It is said to be more aggressive with a higher mortality when found after the age of 40.[8, 47, 48] This is most probably because the tumor has been present for 10 to 20 years at the time of diagnosis; thus there are more invasive tumors in this older age group,[28] and the increased aggressiveness with age may be an artifact.

Younger individuals usually present with a solitary nodule or lump that is noted on routine or self-examination (Fig. 59–4) or with a metastatic node. Papillary carcinomas metastasize to cervical lymph nodes. They are commonly multicentric, particularly in those individuals who received radiation during childhood. Distant metastases to lung, bone, and other tissues do

occur, but they are rare and are found late in the course of the disease.

Survival

Life expectancy does not differ significantly from age-adjusted survival (Fig. 59–5) and it is not adversely altered unless the tumor has invaded the capsule of the thyroid gland and, accordingly, other structures in the neck. These invasive tumors are seldom completely resectable (Fig. 59–6). In contrast to most other carci-

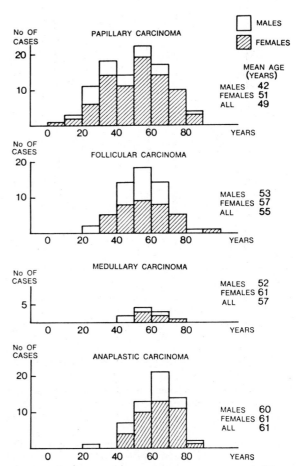

Figure 59–2. Age and sex distribution of patients with different types of thyroid carcinoma. (From Franssila K: Acta Pathol Microbiol Scand (Suppl 225), Section A, 1971.[28])

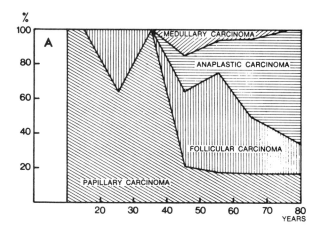

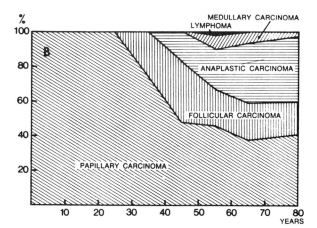

Figure 59–3. Percentage distribution of cases (see Figure 59–2) into histologic types of thyroid cancer in different age groups. (*A*) Distribution for males. (*B*) Distribution for females. (From Franssila K: Acta Pathol Microbiol Scand (Suppl 225), Section A, 1971.[28])

nomas (e.g., breast, stomach, kidney), the presence or absence of lymph node metastases in papillary carcinoma does not appear to affect survival.

Treatment

The treatment of choice for papillary carcinoma is surgical resection. How extensive and how much risk of hypoparathyroidism is acceptable are matters of much debate. In my opinion, total thyroidectomy should not be performed for papillary carcinoma. A near-total thyroidectomy with ipsilateral lobectomy and preservation of the contralateral posterior capsule is probably the treatment of choice if it is performed by a surgeon experienced in this technique who can give 90 to 95 per cent assurance of preservation of parathyroid function. If this cannot be assured, ipsilateral lobectomy and isthmusectomy constitute the treatment of choice when there is no obvious contralateral nodularity at the time of surgery. Many studies have reported no difference in mortality with this more conservative surgical appraoch.[9, 28, 76, 83, 88] Hypoparathyroidism—with continued dangers for hypo- or hypercalcemia, its requirement for frequent and continuous medical follow-up (serum calcium should be determined every 1 to 3 months), and

possible long-term complications (e.g., cataracts, nephrocalcinosis, severe hypo- or hypercalcemia)—is most probably a worse disease with which to live than is papillary carcinoma of the thyroid.

In this same vein, I prefer not to follow or to treat these patients with radioactive iodine. The use of ^{131}I dictates a total thyroidectomy or the use of large doses to destroy residual thyroid tissue in the neck so that one can possibly find metastatic papillary carcinoma. In my experience, papillary carcinoma almost never concentrates the isotope; thus, one exposes the patient to the risks of total thyroidectomy or large doses of radioiodine for a therapeutic procedure that cannot be shown to affect mortality.[47] Recurrences were found to be decreased by ^{131}I therapy, but most of these recurrences were local in the neck and most probably represented residual tumor present at the time of the original surgery. These were usually easily removed surgically without affecting life expectancy.

Papillary carcinoma of the thyroid is a unique tumor that grows so slowly that it seldom results in the death of the patient, and it is thus difficult to show any advantage for any one therapy except for excision of the tumor and grossly involved nodes. More radical surgery or radioiodine does not improve survival and may lead to unnecessary morbidity.

Thyroid hormone in fully suppressive doses should always be administered even after partial thyroidectomy. These tumors are considered TSH-dependent, and the use of thyroid hormone does decrease both recurrences and mortality.[47] Two subclasses of papillary carcinoma deserve special mention.

Occult Papillary Carcinoma

Ranging from microscopic lesions to some that are 1.5 cm in size, these tumors are often incidental findings when thyroidectomy is performed for another reason.

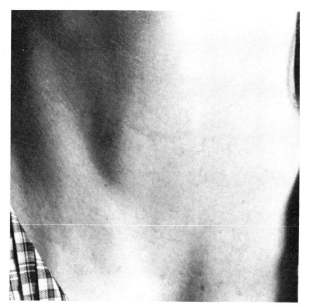

Figure 59–4. Solitary thyroid nodule in a 26-year-old man. The nodule had been noted on routine physical examination a year before, but no growth had been noted in the interval. This patient is further depicted in Figures 59–11 and 59–12.

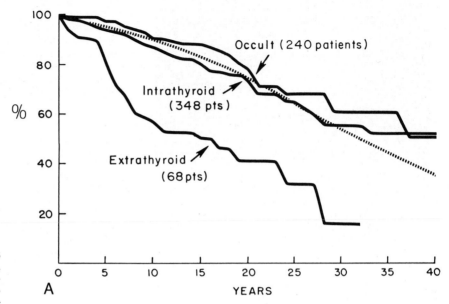

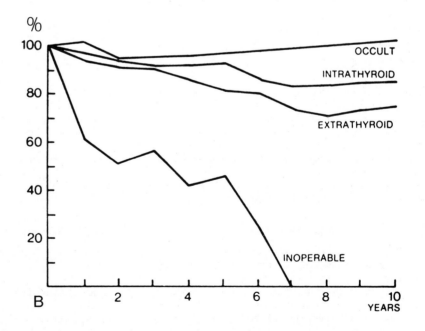

Figure 59–5. Relative survival curves for patients with papillary carcinoma. (*A*) Results in 656 patients. (Extrathyroid indicates direct extension of tumor through the thyroid capsule; most patients had metastases to lymph nodes.) (From Woolner LB, et al: *In* Young S, Inman DR (eds): Thyroid Neoplasia. New York, Academic Press, 1968.[88]) (*B*) Results in 97 patients. (From Franssila K: Acta Pathol Microbiol Scand (Suppl 225), Section A, 1971.[28])

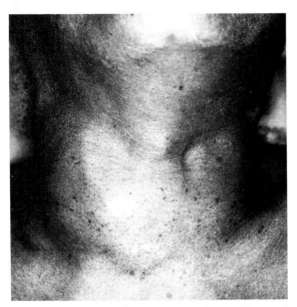

Figure 59–6. A 53-year-old man presented with a history of a thyroid nodule for 4 to 5 years. Within the last 1 to 2 years, there has been definite enlargement, and the patient has experienced ongoing hoarseness. Hard cervical adenopathy was present above the mass. Diagnosis: Invasive papillary carcinoma of the thyroid.

Although these tumors may frequently metastasize to regional nodes, they cause little change in life expectancy and are best treated with lobectomy and removal of ipsilateral involved nodes.[28, 60, 88]

Extracapsular and Inoperable Thyroid Carcinoma

These tumors at the time of original surgery have extended through the capsule of the thyroid gland and thus into vital structures in the neck. Usually, they are not completely resectable or biopsy is done only for diagnosis. These tumors account for most of the mortality from papillary carcinoma within the first 5 years.[83] More aggressive surgical treatment is often attempted, but residual tumor must be left behind. External radiotherapy and/or ^{131}I can often extend life expectancy and change the cause of death in this category.

Follicular Carcinoma

Follicular carcinoma is slightly more malignant than papillary carcinoma and accounts for approximately 30 per cent of all carcinomas of the thyroid gland.[10] It occurs later in life than the papillary type and has a peak incidence in the fifth and sixth decades (Figs. 59–2 and 59–3). It presents as a solitary nodule. The major dilemma is that of differentiation from the follicular adenoma on fine-needle biopsy, on frozen section examination, or even after examination of multiple permanent sections through the capsule of the tumor. Diagnosis of malignancy depends on the demonstration of blood vessel invasion (capsule of the tumor) or invasion of the tumor capsule itself with tumor replacing normal thyroid tissue. Note that this is tumor capsule

invasion, whereas with papillary carcinoma the capsule of the thyroid itself is the important factor in survival. In follicular carcinoma the degree of invasion of the tumor capsule appears to be the most important factor in survival.[28, 88, 89]

Follicular carcinoma metastasizes primarily by the hematogenous route and seldom spreads to the cervical lymph nodes. Survival rates for the various types of follicular carcinoma are shown in Fig. 59–7. The tumor and its metastases usually do concentrate ^{131}I, but usually not until all normal thyroid is removed or destroyed. For these reasons, opinion is more uniform that total or near-total thyroidectomy is the initial treatment of choice with follow-up treatment using [131]I. Thyroid hormone in suppressive doses is mandatory in this tumor also. Following are three important subgroups of follicular carcinoma.

Noninvasive or Microinvasive Tumors

Noninvasive or microinvasive follicular carcinoma can be diagnosed only by examination for blood vessel and tumor capsule invasion on multiple permanent sections. Rarely can this diagnosis be made with confidence on frozen section at the time of surgery. One is then faced with a two-stage thyroidectomy or the use of very large doses of radioiodine to destroy the remaining normal thyroid. If one examines survival (Fig. 59–7), it is difficult to justify further surgery; however, it must be realized that a significant percentage (possibly 20 to 30 per cent) of these persons will have a significant recurrence or distant metastases or will die of this tumor over the next 10 to 20 years. It is not possible to identify those with distant metastases without completing the total thyroidectomy and total body scanning with [131]I.

At this point it is necessary to examine and treat the whole patient—taking into consideration age and life expectancy without follicular carcinoma. Usually, this will weigh in favor of total thyroidectomy and ^{131}I follow-up and treatment with the risk of hypoparathyroidism or recurrent laryngeal nerve damage accepted. It is impossible to fault those who look at the survival curve and elect not to complete the thyroidectomy until or if evidence of distant spread is manifest by follow-up chest x-ray examination, serial liver and bone enzymes, and possibly bone scans. This may be late for those patients with distant metastases, but it avoids the risk for those without these lesions.

Invasive Tumors

Invasive follicular carcinoma can usually be diagnosed by spread through the tumor capsule or by the inability to define a capsule on frozen section; even if this condition is not diagnosed until permanent sections are available, near-total or total thyroidectomy is the treatment of choice. Total body scanning at 2, 6, and 12 months with ^{131}I treatment of residual thyroid or distant metastases is then required. Thyroid hormone in doses sufficient to suppress TSH is mandatory. In spite of this treatment, most of these patients succumb over the next 10 to 20 years and account for most of the mortality from differentiated (papillary and follicular) thyroid carcinoma.

A special instance is the patient who presents with a

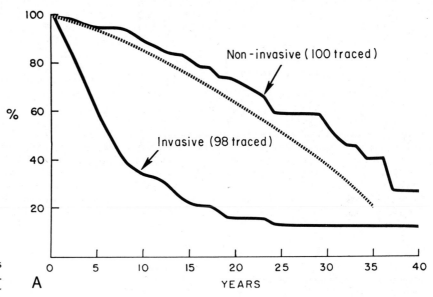

Figure 59–7. Relative survival in patients with follicular carcinoma of the thyroid. (*A*) Results in 198 patients. (From Woolner LB, et al: *In* Young S, Inman DR (eds): Thyroid Neoplasia. New York, Academic Press, 1968.[88]) (*B*) Results in 60 patients. (From Franssila K: Acta Pathol Microbiol Scand (Suppl 225), Section A, 1971.[28])

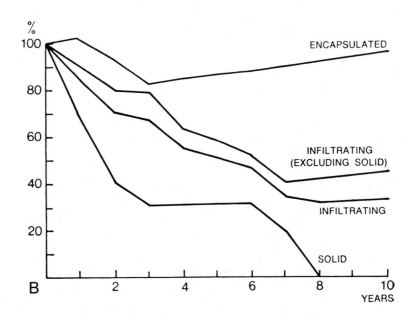

distant metastasis to lung or bone. Even then, if the patient's general health will permit it, survival will be prolonged by thyroidectomy and ^{131}I treatment.

Hürthle Cell Tumors

Hürthle cell tumors exist as both adenomas and carcinomas. It may be extremely difficult to distinguish the benign from malignant varieties, and one may have to follow the patient for the development of distant metastases to be certain. Once this determination has been made, treatment is usually the same as for invasive follicular carcinoma.

Medullary Carcinoma

Medullary carcinoma was first described and characterized in 1959 by Hazard and co-workers.[38] Prior to then, the tumor probably had been classified as an anaplastic carcinoma and accounted for those patients with a survival greater than 1 to 2 years. Medullary carcinoma develops from the parafollicular or C-cells of the thyroid,[86] and thyrocalcitonin serves as a diagnostic marker and means of follow-up.[39, 49] The tumor develops both sporadically and as a familial tumor usually but not always as a part of multiple endocrine adenomatosis syndromes (MEA types IIa and IIb). The components of this familial syndrome are medullary carcinoma, pheochromocytomas, parathyroid hyperplasia, and (in MEA IIb) mucosal neuromas. An intractable diarrhea frequently accompanies metastatic medullary carcinoma.[40, 50]

Sporadic cases usually occur beyond the age of 50, whereas the familial variety is diagnosed much earlier because of studies of the families with pentagastrin-stimulated thyrocalcitonin secretion.[39, 50] The tumor is multifocal, and particularly in the familial variety C-cell hyperplasia may precede or coexist with tumor development.[87]

The tumor spreads to regional nodes and it spreads hematogenously. Survival is usually prolonged over 10

to 20 years (Fig. 59–8). Total thyroidectomy may be curative, and the use of thyrocalcitonin measurements gives a very sensitive method of detecting distant metastatic disease.

Anaplastic Carcinoma

Fortunately, anaplastic carcinoma is the rarest of thyroid carcinomas (less than 5 per cent), developing late in life. It is usually fatal within 6 to 12 months (Fig. 59–9). The history usually reveals that the tumor mass has arisen over a 3- to 6-month period and the mass has extended from the clavicle to the mandible over this period of time (Fig. 59–10). Sometimes, a previous nodule has been present for years, or one finds an area of differentiated carcinoma within the tumor, implying that the tumor transformed from a pre-existing differentiated carcinoma.[58] This remains a matter of debate.

The diagnosis can usually be established by needle biopsy and x-ray therapy initiated immediately. Except for the possibility of a tracheostomy, surgery is of little or no benefit. Although x-ray therapy is only palliative, it is extremely important because it shrinks and decreases the rate of growth of the neck tumor, thus allowing the patient to die from distant metastases. Chemotherapy can be initiated after x-ray treatment, but there is no agent that gives more than a temporary remission.

PATIENT EVALUATION

Most commonly the patient presents because of a "lump" or a nodule in the neck that has been noted during routine physical examination or during shaving or putting on makeup (Fig. 59–4). Usually the nodule will be freely movable on swallowing. Thyroid nodules are usually asymptomatic, and the patient is clinically euthyroid. Knowing the consistency of the nodule is only rarely helpful because most are firm to hard; occasionally a nodule will be so hard that carcinoma is

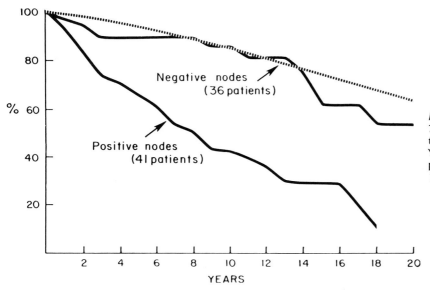

Figure 59–8. Relative survival curves in 77 patients with medullary carcinoma of the thyroid. (From Woolner LB, et al: *In* Young S, Inman DR (eds): Thyroid Neoplasia. New York, Academic Press, 1968.[88])

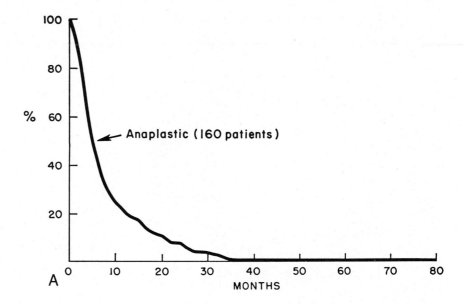

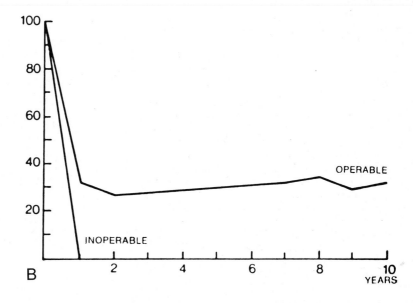

Figure 59–9. Relative survival curves in patients with anaplastic carcinoma of the thyroid. (*A*) Results in 160 patients. (From Woolner LB, et al: In Young S, Inman DR (eds): Thyroid Neoplasia. New York, Academic Press, 1968.[88]) (*B*) Results in 58 patients. (From Franssila K: Acta Pathol Microbiol Scand (Suppl 225), Section A, 1971.[28])

obvious or so soft that a cystic lesion is suspected. A careful examination of the neck for abnormal lymph nodes in the cervical chain above the thyroid, the area of the isthmus, and the supraclavicular areas should be made.

Physical Examination

Examination of the thyroid gland is a part of a general medical examination. Conduct the inspection from the front of the patient. The patient's chin should be in the normal position or slightly raised. Ask the patient to swallow. Diffuse thyroid enlargement can often be visualized as the thyroid is elevated by deglutition. Thyroid nodules can be appreciated by asymmetry in the neck on swallowing.

Palpation of the thyroid can be performed from in front or behind the patient. Initial examination from the front is preferred. Begin with the promontory of the thyroid cartilage, and move the fingers down in the midline. One encounters soft tissue anterior to the cartilage of the trachea; this is the thyroid isthmus. The isthmus is palpable in most normal individuals. After encountering the isthmus, follow it laterally until the lateral lobes are encountered. In most normal persons, very little of the lateral lobes will be palpable; however, in thin individuals, they may be palpable without signifying thyroid enlargement. The normal isthmus usually overlies the first tracheal rings, but it may cross the bottom of the thyroid cartilage and may be confused with visible thyroid enlargement.

Moving behind the patient, reach forward with both

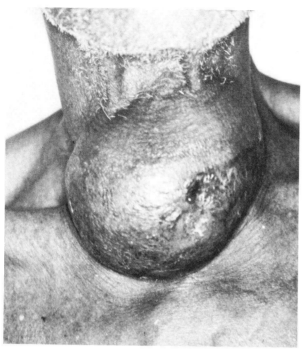

Figure 59–10. An 87-year-old man presented with a history of a rapidly growing tumor mass in the neck over a 5- to 6-month period. A hard vascular mass was noted with little movement on swallowing. Diagnosis: Anaplastic carcinoma of the thyroid confirmed by fine-needle biopsy. Radiation therapy was initiated.

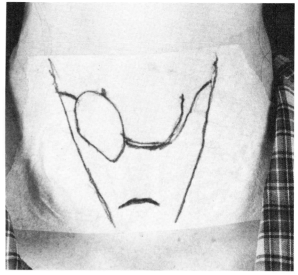

Figure 59–11. Paper tape tracing of thyroid nodule in a 26-year-old man (see Figure 59–4). The thyroid cartilage, isthmus lateral lobes, and sternocleidomastoid muscles are also shown.

hands, identifying the isthmus and lateral lobes as just described. Again, ask the patient to swallow, and the thyroid will pass under the fingers. The left lateral lobe can be best palpated by gently displacing the trachea with the right hand and palpating the left lobe through the sternocleidomastoid with the left hand during swallowing. Repeat this maneuver for the right lobe. Appreciation of slight (one and one-half to two times) thyroid enlargement requires a great deal of experience.

Examine the carotid area carefully for enlarged, hard lymph nodes. The supraclavicular areas should be examined as well. Lymph nodes in the area above the isthmus may also be involved early with metastatic carcinoma. There can be confusion here with a pyramidal lobe, a triangular area of thyroid tissue arising from either the right or left side of the isthmus and pointing toward the midline. The pyramidal lobe is often palpable, with conditions associated with diffuse thyroid enlargement; this finding may be confused with nodules. Small cysts are common in this area also as remnants of the thyroglossal duct.

A useful technique in the observation and follow-up of thyroid nodules is the use of *paper tape tracings* of the nodule size. This technique was adopted from the report of Blum and Rothschild,[5] and examples are shown in Figures 59–11 and 59–12. The tracing can then become a part of the patient's record and is very useful in evaluating for change in size, in referring patients, or in following the long-term course of nodules treated medically or by observation even by multiple examiners. A definite increase in size (>0.5 cm) without pain should probably necessitate surgery. Changes of this magnitude are very difficult to appreciate without the tape tracing.

Treatment Decisions

For many years we have searched for rules that will allow us to select for *surgery* the patients more likely to harbor carcinoma and *observation* or thyroid *hormone suppression* for the others. For example:

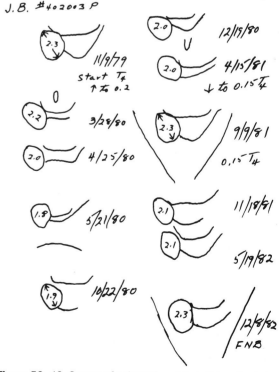

Figure 59–12. Course of a thyroid nodule in the patient shown in Figures 59–4 and 59–11. The nodule was originally warm to scan, solid to ultrasound, and was eventually benign upon fine-needle biopsy. These changes are consistent with a degenerating colloid nodule.

1. All solitary nodules should be removed, and multinodular glands can be observed.

2. Nodules that do not clearly decrease in size after 2 to 18 months of thyroid hormone in suppressive doses should be surgically removed.

3. Nodules that are "cold" to radionuclide scanning (and more recently, solid to ultrasound) should be surgically removed.

With the absolute use of any of these rules, the incidence of carcinoma at surgery would be less than 20 per cent and probably less than 10 per cent and many patients would have unnecessary surgery. The relief that comes in finding that the lesion is benign usually causes both the patient and the physician to avoid asking whether the surgery was really necessary.

These rules also do not take into account the age of the patient, the type of tumor one might expect, the relative risk of surgery, and the presence of coexisting disease that might otherwise limit the life expectancy of the patient or increase the risk of surgery. All of these factors must be considered in the decision for or against surgery.

Although some authors have proposed surgery for all nodules, others have felt that because of the slow growth and good prognosis for most thyroid carcinomas, a period of *observation* and *thyroid suppression* could be recommended for almost all patients. Most of us have attempted to select those patients most likely to have a carcinoma for immediate surgery. In other cases, when carcinoma is unlikely or when there is significant coexisting disease, we choose to observe with or without thyroid hormone suppression. With wider use of the fine-needle biopsy (described later), an even better categorization of risk is possible and it is hoped that fewer patients with benign disease will be sent to surgery.

Factors in Decision-Making

Some factors that currently weigh into this decision will now be discussed. One important factor is the *history of a change in size*. The longer a nodule has been present without change, the more likely it is benign. Although thyroid nodules usually change very slowly, it has always been surprising how many nodules seem to grow from the time of the initial examination to the visit with a consultant a few days later.

Pain. The *sudden onset of pain and tenderness* within a nodule is usually a good sign that it is benign and indicates a recent hemorrhage into a colloid nodule. Carcinomas and adenomas may also grow beyond their blood supply and become hemorrhagic and necrotic, but this is usually a more gradual process and is painless. Nodules that are noted because of a recent onset of localized pain and tenderness can often be observed to decrease in size over the next few weeks or months and may even disappear.

Age and Sex. The age and sex of the patient have often been used to indicate an increased likelihood of carcinoma in children and males younger than 40 years of age in contrast to females. Even in these groups, the majority of nodules considered at "increased risk for carcinoma" will still be benign and the increased risk is more the result of greatly increased incidence of benign nodular disease in females.

Previous Radiation. The history of childhood irradiation to the head and neck calls for a careful thyroid examination and probably a baseline thyroid scan. The finding of an abnormality in either of these examinations can produce great anxiety, which can often only be alleviated by surgery. As already discussed, the incidence of benign nodularity is greatly increased in these patients; the incidence of carcinoma is 7 to 9 per cent. Almost all of the carcinomas are of the occult sclerosing variety, and almost half of the carcinomas found are at a site within the gland other than the nodule for which surgery is performed.[25] These observations make one pause in the decision for surgery, particularly since it involves a total or near total thyroidectomy for a nonfatal lesion. They also raise concerns about how many carcinomas are present in the screened populations or exposed individuals who did not have palpable or scan abnormalities and what the course of this undiscovered disease will be.

Another screening study, not commonly quoted, involved paired examinations of irradiated and non-irradiated individuals. These investigators were unable to demonstrate a significant increase in either nodular disease or carcinoma in the irradiated patients.[56] This again indicates that nodular disease of the thyroid is very common, carcinoma is rare, and the risk of carcinoma from childhood irradiation may be overestimated.

Adenopathy. Pathologic or hard cervical adenopathy is a very useful sign of thyroid malignancy. If it is associated with a nodule in the thyroid or ipsilateral cold area on the scan, thyroid malignancy is very likely. Occasionally no nodularity is observed, the scan is normal, and the diagnosis is established by biopsy of the lymph node. As already discussed and in contrast to other types of cancer, metastases to cervical lymph nodes in papillary carcinoma do not adversely affect prognosis. Medullary or anaplastic carcinoma may also present with pathologic cervical adenopathy, but it usually is associated with an equally impressive thyroid mass.

Other Symptoms. Other signs of possible malignancy such as *hoarseness, dysphagia,* or *dyspnea* are late signs of malignancy and usually indicate that the tumor has extended through the thyroid capsule, that it has invaded other structures in the neck, and that the tumor will not be completely resectable. Rarely, dysphagia or dyspnea may also be seen with large benign goiters.

The history of *intractable and severe diarrhea,* or the presence of mucosal *neuromas* on the tongue associated with a thyroid nodule, should arouse the suspicion of a medullary carcinoma. The family history of death from thyroid cancer (when the type may not be known) or pheochromocytoma should also suggest this tumor.[40, 50]

Hormone Suppression

Thyroid hormone to suppress TSH is no longer commonly used in our clinic for the differential diagnosis of malignancy. Although multiple benign nodules may decrease significantly in size if treated with 0.2 to 0.3 of L-thyroxin (or equivalent) for periods of 6 months to 2 years,[33, 64] this has not been our experience or that of others.[20, 32] Most cold nonfunctioning nodules remain the same size for long periods. It is our feeling that more patients than nodules will disappear in 2 years.

Instead, we attempt to assess the risk of carcinoma on the initial examination (now employing fine-needle biopsy as well) and make a decision for or against surgery. Thyroid hormone in suppressive doses is usually given as therapy with the hope that it might prevent further growth or the development of further nodularity, but not to assess the risk of malignancy.

DIAGNOSTIC TECHNIQUES

The measurement of circulating thyroid hormones and thyroid-binding proteins (serum thyroxin, triiodothyronine (T_3), T_3 resin sponge uptake), and TSH, although excellent tests for determining thyroid function abnormalities, are of so little help in evaluating the usual patient with a thyroid nodule that they should probably be contraindicated. If the clinical examination gives no hint of hyper- or hypothyroidism, these tests are seldom useful because the nodule represents a very small part of the gland and the thyroid-pituitary axis is intact. It will probably never be possible to cease the reflex response of ordering thyroid function studies in the evaluation of the patient with a nodule.

X-ray Examination

Routine x-ray of the neck may sometimes show calcifications in association with a thyroid nodule. These may represent microscopic psammoma bodies that are so numerous as to show a faint, speckled, or cloudy density in the area of the nodule. This finding usually requires soft-tissue films and image intensification, and it seldom is used as a routine diagnostic test. The presence of dense concentric calcification in the nodule usually indicates that the lesion is benign, but it does not totally exclude carcinoma. Tracheal deviation and the presence of substernal goiter on chest films are usually signs of the size of the thyroid gland, but they do not help to determine whether the lesion is benign or malignant.

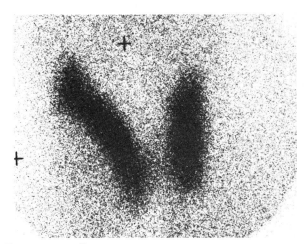

Figure 59–14. $^{99m}TcO_4$ Thyroid scan of a 45-year-old woman who had a thyroid nodule for 3 years. The nodule had been increasing in size, and dysphagia was present. A 2.5 × 4.5 cm mass was noted in the right lobe, but pathologic adenopathy was absent. A fine-needle biopsy proved inconclusive. This was a highly cellular follicular tumor, with minimal atypia. Diagnosis: Follicular carcinoma of the thyroid treated by total thyroidectomy and ^{131}iodine.

Radionuclide Scans

Radionuclide scanning with ^{131}I, ^{123}I, or technetium-labeled pertechnetate ($^{99m}TcO_4$) has been commonly used in the evaluation of thyroid nodules (Figs. 59–13 through 59–17). The advantages and disadvantages of the different isotopes will be covered in the chapter on nuclear medicine (Chapter 61). Nodules must be larger than 1 to 2 cm to be discriminated on the scan. If the nodule is cold, i.e., fails to concentrate the isotope (Figs. 59–14 and 59–15), there is an increased likelihood that it is a carcinoma; in truth, however, virtually 100 per cent of

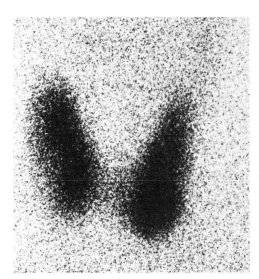

Figure 59–13. $^{99m}TcO_4$ Thyroid scan of a 57-year-old woman with a possible thyroid nodule not confirmed by other examiners. The thyroid scan was normal.

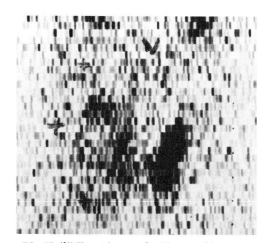

Figure 59–15. ^{131}I Thyroid scan of a 64-year-old woman with a thyroid nodule for "many years." No symptoms were present. Physical examination revealed two 3 × 3 cm nodules in the right lobe that moved with swallowing, and cervical adenopathy was absent. Fine-needle biopsy and aspiration revealed 2 to 3 cm of hemorrhagic fluid with colloid and iron-laden macrophages. Benign follicular cells were also seen. Diagnosis: Colloid nodules—adenomatous goiter.

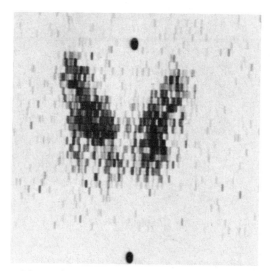

Figure 59–16. [131]I Thyroid scan of a 47-year-old woman with a 3-month history of thyroid enlargement noted by a relative. She was euthyroid, and the thyroid was diffusely enlarged, two to three times normal. Radioimmunologic assay for antithyroglobulin antibodies was positive. The scan shows patchy uptake throughout both lobes. Clinical diagnosis: Hashimoto's thyroiditis.

carcinomas are cold, 85 to 90 per cent of benign nodules are also cold, and more than 90 per cent of nodules are benign—thus radioisotope scanning helps us only occasionally in determining whether a lesion is benign or malignant. Only if the nodule concentrates the isotope to a greater or equal degree with the remainder of the gland does one have assurance that the lesion is benign.

Hot nodules (Fig. 59–17) account for fewer than 10 per cent of scans, and many of these patients are hyperthyroid (by clinical evaluation or by serum measurements of thyroid hormones) and also demonstrate suppression of the remainder of the gland. Although radionuclide scanning remains a routine part of the work-up of thyroid nodules at this time, the more widespread use and experience with fine-needle biopsy should relegate the scan to a secondary test, performed only when the needle biopsy shows a follicular lesion-adenoma or possible carcinoma. For a more detailed analysis of the cost comparison of needle biopsy with scanning or ultrasound, see the article by Van Herle.[80]

Ultrasound

Ultrasonography (Figs. 59–18 through 59–22) has proved to be useful in distinguishing solid from cystic nodules, and simple cysts from complex or mixed solid cystic lesions. This technique can give a better approximation of nodule size than either physical examination or radionuclide scanning.[2, 62, 80] The simple cyst, espe-

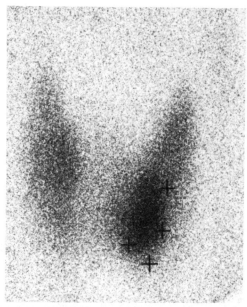

Figure 59–17. [99m]TcO$_4$ Thyroid scan of a 65-year-old woman with a 2 × 2 cm nodule in the left lobe of the thyroid. Clinical and laboratory results proved her to be euthyroid. The scan shows a functioning (hot) nodule in the left lobe with incomplete suppression of the remainder of the thyroid. Diagnosis: Functioning adenoma of the thyroid.

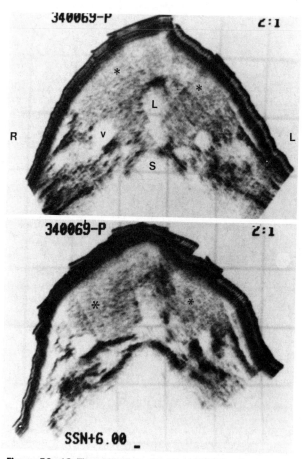

Figure 59–18. Thyroid enlargement in a 38-year-old asymptomatic woman. The patient's thyroid had been enlarged since childhood. Physical examination revealed asymmetric enlargement (the right being greater than the left) of the gland, which was considered three times normal size. Radioisotope scan confirmed diffuse enlargement without cold areas. Transverse echotomograms revealed diffuse enlargement (asterisks). Texture was homogeneous without focal defects. L = Larynx; S = spine; V = vessel; R = right; L = left.

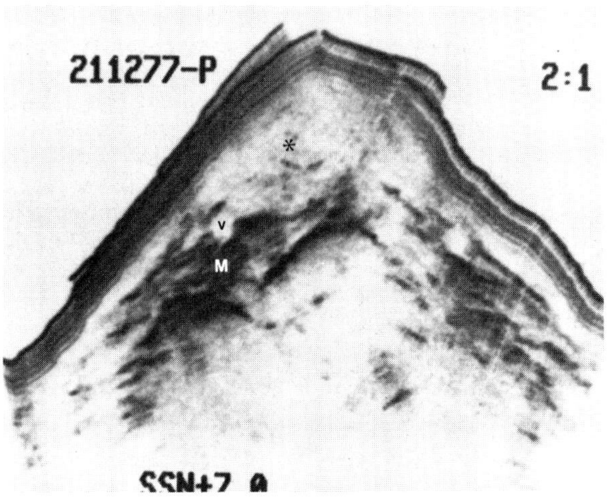

Figure 59–19. This 39-year-old woman has had a 3-cm nodule in the right lobe of the thyroid since 1973. By 1977, the nodule had increased to 4 or 5 cm. Fine-needle biopsy was interpreted as inconclusive, showing fetal or microfollicular adenoma without malignant changes. Transverse echotomograms show a solid nodule (asterisk) in the right lobe. Surgical diagnosis: Benign follicular adenoma. V = vessel; M = muscle.

cially if it is smaller than 4 cm in size, can be assumed to be benign with 96 to 98 per cent accuracy. Because adenomas and carcinomas, especially larger lesions, may undergo cystic degeneration (Fig. 59–21), the larger cystic lesions and complex cysts may be carcinoma in 20 to 25 per cent of the cases. With more routine use of fine-needle biopsy of both cystic and solid nodules, prebiopsy ultrasound may not be necessary and may be reserved for situations in which the biopsy or examination of cyst fluid is suspicious.[80]

Serum Measurements

The measurement of serum thyroglobulin has been useful in detecting residual or metastatic thyroid carcinoma.[79] However, the test has not been helpful in the differentiation of benign from malignant disease or in screening persons who have had head and neck irradiation. One reason may be that many benign thyroid diseases have increased thyroglobulin and small carcinomas localized to the thyroid often do not have elevated thyroglobulin levels.[4, 65]

Thyrocalcitonin levels are very useful in the diagnosis of medullary carcinoma as a means of follow-up for residual or metastatic tumor and for screening of family members for this tumor with the use of pentagastrin stimulation.[39, 40, 50] The relative rarity of this tumor in regard to the frequency of thyroid nodules would make the routine screening of patients with nodules unnecessarily costly unless there is diarrhea, a family history, or some other reason to suspect medullary carcinoma. The dilemma of the patient with proven medullary carcinoma and an elevated thyrocalcitonin without demonstrable residual tumor or metastases is complex and troublesome. Because of the usual long life expectancy with this tumor, I have not favored chemotherapy until metastatic disease is evident or symptomatic.

Biopsy

Fine-needle biopsy of neck masses was first employed in the 1930s by Martin and Ellis,[46] but it was later abandoned because of a large number of false-negative results[6, 30] and because of concerns about spread of tumor in the needle tract.[17] Although the most quoted reference to needle biopsy resulting in tumor spread was written by Crile,[17] more recently he has been routinely recommending needle biopsy before surgery if the lesion is not obviously malignant.[24] Biopsy employing the Vim-Silverman needle has been used by Wang and co-workers.[84] They report excellent results, but needle biopsy was not commonly used in the United States until the mid-1970s.

Beginning in the early 1950s, Scandinavian investigators[23, 68] began to use fine-needle biopsies with a 22- to 27-gauge needle, and evaluation of the cellular specimens was performed by cytopathologic techniques. This technique has gained favor in Canada[82] and the United States[31, 52] only recently.

Fine-needle biopsy is simple, can be performed in the office, is relatively inexpensive (particularly if it replaces the scan and ultrasound), and is safe. The patient is

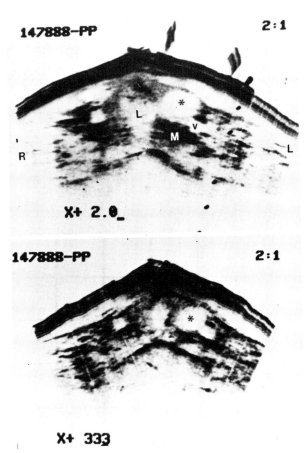

Figure 59–20. This 53-year-old asymptomatic woman had a 1.5 to 2.0 cm nodule in the left lobe of the thyroid. The nodule was cold to isotope scan. Transverse echotomograms show a simple cyst (asterisk). A repeat examination and follow-up sonogram 4 years later revealed no nodule or cyst (not shown). L = Larynx; V = vessel; M = muscle; R = right; L = left.

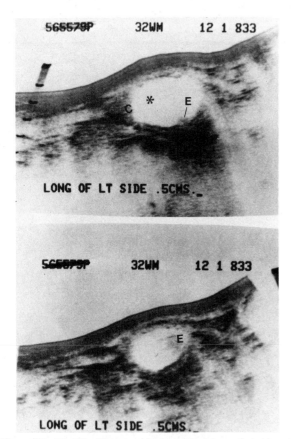

Figure 59–21. This 32-year-old asymptomatic, euthyroid man had a 4 × 5 cm nodule in the left lobe of the thyroid. Isotope scan suggested a cyst, and fine-needle biopsy revealed typical cystic fluid but with many Hürthle cells. A longitudinal ultrasound image made to the left of the midline of the neck shows a sonolucent, round cystic mass (asterisk) with ill-defined margins and internal echoes (E) consistent with a complex cyst. Pathologic diagnosis: Hürthle cell adenoma with ischemic necrosis and cyst formation. H = head; F = feet.

supine with the shoulders on a pillow so that the neck is hyperextended slightly. The skin is infiltrated with local anesthetic. (Others have stated that no anesthetic is necessary; however, since multiple sticks are required to ensure adequate specimen and because patient acceptance is better, I have always employed local anesthetic.) The nodule is entered with a 22- to 27-gauge needle on a dry 20-cc syringe. Four to six insertions with continuous suction on the syringe barrel are made into the nodule to draw cells into the needle. The needle is removed, air is drawn into the syringe, the needle is replaced, and tissue fluid and cells are expressed onto a slide and spread like a blood smear (Fig. 59–23). The slides are immediately fixed with hair spray (Aquanet) and stained with Papanicolaou technique. Four to six slides are made per nodule.[35]

Representative results from the world literature are shown in Table 59–5. Overall, one is able to correctly differentiate benign from malignant lesions 80 to 90 per cent of the time. Another 10 to 15 per cent of nodules must be classified as inconclusive; usually these are highly cellular follicular lesions, adenoma versus carci-

noma. Surgery is usually recommended for these lesions. The false-positive result (interpreted as inconclusive or falsely malignant) is 10 to 15 per cent. The false-negative (malignant lesion interpreted as benign) is 1 to 5 per cent.

The major limiting factor in fine-needle biopsy is that not all pathologists or even cytopathologists have enough experience to interpret thyroid biopsies. Because of this, we started performing biopsies of surgical specimens when direct correlation to more conventional pathologic examination could be made. Over a 2-year period we collected more than 60 cases and assured ourselves that the technique was valid, that we could obtain adequate and representative samples, and that our cytopathologist, Dr. Paul Zaharapoulous, had gained sufficient experience and confidence with examining thyroid biopsies. We have been doing biopsies on nodules in vivo for over a year, and our results in both types of examinations are comparable with those described earlier. We are convinced of the value of fine-needle biopsy and our ability to interpret them correctly. An excellent atlas with many color photographs has been very helpful in presenting information on interpreting needle biopsies of the thyroid.[35]

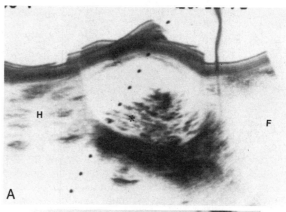

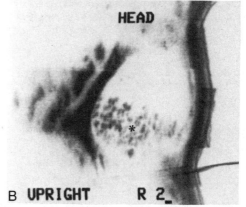

Figure 59–22. This 26-year-old man had a stable thyroid nodule for two years. Over a 3-week period, he experienced pain and tenderness along with a rapid increase in size. A sonogram showed a cystic mass with internal debris (asterisk) in the dependent portion of the lesion on longitudinal images male supine (A) and upright (B). Needle aspiration revealed 25 to 30 ml of typical cystic fluid to be benign. Diagnosis: Recent hemorrhage into benign cyst.

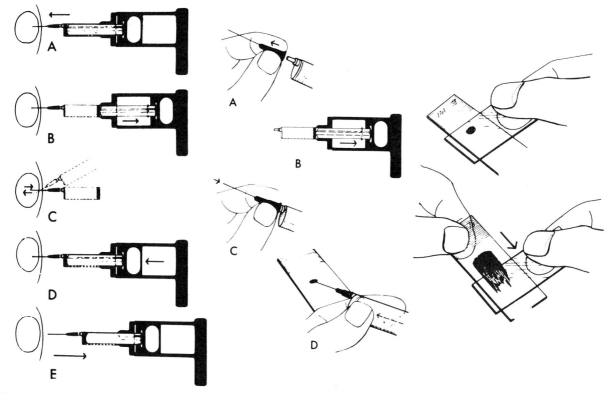

Figure 59–23. Fine-needle biopsy technique of the thyroid. The syringe is attached to a Cameco syringe pistol (Precision Dynamics Corp., Burbank, Cal.). The middle panel shows preparation of slides, and the right panel shows the smearing technique. (From Löwhagen T, et al: Surg Clin North Am 59:3, 1979.)

Assuming that an experienced cytopathologist is at hand, fine-needle biopsy should be a major factor in the decision for surgery in all patients with thyroid nodules unless the nodule is considered to be obviously malignant. Even if anaplastic carcinoma is suspected, a needle biopsy should be performed. Another important exception should be the patient who cannot be considered a surgical candidate because of age or other severe disease. It is sometimes better for the physician not to know that the patient has an inconclusive or suspicious nodule.

The major advantage of fine-needle biopsy is that it offers a histologic basis on which to base a decision for or against surgery and it lends more confidence that a lesion is benign if the physician elects to observe or suppress it. The incidence of carcinoma in nodules sent to surgery increases from 30–40 per cent to 75–85 per cent.[35, 57] The internist or endocrinologist can participate

TABLE 59–5. Results of Fine-Needle Biopsy of the Thyroid Gland*

Year	No. Patient Biopsies	No. Patient Operations	Malignant at Surgery (%)	False-Positive Results (%)	False-Negative Results (%)	Accuracy (%)	Adequate Specimen (%)
1962	449	177	89	0	3	97	98
1975	180	84	67	14	5	95	87
1977	264	131	84	9	9	91	93
1977	33	32†	64	13	6	89	97
1977	150	90	100	0	6	95	92
1978	303	284†	30	0	0.6	99	94
1979	265	—	98	2	0.6	99	92
1979	500	147	44	29	4	82	85
1979	412	412†	47	0	4	97	—
1980	1524	68	90	7	11	90	almost all
1982	156	30	65	0	1	99	95
TOTALS	4236	1455	71%	7%	5%	94%	93%

*Adapted from Rubenfeld S et al: Texas Med 78:41, 1982.[57]
†Studies in which more than 90 per cent of patients who had biopsies underwent surgery, demonstrating no difference from the entire series.

with the surgeon in deciding how much surgery should be done with the probable histologic type of tumor known preoperatively.

The disadvantages and risks are few. The possibility of a false-negative biopsy result is minimized when one considers the biopsy result can be overridden or the course of the nodule followed and rebiopsy or surgery performed at a later date with little increase in risk because of the slow growth of most thyroid cancers. Bleeding has been only a rare and minor complication in contrast to more major bleeding with the Vim-Silverman technique. Although there is concern about infection, particularly with large cysts, this has not been observed. Spread of tumor along needle tracts has been reported with larger needles,[17, 84] but has not been seen with fine-needle biopsy.

In summary, fine-needle biopsy of thyroid nodules is an accurate, safe, and beneficial technique for the preoperative evaluation of thyroid nodules and should be a routine part of the evaluation of thyroid nodules in most patients.

Special thanks to Charles J. Fagan, M.D., Diagnostic Ultrasound, Department of Radiology, University of Texas Medical Branch, for his help in selecting and interpreting the thyroid sonograms; also to Bettye A. Sayle, M.D., Nuclear Medicine, University of Texas Medical Branch, for similar help with the thyroid radioisotope scans; and to Mrs. Ofilia Chlamon for help in preparing the manuscript.

REFERENCES

1. Al-Hindawi AY, Wilson GM: The effect of irradiation on the function and survival of thyroid cells. Clin Sci 28:555, 1965.
2. Ashcraft MW, Van Herle AJ: Management of thyroid nodules I and II. Head Neck Surg 3:216–230, 297–322, 1981.
3. Bastenie PA, Ermans AM, Neve P: Focal lymphocytic thyroiditis in simple goiter: In Bastenie PA, Ermans AM (eds): Thyroiditis and Thyroid Function. Oxford, Pergamon Press, 1972, pp. 143–158.
4. Black EG, Cassoni A, Gimlette TMD, et al: Serum thyroglobulin in thyroid cancer. Lancet 2:443, 1981.
5. Blum M, Rothschild M: Improved nonoperative diagnosis of the solitary "cold" thyroid nodule. JAMA 243:242, 1980.
6. Boehme EJ, Winship T, Lindsay S, et al: An evaluation of needle biopsy of the thyroid gland. Surg Gynecol Obstet 119:831, 1964.
7. Bowens OM, Vander JB: Thyroid nodules and thyroid malignancy. Ann Intern Med 57:245, 1962.
8. Buckwalter JA: Surgical treatment of thyroid carcinoma. Arch Surg 98:579, 1969.
9. Cady B: Surgery of thyroid cancer. World J Surg 5:3, 1981.
10. Cady B, Sedzwick CE, Meissner WA, et al. Changing clinical, pathologic, therapeutic and survival patterns in differentiated thyroid carcinoma. Ann Surg 184:541, 1976.
11. Cantrell RB, Colcock BP: The present-day problem of cancer of the thyroid. J Clin Endocrinol Metab 13:1480, 1953.
12. Cerise EJ, Randall S, Ochsner A: Carcinoma of the thyroid and nontoxic nodular goiter. Surgery 31:552, 1953.
13. Cole WH, Slaughter DP, Roster LJ: Potential dangers of nontoxic nodular goiter. JAMA 127:883, 1945.
14. Conrad RA, Dobyns BM, Sutow WW: Thyroid neoplasia as a late effect of exposure to radioactive iodine in fallout. JAMA 214:316, 1970.
15. Cope O. Dolyns BM, Hamlin E, Hopkirk J: What thyroid nodules are to be feared? J Clin Endocrinol Metab 9:1012, 1949.
16. Crile G, Jr: Cancer of the thyroid. J Clin Endocrinol Metab 10:1152, 1950.
17. Crile G, Jr: The danger of surgical dissemination of papillary carcinoma of the thyroid. Surg Gynecol Obstet 102:161, 1956.
18. DeGroot LJ: Radiation-Associated Thyroid Carcinoma. New York, Grune & Stratton, 1977.
19. DeGroot LJ, Stanbury JB: The Thyroid and Its Diseases, 4th ed. New York, John Wiley & Sons, 1975, p. 648.
20. Ibid., pp. 682–683.
21. Doniach I: The effect of radioactive iodine alone and in combination with methylthiouracil upon tumor production in the rat's thyroid gland. Br J Cancer 7:181, 1953.
22. Duffy BJ, Fitzgerald PJ: Cancer of the thyroid in children. J Clin Endocrinol Metab 10:1296, 1950.
23. Einhorn J, Franzen S: Thin needle biopsy in the diagnosis of thyroid disease. Acta Radiol 58:321, 1962.
24. Esselstyn CB, Crile G, Jr: Needle aspiration and needle biopsy of the thyroid. World J Surg 2:45, 1978.
25. Faves MJ, Schneider AB, Stachwa ME, et al: Thyroid cancer occurring as a late consequence of head and neck irradiation. N Engl J Med 294:1019, 1976.
26. Follis RH, Jr: Studies on the pathogenesis of colloid goiter. Trans Assoc Am Physicians 62:265, 1959.
27. Fortner JG, George PA, Sternberg SS: Induced and spontaneous thyroid cancer in the Syrian (golden) hamster. Endocrinology 66:364, 1960.
28. Franssila K: Value of histologic classification of thyroid cancer. Acta Pathol Microbiol Scand (Suppl 225), Section A, 1971.
29. Frantz VK, Klingerman MM, Harland WA, et al: A comparison of internal and external irradiation on the thyroid gland of the rat. Endocrinology 61:574, 1957.
30. Franzell EL, Foote FW Jr: Papillary cancer of the thyroid. Cancer 11:895, 1958.
31. Gershengorn MC, McClung MR, Chu EW, et al: Fine needle aspiration cytology in the preoperative diagnosis of thyroid nodules. Ann Intern Med 87:265, 1977.
32. Glassford GH, Fowler EF, Cole WH: The treatment of non-toxic nodular goiter with desiccated thyroid. Surgery 58:621, 1965.
33. Greer MA, Astwood EB: Treatment of simple goiter with thyroid. J Endocrinol Metab 13:1312, 1953.
34. Greer MA, Studer H, Kendall JW: Studies on the pathogenesis of colloid goiter. Endocrinology 81:623, 1967.
35. Hamburger JI, Miller JM, Kini SR: Clinical-Pathological Evaluation of Thyroid Nodules: Handbook and Atlas. Southfield, Mich., Northland Thyroid Laboratory, 1979, pp. 76–77.
36. Harmen MH: Application of TNM classification to malignant tumors of the thyroid gland. In Hedinger CE (ed): Berlin and New York, Springer-Verlag, 1969, p. 64.
37. Hazard JB, Kauffman N: A survey of thyroid glands in a so-called goiter area. Am J Clin Pathol 22:860, 1952.
38. Hazard JB, Hawk WA, Crile G Jr: Medullary (solid) carcinoma of the thyroid: Clinicopathologic entity. J Clin Endocrinol Metab 19:152, 1959.
39. Hennessay JF, Wells SA, Ontjes DA, Cooper CW: A comparison of pentagastrin injection and calcium infusion as provocative agents for the detection of medullary carcinoma of the thyroid. J Clin Endocrinol Metab 39:487, 1974.
40. Hill CS, Ibanez ML, Saaman NA, et al: Medullary carcinoma of the thyroid gland. Medicine 52:141, 1973.
41. Hinton JW, Lord JW Jr: Is surgery indicated in all cases of nodular goiter, toxic and nontoxic? JAMA 129:605, 1945.
42. Hoffman GL: The solitary thyroid nodule: A reassessment. Arch Surg 105:379, 1972.
43. Jaffe RH: Variation in the weight of the thyroid gland and frequency of its abnormal enlargement in the region of Chicago. Arch Pathol 10:887, 1930.
44. Lakey FH, Hare HF: Malignancy in adenomas of the thyroid. JAMA 145:689, 1951.
45. Langer P: Antithyroid action in rats of small doses of some naturally occurring compounds. Endocrinology 79:1117, 1966.
46. Martin HE, Ellis EB: Biopsy of needle puncture and aspiration. Ann Surg 92:169, 1930.
47. Mazzaferri EL, Young RL, Ortel JE, et al: Papillary thyroid carcinoma: The impact of therapy in 576 patients. Medicine 56:171, 1977.
48. McDermott WV Jr, Morgan WS, Hamlin E Jr, Cope O: Cancer of the thyroid. J Clin Endocrinol Metab 14:1336, 1953.
49. Melvin KE, Tashjian AH Jr: The syndrome of excessive thyrocalcitonin produced by medullary carcinoma of the thyroid. Proc Natl Acad Sci 59:1216, 1968.
50. Melvin KE, Tashjian AH, Miller HH: Studies on familial (medullary) thyroid carcinoma. Recent Prog Horm Res 28:339, 1972.
51. Miller JM: Carcinoma and thyroid nodules. N Engl J Med 252:247, 1955.
52. Miller JM, Hamburger JI, Kine S: Diagnosis of thyroid nodules: Use of fine needle aspiration and needle biopsy. JAMA 241:481, 1979.
53. Mortensen JD, Woolner LB, Bennett WA: Gross and microscopic findings in clinically normal thyroid glands. J Clin Endocrinol Metab 15:1270, 1955.
54. Nishiyama RH, Ludwig WK, Thompson RW: The prevalence of small papillary thyroid carcinomas in 100 consecutive necropsies in an American population. In DeGroot LJ (ed): Radiation-Associated

Thyroid Carcinoma. New York, Grune & Stratton, 1977, pp. 123–136.

55. Purves HD, Griesbach WE, Kennedy TH: Studies in experimental goiter: Malignant change in a transplantable tumor. Br J Cancer 5:301, 1951.
56. Royce POL, MacKay BR, DiSabella PM: Value of post-irradiation screening for thyroid nodules. JAMA 242:2675, 1979.
57. Rubenfeld S, Wheeler TH, Spjut HJ: Fine needle aspiration biopsy of thyroid nodules. Texas Med 78:41, 1982.
58. Russell WO, Ibanez ML, Clark RL, et al: Thyroid carcinoma: Classification, intraglandular dissemination, and clinicopathological study based on whole organ sections of 80 glands. Cancer 16:1425, 1963.
59. Sampson RJ, Woolner LB, Bahn RC, Kurland LT: Occult thyroid carcinoma in Olmstead County, Minn.: Prevalence at autopsy compared with that in Hiroshima and Nagasaki, Japan. Cancer 34:2072, 1974.
60. Sampson RJ: Prevalence and significance of occult thyroid cancer. In DeGroot LJ (ed): Radiation-Associated Thyroid Carcinoma. New York, Grune & Stratton, 1977.
61. Sampson RJ: Comment on the natural history of occult thyroid carcinoma. In DeGroot LJ (ed): Radiation-Association Thyroid Carcinoma. New York, Grune & Stratton, 1977.
62. Scheible W, Leopold GR, Woo VL, et al: High-resolution real-time ultrasonography of thyroid nodules. Radiology 133:413, 1979.
63. Schlesinger MJ, Gorgill SL, Saxe IH: Studies in nodular goiter. JAMA 110:1638, 1938.
64. Schneeber NG, Stahl TJ, Modia G, et al: Regression of goiter by whole thyroid or triiodothyronine. Metabolism 11:1054, 1962.
65. Schneider AB, Favas MJ, Strachura ME, et al: Plasma thyroglobulin in detecting thyroid carcinoma after childhood head and neck irradiation. Ann Intern Med 86:29, 1977.
66. Scholler RT, Stevenson JK: Development of carcinoma of the thyroid in iodine deficient mice. Cancer 19:1063, 1966.
67. Silverberg E, Lubera JA: A review of American Cancer Society estimates of cancer cases and deaths. Ca 33:2, 1983.
68. Soderstom N: Puncture of goiters for aspiration biopsy: A preliminary report. Acta Med Scand 144:237, 1952.
69. Sokal JE: Occurrence of thyroid cancer. N Engl J Med 249:393, 1953.
70. Sokal JE: A long-term follow-up of non-toxic nodular goiter. AMA Arch Intern Med 99:60, 1957.
71. Sokal JE: The problem of malignancy in nodular goiter—recapitulation and challenge. JAMA 170:405, 1959.
72. Staffer RP, Welch JW, Hellwig CA, et al: Nodular goiter. AMA Arch Intern Med 106:10, 1960.
73. Stanbury, JB: Familial Goiter. In Stanburg JB, Wyngaarden JB, Fredrickson DS (eds): The Metabolic Basis of Inherited Disease, vol IV. New York, McGraw-Hill, 1978, pp. 206–239.
74. Studer HR, et al: Transformation of normal follicles into thyrotropin-refractory "cold" follicles in the aging mouse thyroid gland. Endocrinology 102:1576, 1978.
75. Taylor S: The evolution of nodular goiter. J Clin Endocrinol Metab 13:1232, 1953.
76. Tollefsen HR, De Casse JJ: Papillary carcinoma of the thyroid. Am J Surg 106:728, 1963.
77. Vander JB, Gaston EA, Dawber TR: Significance of solitary nontoxic thyroid nodules. N Engl J Med 251:970, 1954.
78. Ibid: Final report of a 15-year study of the incidence of thyroid malignancy. Ann Intern Med 69:537, 1968.
79. Van Herle AJ: Serum thyroglobulin levels in patients with differentiated thyroid carcinoma. Ann Radiol 20:743, 1977.
80. Van Herle AJ, Rich, P. Britt-Marie Ljung E, et al: The thyroid nodule. Ann Intern Med 96:221, 1982.
81. Veith FJ, Brooks JR, Grigsby WP, Selenkow HA: The nodular thyroid gland and cancer. N Engl J Med 270:431, 1964.
82. Walfish PG, Hazani E, Strawbridge H, et al: Combined ultrasound and needle aspiration cytology in the assessment and management of hypofunctioning thyroid nodules. Ann Intern Med 87:270, 1977.
83. Wanebo HJ, Andrews W, Kaiser DL: Thyroid cancer: Some basic considerations. Ca 33:87, 1983.
84. Wang C, Vickery AL Jr, Maloof F: Needle biopsy of thyroid nodules. Surg Gynecol Obstet 143:365, 1976.
85. Weiss ES, Rallison ML, London WT, et al: Thyroid nodularity in southwestern Utah school children exposed to fallout radiation. Am J Public Health 61:241, 1971.
86. Williams ED: Histogenesis of medullary carcinoma of the thyroid. J Clin Pathol 19:114, 1966.
87. Wolfe HE, Melvin KE, Cervi-Skinner SJ, et al: C-cell hyperplasia preceding medullary thyroid carcinoma. N Engl J Med 289:437, 1973.
88. Woolner LB, Beahrs OH, Black BM, et al: Thyroid carcinoma: General considerations and follow-ups of 1181 cases. In Young S, Inman, DR (eds): Thyroid Neoplasia, New York, Academic Press, 1968, pp. 51–79.
89. Young RL, Mazzaferri EL, Rahe AJ, et al: Pure follicular carcinoma: Impact of therapy in 214 patients. J Nucl Med 21:733, 1980.
90. Zimmerman LM, Shubik P, Baserga R, et al: Experimental production of thyroid tumors by alternating hyperplasia and involution. J Clin Endocrinol Metab 14:1367, 1954.

CHAPTER 60

Pathology of Thyroid Tumors

Virginia A. LiVolsi, M.D. • Maria J. Merino, M.D.

The thyroid gland is divided into follicles, oval or round sacs containing the glycoprotein colloid. The average follicle, measuring 200 nm in diameter, is lined by a single layer of low cuboidal epithelium. Twenty to 40 follicles surrounded by connective tissue and supplied by a lobular artery comprise a thyroid *lobule*.[54] This lobular architecture of the thyroid is maintained or accentuated in most non-neoplastic disorders, which generally involve the gland diffusely (i.e., thyroiditis). In the presence of neoplasms, the lobulation is destroyed. Scarring and distortion occur in adenomatous goiter, so that in this condition, the lobular configuration is obscured also.[102]

Ultrastructural studies have shown that normal follicles are surrounded by a rich network of capillaries and lymphatics.[44, 60] The *follicular cells* are enclosed by a basal lamina; within these are found the *parafollicular* or *C-cells*, the source of calcitonin.[20, 40] The latter show the ultrastructural features of *neuroendocrine cells*, including numerous membrane-bound secretory granules that contain immunoreactive calcitonin. This chapter discusses the pathologic changes that occur in the thyroid and that lead to the production of nodules. Since most thyroid neoplasms present as nodules, the differential diagnosis of such lesions includes not only neoplasms but also other conditions that produce nodules and mimic thyroid neoplasms.

The classification of thyroid nodules used in this chapter is listed in Table 60–1.

GOITER

"Goiter" describes any enlargement of the thyroid; it may be diffuse or nodular, malignant or benign. Most often, goiter describes a benign process. The causes of goiter include inborn errors of metabolism, iodine deficiency, or goitrogens, each of which produces an increase in thyrotropin (TSH) production from the pituitary. Increased cellular activity and growth of the gland (hyperplasia) occur in an attempt to attain a euthyroid state.

Of concern to the subject of thyroid neoplasms are those thyroid enlargements that result in *nodular* goiter. The pathogenesis of simple, or nontoxic, nodular goiter is not understood because all follicular epithelial cells presumably respond to normal regulatory mechanisms in a similar fashion. Generation of follicles is necessary for the development of a goiter. Some follicular epithelial cells may possess an ability to multiply more rapidly than others. If this occurs in several foci in the gland, and if following this generation of new follicles there is stromal reaction, nodules result. Less rapidly replicating areas might undergo involution and further nodularity ensues.[102]

Expansion of these nodules impinges upon blood supply, causing necrosis and subsequent fibrosis. The replicating follicles become entrapped in this new connective tissue, and gross nodularity results. Most adenomatous follicular lesions of the thyroid are thus polyclonal and heterogeneous. True monoclonal neoplasms (adenomas) are extremely rare.[102]

Although nodular goiter is a process that involves the entire thyroid, the nodularity may be asymmetric and a single large nodule may dominate. In such cases, distinguishing a true neoplasm from an adenomatous nodule may not be possible.

By convention, "adenoma" describes a solitary lesion of uniform structure that is encapsulated and compresses the adjacent parenchyma. "Adenomatous nodule" defines a poorly or non-encapsulated nodule of varied architecture that is one of many in an abnormal gland. Biologically, most follicular lesions represent non-neoplastic adenomatous nodules.[102]

Grossly, both adenomas and adenomatous nodules are circumscribed and demarcated from surrounding tissue. Both may appear translucent or fleshy. Hemorrhage, scarring, and cystic degeneration can be seen in both.

Histologically, the adenomatous nodule displays a variable pattern of small and large follicles of irregular shape. The cells are flat to columnar and contain small uniform nuclei. The adenoma is cellular with uniform architecture ranging from microfollicular to trabecular to solid. Rarely, macrofollicles or spindle cell lesions are encountered. An occasional adenoma will show several patterns.[5, 10, 76, 78]

TABLE 60–1. Classification of Thyroid Tumors

Benign
   Adenomatous nodule
   Adenoma
Malignant
   Papillary carcinoma
   Follicular carcinoma
   Medullary carcinoma
   Anaplastic carcinoma
   Malignant lymphoma
   Metastatic tumors to the thyroid

Both adenomatous nodules and adenomas can undergo degenerative changes with necrosis, hemorrhage, and fibrosis. Calcification may occur. Cyst formation is seen commonly, especially in adenomatous nodules.[5, 76] These cystic foci may show moderate to marked degenerative change with papillary features and may be confused with papillary carcinoma.

ATYPICAL ADENOMA

Atypical adenoma, a term which we consider to be confusing, has been used to describe two distinct entities:

1. Follicular neoplasms containing abnormal features, i.e.; many mitoses, bizarre nuclei, necrosis, but without demonstrable capsular or vascular invasion.

2. Spindle cell encapsulated tumors, which probably represent variants of medullary thyroid carcinoma.[42, 78, 81]

Because the biology of these two types of lesions is different, we feel they should be classified accordingly. Follicular neoplasms that show unusual or disturbing histologic features but that do not fulfill acceptable criteria for malignancy are diagnosed as "follicular adenoma with atypical features." Those spindle cell lesions that are medullary carcinomas are diagnosed as such. (In some cases, immunohistochemical localization of calcitonin may be needed to appropriately categorize a particular tumor.)

MALIGNANT THYROID NEOPLASMS

Malignant neoplasms of the thyroid may originate from:

1. *Follicular epithelium* (papillary, follicular, and anaplastic carcinoma).

2. *Parafollicular* or *C-cells* (medullary carcinoma and some anaplastic cancers).

3. *Nonepithelial elements* (primary malignant lymphoma of the thyroid).

Most (85 per cent) of thyroid cancers arise from follicular epithelium and are well differentiated. The prognosis of the majority of thyroid tumors is excellent, with most such neoplasms exhibiting indolent biologic behavior.

The prognosis of thyroid cancer, however, depends not only on the histologic type; age, sex, tumor size, extension of the lesion into perithyroidal (non-nodal) tissues, and presence of metastasis also represent important prognostic variables.[18, 28, 49, 74, 75, 110]

The pathologic diagnosis of thyroid neoplasms may involve a variety of techniques: fine-needle aspiration cytology, needle-core biopsy, or direct surgical intervention. Poorly differentiated neoplasms are usually easily recognized as malignancies, although their exact histogenesis may require ancillary diagnostic techniques. Well-differentiated tumors often require the evaluation of many sections of the periphery of the neoplasm to detect invasive properties and infiltrative growth patterns. Cytology, needle biopsy, and even frozen sections may be inadequate for the diagnosis of some well-differentiated tumors, especially lesions with a predominantly follicular growth pattern. In such cases, appropriate fixation and processing for histologic examination are required for diagnosis.

Immunohistochemistry (especially immunoperoxidase staining) techniques for localization of calcitonin and thyroglobulin can be useful in diagnosing thyroid tumors demonstrating unusual histology or in aiding recognition of metastases from thyroid cancers.[19, 20]

Papillary Carcinoma

Papillary cancer is the most common form of thyroid cancer, comprising 75 to 80 per cent of all primary tumors of the thyroid.[28, 77, 104] Its name describes the most characteristic feature of this tumor: the presence of papillary fronds. However, most papillary cancers contain follicular areas; we consider such lesions papillary, since their biologic behavior follows that of papillary carcinoma and differs from true follicular cancer (described later in this chapter).

The tumors affect females more frequently than males (ratio of 4:1). Although it is diagnosed predominantly between the third and fifth decades of life, papillary cancer is the most common thyroid neoplasm occurring in children.[28, 62, 94]

Although the etiology of these tumors is not completely understood, a relationship to exposure of the thyroid to ionizing radiation is well documented.[4, 18, 24, 96] Experimentally, in animals papillary cancers may appear after prolonged and continuous stimulation of the gland by thyroid-stimulating hormone (TSH), which promotes thyroid cell proliferation—some of which may eventually undergo malignant transformation.[83, 93]

Clinically, these neoplasms are frequently identified by palpation of a nodule or an area of irregular induration in the thyroid. Occasionally, occult papillary cancers initially present with one or more enlarged cervical lymph nodes (i.e., metastasis). A "cold" nonfunctional nodule is usually reported when radionuclide studies using ^{99m}technetium pertechnetate, ^{123}iodine, or ^{131}iodine, are performed. However, the variable vascularity and presence of degenerative changes may lead to erroneous interpretations of the thyroid scans. Approximately 15 to 20 per cent of cold nodules are thyroid carcinomas.[2]

Papillary cancers are divided into three categories by gross characteristics: (1) occult, (2) intrathyroidal, and (3) extrathyroidal.[39, 110, 111] The "occult" form of papillary cancer is usually very small (measuring 1.5 cm), although the majority of the tumors measure less than 1 cm and generally cannot be palpated. This type of malignancy may only be found after extensive sectioning of the gland.[112]

Grossly, most papillary cancers present as white-gray, firm, non-encapsulated tumor masses located anywhere in the gland, often near the capsule. The center of the tumor shows fibrosis and scarring. Hemorrhage, necrosis, and cystic degeneration may be present in larger tumors. Tumors that extend into perithyroidal soft tissues often are large masses with extensive necrosis.

Histologically, the major feature of papillary cancer is the presence of papillary fronds composed of stalks of fibroconnective tissue lined by a row of cuboidal cells, in which characteristic, ground-glass, "Orphan Annie" or clear nuclei are present (Fig. 60–1). The clear nucleus consists of a round, smooth nuclear membrane with

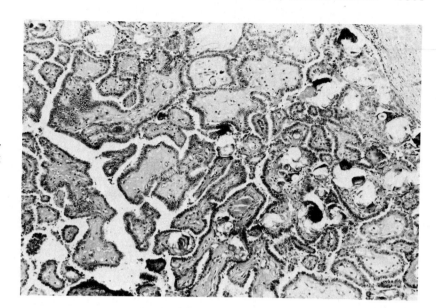

Figure 60–1. Characteristic papillary fronds of papillary cancer containing psammoma bodies. (H&E, ×200)

condensation of the chromatin in its periphery, giving the center of the nucleus an empty washed-out appearance.[36] The papillae range in size from small to large, and edematous ones may contain lymphocytes or histiocytes in their stroma. Foci of sclerosis with deposits of calcium may be present in many areas. A specific type of calcification, the concentrically laminated psammoma body, is found in approximately 40 to 50 per cent of papillary cancers (Fig. 60–2). Psammoma bodies are very rare in other thyroid neoplasms or benign conditions, and they probably originate from degenerated tumor papillae.[50] Squamous metaplasia may be present in about one third of tumors and is generally considered to be benign.[64] A lymphoplasmacytic inflammatory (perhaps immunologic) response is frequently seen at the invasive edges of papillary cancers. Occasionally, such

an infiltration may be present within the neoplastic papillae.[28]

Most papillary cancers are composed of an admixture of papillae and follicles; some contain solid areas of tumor. The follicles contain abundant colloid and are lined by uniform cuboidal cells in which typical ground-glass nuclei are identified (Figs. 60–3 and 60–4). Occasional lesions are composed solely of follicles; in this follicular variant of the papillary cancer, papillae are not present in the primary tumor but can be present in metastases.[12, 29] Biologically, the follicular variant behaves like papillary cancer, not like true follicular carcinoma. Hence its recognition as an entity is important.

In mixed papillary-follicular lesions, the proportion of papillary to follicular elements carries little if any prognostic significance because these lesions follow the same

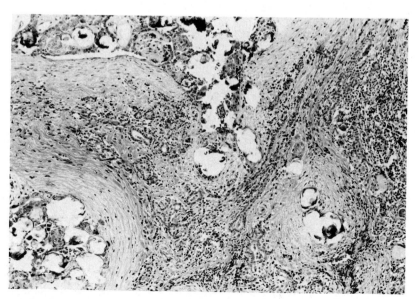

Figure 60–2. Invasive papillary cancer showing psammoma bodies, focal squamous metaplasia, and lymphoplasmacytic response. (H&E, ×200)

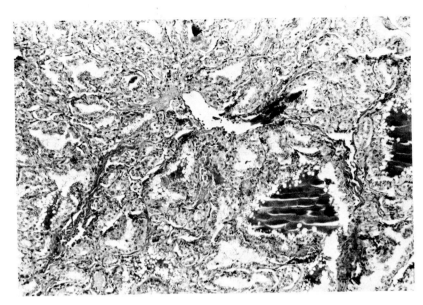

Figure 60–3. Follicular variant of papillary cancer. Note the absence of well-formed papillae. Follicles containing colloid are present. (H&E, ×200)

pattern of spread and clinical behavior as pure papillary cancers.

In some papillary tumors, large, tall eosinophilic cells are recognized. This pink, or eosinophilic, variant of papillary cancer can be seen in young individuals, but it is associated with larger tumors and carries a poorer prognosis when it affects older patients.[106]

The presence of multifocal lesions within the same gland has been described in up to 75 per cent of cases.[13] Whether these findings represent multicentric origin of the tumor or intraglandular metastasis has been debated; the studies of Fialkow suggest the latter as more likely.[26]

The differential diagnosis of papillary carcinoma includes (1) papillary hyperplasia seen in adenomatous goiter or Graves' disease, and (2) pure follicular carcinoma.

The main diagnostic features present in papillary cancers, but absent in any of the other conditions, are (1) the ground-glass nuclei, (2) psammoma bodies, and (3) well-formed fibrovascular cores within papillae. In Graves' disease there is preservation of the lobular architecture, which disappears in papillary carcinoma; follicular cancers lack the ground-glass nuclei.

The prognosis of papillary carcinoma is excellent. Many authors feel that the patient's age at diagnosis and sex, plus the presence or absence of transcapsular spread, are the most important factors.[28, 30, 49, 74, 75, 95] Younger patients enjoy a better prognosis. Papillary cancer seems to have a worse prognosis in men than in women. The biologically indolent course of papillary cancer requires life-long follow-up. Papillary cancers may recur locally, and they invade local adjacent structures as well as metastasize to regional lymph nodes. Dissemination through the blood stream occurs in fewer than 5 per cent of cases. Recurrences have been reported more frequently in larger tumors or in those showing vascular invasion or extrathyroidal spread. Growth pat-

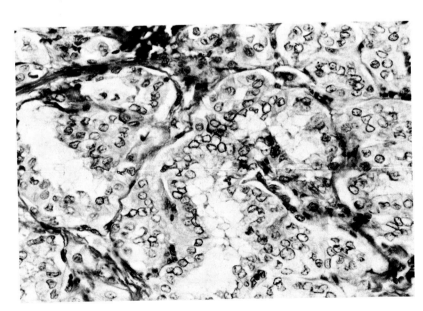

Figure 60–4. Characteristic "ground-glass" nuclei of papillary carcinoma. (H&E, ×400)

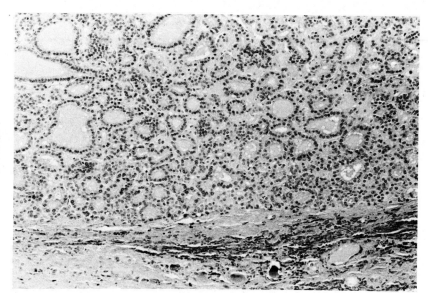

Figure 60–5. Follicular neoplasm of thyroid is shown. The grossly encapsulated tumor showed microscopic encapsulation, also seen here. In other areas, vascular invasion was noted. (H&E, ×200)

tern, psammoma bodies, clear nuclei, squamous metaplasia, or lymphocytic infiltration does not appear to affect prognosis.[28, 49]

The treatment of choice for papillary cancer ranges from total thyroidectomy to less aggressive approaches. Lobectomy and isthmusectomy, which may or may not be followed by radioiodine ablation of the residual thyroid tissue, have been used.[13, 18, 23, 74, 75, 105] Surgery alone and subsequent lifelong thyroid suppressive medication have been advocated, especially for small tumors or those found incidentally.

Follicular Carcinoma

About 5 to 10 per cent of thyroid neoplasms are follicular carcinomas that occur more commonly in women than in men. This tumor occurs more frequently in individuals living in endemic goiter regions.[16, 28, 65]

Grossly, follicular carcinoma grows in either an expansile or an infiltrative fashion. The grossly encapsulated lesions resemble adenomas. Focally scarring calcification and cystic change may be noted. Obvious gross extension of the tumor beyond its capsule or into veins will be seen in the infiltrative variety.[16, 28, 55, 65, 111]

Histologically, most follicular carcinomas show a microfollicular pattern, although trabecular or solid areas can be found (Figs. 60–5 and 60–6). In predominantly solid tumors, thyroglobulin localization may be required to define the tumor type.

Distinction between follicular adenoma and encapsulated follicular carcinoma may be difficult and may require evaluation of numerous sections from the tumor-capsule-thyroid interface (Fig. 60–6). A follicular carcinoma invades into or beyond its capsule or invades veins at the edge of the tumor.[42, 55, 61] Well-differentiated follicular carcinomas may display hypercellularity or many mitoses. Such features should raise the suspicion

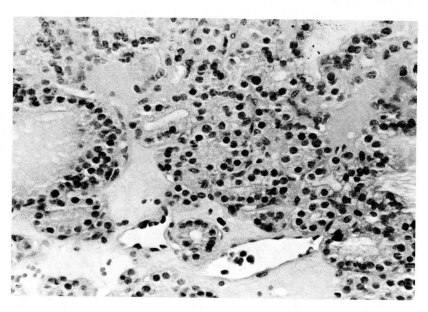

Figure 60–6. Center of a well-differentiated follicular lesion; based on this type of material, no prediction as to biologic behavior can be made. The tumor-thyroid-capsule interface must be examined. Same case as in Figure 60–5, well-differentiated follicular carcinoma. (H&E, ×300)

of carcinoma, but the definitive diagnosis rests on the detection of invasion.[55]

A follicular neoplasm that is minimally invasive (i.e., requires extensive search for fulfillment of definitive diagnostic criteria) is associated with a good prognosis (85 per cent or more survival at 5 years). Some tumors of this type, however, may recur or metastasize after many years.[28, 55, 110, 111]

"Obvious" follicular carcinomas (those that are grossly recognized as malignant) often show numerous mitoses, hypercellularity, and necrosis. Infiltration of veins or normal tissues is detected readily.[65] Such lesions are associated with a poor prognosis.

Follicular carcinoma rarely, if ever, spreads to lymph nodes (except by direct extension).[29, 55] This tumor metastasizes via the blood stream most often to lungs, bone, and brain. This metastatic behavior contrasts that of predominantly follicular variants of papillary cancer, which do, of course, spread embolically to lymph nodes.

We consider Hürthle (oxyphilic) cell tumors to represent variants of follicular tumors.[6, 34, 97] We recognize benign and malignant types. Such neoplasms can be distinguished as carcinoma using the same criteria (capsular or vascular invasion) as are used to differentiate benign from malignant non–Hürthle cell follicular neoplasms. Lesions composed solely of Hürthle cells, however, more frequently fulfill the criteria for malignancy than ordinary follicular tumors. Occasional examples of papillary cancers composed of oxyphil cells can be identified. These usually behave as papillary tumors in their patterns of spread.

Medullary Carcinoma

Medullary carcinoma, which is derived from parafollicular cells, comprises about 5 to 10 per cent of thyroid cancers. It has attracted considerable interest since its description because (1) it may be found in patients with other endocrine or neural lesions (10 to 20 per cent), (2) it may be familial (10 to 20 per cent), and (3) it produces large quantities of the parafollicular cell hormone, calcitonin, which can be measured giving diagnostic and prognostic information.[40, 41, 66, 79, 101]

The usual sporadic form of medullary carcinoma occurs in middle-aged to elderly patients and arises unifocally. Familial medullary carcinoma is found in younger individuals, shows multicentricity and bilaterality, and is associated with the precursor lesion, C-cell hyperplasia. Parathyroid hyperplasia and pheochromocytoma (often multiple) or bilateral adrenal medullary hyperplasia are the associated endocrine lesions in classic Sipple's syndrome (Multiple Endocrine Neoplasia, type 2:MEN-2).[3] Variant syndromes include the triad of medullary carcinoma, pheochromocytoma, and mucosal neuromas (MEN-2b or 3); medullary carcinoma, pheochromocytoma, and ganglioneuromatosis of the intestines; and MEN-2b complex associated with Marfanoid habitus.[11, 66, 79, 101]

Grossly, medullary carcinomas are firm, are gray to yellow, and may appear circumscribed or obviously invasive.

Histologically, a variety of patterns can be seen: spindled cells arranged in a rich vascular network (Figs. 60–7 and 60–8), round uniform cells displaying an organoid pattern, or combinations of these patterns.[11, 20, 40, 56, 66, 80, 82, 88, 90] Giant cell variants may occur.[80, 82, 88]

Occasionally papillae or follicle formation may be seen; this does not imply papillary or follicular cancer.[56] Stromal amyloid, which represents secretory products (probably procalcitonin) of the tumor cells, is found in the primary tumor and in metastases. If searched for with special stains, amyloid can be found in about 85 to 90 per cent of medullary cancers. Occasionally, the amyloid may be so extensive as to obscure the cells of the neoplasm. Ultrastructural and immunohistochemical studies indicate that amyloid is not required for the diagnosis.[47, 88, 90–92]

Medullary carcinoma invades lymphatics and veins. Regional node metastases are found in over 50 per cent of cases. Blood-borne metastases to lung, liver and bone are common also. The degree of biologic malignancy varies greatly, with some medullary carcinomas recurring locally or regionally after many years, and others following a rapidly fatal course with widespread metastases. It is difficult to predict biologic potential from histologic appearance; however, most tumors that behave in an aggressive fashion show necrosis, considerable pleomorphism, and many mitoses.[47, 57, 79, 101]

Anaplastic Carcinoma

Anaplastic (undifferentiated) carcinoma of the thyroid comprises about 10 per cent of all thyroid malignancies and appears to occur more frequently in endemic goiter areas. Elderly patients (over age 50), especially women, are affected.[1, 27, 43, 89, 104]

Origin in abnormal thyroids has been implicated, in that 80 per cent of patients note a long history of "goiter." Histologically, the pre-existing goiter may represent adenomatous goiter, adenoma, or well-differentiated carcinoma (follicular or papillary). This association both by history and histology has led to the theory of "transformation" of a benign or low-grade malignant neoplasm. The incidence of this transformation is not known, but judging from the number of nodules detected clinically and the rarity of anaplastic carcinoma, transformation must represent a rare event.[1, 27, 43, 59, 89, 104]

Grossly, anaplastic carcinomas present as large masses that freely infiltrate extrathyroidal tissues (trachea, soft tissue, vessels). The tumor is white-tan and fleshy with zones of hemorrhage and necrosis. In one portion of the tumor, an encapsulated nodule representing a pre-existing low-grade lesion may be found.[1, 27, 89]

Microscopically, anaplastic carcinomas have been divided into giant cell, spindle cell, and small cell types. (We believe that small cell carcinoma is so rare as to be practically nonexistent.) Most examples of purported small cell carcinoma represent malignant lymphoma, medullary carcinoma without amyloid, or metastatic small cell carcinoma from another site, i.e., lung.[71] In giant and spindle cell carcinoma, the spindle cell component is always malignant and resembles fibrosarcoma or malignant fibrous histiocytoma. In most cases, the giant cells are also malignant resembling pleomorphic rhabdomyosarcoma (Figs. 60–9 and 60–10) or fibrous histiocytoma.[1, 27, 89] In all varieties of anaplastic carcinoma, abnormal mitoses are numerous, necrosis is common, and infiltration of thyroid and soft tissue is easily recognized. Squamous differentiation may occur in anaplastic carcinoma as well as in well-differentiated tumors. Pure squamous cell carcinoma can apparently

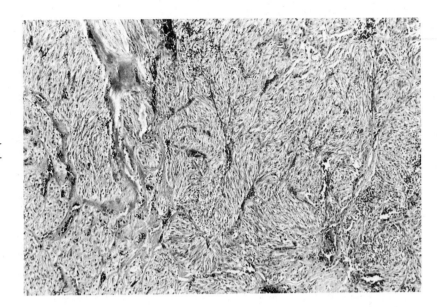

Figure 60–7. Medullary thyroid carcinoma, spindle cell type. Note vascularity. (H&E, ×200)

arise in the thyroid; its behavior mimics that of anaplastic carcinoma.[37, 46, 48, 72, 86, 89, 104] It is essential to distinguish primary squamous carcinoma from the more common metastatic type arising in larynx, esophagus, or lung.

Anaplastic carcinoma has been associated with a dismal prognosis, with most patients dead within one year. Death by suffocation or exsanguination caused by locally uncontrollable tumor growth is common.[59, 89, 98, 104]

Of interest from a pathologic and epidemiologic standpoint is the apparent decrease in incidence of anaplastic carcinoma in recent years. Causes for this include supplementation of iodine-deficient diets in endemic goiter regions and the recognition of many cases of "anaplastic carcinoma" as tumors of other types, i.e., malignant lymphoma.[14, 15, 21, 45]

Malignant Lymphoma

Primary malignant lymphoma of the thyroid, for many years, was not recognized as an entity; instead,

these tumors were classified as "epithelial neoplasms of anaplastic type." With the development of new techniques such as electron microscopy and immunohistology (immunoperoxidase), it became evident that primary thyroid lymphomas do exist and that all variants of lymphoma can occur in this gland.[7, 14, 31, 63, 73, 113]

The tumors occur in patients over the age of 50 and affect predominantly the female population in a ratio of 3:1. Clinically, the tumors present as rapidly enlarging neck masses of variable sizes that can compress adjacent structures and produce associated symptoms such as hoarseness, dysphagia, and respiratory distress.[113] Since these patients often have a history of goiter, this rapid growth mimics clinically the development of anaplastic carcinoma.

The majority of thyroid lymphomas develop in the abnormal setting of Hashimoto's thyroiditis.[14, 63] Hence, laboratory tests may show hypothyroidism; this is especially true if the tumor has replaced and destroyed a large portion of the gland. Thyroid scans show either single or multiple cold nodules.

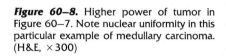

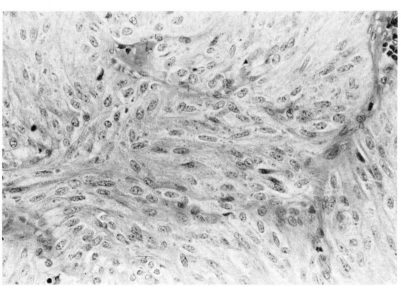

Figure 60–8. Higher power of tumor in Figure 60–7. Note nuclear uniformity in this particular example of medullary carcinoma. (H&E, ×300)

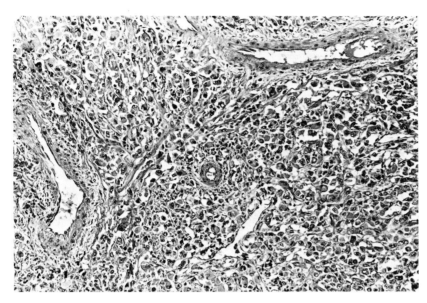

Figure 60–9. Anaplastic carcinoma is shown. This rapidly growing mass in a 70-year-old woman shows the giant cell pattern of this type of neoplasm. (H&E, ×150)

Grossly, thyroid lymphomas may be unilateral or may involve the entire gland. They appear as large, bulky tumor masses that on cut section show the characteristic tan-yellowish and "fish flesh" appearance of lymphomas. Focally, areas of necrosis are often present. Commonly, the tumor extends beyond the capsule into soft tissue and muscle. Regional lymph nodes may be involved.[7, 14, 25, 31, 58, 63, 73, 100, 113]

Histologically, all variants of malignant lymphomas have been reported to originate in the thyroid, but the non-Hodgkin's B-cell type predominates (Figs. 60–11 and 60–12). The most common subtypes of primary thyroid lymphomas are (1) the large noncleaved follicular center cell type, or B-cell immunoblastic sarcoma (histiocytic lymphoma), and (2) the small noncleaved cell type (poorly differentiated malignant lymphoma).[69, 70, 103, 113] Most of these tumors grow in a diffuse pattern, although occasionally nodular lymphomas are seen.

The normal thyroid architecture is obliterated by the diffusely infiltrative process, but remnants of atrophic follicles or single eosinophilic epithelial cells may be identified (Fig. 60–11). Mitoses as well as foci of necrosis are common (Fig. 60–12). When nontumoral parenchyma is sampled, changes of Hashimoto's thyroiditis are usually recognized.

The differential diagnosis of primary malignant lymphomas is with anaplastic epithelial carcinomas, both giant cell and so-called small cell type.[9, 37, 48, 59, 71, 72, 78, 86, 89, 104] Electron microscopy and immunoperoxidase staining are helpful in making the distinction between the two entities. Ultrastructural studies of the epithelial neoplasms show prominent basement membrane and desmosomal attachments. Lymphomas lack these features.[9] Immunoperoxidase stains for surface immunoglobulins may give variable results, but in many cases this technique confirms the B-cell nature of these neoplasms and their monoclonality.[103]

The treatment of primary malignant lymphomas of

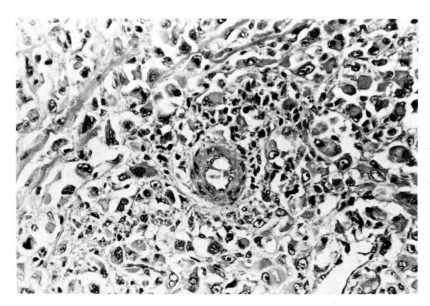

Figure 60–10. At higher power, giant cells show abundant cytoplasm and eccentric nuclei; eosinophilia of cytoplasm recapitulated rhabdomyoblastic differentiation. (H&E, ×400)

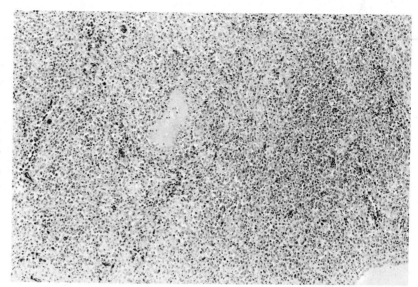

Figure 60–11. The normal thyroid parenchyma has been destroyed by a diffusely infiltrative malignant process consistent with malignant lymphoma. (H&E, ×100)

the thyroid consists of surgery for diagnosis or for decompression of the neck organs; adjuvant radiation and/or chemotherapy is usually given, depending on subtype of tumor and stage of disease.[7, 31, 58, 63, 73, 100, 113]

The prognosis of thyroid lymphomas depends upon stage of disease and type of lymphoma, with small cell tumors associated with a good prognosis and patients with immunoblastic sarcoma having a 30 to 40 per cent 5-year survival rate.[14, 113] In contrast, anaplastic carcinomas are associated with a dismal prognosis.[37, 48, 59, 71, 72, 86, 104]

The thyroid may be affected occasionally by other types of hematopoietic neoplasms: granulocytic sarcoma and plasmacytoma.

Granulocytic sarcomas or "chloromas" are tumors composed of immature myeloid precursor cells in an extramedullary site. They involve the thyroid very rarely, but may represent the initial manifestation of a leukemic process.[87]

Plasmacytomas (tumors composed solely of plasma cells) are also rare in the thyroid. Solitary lesions isolated to the gland can be successfully treated by surgery.[8, 84] The pathologist and clinician must be aware that such a lesion may represent an early manifestation of systemic myeloma.

Metastatic Tumors

The thyroid gland is rarely affected by metastatic spread of other tumors despite the fact that the thyroid is one of the most richly vascularized organs. No satisfactory biologic reason for the low metastatic rate is known.

Metastatic spread to the thyroid can occur in two ways: (1) by direct extension of tumors of the neck (i.e., squamous cell carcinoma of the larynx) or (2) by vascular or lymphatic spread from a distant site.[65]

Some authors note that metastatic tumors are found

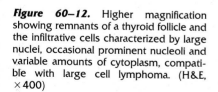

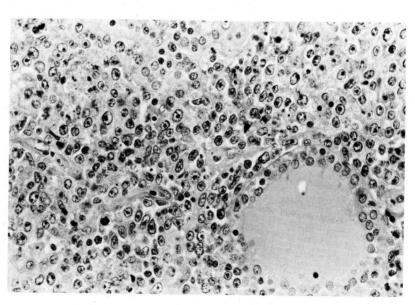

Figure 60–12. Higher magnification showing remnants of a thyroid follicle and the infiltrative cells characterized by large nuclei, occasional prominent nucleoli and variable amounts of cytoplasm, compatible with large cell lymphoma. (H&E, ×400)

with greater frequency in adenomatous glands.[85, 99] Architectural and vascular alterations in such a thyroid may favor the deposits of tumor emboli. The most common tumors to metastasize to the thyroid are malignant melanoma and carcinomas of the kidney, lung, breast, and colon.[17, 22, 38, 78, 85, 99]

In surgical material, the clinical significance of metastatic involvement of the thyroid resides in these lesions that mimic primary tumors. A history of a known cancer is useful, but may be lacking. The time interval between diagnosis of the primary lesion and the thyroid metastasis may be unexpectedly long. The Mayo Clinic study[17] disclosed that this interval averaged 82 months in five patients with kidney cancer metastatic to the thyroid. If a patient with a known malignancy presents with a thyroid mass and if the histologic pattern is compatible with a primary in the gland, the pathologist must be cautious in interpreting the lesion. Review of previous material may be essential in these cases.[22]

NEEDLE BIOPSY AND FINE-NEEDLE ASPIRATION CYTOLOGY

Two techniques have become standard procedure in the evaluation of patients with thyroid nodules: core-needle biopsy and fine-needle aspiration cytology.

The needle core biopsy produces a piece of tissue that is evaluated *histologically.*[107, 109] For documenting the diagnosis of thyroiditis, such a technique might prove useful but is often not necessary. When needle core biopsy is used to obtain diagnostic material from a thyroid nodule, the reported results are excellent. The diagnosis of papillary, medullary, and anaplastic carcinomas can be rendered readily. In follicular tumors, however, the absence of the diagnostic clue (tumor-capsule-thyroid interface) often makes definitive diagnosis difficult, especially in well-differentiated tumors.

Similar results have been described for fine-needle aspiration cytology.[32, 33, 67, 108] Ease of performance and virtual absence of complications have made this technique a widely acceptable one. For papillary, medullary, and anaplastic cancers, this method proves accurate in a very high percentage of cases. It has become apparent that increasing experience has improved diagnostic accuracy.[35] However, for follicular lesions, the problems of relying upon cytologic (mostly nuclear) details have not been easily overcome. Although some pathologists and cytologists believe they can distinguish among adenomatous nodule, follicular adenoma, and follicular carcinoma readily,[32, 33, 35, 67, 108] others find this distinction difficult. We concur with the latter group, since the cytologic features of well-differentiated follicular cancers so closely resemble those of adenomas and adenomatous nodules (Fig. 60–6). Although some authors have indicated the accuracy of cytology,[35] recent studies attempting to define cytologic differences between benign and malignant follicular thyroid lesions by use of scanning electron microscopy, image analysis, and flow cytometry have disclosed that even with such refined techniques a diagnostic differentiation among follicular tumors is not easily obtained.[51–53, 68]

However, we recognize that most thyroid nodules display a follicular pattern and that the majority of these represent adenomatous nodules. Therefore, interpretation of a fine-needle aspiration cytology specimen of a follicular lesion as "adenomatous nodule" or "adenoma" will be correct in over 90 per cent of cases. The false-negative rate is low enough to be acceptable.

In practice, follicular lesions that on cytologic examination appear cellular or show nuclear irregularity or pleomorphism are diagnosed as "atypical." Now the pathologist is unsure, the odds have changed, the problem is returned to the clinician, and most patients with such a diagnosis will undergo surgery.

In conclusion, aspiration cytology or needle biopsy of thyroid nodules serves to confirm or to exclude the diagnosis of papillary, medullary, and, rarely, anaplastic carcinoma. If the nodule is follicular and not atypical, the clinician can assume it is a benign lesion, in which case nonsurgical therapy or watchful waiting usually suffices.

REFERENCES

1. Aldinger KA, Samaaan NA, Ibanez M, Hill CS: Anaplastic carcinoma of the thyroid: A review of 84 cases of spindle and giant cell carcinoma of the thyroid. Cancer 41:2267, 1978.
2. Arnold JE, Pinsky S: Comparison of ^{99m}Tc and ^{123}I for thyroid imaging. J Nucl Med 17:261, 1976.
3. Bigner SH, Mendelsohn G, Wells SA, et al: Medullary carcinoma of the thyroid in the multiple endocrine neoplasia IIA syndrome. Am J Surg Pathol 5:459, 1979.
4. Block MA, Miller MJ, Horn RC: Carcinoma of the thyroid after external radiation to the neck in adults. Am J Surg 118:764, 1969.
5. Bocker W, Dralle H, Koch G, et al: Immunohistochemical and electron microscope analysis of adenomas of the thyroid gland: II. Adenomas with specific cytological differentiation. Virchows Arch [A] (Pathol Anat) 380:205, 1978.
6. Bondeson L, Bondeson A-G, Ljungberg O, Tibblin S: Oxyphil tumors of the thyroid. Ann Surg 194:677, 1981.
7. Burke JS, Butler JJ, Fuller LM: Malignant lymphomas of the thyroid: A clinicopathologic study of 35 patients including ultrastructural observations. Cancer 39:1587, 1977.
8. Buss D, Marshall RB, Holleman IL, Myers RT: Malignant lymphoma of the thyroid gland with plasma cell differentiation (plasmacytoma). Cancer 46:2671, 1980.
9. Cameron RD, Seemayer TA, Wang NS, et al: Small cell malignant tumors of the thyroid. Human Pathol 6:731, 1975.
10. Campbell WL, Santiago HE, Perzin KH, Johnson PM: The autonomous thyroid nodule: Correlation of scan appearance and histopathology. Radiology 107:133, 1973.
11. Carney JA, Sizemore GW, Hayles AB: C-cell disease of the thyroid gland in multiple endocrine neoplasia, type 2b. Cancer 44:2173, 1979.
12. Chen KTK, Rosai J: Follicular variant of thyroid papillary carcinoma: A clinicopathologic study of six cases. Am J Surg Pathol 1:123, 1977.
13. Clark RL, White EC, Russell WO: Total thyroidectomy for cancer of the thyroid: Significance of intraglandular dissemination. Ann Surg 149:858, 1959.
14. Compagno J, Oertel JE: Malignant lymphoma and other lymphoproliferative disorders of the thyroid gland: A clinicopathologic study of 245 cases. Am J Clin Pathol 74:1–11, 1980.
15. Cox MT: Malignant lymphoma of the thyroid. J Clin Pathol 17:591, 1964.
16. Cuello C, Correa P, Eisenberg H: Geographic pathology of thyroid carcinoma. Cancer 23:230, 1969.
17. Czech JM, Lichtor TR, Carney JA, van Heerden JA: Neoplasms metastatic to the thyroid. Surg Gynecol Obstet 155:503, 1982.
18. DeGroot LJ, Reilly M, Pinnameneni K, Refetoff S: Retrospective and prospective study of radiation-induced thyroid disease. Am J Med 74:852, 1983.
19. De Lellis RA, Sternberger LA, Mann RB, et al: Immunoperoxidase techniques in diagnostic pathology. Am J Clin Pathol 71:483, 1979.
20. De Lellis RA, Wolfe HJ: The pathobiology of the human calcitonin (C)-cell: A review. Pathol Ann 16: (Part 2) 25, 1981.
21. Devine RM, Edis AJ, Banks PM: Primary lymphoma of the thyroid: A review of the Mayo Clinic experience. World J Surg 5:33, 1981.

22. Elliott RS, Frantz VK: Metastatic carcinoma masquerading as primary thyroid cancers. Ann Surg 151:551, 1960.

23. Esselstyn CB, Crile G: Indications for surgical therapy in thyroid disease. Semin Nucl Med 1:474, 1971.

24. Favus MJ, Schneider AB, Stachura ME, et al: Thyroid cancer occurring as a late consequence of head and neck irradiation. N Engl J Med 294:1019, 1976.

25. Feigin GA, Buss DH, Paschal B, et al: Hodgkin's disease manifested as a thyroid nodule. Human Pathol 13:774, 1982.

26. Fialkow PJ: The origin and development of human tumors studied with cell markers. N Engl J Med 291:26, 1974.

27. Fisher ER, Gregorio R, Shoemaker R, et al: The derivation of so-called "giant-cell" and "spindle-cell" undifferentiated thyroid neoplasms. Am J Clin Pathol 61:680, 1974.

28. Franssila K: Value of histologic classification of thyroid cancer. Acta Pathol Microbiol Scand (Suppl) 225:5, 1971.

29. Franssila KO: Is the differentiation between papillary and follicular thyroid carcinoma valid? Cancer 32:853, 1973.

30. Franssila KO: Prognosis in thyroid carcinoma. Cancer 36:1138, 1975.

31. Freeman C, Berg J, Cutler SJ: Occurrence and prognosis of extranodal lymphomas. Cancer 29:252, 1977.

32. Friedman M, Shimaoka K, Getaz P: Needle aspiration of 310 thyroid lesions. Acta Cytol 23:194, 1979.

33. Gershengorn MC, McClung MR, Chu EW, et al: Fine needle aspiration cytology in the preoperative diagnosis of thyroid nodules. Ann Intern Med 87:265, 1977.

34. Gundry SR, Burney RE, Thompson NW, Lloyd R: Total thyroidectomy for Hürthle cell neoplasms of the thyroid. Arch Surg 118:529, 1983.

35. Hamburger J, Miller JM, Kini SR: Clinical-Pathological Evaluation of Thyroid Nodules. Southfield, Mich., Associated Endocrinologists, 1979.

36. Hapke MR, Dehner LP: The optically clear nucleus: A reliable sign of papillary carcinoma of the thyroid. Am J Surg Pathol 3:31, 1979.

37. Harada T, Shimaoka K, Yakamuru K, Ito K: Squamous cell carcinoma of the thyroid gland—transition from adenocarcinoma. J Surg Oncol 19:36, 1982.

38. Harcourt-Webster JN: Secondary neoplasm of the thyroid presenting as a goitre. J Clin Pathol 18:282, 1965.

39. Hawk WA, Hazard JB: The many appearance of papillary carcinoma of the thyroid. Cleve Clin Q 43:207, 1977.

40. Hazard JB: The C-cells (parafollicular cells) of the thyroid gland and medullary thyroid carcinoma: A review. Am J Pathol 88:214, 1977.

41. Hazard JB, Hawk WA, Crile G: Medullary (solid) carcinoma of the thyroid—a clinicopathologic entity. J Clin Endocrinol Metab 19:152, 1959.

42. Hazard JB, Kenyon R: Atypical adenoma of the thyroid. Arch Pathol 58:554, 1954.

43. Hedinger CE: Thyroid Cancer. Heidelberg, Springer-Verlag, Inc., 1969.

44. Heimann P: Ultrastructure of human thyroid. Acta Endocrinol 53 (Suppl): 110, 1966.

45. Heimann R, Vannineuse A, De Sloover C, Dor P: Malignant lymphomas and undifferentiated small cell carcinoma of the thyroid: A clinicopathological review in light of the Kiel classification for malignant lymphomas. Histopathology 2:201, 1978.

46. Huang TY, Assor D: Primary squamous cell carcinoma of the thyroid gland. Am J Clin Pathol 55:93, 1971.

47. Ibanez ML: Medullary carcinoma of the thyroid gland. Pathol Ann 9:263, 1974.

48. Jao W, Gould VE: Ultrastructure of anaplastic (spindle and giant cell) carcinoma of the thyroid. Cancer 35:1280, 1975.

49. Johannessen JV, Sobrinho-Simoes M: Well-differentiated thyroid tumors. Pathol Ann 18 (Part 1):255, 1983.

50. Johannessen J, Sobrinho-Simoes M: The origin and significance of thyroid psammoma bodies. Lab Invest 43:287, 1980.

51. Johannessen JV, Sobrinho-Simoes M: Follicular carcinoma of the human thyroid gland: An ultrastructural study with emphasis on scanning electron microscopy. Diagn Histopathol 5:113, 1981.

52. Johannessen JV, Sobrinho-Simoes M, Finseth I, Pilstrom L: Ultrastructural morphometry of thyroid neoplasms. Am J Clin Pathol 79:162, 1983.

53. Johannessen JV, Sobrinho-Simoes M, Lindmo T, Tangen KO: The diagnostic value of flow cytometric DNA measurements in selected disorders of the human thyroid. Am J Clin Pathol 77:20, 1982.

54. Johnson N: The blood supply of the thyroid gland: I. The normal gland. Aust N Zeal J Surg 23:95, 1953.

55. Kahn NF, Perzin KH: Follicular carcinoma of the thyroid. Pathol Ann 18 (Part 1):221, 1983.

56. Kakudo K, Miyauchi A, Takai S, et al: C-cell carcinoma of the thyroid: Papillary type. Acta Pathol Jpn 29:653, 1979.

57. Kakudo K, Miyauchi A, Ogihara T, et al: Medullary carcinoma of the thyroid: Giant cell type. Arch Pathol Lab Med 102:445, 1978.

58. Kapadia SB, Dekker A, Cheng VS, et al: Malignant lymphoma of the thyroid gland: A clinicopathologic study. Head Neck Surg 4:270, 1982.

59. Kapp DS, LiVolsi VA, Sanders MM: Anaplastic carcinoma following well-differentiated thyroid cancer: Etiological considerations. Yale J Biol Med 55:521, 1982.

60. Klinck GH, Oertel JE, Winship T: Ultrastructure of normal human thyroid. Lab Invest 22:2, 1970.

61. Lang W, Atay Z, Stauch G, Kienzle E: The differentiation of atypical adenomas and encapsulated follicular carcinomas in the thyroid gland. Virchows Arch [A] (Pathol Anat) 385:125, 1980.

62. Liechtly RD, Safaie-Shirazi S, Soper RT: Carcinoma of the thyroid in children. Surg Gynecol Obstet 134:595, 1972.

63. Lindsay S, Dailey ME: Malignant lymphoma of the thyroid gland and its relation to Hashimoto's disease: A clinical and pathological study of 8 patients. J Clin Endocrinol Metab 15:1332, 1955.

64. LiVolsi VA, Merino MJ: Squamous cells in the human gland. Am J Surg Pathol 2:133, 1978.

65. LiVolsi VA: Pathology. In Greenberg LL (ed): Thyroid Cancer, West Palm Beach, Fla., CRC Press, 1978, pp. 85–141.

66. LiVolsi VA: Calcitonin: The hormone and its significance. Progr Surg Pathol 1:71, 1980.

67. Löwhagen T, Granberg PO, Lundell G, et al: Aspiration biopsy cytology (ABC) in nodules of the thyroid gland suspected to be malignant. Surg Clin North Am 59:3, 1979.

68. Luck JB, Mumaw VC, Frable WJ: Video plan image analysis on fine needle aspiration biopsies of the thyroid gland. Acta Cytol 25:718, 1981.

69. Lukes RJ, Collins RD: New approaches to the classification of the lymphomata. Br J Cancer 31 (Suppl II):1–18, 1975.

70. Lukes RJ, Parker JW, Taylor CR, et al: Immunologic approach to non-Hodgkin's lymphomas and related leukemias: Analysis of the results of multiparameter studies of 425 cases. Semin Hematol 15:322, 1978.

71. Luna MA, Mackay B, Hill CS, et al: Malignant small cell tumor of the thyroid. Ultrastructural Pathol 1:265, 1980.

72. Mahoney JP, Saffos RO, Rhatigan RM: Follicular adenocanthoma of the thyroid gland. Histopathol 4:547, 1980.

73. Maurer R, Taylor C, Terry R, Lukes R: Non-Hodgkin's lymphomas of the thyroid. Virchows Arch [A] (Pathol Anat) 383:293, 1979.

74. Mazzaferri EL, Young RL: Papillary thyroid carcinoma: A 10-year followup report of the impact of therapy in 576 patients. Am J Med 70:511, 1981.

75. Mazzaferri EL, Young RL, Oertel JE, et al: Papillary thyroid carcinoma: The impact of therapy in 576 patients. Medicine 56:171, 1977.

76. Meissner WA: Surgical Pathology. In Sedgwick CE (ed): Surgery of the Thyroid Gland. Philadelphia, W.B. Saunders Co., 1974, pp. 24–53.

77. Meissner WA, Adler A: Papillary carcinoma of the thyroid: A study of the pathology of 226 cases. Arch Pathol 66:518, 1958.

78. Meissner WA, Warren S: Tumors of the Thyroid Gland. In Atlas of Tumor Pathology, second series, Fasc. IV. Washington, D.C., Armed Forces Institute of Pathology, 1969.

79. Melvin KEW, Tashjian AH, Miller HH: Studies in familial (medullary) thyroid carcinoma. Recent Progr Horm Res 28:399, 1972.

80. Mendelsohn G, Bigner SH, Eggleston JC, et al: Anaplastic variants of medullary thyroid carcinoma. Am J Surg Pathol 4:333, 1980.

81. Mendelsohn G, Oertel JE: Encapsulated medullary thyroid carcinomas: Differentiation from atypical adenomas by calcitonin immunohistochemistry. Lab Invest 44:43A, 1981.

82. Mendelsohn G, Pressig SH, Eggleston JC, et al: Unusual morphologic variants of medullary thyroid carcinoma. Lab Invest 40:273A, 1979.

83. Money WL: Chemical carcinogenesis and sex hormones in experimental thyroid tumours. In Hedinger CE (ed): Thyroid Cancer. Heidelberg, Springer-Verlag, Inc., 1969, pp. 140–149.

84. More MRS, Dawson DW, Ralston AS, Craig I: Plasmacytoma of the thyroid. J Clin Pathol 21:661, 1968.

85. Mortensen JO, Woolner LB, Bennett WA: Secondary malignant tumors of the thyroid gland. Cancer 9:306, 1956.

86. Newland JR, Mackay B, Hill CS, Hickey RC: Anaplastic thyroid carcinoma: An ultrastructural study of 10 cases. Ultrastructural Pathol 2:121, 1981.

87. Nieman RS, Barcos M, Bernard C, et al: Granulocytic sarcoma: A clinicopathologic study of 61 biopsied cases. Cancer 48:1426, 1981.

88. Nieuwenhuijzen-Kruseman AC, Bosman FT, van Bergen Hene-

gouw JC, et al: Medullary differentiation of anaplastic thyroid carcinoma. Am J Clin Pathol 77:541, 1982.

89. Nishiyama RH, Dunn E, Thompson NW: Anaplastic spindle-cell and giant-cell tumors of the thyroid gland. Cancer 30:113, 1972.
90. Normann T, Gautvik KM, Johannessen JV, Brennhovd IO: Medullary carcinoma of the thyroid in Norway: Clinical course and endocrinological aspects. Acta Endocrinol 83:71, 1977.
91. Normann T, Johannessen JV: Cell types in medullary thyroid carcinoma. Acta Pathol Microbiol Scand 85:561, 1977.
92. Normann T, Johannessen JV, Gautvik KM: Medullary carcinoma of the thyroid. Cancer 38:366, 1976.
93. Olen E, Klinck GH: Hyperthyroidism and thyroid cancer. Arch Pathol 81:531, 1966.
94. Roeher HD, Daum R, Pieper M, Rudolph HJ: Juvenile thyroid carcinoma. J Pediatr Surg 7:27, 1972.
95. Russell MA, Gilbert EF, Jaeschke WF: Prognostic features of thyroid cancer: A long-term pathologic follow-up of 68 cases. Cancer 36:553, 1975.
96. Sampson RJ, Key CR, Buncher CR, Tijima S: Thyroid carcinoma in Hiroshima and Nagasaki: I. Prevalence of thyroid carcinoma at autopsy. JAMA 209:65, 1969.
97. Savino D, Sibley RK, Sumner H: Significance of Hürthle cells in thyroid neoplasms: Reexamination of an old but persistent problem. Lab Invest 44:59A, 1981.
98. Silverberg SG, Hutter RVP, Foote FW: Fatal carcinoma of the thyroid: Histology, metastases and causes of death. Cancer 25:792, 1970.
99. Silverberg SG, Vidone RA: Metastatic tumors in the thyroid. Pacif Med Surg 74:175, 1966
100. Sirota DK, Segal RL: Primary lymphoma of the thyroid gland. JAMA 242:1743, 1979.
101. Stepanas AV, Samaan NA, Hill CS, Hickey RC: Medullary thyroid carcinoma: Importance of serial serum calcitonin measurement. Cancer 43:825, 1979.

102. Studer H, Ramelli F: Simple goiter and its variants: Euthyroid and hyperthyroid multinodular goiters. Endocr Rev 3:40, 1982.
103. Taylor CR: Immunohistologic studies of lymphoma: Past, present, and future. J Histochem Cytochem 28:777, 1980.
104. Tollefsen HR, DeCosse JJ, Hutter RVP: Papillary carcinoma of the thyroid: A clinical and pathological study of 70 fatal cases. Cancer 17:1035, 1964.
105. Tollefsen HR, Shah JP, Huvos AG: Papillary carcinoma of the thyroid. Recurrence in the thyroid gland after initial surgical treatment. Am J Surg 124:468, 1972.
106. Tscholl-Ducommun J, Hedinger CH: Papillary thyroid carcinoma, morphology and prognosis. Virch Arch [A] (Pathol Anat) 396:19, 1982.
107. Vickery AL: Needle biopsy pathology. Clin Endocrinol Metab 10:275, 1981.
108. Walfish PG, Hazani E, Strawbridge HTG, et al: A prospective study of combined ultrasonography and needle aspiration biopsy in the assessment of the hypofunctioning thyroid nodule. Surgery 82:474, 1977.
109. Wang CA, Vickery AL, Maloof F: Needle biopsy of the thyroid. Surg Gynecol Obstet 143:365, 1976.
110. Woolner LB: Thyroid carcinoma: Pathologic classification with data on prognosis. Semin Nucl Med 1:481, 1971.
111. Woolner LB, Beahrs OH, Black BM, et al: Classification and prognosis of thyroid carcinoma: A study of 885 cases observed in a 30-year period. Am J Surg 102:354, 1961.
112. Woolner LB, Lemmon ML, Beahrs OH, et al: Occult papillary carcinoma of the thyroid gland: A study of 140 cases observed in a 30-year period. J Clin Endocrinol Metab 20:89, 1960.
113. Woolner LB, McConahey WM, Beahrs OH, Black BM: Primary malignant lymphomas of the thyroid: Review of forty-six cases. Am J Surg 111:502, 1966.

CHAPTER 61

Nuclear Medicine Therapy of Thyroid Cancer

William H. Blahd, M.D.

The concentration of radioactive iodine (radioiodine) in metastatic thyroid cancer was first demonstrated by Keston and associates[33] in 1942. However, it was not until the late 1940s and early 1950s, when radioiodine became generally available, that significant experience was obtained in its use in the treatment of thyroid cancer. Early studies by Fitzgerald and Foote[18] demonstrated that only one half of well-differentiated thyroid cancers concentrated radioiodine. Subsequently, Rawson and his colleagues[50] observed that thyroid cancer metastases rarely concentrated radioiodine in euthyroid patients, but that hypothyroidism induced by surgical or radioiodine ablation of residual normal thyroid tissue was necessary before significant concentration of radioiodine occurred. Pochin[45] reported that significant radioiodine concentration occurred in 50 to 80 per cent of patients with well-differentiated thyroid carcinoma following the ablation of thyroid tissue. By the administration of large doses of radioiodine, he was able to eradicate all evidence of cancer in 15 of 192 patients who had inoperable metastatic disease. Subsequently, other investigators have shown improved survival in patients with distant metastases who were treated with radioiodine.[11, 24, 32, 37, 39, 40, 54, 55]

Efficient uptake of and response to radioiodine are observed in tumors that are of the differentiated cell type, such as papillary or follicular, whereas undifferentiated tumors and Hürthle cell and medullary carcinomas rarely concentrate radioiodine. Effective tumor uptake is approximately 0.5 per cent of the dose per gram, with a biologic half-life of approximately 4 days.[46] From the administration of 150 mCi ^{131}I, a tumor will receive about 25,000 rad, or five times the absorbed dose that can be delivered by a course of external radiation therapy. Moreover, this dose will be delivered to every functional metastasis, regardless of its size or location in the body, and tumor tissue will receive several hundred times the radiation exposure received by the rest of the body.

RADIOIODINE ABLATION OF RESIDUAL THYROID TISSUE

Although the majority of thyroid adenocarcinomas can be removed surgically, there is often uncertainty as to the completeness of the resection and the presence of local or distant histologic metastases, despite the absence of clinically detectable abnormalities. There is mounting evidence indicating an increased rate of survival and a decreased rate of tumor recurrence in patients who have received radioiodine therapy. It would appear to be prudent, therefore, to ablate with radioiodine any residual thyroid tissue that has not been removed surgically, for the complete ablation of all normal thyroid tissue usually ensures rapid radioiodine uptake in remaining tumor deposits and tumor metastases.

Ablation of small thyroid remnants after near-total thyroidectomy may be accomplished by the administration of 75 to 150 mCi of radioiodine, regardless of the amount of thyroid tissue remaining and the percentage of uptake.[34] Ablation of thyroid remnants is usually carried out 3 to 6 weeks after thyroidectomy. Whole-body imaging with radioiodine should be performed routinely prior to ablation. If residual cancer or metastases are detected, radioiodine treatment rather than ablation must be considered. Approximately 4 to 6 months after ablation, whole-body imaging is performed again to assess the completeness of ablation and to determine whether any residual thyroid cancer or metastases are capable of concentrating radioiodine. Subsequent management is based on the results of the imaging procedure.

RADIOIODINE TREATMENT

The objective of the treatment of thyroid cancer with radioactive iodine is to destroy functioning thyroid cancer tissue. The following criteria should be considered in the evaluation of patients with well-differentiated thyroid cancer for radioiodine treatment:[31]

1. Inoperable primary cancer.
2. Residual postoperative thyroid cancer in cervical region.
3. Metastases to cervical or mediastinal lymph nodes.
4. Distant metastases.
5. Recurrent thyroid cancer.

Prior to radioiodine therapy, the ability of residual or metastatic thyroid cancer to concentrate radioiodine is evaluated by radioiodine imaging procedures. If thyroid hormone has been administered, it must be discontinued. Studies have shown that withdrawal of triiodothyronine (T_3) replacement for 2 weeks gives as good a radioiodine uptake in functional metastases as withdrawal of T_3 for 4 weeks.[20, 29] The shorter period of withdrawal minimizes the period of hypothyroidism. Accordingly, patients are switched from suppression therapy with L-thyroxine to a comparable dose of T_3 for 2 to 4 weeks to allow disposal of the thyroxine. This is followed by 2 weeks of withdrawal of T_3, which is cleared from the body much more rapidly than thyroxine. Serum thyroid-stimulating hormone (TSH) concentration is measured before radioiodine imaging is begun. Optimally, serum TSH levels exceed 40 µU/ml. Measurement of serum TSH may help to identify the rare individual who does not respond to the brief period of T_3 withdrawal. In such cases, the administration of exogenous bovine TSH is necessary.

Bovine TSH is given to increase the accumulation of radioiodine in thyroid cancer metastases. Even after the thyroid gland has been removed or ablated, injection of bovine TSH will occasionally result in a significant increase in radioiodine uptake by functioning thyroid cancer metastases.[5] Presumably, the tumors in such patients produce sufficient thyroid hormone to suppress endogenous TSH. However, the administration of bovine TSH is not without complications, for sensitivity reactions may occur in as many as 40 per cent of patients who receive repeated courses.[35] Controversy also exists as to whether or not exogenous TSH is significantly additive to the endogenous TSH levels that ordinarily follow a period of withdrawal of thyroid hormone.[27] Furthermore, because repeated administration of exogenous TSH may result in the development of immunoreactive and neutralizing anti-TSH antibodies, it is recommended that its use be limited to the initial diagnostic studies and therapy.[41]

Patients undergoing radioiodine treatment or ablation or whole-body imaging with radioiodine also must be protected from contamination from iodine-containing medications and x-ray contrast media. In addition, some investigators recommend a low-iodine diet for at least a week prior to radioiodine therapy.[21]

Once adequate tumor uptake has been ensured by radioiodine imaging studies, therapeutic doses of radioiodine are administered. Most investigators recommend a fixed amount of radioiodine that varies from 100 to 200 mCi, depending on the extent of tumor distribution.[3, 8, 17, 38, 46] This dose range has been found empirically to be without significant complications in the majority of patients. To estimate the radiation dose prior to treatment Hurley and Becker[31] recommend the use of a quantitative technique that is based on a rough estimate of tumor mass, as determined from radioiodine images obtained with a rectilinear scanner. Quantitative uptake is determined with a scintillation probe or a camera interfaced with a computer. The effective half-life of radioiodine in the tumor is determined from sequential measurements obtained over a period of 3 to 7 days. The radiation dose to the tumor per millicurie of radioiodine administered then can be calculated based on MIRD* dosimetry:

*Report of Medical Internal Radiation Dose Committee, Society of Nuclear Medicine, 1968, New York, N. Y.

$$rad/mCi = \frac{t\frac{1}{2} \text{ eff (days)} \times \% \text{ tumor uptake (t = 0)} \times 152}{\text{estimated tumor mass (gm)}}$$

If the calculated dose to the tumor is less than 5000 rad, other means of therapy must be considered.

Therapy doses are given at intervals of 4 to 6 months until no clinical or radioiodine imaging evidence of functioning tumor tissue is demonstrable.

Complications

Serious complications as a result of radiation damage to normal tissues following the administration of 200 mCi of radioiodine or less are uncommon and rarely interfere with therapeutic endeavors.[3, 8, 9, 17, 38] They are more common after large single treatments or when large cumulative amounts of radioiodine have been given.[6, 46] Whole-body radiation from usual therapeutic doses of radioiodine is estimated at 20 to 40 rad. Transient radiation thyroiditis may occur, persisting for 2 to 3 weeks, and occasionally swelling of the parotid or submaxillary salivary glands may be observed shortly after therapy and may persist for several days. Bone marrow depression is uncommon with usual dosage regimens, except when bone metastases are present.[17] Pulmonary fibrosis has been reported in patients with pulmonary metastases after repeated administration of large therapeutic doses.[48] Fifteen cases of leukemia have been reported in the medical literature, an incidence that is slightly greater than the expected natural incidence.[53] The majority of such patients had received large total cumulative radioiodine doses. The transformation of previously differentiated tumors to rapidly growing anaplastic cancers may occur in a small percentage of patients.[42] This transformation is known to occur spontaneously in untreated adenocarcinomas; thus, there appears to be no evidence to implicate radiation as the cause of tumor transformation.

Treatment Follow-up and Management

Following total thyroid cancer ablation, radioiodine imaging with test doses of 5 mCi of ^{131}I is performed at yearly intervals for 3 years and biennially thereafter for a minimum of 10 years (Table 61–1). If there is tumor recurrence, the patient is re-treated. If there is persistent or progressive disease with undetectable or inadequate uptake of radioiodine, suppressive amounts of thyroxine are resumed and the patient is evaluated for treatment with external radiation therapy or chemotherapy.

Long-term follow-up is important in the management of patients with thyroid cancer. The recurrence of tumor following radioiodine ablation of all functioning tumor tissue has been observed in more than 50 per cent of patients who had tumor metastases and in 25 per cent of patients who did not have metastases.[34] Recurrences have been observed after 5 to 10 years of negative diagnostic studies.[34, 38] In view of the possibility of late recurrence, all patients in whom total radioiodine ablation has been obtained should be followed by means of diagnostic imaging studies for at least 10 years to ensure that they remain free of recurrent tumor. In most instances, recurrence occurs at the same site and responds to treatment with radioiodine.

Because pituitary thyrotropin is an important growth factor for thyroid follicular cells, suppression of TSH by the administration of thyroid hormone appears to be an effective way of preventing recurrence in patients fol-

TABLE 61–1. Diagnostic, Therapeutic, and Follow-up Procedures Following Tumor Ablation*

Diagnostic Procedure after Thyroidectomy
1. Switch from thyroxine suppression therapy to T_3 (50–75 μg daily) for 2 to 4 weeks; then discontinue T_3 for 2 weeks
2. Give 10 units of TSH daily for 3 days†
3. Give 5 mCi ^{131}I orally 24 hr after last TSH injection
4. Scan neck and body 48 hr after ^{131}I dose

Therapeutic Procedure
1. Repeat steps 1 and 2 of diagnostic procedure
2. Give 100 to 200 mCi ^{131}I orally 24 hr after last TSH injection
3. Scan neck and body 3 to 5 days after ^{131}I dose

Follow-up Procedure
1. Repeat diagnostic procedure yearly for 3 years and every 2 years, thereafter for a total of 10 years
2. Re-treat according to the therapeutic procedure above if functioning metastases are detected
3. Prescribe thyroid hormone suppression therapy after and between ^{131}I diagnostic and therapeutic procedures

*Modified from Krishnamurthy GT, Blahd WH: Cancer *40*:195, 1977.
†TSH should be administered if prediagnostic or pretherapy serum TSH levels do not rise to at least 20 μU/ml.

lowing surgical or radioiodine therapy of well-differentiated carcinoma.[39, 55] In a few instances, metastatic thyroid carcinoma has transiently regressed after treatment with thyroid hormone.[14]

The mean dose of thyroxine required to obliterate TSH secretion is approximately 220 μg. This is only about 25 to 70 μg greater than the mean replacement dose of thyroxine in adults. The dose must be adjusted for each patient because excessive doses of thyroxine may cause disturbing symptoms of thyrotoxicosis, exert deleterious effects on the heart, and result in demineralization of bone if continued chronically.[28]

The radioimmunoassay systems for the measurement of TSH concentration are not sufficiently sensitive to demonstrate low levels; therefore, the suppression of TSH response to thyrotropin-releasing hormone (TRH) may be a useful guide in the follow-up management of patients with thyroid cancer.[30, 36]

Use of Serum Thyroglobulin

Although whole-body imaging with radioiodine has been considered to be the most sensitive means of detecting recurrent disease, it is a formidable procedure requiring withdrawal of thyroid hormone and periods of symptomatic hypothyroidism. Recent reports suggest that the determination of serum thyroglobulin (Tg) may be as sensitive in the detection of recurrent thyroid cancer as whole-body imaging, and that it may supplement or even replace routine whole-body imaging in the management and follow-up of patients who appear to be in remission.[1, 7, 12, 19]

Thyroglobulin is a large glycoprotein molecule that is found in normal thyroid gland follicular tissue. In the course of thyroid hormone secretion, small amounts of Tg are secreted and can be detected in low concentration in the blood of most normal individuals by sensitive radioimmunoassay systems. The great majority of differentiated thyroid carcinomas secrete Tg, including some, such as the Hürthle cell variant of follicular carcinoma, that may not concentrate radioiodine and therefore are not detectable by means of whole-body imaging.[1, 16] Medullary and anaplastic carcinomas do not secrete Tg. Patients with differentiated thyroid carcinoma may have elevated serum Tg preoperatively, but similar elevations are often found in patients with benign thyroid neoplasms. Consequently, serum Tg concentrations are of little help in the preoperative evaluation of thyroid cancer, but they are a useful marker for metastatic disease in patients who have had total thyroid gland removal.[1, 2, 44, 51]

Serial monitoring of thyroglobulin can detect residual tumor tissue, metastases, or the recurrence of disease. A significantly elevated level in a patient receiving thyroid hormone suppression therapy is a clear indication for a radioiodine body scan. Low levels appear to exclude the presence of residual or recurrent thyroid carcinoma.[10] Borderline serum thyroglobulin levels should be restudied after withdrawal of thyroid hormone. The subsequent elevation of serum TSH has a stimulatory effect on functional thyroid tumor tissue, and elevated thyroglobulin levels under these circumstances are indicative of the presence of tumor tissue. Patients with bone and lung metastases have the highest Tg concentrations, and those with metastases to the lymph nodes have the lowest. In some patients, elevated thyroglobulin levels have been observed when radioiodine body scans were negative, but generally, there is a good correlation between abnormal scans and elevated thyroglobulin levels. Rarely, the scan is positive, and the serum thyroglobulin is negative. In general, the measurement of serum thyroglobulin complements radioiodine body imaging in the management of patients with differentiated thyroid cancer.

Results of Radioiodine Treatment

Despite 30 years of experience, the therapeutic efficacy of radioiodine in the management of thyroid cancer remains controversial. There are several possible explanations for this circumstance. Of primary consideration is the fact that relatively few patients have been treated with radioiodine. Conservative estimates place this figure at approximately 5000. Only a small number have been followed for a period that is sufficient for evaluation of long-term therapeutic benefit. This situation exists because of the remarkable longevity of many thyroid cancer patients. Evaluation is further confounded by the multiple and combined forms of adjunctive therapy that have been employed in most reported series.[9]

A number of reports that have appeared in recent years would tend to support the therapeutic efficacy of radioiodine therapy.[11, 24, 32, 37–40, 54, 55] In a large group of patients with papillary and follicular carcinoma, Varma and colleagues[54] observed that surgery combined with radioiodine therapy significantly improved the rate of survival in patients over 40 years of age when compared with a series of 50 patients who were treated with surgery only. They also observed a 20-fold increase in the death rate when total radioiodine ablation of tumor tissue was not achieved.

Maheshwari and co-workers[38] reported 70 per cent complete remission and 30 per cent partial response or recurrence of disease in a study of 352 thyroid cancer patients who received radioiodine therapy. Forty-four patients (12.5 per cent) were unresponsive to radioiodine and died of progressive thyroid cancer; all were over 40 years of age at the time of initial diagnosis.

Using recurrence of papillary cancer as an index of response, Mazzaferri and Young[39] observed a 6.4 per cent recurrence rate at 10 years and only 11 deaths in a group of 114 patients who received radioiodine and thyroid hormone therapy postoperatively. In those patients who received only thyroid hormone postoperatively, the recurrence rate was 13 per cent, and in those patients who received no postoperative therapy, the recurrence rate was 40 per cent, with a mortality rate of 10 per cent. In patients with small primary papillary tumors (less than 1.5 cm in diameter) in whom less than total thyroidectomy was performed and who only received postoperative therapy with thyroid hormone, results did not differ statistically from the results achieved with radioiodine therapy. On the other hand, in 214 patients with follicular thyroid carcinoma, the lowest recurrence rate was observed in patients treated with total thyroidectomy, radioiodine, and thyroid hormone.[55]

In some patients, no therapeutic benefit is obtained with radioiodine therapy, whereas in others, large and disseminated tumor masses disappear, and no evidence of recurrence of tumor tissue can be demonstrated after 20 years of follow-up. In view of this variability in response, it is important that radioiodine therapy be used judiciously in the appropriate clinical situation and for the histologic type of tumor that can be expected to be clinically responsive. In this regard, there are several case reports of beneficial effects of ^{131}I on medullary thyroid carcinoma.[15, 25] Presumably, the malignant parafollicular cells are sensitive to the particulate radiation of the radioiodine trapped by adjacent functioning follicular cells. In two cases, metastatic medullary carcinoma was believed to concentrate [131]I.[43, 49] Therapy with ^{131}I for medullary thyroid carcinoma remains experimental.

One may conclude from the foregoing discussion that postoperative radioiodine ablation therapy is efficacious in the management of patients with adenocarcinoma of the thyroid. It is also clear that the risk of death from residual postoperative tumor or the continued spread of inoperable tumor is considerably greater than the hazards attributed to radioiodine therapy.

EXTERNAL RADIATION

Conventional radiation therapy may be detrimental to the success of radioiodine therapy in thyroid adenocarcinomas and should not precede therapeutic efforts with radioiodine.[26] External radiation therapy in the management of thyroid cancer has been reserved for anaplastic carcinoma and lymphoma. It is of questionable value in Hürthle cell and medullary carcinomas. Therapy is best given with high-energy electrons.[23] Recent reports[13] have documented beneficial results with 3500 to 7000 rad for treatment of local recurrences of differentiated thyroid cancers that did not take up [131]I.

CHEMOTHERAPY

Doxorubicin and bleomycin are active as single agents in thyroid cancer.[4, 22, 47, 52] Twenty-three other single agents and 25 drug combinations have been tested for activity, but the results are inconclusive because of the small number of patients treated.[47]

REFERENCES

1. Ashcraft MW, Van Herle AJ: The comparative value of serum thyroglobulin measurements and iodine 131 total body scans in the follow-up study of patients with treated differentiated thyroid cancer. Am J Med 71:806, 1981.
2. Barsano CP, et al: Serum thyroglobulin in the management of patients with thyroid cancer. Arch Intern Med 142:763, 1982.
3. Beierwaltes WH: The treatment of thyroid carcinoma with radioactive iodine. Semin Nucl Med 8:79, 1978.
4. Benker G, Reinwein D: Results of chemotherapy in thyroid cancer. Dtsch Med Wochenschr 108:403, 1983.
5. Benua RS, Sonenberg M, Leeper RD, Rawson RW: An 18-year study of the use of beef thyrotropin to increase I-131 uptake in metastatic thyroid cancer. J Nucl Med 5:796, 1964.
6. Benua RS, Cicale NR, Sonenberg M, Rawson RW: The relation of radioiodine dosimetry to results and complications in the treatment of metastatic thyroid cancer. Am J Roentgenol 87:171, 1962.
7. Black EG, Gimlette TMD, Maisey MN, et al: Serum thyroglobulin in thyroid cancer. Lancet 2:443, 1981.
8. Blahd WH: Treatment of malignant thyroid disease. Semin Nucl Med 9:95, 1979.
9. Blahd WH, Nordyke RA, Bauer FK: Radioactive iodine (I-131) in the postoperative treatment of thyroid cancer. Cancer 13:745, 1960.
10. Blahd WH, Drickman MV, Porter CW, et al: Serum thyroglobulin, a monitor of differentiated thyroid carcinoma in patients receiving thyroid hormone suppression therapy. J Nucl Med 25:673, 1984.
11. Bricout P, Kibler RS: Experience in the management of thyroid carcinoma by I-131. A report of 39 cases. J Can Assoc Radiol 24:323, 1973.
12. Charles MA, Dodson LE Jr, Waldeck N, et al: Serum thyroglobulin levels predict total body iodine scan findings in patients with treated well-differentiated thyroid carcinoma. Am J Med 69:401, 1980.
13. Chung CT, Sagerman RH, Ryoo MC, et al: External irradiation for malignant tumors. Radiology 136:753, 1980.
14. Crile G Jr: Endocrine dependency of papillary carcinomas of the thyroid. JAMA 195:101, 1966.
15. Deftos LJ, Stein MF: Radioiodine as an adjunct to the surgical treatment of medullary thyroid carcinoma. J Clin Endocrinol Metab 50:967, 1980.
16. Echenique RL, Kasi L, Haynie TP, et al: Critical evaluation of serum thyroglobulin levels and I-131 scans in post-therapy patients with differentiated thyroid carcinoma: Concise communication. J Nucl Med 23:235, 1982.
17. Edmonds CJ: Treatment of thyroid cancer. Clin Endocrinol Metab 8:223, 1979.
18. Fitzgerald PJ, Foote FW Jr: The function of various types of thyroid carcinoma as revealed by the radioautographic demonstration of radioactive iodine (I-131). J Clin Endocrinol 9:1153, 1949.
19. Fui ST, Hoffenberg R, Maisey MN, Black EG: Serum thyroglobulin concentrations and whole-body radioiodine scan in follow-up of differentiated thyroid cancer after thyroid ablation. Br Med J 2:298, 1979.
20. Goldman JM, Line BR, Aamodt RL, Robbins J: Influence of triiodothyronine withdrawal time on I-131 uptake postthyroidectomy for thyroid cancer. J Clin Endocrinol Metab 50:734, 1980.
21. Goslings BM: Effect of a low iodine diet on I-131 therapy in follicular thyroid carcinomata. J Endocrinol 64:30, 1974.
22. Gottlieb JA, Hill CS Jr: Chemotherapy of thyroid cancer with adriamycin. N Engl J Med 290:193, 1974.
23. Halnan KE: The non-surgical treatment of thyroid cancer. Br J Surg 62:769, 1975.
24. Haynie TP, Nofal MM, Beierwaltes WH: Treatment of thyroid carcinoma with I-131. JAMA 183:303, 1963.
25. Hellman DE, Kartchner MV, Antwerp JD, et al: Radioiodine in the treatment of medullary carcinoma of the thyroid. J Clin Endocrinol Metab 48:451, 1979.

26. Henk JM, Kirkman S, Owen GM: Whole-body scanning and I-131 therapy in the management of thyroid carcinoma. Br J Radiol 45:369, 1972.
27. Hershman JM, Edwards CL: Serum thyrotropin (TSH) levels after thyroid ablation compared with TSH levels after exogenous bovine TSH: Implications for I-131 treatment of thyroid carcinoma. J Clin Endocrinol Metab 34:814, 1972.
28. Hershman JM, Blahd WH, Gordon HE: Thyroid gland. In Haskell CM (ed): Cancer Treatment. Philadelphia, W. B. Saunders Co., 1980.
29. Hilts SV, Hellman D, Anderson J, et al: Serial TSH determination after T3 withdrawal or thyroidectomy in the therapy of thyroid carcinoma. J Nucl Med 20:928, 1979.
30. Hoffman DP, Surks MI, Oppenheimer JH, Weitzman ED: Response to thyrotropin releasing hormone: An objective criterion for the adequacy of thyrotropin suppression therapy. J Clin Endocrinol Metab 44:892, 1977.
31. Hurley JR, Becker DV: The use of radioactive iodine in the management of thyroid cancer. In Freeman LM, Weissmann HS (eds): Nuclear Medicine Annual. New York, Raven Press, 1983.
32. Jackson GL, Blosser NM: Surgical and radio-iodine therapy in thyroid carcinoma. Penn Med 74:77, 1971.
33. Keston AS, Ball RP, Frantz VK, Palmer WW: Storage of radioactive iodine in a metastasis from thyroid carcinoma. Science 95:362, 1942.
34. Krishnamurthy GT, Blahd WH: Radioiodine I-131 therapy in the management of thyroid cancer. Cancer 40:195, 1977.
35. Krishnamurthy GT: Human reaction to bovine TSH: Concise communication. J Nucl Med 19:284, 1978.
36. Krugman LG, Hershman JM: TRH test as an index of suppression compared with the thyroid radioiodine uptake in euthyroid goitrous patients treated with thyroxine. J Clin Endocrinol Metab 47:78, 1978.
37. Leeper RC: The effect of I-131 therapy on survival of patients with metastatic papillary or follicular thyroid carcinoma. J Clin Endocrinol Metab 36:1143, 1973.
38. Maheshwari YK, Hill CS Jr, Haynie TP III, et al: I-131 therapy in differentiated thyroid carcinoma. Cancer 47:664, 1981.
39. Mazzaferri EL, Young RL: Papillary thyroid carcinoma: A 10 year follow-up report of the impact of therapy in 576 patients. Am J Med 70:511, 1981.
40. McGowan DK, Adler RA, Ghaed N, et al: Low dose radioiodide thyroid ablation in postsurgical patients with thyroid cancer. Am J Med 61:52, 1976.
41. Melmed S, Harada A, Hershman JM, et al: Neutralizing antibodies to bovine thyrotropin in immunized patients with thyroid cancer. J Clin Endocrinol Metab 51:358, 1980.
42. Nishiyama RH, Dunn EL, Thompson NW: Anaplastic spindle-cell and giant-cell tumors of the thyroid gland. Cancer 30:113, 1972.
43. Nusynowitz MD, Pollard E, Benedetto AR, et al: Treatment of medullary carcinoma of the thyroid with I-131. J Nucl Med 23:143, 1982.
44. Pacini F, Pinchera A, Giani C, et al: Serum thyroglobulin concentrations and I-131 whole body scans in the diagnosis of metastases from differentiated thyroid carcinoma (after thyroidectomy). Clin Endocrinol 13:107, 1980.
45. Pochin EE: Prospects from the treatment of thyroid carcinoma with radioiodine. Clin Radiol 18:113, 1967.
46. Pochin EE: Radioiodine therapy of thyroid cancer. Semin Nucl Med 1:503, 1971.
47. Poster DS, Bruno S, Penta J, et al: Current status of chemotherapy in the treatment of advanced carcinoma of the thyroid gland. Cancer Clin Trials 4:301, 1981.
48. Rall JE, Alpers JB, Lewallen CG, et al: Radiation pneumonitis and fibrosis: A complication of radioiodine treatment of pulmonary metastases from cancer of the thyroid. J Clin Endocrinol Metab 17:1263, 1957.
49. Rasmusson B, Hansen HS: Treatment of medullary carcinoma of the thyroid. Value of calcitonin as tumour marker. Acta Radiol Oncol Radiat Phys Biol 18:521, 1979.
50. Rawson RW, Marinelli LD, Skanse BN, et al: The effect of total thyroidectomy on the function of metastatic thyroid cancer. J Clin Endocrinol 8:826, 1948.
51. Schneider AB, et al: Sequential serum thyroglobulin determinations, I-131 scans, and I-131 uptakes after triiodothyronine withdrawal in patients with thyroid cancer. J Clin Endocrinol Metab 53:1199, 1981.
52. Shimaoka K: Adjunctive management of thyroid cancer: Chemotherapy. J Surg Oncol 15:283, 1980.
53. Siemsen JK: Leukemia following cancericidal doses of radioiodine. J Nucl Med 11:400, 1970.
54. Varma VM, Beierwaltes WH, Nofal MM, et al: Treatment of thyroid cancer. Death rates after surgery and after surgery followed by sodium iodide I-131. JAMA 214:1437, 1970.
55. Young RL, Mazzaferri EL, Rahe AJ, Dorfman SG: Pure follicular thyroid carcinoma: Impact of therapy in 214 patients. J Nucl Med 21:733, 1980.

CHAPTER 62

Surgical Therapy of Thyroid Tumors

Melvin A. Block, M.D., Ph.D.

This discussion of the surgical therapy for thyroid tumors will attempt to be as comprehensive as feasible, providing the author's personal experience and preferences but also including other practices and policies. Both benign and malignant lesions will be discussed, and are categorized in Table 62–1. The objective is to provide working knowledge that can be modified to personal practices.

A HISTORICAL PERSPECTIVE

During the modern era of surgery, not much more than 100 years in duration, surgical attention to the thyroid was given initially to the management of hyperthyroidism and the huge colloid goiters because

TABLE 62–1. A Classification of Thyroid Tumors

I. Benign thyroid tumors
  A. Nodules in euthyroid patient
    1. Nodular hyperplasia
    2. Adenomas
    3. Indeterminate for possible low-grade carcinoma
  B. Associated with hyperthyroidism
    1. Graves' disease without or with nodules
    2. Toxic nodular goiter
    3. Autonomous functioning nodule
  C. Cysts
    1. Associated with nodules (majority are benign)
    2. Simple cyst
    3. Thyroglossal duct cyst
  D. Thyroiditis, with or without associated nodule
II. Malignant thyroid tumors
  A. Carcinoma
    1. Papillary (includes occult, associated with anaplastic carcinoma)
    2. Follicular
      Well-encapsulated, low-grade
      Angioinvasive
      Hürthle cell
      Miscellaneous, including occult, associated with anaplastic carcinoma
    3. Medullary
      Hereditary
      Sporadic
    4. Anaplastic
  B. Lymphoma
  C. Metastatic

these were the most common problems. Coincident with the development of the needed tools of anesthesia and certain surgical instruments, particularly the hemostat, thyroid surgery became possible, and the thyroid was one of the organs to attract early surgical attention.[42] Following the development of nonsurgical measures to control most cases of hyperthyroidism and colloid goiters, resulting from the availability of radioactive iodine and the institution of iodine intake to prevent colloid goiter, surgical attention was directed to nodules, both benign and malignant, but with emphasis on the latter.

In the 1940s and 1950s, attempts were initiated to determine the frequency of carcinoma-producing thyroid nodules and criteria for operation for thyroid nodules. Thyroid scans, using radioactive iodine, became available and assumed a frequently used role in identifying hypofunctional abnormalities of the thyroid gland. However, it soon became evident that this procedure is of little help in separating the malignant from the more numerous benign thyroid nodules.

After reports of an incidence of carcinoma in approximately 24 per cent of the single thyroid nodules, further reflection and analysis led to the realization that such figures could result only from highly selected series.[46, 61] Comprehensive studies, such as those from consecutive autopsies or unselected patient groups, placed the incidence at a figure of approximately 4 per cent.[61] Further contemplation showed that the number of annual deaths from thyroid carcinoma is low, making the specter of thyroid carcinoma as a major cause of death illogical. Nevertheless, the occurrence of death and morbidity from thyroid carcinoma, even though infrequent, could not be overlooked when it became evident that early recognition of disease could prevent such an outcome. Furthermore, death occurring many years after initial recognition called attention to the lack of early recognition of thyroid carcinoma and appropriately prompt surgery.

These observations have continued to be basic considerations in the search during the past two decades for:

1. Procedures that accurately detect thyroid carcinoma without resorting to wholesale surgery for thyroid nodules.

2. Operative procedures that adapt to the thyroid carcinoma at hand to permit control without significant technical complications.[7]

These developments did result in a significant reduction in the numbers of thyroid operations performed and were reflected in the change of the name of the American Goiter Association to the American Thyroid Association.

During the course of the preceding events, there occurred an increased frequency of thyroid carcinoma, and this complicated the efforts to finalize the management of thyroid nodules and carcinoma.[64] It was documented that external radiation therapy to the head and neck given to infants, as well as to patients of all ages, was a factor in this increased frequency of thyroid carcinoma.[29] This factor must be included even now in policies for treatment of thyroid nodules.

The past decade has marked further attempts to improve selectivity in surgery for thyroid nodules. Ultrasonography was initially considered to be valuable because cystic degenerating thyroid nodules are usually benign, but the procedure has been discarded as too imprecise (error rate for characterizing thyroid nodules as solid or cystic has been too high with equipment available, and some cystic nodules are malignant).

Needle biopsy techniques have slowly been shown to provide nearly the desired selection of patients with thyroid nodules for operation.[6, 20, 43, 54, 67, 73] There are significant limitations, including the inability to differentiate certain cellular nodules into benign or low-grade follicular carcinoma. Furthermore, this procedure requires participation by an experienced thyroid cytologist—this is currently the limiting factor in the uniform adoption of this technique by physicians everywhere.

Although there has been increasing agreement in policies for the extent of operation for thyroid carcinoma, the precise indications for total thyroidectomy for thyroid carcinoma have not evolved. Data derived from prospective statistically valid studies are not available to stipulate the extent of operation or other treatment, such as the employment of radioactive iodine postoperatively, for each pathologic variety or each clinical pattern of thyroid carcinoma. Current practices in treating thyroid carcinoma are based, for the most part, on a hodgepodge of retrospective studies. Never-

theless, much information is available, and an attempt will be made to utilize this information in outlining guidelines to follow currently in the surgical treatment of thyroid nodules and carcinoma.[8]

SURGICAL ANATOMY

Not only must the thyroid surgeon be familiar with the anatomic features in and around the thyroid gland, but this knowledge must be precise for several critical areas. One of these areas is the region of the *upper pole of each lobe* of the thyroid gland (Fig. 62–1). Care must be exerted here to avoid injury to the external branch of the superior laryngeal nerve, to an upper parathyroid gland that often is located immediately posterior to the upper pole of the thyroid gland, and to the recurrent laryngeal nerve that enters the larynx at the infralateral cornu of the laryngeal cartilage. The external branch of the superior laryngeal nerve is adjacent to the superior thyroid vessels. Loss of the nerve results in a weak voice. Preservation of this nerve is achieved best by restricting dissection to the vessels and by dividing the vessels over the thyroid gland itself rather than cephalad to the upper pole of the thyroid gland. These precautions assure protection of the superior laryngeal nerve when permitted by the disease process at hand. The superior parathyroid gland is frequently located posterior to the upper pole of the thyroid gland. This gland can often be preserved best by delay of dissection of this area until the anatomic features of the posterolateral aspect of the thyroid gland are better visualized and the lobe itself is reflected medially. In particular, the blood supply to the superior parathyroid gland originates primarily from the superior thyroid vessels and must be preserved. More posteriorly, located under the superior pole of the thyroid gland, is the posterolateral cornu of the laryngeal cartilage, which marks the entrance of the recurrent laryngeal nerve into the larynx. Caudad to this point, this nerve is closely attached to the undersurface of the superior pole of the thyroid lobe

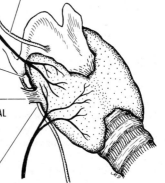

EXTERNAL BRANCH OF SUPERIOR LARYNGEAL NERVE, CLOSE TO SUPERIOR LARYNGEAL VESSELS

UPPER PARATHYROID GLAND, OFTEN POSTERIOR TO UPPER POLE THYROID LOBE

POSTERIOR SUSPENSORY LIGAMENT UNDER WHICH RECURRENT LARYNGEAL NERVE PASSES TO ENTER LARYNX AT POSTERIOR LATERAL CORNU

Figure 62–1. Anatomic features at the upper pole of each lobe of thyroid are critical in surgical procedures on this gland.

RECURRENT LARYNGEAL NERVE, LOCATED CLOSELY ADJACENT TO POSTERIOR ASPECT OF UPPER POLE THYROID, PLACING NERVE IN JEOPARDY DURING DISSECTION IN THIS REGION

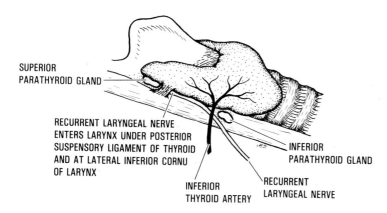

SUPERIOR
PARATHYROID GLAND

RECURRENT LARYNGEAL NERVE
ENTERS LARYNX UNDER POSTERIOR
SUSPENSORY LIGAMENT OF THYROID
AND AT LATERAL INFERIOR CORNU
OF LARYNX

INFERIOR
PARATHYROID GLAND

INFERIOR
THYROID ARTERY

RECURRENT
LARYNGEAL NERVE

Figure 62–2. Anatomic features in the tracheoesophageal groove are critical in operative procedures on the thyroid gland.

and is covered by the posterior suspensory ligament. It is here that the nerve is most likely to be injured in mobilizing the thyroid lobe for lobectomy.

A second critical anatomic area in surgery of the thyroid lobe is the *posterolateral region,* including the *tracheoesophageal groove* (Fig. 62–2). The anatomic key to this location is the inferior thyroid artery, which usually divides into two branches before entering the surface of the thyroid gland. This artery is readily identified in most patients, often by palpation after dividing an overlying middle thyroid vein. It is possible to confuse the inferior thyroid artery with the recurrent laryngeal nerve; therefore, the artery is never divided until this nerve is definitely identified. The nerve customarily forms a triangle with the inferior thyroid artery and the tracheoesophageal junction as the thyroid lobe is retracted medially, as depicted in Figure 62–2. Thus, once the artery is identified, the nerve can be located with relative ease. Once the nerve has been seen at this point, its course to the larynx along the undersurface of the upper pole of the thyroid lobe can be projected by palpating the inferolateral corner of the laryngeal cartilage. The dissection along the inferior thyroid artery must be conducted with care because the inferior parathyroid gland is customarily located in those tissues. Parathyroid glands are identified by their color, which is a darker yellow-brown in contrast to fat, and a well-defined thin fascial capsule containing minute blood vessels. The parathyroid glands and their blood supply are tenuous and easily injured by manipulation and repeated sponging. A thyroid lobectomy consists, in essence, of the separation of thyroid tissue from adjacent laryngeal nerves (recurrent and external branch of superior) and parathyroid glands, removing regional lymph nodes with the gland on the basis of gross findings and the disease being treated.

The tremendous variations in the number and location of branches of the recurrent laryngeal nerve, as well as variations in the location of the inferior thyroid artery and its relation to the recurrent laryngeal nerve, have been emphasized in a monograph by Rustad.[69] In a study of the dissection of 100 cadavers (200 nerves), Rustad categorized anatomic arrangements into 11 groups, pointing out the need for awareness on the part of the surgeon of the multiple anatomic possibilities. Of the 200 nerves, 86 (43 per cent) divided at the thyroid level. Of these, 21 divided high at the superior thyroid level, with 65 at the lower level. Thus, in at least one

third of patients, a potential exists for damage to a branch of a nerve. The surgeon may preserve one branch of the recurrent laryngeal nerve and yet injure others. The precise effect of injury to one of the branches of the recurrent laryngeal nerve has not been well documented, but Rustad expresses the opinion that this may cause voice fatigue postoperatively. At any rate, divisions or branches of the recurrent laryngeal nerve may vary in size, resulting in the potential for misinterpretation of preserved nerves and injury to significant nerves. In general, no structure between the carotid sheath and thyroid gland should be divided, except the middle thyroid vein, until the recurrent laryngeal nerve and its divisions, when present, have been definitely identified. Of the 200 nerves, nine had three divisions, seven had four divisions, two had five divisions, and one had six divisions. Thus, nearly 10 per cent of the nerves contained more than two divisions. Anatomic variations on one side of the neck could not be expected to be duplicated on the contralateral side. In no instance was the nerve located within the thyroid gland. It should be pointed out that nodules of a multinodular thyroid gland can extend from the thyroid lobe and can envelope the nerve, adding to the technical difficulty in preserving the nerve. The locations, appearance, and variations of the recurrent laryngeal nerve must be familiar to the thyroid surgeon (Fig. 62–3).

A third anatomic region of particular significance in thyroid surgery is the *anterior superior mediastinum* (Fig. 62–4). Within this location are the recurrent laryngeal nerves on each side, superior extensions of thymic lobes, and lymph node–bearing tissue. If thymic tissue extends cephalad to the proximity of the thyroid gland, parathyroid glands often (approximately 20 per cent of cases) are located within or on the surface of this thymic tissue.[72] In operative procedures for thyroid carcinoma, removal of the lymph node–bearing tissue in the anterior superior mediastinum, but with preservation of the recurrent laryngeal nerves and parathyroid glands, is desired. Lymph nodes characteristically surround the recurrent laryngeal nerves, but even when containing mestastases from well-differentiated thyroid carcinoma, they can be separated from the nerves.

Thyroid malignancy invades, on occasion, adjacent anatomic structures. This usually initially involves overlying strap muscles. These muscles are removed with the lobe in such cases.

Remnants of thyroid tissue can be present outside the

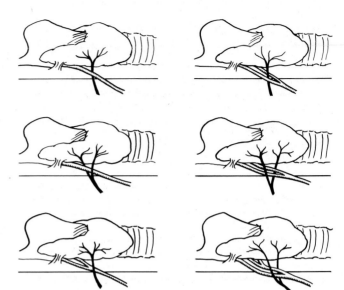

Figure 62–3. Examples of common anatomic variations of the recurrent laryngeal nerve and inferior thyroid artery.

thyroid gland proper, along the tract of the embryologic descent of the thyroid gland from the base of the tongue to the lower anterior neck. This can result in thyroglossal duct cysts along the anterior midline of the neck and varying amounts of pyramidal lobes extending cephalad from the isthmus of the thyroid gland. Rarely, isolated clumps of thyroid tissue are present outside the thyroid gland proper in the anterior neck.[21]

TREATMENT PROCEDURES

Benign Tumors

Basic factors in the management of miscellaneous benign tumors will be considered briefly before devoting major attention to the surgical treatment of thyroid nodules of undetermined etiology and thyroid malignancy.

Thyroglossal duct cysts characteristically occur in the upper midline cephalad to the larynx or over the larynx. They can first be evident at any age and frequently are involved by inflammation. Cure requires excision, using a short transverse incision over the lesion, separating the lesion from adjacent structures, isolating its fibrous tract through or adjacent to the central segment of the hyoid bone, and removing this central segment of the bone as the tract is isolated at its origin at the base of the tongue. The final excision of the tract is performed with the finger of one hand of the surgeon placed in the patient's mouth at the base of the tongue. Divided structures are resutured in closing the wound. Rarely, carcinoma, usually the papillary variety, is associated with a thyroglossal duct cyst. Unless palpable cervical lymphadenopathy is present, no further treatment is needed.

Hyperthyroidism of the Graves' type requires subtotal thyroidectomy to reduce thyroid hormone output to

Figure 62–4. Anatomic features in anterior superior mediastinum are critical in operative procedures on the thyroid gland.

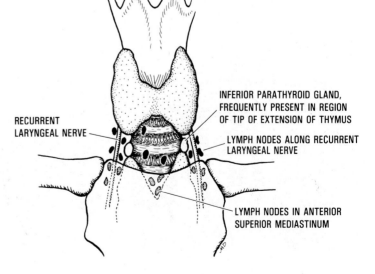

RECURRENT LARYNGEAL NERVE

INFERIOR PARATHYROID GLAND, FREQUENTLY PRESENT IN REGION OF TIP OF EXTENSION OF THYMUS

LYMPH NODES ALONG RECURRENT LARYNGEAL NERVE

LYMPH NODES IN ANTERIOR SUPERIOR MEDIASTINUM

euthyroid levels. I remove all but an estimated 3 gm of each lobe of the thyroid, or preserve a total of approximately 6 gm of thyroid tissue from one lobe with contralateral total lobectomy. This permits preservation of parathyroid function and recurrent laryngeal nerves while minimizing recurrence, accepting hypothyroidism in approximately 20 per cent of patients. The hypothyroidism usually appears within 1 year but can occur a number of years later. Other surgeons preserve more thyroid tissue and accept a higher recurrence rate but a lower incidence of hypothyroidism, and still others advocate a total thyroidectomy and accept the uniform occurrence of hypothyroidism.[60] If the patient desires that radioactive iodine never be needed for recurrent hyperthyroidism, a total or more complete thyroidectomy is needed.

Hyperthyroidism of the toxic nodular variety is treated by partial thyroidectomy, preserving approximately 7 gm of thyroid tissue of each lobe in most cases. This readily controls hyperthyroidism with absence of parathyroid or nerve complications, but it is followed by a high (as much as a 45 per cent) incidence of hypothyroidism.

A *single toxic autonomous nodule* is managed by total lobectomy of the involved thyroid gland. Although it is recognized that hyperfunctioning micronodules are usually present in remaining thyroid tissue, this does not appear to be a problem from the standpoint of recurrence.[62]

Chronic lymphocytic thyroiditis rarely requires operation unless the size of the gland becomes excessively large, becomes symptomatic, and does not respond to thyroid hormone therapy. In such cases, bilateral subtotal thyroidectomy is preferred. Nodules coexistent with chronic lymphocytic thyroiditis are managed on the basis of their individual features.[11]

Nodules under surgical consideration because of a *suspicion of carcinoma* provide the largest thyroid problem to surgeons from the numerical standpoint. Fortunately, needle biopsy techniques now frequently provide a preoperative diagnosis of carcinoma, suspicion for carcinoma, or benignancy for guidance in the surgical approach. There are, however, indeterminate cases, approximating 20 per cent of fine-needle aspiration studies, in which carcinoma (usually the low-grade,

well-differentiated type) is present in 20 to 60 per cent of reports.[10] Such cases usually deserve operation. For another group, approximating 7 to 10 per cent of studies, the aspirate is inadequate for diagnosis and decision-making for treatment on the basis of factors other than the needle biopsy is required. Further details concerning the clinical evaluation of thyroid nodules are considered in Chapter 59.

Certain nodules, even benign, deserve operation on the basis of size, failure to respond to medical therapy, persistent symptoms, previous external radiation therapy, or the patient's desire. *Cystic nodules* are usually benign degenerating nodules, but are rarely malignant; an attempt is made to delineate treatment by needle biopsy of the solid component.[63] The rare true thyroid cyst is usually controlled by aspiration.

The operative procedure for a benign thyroid lesion is usually a total lobectomy, this procedure often being easier and safer than a partial lobectomy. Lobectomy also ensures better results if malignancy is later identified.[70, 71] For lesions indeterminate by needle biopsy, removal of the isthmus and a portion (one half to three fourths) of the contralateral thyroid lobe is justified. This permits study of significant amounts of extranodular tissue for evidence of multicentricity if carcinoma is identified later by study of permanent sections from the nodule. Also, by removing additional thyroid tissue, the likelihood of development of additional benign nodules may be reduced (Fig. 62–5).

Previous external radiation therapy predisposes to the development of thyroid nodules as well as other neoplasms in the anatomic area (skin, parathyroid, salivary gland).[19, 29] Although the majority of thyroid nodules with this background are benign (carcinoma is present in 3 per cent of single nodules and 18 per cent of multinodular glands), incidental carcinomas do occur.[30] If thyroid nodules do occur, it is valuable to determine their nature by needle biopsy to more precisely direct the operation and to discuss more definitely the operative procedure with the patient. Some surgeons advocate operation for such patients, even though the nodule is benign by preoperative studies, because of the possible presence of an incidental carcinoma elsewhere in the thyroid and to resolve early the matter of therapy.

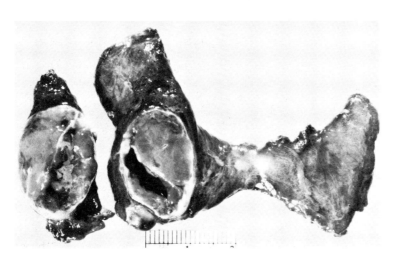

Figure 62–5. Right lobectomy with a partial left lobectomy of the thyroid performed for a nodule in the right lobe. In the operation for a thyroid nodule that is suspect for carcinoma, lobectomy with partial contralateral lobectomy is performed to assess multicentricity, possibly reduce the recurrence of benign nodules, and reduce thyroid volume if radioactive iodine therapy should be needed later.

Incidental carcinomas occur in patients with "hot" thyroid nodules (two of the cases of De Groot and associates).[30] For patients undergoing operations for nodules that are indeterminate for one reason or another, near-total thyroidectomy is preferred, removing the thyroid lobe on the side of the nodule and removing all but a few grams of tissue on the contralateral side, to minimize damage to the parathyroid glands and recurrent laryngeal nerves.[29] This rather aggressive operation for thyroid nodules associated with previous radiation therapy is based on the frequent multicentricity of thyroid carcinomas and nodules, the significant frequency of incidental carcinoma, and the planned use postoperatively of thyroid hormone therapy.[30] The possible later occurrence of carcinoma in the remnant of thyroid tissue preserved is a moot point at this time. Of interest is the finding of thyroid carcinoma invading parathyroid glands in 17 per cent of cases reported by De Groot and associates.[30] If carcinoma is identified, operative procedures conform to the malignancy present and its extent.

Malignant Tumors

In determining operative procedures for the treatment of thyroid carcinoma, two major considerations are basic:

1. The histologic variety of carcinoma, which identifies its biologic characteristics.

2. The evident anatomic spread of carcinoma, which directs the extent of operation for removal and which also reflects biologic characteristics.

Other factors include, of course, the general health status of the patient, the patient's personal desires, and the skill of the surgeon.

Histologic varieties of thyroid carcinomas used in governing the extent of operation include:

1. Well-differentiated thyroid carcinomas.

2. Medullary thyroid carcinomas.

3. Undifferentiated or anaplastic carcinomas.

Miscellaneous and unusual malignancies include:

1. Lymphomas.

2. Metastatic malignancy.

The level of preoperative diagnosis is now also important in directing operation. The use of needle biopsy techniques improves and alters the plan for operation, as follows:

1. Combining a specific histologic diagnosis of the thyroid carcinoma provided by a preoperative needle biopsy with the findings by physical examination, as well as operative findings, projects the extent of operation, which can be discussed with the patient preoperatively.

2. A preoperative diagnosis of an indeterminate or unsatisfactory needle biopsy currently directs us to perform a total lobectomy for the side containing the nodule and a contralateral partial lobectomy. This is an effort to ensure wide removal of the lesion under suspicion with removal of sufficient extranodular thyroid tissue to assess the factor of multicentricity in determining advisability of later reoperation for total thyroidectomy if carcinoma is identified only by the study postoperatively of permanent sections. Isthmus nodules are usually treated surgically by a partial or subtotal resection of each thyroid lobe with the thyroid isthmus. A large number of thyroid nodules that are indeterminate by needle biopsy prove to be low-grade well-differentiated carcinomas, recognized only by careful cytologic study and adequate examinations for capsular and vascular invasion of permanent sections.

3. Thyroid nodules found to be benign by needle biopsy but for which operation is indicated because of their large size are treated by lobectomy, with the extent of contralateral lobectomy being dependent on the presence of additional nodules in this lobe and the desire to limit the likelihood of later development of more benign nodules. Studies have indicated that, following operation for a benign thyroid nodule, approximately 15 per cent of patients will develop additional thyroid nodules in remaining thyroid tissue within 10 years.[51] The influence of suppressive doses of thyroid hormone in minimizing recurrent benign thyroid nodules is not well established.[38, 66] Obviously, the age of the patient will influence the likelihood of the development of recurrent thyroid nodules and, therefore, the need for considering suppression therapy with thyroid hormone.

Much discussion and apparent dispute has occurred in relation to the preferred or indicated operative procedure for thyroid carcinomas, particularly the well-differentiated varieties. This persists to this date.[8, 24] Arguments for and against total thyroidectomy as the basic operation continue. Similarly, support for lobectomy as the preferred operation for thyroid carcinoma persists.[22, 33, 36, 46] Another confusing factor in utilizing retrospective studies to develop recommended plans for therapy is the mixing of the frequency of carcinoma occurring later in lateral cervical lymph nodes with the frequency of carcinoma occurring later (including both actual recurrence and new lesions) in the remaining thyroid gland in order to conclude whether or not total or less than total thyroidectomy should be advocated for thyroid carcinoma.[57, 58] Our position has been to emphasize selectivity in the operative treatment for thyroid carcinoma, using the two major factors (histologic variety and gross extent of tumor) as the determinants. It is likely that most surgeons do, in practice, select the operative procedure on the basis of these factors.

There is a need for precise, controlled, prospective studies to develop optimal policies for the operative treatment for thyroid carcinoma. The relative rarity of thyroid carcinoma and difficulties in organizing a large number of surgeons to follow necessary protocols for such studies make unlikely the availability of such information in the near future. In the meantime, it is necessary to depend on isolated studies by different investigators to provide guidelines for the treatment of thyroid carcinoma. An attempt will be made to incorporate conclusions available from such studies in outlining working policies for the treatment of thyroid carcinomas.

Well-Differentiated Thyroid Carcinoma

Papillary and follicular thyroid carcinomas can be combined, to a limited extent, as well-differentiated thyroid carcinomas in regard to operative treatment. These two varieties compose the majority of thyroid carcinomas (approximately 90 per cent). However, there are distinctive factors for these two categories, including the following:

1. All lesions containing any papillary content microscopically can be considered, from a practical standpoint, to be papillary carcinomas for treatment.

2. Follicular thyroid carcinoma includes two major and distinctive varieties: the *low-grade, well-encapsulated* and the *high-grade angioinvasive* carcinomas. *Hürthle cell thyroid carcinomas* also have distinctive features and may be included in this category.

Papillary Carcinoma

Papillary carcinoma biologically demonstrates the following major characteristics:

1. Slow growth of the primary lesion.

2. A predisposition for multicentricity in the thyroid gland as multiple primary foci of carcinoma or intrathyroidal metastases by lymphatic spread. Previous external radiation therapy to the head and neck appears to increase the likelihood of multicentricity of thyroid carcinoma.[30]

3. A predisposition to spread to cervical and superior mediastinal lymph nodes. This may be the first clinical evidence of the carcinoma. However, the carcinoma tends to remain within the nodes and not penetrate outside the cervical lymph node capsule. This permits conservation in cervical lymph node dissection by preservation of the structures accomplished in a modified cervical lymph node dissection.

4. Lack of a predisposition for distant metastases by the vascular route.

5. Frequent uptake by radioactive iodine, making this substance feasible for diagnostic and therapeutic purposes.

However, each papillary carcinoma is a law unto itself and must be managed on the basis of its demonstrated characteristics and extent. In most cases, it is slow-growing and patients can live with the carcinoma for decades, with death occurring only after a usual lifetime, even if it remains untreated. In other cases, however, the carcinoma behaves more aggressively, metastasizes widely, and can kill in a few years.

PROGNOSIS

Important factors determining the outlook for papillary thyroid carcinoma and, thereby, influencing extent of operation, include the age of the patient and the size of the lesion. This neoplasm is much more virulent, especially in terms of local invasion, in patients over the age of 40 years.[23] In young adults, lymph node metastases can be evident for a number of years and may not significantly influence prognosis. However, in patients over 40 years of age, the papillary thyroid carcinoma tends to invade surrounding tissues at its primary origin in the thyroid and at the site of metastasis.

In general, primary lesions under 1.5 cm in diameter, if isolated, rarely show late metastases. In these cases the disease is controlled by conservative operations, namely, thyroid lobectomy.[46]

INDICATIONS FOR SURGERY

In surgery for thyroid carcinoma, major consideration must be given to the extent of the procedure as it relates to the thyroid gland, removal of central lymph nodes, and the removal of lateral cervical lymph nodes. A major controversy, or at least discussion, concerns the *extent of thyroid removal* for papillary thyroid carcinoma. This relates primarily to the justification or indications for total thyroidectomy, as noted previously. Considerations, thought to be objective, can be summarized as follows:

1. Gross or proved biopsy presence of bilateral papillary thyroid carcinoma deserves total thyroidectomy.

2. Previous external radiation therapy to the head and neck justifies total thyroidectomy because of the evidence of increased multicentricity.

3. For single papillary carcinomas larger than 1.5 cm, evidence indicates that the incidence of later papillary carcinoma in the contralateral lobe approximates 5 to 10 per cent. This, then, permits a judgment decision on the part of the surgeon based on his or her surgical skill in performing a total thyroidectomy with minimal risk of permanent hypoparathyroidism or laryngeal nerve damage, the given patient's anatomic situation in relation to the ease in preserving these important anatomic structures, and the patient's medical status and attitude. In general, the larger the primary carcinoma, the greater the justification for total thyroidectomy on the basis of retrospective studies.[22, 76]

4. If papillary thyroid carcinoma is recognized only postoperatively following study of permanent sections, the question then may arise as to the justification for reoperation to complete a total thyroidectomy. Empirically, we have based this decision primarily on evidence of multicentricity of carcinoma in the thyroid tissue removed or the finding of lymph node metastases; therefore, at the initial operation for thyroid nodule under suspicion for carcinoma we remove the isthmus as well as one half or more of the contralateral lobe to provide tissue for the assessment of multicentricity. Other factors such as the patient's age and the degree of microscopic differentiation enter also into decision-making for or against reoperation to complete total thyroidectomy. Near-total thyroidectomy can be a compromise in that only one to several grams of thyroid tissue are preserved on the side contralateral to the carcinoma to preserve parathyroid glands and the laryngeal nerve.

5. If the primary papillary thyroid carcinoma is less than 1.5 cm in diameter, evidence available indicates that lobectomy alone suffices for treatment.[46] In this situation, as well as that listed in the preceding paragraph, regional central lymph nodes can be removed at the initial operation as biopsies to assist in decision-making.

6. If there is evidence of cervical lymph node metastases, or certainly if there is evidence of distant metastases, total or near-total thyroidectomy is justified.[5, 45] This permits the use of radioactive iodine therapy, which may be needed in this situation. However, a spectrum of disease, for which extent of thyroid removal should be matched, exists. The primary carcinoma can be single and occult and may result in regional or lateral cervical lymph node metastases. Lymph node metastases may be present only in adjacent lymph nodes. On the other hand, the presence of lymph node metastases does, in general, signify more extensive carcinoma.

7. In general, total thyroidectomy with appropriate

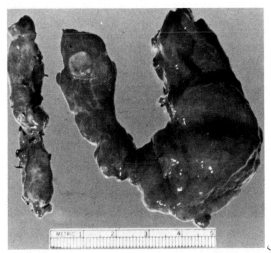

Figure 62–6. Following lobectomy and partial contralateral lobectomy for a thyroid nodule suspect of carcinoma (specimen at right), the finding of multicentric well-differentiated carcinoma justifies removal of the remaining thyroid (at left). Foci of carcinoma may be present in this remnant.

cervical lymph node dissection provides the best prognosis for well-differentiated thyroid carcinoma of the papillary and angioinvasive follicular types, particularly in situations in which thyroid and lymph node involvement is extensive.[3, 23, 25, 57, 70] It remains preferable to perform adequately extensive procedures early for thyroid carcinoma rather than late when reoperation is associated with reduced opportunities to control the carcinoma and greater risks for technical complications.[1]

As previously noted, *near-total thyroidectomy* is an extremely important alternative to *total thyroidectomy*, the objective being preservation of parathyroid glands and the recurrent laryngeal nerve on at least one side of the neck. With this procedure, the option remains of eradicating residual thyroid tissue later with radioactive iodine (Fig. 62–6).

In recent years, several reports have recommended the uniform performance of total thyroidectomy in all cases of well-differentiated thyroid carcinoma on the basis of better results, particularly if radioactive iodine is used.[24, 57, 58, 70] However, all these reports have serious limitations or deficiencies, and in our opinion, they should not be used to mandate routine total thyroidectomy over its selective use.[8] Thus, Mazzaferri and associates report that recurrence is less common after total thyroidectomy for papillary carcinoma, yet in their study the recurrences were primarily in lateral cervical lymph nodes and the operation was associated with a high complications rate.[57, 58] Clark and Way, in recommending total thyroidectomy, used data based on a high incidence of patients having had previous external radiation therapy and included a substantial number of cases in which no carcinoma was present.[24] Samaan and associates urged total thyroidectomy, and yet their data lumped all well-differentiated thyroid carcinoma without any selectivity, provided no details correlating location of recurrences with histologic type or extent of initial disease or extent of initial operation, and were associated with unacceptable complication rates.[70]

Cervical lymph node removal can be considered from the standpoint of the central and lateral cervical nodes. The centrally located nodes are most important and include nodes in the tracheoesophageal grooves and anterior superior mediastinum. A chain of these nodes is located along the recurrent laryngeal nerves. In general, nodes in the ipsilateral tracheoesophageal groove and the anterior superior mediastinum are removed in continuity with lobectomy for thyroid carcinoma. Those centrally located lymph nodes are most likely to produce problems if invasion beyond their capsule occurs because of the presence in this anatomic location of vital structures.

At the time of operation, frozen section study of grossly suspicious lymph nodes can be used to confirm the diagnosis and in decision-making for lateral cervical lymph node removal.[55]

Lateral cervical lymph node removal is the least important of operative procedures for papillary thyroid carcinoma, but it can be significant in a few cases in preventing involvement by direct invasion of important structures and in removing a focus for peripheral dissemination. Experience has demonstrated, however, that "prophylactic" lateral cervical lymph node dissection does not improve prognosis over removal of these nodes when they are palpably enlarged.[47] Despite this evidence, there are reports purporting to show that the prognosis is improved, primarily on the basis of reduced recurrence, by the use of radioactive iodine to eliminate occult metastases in those lymph nodes, as evidenced by postoperative scans and elevated uptake of radioactive iodine.[57, 58] Confusing the importance of eradication of metastatic carcinoma in the central neck and peripheral tissues with the eradication of occult metastases in lateral cervical lymph nodes may be responsible for such concepts.

Removal of lymph nodes adjacent to the jugular vein in the midpoint of the neck as a biopsy procedure at the time of operation may be a compromise procedure in deciding whether or not to remove lateral cervical nodes. This can be particularly useful for patients without palpable cervical lymphadenopathy but with large primary papillary thyroid carcinomas and thick necks, making palpation of enlarged lymph nodes difficult. We have followed this policy for a number of years, using frozen section study of those node biopsies as a criterion in determining the need for modified lateral cervical lymph node dissections in an effort to minimize the need for later reoperation.[4] The potential morbidity associated with reoperation for a disease that should be controllable by operation justifies efforts to match the magnitude of operation to the extent of disease present.

Unless there is gross evidence of invasion by metastatic carcinoma beyond lymph node capsules, lateral cervical lymph node dissection can be modified from the classical, or "radical," procedure.[16] Preservation of the sternocleidomastoid muscle, spinal accessory nerve, internal jugular and posterior jugular veins, and the omission of submaxillary triangle dissection reduces morbidity and permits adequacy of lateral cervical lymph node dissection for most patients. In the elderly patient with lateral cervical lymph node metastases invading outside lymph nodes, modification of the classical lymph node dissection may not be feasible. Conservatism in avoiding morbidity from total thyroidectomy is justified in this situation, but a few cases have proved ultimately to be fatal as a result of distant metastases.[2, 53a, 59]

Follicular Carcinoma

Detailed studies specifically of follicular thyroid carcinoma have not been accomplished to the degree reported for papillary carcinoma. My personal experience with this entity will be used primarily in this discussion.

RECOGNITION

Well-Differentiated, Low-Grade, Encapsulated Follicular Thyroid Carcinoma. This type of carcinoma is of concern primarily from standpoints of precise diagnosis, size, and the potential for blood-borne distant metastases. The approximation to cytologic normality makes recognition of this carcinoma difficult for pathologists, and there have been surprises when metastatic thyroid carcinoma occurs in a few cases. Experience in the pathologic study of multiple sections for evidence of capsular or vascular invasion is needed to recognize this lesion in the thyroid gland.[48, 53] From the surgical standpoint, lobectomy suffices in nearly all cases. Of course, total thyroidectomy is needed if metastasis does occur, justifying the use of radioactive iodine.

High-Grade, Angioinvasive, Follicular Thyroid Carcinomas. These are associated with a poor prognosis. A predisposition for local invasion, in particular, produces difficulty in surgery for this entity. In addition, there is a high incidence of metastases to cervical lymph nodes and distant sites. Therefore, total thyroidectomy, removal of central lymph nodes on the side of the lesion, and appropriate lateral cervical lymph node dissection are indicated.

Hürthle Cell Carcinomas. These can be considered as a variety of follicular thyroid carcinoma, although this can be disputed. This must be differentiated from Hürthle cell adenomas, a task that can be difficult, especially for inexperienced pathologists. The University of Michigan and M. D. Anderson Hospital and Tumor Institute experiences have emphasized the high incidence of bilaterality of the lesion, its lethal potential in long-term studies, and the justification for total thyroidectomy and approximate lymph node dissection when this entity is recognized.[41, 70] Needle biopsy studies now permit recognition of this entity preoperatively with a planned operation when possible. If the lesion is recognized only postoperatively by study of permanent sections, a decision relative to the need for reoperation to complete total thyroidectomy is necessary. Experience of the M. D. Anderson Hospital and Tumor Institute places Hürthle cell carcinomas as the most aggressive of all well-differentiated thyroid carcinomas.[70]

SPECIAL CASES

There are many vagaries of well-differentiated follicular thyroid carcinoma. Some specific types will be considered here.

Minimal or Occult Carcinomas. These have been mentioned earlier. In general, lobectomy or conservative removal of thyroid tissue is justified. For the few cases producing clinically evident cervical lymph node metastases, near-total or total thyroidectomy with an appropriate cervical lymph node dissection is justified.

Incidental Thyroid Carcinoma. The incidental finding of a microscopic or otherwise occult well-differentiated thyroid carcinoma in thyroid tissue removed for a benign nodule probably is related to the recognized occurrence of thyroid carcinoma in a subclinical state in routine autopsy studies. It requires no additional operation other than those noted for minimal or occult thyroid carcinoma.[9] This probably occurs with an increased frequency in patients who have received previous external radiation therapy to the head and neck. There may be an increased frequency of incidental thyroid carcinoma in patients with autonomous functioning nodules, but this is unlikely.

It is plausible to include in this category cases of minute carcinomas recognized by needle biopsy of questionable irregularities of the surface of the thyroid gland. Thus, we identified a single 4-mm papillary thyroid carcinoma by fine-needle aspiration biopsy in a 23-year-old patient.

Associated Anaplastic Thyroid Carcinoma. In a few cases (no more than 5 per cent of well-differentiated thyroid carcinomas) anaplastic thyroid carcinoma is present concomitantly. The clinical course for such patients is determined by the anaplastic carcinoma, making aggressive surgery justified for such patients. These cases may account for some instances in which well-differentiated carcinoma becomes anaplastic carcinoma at a later time.[44]

PROGNOSIS

The prognosis for well-differentiated follicular thyroid carcinomas depends on the following:
1. The histologic variety.
2. Demonstrated extent of malignancy.
3. Age of patient (prognosis is worse for patients over 40 years of age).
4. Adequacy of initial operation.
5. Presence of residual carcinoma or metastases.

In general, the outlook for papillary thyroid carcinoma relates to the size of the primary lesion and its invasive characteristics.[22, 57, 76] Comprehensive reviews of a long-term experience at the Mayo Clinic document survival for treated noninvasive papillary thyroid carcinoma to approximate that of the normal population, whereas invasive carcinoma larger than 5 cm in diameter in patients over 50 years of age had a mortality rate approaching 30 per cent for follow-up periods as long as 25 years.[59, 76] The overall mortality rate appears to be around 5 to 7 per cent and has improved with more aggressive but selective surgery in recent years.[5, 56]

The outlook for thyroid carcinoma is related to the presence of distant metastases at the time of initial diagnosis; death from this disease rarely occurs in the absence of this situation.[56] This factor is particularly true for follicular thyroid carcinoma, in which the high mortality rate is restricted to those with distant metastases for the low-grade encapsulated variety.[76] Angioinvasive follicular carcinoma and Hürthle cell carcinomas are associated with the worst prognosis for well-differentiated thyroid carcinomas. The long-term experience of the Mayo Clinic indicates an overall mortality rate of 17.2 per cent for follicular thyroid carcinomas.[59]

Medullary Thyroid Carcinoma

Surgery for medullary carcinoma includes total thyroidectomy, with the extent of lymph node dissection dependent on whether the case is the hereditary or sporadic variety and the stage at the time of detection.[13, 18] The production of the tumoral agent *calcitonin* permits detection and postoperative monitoring for the presence of this variety of thyroid carcinoma. The delineation of this thyroid carcinoma into *sporadic* and *hereditary* categories is critical (Table 62–2).[12]

Sporadic Medullary Thyroid Carcinoma. This type is currently recognized after palpable nodules appear in the thyroid gland. This variety does not appear to be associated with other endocrine tumors. Currently, total thyroidectomy is the preferred operation because it is not always possible to eliminate the hereditary variety, which is uniformly bilateral. The frequency of cervical lymph node metastases and the aggressive nature of this carcinoma justify concomitant central and lateral cervical lymph node dissection. The lateral cervical lymph node dissection is the classical procedure for cases with palpable and locally invasive metastases and modified for patients not exhibiting palpable lymphadenopathy.

Hereditary Medullary Thyroid Carcinoma. This carcinoma is uniformly bilateral and is transmitted as an autosomal dominant trait with penetrance, resulting in at least a 50 per cent occurrence in the affected family (Fig. 62–7). It occurs in two multiple endocrine neoplasia (MEN) forms: the *MEN 2a* and *MEN 2b syndromes.*

Pheochromocytomas can occur in both the MEN 2a and 2b varieties and should be eliminated by tests before the medullary thyroid carcinoma is treated surgically. If pheochromocytomas are present, surgery on the adrenal glands is initiated. Other components of the MEN 2 syndromes include hyperparathyroidism in the MEN 2a, mucosal neuromas in the MEN 2b, and Cushing's syndrome. These additional endocrine lesions are sporadically present with the medullary thyroid carcinoma.

The MEN 2a syndrome usually is evident later in life than the MEN 2b type. In the MEN 2b syndrome, the presence of neuromas and the Marfinoid habitus make diagnosis evident in infancy. The MEN 2b syndrome has a worse prognosis than the MEN 2a variety and

TABLE 62–2. Distinctive Clinical Features of Hereditary and Sporadic Forms of Medullary Thyroid Carcinoma

Clinical Feature	Hereditary Form	Sporadic Form
Bilaterality	Always bilateral	Unilateral
C-cell hyperplasia outside primary carcinoma	Uniformly present	Absent
Other endocrine diseases	MEN 2a, MEN 2b present Pheochromocytoma, Cushing's syndrome in some patients Hyperparathyroidism only in MEN 2a Mucosal neuromas only in MEN 2b	Absent
Usual clinical recognition	Screening family members for elevated serum calcitonin, palpable nodule, thyroid carcinoma in some	Palpable nodule in thyroid in all cases

requires diagnostic and therapeutic considerations in childhood. The MEN 2a syndrome differs from the MEN 2b syndrome in that, in some cases, parathyroid hyperplasia and potential hyperparathyroidism are present. The surgeon, therefore, must be alert for enlarged parathyroid glands in operations for the MEN 2a syndrome.

INDICATIONS FOR SURGERY

The extent of operation for medullary thyroid carcinomas depends, from the standpoint of the cervical node dissection, on the stage of recognition. The presence of a palpable thyroid nodule uniformly is associated with lateral cervical node metastases and requires total thyroidectomy with bilateral central and lateral cervical node dissection. The lateral cervical lymph node dissection is either classical or modified, depending on evidence for invasion of metastases outside the lymph nodes.

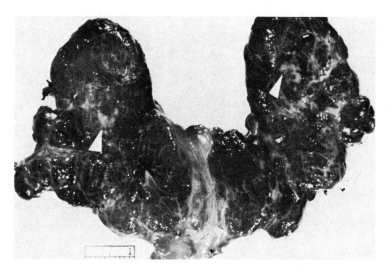

Figure 62–7. This bilateral minute medullary thyroid carcinoma (arrows) in the hereditary form had been detected by screening with provocative tests for elevated levels of serum calcitonin.

DIAGNOSIS

The diagnosis of hereditary medullary thyroid carcinoma can be established before there is clinical evidence of a thyroid lesion otherwise and even at the stage of parafollicular or C-cell hyperplasia.[75] This acuity of detection is achieved by screening members of affected families with radioimmunoassay for elevated serum levels of calcitonin, provocation with pentagastrin being utilized if basal levels are normal. In such cases it is rare for cervical lymph node metastases to be present. Therefore, we perform a total thyroidectomy and biopsy of midjugular lymph nodes in these cases, accomplishing cervical lymph node dissections only if these lymph nodes contain metastases by the study of frozen section at the time of operation. Inasmuch as elevated levels of serum calcitonin can appear in childhood, this procedure may be needed at this age level. In the MEN 2b syndrome, this procedure is needed in infancy to prevent the rapid progression of disease that is characteristic of this entity.

It is only in patients for whom medullary thyroid carcinoma is detected by screening affected families for elevation of serum calcitonin after provocative tests that we uniformly have found postoperative serum calcitonin levels to be normal.[12, 50] In both hereditary and sporadic forms of clinically evident medullary thyroid carcinoma, serum calcitonin levels remain elevated in the majority of patients, despite total thyroidectomy and bilateral cervical lymph node dissection (Fig. 62–8).[15, 50]

The degree of elevation of serum calcitonin has a general correlation with the extent of residual disease. It is rare, if ever, that metastases can be identified and be isolated so that further operation for their removal is justified. Periodic, usually annual, re-evaluation with determinations of serum calcitonin are performed. The location of metastases of medullary thyroid carcinoma can be identified by uptake of certain radioactive agents, such as thallium 201.

In the MEN 2a form of medullary thyroid carcinoma, hyperplasia of parathyroid glands can occur. Clinically evident hyperparathyroidism is rare, however. At the time of operation, enlarged parathyroid glands that are encountered are removed.[14] Emphasis is placed on preservation of parathyroid tissue, however. If clinical hyperparathyroidism occurs, it is probably best to perform a subtotal parathyroidectomy in view of the high frequency of multiple gland involvement. Hyperparathyroidism has not been encountered in the sporadic or MEN 2b forms of medullary thyroid carcinoma.

PROGNOSIS

The prognosis after treatment for medullary thyroid carcinoma lies between the good outlook for well-differentiated thyroid carcinoma and the extremely poor results for anaplastic carcinoma. The expectations following treatment vary with the stage of recognition and are improving greatly with increased appreciation of the behavior of the disease. For the hereditary form, recognized only by screening for elevated levels of serum calcitonin, operation provides complete control of the disease.[12, 50] In the past, sporadic medullary thyroid carcinoma carried a mortality rate of approximately 50 per cent, but this appears to be improving greatly with more aggressive early surgical treatment.[50] Patients, following operation, may show persistent elevation of serum calcitonin indefinitely without great change or clinical evidence of disease over a period of years. There is evidence that radioactive iodine and external radiation therapy may be of benefit for some patients with medullary thyroid carcinoma.[28, 40] Tricyclic antidepressants, such as imipramine and amoxapine, have been found to be of help in controlling diarrhea related to extensive medullary thyroid carcinoma.

Anaplastic Thyroid Carcinoma

This variety characteristically occurs in elderly patients who have recognized the presence of a thyroid nodule which, without apparent cause, abruptly enlarges and rapidly invades all surrounding tissue, including other portions of the thyroid. There is evidence that this frequently represents a transformation from a well-differentiated thyroid carcinoma.[44] It is only with early recognition and extensive operation that these patients can be provided surgical help. In most cases, the situation is unresectable from the standpoint of control of local disease at the time of recognition. If resectable, a total thyroidectomy and appropriate unilateral or bilateral cervical lymph node dissection are performed.

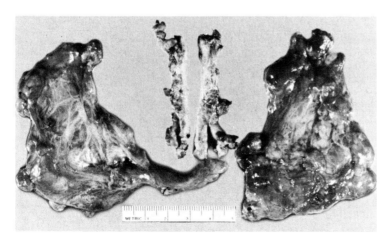

Figure 62–8. Elevated levels of serum calcitonin in a patient with hereditary medullary thyroid carcinoma who had undergone previous bilateral subtotal thyroid lobectomy led to removal of the remnants of each thyroid lobe (two small specimens in center) and bilateral modified cervical lymph node dissection (specimens on each side). Nevertheless, serum calcitonin levels remained elevated postoperatively.

A biopsy is often the only surgical procedure that is feasible for diagnosis of anaplastic thyroid carcinoma. It is important to establish the diagnosis and be sure that the thyroid lesion is not a lymphoma or thyroiditis. Fine-needle aspiration biopsy may not conclusively make this differentiation, making a cutting-needle biopsy or open biopsy under local anesthetic necessary. The response of treatment with other modalities has been poor.[39, 68] Survival from anaplastic thyroid carcinoma is rare and depends on early diagnosis, which is usually made inadvertently. On occasion, anaplastic thyroid carcinoma is associated with well-differentiated thyroid carcinoma. In this latter structure, survival can be achieved by early recognition and treatment of this entity.

Primary Lymphoma

This rare lesion usually appears as a rapidly enlarging, firm thyroid mass in middle-aged or older women.[31] It appears to be a distinct entity inasmuch as involvement of the thyroid gland in generalized lymphoma is especially rare. Tracheal and esophageal compression produces symptoms. *Small cell anaplastic thyroid carcinoma* probably is a lymphoma and should be treated as such. Primary Hodgkin's disease of the thyroid gland is particularly rare.[27] Lymphoma may be restricted to one lobe of the thyroid gland. *Plasmacytomas* are rare, appear to be restricted to the thyroid gland when in this location, and are controlled by the operative procedure on the thyroid gland.

DIAGNOSIS AND TREATMENT

Histologic diagnosis of lymphoma is necessary in order to institute treatment. Because fine needle aspiration biopsies may not definitely provide this evidence, large cutting needle biopsy, open biopsy, or even lobectomy may be required before the diagnosis can be firmly established.[52]

Evidence indicates that both surgery and radiation therapy provide appropriate treatment for primary lymphoma of the thyroid gland. If the diagnosis can be established by biopsy, radiation therapy is appropriate. The extent of involvement determines the extent of therapy, with the disease varying from involvement of one lobe of the thyroid only to involvement of the entire thyroid with invasion of surrounding tissue and presence in regional lymph nodes. If operation is performed, postoperative external radiation therapy appears justified.

PROGNOSIS

The prognosis of lymphoma of the thyroid gland is determined by the extent of involvement. Devine and associates report that the 5-year survival rate is 86 per cent for patients with primary lymphoma that is restricted to the thyroid gland.[31] For patients in whom primary thyroid lymphoma invaded surrounding tissue or involved regional lymph nodes, the 5-year survival rate was reduced to 38 per cent. If thyroid lymphoma is a part of a generalized disease, the outlook is poor.

Metastatic Thyroid Carcinoma

Metastatic malignancy to the thyroid gland is uncommon but must be considered in the management of thyroid nodules. This cause for thyroid enlargement is easily recognized in most cases because the thyroid gland is only one of many sites of metastatic carcinomas. However, on occasion the metastasis to the thyroid appears clinically as an isolated event and requires alertness to recognize the lesion as a metastasis. This latter situation is particularly true for metastatic renal cell carcinoma, which may become evident in the thyroid gland many years or even decades after original treatment of the renal carcinoma. It is possible to recognize metastatic lesions by fine-needle aspiration biopsies of the thyroid gland. Recognition of a thyroid nodule as a metastasis is important inasmuch as surgery for such a lesion is of no real help for these patients.

SURGICAL TECHNIQUES

Pertinent technical aspects of basic operative procedures on the thyroid gland will be discussed. Important anatomic features involved in these operations have been presented under the surgical anatomy section of this chapter.

Surgical Exposure of the Thyroid Gland

A low anterior cervical transverse incision, placed in a skin crease, is usually employed to expose the thyroid gland. With the patient's head moderately hyperextended by placing a towel roll or similar object under shoulders and a "doughnut" under the patient's head, the thyroid gland is brought up from the submanubrial region and access is maximally provided. This arrangement also reduces posterior cervical pain by preventing excess strain on the posterior cervical muscles, yet shifting the neck forward.

The incision is placed low in the neck, cephalad to the level of the clavicles, resulting in an incision in an inconspicuous location. The usual incision extends from the anterior margin of the sternocleidomastoid muscle on one side of the neck to a similar location on the opposite side of the neck. This is a shorter incision than has been used in the past, provides better cosmetic results, but must be extended for large masses. In the case of a small thyroid nodule in a patient with a thin neck, a very short incision can be used, no more than an inch or so long, but this must be placed directly over the thyroid gland; this is a higher location in the neck and requires great familiarity with the anatomy involved in the procedure (Fig. 62–9A and B). The incision is carried through the underlying subcutaneous tissues, platysma muscle, and fascia in the midline. The anterior jugular vein should not be injured or divided in making the incision.

After the incision is made, the flaps are reflected superiorly and inferiorly, the flaps held under traction as sharp dissection is used initially to develop the proper anatomic plane for the flap after which blunt dissection with the finger completes the development of the flap (Figs. 62–10 and 62–11). Several veins usually require division in making the superior flap; otherwise, the dissection can be placed in a relatively avascular plane.

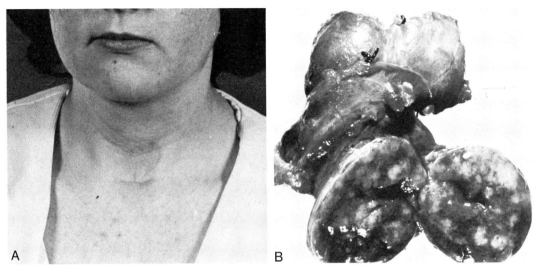

Figure 62–9. A short transverse cervical incision (A) placed over the thyroid gland can permit lobectomy and excision of the isthmus and a part of the contralateral lobe for a thyroid nodule. (B) Operative specimen.

Superiorly, the flap should extend above the entire width of the thyroid cartilage. Inferiorly, the flap is freed over the sternoclavicular juncture. Subcutaneous veins at this level may require division.

The reflected skin flaps are maintained in position by retraction, such as with a Beckman retractor. The fascia is opened in the midline between strap muscles, extending from over the thyroid cartilage down to the sternal notch. Exposure of the thyroid gland is maximized by mobilizing the flaps laterally off the anterior margins of the sternocleidomastoid muscles and by freeing strap muscles superiorly from underlying structures. It is only rarely necessary to divide strap muscles to better expose the thyroid gland and the tracheoesophageal grooves, but this is a matter of personal preference.

The thyroid gland is exposed by gently separating overlying strap muscles from each lobe (Fig. 62–12). The strap muscles are retracted as the thyroid lobe is pushed posteriorly, separating areolar tissues gently and avoiding injury to veins in the surface of the thyroid gland. If strap muscles are adherent to a nodule suspicious for or identified as carcinoma, the strap muscles are divided so as to remove the muscles with the thyroid gland and thus permit removal of the carcinoma intact.

Each lobe of the thyroid lobe and the isthmus are carefully examined for abnormalities. An assessment is made for lymphadenopathy in the tracheoesophageal grooves, anterior superior mediastinum, and lateral neck. Excision of enlarged lymph nodes for frozen section study for metastases is carried out selectively on the basis of need for such information diagnostically or for determining the extent of operation. We prefer to remove enlarged lymph nodes in the tracheoesophageal grooves and anterior superior mediastinum en bloc with the thyroid lobe, or thyroid gland, when carcinoma is evident or suspected (see Figs. 62–2 and 62–4).

Thyroid Lobectomy

The basic operative procedure on the thyroid gland is lobectomy. Mobilization of the thyroid lobe may be initiated by dividing the isthmus initially, but most surgeons first mobilize the medial aspect of the upper pole and then the lateral aspect of the lobe (Fig. 62–13). As the medial aspect of the superior pole of the lobe is mobilized, areolar tissue containing small vessels is

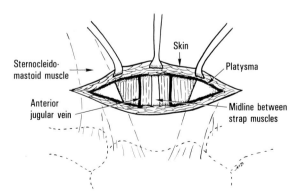

Figure 62–10. Transverse incision in lower anterior neck carried through platysma muscle, preserving anterior jugular veins.

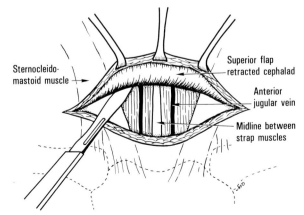

Figure 62–11. Elevating superior incision flap by dissecting at the level between platysma muscle and underlying fascia over strap muscles.

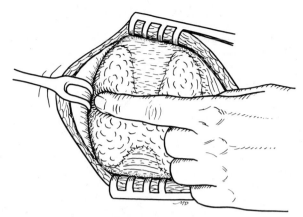

Figure 62–12. Mobilizing right lobe of thyroid gland by careful blunt separation of thyroid lobe from areolar tissue. The index finger pushes the thyroid lobe away from the retracted strap muscles to avoid injury to veins on the thyroid lobe.

divided in segments, occluding vessels with fine suture. Then, with retraction of the strap muscles at the cephalad end of the wound, branches of the superior thyroid vessels are isolated and divided. Maintaining this dissection adjacent to the thyroid tissue or dividing those major vessels over the surface of the upper pole of the thyroid gland avoids injury to the external branch of the superior laryngeal nerve, which is located more medially. The branches of the superior thyroid vessels must be securely occluded to avoid later hemorrhage; the level of division of these vessels is also determined by gross evidence of the extent of carcinoma at this level.

Before proceeding with dissection along the medial aspect of the upper pole of the thyroid lobe, or before the superior thyroid vessels are divided, the surgeon should identify the location of entry of the recurrent laryngeal nerve into the larynx. Palpation of the inferior lateral cornu of the laryngeal cartilage (Fig. 62–1) identifies the location of entry of the recurrent laryngeal nerve into the larynx; dissection cephalad to this level avoids injury to this nerve.

Before dissection is conducted along the posterior aspect of the superior pole of the thyroid lobe, it is helpful to mobilize the entire lobe laterally. Thereby, visualization of the posterior aspect of the upper pole of the thyroid lobe is improved and permits preservation, when appropriate, of the upper parathyroid gland when it is situated at this location, which is often the case.

The posterolateral aspect of the thyroid lobe (the tracheoesophageal groove region) is exposed by medial retraction of the lobe by the fingers of the assistant or the surgeon. This form of retraction is preferred to the use of instruments, which can tear tissue, aggravate bleeding, and disseminate carcinoma (Fig. 62–14). Lateral retraction of muscles is provided with the use of retractors. Areolar tissue in the tracheoesophageal groove is separated to permit visualization of structures in this groove. During the dissection, alertness is exercised for the presence of parathyroid glands and the recurrent laryngeal nerve.

Clarification of structures in the tracheoesophageal groove is achieved by early identification of the inferior thyroid artery and placement of a suture around it for use in retracting the artery. The artery is not divided at this time in order to permit its use in identifying the recurrent laryngeal nerve, to avoid deprivation of arterial blood to parathyroid glands at this level, and to avoid a mistake of incorrectly interpreting the artery for the nerve and inadvertently dividing the nerve. The recurrent laryngeal nerve is best identified posterior to the inferior pole of the thyroid lobe, where it is a centimeter or more separated from the thyroid lobe, running cephalad and anteriorly to pass under, over, or through branches of the inferior thyroid artery and then to run cephalad immediately adjacent to the posterior surface of the upper pole of the thyroid lobe (Figs. 62–2 and 62–3). Once the recurrent laryngeal nerve is identified inferiorly, its course superiorly can be projected by palpating the inferior lateral cornu of the thyroid cartilage to determine the point of the nerve's entry into the larynx. Confirmation of the nerve can be accomplished by following the structure caudad to demonstrate its origin from the mediastinum. During the dissection in these tissues adjacent to and caudad to the inferior thyroid artery, attention also is given to identifying and preserving, if possible, the inferior parathyroid gland, which may be in this location.

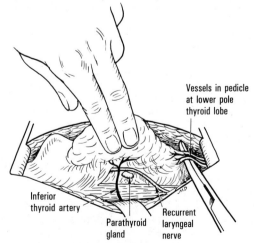

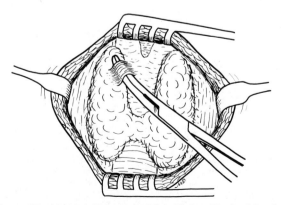

Figure 62–13. Mobilizing right lobe of thyroid gland by first dividing areolar tissue at the medial aspect of the upper pole. The presence of small vessels requires ligatures on the pedicles.

Figure 62–14. Mobilizing and dividing blood vessels and tissue at the lower pole of the right lobe of the thyroid gland. This is done after identification of the recurrent laryngeal nerve.

Once the anatomic details of the tracheoesophageal groove have been clarified, as noted in the preceding paragraph, mobilization of the thyroid lobe can commence. The tissues caudad to the inferior pole can be divided first, thereby occluding the inferior thyroid and thyroid ima vessels (Fig. 62–14). In so doing, attention is given to preservation of the inferior parathyroid gland, which may be in this location. If a tongue of the thymus projects into the anterior superior mediastinum and approaches the inferior pole of the thyroid lobe, the inferior parathyroid gland often is situated anterior, posterior, or within this tip of thymic tissue. In mobilizing the inferior pole of the thyroid gland, lymph node–bearing tissue in the anterior superior mediastinum is mobilized medial to the recurrent laryngeal nerve and removed en bloc with the thyroid lobe (Fig. 62–4).

The thyroid lobe is further mobilized by the dissection proceeding cephalad, dividing tissues adjacent to the posterolateral aspect of the lobe, preserving the recurrent laryngeal nerve and parathyroid glands. The inferior thyroid artery or its branches are divided as encountered. Lymph node–bearing tissue in the tracheoesophageal groove is mobilized and removed en bloc with the thyroid lobe, but the important anatomic structures are preserved. As the thyroid lobe is mobilized, the tissues are divided in segments, and blood vessels in these segments are occluded with suture.

As the dissection proceeds cephalad to the level of the superior pole of the thyroid gland, the recurrent laryngeal nerve lies close to the undersurface of the thyroid gland. It is at this level, or where the nerve makes turns before entering the larynx, that the nerve is in greatest jeopardy for injury. Here the dissection consists primarily of freeing the nerve from the thyroid gland.

It is posterior to the upper pole of the thyroid lobe, particularly cephalad to the inferior lateral cornu of the larynx, that attention is provided to preserving the superior parathyroid gland, often evident in this position. The mobilization of the upper pole of the thyroid lobe is then completed.

Particular care must be exerted in the dissection at the inferior cornu of the larynx (Fig. 62–2). The posterior suspensory ligament of the thyroid gland at this point is surrounded by small blood vessels, the recurrent laryngeal nerve may make turns before entering the larynx at this point, and thyroid tissue may project posteriorly over these structures to increase technical difficulties. If it is necessary to preserve a small amount of thyroid tissue at this location to ensure viability of the recurrent laryngeal nerve and parathyroid gland, this compromise to a total thyroid lobectomy is justified.

The thyroid lobe now can be reflected medially off the trachea, as sharp dissection divides areolar tissue between the trachea and thyroid gland. It is extremely rare for thyroid carcinoma to invade the anterior aspect of the trachea, permitting the use of sharp dissection at this location. The thyroid isthmus along with the lobe of thyroid gland are thereby freed.

Tissues inferior and superior to the thyroid isthmus are mobilized with the thyroid gland. Cephalad, the pyramidal lobe of thyroid, along with the thyroglossal duct tract as high as feasible, are identified and removed en bloc with the thyroid lobe and isthmus. Vessels surrounding the pyramidal lobe are isolated and divided and are occluded with sutures.

A decision is then made as to the location for division of thyroid tissue. Commonly, the division occurs at the junction of the isthmus and contralateral lobe. However, we usually remove one half or more of the contralateral lobe for the following reasons:

1. If a nodule in the excised thyroid lobe is reported by pathologists to be carcinoma on the basis of study of permanent section several days postoperatively, additional tissue is available to assess multicentricity and the advisability of reoperation to remove the residual thyroid tissue.

2. In the case of benign thyroid nodules, recurrence of benign nodules in remaining thyroid tissue occurs in long-term studies at a frequency of approximately 15 per cent after 10 years and at a greater frequency after longer follow-up periods.[51] Removal of additional thyroid tissue in the contralateral lobe may reduce this recurrence rate.

3. If radioactive iodine is to be administered postoperatively for any reason, the dose required will be reduced.

Mobilization of the contralateral lobe is accomplished to the degree required to remove the selected amount of the lobe. Following division of the contralateral thyroid lobe, hemostasis is obtained and the cut surface of thyroid remnant is sutured against the fascia along the lateral aspect of the trachea, using interrupted suture ligatures (Fig. 62–15). This obliterates the raw surface of divided thyroid tissues and prevents the surface from adhering to surrounding tissues. Bleeding points, present often on the exposed surface of the trachea, are occluded by electrocautery or suture ligatures. Hemostasis throughout the wound is then secured.

A soft rubber drain is usually placed in the wound and brought to the outside at the lateral end of the incision. The objective of this drainage is to prevent the later accumulation of serous fluid, which may require removal. The wound is then closed by approximating layers anatomically. Skin edges can be reapproximated by a running subcuticular suture.

Thyroid nodules extending under the manubrium can nearly always be removed through the cervical incision. In particular, substernal goiters justify removal because

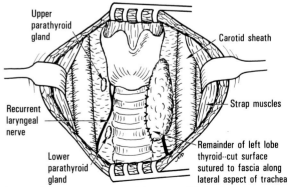

Figure 62–15. Appearance of the wound following right lobectomy and partial left lobectomy of the thyroid gland. Intact recurrent laryngeal nerves and parathyroid glands are evident.

of the significant occurrence of compression symptoms and carcinoma.

Total Thyroidectomy

Total thyroidectomy involves a dissection as outlined for lobectomy, except a decision must be made of the extent of dissection in the contralateral tracheoesophageal groove. Extensive dissection of the contralateral tracheoesophageal groove is omitted except for patients with widespread bilateral thyroid carcinoma. If evidence is not adequate at operation for carcinoma of the contralateral lobe, or if the carcinoma is minimal, the dissection laterally follows closely the lateral surface of the thyroid gland after identifying the course of the recurrent laryngeal nerve to permit its preservation. Limiting dissection of the contralateral tracheoesophageal groove minimizes damage to parathyroid glands in this location.

Near-Total and Subtotal Thyroidectomy

In both types of thyroidectomy procedures, thyroid tissue of the posterior aspect of the contralateral thyroid lobe is preserved to prevent damage to the vital structures in the tracheoesophageal groove. In near-total thyroidectomy a few grams of thyroid tissue are preserved, and dissection in the contralateral tracheoesophageal groove is avoided. More tissue is preserved in a subtotal thyroidectomy, consisting of an estimated 3 gm more of one lobe, the amount of residual thyroid tissue not exceeding one fourth of a lobe.

Near-total thyroidectomy minimizes complications from total thyroidectomy, yet retains most of the advantages over total thyroidectomy. Thus, it should have a significant role in thyroid surgery, especially in patients with minimal or no gross evidence of carcinoma in the contralateral thyroid lobe and in lymph nodes in this tracheoesophageal groove.

Cervical Lymph Node Dissection

Removal of central lymph nodes in the tracheoesophageal grooves and anterior superior mediastinum have been discussed earlier. These are the most important locations for lymph node removal. Lymph nodes are located around the recurrent laryngeal nerves, and when involved by metastatic carcinoma they can enclose this nerve (Fig. 62–4). Nevertheless, it is frequently possible to remove these nodes and preserve nerve function, particularly in the case of well-differentiated thyroid carcinoma in a patient with normal vocal cord function preoperatively.

Lateral cervical lymph node dissections have been alluded to previously in this section and are discussed in more detail in Part IX of this book. To be emphasized in modified lateral neck dissection are preservation of the spinal accessory nerve (but removal of lymph nodes along the nerve) (Fig. 62–16) and the hypoglossal nerve. The lateral jugular vein can often be preserved to minimize postoperative edema in the neck. Usually, the internal jugular vein is preserved, particularly on the side of least involvement if bilateral lateral cervical lymph node dissection is performed.

Extended Resections

Rarely, well-differentiated or medullary thyroid carcinoma invades a short segment of trachea or esophagus and yet is otherwise operable at the time of the primary operation or at the time of reoperation for recurrence. In such cases, the carotid sheath has remained free of invasion. On occasion, extension of thyroid carcinoma into the larynx requires laryngectomy for adequate removal. The laryngectomy may be total or involve partial removal of part of the cricoid cartilage.[32, 37]

The preoperative assessment for operability in such cases of extensive thyroid carcinoma requires bronchoscopy and esophagoscopy. Computerized tomography can also be of value. After resection of a limited segment of trachea, reconstruction can be accomplished by end-to-end anastomosis. It is reported that the resection can include up to 10 tracheal cartilaginous rings.[49] Intraluminal spread into the trachea can also be treated palliatively with a laser.

Mediastinal extension of thyroid carcinoma is usually restricted to the anterior superior mediastinum and can

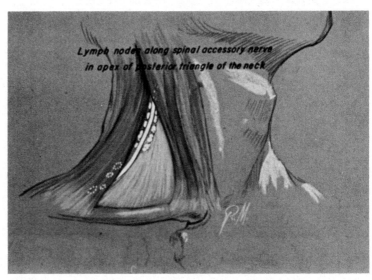

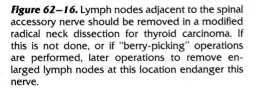

Figure 62–16. Lymph nodes adjacent to the spinal accessory nerve should be removed in a modified radical neck dissection for thyroid carcinoma. If this is not done, or if "berry-picking" operations are performed, later operations to remove enlarged lymph nodes at this location endanger this nerve.

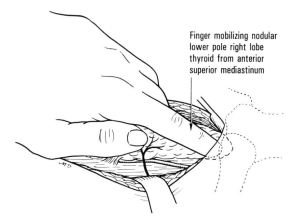

Finger mobilizing nodular lower pole right lobe thyroid from anterior superior mediastinum

Figure 62–17. Mobilizing nodular lower pole of the right lobe of the thyroid from the anterior superior mediastinum. Division of structures is initiated after identification of the recurrent laryngeal nerve. The surgeon's index finger carefully facilitates mobilization of the lobe, descending into the anterior superior mediastinum.

be removed through the neck incision (Fig. 62–17). Rarely, recurrence of well-differentiated thyroid carcinoma is located at more caudad levels and can be removed after a median sternotomy.[4]

A few patients can be salvaged by these extended operative procedures for local invasion by well-differentiated or medullary thyroid carcinoma.

PREVENTION AND MANAGEMENT OF POSTOPERATIVE COMPLICATIONS

Technical complications unique to thyroid operations relate to injury to the recurrent laryngeal nerve, external branch of the superior laryngeal nerve, and the parathyroid glands. Prevention of damage to those structures has been emphasized during the previous discussion concerning the operative procedures of thyroid lobectomy. Anatomic familiarity permits recognition and preservation of structures and obviates complications.

Loss of nerve function can be temporary and is related to stretching or handling of nerves. Loss of function of the ipsilateral vocal cord results from injury to the recurrent laryngeal nerve. This is manifested by a raspy voice. Recovery can occur in a period of weeks to many months. There can be no substitute for identification and preservation of the recurrent laryngeal nerve in thyroid surgery.[65] If division of the recurrent laryngeal nerve is recognized, it should be repaired immediately. Immediate repair is not likely to produce a normal voice, but vocal cord atrophy can be minimized.[35] Permanent loss of function can be treated by injections of Teflon and other materials into the vocal cord to permit better approximation of the cords. If bilateral recurrent laryngeal nerve injury occurs, airway compromise usually requires a tracheostomy immediately or within a few hours postoperatively. The tracheostomy is temporary in the case of transient nerve damage. The preoperative assessment of vocal cord function is needed to evaluate pre-existing loss of vocal cord function from carcinoma or other causes.

The parathyroid glands are fragile and possess a tenuous blood supply. Excessive sponging of their surface or manipulation alone results in at least a temporary loss of parathyroid function.[17, 34] Significant hypocalcemia is manifested early by parasthesia of the hands and a positive Chvostek sign. The slow intravenous administration of calcium gluconate (10 or 20 ml of 10 per cent solution) will rapidly correct this situation. Oral administration of calcium (such as Os-Cal 500, two or three tablets three or four times daily) will usually control temporary hypocalcemia. The patient is weaned off the medication as serum calcium levels return to normal. Permanent hypoparathyroidism results in low serum calcium levels (below 6.5 mg per 100 ml) and the need for administration of vitamin D. Young patients are more sensitive to hypocalcemia, and their clinical manifestations are more severe.

Autotransplantation of parathyroid tissue can prevent permanent hypoparathyroidism.[74] If parathyroid tissue appears questionably viable, especially in a patient undergoing total thyroidectomy, which increases the risk of hypoparathyroidism, immediate autotransplantation or appropriate freezing of the parathyroid tissue for later autotransplantation, if needed, are desired. Confirmation of parathyroid tissue is accomplished by frozen section study of a minute biopsy. The parathyroid tissue is then cut into fine slices, which are individually placed in pockets in muscle of the sternocleidomastoid muscle or a forearm muscle. If the patient possesses no parathyroid tissue except for that which is autotransplanted, medical treatment is required for at least several months while the function of transplanted parathyroid tissue develops. Liberal use of parathyroid gland autotransplantation should reduce the frequency of permanent hypoparathyroidism following total thyroidectomy for carcinoma. However, this procedure is not always successful and involves expense and intricacies of medical management during at least a temporary period of hypoparathyroidism; therefore, parathyroid autotransplantation should not be a substitute for careful and selective thyroid operations.

REOPERATION FOR RECURRENT DISEASE

In recent years emphasis has been placed on early complete and adequate operations, instead of minimal initial procedures, with reoperation carried out for recurrent disease when it becomes evident. For patients with extensive lesions, early extensive operations have provided better results in regard to morbidity, mortality, and recurrent disease. "Berry-picking" operations for clinically evident metastases of well-differentiated thyroid carcinoma to cervical lymph nodes usually result in the need later for reoperation for recurrence or additional metastases with attendant increased morbidity.

Decision-making for the need of reoperation in the case of well-differentiated thyroid carcinoma recognized only postoperatively by study of permanent sections has been discussed previously. In general, this matter is individualized on the basis of the type of carcinoma, its size, and evidence for multicentricity in the tissue removed. Additional operation for well-differentiated encapsulated follicular carcinomas is not considered necessary. A papillary thyroid carcinoma more than 2 cm in diameter with additional foci in the thyroid gland removed is a situation in which experience to date appears to justify reoperation to remove remaining thyroid tissue. Reoperation can be delayed in such cases for 6 months or more to permit surgery in a less technically difficult situation.

Clinically recurrent thyroid carcinoma in the neck is best treated by reoperation whenever anatomically feasible. The response to radioactive iodine and other medical modalities is improved with maximal removal of thyroid carcinoma in the neck.[3] It is rare that operative removal of metastatic lesions outside the neck proves beneficial. Isolated metastases of well-differentiated thyroid carcinoma in the mediastinum warrant removal.

CURRENT CHALLENGES

There is virtually nothing in medicine and surgery that cannot be improved. Needed in surgery of thyroid tumors, particularly thyroid carcinoma, are data from statistically valid prospective randomized studies of the treatment alternatives for each variety of thyroid carcinoma. The clinical situation in which total thyroidectomy (or near-total thyroidectomy) should be selected in the treatment of well-differentiated thyroid carcinoma awaits substantiation. The clinical situation in which a residual remnant of thyroid tissue should be eradicated following less than total thyroidectomy for well-differentiated thyroid carcinoma requires precise definition. The place of postoperative radioactive iodine should be based on established data.

Medullary thyroid carcinoma with its unique hereditary form and tumoral marker (calcitonin) provides a unique tool for the study of basic factors in the etiology of cancer. Factors determining which members of a family will develop the cancer should be determinable with basic studies and techniques in molecular biology.

The management of benign thyroid nodules in terms of control and prevention lacks precision. It is important to determine which nodules can be expected to respond to suppression with thyroid hormone.

REFERENCES

1. Beahrs OH, Vandertoll DJ: Complications of secondary thyroidectomy. Surg Gynecol Obstet 117:535, 1963.
2. Beierwaltes WH: Personal Communication.
3. Beierwaltes WH, Nishiyama RH, Thompson NW, et al: Survival time and "cure" in papillary and follicular thyroid carcinoma with distant metastases: Statistics following University of Michigan therapy. J Nucl Med 23:561, 1982.
4. Block MA: Well-differentiated carcinoma of the thyroid. Curr Probl Cancer 3:32, 1979.
5. Block MA: Thyroid carcinoma with cervical lymph node metastases: Effectiveness of total thyroidectomy and neck dissection. Am J Surg 122:458, 1971.
6. Block MA: Fine needle aspiration and lesions of the thyroid. Int Adv Surg Oncol 5:1, 1982.
7. Block MA: Management of carcinoma of the thyroid. Ann Surg 185:133, 1977.
8. Block MA: Surgery of thyroid nodules and malignancy. Curr Probl Surg 20:134, 1983.
9. Block MA, Brush BE, Horn RC: The incidental carcinoma found in surgery for thyroid nodules. Arch Surg 80:715, 1960.
10. Block MA, Dailey GE, Robb JA: Thyroid nodules indeterminate by needle biopsy: Surgical management. Am J Surg 146:72, 1983.
11. Block MA, Horn RC, Miller JM: Unilateral thyroid nodules with lymphocyte thyroiditis. Arch Surg 87:280, 1963.
12. Block MA, Jackson CE, Greenawald RA, et al: Clinical characteristics distinguishing hereditary from sporadic medullary thyroid carcinoma. Arch Surg 115:142, 1980.
13. Block MA, Jackson LE, Tashjian AH Jr: Medullary thyroid carcinoma detected by serum calcitonin assay. Arch Surg 104:579, 1972.
14. Block MA, Jackson CE, Tashjian AH Jr: Management of parathyroid glands in surgery for medullary thyroid carcinoma. Arch Surg 110:617, 1975.
15. Block MA, Jackson CE, Tashjian AH Jr: Management of occult medullary thyroid carcinoma: Evidenced only by serum calcitonin level elevations after apparently adequate neck operation. Arch Surg 113:368, 1978.
16. Block MA, Miller JM: Modified neck dissection for thyroid carcinoma. Am J Surg 101:349, 1961.
17. Block MA, Miller JM, Horn RC Jr: Minimizing hypoparathyroidism after extended surgery for carcinoma of the thyroid. Surg Gynecol Obstet 123:501, 1966.
18. Block MA, Miller JM, Horn RC Jr: Medullary thyroid carcinoma of the thyroid: Surgical implications. Arch Surg 96:521, 1968.
19. Block MA, Miller JM, Horn RC: Carcinoma of the thyroid after external radiation to the neck in adults. Am J Surg 118:764, 1969.
20. Block MA, Miller JM, Kini SR: The potential impact of needle biopsy on surgery for thyroid nodules. World J Surg 4:739, 1980.
21. Block MA, Wylie JH, Patton RB, Miller JM: Does benign thyroid tissue occur in the lateral part of the neck? Am J Surg 112:476, 1966.
22. Buckwalter JA, Thomas CG Jr: Selection of surgical treatment for well-differentiated thyroid carcinoma. Ann Surg 176:565, 1972.
23. Cady B, Sedgwick CE, Meissner WA, et al: Changing clinical, pathologic, therapeutic, and survival patterns in differentiated thyroid carcinoma. Ann Surg 184:541, 1976.
24. Clark OH, Way LW: Total thyroidectomy: The treatment of choice for patients with thyroid cancer. Ann Surg 19:362, 1982.
25. Cody HS III, Shah JP: Locally invasive, well-differentiated thyroid cancer: 22 years' experience at Memorial Sloan-Kettering Cancer Center. Am J Surg 142:480, 1981.
26. Cole WH, Slaughter OP, Rossiter LJ: Potential dangers of nontoxic nodular goiter. JAMA 127:883, 1945.
27. De Baets M, Vanholder R, Eeckhaut W, et al: Primary Hodgkin's disease of the thyroid. Acta Haematol 68:54, 1981.
28. Deftos LJ, Stein MF: Radioiodine as an adjunct to the surgical treatment of medullary thyroid carcinoma. J Clin Endocrinol Metab 50:967, 1980.
29. De Groot LJ, Frohman LA, Kaplan EL, Refetoff S (eds): Radiation-Associated Thyroid Carcinoma. New York, Grune & Stratton, 1977, p 537.
30. De Groot LJ, Reilly M, Pinnameneni K, Refetoff S: Retrospective and prospective study of radiation-induced thyroid disease. Am J Med 74:852, 1983.
31. Devine RM, Edis AJ, Banks PM: Primary lymphoma of the thyroid: A review of the Mayo Clinic experience through 1978. World J Surg 5:33, 1981.
32. Djalilian M, Beahrs OH, Devine KD, et al: Intraluminal involvement of the larynx and trachea by thyroid cancer. Am J Surg 128:500, 1974.
33. Duffield RGM, Lowe D, Burnand KG: Treatment of well-differentiated carcinoma of the thyroid based on initial surgery. Br J Surg 69:426, 1982.
34. Edis AJ: Prevention and management of complications associated with thyroid and parathyroid surgery. Surg Clin North Am 59:83, 1979.
35. Ezaki H, Ushio H, Hayada Y, Takeichi N: Recurrent laryngeal nerve anastomosis following thyroid surgery. World J Surg 6:342, 1982.
36. Farrar WB, Cooperman M, James AG: Surgical management of papillary and follicular carcinoma of the thyroid. Ann Surg 192:701, 1980.
37. Friedman M, Shelton VK, Skolnik EM, et al: Laryngotracheal invasion by thyroid carcinomas. Ann Otol Rhinol Laryngol 91:363, 1982.
38. Gemsenjager E, Heitz PV, Staub JJ, et al: Surgical aspects of thyroid autonomy in multinodular goiter. World J Surg 7:363, 1983.
39. Goldman JM, Goren EN, Cohen MH, et al: Anaplastic thyroid carcinoma long-term survival after radical surgery. J Surg Oncol 14:389, 1980.
40. Greenfield LD, Vemahi A, George EW III, et al: The role of radiation therapy in the treatment of medullary thyroid cancer. Contemp Surg 18:59, 1981.
41. Gundry SR, Burney RE, Thompson NW, Lloyd R: Total thyroidectomy for Hürthle cell neoplasm of the thyroid. Arch Surg 118:529, 1983.
42. Halsted WS: The operative story of goiter. Johns Hopkins Hosp Rep 19:71, 1929.

43. Hamburger JI, Miller JM, Kini SR: Clinical Pathological Evaluation of Thyroid Nodules: Handbook and Atlas. Southfield, Michigan, private publication by Joel Hamburger, 1979.
44. Haranda T, Ito K, Shimaoka K, et al: Fatal thyroid carcinoma: Anaplastic transformation of adenocarcinomas. Cancer 39:2588, 1977.
45. Harness JK, Thompson NW, Sisson JC, Beierwaltes WH: Differentiated thyroid carcinomas. Treatment of distant metastases. Arch Surg 108:410, 1974.
46. Hubert JP, Kiernan JP, Beahrs OH, et al: Occult papillary carcinoma of the thyroid. Arch Surg 115:394, 1980.
47. Hutter RVP, Frazell EL, Foote FW Jr: Elective radical neck dissection: An assessment of its use in the management of papillary thyroid cancer. Cancer 20:87, 1970.
48. Ida F: Surgical significance of capsule invasion of adenoma of the thyroid. Surg Gynecol Obstet 144:710, 1977.
49. Ishinara T, Yamazahi S, Kubayashi K, et al: Resection of the trachea infiltrated by thyroid carcinoma. Ann Surg 195:4961, 1982.
50. Jackson CE, Talpos GB, Kambouris A, et al: The clinical course following definitive surgery for medullary thyroid carcinoma. Presented at Fourth Annual Meeting, American Association of Endocrine Surgeons, San Francisco, April 19, 1983.
51. Jenny H, Block MA, Horn RC, Miller JM: Recurrence following surgery for benign thyroid nodules. Arch Surg 92:525, 1966.
52. Kini SR, Miller JM, Hamburger JI: Problems in the cytologic diagnosis of the "cold" thyroid nodule in patients with lymphocytic thyroiditis. Acta Cytol 25:506, 1981.
53. Lang W, Georgii A, Stauch G, Keinzle E: The differentiation of atypical adenomas and encapsulated follicular carcinomas in the thyroid gland. Virchows Arch (Pathol Anat) 385:125, 1980.
53a. Lloyd RV, Beierwaltes WH: Occult sclerosing carcinoma of the thyroid: Potential for aggressive biologic behavior. Southern Med J 76:437, 1983.
54. Löwhagen T, Willems JS, Lundell G, et al: Aspiration biopsy cytology in diagnosis of thyroid cancer. World J Surg 5:61, 1981.
55. Maitland A, Rosen IB: New operative strategy for thyroid cancer duct cervical node sampling. Presented at Fourth Annual Meeting, American Association of Endocrine Surgeons, San Francisco, California, April 19, 1983.
56. Mazzaferri EL: Papillary and follicular thyroid cancer: A selective approach to diagnosis and treatment. Annu Rev Med 32:73, 1981.
57. Mazzaferri EL, Young RL: Papillary thyroid carcinoma: A 10-year follow-up report of the impact of therapy in 576 patients. Am J Med 70:511, 1981.
58. Mazzaferri EL, Young RL, Oertel JE, et al: Papillary thyroid carcinoma: The impact of therapy in 576 patients. Medicine 56:171, 1977.
59. McConahey WM: Reassessment of the Mayo Clinic experience with well-differentiated thyroid carcinoma. Presented at the American Thyroid Association Clinical Day Program, Minneapolis, Sept. 16, 1981.
60. Mickie W, Beck JS, Pollet JE: Prevention and management of hypothyroidism after thyroidectomy for thyrotoxicosis. World J Surg 2:307, 1978.
61. Miller JM: Carcinoma and thyroid nodules: The problems in an endemic goiter area. N Engl Med 252:247, 1955.
62. Miller JM, Block MA: The autonomous functioning thyroid nodule. Arch Surg 96:386, 1968.
63. Miller JM, Hamburger JI, Taylor CI: Is needle aspiration of the cystic thyroid nodule effective and safe treatment? In Hamburger JI, Miller JM (eds): Controversies in Clinical Thyroidology. New York, Springer Verlag, 1981, p. 209.
64. Miller JM, Horn RC, Block MA: The increasing incidence of carcinoma of the thyroid in a surgical practice. JAMA 17:1176, 1959.
65. Nemiroff PM, Katz AD: Extralaryngeal divisions of the recurrent laryngeal nerve. Am J Surg 114:468, 1982.
66. Persson CPA, Johansson H, Westermark K, Karlsson FA: Nodular goiter—is thyroxine medication of any value? World J Surg 6:391, 1982.
67. Rosen IB, Wallace C, Strawbridge HG, Walfish PG: Reevaluation of needle aspiration cytology in the detection of thyroid cancer. Surgery 90:747, 1981.
68. Rossi R, Cady B, Meissner WA, et al: Prognosis of undifferentiated carcinoma and lymphoma of the thyroid. Am J Surg 135:589, 1978.
69. Rustad WH: The Recurrent Laryngeal Nerves in Thyroid Surgery. Springfield, Ill., Charles C Thomas, 1956.
70. Samaan NA, Maheshwari S, Hill CS Jr, et al: Impact of therapy for differentiated carcinoma of the thyroid: An analysis of 706 cases. J Clin Endocrinol Metab 56:1131, 1983.
71. Sawyer JL, Block MA, Bowman HE: Results of surgical management of carcinoma of the thyroid. Mich State Med Soc 56:468, 1957.
72. Wang C: The anatomic basis of parathyroid surgery. Ann Surg 183:271, 1976.
73. Wang C, Vickery AL, Maloof F: Needle biopsy of the thyroid. Surg Gynecol Obstet 143:365, 1976.
74. Wells SA Jr, Ross AJ III, Dale JK, Gray RS: Transplantation of the parathyroid glands: Current status. Surg Clin North Am 59:167, 1979.
75. Wolfe HJ, Melvin KEW, Cerri-Skinner SJ, et al: C-cell hyperplasia preceding medullary thyroid carcinoma. N Engl J Med 289:437, 1973.
76. Woolner LB, Beahrs OH, Black BM, et al: Thyroid carcinoma: General considerations and follow-up data on 1181 cases. In Young S, Inman DR (eds): Thyroid Neoplasia: Proceedings of the 2nd Surgical Cancer Research Foundation Symposium. London, Academic Press, 1968, p 51.

CHAPTER 63

Clinical Evaluation of Parathyroid Tumors

Neil A. Breslau, M.D. • **Charles Y. C. Pak, M.D.**

HISTORICAL ASPECTS

The diagnosis of primary hyperparathyroidism (PHPT) with appropriate surgical intervention was first accomplished in the mid-1920s in Vienna and Boston. The saga of how the Austrian group relying on the classical techniques of European anatomic pathology and the American investigators emphasizing the physiologic approach finally discovered this disorder is beautifully recounted by Albright.[1] The highlights of these endeavors are summarized in Table 63–1.

Initially, PHPT was regarded as a rare and severe disease of bone, "osteitis fibrosa cystica." Subsequently in the 1940s and 1950s, Albright's group recognized a different clinical presentation of PHPT in patients with

TABLE 63–1. History of the Recognition of Primary Hyperparathyroidism

Year	Event
European Pathologic Approach	
1880	Sandstrom discovers parathyroid glands.
1891	Von Recklinghausen describes osteitis fibrosa cystica.
1903	Askanazy describes parathyroid tumor in a case of osteitis fibrosa cystica.
1906	Erdheim discovers relationship between parathyroid glands and bone disease, but believes parathyroid enlargement is compensatory and beneficial.
1915	Schlagenhaufer maintains that parathyroid tumors in osteitis fibrosa cystica are primary.
1925	Mandl removes parathyroid tumor from "Albert the tramcar conductor," and the patient's osteitis fibrosa cystica improves.
American Physiologic Approach	
1900	Loeb finds that calcium in body fluids keeps muscles from constantly contracting.
1909	MacCallum and Voegtlin find that serum calcium is low in hypoparathyroidism and that calcium infusion can prevent tetany.
1924	Hanson and Collip independently extract the active principle of parathyroid glands and can test for its presence by measuring serum calcium. Collip observes that excessive parathyroid extract causes hypercalcemia in dogs.
1925	Greenwald finds that parathyroid extract causes negative calcium balance in dogs.
1926	DuBois makes the first diagnosis of primary hyperparathyroidism in America in Captain Charles Martell on the basis of bone disease, high serum calcium, and negative calcium balance. On the seventh parathyroid exploration, Dr. Edward Churchill finds a retrosternal parathyroid adenoma.

renal stones but without evidence of overt bone disease.[2, 19] It soon became clear that renal stones were a far more frequent complication of PHPT than overt osteitis, being the presenting complaint in as many as 50 per cent of patients in some series.[15] In recent years, routine screening of serum calcium (Ca) by automated clinical chemistry techniques has contributed to an increased rate of detection of PHPT in the population. For example, introduction of multichannel screening at the Mayo Clinic has resulted in a fourfold increase in the diagnosis of PHPT among local residents.[35] As cases are discovered earlier in their course, the typical clinical presentation has become more subtle. Again, in reviews of the Mayo Clinic data,[35] it was noted that patients whose PHPT was diagnosed after Ca screening began had a dramatically lower frequency of urolithiasis, 51 per cent before screening versus 4 per cent afterward. Over half the cases of PHPT currently diagnosed are totally asymptomatic.[7, 35] The issue of whether to treat or follow the increasing number of patients presenting with mild asymptomatic disease is one of the most important areas under current investigation.[36, 38]

INCIDENCE, EPIDEMIOLOGY, AND ETIOLOGY

Primary hyperparathyroidism is now recognized as being quite common. Epidemiologic studies report overall incidence rates of 25 to 28 cases per 100,000 population per year.[36, 51] The annual incidence rate increases sharply beyond the age of 40 years, and after age 60 it reaches almost 200 cases per 100,000 in women and 100 cases per 100,000 in men. More than 60,000 new cases of PHPT occur each year in the United States. Greater than 85 per cent of diagnosed patients are between the ages of 30 and 70 years. At all ages, females with PHPT outnumber males by a factor of 2:1.[12]

The etiology of PHPT in patients with sporadic parathyroid adenomas and primary hyperplasia is unknown. Some authors have suggested that PHPT may at times represent the consequence of long-term adaption to forces tending to drive the serum Ca downward.[57, 63] They cite as evidence the increasing frequency of four-gland hyperplasia as opposed to a single parathyroid adenoma with the advent of earlier diagnosis. Additional support for this concept derives from the development of autonomous hyperparathyroidism in cases of long-standing secondary hyperparathyroidism, as has been reported to occur in renal failure,[57] steatorrhea,[21] and nephrolithiasis due to renal hypercalciuria.[47] There are also an increasing number of reports in the literature suggesting that prior head and neck irradiation is associated with an increased incidence of PHPT, usually resulting from a parathyroid adenoma.[16, 76] Parathyroid carcinoma in this setting has not been reported.

The etiology of chief cell hyperplasia in patients with familial hyperparathyroidism, multiple endocrine neoplasia type I (MEN I), and multiple endocrine neoplasia type II (MEN II) remains unclear.[12] A major difficulty with the APUD (apocrine *a*mine *p*recursor *u*ptake and *de*carboxylation) hypothesis with respect to the parathyroid lesion is the lack of evidence that parathyroid cells are neuroectodermal in origin. Other theories have been proposed concerning parathyroid stimulation under the influence of humoral factors such as calcitonin from medullary carcinoma of the thyroid (which might induce transient hypocalcemia) or catecholamines from pheochromocytoma (direct stimulus to parathyroid hormone [PTH] secretion).[63] These theories lack direct support.

CLASSIFICATION

In most series, a single parathyroid adenoma is found in greater than 80 per cent of patients with PHPT (Table 63–2).[12] In our own more recent series, a single parathyroid adenoma was the cause of PHPT in 67 per cent of the patients, with primary chief cell hyperplasia identified in 33 per cent.[55] As is the case with other endocrine tissues, it is difficult to distinguish histologically between normal tissue, hyperplasia, adenoma, or carcinoma. The major clinical problem lies in distinguishing adenoma from primary chief cell hyperplasia. Typical parathyroid adenomas weigh between 0.5 and 5 gm, although rarely they may be as large as 10 to 25 gm. The diagnosis of parathyroid adenoma is ensured if there is a single enlarged gland, surrounded by a clearly defined capsule, with an external rim of compressed normal parathyroid tissue and if the uninvolved glands are atrophic. Often, however, a single hyperplastic gland cannot be distinguished grossly or histologically from an adenomatous gland. This finding, coupled with the fact that the four parathyroid glands are frequently unequally involved by the hyperplastic process, defines the nature of the clinical problem. The situation is further complicated by the presence of supernumerary parathyroid glands (fifth or sixth gland) in 2 to 6 per cent of the population.[64] Supernumerary glands should

TABLE 63–2. Classification of Parathyroid Lesions in 1076 Patients with Primary Hyperparathyroidism*

Lesion	Per Cent
Adenoma	
Single	84%
"Double" or "nodular hyperplasia"	2%
Hyperplasia	
Chief cell	9%
Clear cell	2%
Carcinoma	3%

*Adapted from Broadus AE: Mineral metabolism. *In* Felig P, Baxter JD, Broadus AE, Frohman LA (eds): Endocrinology and Metabolism. New York, McGraw-Hill Book Company, 1981, p. 1019.[12]

be suspected as the site of pathology when a patient with a secure diagnosis of hyperparathyroidism has one of these conditions:

1. Four normal parathyroid glands present, as proven by biopsy.
2. Persistent hypercalcemia following subtotal parathyroidectomy for chief cell hyperplasia.
3. Persistent hypercalcemia after a single adenoma is removed and biopsy of the "three remaining" normal glands.

Up to 1 to 2 per cent of patients with PHPT may harbor a second parathyroid adenoma.[64] The location of hyperfunctioning supernumerary parathyroid glands appears to be variable, but most of them are located in the anterior mediastinum, often within the thymus.

There are two variants of primary parathyroid hyperplasia that occur sporadically. In *clear cell hyperplasia*, all four glands are involved and the cells have a monotonously empty-looking appearance. This lesion is rare and has not been observed in familial disease or in states of secondary hyperparathyroidism. Primary *chief cell hyperplasia* is more common. Occasionally the hyperplastic tissue contains nodules of hyperplastic cells ("nodular hyperplasia"). It is possible that multiple adenomas reported in the past may have represented unappreciated chief cell hyperplasia. Chief cell hyperplasia is the predominant, if not the sole, lesion which occurs in patients with MEN I and II. It is also the typical lesion in patients with familial hyperparathyroidism without other demonstrable elements of the multiple glandular syndromes and in patients with secondary hyperparathyroidism, as in renal disease. All such patients require subtotal parathyroidectomy (three and one-half glands removed), with or without parathyroid autotransplantation.[20]

According to most series, 3 per cent or fewer cases of PHPT are due to *parathyroid carcinoma.*[37] More than 90 per cent of parathyroid carcinomas are functional and associated with the clinical diagnosis of PHPT.[12] The lesion typically grows and invades slowly and metastasizes by local lymphatic spread. Rarely, the lesion is nonfunctional, or it pursues a fulminant course with widespread hematogenous metastases. The clinical presentation is often, but not always, more severe and more rapidly progressive than is noted in the average patient with PHPT.[65] The lesion is recognized grossly by adherence to surrounding tissue and/or by local metastases and histologically by the presence of fibrosis, mitotic figures, and capsular or blood vessel invasion by the malignant cells.[65] The routine use of automated serum Ca determinations has led to earlier detection of this malignancy while it is often still quite localized. Therefore, en bloc local excision with removal of any involved structures to ensure clear margins is adequate primary treatment.[37] The presence of nodal metastasis would, of course, require radical neck dissection. Postoperatively, patients should be closely followed with serial serum Ca determinations to detect any recurrence or distant metastasis. These recurrences can usually be managed successfully by repeated local excision of recurrences and palliative resection of functioning metastases.[30] Occasionally, the nature of the process goes unrecognized and the patient is subjected to multiple neck explorations for "recurrent" PHPT.

CLINICAL PRESENTATION

A convenient means of recalling the various ways PHPT may present involves "the six moans of hyperparathyroidism":[12] (1) stones, (2) bones, (3) groans (abdominal symptoms), (4) ions (asymptomatic hypercalcemia), (5) neurons (neuromuscular and psychiatric presentations), and (6) hormones (to emphasize the occurrence of PHPT as part of multiple endocrine neoplasia syndromes).

Another approach is to consider the spectrum of PHPT presented in Table 63–3.[15] The three categories listed in the table are somewhat artificial, but are designed to describe the framework within which typical patients with PHPT present clinically. The table does not intend to imply that there are three discrete clinical forms of PHPT, for the disease clearly represents a continuum and a number of patients present with features included in more than one of these categories. The scheme is useful, however, because it depicts the principal ways in which patients with PHPT present clinically. In modern-day practice, "stones" account for 25 to 30 per cent of cases; the "groan" category (which is meant to include abdominal symptoms, nonspecific complaints, and asymptomatic cases) accounts for 50 to 70 per cent of cases; and the "bone" category represents only some 5 per cent of patients. An important point with respect to natural history of the disease is that, in general, evolution or progression from left to right in the table does not occur. Rather, patients tend to present and remain predominantly within one category when followed over time. This chapter will present the specific stone and bone complications of PHPT, followed by a discussion of the nonspecific manifestations of the disease and the asymptomatic presentation ("groans").

Predominant Presentations

Nephrolithiasis

The typical patient with PHPT that is complicated by renal stones presents with a history of chronicity (often years), mild hypercalcemia, mildly to moderately abnormal parathyroid function tests, and a modest parathyroid mass at surgery (Fig. 63–1)[42, 43] The hypercalciuria is pronounced with respect to the modestly elevated

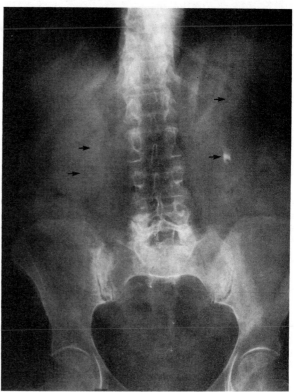

Figure 63–1. Roentgenographic examination of the abdomen (KUB) revealing two small stones in the right kidney, a small stone in the upper pole of the left kidney, and an early staghorn calculus in the lower pole of the left kidney. The patient, a 65-year-old female with primary hyperparathyroidism, had had mild hypercalcemia with significant hypercalciuria for at least 8 years. She had been completely unaware of the kidney stones, which were revealed on a routine admission evaluation.

serum Ca level (which may intermittently fall within the normal range), thus making this presentation of PHPT difficult to distinguish from idiopathic hypercalciuria. Patients with PHPT may form pure calcium phosphate stones, calcium oxalate stones, or mixed calcium stones. Hypercalciuria is an important, though not the sole, factor involved in renal stone disease. Approximately two thirds of patients with PHPT have demonstrable hypercalciuria, but statistical relationships between the quantity of Ca excreted and stone formation in hyperparathyroid patients have been difficult to establish. Peacock found that hyperparathyroid patients presenting with a history of renal stones uniformly displayed an increase in intestinal Ca absorption, whereas patients presenting with "other" (non-stone) presentations displayed widely varying patterns of Ca absorption.[59] Broadus and colleagues found that the hyperparathyroid patients with marked elevations in serum $1,25-(OH)_2D$, intestinal hyperabsorption of calcium, and resultant hypercalciuria were the most prone to stone disease.[11] The greater intestinal absorption of Ca with associated parathyroid suppression could explain the tendency for smaller parathyroid glands and disproportionate hypercalciuria in these patients. It remains unexplained why certain patients with PHPT have normal or near-normal circulating levels of

TABLE 63–3. Spectrum of Primary Hyperparathyroidism*

	Stones	Groans	Bones
History	Chronic	Indeterminate	Subacute
Serum calcium	Mild	11–12 mg/dl	Severe
iPTH, NcAMP	1+†	1+ to 2+	3+ to 4+
Parathyroid mass	1 gm	Indeterminate	5 gm
Differential diagnosis	Idiopathic hypercalciuria	Multiple	Cancer

*From Broadus AE: Primary hyperparathyroidism viewed as a bihormonal disease process. Miner Electrolyte Metab 8:199, 1982.

†The plus scale indicates increasing quantitative degrees of abnormality.

Abbreviations: iPTH = Immunoreactive PTH; NcAMP = nephrogenous cyclic AMP.

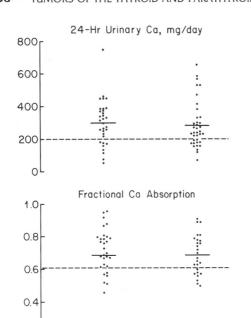

Figure 63–2. Urinary calcium (Ca) and fractional Ca absorption in surgically proven primary hyperparathyroidism with and without stones. Dashed line = Upper normal limits for urinary Ca and fractional Ca absorption; solid line = mean values.

$1,25-(OH)_2D$ while others have marked elevations in the circulating level of the active metabolite. Moreover, our own group was unable to confirm any differences between stone-forming (N = 32) and non–stone-forming (N = 37) hyperparathyroid patients with respect to serum $1,25-(OH)_2D$, fractional intestinal Ca absorption, or urinary calcium excretion (Fig. 63–2).[55]

Thus, many patients with PHPT do not form stones despite hypercalciuria and despite the passage of urine that is supersaturated with respect to brushite and calcium oxalate. In patients who do form stones, there may be an increased renal excretion of certain noncrystalline substances that facilitate stone formation by enhancing spontaneous nucleation of calcium phosphate and calcium oxalate. This "promoter" of nucleation has not been characterized. There may be a deficiency of urinary inhibitors as well. A low pyrophosphate and citrate excretion has been reported in stone-forming patients with PHPT. Whatever the major risk factors for stone formation may be, nephrolithiasis generally ceases following successful parathyroidectomy.[17, 48]

Bone Disease

The typical patient with overt hyperparathyroid bone disease has a more subacute history, moderate to severe hypercalcemia, markedly abnormal parathyroid function tests, and a large mass of abnormal parathyroid tissue.[42, 43] The major clinical problem within this category is that of differential diagnosis between patients with severe PHPT and those with hypercalcemia of malignancy.

The classical bone disease of PHPT is *osteitis fibrosa cystica*. This disorder is characterized by bone pain, pathologic fractures of long bones and crush fractures of the spine, and skeletal deformities. Radiologically, it is characterized by "demineralization," erosion of outer and inner cortical surfaces, fractures and deformities, locally destructive lesions, chondrocalcinosis, and soft-tissue calcifications. The demineralization is patchy rather than homogeneous, as typified by the "moth-eaten" appearance of the skull (Fig. 63–3). The outer cortical erosions are referred to as *subperiosteal resorption* and are best demonstrated on the radial aspect of the middle phalanges of the hands, using fine-detailed radiography (Fig. 63–4).

The locally destructive lesions comprise two types of cystic lesions: true bone cysts and "brown tumors." The former are true fluid-filled cysts; the latter are composed largely of osteoclasts, intermixed with poorly mineralized woven bone, and are sometimes referred to as *osteoclastomas*. These two lesions have the same radiologic appearance, but bone cysts remain indefinitely after successful surgery, whereas brown tumors resolve and remineralize (Fig. 63–5). The subperiosteal resorption and bony demineralization are also reversible.[41]

Classic radiographic findings of osteitis fibrosa cystica are considered to be diagnostic of PHPT. Histologically, this lesion is associated with extensive fibrosis, with replacement of normal marrow and bone cell elements. Although fewer than 5 per cent of patients with PHPT present with bone-related symptoms as their chief complaint, the radiologic diagnosis of osteitis fibrosa cystica may be made in 10 to 15 per cent.

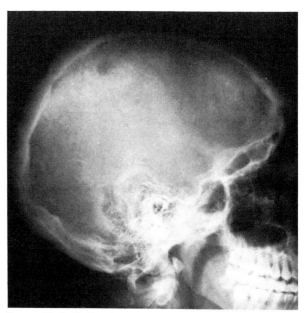

Figure 63–3. Skull radiograph of a patient with hyperparathyroidism demonstrating "salt-and-pepper" or "moth-eaten" appearance of the skull. A marble-size brown tumor is also visible near the top of the skull. (Courtesy of Dr. Geral Dietz, Associate Professor of Clinical Radiology, University of Texas Health Science Center at Dallas, Southwestern Medical School.)

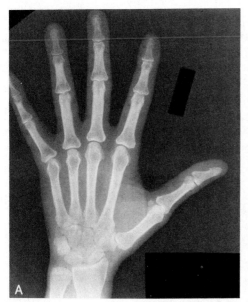
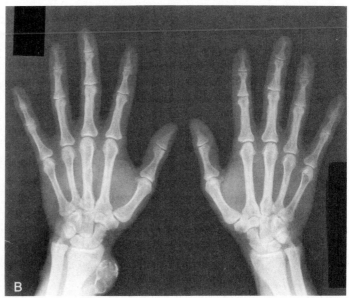

Figure 63–4. (A) Radiogram of a normal hand for comparison. (B) Hand films from a patient with end-stage renal disease and severe secondary hyperparathyroidism. Subperiosteal resorption is best seen on the radial aspect of the midphalanx of the second and third digit of each hand. There is considerable loss of the distal phalangeal tufts. A brown tumor is present at the midregion of the third left metacarpal. Incidentally noted is a calcification of the arteriovenous fistula site near the left wrist. (Courtesy of Dr. Geral Dietz, Associate Professor of Clinical Radiology, University of Texas Health Science Center at Dallas, Southwestern Medical School.)

The pathogenesis of osteitis fibrosa cystica is not clearly defined. It appears to be a complication of severe and rapidly progressive PHPT associated with large adenomas and high PTH levels.[42, 43] Indeed, such a presentation is typical of patients harboring a parathyroid carcinoma.[65] Bone disease resembling osteoporosis may result from a mild to moderate stimulation of PTH secretion for a prolonged period, especially in white postmenopausal women.[52] In a series reported in 1973, osteopenia of the spine was noted in 20 per cent and in the hands of 36 per cent of patients with PHPT.[29] For patients with this milder "osteopenic" form of bone disease, the biochemical presentation may be similar to that of stone-formers.

Figure 63–5. (A) Subperiosteal resorption, loss of terminal tufts, and brown tumors noted in the second and third digits of a patient with primary hyperparathyroidism. (B) Repeat film of the same digits after successful parathyroidectomy. Note the improved density, sharper cortical margins, and sclerotic areas where the two brown tumors have been "filled in."

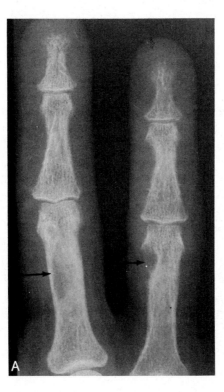
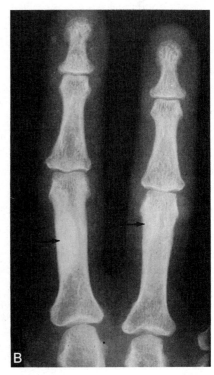

Abdominal and Nonspecific Conditions

The typical patient with the "groan", or nonspecific, presentation is in all ways intermediate in the spectrum of PHPT (Table 3). The main clinical problems within this category do not have to do with confirmation of diagnosis, which is usually readily achievable with modern diagnostic techniques, but with the requirement that the diagnosis be considered in so many clinical settings and with uncertainties regarding the recommendation of neck exploration on the basis of such nonspecific manifestations of the disorder.

Peptic Ulcer. Peptic ulcer disease occurs with increased frequency in patients with PHPT[3] i.e., in 14 per cent of patients compared with estimates of 2 to 3 per cent in the general adult population. Peptic ulcer disease may result from the stimulation of the secretion of gastrin and of hydrochloric acid by hypercalcemia.[3] In any patient with PHPT and peptic ulcer disease, the possibility of Zollinger-Ellison syndrome should be considered (gastrinomas may coexist with PHPT in multiple endocrine neoplasia type I). Patients with Zollinger-Ellison syndrome usually have very high gastrin levels (>150 pg/ml), but in questionable cases this measurement should be repeated following parathyroidectomy. Although symptoms and objective findings of acid-peptic disease are generally said to improve postparathyroidectomy, this impression is based on surprisingly little systematic evidence.

Pancreatitis. Acute or chronic pancreatitis occurs in approximately 2 per cent of patients with PHPT. The frequency of pancreatitis is much higher in patients with severe PHPT or "parathyroid crisis," in whom an incidence of 30 per cent or more has been reported.[33] The pathogenesis of pancreatitis as it occurs in PHPT is unknown, but it has been proposed that pancreatic obstruction or injury occur due to ductal calculi and parenchymal calcifications. Substantial clinical improvement in abdominal symptoms has been observed following successful parathyroidectomy.[49] Other nonspecific gastrointestinal symptoms that may accompany PHPT and resolve after parathyroidectomy include diffuse, ill-defined abdominal pain; constipation; anorexia; weight loss; nausea; and vomiting.

Hypertension. Hypertension occurs in 20 to 50 per cent of patients with PHPT, which equals or exceeds by several fold the occurrence of essential hypertension in 20 per cent of the adult population in the United States.[7, 35, 43] The mechanism for the hypertension has not been well defined. In any patient with PHPT and hypertension, the possibility of pheochromocytoma (as occurs in MEN II) must be considered but is rare.[66] The reported influence of surgical correction of PHPT on blood pressure has been widely divergent, and it is impossible to predict whether blood pressure will improve in a given patient following parathyroidectomy.[12]

Neuromuscular and Psychiatric Presentations

The importance of neurologic findings in PHPT has been emphasized by the National Institutes of Health group.[58] The most common symptoms were weakness and fatigability, particularly in the proximal muscles of the lower extremities. Physical findings included muscular weakness, muscle atrophy, hyperflexia, and pe-

culiar fine fasciculations of the tongue. Sensory abnormalities were rare. Neurologic deficits were found in 14 of 16 patients with PHPT.[58] Detailed evaluation of the patients by electromyography, determination of nerve conduction time, and muscle biopsies were consistent with neuropathy rather than myopathy. These neuropathic abnormalities were completely reversible following successful parathyroidectomy.[58] A similar reversible neuromuscular syndrome has been described in patients with secondary hyperparathyroidism.[44] Central nervous system manifestations may include lethargy, confusion, and obtundation accompanying hypercalcemia. Psychoneurotic symptoms including depression, personality change, memory loss, or overtly psychotic behavior have also been described in PHPT; these symptoms may or may not resolve with successful parathyroidectomy.

Patients with PHPT may complain of joint pains. Skeletal fractures are commonly associated with degenerative osteoarthritis in contiguous weight-bearing joints. Both gouty arthritis and pseudogout have been reported to occur with an increased frequency in PHPT. The renal clearance of uric acid is reduced in this disorder, and hyperuricemia is common.[43]

Asymptomatic Derangements

Although the triad of nephrolithiasis, bone disease, and peptic ulcer disease continues to comprise the principal symptomatology, there has been a major change in the clinical presentation of PHPT during the past 10 to 15 years. This changing trend, probably the result of earlier detection through routine analysis of serum Ca and from availability of improved diagnostic techniques, has resulted in a larger fraction of patients (>50 per cent) who present without symptoms. The increased frequency of diagnosis of asymptomatic PHPT presents a new therapeutic challenge. Although the need for surgical parathyroidectomy in symptomatic PHPT is well recognized, the role of surgery in the asymptomatic form has not been established. The Mayo Clinic group in a 10-year follow-up study found that only 25 per cent of patients who presented asymptomatically went on to develop surgical indications (including serum Ca levels greater than 11.0 mg/dl, roentgenographic evidence of bone disease, decreased renal function, metabolically active or infected renal lithiasis, impracticality for prolonged observation, or gastrointestinal complications).[67] Thus, fully 75 per cent of patients who presented asymptomatically did not develop a surgical indication over a 10-year period. Unfortunately, it was not possible to predict from the initial presentation which patients would ultimately require surgery and which would not. Some investigators have suggested that perhaps all patients in whom the diagnosis of PHPT is made should be operated upon either because of concern about insidious spinal bone mineral loss[36, 68] or because of progressive renal impairment of uncertain etiology which may occur in up to 5 per cent of patients.[18]

We have found that a search for certain physiologic derangements indicative of PTH excess may help to identify asymptomatic patients who might benefit from parathyroid surgery.[38] These derangements may include hypercalciuria, negative Ca balance (e.g., a high fasting urinary Ca, urinary Ca exceeding absorbed Ca, and a

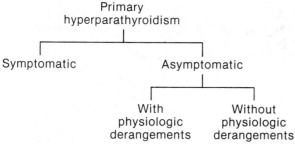

```
              Primary
         hyperparathyroidism
                 |
        ┌────────┴────────┐
   Symptomatic        Asymptomatic
                     ┌─────┴─────┐
                   With        Without
                physiologic   physiologic
               derangements  derangements
```

Figure 63–6. Classification of primary hyperparathyroidism.

low bone density), and reduced endogenous creatinine clearance of less than 65 ml/min. These deleterious effects of PTH excess form the basis for the further separation of the asymptomatic group, since they are present in some but not all patients with asymptomatic PHPT (Fig. 63–6).

Parathyroidectomy is probably indicated in the subgroup with physiologic derangements because these derangements may herald the eventual development of symptoms, are also present in the symptomatic group, and may be corrected largely by parathyroid surgery.[38] The need for parathyroid exploration in the asymptomatic patients without physiologic derangements is not established. Preliminary data in six of these patients show a lack of progression of the disease over 4 to 6 years of follow-up. Assessment of bone histomorphometry revealed that 75 per cent of asymptomatic hyperparathyroid patients with physiologic derangements had abnormalities of bone (increased resorption surface, increased bone turnover) whereas only 11 per cent of the group without derangements had bony abnormalities (unpublished observation). Further characterization and long-term follow-up will be required before it is known whether the asymptomatic hyperparathyroid patients without physiologic derangements represent an early stage of the disease or a pathogenetically unique subset characterized by skeletal resistance to PTH and an exaggerated renal tubular reabsorption of Ca. This group, which comprises 10 per cent of patients with PHPT, probably does not have familial hypocalciuric hypercalcemia (see later), since there was no hypermagnesemia or family history of hypercalcemia.

Familial Hypercalcemic Syndromes

Primary hyperparathyroidism may be part of or confused with certain familial hypercalcemic syndromes. All of these syndromes are inherited in an autosomal dominant pattern. Multiple endocrine neoplasia type I (MEN I) consists of neoplasms of the pituitary, parathyroids, and pancreas ("the three P's").[79] There are two variants of multiple endocrine neoplasia type II (MEN II). The key features of MEN IIA are medullary carcinoma of the thyroid, hyperparathyroidism, and pheochromocytoma.[39] The key features of MEN IIB are mucosal neuromas, marfanoid skeletal deformities, medullary carcinoma of the thyroid and pheochromocytomas.[40] Hyperparathyroidism usually does not occur in patients with MEN IIB. Familial hyperparathyroidism, inherited in an autosomal dominant pattern but in

the absence of other features of MEN I or MEN II, has also been reported.[31]

For each of the preceding familial hypercalcemic syndromes, the usual sequelae of PHPT may develop. Parathyroid surgery would then be appropriate. However, in the syndrome of familial hypocalciuric hypercalcemia (FHH), surgery is generally not indicated. This complex syndrome has been extensively investigated by Marx and co-workers.[46] The mode of inheritance is autosomal dominant, and 50 per cent of offspring in affected families will develop hypercalcemia before the age of 10 years. Despite mean serum Ca values in the range of 12 mg/dl, patients with FHH typically lack the characteristic manifestations of PHPT, such as kidney stones, bone disease, or peptic ulcers. Features of MEN I or MEN II also do not occur. A key feature of FHH is a clear-cut reduction in the fractional excretion of both calcium and magnesium, so that these patients display a proportional degree of hypercalcemia and hypermagnesemia. Mean 24-hour urine Ca excretion is in the range of 100 mg (compared with the daily output characteristic of PHPT of greater than 300 mg) and the calcium to creatinine clearance ratio is less than 0.01. Despite the enhanced renal reabsorption of divalent cations, values for serum PTH and urinary cyclic AMP are usually in the mid- to high-normal range and occasionally are frankly elevated. Parathyroid hyperplasia has been reported in a few patients who have undergone parathyroid exploration. These observations suggest abnormal Ca transport occurs at a minimum of two sites: kidney and parathyroid glands. Subtotal parathyroidectomy generally does not abolish the hypercalcemia, although total parathyroidectomy may cause hypoparathyroidism. Since patients with FHH are usually asymptomatic, careful follow-up seems more appropriate than attempts at surgery.

HISTORY AND PHYSICAL EXAMINATION

The first step in diagnosing PHPT is a careful history aimed at uncovering the typical manifestations. On physical examination one may observe band keratopathy, which can appear as a moth-eaten, irregular calcium deposit located at the medial and lateral limbic regions of the cornea or as a hazy band across the cornea (Fig. 63–7). Small conjunctival calcifications surrounded by erythema may also be noted. Subtle neuromuscular findings, including proximal muscle weakness in the lower extremities, and peculiar fine fasciculation in the tongue can sometimes be demonstrated. Bone tenderness, an indication of bone involvement, should be specifically searched for and is most readily appreciated by applying moderate thumb pressure to the distal tibia or iliac crest.

Routine Laboratory Tests

The classical laboratory findings in PHPT are hypercalcemia and hypophosphatemia. An elevated mean serum Ca level in the absence of malignancy, sarcoidosis, hypervitaminosis D, hyperthyroidism, thiazides, hypocalciuria, milk-alkali syndrome, or immobilization is still the best test for PHPT. If the hypercalcemia can be demonstrated to have been present for 12 months or

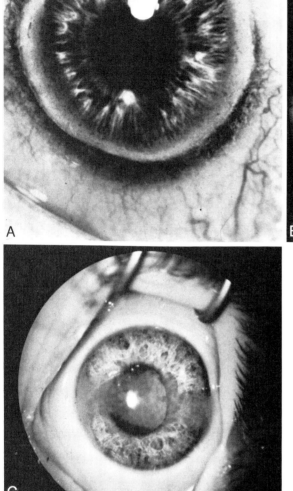

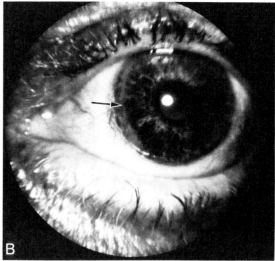

Figure 63–7. (*A*) Arcus senilis should not be confused with band keratopathy. Arcus senilis appears as a dense, whitish-gray band completely surrounding the cornea. It may be seen in normal individuals as a component of aging and in patients with hypercholesterolemia. This circular band is composed of cholesterol esters and has nothing to do with hyperparathyroidism.

(*B*) In hyperparathyroidism, but also in other hypercalcemic conditions such as sarcoidosis, vitamin D intoxication or milk-alkali syndrome, calcium phosphates and carbonates may precipitate, primarily beneath the corneal epithelium. This may appear as a moth-eaten irregular deposit in the medical limbic region of the cornea as shown above.

(*C*) In more classical, advanced band keratopathy, the calcium salts may deposit in a plane corresponding to the interpalpebral tissue. This appears as a hazy band across the cornea. (Courtesy of Deborah Elkins. Medical Photographer, Department of Ophthalmology, University of Texas Health Science Center at Dallas, Southwestern Medical School.)

more, or if it is associated with elements of the diagnostic triad (stones, bone fractures, or ulcers), the diagnosis is virtually ensured. Following a careful history and physical examination, routine serum chemistry, a complete blood count, serum protein electrophoresis, thyroid function tests, 24-hour urine Ca, and radiographic evaluation of the chest, hands, and kidneys may be the only tests required to rule out other potential causes of hypercalcemia. The presence of localized bone pain would warrant a skeletal survey or bone scan.

Owing to the phosphaturic effect of PTH, hypophosphatemia is commonly observed in PHPT. In the absence of renal impairment, hypophosphatemia (based on age- and sex-matched control ranges) is demonstrable in approximately 70 per cent of patients with PHPT.[12] During the past decade, Bijvoet and his associates in Holland have introduced the determination of the renal phosphorus threshold, or the ratio of maximal tubular reabsorption of phosphorus to the glomerular filtration rate (TmP/GFR), as a measure of renal phosphate handling.[5, 78] The TmP/GFR may be regarded as the "set point" of renal phosphate reabsorption. It is this set point that is the principal determinant of the serum phosphorus concentration under steady-state conditions. In essence, PTH influences this system by resetting the TmP/GFR at a lower level. The required samples are timed or spot-fasting morning urine and serum specimens, and each of these is analyzed for phosphate and creatinine content. The fractional excretion of phosphate (or TRP) is calculated and the TmP is derived from a nomogram (Fig. 63–8).[78]

For adults, the normal range for TmP/GFR is 2.5 to 4.2 mg/dl. Based on age- and sex-matched control ranges, reduced values for TmP/GFR are observed in 80 per cent or more of patients with PHPT and values above 3 mg/dl are rare.[13] Since PTH also increases renal bicarbonate excretion and tends to produce a mild hyperchloremic acidosis, some authors have used the chloride: phosphate ratio as a diagnostic parameter.[56] Ratios greater than 33 were observed in the majority of patients with PHPT and were rarely found in patients with other causes of hypercalcemia.[56] These findings and the utility of the chloride:phosphate ratio have been challenged.[53]

Other miscellaneous laboratory abnormalities that occasionally may be noted in PHPT include increased

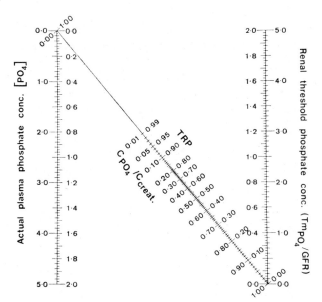

Figure 63–8. Nomogram for derivation of renal threshold phosphate concentration.

serum alkaline phosphatase activity, hypomagnesemia, modest hyperuricemia, an increased sedimentation rate, and a mild nonspecific anemia.[43]

Serum PTH Measurement

The *definitive* diagnosis of PHPT rests on the simultaneous demonstration of hypercalcemia together with an index of abnormal or inappropriate parathyroid function. Parathyroid function is best evaluated by measurement of serum immunoreactive PTH and urinary cyclic adenosine monophosphate (cylic AMP).

The determination of the serum immunoreactive PTH potentially provides the most direct measure of parathyroid function. However, several problems have limited the reliability of this measurement and caused discrepant results from different laboratories. These problems have included:

1. The general unavailability of homologous (i.e., antihuman PTH) antiserums, which limits sensitivity.

2. The immunoheterogeneity of circulating PTH.

3. The lack of standardized reagents and assay procedures for interlaboratory use.

There are multiple forms and/or fragments of PTH in the peripheral circulation. Carboxy-terminal fragments constitute approximately 80 per cent of the immunoreactive material in serum.[45] These fragments are biologically inactive, are derived principally from peripheral metabolism of the intact hormone, have a relatively long circulating half-time, and are eliminated from the circulation entirely by glomerular filtration. Carboxy-terminal radioimmunoassays provide information of a relatively time-integrated character, which may provide greater sensitivity in picking up hyperparathyroidism, but they must be carefully interpreted with respect to the degree of renal function. In renal failure, impaired clearance of carboxy-terminal fragments may result in a high serum immunoreactive PTH level with little bearing on the degree of parathyroid hypertrophy present or the level of biologically active hormone.

The active, intact hormone accounts for only some 10 to 15 per cent of the immunoreactive material in serum, has a short circulating half-time, and is metabolized by a number of peripheral tissues. Amino-terminal radioimmunoassays measure the intact hormone and possibly some short-lived amino-terminal fragments. Since they do not recognize the abundant but inactive carboxy-terminal fragments, they are more sensitive to fluctuations in parathyroid secretory rates and are more useful in accurately assessing parathyroid function in patients with renal failure.[34] Until recently, the problem with amino-terminal radioimmunoassays had been their insensitivity, often resulting in a failure to detect any serum PTH in normal subjects and even in some patients with proven PHPT. With most reliable PTH radioimmunoassays, there is an inverse correlation between serum PTH levels and the serum Ca in normal subjects, so that at higher serum Ca levels the circulating PTH becomes low or undetectable. A "normal" level of PTH at a high serum Ca may be inappropriate and may signify PHPT. For this reason, it is essential that radioimmunoassays be sufficiently sensitive to detect normal PTH levels. An amino-terminal antiserum has been developed in chickens against synthetic human PTH 1-34 that is sufficiently sensitive to measure immunoreactive PTH in over 90 per cent of normal subjects.[69] This assay apparently measures only the biologically active hormone, since normal values are less than 30 pg/ml (comparable with values obtained in laborious cytochemical bioassays).[32] Moreover, absolute elevations in serum PTH have been found in 93 per cent of patients with surgically confirmed PHPT. The amino-terminal assay may be particularly useful in chronic renal failure, where it appears to segregate patients with osteitis fibrosa from patients with renal failure who do not show severe bone disease.[28] This assay is now commercially available from the Nichols Institute (Los Angeles). Whichever radioimmunoassay is used, the physician should know and understand the characteristics and track record of that particular assay system and should interpret the serum PTH level with respect to serum Ca and level of renal function.

Urinary Cyclic AMP Measurement

Another discriminating test that has proved useful in the diagnosis of PHPT involves the measurement of urinary cyclic AMP.[10, 54] This test is based on the fact that PTH is a potent stimulus for renal adenylate cyclase and the cyclic AMP so formed is rapidly excreted in the urine, probably because of the permeability characteristics of the tubular membrane near the site of nucleotide synthesis. No other hormone system shares these features. The measurement of urinary cyclic AMP has certain advantages over the radioimmunoassay for PTH as a test of parathyroid function, since it reflects the biological activity of PTH and it represents an "integrated" measure of PTH level over the period of urine collection rather than at a single moment in time.

The total urinary cyclic AMP is the sum of a filtered component from plasma and a nephrogenous component produced within the kidney. Under normal circumstances, approximately 40 per cent of total cyclic AMP consists of the nephrogenous fraction, most of which is produced under the influence of PTH. In conditions of

PTH excess, the amount of filtered cyclic AMP is not altered, which indicates that any nucleotide produced outside the kidney under the influence of PTH does not contribute significantly to the urinary cyclic AMP. However, the PTH-dependent nephrogenous fraction is significantly increased in the hyperparathyroid state. Thus, assessment of nephrogenous cyclic AMP is superior to total urinary cyclic AMP as a measure of parathyroid function, since it is unaffected by other hormonal influences. However, because of the relative constancy of the filtered fraction when renal function is normal, measurement of total urinary cyclic AMP, expressed in relation to the glomerular filtration rate, yields qualitatively similar data to the nephrogenous cyclic AMP. The expression of total cyclic AMP as a function of glomerular filtration rate may be calculated simply as the product of urinary cyclic AMP in nmol/mg creatinine and serum creatinine in mg/dl, to yield a value expressed as nmol/100 ml glomerular filtrate. Although measurement of nephrogenous cyclic AMP is technically somewhat demanding, the measurement of total cyclic AMP in urine is extremely simple and well within the reach of a routine endocrine laboratory.

Measurement of nephrogenous cyclic AMP, which is abnormal in about 97 per cent of patients,[10] provides the most reliable and specific diagnosis of PHPT. Measurement of total urinary cyclic AMP expressed per 100 ml glomerular filtration is almost as reliable (increased in 94 per cent of patients).[10, 54] The urinary cyclic AMP is such a rapid and sensitive index of parathyroid function that if the appropriate technology is available, intraoperative measurements of urinary cyclic AMP may serve as a guide to completeness of parathyroid surgery.[73] Results for urinary cyclic AMP determinations are valid down to levels of glomerular filtration rate in the range of 25 ml/min, but have not been validated in patients with more advanced azotemia.[13] Another cautionary note is that because urinary cyclic AMP measurements reflect subtle alterations in parathyroid function, levels detected will be influenced by dietary calcium intake. For example, the oral administration of the quantity of calcium present in an average calcium-containing meal results in a 30 per cent suppression of nephrogenous cyclic AMP in normal subjects.[13] One study found that in patients with PHPT, results for total cyclic AMP excretion were elevated in 96 per cent on a restricted Ca diet but only in 72 per cent on a high-normal Ca diet.[14] Clearly, patients suspected of having PHPT should be studied on a restricted Ca intake (400 mg daily).

DIFFERENTIAL DIAGNOSIS

Differential diagnosis involves distinguishing the hypercalcemia of PHPT from hypercalcemia due to other causes. Three causes of hypercalcemia that should be considered include malignancy, sarcoidosis, and thiazide therapy. *Hypercalcemia complicating malignant disease* is a poor prognostic sign and correlates with extensive disease that is generally readily apparent. Hypercalcemia tends to be greater than 13 mg/dl, of acute onset, and unstable. Radiologic evidence of osteitis fibrosa cystica or kidney stones is rare in patients with malignancy. Although detectable or occasionally slightly ele-

vated serum levels of immunoreactive PTH have been variously reported by different laboratories in patients with malignant disease and hypercalcemia, these levels are usually discordant with the degree of hypercalcemia; that is, patients with severe PHPT and comparable levels of serum Ca generally have serum PTH levels that are much higher. Despite relatively "normal" PTH levels, patients with malignancy who appear to have a humoral basis for their hypercalcemia display a reduction in TmP/GFR and elevated levels of urinary cyclic AMP.[74] A reduction in circulating 1,25-dihydroxyvitamin D was regularly observed in these patients; this finding is in sharp contrast to the elevated levels of this metabolite found in patients with PHPT (Fig. 63–9).[9, 74] This latter test may prove to be the most reliable laboratory means of distinguishing PHPT from humoral hypercalcemia of malignancy, except for some patients with lymphoma who also appear to have elevated 1,25-dihydroxyvitamin D levels (Fig. 63–9).[9]

Sarcoidosis, like PHPT, may present with hypercalcemia, hypercalciuria, and kidney stones in association with increased serum 1,25-dihydroxyvitamin D levels (Fig. 63–10). The granulomatous tissue is believed capable of producing this vitamin D metabolite, which is the probable cause for abnormal calcium metabolism in sarcoidosis.[4] A history of cough or shortness of breath, chest radiograph revealing bilateral hilar adenopathy or diffuse fibronodular infiltrate, and serum protein electrophoresis revealing high total protein with increased globulin would suggest the diagnosis. Serum PTH and urinary cyclic AMP would be suppressed because of the enhanced intestinal Ca absorption. If doubt persists, the glucocorticoid suppression test may be used to distinguish sarcoidosis from PHPT.[8] In response to prednisone, 50 mg daily for a week, there are marked reductions in serum Ca, urine Ca, 1,25-$(OH)_2$D and intestinal Ca absorption in patients with sarcoidosis, but not in patients with PHPT.[8]

Thiazide diuretics may cause hypercalcemia because of volume contraction and a direct stimulation of distal renal tubular Ca reabsorption. In normal subjects, serum

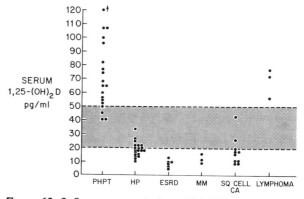

Figure 63–9. Serum concentrations 1,25-$(OH)_2$ vitamin D in patients with parathyroid disorders, renal failure, or hypercalcemia of malignancy. The cross-hatched area represents the normal range of 1,25-$(OH)_2$ vitamin D (20–50 pg/ml). PHPT = primary hyperparathyroidism; HP = hypoparathyroidism and pseudohypoparathyroidism; ESRD = end stage renal disease; MM = multiple myeloma; SQ CELL CA = squamous cell carcinoma of head, neck, or lungs.

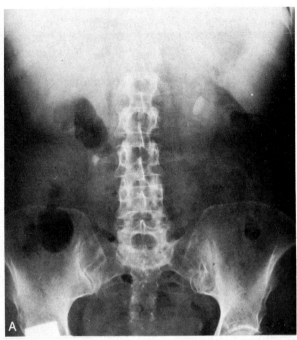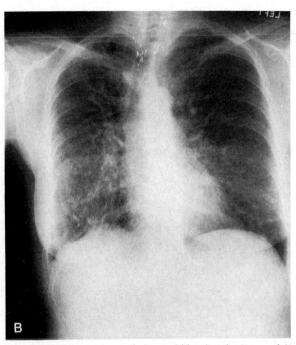

Figure 63–10. (*A*) A 51-year-old patient had passed several kidney stones in the presence of elevated blood and urinary calcium levels. The abdominal flat plate confirmed the presence of multiple kidney stones bilaterally. Serum iPTH was inappropriately elevated for the degree of hypercalcemia. Serum calcium failed to suppress after a week of prednisone treatment. The diagnosis of primary hyperparathyroidism was made. At surgery, two hyperplastic parathyroid glands were removed from the superior position, but the inferior parathyroids could not be found because of a cluster of lymph nodes extending into the mediastinum. These lymph nodes were later found to contain noncaseating granulomas.

(*B*) Hypercalcemia, hypercalciuria, and kidney stone formation persisted after parathyroidectomy. Chest radiogram revealed extensive bilateral fibronodular disease consistent with the patient's complaints of dyspnea and cough. Serum iPTH was now suppressed, and in response to prednisone challenge there were significant decreases in serum and urine calcium concentration, 1,25-(OH)₂ vitamin D level, and intestinal calcium absorption. The continued stone formation was attributed to sarcoidosis, and the patient has responded very well to dietary calcium restriction.

Ca usually does not rise to higher than 10.5 to 11.0 mg/dl.[75] Ionized Ca generally is normal,[50] and parathyroid function normal or suppressed.[75] Increased total Ca is typically self-limited, may occur at various times of therapy, and subsides within 2 weeks of thiazide withdrawal. Therefore, PHPT should be suspected if there is increased ionized Ca, increased serum PTH or urinary cyclic AMP, or persistence of hypercalcemia 2 weeks after thiazide therapy has been discontinued.

PREOPERATIVE LOCALIZATION STUDIES

From the standpoint of the parathyroid surgeon, a procedure that could identify the parathyroid glands preoperatively and indicate which glands were diseased would be valuable. A variety of noninvasive and invasive techniques have been introduced in an attempt to provide this information.[22, 26, 27]

Noninvasive Techniques

Noninvasive techniques for localization of abnormal parathyroid tissue have included (1) neck massage with measurement of serum PTH, (2) [⁷⁵Se] selenomethionine scanning, (3) cervical esophagography, (4) computed tomography (CT), and (5) ultrasonography.

Neck Massage and Hormone Measurement. It was initially reported that both adenomatous and hyper-

plastic parathyroid tissue could be localized by measuring increases in peripheral circulating levels of the hormone following neck massage.[62] This observation has not been confirmed.[72]

Selenomethionine. Ten to 15 years ago, there was a flurry of interest in the use of an amino acid analogue, selenomethionine, which tended to be concentrated in the parathyroids.[60] This radionuclide scan was not always reliable, primarily because of difficulty in scanning the appropriate plane of the neck and because of some thyroid uptake.[22] Unfortunately, only large tumors could be identified with this technique and it has not been used in recent years with any great success.

Cervical Esophagography. In one report, cervical esophagograms led to the accurate preoperative localization of 19 of 20 consecutively studied parathyroid adenomas in patients with PHPT.[71] Others have found that the yield with cine-esophagographic examination was too low, with a 30 per cent accuracy at best.[27]

Computed Tomography. Computed tomography of the neck and mediastinum has been performed for parathyroid localization.[24, 70] The initial results in finding cervical adenomas have not been encouraging, but recent improvements in equipment may produce better results in the future. The CT scanner is successful in detecting mediastinal adenomas of 15 mm in diameter (the normal parathyroid being 5 mm in diameter).[27] It is better than ultrasound for detecting lesions behind the osseous sternum.

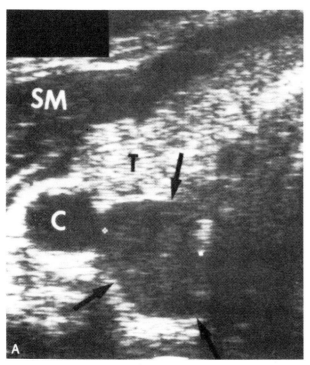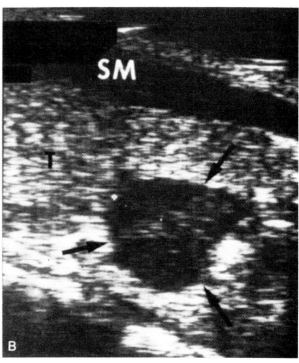

Figure 63–11. An example of high-resolution parathyroid sonography. Right transverse (*A*) and parasagittal (*B*) sonograms. Thyroid (T) and typical hypoechoic 1 cm parathyroid adenoma posteriorly (arrows). Carotid artery (*C*), anterior strap muscles (SM). (From Reading CC, Charboneau JW, James EM, et al: AJR *139*:539, 1982; copyright, The Williams & Wilkins Co.)

Ultrasonography. Considerable success has been achieved with the addition of high-resolution real-time (also called "small parts") ultrasonography to the localization armamentarium (Figs. 63–11 and 63–12).[27, 61, 77] This technique has proved sufficiently sensitive to detect 70 to 80 per cent of abnormal parathyroid glands in the neck, including glands down to 5 mm in diameter. Three distinct groups of patients may benefit from this procedure:

1. Those with a new diagnosis of PHPT who are undergoing primary cervical exploration. Sonography may be helpful to the surgeon by precisely localizing an enlarged parathyroid gland. However, since in the hands of an experienced parathyroid surgeon a cure rate of more than 90 per cent can be expected, high-resolution sonography probably will not identify any additional lesions that would not have been discovered operatively.[77]

2. Those undergoing a repeat cervical exploration. Reoperations are notoriously difficult, having both an increased complication rate and a decreased success rate. Therefore, precise preoperative sonographic localization should be most helpful. With sonography, 16 of 20 abnormal parathyroid glands in such patients were correctly identified for a sensitivity of 80 per cent.[61]

3. Those with severe hypercalcemia, a potential surgical emergency. If a parathyroid adenoma is present, it should be removed immediately. There are numerous other etiologies of hypercalcemia, among which are neoplasm, sarcoid, and drug-induced causes. A positive sonographic examination that identifies a parathyroid adenoma may simplify or shorten the work-up of these patients.

Because of the high accuracy, noninvasiveness, and relatively low cost (less than $130 per examination) of high-resolution sonography, it has become the procedure of choice for preoperative localization of enlarged parathyroid glands at the Mayo Clinic[61] and the Massachusetts General Hospital.[27] It remains to be determined whether the procedure will influence the surgical success rate.

Invasive Techniques

Invasive techniques for localizing parathyroid lesions include (1) angiography and (2) thyroid venous sampling.[6, 23] Performance of these techniques requires a great deal of angiographic skill and experience. They should not be attempted in institutions where they are not regularly performed.

Angiography. In patients to be catheterized prior to parathyroid re-exploration, cervical arteriography is initially performed in order to outline the distorted venous anatomy prior to attempted selective venous catheterization (Figs. 63–13 and 63–14).

Thyroid Vein Sampling. A two- to fourfold "step-up" in PTH concentrations over peripheral circulating levels is regarded as significant. The most common cause of failure in selective venous catheterization is the inability to obtain representative inferior thyroid vein samples for PTH determination. The inferior thyroid venous anatomy is anomalous in approximately 15 per cent of patients and is often markedly distorted in patients who have undergone previous neck exploration.

Accurate differential and localizing information is

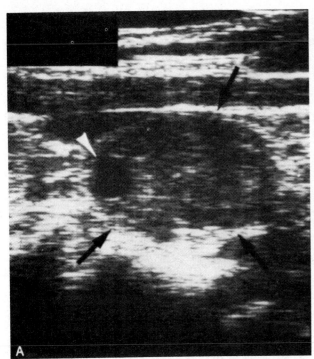
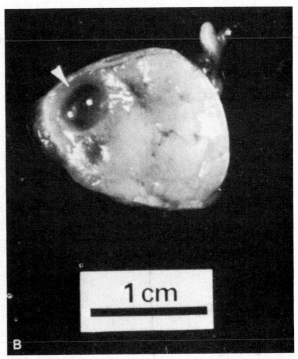

Figure 63–12. The sensitivity of high-resolution parathyroid sonography is well illustrated. Parasagittal sonogram (*A*) and pathologic specimen (*B*) of 1.5-cm parathyroid adenoma (arrows). Note the 3-mm internal cystic component in cranial pole (arrowhead). (From Reading CC, Charboneau JW, James EM, et al: AJR *139*:539, 1982; copyright, The Williams & Wilkins Co.)

obtained by experienced angiographers in approximately 80 to 90 per cent of patients who have not undergone prior neck exploration and in approximately 70 per cent of patients who have previously undergone exploration.[6, 23] At the NIH, this is the procedure of choice for patients with prior unsuccessful neck explo-

ration, patients in poor general medical condition with PHPT of sufficient severity to require surgery, and in patients with known malignant disease suspected of having coincident PHPT. However, several authorities have reported transient cortical blindness and more serious neurologic complications as a result of thyro-

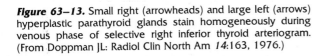
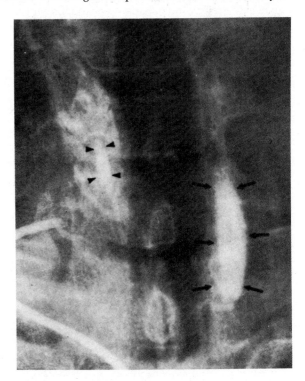

Figure 63–13. Small right (arrowheads) and large left (arrows) hyperplastic parathyroid glands stain homogeneously during venous phase of selective right inferior thyroid arteriogram. (From Doppman JL: Radiol Clin North Am *14*:163, 1976.)

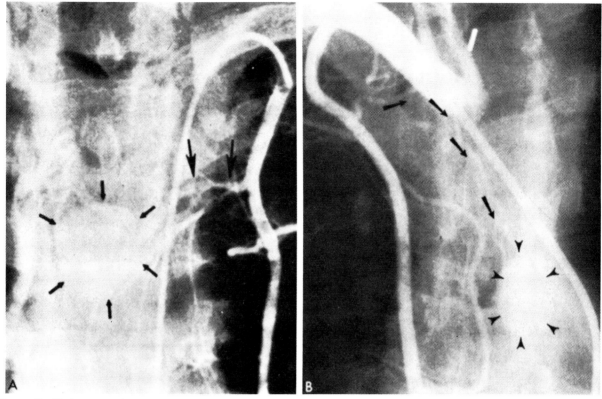

Figure 63–14. Arteriographic demonstration of mediastinal parathyroid adenomas supplied by thymic branch of left (*A*) and right (*B*) internal mammary artery. (From Doppman JL: Radiol Clin North Am *14*:163, 1976.)

cervical arteriographic examination.[25, 27, 77] Therefore, this procedure should not be performed routinely in patients with newly diagnosed PHPT. For some patients requiring re-explorations, noninvasive ultrasonography may obviate the need for angiography.

REFERENCES

1. Albright F: A page out of the history of hyperparathyroidism. J Clin Endocrinol Metab 8:637, 1948.
2. Axelrod L: Bones, stones and hormones: The contributions of Fuller Albright. N Engl J Med 283:964, 1970.
3. Barreras RF: Calcium and gastric secretion. Gastroenterology 64:1168, 1973.
4. Bell NH, Stern PH, Pantzer E, et al: Evidence that increased circulating 1,25−(OH)$_2$D is the probable cause for abnormal calcium metabolism in sarcoidosis. J Clin Invest 64:218, 1979.
5. Bijvoet OLM: Kidney function in calcium and phosphate metabolism. In Avioli LV, Krane SM (eds): Metabolic Bone Disease Vol I. New York, Academic Press, 1977, p. 49.
6. Bilezikian JP, Doppman JL, Shimkin PM, et al: Preoperative localization of abnormal parathyroid tissue: Cumulative experience with venous sampling and arteriography. Am J Med 55:505, 1973.
7. Bone HG III, Snyder WH III, Pak CYC: Diagnosis of hyperparathyroidism. Ann Rev Med 28:111, 1977.
8. Breslau NA, Zerwekh JE, Nicar MJ, Pak CYC: Effects of short-term glucocorticoid administration in primary hyperparathyroidism: Comparison to sarcoidosis. J Clin Endocrinol Metab 54:824, 1982.
9. Breslau NA, McGuire J, Zerwekh JE, et al: Hypercalcemia associated with increased serum 1,25-dihydroxyvitamin D in three patients with lymphoma. Ann Intern Med 100:1, 1984.
10. Broadus AE, Mahaffey JE, Bartter FC, Neer RM: Nephrogenous cyclic adenosine monophosphate as a parathyroid function test. J Clin Invest 60:771, 1977.
11. Broadus AE, Horst RL, Lang R, et al: The importance of circulating 1,25-dihydroxyvitamin D in the pathogenesis of hypercalciuria and renal stone formation in primary hyperparathyroidism. N Engl J Med 302:421, 1980.
12. Broadus AE: Mineral metabolism. In Felig P, Baxter JD, Broadus AE, Frohman LA) (eds): Endocrinology and Metabolism. New York, McGraw-Hill Book Company, 1981, p. 1019.
13. Broadus AE, Rasmussen H: Clinical evaluation of parathyroid function. Am J Med 70:495, 1981.
14. Broadus AE, Lang R, Kliger AS: The influence of calcium intake and the status of intestinal calcium absorption on the diagnostic utility of measurements of 24-hour cyclic adenosine 3', 5'-monophosphate excretion; J Clin Endocrinol Metab 52:1085, 1981.
15. Broadus AE: Primary hyperparathyroidism viewed as a bihormonal disease process. Miner Electrolyte Metab 8:199, 1982.
16. Christensson T: Hyperparathyroidism and radiation therapy. Ann Intern Med 89:216, 1978.
17. Coe FL: Nephrolithiasis: Pathogenesis and Treatment. Chicago, Year Book Medical Publishers, 1978, p. 46.
18. Coe FL, Favus MJ: Does mild, asymptomatic hyperparathyroidism require surgery? N Engl J Med 302:224, 1980.
19. Cope O: The story of hyperparathyroidism at the Massachusetts General Hospital. N Engl J Med 274:1174, 1966.
20. Cope O: Hyperparathyroidism—too little, too much surgery? N Engl J Med 295:100, 1976.
21. Davies DR, Dent CE, Willcox A: Hyperparathyroidism and steatorrhea. Br Med J: 2:1133, 1956.
22. Dobben GD, Valvassori GE: Radiologic diagnosis of hyperparathyroidism. Otolaryngol Clin North Am 13:147, 1980.
23. Doppman JL: Parathyroid localization: Arteriography and venous sampling. Radiol Clin North Am 14:163, 1976.
24. Doppman JL, et al: Computed tomography for parathyroid localization. J Comp Assist Tomogr 1:30, 1977.
25. Edis AJ, Sheedy PF II, Beahrs OH, Van Heerden JA: Results of reoperation for hyperparathyroidism, with evaluation of preoperative localization studies. Surgery 84:384, 1978.
26. Egdahl RH: Preoperative parathyroid localization. N Engl J Med 301:548, 1979.
27. Egdahl RH, Wang C-A: Case records of the Massachusetts General Hospital. N Engl J Med 304:1284, 1981.
28. Endres D, Brickman A, Goodman W, et al: N- and C-terminal PTH

radioimmunoassays in assessment of renal osteodystrophy. Kidney Int 21:132, 1982.

29. Genant HK, Heck LL, Lanzl LH, et al: Primary hyperparathyroidism: A comprehensive study of clinical, biochemical, and radiological manifestations. Radiology 109:513, 1973.

30. Gogas J, Kalos A, Skalkeas G: Functioning metastatic parathyroid carcinoma. Am Surg 41:419, 1975.

31. Goldsmith RE, Sizemore GW, Chen IW, et al: Familial hyperparathyroidism. Ann Intern Med 84:36, 1976.

32. Goltzman D, Henderson B, Loveridge N: Cytochemical bioassay of parathyroid hormone. J Clin Invest 65:1309, 1980.

33. Habener JF, Potts JT: Parathyroid physiology and primary hyperparathyroidism. In Aviolo LV, Krane SM (eds): Metabolic Bone Disease, Vol. II New York, Academic Press, 1978, p. 1.

34. Habener JF, Segre GV: Parathyroid hormone radioimmunoassay. Ann Intern Med 91:782, 1979.

35. Heath H, III, Hodgson SF, Kennedy MA: Primary hyperparathyroidism: Incidence, morbidity and potential economic impact in a community. N Engl J Med 302:189, 1980.

36. Hodgson SF, Heath H III: Asymptomatic primary hyperparathyroidism: Treat or follow? Mayo Clin Proc 56:521, 1981.

37. Jarman WT, Myers RT, Marshall RB: Carcinoma of the parathyroid. Arch Surg 113:123, 1978.

38. Kaplan RA, Snyder WH, Stewart A, Pak CYC: Metabolic effects of parathyroidectomy in asymptomatic primary hyperparathyroidism. J Clin Endocrinol Metab 42:415, 1976.

39. Keiser HR, Beaven MA, Doppman J, et al: Sipple's syndrome: Medullary thyroid carcinoma, pheochromocytoma, and parathyroid disease. Ann Intern Med 78:561, 1973.

40. Khairi MR, Dexter RN, Burzynski NJ, Johnston CC: Mucosal neuroma, pheochromocytoma and medullary thyroid carcinoma: Multiple endocrine neoplasia type 3. Medicine 54:89, 1975.

41. Leppla DC, Northcutt C, Snyder W, Pak CYC: Sequential changes in bone density before and after parathyroidectomy in primary hyperparathyroidism. Invest Radiol 17:604, 1982.

42. Lloyd HM: Primary hyperparathyroidism: An analysis of the role of the parathyroid tumor. Medicine 47:53, 1968.

43. Mallette LE, Bilezikian JP, Heath DA, Aurbach GD: Primary hyperparathyroidism: Clinical and biochemical features. Medicine 53:127, 1974.

44. Mallette LE, Patten BM, Engel WK: Neuromuscular disease in secondary hyperparathyroidism. Ann Intern Med 82:474, 1975.

45. Martin KJ, Hruska KA, Freitag JJ, et al: The peripheral metabolism of parathyroid hormone. N Engl J Med 301:1092, 1979.

46. Marx SJ, Spiegel AM, Levine MA, et al: Familial hypocalciuric hypercalcemia: The relation to primary parathyroid hyperplasia. N Engl J Med 307:416, 1982.

47. Maschio G, Vecchioni R, Tessitore N: Recurrence of autonomous hyperparathyroidism in calcium nephrolithiasis. Am J Med 69:607, 1980.

48. McGeown MG: Effect of parathyroidectomy on the incidence of renal calculi. Lancet 1:586, 1961.

49. Mixter CG, Keynes WM, Chir M, Cope O: Further experience with pancreatitis as a diagnostic clue to hyperparathyroidism. N Engl J Med 266:265, 1962.

50. Mohamadi M, Bivins L, Becker K: Effect of thiazides on serum calcium. Clin Pharmacol Ther 26:390, 1979.

51. Mundy GR, Cove DH, Fisken R: Primary hyperparathyroidism: Changes in the pattern of clinical presentation. Lancet 1:1317, 1980.

52. Pak CYC, Stewart A, Kaplan R, et al: Photon absorptiometric analysis of bone density in primary hyperparathyroidism. Lancet 2:7, 1975.

53. Pak CYC, Townsend J: Chloride/phosphate ratio in primary hyperparathyroidism. Ann Intern Med 85:830, 1976.

54. Pak CYC: Use of cyclic nucleotides in detection of disturbed parathyroid function: Advances in Cyclic Nucleotide Research, Vol 12. In Hamet P, Sands H (eds): New York, Raven Press, 1980, p. 393.

55. Pak CYC, Nicar MJ, Peterson R, et al: A lack of unique pathophysiologic background for nephrolithiasis of primary hyperparathyroidism. J Clin Endocrinol Metab 53:536, 1981.

56. Palmer FJ, Nelson JC, Bacchus H: The chloride-phosphate ratio in hypercalcemia. Ann Intern Med 80:200, 1974.

57. Paloyan E, Lawrence AM: Primary vs. secondary hyperparathyroidism: Time for reappraisal. Arch Intern Med 140:171, 1980.

58. Patten BM, Bilezikian JP, Mallette LE, et al: Neuromuscular disease in primary hyperparathyroidism. Ann Intern Med 80:182, 1974.

59. Peacock M: Renal stone disease and bone disease in primary hyperparathyroidism and their relationship to the action of parathyroid hormone on calcium absorption. In Talmage RV, Owen M, Parsons JA (eds): Calcium Regulating Hormones: Proceedings of 5th Parathyroid Conference. Amsterdam, Excerpta Medica, 1975, p. 78.

60. Potchen EJ, Watts HG, Awwad HK: Parathyroid scintiscanning. Radiol Clin North Am 5:267, 1967.

61. Reading CC, Charboneau JW, James EM, et al: High resolution parathyroid sonography. AJR 139:539, 1982.

62. Reiss E, Canterbury JM: Primary hyperparathyroidism: Application of radioimmunoassay to differentiation of adenoma and hyperplasia and to preoperative localization of hyperfunctioning parathyroid glands. N Engl J Med 280:1381, 1969.

63. Reiss E, Canterbury JM: Genesis of hyperparathyroidism. Am J Med 50:679, 1971.

64. Russell CF, Grant CS; van Heerden JA: Hyperfunctioning supernumerary parathyroid glands: An occasional cause of hyperparathyroidism. Mayo Clin Proc 57:121, 1982.

65. Schantz A, Castleman B: Parathyroid carcinoma: A study of 70 cases. Cancer 31:600, 1973.

66. Scholz DA: Hypertension and hyperparathyroidism. Arch Intern Med 137:1123, 1977.

67. Scholz DA, Purnell DC: Asymptomatic primary hyperparathyroidism: 10-year prospective study. Mayo Clin Proc 56:473, 1981.

68. Seeman E, Wahner HW, Offord KP, et al: Differential effects of endocrine dysfunction on the axial and the appendicular skeleton. J Clin Invest 69:1302, 1982.

69. Segre GV, Harris ST, Tully G, Neer R: Amino-terminal radioimmunoassay for human parathyroid hormone. Program of 63rd Annual Meeting of the Endocrine Society, Cincinnati, June 1981, p. 228 (abstract 584).

70. Shimshak RR, Shoenrock GJ, Taekman HP, et al: Pre-operative localization of a parathyroid adenoma using computed tomography and thyroid scanning: Case report. J Comp Assist Tomogr 3:117, 1979.

71. Sofianides T, Yu-Shang C, Leary JS, et al: Localization of parathyroid adenomas by cervical esophogram. J Clin Endocrinol Metab 46:587, 1978.

72. Spiegel AM, Doppman JL, Marx SJ, et al: Preoperative localization of abnormal parathyroid: Neck massage versus arteriography and selective venous sampling. Ann Intern Med 89:935, 1978.

73. Spiegel AM, Eastman ST, Altie MF, et al: Intraoperative measurements of urinary cyclic AMP to guide surgery for primary hyperparathyroidism. N Engl J Med 303:1457, 1980.

74. Stewart AF, Horst RL, Deftos LJ, et al: Biochemical evaluation of patients with malignancy-associated hypercalcemia: evidence for humoral and non-humoral groups. N Engl J Med 303:1377, 1980.

75. Stote RM, Smith LH, Wilson DM, et al: Hydrochlorothiazide effects on serum calcium and immunoreactive PTH concentrations. Ann Intern Med 77:587, 1972.

76. Tisell LE, Carlsson S, Lindberg S, Ragnhult I: Autonomous hyperparathyroidism: A possible late complication of neck radiotherapy. Acta Chir Scand 142:367, 1976.

77. Van Heerden JA, Meredith JE, Karsell PR, et al: Small-part ultrasonography in primary hyperparathyroidism: Initial experience. Ann Surg 195:774, 1982.

78. Walton RJ, Bijvoet OLM: Nomogram for derivation of renal threshold phosphate concentration. Lancet 2:309, 1975.

79. Wermer P: Genetic aspects of adenomatosis of endocrine glands. Am J Med 16:363, 1954.

CHAPTER 64

Pathology of Parathyroid Tumors

Ronald H. Nishiyama, M.D.

Tumors of the parathyroid glands are difficult to recognize morphologically, and controversy prevails in the histologic diagnosis of adenomas, the most common cause of primary hyperparathyroidism. Carcinomas of the parathyroid glands are also difficult to define histologically. The difficulty in differentiating parathyroid neoplasia from hyperplasia necessitates a description of many of the clinical syndromes characterized by hyperparathyroidism and neoplastic or non-neoplastic enlargement (tumors) of the parathyroid glands.

THE NORMAL PARATHYROID GLAND

The normal weight, size, and fat content of a parathyroid gland remain uncertain. The weight of a normal gland has been recorded to be as low as 40 mg, and a limit of 50 to 60 mg has been suggested.[3]

A recent study demonstrated that the weights of normal parathyroid glands have a skewed distribution. The mean total weight in the study was 29.5 ± 17.8 mg, with an upper limit of 65 mg. However, the actual value for the 97.5 percentile was 75 mg, and this correlates with the operative findings in primary hyperparathyroidism.[3]

Chronic illnesses, race, and individual variations affect the weights of the glands. Patients with chronic illnesses have lower total weights, and males and black patients have higher total weights. Glands removed from the same patients may show wide variations in weights. One gland is often much smaller, and at times, both glands are small.

Almost no studies of normal parathyroid glands include the dimensions of the glands. Normal dimensions of 3 to 6 mm in length, 2 to 4 mm in width, and 0.5 to 2 mm in thickness have been proposed, as well as an average of three dimensions of $5 \times 3 \times 1$ mm. Normal glands as large as 12 mm and larger have been reported.[11, 62]

Glandular weight is accepted as a better measure of size than glandular dimensions. For the surgeon, knowledge of normal dimensions of parathyroid glands would be extremely useful. For practical purposes, enlargement of parathyroid glands is determined in the operating room by size rather than by weight, for the determination of weight or density necessitates removal of glands, and this may not be indicated.

The stromal fat content of parathyroid glands is the hallmark in the evaluation of the functional status of the glands. Detailed studies of normal glands have demonstrated wide variations in fat content.[16, 19] The accepted percentage of normal fat content is 50 per cent. A recent study indicates that greater than 75 per cent of normal parathyroid glands have less than 30 per cent stromal fat; 50 per cent have less than 10 per cent; and only a small number have 40 per cent. Another study recorded an average fat content of 17 per cent. Only one patient had more than 50 per cent fat, and 16 per cent of patients had more than 30 per cent. Nearly one third of the patients had less than 10 per cent fat. With these data, measurement of stromal fat content has become nearly useless as an indicator of function.[16, 19]

Parathyroid glands in children and adolescents contain little fat. After adolescence, stromal fat progressively increases until 25 to 30 years of age. After that, fat content is largely determined by constitutional factors. Women have a tendency to have higher parathyroid fat content. Stromal fat is also related to total body fat.[27]

The cellular content of the normal gland is dominated by chief cells. Water-clear cells are rare. Oxyphilic and transitional oxyphilic cells are rare in the young and tend to increase with age. Oxyphils are more common in adults over 40 years of age. Nodules of oxyphils are more commonly seen in patients with parathyroid hyperplasia secondary to renal failure.

PRIMARY HYPERPARATHYROIDISM: SINGLE AND MULTIPLE GLANDULAR ENLARGEMENT

A reflection of the lack of precision in the histologic differentiation of parathyroid adenomas from primary parathyroid hyperplasia is the greater prevalence of the description of the pathologic features of primary hyperparathyroidism in terms of single or multiple enlargement of parathyroid glands or to "single gland" or "multiple gland" disease.[20, 48, 54, 66] None of the morphologic criteria that distinguish adenoma from hyperplasia have survived the test of time or use in the pathologic evaluation of a large number of cases.

A parathyroid "adenoma" is characterized by enlargement of one parathyroid gland with a recognizable rim of normal tissue and usually a monomorphic proliferation of chief cells. Fifty to 70 per cent of "adenomas" have been reported to possess a rim of normal tissue when adequate samples of tissue are examined[27] (Figs. 64–1 to 64–3). This rim is often absent in permanent histologic sections and in samples of tissue taken for

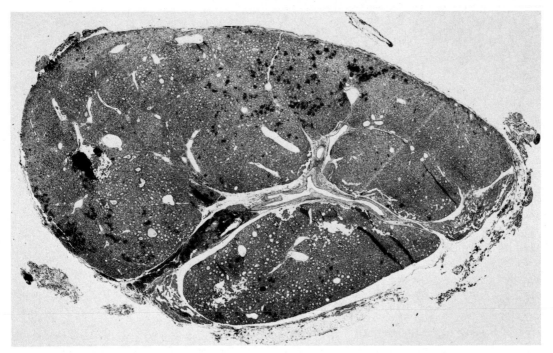

Figure 64–1. Adenoma with a small rim of normal tissue at the lower margin. (H&E, ×25)

Figure 64–2. Adenoma with a rim of normal parathyroid tissue. (H&E, ×160)

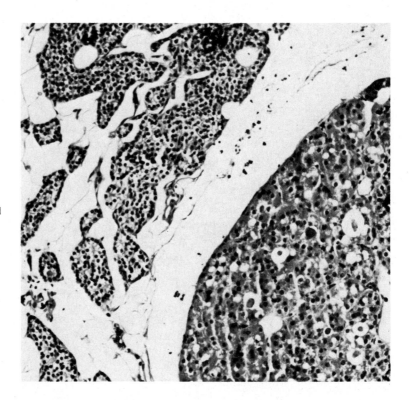

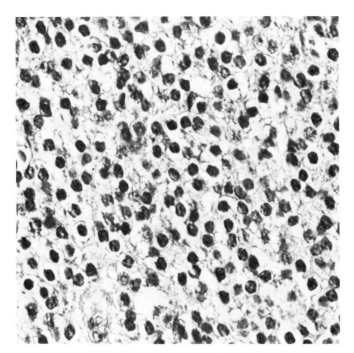

Figure 64–3. Monomorphic chief cells in an adenoma. (H&E, ×400)

frozen sections. In addition, the concept of nodular hyperplasia of parathyroid glands, in which hyperplastic nodules may expand to form a "normal rim," has nearly negated the use of the "normal rim" in the diagnosis of parathyroid adenoma.[4, 5, 33]

The cellular composition of an enlarged parathyroid gland cannot be used to distinguish an adenoma from a hyperplastic gland. In both, the glands contain a mixture of cells; however, cellular pleomorphism is seen more often in adenomas (Fig. 64–4). Pleomorphic cells are more common in adenomas than in hyperplastic or carcinomatous glands, but mitotic figures are rare in adenomas and more easily found in carcinomas.[36]

A distinctive "adenoma" is the oxyphilic form. Most oxyphilic "adenomas" are nonfunctional and are incidental findings at autopsy. Functional oxyphilic "adenomas" have been reported, although most are composed of a mixture of cells. Oxyphilic cells can produce parathormone, and "adenomas," composed predominantly of oxyphilic cells, can cause clinical hyperparathyroidism.[3, 45, 47]

Approximately 80 per cent of the clinical cases of

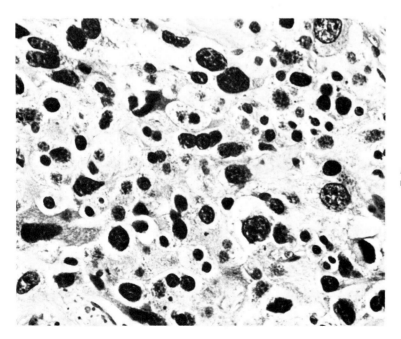

Figure 64–4. Nuclear pleomorphism in an adenoma. (H&E, ×400)

primary hyperparathyroidism are associated with enlargement of a single parathyroid gland. In spite of the difficulty of defining an adenoma, removal of the enlarged gland usually results in cures and a very low incidence of recurrent or persistent hyperparathyroidism. In most cases, a normal-sized gland is removed, or biopsies are taken of the normal-sized glands to confirm the presence of normal parathyroid tissue to aid in establishing the histologic diagnosis of an adenoma.[20, 22, 48]

The absence of fat is useful in the recognition of abnormal parathyroid tissue, provided that the sample is sufficient. However, the problem arises in the histologic evaluation of the normal parathyroid glands and the small biopsies that are taken of normal-sized or slightly enlarged glands.[20, 66] Many appear hypercellular because of the uneven distribution of stromal fat and because pathologists may not be familiar with the normal content of stromal fat. Also, stromal fat is distorted when frozen, and frozen sections may appear misleadingly hypercellular.

The surgeon, then, is responsible for the recognition of abnormal parathyroid tissue by evaluating the sizes of the glands at the time of operation. However, even this procedure is not foolproof.

Problems are more common in primary hyperparathyroidism that is caused by multiple enlargement or primary hyperplasia of parathyroid glands. The incidence varies from 3 to 65 per cent. The rate most commonly reported ranges between 15 and 20 per cent.[54]

The usual case is characterized by obvious enlargement of four glands. The most common histologic finding is chief cell hyperplasia, with a predominance of chief cells, although a mixture of cell types is more characteristic. However, hyperplastic glands cannot be differentiated from adenomas by their cellular composition, although nodularity in a cellular gland is more characteristic of a hyperplastic parathyroid gland[36] (Fig. 64–5). Clear cell hyperplasia is distinctive, but for some unknown reason has become rare.[11, 15]

The treatment of primary hyperparathyroidism was complicated when microscopic hyperplasia was described in the normal-sized glands or in slightly enlarged glands in cases of "single gland" disease.[7, 28, 55, 66] Routine or prophylactic subtotal parathyroidectomy in the treatment of all cases of primary hyperparathyroidism was then recommended to reduce the incidence of recurrent or persistent hyperparathyroidism. Asymmetric enlargement of parathyroid glands is common, and microscopic hyperplasia in parathyroid glands can be present without clinical disease.[7, 8, 30]

The most important factor in the discrepancy between the incidences of hyperplasia and adenoma in primary hyperparathyroidism is the difficulty in distinguishing minimally enlarged normal glands from hyperplastic glands. Data support the concept that mild enlargement (40 to 70 mg) and histologic hyperplasia in a normal-sized parathyroid gland do not correlate with hyperfunction. In one study, 50 per cent of parathyroid glands, weighing between 40 and 70 gm and considered

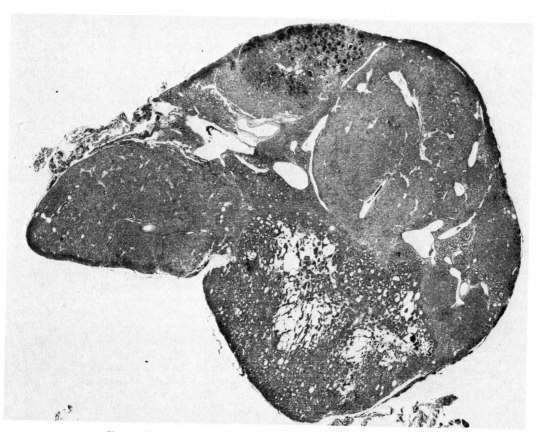

Figure 64–5. Primary hyperplasia with slight nodularity. (H&E, ×25)

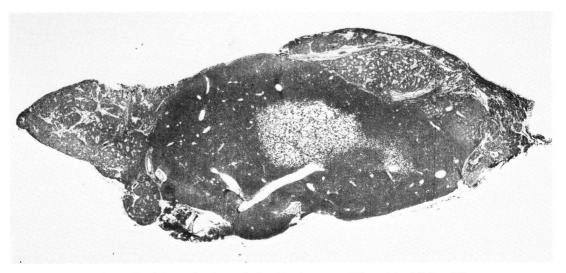

Figure 64–6. Secondary hyperplasia with a large oxyphilic nodule. (H&E, ×25)

abnormal, were considered to be histologically hyperplastic. When these glands were defined to be normal for weight, the frequency of histologic hyperplasia dropped to 22 per cent.[21]

The frequency of "multiple gland" disease was overestimated by about 30 per cent by including normal-sized or minimally enlarged glands (less than 70 mg) that were histologically hypercellular. Caution is, therefore, advised in removing parathyroid glands that are minimally enlarged (70 mg), except in familial hyperparathyroidism and multiple endocrinopathic syndromes and unless no single gland is obviously enlarged or abnormal.[21]

The following criteria have been adopted to identify multiple adenomas:

1. The finding of more than one enlarged parathyroid gland that is histologically hyperplastic.

2. Operative confirmation that the remaining parathyroid glands are normal in size, consistency, and color and that at least one or more are histologically normal.

3. Neither clinical evidence nor family history of multiple endocrine neoplasia (MEN) syndromes or familial hyperparathyroidism.

4. Permanent cure of hypercalcemia by excision of the enlarged parathyroid glands.[29, 61]

On the basis of these criteria, 43 cases of multiple adenomas were found among 2262 cases of primary hyperparathyroidism (1.9 per cent). In a contrasting study, 13 patients with double adenomas found at the Massachusetts General Hospital through 1958, six eventually proved to have primary hyperplasia, and the diagnosis was not firmly established in the remaining seven patients.[63]

Lipid stains for intracellular fat in parenchymal cells have been used in an attempt to refine the histologic assessment of normal, hyperplastic, and adenomatous parathyroid tissue. The intracellular content of lipid is less in abnormal parathyroid tissue, and the lipid stains supposedly allow rapid and easy differentiation of hyperplastic and adenomatous parathyroid tissue from normal tissue on frozen sections. However, contradictory and nonuniform results have been reported, and longer and more extensive use of the method is probably required to establish its effectiveness in the evaluation of the functional status of parathyroid tissue.[17, 18, 35, 38, 49, 58]

SECONDARY PARATHYROID HYPERPLASIA

The most common cause of secondary parathyroid hyperplasia is chronic renal failure (Fig. 64–6). Chronic hypocalcemia and hyperphosphatemia result in prolonged stimulation and enlargement of the parathyroid glands with concomitant hypercalcemia and increased serum levels of parathormone. The usual indications for parathyroidectomy are severe bone disease, bone pain, metastatic calcification and intractable pruritus.[11]

Asymmetric enlargement of the parathyroid glands, as in primary hyperplasia, is common. However, in contrast to primary hyperplasia, the enlargement is more obvious. In one group of patients, the smallest gland weighed 250 mg.[6]

Comparative studies of parathyroid glands in primary and secondary hyperplasia have demonstrated that there are no microscopic changes that differentiate the two conditions. Fibrosis and nodularity, however, appear to be more prominent in enlarged parathyroid glands removed from patients with prolonged renal failure. No well-documented case of a parathyroid adenoma in secondary hyperparathyroidism has been reported.[6]

"Tertiary hyperparathyroidism" is a concept that implies that one or more secondarily hyperplastic parathyroid glands become autonomous in their function. Parathyroid autonomy is clinically documented by determination of suppressibility of parathyroid function before and after calcium loading. Parathyroid function in many patients with chronic renal failure is suppressible, but a few have nonsuppressible or "tertiary hyperparathyroidism." In addition, persistent hypercalcemia after renal transplantation, as long as 7 years, had added impetus to this concept.[6, 32]

However, tertiary hyperparathyroidism as a clinical and pathologic entity is suspect. Except in rare instances, the hypercalcemia subsides, and in patients treated by subtotal parathyroidectomy for nonsuppressible secondary hyperparathyroidism, parathyroid function becomes suppressed. These phenomena have been related to the total mass of parathyroid tissue. In renal transplantation, parathyroid tissue, far in excess of the patient's needs, persists, and in the other, the mass has been considerably reduced.[6] No distinctive morphologic changes in the parathyroid glands have been described for tertiary hyperparathyroidism.

ABERRANT, ECTOPIC, AND SUPERNUMERARY PARATHYROID TUMORS

A study of the surgical anatomy of primary hyperparathyroidism has demonstrated that many adenomas are found in abnormal locations.[57] It is well known that large parathyroid tumors can migrate to an abnormal location in the neck. Aberrant parathyroid tumors are those that have been displaced in the neck from their normal anatomic sites to abnormal positions. Ectopic parathyroid tumors are those that are found in an unexpected anatomic location because of abnormal embryologic development.

An analysis of 216 patients with single adenomas showed that 39 per cent of adenomas of the right superior gland and 36 per cent of left superior adenomas were in abnormal anatomic locations. The adenomas were large, with mean weights of 4.6 gm and 5.1 gm,

respectively. The superior adenomas had been displaced to retropharyngeal, retroesophageal, paraesophageal, tracheoesophageal, and superior posterior mediastinal locations. Only one, located lateral to the carotid sheath and in the scalene fat pad, was considered to have developed in an ectopic gland.

Adenomas of the inferior parathyroid glands were also found in abnormal locations, although not as frequently as the superior ones. Twelve per cent of right inferior adenomas and 16 per cent of left inferior adenomas were within the thymus and carotid sheath. Only five adenomas (2 per cent) were intrathyroidal in location (Fig. 64–7). All were within the inferior poles of thyroid glands and were considered to have developed in ectopic inferior parathyroid glands.

The most common cause of recurrent or persistent hyperparathyroidism is an adenoma in an abnormal anatomic location.[9, 12, 46, 63] The surgeon must be cognizant of the high probability of displacement of parathyroid tumors from their normal anatomic locations to aberrant sites in order to reduce the need for re-explorations of the neck for recurrent or persistent adenomas.

Mediastinal parathyroid tumors are either parathyroid adenomas or hyperplastic parathyroid glands that have migrated into the mediastinum or that develop in ectopic glands. The migrating tumors usually involve the superior glands, retain a vascular pedicle from the neck, and are usually accessible from the neck. The ectopic tumors occur in glands that develop in the chest, usually within the thymus or in relation to the great vessels,

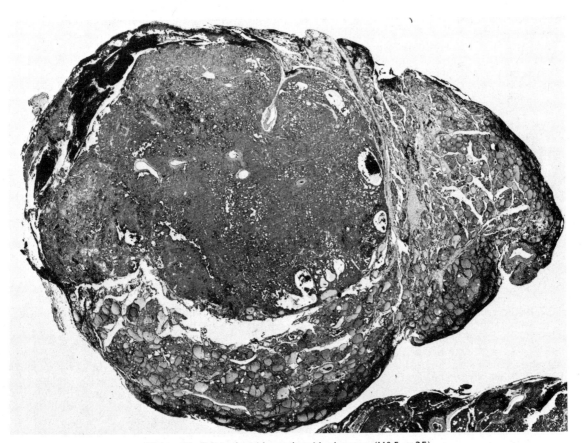

Figure 64–7. Intrathyroid parathyroid adenoma. (H&E, ×25)

and arise in inferior parathyroid glands that have descended into the chest during embryologic development or in supernumerary glands. These adenomas usually require mediastinotomies for removal.

An analysis of mediastinal parathyroid tumors showed an incidence of 1.4 per cent in 2770 patients with primary hyperparathyroidism.[50] Seventy per cent were within the thymus, and all except one were considered to have developed in an ectopic inferior or a supernumerary gland. One paraesophageal tumor in the posterior mediastinum was thought to be a migrating superior gland tumor. Twenty-one per cent of the tumors developed in supernumerary (fifth) glands. Other studies have confirmed the rare requirement of a mediastinotomy for removal of mediastinal parathyroid tumors. The vast majority can be removed through a cervical incision.[43, 53]

A preponderance of humans (80 to 97 per cent) have four parathyroid glands. The prevalence of supernumerary parathyroid gland varies from 2.5 to 13 per cent. Grimelius and associates report a prevalence of 13 per cent, and in their study, 5 per cent were "true" supernumerary glands, and 8 per cent were divided or rudimentary glands. Divided glands are defined as groups of glands in the same site, and rudimentary glands are very small glands located close to normal parathyroid glands.[27]

The usual location of a fifth gland is below the thyroid gland near the thymus or the thyrothymic ligament. Bilobated or multilobated parathyroid glands are more often associated with supernumery glands and when found should alert the surgeon to the possible presence of a supernumerary gland.[27]

In two large studies, 21 of 2777 patients (0.75 per cent) with primary hyperparathyroidism had functioning supernumerary parathyroid tumors.[51, 64] Fourteen patients had tumors in the anterior mediastinum, and of these, 11 were in the thymus. Two were within a thymic remnant in the neck; three were in relation to the aorta and great vessels; two were within the thyroid gland; two were in the area of the carotid sheath; and one was in the right middle neck. Nearly all these patients had one enlarged parathyroid gland, which was the supernumerary one, and all had at least four normal parathyroid glands, proven by biopsies, within the neck.

CARCINOMA OF THE PARATHYROID GLAND

Carcinomas of the parathyroid gland are rare. An accurate assessment of their prevalence is impossible because of the difficulty in establishing the histologic diagnosis.

Clinical manifestations of parathyroid carcinomas are helpful in establishing the diagnosis. They are more common in males, and benign causes of primary hyperparathyroidism are more common in females. A palpable mass in the neck associated with hypercalcemia is highly suggestive. Serum levels of calcium tend to be higher in patients with carcinomas.[2, 31, 59]

The observations of the surgeon are vital. Most carcinomas are grossly distinctive. They are hard and are surrounded by dense fibrous connective tissue, resulting in a white mass, often adherent to or invading adjacent structures. This inflammation-like reaction is considered by experienced surgeons to be virtually diagnostic.

The principle histologic features that have been proposed to distinguish parathyroid carcinomas from adenomas are a trabecular pattern, mitotic figures, thick fibrous bands, and capsular and blood vascular invasion[52] (Figs. 64-8 and 64-9). Only a few of the changes are seen in most cases, and with the exception of the finding of mitotic figures, the other changes, by themselves, are not helpful. A retrospective application of the proposed criteria concluded that the histologic appearance, coupled with certain clinical observations, can aid in establishing a diagnosis of parathyroid carcinoma but, short of actual metastasis, is rarely successful in establishing the diagnosis with certainty.[34]

Death is caused by persistent hypercalcemia and its sequelae. The best hope for cure is complete removal of the neoplasm at the time of the first operation. Operations for recurrent carcinomas or metastases are never curative, although repeated operations have aided in the control of hypercalcemia.[25]

The prognosis for parathyroid carcinomas is poor. In the two largest reported groups of patients, the cumulative 5- and 10-year survival rates were 50 and 13 per cent, respectively. In another, only 29 per cent were alive and without disease after 5 years.[52]

LIPOADENOMA

A rare cause of hyperparathyroidism is a distinctive tumor composed of parenchymal cells separated by large amounts of adipose tissue and, rarely, by a myxoid and fibrillar stroma (Fig. 64-10). These tumors are usually solitary and large and may be functional or nonfunctional. The majority of the tumors recorded in the literature have been functional.[1, 26, 37, 44, 65] Several terms have been used to describe this lesion: "lipoadenoma," "hamartoma," and "parathyroid adenomas with unusual stroma." Lipoadenoma is probably the most acceptable designation.

The presence of fat may cause some difficulty in interpretation. Confusion with a normal parathyroid gland is possible, but the size of the lesion makes the diagnosis obvious.

PARATHYROID CYSTS

Parathyroid cysts of clinical significance usually present as palpable asymptomatic masses in the neck. A preoperative diagnosis is rarely made unless the cyst is functional.

Confusion with a thyroid nodule is common. Aspiration of a cyst and examination of the fluid may be helpful. An aspirate composed of clear and colorless fluid is suggestive, and the finding of high levels of parathyroid hormone and low levels of thyroid hormone in the fluid supports the diagnosis.

The cysts are usually solitary and unilocular and are often located low in the neck, often near the inferior portion of the thyroid gland. The wall is thin, smooth, and semitransparent and may be loosely attached to the thyroid gland or at times may be within it. The lining

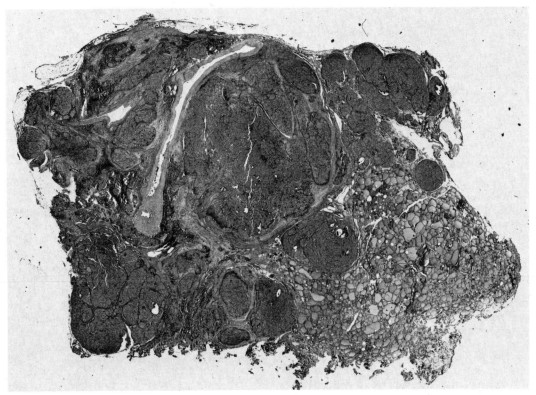

Figure 64–8. Parathyroid carcinoma invading thyroid gland. (H&E, ×25)

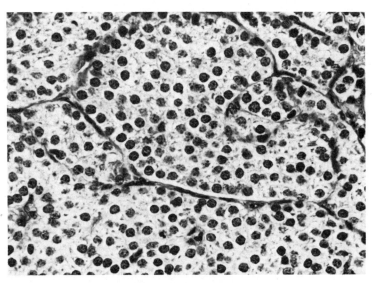

Figure 64–9. Parathyroid carcinoma with large chief cells but no nuclear pleomorphism or mitotic figures. (H&E, ×400)

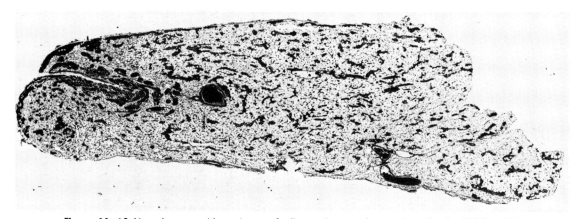

Figure 64–10. Lipoadenoma with a mixture of adipose tissue and parenchymal cells. (H&E, ×25)

of the cyst is cuboidal or low columnar in type, and the cells stain positively for glycogen. The presence of parathyroid cells within the wall is diagnostic[13] (Fig. 64–11).

The prevailing theories for the pathogenesis of these cysts are enlargement or coalescence of microcysts common in normal parathyroid glands, retention of parathormone, persistence of embryologic remnants (Kursteiner's canals), and cystic degeneration of an adenoma.[13] A few cysts are functional, and under these circumstances, cystic degeneration of an adenoma or cystic parathyroid hyperplasia must be considered. Microcysts in an adenoma and in hyperplastic glands are not unusual; however, macrocysts are rare. Macrocystic changes resulting in cystic adenomas and in cystic hyperplastic glands have been reported. The involvement of hyperplastic glands have varied from one to all four glands.[14, 23] This emphasizes the importance of identifying all the parathyroid glands before concluding that a "true" parathyroid cyst is the cause of clinical hyperparathyroidism.

FAMILIAL HYPERPARATHYROIDISM

Familial hyperparathyroidism is most commonly seen in the familial multiple endocrine neoplasia (MEN) syndromes.[60] Multiple endocrine neoplasia, type I (MEN-I), predominantly involves the parathyroid glands (hyperplasia), pancreatic islets (islet cell tumors), and the anterior pituitary glands (hyperplasia, adenomas). Ninety-seven per cent of patients have primary hyperparathyroidism. The Zollinger-Ellison syndrome is one phenotypic expression of MEN-I.[42]

The pathologic changes described in parathyroid glands removed from patients with the MEN-I syndrome varies. Primary hyperplasia occurred in 69 per cent of one large group of patients, a single adenoma was found in 27 per cent, and two adenomas were found in 4 per cent.[60]

An opposing concept is that parathyroid hyperplasia is the rule in MEN-I. Asymmetric enlargement of the parathyroid glands is more common in MEN-I and may result in erroneous gross diagnoses of adenoma or

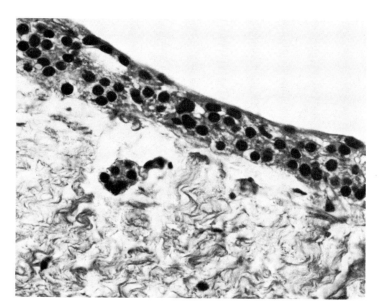

Figure 64–11. Wall of parathyroid cyst, composed of parathyroid cells and fibrous connective tissue. (H&E, ×400)

adenomas. Biopsies of normal-sized glands in such cases show microscopic hyperplasia in all patients.[39, 56]

Data in the literature would support the latter concept. In the group of patients in whom only the one or two enlarged glands were removed, the rate of recurrence was 76 per cent. The remaining patients developed persistent or recurrent hyperparathyroidism. In retrospect, most of the patients with postoperative hypercalcemia had parathyroid hyperplasia. Persistent postoperative hypercalcemia in MEN-I also results from the higher than normal incidence of supernumerary parathyroid glands (15 versus 6 per cent).[60]

Multiple endocrine neoplasia, type IIA (MEN-IIA), affects the C-cells of thyroid gland (C-cell hyperplasia, medullary carcinoma), the adrenal medulla (adrenal medullary hyperplasia, pheochromocytomas), and the parathyroid glands. Primary hyperparathyroidism develops in up to 30 per cent of these patients.[42] Subtle parathyroid hyperfunction, however, is nearly universal in adult patients. The parathyroid hyperplasia is commonly encountered as an incidental finding at the time of thyroidectomy for medullary thyroid carcinomas. In such patients, parathyroid tissue is conserved, and only enlarged glands are removed. A subtotal parathyroidectomy is recommended only for the treatment of clinically evident hyperparathyroidism.

Multiple endocrine neoplasia, type IIB (MEN-IIB), syndrome has all the elements of MEN-IIA in addition to neurogenous lesions (mucosal neuromas, intestinal ganglioneuromatosis, hypertrophy of corneal nerves), a Marfinoid habitus, and distinctive facies.[42]

The histologic appearance of the parathyroid glands varies from normal to mild hyperplasia to frank hyperplasia. The hyperplasia is age-dependent and is rarely associated with clinically or biochemically overt hyperparathyroidism.[10]

The recognition of familial hypocalciuric hypercalcemia (FHH) has contributed enormously to better treatment of patients with familial hyperparathyroidism.[24, 41] The principal features of this syndrome are (1) hypercalcemia without other endocrine changes of MEN-I; (2) hypercalcemia that is recognized before 10 years of age; (3) hypercalcemia with related hyperthyroidism; and (4) the inability to remain normocalcemic after parathyroidectomy.[42]

A related syndrome is neonatal severe primary hyperparathyroidism, which is characterized by hypercalcemia, muscular hypotonia, poor mineralization of bones, and a high mortality rate. This syndrome may be the most pathologic nonlethal expression of a phenotype related to FHH.[40]

Mild hyperplasia of parathyroid glands is characteristic of FHH.

No treatment is recommended for most patients. The lifelong hypercalcemia in this disorder results in little morbidity, and persistent hypercalcemia is likely after subtotal or total parathyroidectomy.

The parathyroid glands in severe neonatal hyperparathyroidism are hyperplastic, and in this syndrome total parathyroidectomy is recommended.

REFERENCES

1. Abul-Haj SK, Conklin H, Hewitt WC: Functioning lipoadenoma of the parathyroid gland. Report of a unique case. N Engl J Med 266:121, 1962.
2. Aldinger KA, Hickey RC, Ibanez ML, Samaan NA: Parathyroid carcinoma: A clinical study of seven cases of functioning and two cases of non-functioning parathyroid cancer. Cancer 49:388, 1982.
3. Allen TB, Thorburn KM: The oxyphil cell in abnormal parathyroid glands. A study of 114 cases. Arch Pathol Lab Med 105:421, 1981.
4. Black WC, Haff RC: The surgical pathology of parathyroid chief cell hyperplasia. Am J Clin Pathol 53:565, 1970.
5. Black WC, Utley JR: The differential diagnosis of parathyroid adenoma and chief cell hyperplasia. Am J Clin Pathol 49:761, 1968.
6. Black WC, Slatopolsky E, Elkan I, Hoffstein P: Parathyroid morphology in suppressible and nonsuppressible renal hyperparathyroidism. Lab Invest 23:497, 1970.
7. Block MA, Greenawald K, Horn RC, Frame B: Involvement of multiple parathyroids in hyperparathyroidism. Surgical Aspects. Am J Surg 114:530, 1967.
8. Block MA, Frame B, Jackson CE, et al: Primary diffuse microscopical hyperplasia of the parathyroid glands. Surgical Importance. Arch Surg 111:348, 1976.
9. Brennan MF, Marx SJ, Doppman J, et al: Results of reoperation for persistent and recurrent hyperparathyroidism. Ann Surg 194:671, 1981.
10. Carney JA, Roth SI, Heath H III, et al: The parathyroid glands in multiple endocrine neoplasia type 2b. Am J Pathol 99:387, 1980.
11. Castleman B, Roth SI: Tumors of the Parathyroid Glands. Atlas of Tumor Pathology, Second Series, Fasicle 14, AFIP, 1978.
12. Clark O, Taylor S: Persistent and recurrent hyperparathyroidism. Br J Surg 59:555, 1972.
13. Clark OH: Parathyroid cysts. Am J Surg 135:395, 1978.
14. Clark OH: Hyperparathyroidism due to primary cystic parathyroid hyperplasia. Arch Surg 113:748, 1979.
15. Cope O, Keynes WM, Roth SI, Castleman B: Primary chief-cell hyperplasia of the parathyroid glands: A new entity in the surgery of hyperparathyroidism. Ann Surg 148:375, 1958.
16. Dekker A, Dunsford HA, Geyer SJ: The normal parathyroid gland at autopsy: The significance of stromal fat in adult patients. J Pathol 128:127, 1979.
17. Dekker A, Watson CG, Barnes L Jr: The pathologic assessment of primary hyperparathyroidism and its impact on therapy. A prospective evaluation of 50 cases with oil-red-0-stain. Ann Surg 190:671, 1979.
18. Dufour DR, Durkowski C: Sudan IV stain. Its limitations in evaluating parathyroid functional status. Arch Pathol Lab Med 106:224, 1982.
19. Dufour DR, Wilkerson SY: The normal parathyroid revisited: Percentage of stromal fat. Human Pathol 13:717, 1982.
20. Edis AJ: Surgical anatomy and technique of neck exploration for primary hyperparathyroidism. Surg Clin North Am 57:495, 1977.
21. Edis AJ, Beahrs OH, van Heerden JA, Akwari OE: "Conservative" versus "liberal" approach to parathyroid neck exploration. Surgery 82:466, 1977.
22. Esselstyn CB: Parathyroid surgery: How many glands should be excised? Is there still a controversy? Surg Clin North Am 59:77, 1979.
23. Fallon MD, Haines JW, Teitelbaum SL: Cystic parathyroid gland hyperplasia—Hyperparathyroidism presenting as a neck mass. Am J Clin Pathol 77:104, 1982.
24. Familial hypocalciuric hypercalcaemia (editorial). Lancet 1:488, 1982.
25. Flye MW, Brennan MF: Surgical resection of metastatic parathyroid carcinoma. Ann Surg 193:425, 1981.
26. Geelhoed GW: Parathyroid adenolipoma: Clinical and morphologic features. Surgery 92:806, 1982.
27. Grimelius L, Akerstrom G, Johansson H, Bergstrom R: Anatomy and histopathology of human parathyroid gland. Pathol Annu 16:1, 1981.
28. Haff RC, Ballinger WF: Causes of recurrent hypercalcemia after parathyroidectomy for primary hyperparathyroidism. Ann Surg 173:884, 1971.
29. Harness JK, Ramsburg SR, Nishiyama RH, Thompson NW: Multiple adenomas of the parathyroid: Do they exist? Arch Surg 114:468, 1979.
30. Harrison TS, Duaete B, Reitz RE, et al: Primary hyperparathyroidism. Four-to eight-year postoperative follow-up demonstrating persistent functional insignificance of microscopic parathyroid hyperplasia and decreased autonomy of parathyroid hormone release. Ann Surg 194:429, 1981.
31. Holmes EC, Morton DL, Ketcham AS: Parathyroid carcinoma: A collective review. Ann Surg 169:631, 1969.
32. Hyperparathyroidism after renal transplantation (editorial). Lancet 1:343, 1977.
33. Kay S: The abnormal parathyroid. Hum Pathol 7:127, 1976.
34. Kay S, Hume DM: Carcinoma of the parathyroid gland. How reliable are the clinical and histologic features? Arch Pathol 96:316, 1973.

35. King DT, Hirose FM: Chief cell intracytoplasmic fat used to evaluate parathyroid disease by frozen section. Arch Pathol Lab Med *103*:609, 1979.

36. Lawrence DAS: A histological comparison of adenomatous and hyperplastic parathyroid glands. J Clin Pathol *31*:626, 1978.

37. LeGolvan DP, Moore BP, Nishiyama RH: Parathyroid hamartoma. Report of two cases and review of the literature. Am J Clin Pathol *67*:31, 1977.

38. Ljungberg O, Tibblin S: Preoperative fat staining of frozen sections in primary hyperparathyroidism. Am J Pathol *95*:633, 1979.

39. Majewski JT, Wilson SD: The MEA-I Syndrome: An all-or-none phenomenon? Surgery *86*:475, 1979.

40. Marx SJ, Attie MF, Spiegel AM, et al: An association between neonatal severe primary hyperparathyroidism and familial hypocalciuric hypercalcemia in three kindreds. N Engl J Med *306*:257, 1982.

41. Marx SJ, Spiegel AM, Brown EM, Aurbach GD: Family studies in patients with primary parathyroid hyperplasia. Am J Med *62*:698, 1977.

42. Marx SJ, Spiegel AM, Levine MA, et al: Familial hypocalciuric hypercalcemia. The relation to primary parathyroid hyperplasia. N Engl J Med *307*:416, 1982.

43. Nathaniels EK, Nathaniels AM, Wang C: Mediastinal parathyroid tumors: A clinical and pathological study of 84 cases. Ann Surg *171*:165, 1970.

44. Ober WB, Kaiser GA: Hamartoma of the parathyroid. Cancer *11*:601, 1958.

45. Ordonez NG, Ibanez ML, MacKay B, et al: Functioning oxyphil cell adenomas of parathyroid gland: Immunoperoxidase evidence of hormonal activity in oxyphil cells. Am J Clin Pathol *78*:681, 1982.

46. Organ CH Jr, Albano WA: Surgical management of recurrent and persistent hyperparathyroidism. Surg Gynecol Obstet *151*:237, 1980.

47. Poole GV Jr, Albertson DA, Marshall RB, Myers RT: Oxyphil cell adenoma and hyperparathyroidism. Surgery *92*:799, 1982.

48. Purnell DC, Scholz DA, Beahrs OH: Hyperparathyroidism due to single gland enlargement. Arch Surg *112*:369, 1977.

49. Roth SI, Gallagher MJ: The rapid identification of "normal" parathyroid glands by the presence of intracellular fat. Am J Pathol *84*:521, 1976.

50. Russell CF, Edis AJ, Scholz DA, et al: Mediastinal parathyroid tumors. Experience with 38 tumors requiring mediastinotomy for removal. Ann Surg *193*:805, 1981.

51. Russell CF, Grant CS, van Heerden JA: Hyperfunctioning supernumerary parathyroid glands. An occasional cause of hyperparathyroidism. Mayo Clin Proc *57*:121, 1982.

52. Schantz A, Castleman B: Parathyroid carcinoma. A study of 70 cases. Cancer *31*:600, 1973.

53. Scholz DA, Purnell DC, Woolner LB, Clagett OT: Mediastinal hyperfunctioning parathyroid tumors: Review of 14 cases. Ann Surg *178*:173, 1973.

54. Scholz DA, Purnell DC, Edis AJ, et al: Primary hyperparathyroidism with multiple parathyroid gland enlargement. Review of 53 cases. Mayo Clin Proc *53*:792, 1978.

55. Straus FH II, Paloyan E: The pathology of hyperparathyroidism. Surg Clin North Am *49*:27, 1969.

56. Thompson NW: Surgical Considerations in the MEA I Syndrome. Endocrine Surgery. London, Butterworth & Co. (Publishers), Ltd., 1983.

57. Thompson NW, Eckhauser FE, Harness JK: The anatomy of primary hyperparathyroidism. Surgery *92*:814, 1982.

58. Tibblin S, Bondeson A, Ljungberg O: Unilateral parathyroidectomy in hyperparathyroidism due to single adenoma. Ann Surg *195*:245, 1982.

59. van Heerden JA, Weiland LH, ReMine WH, et al: Cancer of the parathyroid glands. Arch Surg *114*:475, 1979.

60. van Heerden JA, Kent RB, Sizemore GW, et al: Primary hyperparathyroidism in patients with multiple endocrine neoplasia syndromes. Surgical experience. Arch Surg *118*:533, 1983.

61. Verdonk CA, Edis AJ: Parathyroid "double adenomas": Fact or fiction? Surgery *90*:523, 1982.

62. Wang C: The anatomic basis of parathyroid surgery. Ann Surg *183*:271, 1976.

63. Wang C: Parathyroid re-exploration. A clinical and pathological study of 112 cases. Ann Surg *186*:140, 1977.

64. Wang C, Mahaffey JE, Axelrod L, Perlman JA: Hyperfunctioning supernumerary parathyroid glands. Surg Gynecol Obstet *148*:711, 1979.

65. Weiland LH, Garrison RC, ReMine WH, Scholz DA: Lipoadenoma of the parathyroid gland. Am J Surg Pathol *2*:3, 1978.

66. Wells SA Jr, Leight GS, Ross AJ: Primary hyperparathyroidism. Curr Probl Surg *17*:439, 1980.

CHAPTER 65

Surgical Therapy of Parathyroid Tumors

Gregorio A. Sicard, M.D.

HISTORICAL PERSPECTIVE

Hyperparathyroidism, a disorder of the parathyroid glands characterized by the abnormal secretion of parathyroid hormone, is currently the leading cause of hypercalcemia in nonhospitalized patients and is the second most common cause of hypercalcemia, after malignancy, in hospitalized patients. In 1891 von Recklinghausen recognized the clinical impact of hyperparathyroidism and described *osteitis fibrosa cystica* as the pathognomonic bone lesions of this entity. The association between bone disease and parathyroid gland abnormalities was originally described by Askanazy in 1904 in a woman with pain in the extremities and spontaneous fractures, although he did not appreciate the etiologic significance. At autopsy this patient was found to have generalized osteitis fibrosa cystica as previously described by von Recklinghausen. Schlagenhaufer, in 1915, proposed the association between parathyroid tumors and *secondary* changes in the skeleton. In 1926 Mandl surgically removed a parathyroid tumor in a patient with hypercalcemia, hypercalciuria, and radiologic changes of osteitis fibrosa cystica and demonstrated postoperative regression of the bone and biochemical abnormalities. Unfortunately, the patient's bone disease recurred within 6 years, resulting in his death. Barr and collaborators in 1929 reported permanent resolution of hypercalcemia and regression of bone abnormalities in a patient with severe hyperparathyroidism after surgical removal of a parathyroid adenoma. This procedure, performed by Dr. I. Y. Olch at Washington University, was the first successful parathyroidectomy performed in the United States.

The metabolic studies reported by Albright and Aub[2] in 1934 described the physiologic abnormalities in calcium and phosphorus metabolism and their effect on the renal function of patients with hyperparathyroidism. These elegant studies, along with the surgical reports by Churchill and Cope,[15] established hyperparathyroidism as a clinical entity.

EPIDEMIOLOGY

The incidence of primary hyperparathyroidism has been reported between 25 and 50 per 100,000 population per year.[41, 56] The highest incidence occurs in women in the fourth to the sixth decades of life, approaching 200 cases per 100,000 population per year.

Once a diagnosis of primary hyperparathyroidism has been established, appropriate management still remains controversial. In patients with symptomatic hyperparathyroidism or patients with a serum calcium level of 11 mg/dl or greater, surgery remains the treatment of choice. On the other hand, the management of patients with mild or biochemical hyperparathyroidism has been the source of controversy. Heath and collaborators[41] tried to assess the natural history of hyperparathyroidism in a prospective study of 147 patients with the provisional diagnosis of asymptomatic hyperparathyroidism. Their results suggest that the natural history of patients with mild hyperparathyroidism is such that approximately 20 per cent of these patients will require surgical therapy during the first 10 years of their follow-up. Unfortunately, it was not possible to predict which patients would require operative therapy prior to the development of complications. The lack of patient compliance to periodic follow-up was also a major problem in their study. Furthermore, a prolonged period of observation with frequent tests may not be cost-effective. In patients with mild episodic hypercalcemia (< 11 mg/dl) without significant hypercalciuria, a period of follow-up and retesting after 6 months is acceptable. If hypercalcemia persists and elevated serum parathormone is demonstrated, then surgical therapy is indicated. Approximately 26 per cent of patients with asymptomatic hyperparathyroidism will develop significant complications related to the disease in 10 years.[67] Similarly, there is data to support that complications of hyperparathyroidism, mainly renal dysfunction, may be irreversible once established.[60] The low mortality and morbidity rates, as well as the cost effectiveness,[41] of parathyroidectomy establishes the surgical approach for asymptomatic hyperparathyroidism as the *current* treatment modality of choice.

EMBRYOLOGIC CONSIDERATIONS

In humans the *superior parathyroid glands* arise from the fourth pharyngeal pouch and share the embryoanatomic region with the lateral thyroid complex. Because of their anatomic proximity to the thyroid gland and the short caudal migration of the thyroid, superior glands are rarely ectopic, although occasionally they may become completely enclosed within the thyroid parenchyma or may migrate to the superior *posterior mediastinum*.

The *inferior parathyroid glands* share the third branchial pouch with the thymus, and during embryologic maturation they descend caudally to the inferior aspect of the neck. The variability of this migration is responsible for the extremely wide anatomic distribution of the inferior parathyroid glands in the adult. When the inferior glands migrate to the superior mediastinum, they are commonly located in an anterior position and receive their blood supply from the inferior thyroid artery or from a branch of the internal mammary artery. Anomalies in anatomic position and number are very common in the parathyroid glands, especially in the inferior glands. Ectopic glands or accessory glands can be found in any region of the neck and thorax (angle of the jaw, anterior mediastinum, posterior mediastinum, retroesophageal region, pericardium), making their identification difficult during parathyroidectomy.

ANATOMIC CONSIDERATIONS

A thorough understanding of the embryologic development and normal anatomy of the parathyroid glands is of utmost importance in planning the surgical approach to hyperparathyroidism. Similarly, familiarity with the gross appearance of normal and abnormal parathyroid glands gives a clue to the surgeon on the number of glands to excise. Humans usually have four parathyroid glands, although various series have reported the incidence of supernumerary parathyroid glands to range from 2.5 to 6.5 per cent.[3, 36, 78] The clinical significance of supernumerary parathyroid glands in recurrent or persistent hyperparathyroidism after subtotal parathyroidectomy has been reported.[28] Similarly, Wells and collaborators[86] reported a 38 per cent incidence of persistent hypercalcemia in patients with secondary hyperparathyroidism who had undergone total parathyroidectomy and autotransplantation to the forearm. They speculated that the persistent hypercalcemia was secondary to residual parathyroid tissue in the neck despite a four-gland parathyroidectomy. Akerstrom and collaborators[1] reported the anatomic distribution of parathyroid glands in an autopsy study of 503 cases. In 18 (3 per cent) of 503 cases only three glands were found, but the total weight was less than the usual total glandular weight, suggesting that the fourth gland was not identified. In 421 (84 per cent) of 503 cases four glands were identified, and in 64 cases (13 per cent) more than four glands were found. In 11 of the 64 cases, the supernumerary gland was very small, weighing less than 5 mg, and was usually found in close proximity to a normal gland. In 32 cases the supernumerary gland consisted of a split gland lying very close to another, but they were clearly separated from each other. Supernumerary glands weighing more than 5 mg and found not to be in close proximity to other glands were found in 24 (5 per cent) of 503 cases. More important was the finding that in two thirds of the cases with supernumerary glands, the gland was found inferior to the thyroid gland and in close association with the thyroid ligament or in the thymus gland itself. The importance of this finding will be further discussed in the surgical approach to hyperparathyroidism.

PATHOLOGY

Adenoma

Parathyroid adenoma is the most common histologic diagnosis in primary spontaneous hyperparathyroidism. Although the frequency of adenomas in primary hyperparathyroidism has varied from 51 to 96 per cent, most series report frequencies of 80 to 90 per cent (Table 65–1). This discrepancy has important clinical implications and has been the subject of much debate.[25] Although parathyroid adenomas are usually single, multiple adenomas have also been described.[10]

The controversy regarding histologic characterization of abnormal parathyroid tissue has led various authors to classify abnormalities in parathyroid glands as single- or multiple-gland enlargement.[10, 57, 85] Wells and collaborators[85] reported an incidence of 65 per cent of single-gland enlargement and 15, 10, and 10 per cent for two, three, and four enlarged parathyroids, respectively, in 100 consecutive patients operated on for primary hyperparathyroidism. Similarly, Paloyan and associates[57] found a 60 per cent incidence of single-gland

TABLE 65–1. Histologic Diagnosis of Selected Series of Primary Hyperparathyroidism

Author	Number of Patients	Single Adenoma	Multiple Adenoma	Hyperplasia	Carcinoma	No Diagnosis
Cope et al., 1958[18]	206	76%	5%	11%	4%	4%
Cope, 1966[17]	343	77%	4%	15%	4%	—
Hoehn et al., 1969[42]	813	92%	—	7%	1%	—
Haff and Ballinger, 1971[40]	47	51%	—	49%	—	—
Goldman et al., 1971[38]	300	92%	4%	3%	1%	—
Paloyan et al., 1973[58]	84	33%	—	65%	2%	—
Esselstyn et al., 1974[30]	100	51%	—	49%	—	—
Wang, 1976[78]	525	80%	2%	15%	3%	—
Taylor, 1977[76]	102	73%	—	26%	3%	—
Kelly, 1980[46]	242	88%	—	11%	1%	—
McGarity et al., 1981[54]	100*	50%	—	46%	2%	2%
	93†	76%	—	19%	3%	2%

*Histologic examination of four glands.
†Histologic examination of less than four glands.
Source: Modified from Sicard GA, Wells SA: Tumors of the parathyroid gland. *In* Moossa AR (ed): Comprehensive Textbook of Oncology. Baltimore, Williams & Wilkins Co. (in press). Used with permission.

disease and a 39 per cent incidence of multiple-gland disease, with only 13 per cent having four-gland enlargement. The significant incidence of multiple-gland enlargement as well as the frequent bilaterality of this finding stresses the importance of bilateral neck exploration during parathyroidectomy, regardless of the histologic appearance in frozen section.

Hyperplasia

The frequency of primary chief cell hyperplasia in primary hyperparathyroidism varies from 11 to 65 per cent, the higher incidence being more common in series of patients with hereditary hyperparathyroidism. This histologic entity was originally described by Cope and associates in 1958.[18] A second histologic form of parathyroid hyperplasia is that of water clear cell hyperplasia. Histologically, water clear cell hyperplasia is characterized by the presence of large cells with clear cytoplasm and a high glycogen content. Wang and collaborators[80] found 20 (19 per cent) cases of water clear cell hyperplasia in 104 patients treated at the Massachusetts General Hospital between 1933 and 1978 for primary parathyroid hyperplasia. Water clear cell hyperplasia has decreased in incidence since its original description and now is associated with less than 5 per cent of cases of parathyroid tumors.

Parathyroid Carcinoma

Parathyroid carcinoma is a very rare lesion and represents 0 to 4 per cent of reported series of parathyroid neoplasms (Table 65–1). Histologic diagnosis of parathyroid carcinoma is difficult when the disease is limited to the affected parathyroid gland. The presence of mitotic figures or vascular invasion of parathyroid cells does not necessarily constitute proof of malignancy in parathyroid carcinoma. The diagnosis of parathyroid carcinoma is usually made in a markedly hypercalcemic patient with a parathyroid tumor that is locally invasive or metastatic and is associated with marked elevation of serum parathormone. Parathyroid carcinoma can metastasize to lymph nodes, lung, and liver, although most patients die from complications of persistent hypercalcemia rather than from distant organ involvement.[4]

Parathyroid carcinomas tend to affect females and males equally, are palpable in 50 per cent of the cases, and are associated with severe hypercalcemia (more than 15 mg/dl). On the other hand, benign parathyroid tumors are rarely palpable, are found frequently in females, and usually are associated with mild forms of hypercalcemia.

DIAGNOSIS

General Tests

Hypercalcemia remains the most constant finding in the diagnosis of primary hyperparathyroidism. Although in hospitalized patients malignancy continues to be the single most common cause of hypercalcemia, primary hyperparathyroidism is the second. Because of normal daily fluctuations of serum calcium, it is impor-

tant to have obtained several elevated calcium levels prior to pursuing more extensive and expensive diagnostic tests. Alterations in serum proteins (such as albumin) can also influence the total serum calcium level and should be closely monitored.

The two main fractions of plasma calcium are the *calcium bound to proteins* and various organic acids and *ionized calcium*, which is the physiologically active fraction. Ionized calcium is regulated by parathyroid hormone and therefore is the elevated fraction in primary hyperparathyroidism. Elevation of this fraction constitutes evidence of primary hyperparathyroidism and is an indication for pursuing more specific diagnostic tests (parathormone assay).

Hypercalciuria and hypophosphatemia, although useful in the diagnosis of primary hyperparathyroidism, are less specific than hypercalcemia and therefore are of lesser diagnostic value. Similarly, elevations in alkaline phosphatase and urinary hydroxyproline, found in primary hyperparathyroidism with severe bone involvement, are not specific for hyperparathyroidism. Other electrolyte abnormalities like hyperchloremic acidosis and decreased serum bicarbonate can be present in hyperparathyroidism but are not specific for the disease.

Specific Tests for Parathyroid Function

Tubular Reabsorption of Phosphate. In patients with primary hyperparathyroidism the tubular reabsorption of phosphate (TRP) is markedly decreased when compared with normal patients. This abnormality reflects the effect of parathyroid hormone (PTH) in the tubular handling of phosphates. Unfortunately, normal patients or patients with diseases such as multiple myeloma and gout can have abnormal excretion of phosphorus, making it a nonspecific test in the diagnosis of primary hyperparathyroidism.

Radioimmunoassay for Parathyroid Hormone (iPTH). Serum parathyroid hormone determined by radioimmunoassay technique remains the single most *specific* test in the diagnosis of hyperparathyroidism. An abnormal elevation of PTH in relation to the serum calcium concentration remains the sine qua non for the diagnosis of hyperparathyroidism. Radioimmunoassays that employ antisera that measure the *carboxy terminal* portion of the PTH molecule give more reproducible results than those that measure the *amino terminal* portion of the PTH molecule. The assay that measures the carboxy terminal portion of PTH can determine the difference between normal subjects and hyperparathyroid patients in 95 per cent of the cases. Familiarization with the variability of the radioimmunoassay utilized in the specific diagnostic laboratory is important for surgeons who treat patients with parathyroid disease.

Radiologic Studies. Radiologic changes in bone in patients with primary hyperparathyroidism can be very subtle but diagnostic. The earliest x-ray skeletal change in primary hyperparathyroidism is subperiosteal resorption, which is most commonly found in the phalanges of the hand and the distal third of the clavicle (Figs. 65–1 and 65–2). Similarly, skull x-rays can give a salt-and-pepper appearance to the calvarium owing to demineralization. Bone cysts (brown tumors) and osteoclastomas can also be found in the central medullary part of the shaft of long bones, phalanges (Fig. 65–1), metacarpals,

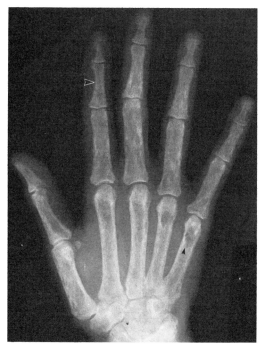

Figure 65–1. Hand radiograph from a patient with secondary hyperparathyroidism. Note marked subperiosteal reabsorption of middle phalanx index finger (large arrow) and bone cyst in fifth metacarpal (small arrow).

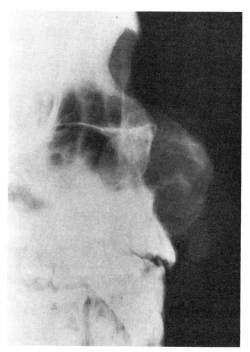

Figure 65–3. Facial bone film. Brown tumor of maxilla in patient with secondary hyperparathyroidism.

ribs, and maxilla (Fig. 65–3). Other radiologic studies such as sonography, computerized tomography, and selective arteriography or venous drainage for PTH determination have no place in the initial diagnosis of hyperparathyroidism but can be useful localization studies in recurrent or persistent hyperparathyroidism (see section on Reoperative Parathyroid Surgery).

Isotopic Studies. The results of scanning techniques to localize abnormal parathyroid tissue have been disappointing. Initially, the technique for scanning was

that of methionine combined with selenium-75. Only cases with large parathyroid adenoma have been shown by this technique, and for practical purposes, the intravenous [^{75}Se]selenomethionine technique has been abandoned. Intra-arterial injections of ^{75}Se and selenomethionine have been useful in identifying abnormal parathyroid tissue but should be reserved only for those patients undergoing arteriography after previously unsuccessful parathyroid surgery (see section on Reoperative Parathyroid Surgery).

SURGICAL TREATMENT OF HYPERPARATHYROIDISM

Once the diagnosis of primary hyperparathyroidism has been established, surgical therapy remains the treatment modality of choice. Although most patients with primary hyperparathyroidism have a parathyroid adenoma as the pathologic cause, parathyroid hyperplasia, commonly found in patients with hereditary hyperparathyroidism, can also be an etiologic factor. A complete history along with a careful search for physical findings associated with some of the multiple endocrinopathies can alert the surgeon to the possibility that the hyperparathyroidism may be caused by four-gland hyperplasia. This type of careful preoperative assessment can diminish the incidence of persistent or recurrent hyperparathyroidism. Similarly, patients with elevated serum creatinine or end-stage renal disease commonly have secondary hyperparathyroidism, which is associated with four-gland hyperplasia. Patients who have undergone a successful renal transplantation can have tertiary hyperparathyroidism, which can be caused by either diffuse four-gland hyperplasia or a nonsuppressible adenoma, although the hyperplasia is more common.

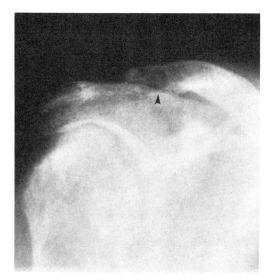

Figure 65–2. Shoulder film from patient with secondary hyperparathyroidism. Note subperiosteal reabsorption and bone cyst in distal third of the clavicle.

Surgical Technique

The patient is operated on in the supine position with hyperextension of the neck to provide access from the base of the tongue to the superior mediastinum. A low cervical incision (Kocher) is made two fingerbreadths above the suprasternal notch, usually over a natural skin crease, and is carried down through the platysma. A superior flap is elevated between the platysma and the strap muscles superiorly to the level of the thyroid cartilage and laterally to the medial border of the sternocleidomastoid muscle. The inferior flap is elevated to the sternal notch. The strap muscles are separated in the midline (Fig. 65–4). In the initial exploration of hyperparathyroidism, division of the strap muscle is rarely necessary. A plane of dissection posterior to the strap muscles and close to the thyroid capsule is entered, ascertaining that the thyroid parenchyma is not violated to avoid excessive bleeding, which may stain the parathyroid glands a darker color, making them difficult to distinguish from fat, lymph nodes, or other surrounding structures. The parathyroid glands are usually distinguished by their yellowish brown color, and in a bloodless field they should be identified easily by a trained surgeon. The thyroid gland is then retracted medially until the middle thyroid vein is identified (Fig. 65–5). This vein is ligated and divided, allowing for further medial retraction of the thyroid lobe. Ligation of the superior or inferior thyroid artery is not necessary in order to adequately rotate the thyroid lobe medially during routine parathyroidectomy. Careful dissection is performed in the area superior and inferior to the inferior thyroid artery, separating the thyroid gland from the inferior aspect of the strap muscles and exposing the usual anatomic location of the parathyroid glands. The next step prior to searching for the parathyroid glands is the identification of the recurrent laryngeal nerve, which is commonly found in the tracheoesophageal groove. This nerve should be identified low and traced up to its entry point into the trachea to avoid injury during mobilization and resection of the superior parathyroid glands (Fig. 65–5).

A *systematic* search of parathyroid glands remains the most logical approach and should provide a high success rate of identification of abnormal parathyroid tissue. The inferior glands are usually searched for initially. The inferior parathyroid glands tend to be larger, they are located anteriorly, and their anatomic location is less constant. The inferior glands are commonly found adjacent to the inferior pole of the thyroid or in the thymic fat that extends from the inferior portion of the thyroid gland to the superior mediastinum. The superior parathyroid glands are commonly found just superior to the entrance of the inferior thyroid artery into the inferior

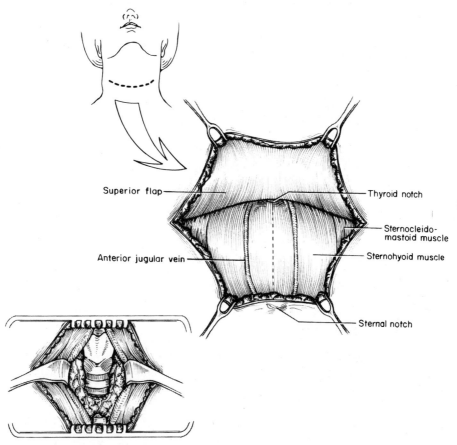

Figure 65–4. In this initial stage of parathyroid surgery, a superior flap is elevated between the platysma and the strap muscles. The inferior flap is elevated to the sternal notch, and the strap muscles are separated in the midline.

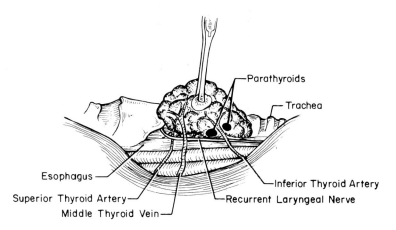

Parathyroids

Trachea

Esophagus

Superior Thyroid Artery

Middle Thyroid Vein

Inferior Thyroid Artery

Recurrent Laryngeal Nerve

Figure 65–5. In order to locate and expose the parathyroid glands, the thyroid gland is retracted medially. Once the middle thyroid vein is identified, it is ligated to allow further retraction of the thyroid gland. Care must be taken not to injure the recurrent laryngeal nerve.

pole of the thyroid gland and near the entrance of the recurrent laryngeal nerve into the larynx.[85] If the glands are not easily identified, extensive *systematic* exploration of the neck is performed from the hyoid bone superiorly, to the superior anterior mediastinum inferiorly, to the carotid sheath laterally, and to the tracheoesophageal groove and retroesophageal area posteriorly. Careful observation for an abnormally large vascular pedicle arising from the inferior thyroid artery can lead to abnormal parathyroid glands, especially those in ectopic locations.

Once a complete neck exploration has been performed, the next step should be the removal of the contents of the anterior superior mediastinum, which can harbor abnormal parathyroid tissue (usually the inferior glands). If the abnormal gland has not been found, then a careful evaluation of the ipsilateral thyroid lobe is important because abnormal intrathyroidal tumors can be found in 5 to 8 per cent of patients with hyperparathyroidism.[9, 73] Under all circumstances, all glands should be visually *identified*, and a small biopsy sample is taken for frozen section verification of parathyroid tissue prior to excision. Biopsy of a normal parathyroid gland must be performed after minimal mobilization of the gland and is taken away from the hilum to avoid devascularization. Complete removal of any gland *is not performed* until all glands have been

identified both *visually* and *histologically*. If four normal glands are identified in a patient with hyperparathyroidism, the thymus and superior anterior mediastinum contents should be inspected carefully because this area remains a common location for ectopic supernumerary parathyroid glands (Fig. 65–6). Some surgeons advise the *routine* evacuation of the superior mediastinal contents in order to decrease the incidence of recurrent or persistent hyperparathyroidism in patients with supernumerary parathyroid glands. Superior parathyroid glands can migrate to the superior posterior mediastinum and can be found in the retroesophageal space, although the second most common abnormal location of abnormal parathyroid tissue remains intrathyroidal tumors. Commonly, the abnormal gland can be palpated in a normal-size thyroid lobe, but it may be difficult in an enlarged thyroid gland. If extensive exploration of the neck, including opening of the carotid sheath, still fails to identify a fourth parathyroid gland, then blind unilateral thyroid lobectomy on the side of the missing gland is indicated.

If despite all these maneuvers the abnormal gland still has not been found, the remaining normal glands should *not* be excised but are marked with stainless steel clips for identification at the time of re-exploration. A median sternotomy should *not* be performed at the time of the original exploration. If four normal glands

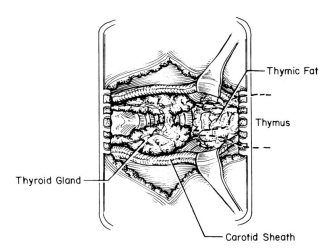

Thymic Fat

Thymus

Thyroid Gland

Carotid Sheath

Figure 65–6. The thymus and superior anterior mediastinum contents are common locations for supernumerary parathyroid glands.

TABLE 65–2. Recommended Surgical Approach in the Treatment of Parathyroid Disease

Parathyroid Disease	Recommended Treatments	Comments
Primary hyperparathyroidism		
Single adenoma	Biopsy all four glands for histologic verification	
	Excise adenoma	
Multiple adenoma	Biopsy all four glands for histologic verification	If three glands enlarged, cryopreservation is recommended
	Excise all enlarged glands	
Four-gland hyperplasia	Biopsy all glands for histologic verification	Cryopreservation of at least 100 mg tissue
	Total parathyroidectomy and autotransplantation	Some authors recommend subtotal parathyroidectomy
Secondary hyperparathyroidism	Biopsy all glands	Cryopreservation of at least 100 mg tissue
	Total parathyroidectomy and autotransplant	Some authors recommend subtotal parathyroidectomy
Persistent or recurrent hyperparathyroidism		
With enlarged gland only, tissue present in neck	Excision and immediate forearm muscle autotransplant	Cryopreservation of at least 100 mg tissue
With unknown number of glands in neck	Excision of enlarged gland and cryopreservation	Delayed autograft of cryopreserved tissue if patient remains hypoparathyroid 1 to 3 months after surgery

are found and the superior anterior mediastinal fat has been properly evacuated, then the neck should be closed. Should the patient remain hyperparathyroid, then reoperative localization studies should be done. Once all glands have been visualized and biopsied and the pathologist has identified histologically all parathyroid glands, then resection should be carried out, based on the clinical entity responsible for the primary hyperparathyroidism and the number of enlarged glands (Table 65–2). The operative options will be further discussed in the sections to follow.

Primary Hyperparathyroidism

Most patients with spontaneous primary hyperparathyroidism have single-gland enlargement; thus, the identification of all the glands and biopsy and histologic verification are then followed by removal of the enlarged gland. Occasionally, multiple adenomas are found in patients with primary hyperparathyroidism. The incidence of multiple adenomas is between 5 and 25 per cent,[9, 57, 85] which stresses the importance of bilateral neck exploration and identification of *all four glands* prior to ending the neck exploration. In patients with multiple adenomas, we recommend visual and histologic identification of all parathyroid glands, followed by excision of the enlarged glands. The normal glands should be carefully marked with a stainless steel clip. These patients represent an unusual group of primary hyperparathyroidism, and close long-term follow-up is necessary because the true incidence of recurrent disease in this subgroup has not been defined as well as with other forms of parathyroid gland enlargement.

In patients with four-gland enlargement, subtotal parathyroidectomy or total parathyroidectomy and forearm autotransplant are the two therapeutic options. Total parathyroidectomy and forearm autotransplantation is the preferred procedure because it avoids the

risk of permanent devascularization of the parathyroid remnants left in subtotal parathyroidectomy and eliminates the morbidity associated with neck re-exploration in those cases of recurrent hyperparathyroidism. Furthermore, patients with four-gland enlargement should be carefully screened for familial hyperparathyroidism or other forms of hereditary hyperparathyroidism, such as multiple endocrine neoplasia (MEN) type 1 or 2. The frequency of hyperparathyroidism in MEN type 1 seems to be much higher (95 versus 30 per cent) than in MEN type 2.[77]

In patients with hereditary hyperparathyroidism treated with subtotal parathyroidectomy the incidence of recurrence or persistent hyperparathyroidism is extremely high. Various series report recurrence or persistent rates between 25 and 38 per cent in patients with MEN type 1.[69] Similarly, Marx and collaborators[51] reported an incidence of recurrence or persistent hypercalcemia in 85 per cent of patients with familial hypercalcemic hypocalciuric hyperparathyroidism (FHHH) treated with subtotal parathyroidectomy. The high recurrence and persistence rates in this group of patients with primary hyperparathyroidism have led Wells and collaborators[83] to propose total parathyroidectomy and forearm autotransplantation in patients with hereditary hyperparathyroidism in order to eliminate persistent disease and to allow safer therapy of recurrence by excision of tissue in the forearm. The technique for forearm autotransplantation will be described in the following section (Surgical Therapy of Secondary Hyperparathyroidism).

Secondary Hyperparathyroidism

Etiology

Despite aggressive medical management in patients with renal osteodystrophy, a large number of patients will develop significant secondary hyperparathyroid-

TABLE 65–3. Clinical Features of Surgically Treated Secondary Hyperparathyroidism

Author	Number of Patients	Bone Abnormalities and Bone Pain	Pruritus	Soft-Tissue Calcifications	Vascular Calcifications
Glassford et al., 1976[37]	16	46%	65%	—	—
Cordell et al., 1979[19]	44	52%	27%	20%	—
Diethelm et al., 1981[21]	61	80%	65%	34%	—
Mozes et al., 1980[55]	16	94%	13%	13%	—
Rothmund and Wagner, 1983[61]	46	85%	57%	—	—
Sicard et al., 1980[70]	14	100%	50%	—	50%
Wilson et al., 1971[88]	28	86%	61%	36%	50%
Max et al., 1981[53]	16	56%	19%	—	19%
Swanson et al., 1979[75]	20	90%	80%	—	10%

Source: Modified from Sicard GA, Wells SA: Surgical treatment of secondary hyperparathyroidism. *In* Kaplan EL (ed): Surgery of the Thyroid and Parathyroid Glands. New York, Churchill Livingstone, 1983, p. 245. Used with permission.

ism. It has been estimated that the incidence of secondary hyperparathyroidism in the chronic renal failure population ranges from 20 to 90 per cent. The primary factor associated with the development of secondary hyperparathyroidism in chronic renal insufficiency remains the alterations in phosphate and calcium metabolism. Other pathophysiologic abnormalities described in patients with chronic renal failure include (1) diminished production of 1,25-dihydroxycholecalciferol, (2) abnormal degradation of parathyroid hormone by the kidney, and (3) skeletal resistance to the action of parathormone. Regardless of the mechanism responsible, persistent excessive PTH secretion remains the prominent feature in the development of severe bone disease characteristic of parathyroid disease in chronic renal failure.

Clinical Presentation

The most common clinical presentation of secondary hyperparathyroidism is *symptomatic* or *asymptomatic progressive bone disease* in a patient with elevated alkaline phosphatase and serum parathormone levels. Other clinical presentations include soft-tissue and vascular calcifications, intractable pruritus, and rarely neuromuscular abnormalities (Table 65–3). The main clinical indications for surgical treatment in secondary hyperparathyroidism are marked progression of bone disease that is either symptomatic or asymptomatic, persistent hypercalcemia, intractable pruritus not responsive to dialysis or aggressive medical therapy, progressive soft-tissue calcifications, calcium-phosphate product higher than (75:80) despite adequate restriction of phosphate intake, and progressive vascular calcifications (calciphylaxis).

Surgical Procedures

Three procedures have been proposed in the surgical treatment of secondary hyperparathyroidism:
1. Subtotal parathyroidectomy.
2. Total parathyroidectomy.
3. Total parathyroidectomy with autotransplantation.
Although *total parathyroidectomy without autotransplantation* was originally proposed as a means of abrogating all functional parathyroid tissue, the progression of osteomalacia as well as the difficulties encountered in

the management of permanent hypoparathyroidism, especially in patients undergoing successful renal transplantation, has made this procedure unpopular.[31, 47]

SUBTOTAL PARATHYROIDECTOMY

Subtotal (near-total) parathyroidectomy remains a popular procedure. The results of this technique have been favorable, although recurrent and persistent rates of 10 to 20 per cent have been reported. Furthermore, because four-gland enlargement is the rule in secondary hyperparathyroidism, partial excision of a markedly enlarged fourth gland, in an attempt to leave 50 to 100 mg of functional parathyroid tissue, can be rather difficult and may lead to devascularization of the remnant and permanent hypoparathyroidism.

TOTAL PARATHYROIDECTOMY
WITH FOREARM AUTOTRANSPLANTATION

The use of total parathyroidectomy and forearm autotransplantation in patients with renal osteodystrophy has been reported by Wells and associates[86] as an improvement over subtotal parathyroidectomy because recurrent hyperparathyroidism can be treated more effectively by reoperation in the forearm than by reexploration of the neck. The indications for total parathyroidectomy and autotransplant are shown in Table 65–4. Compared to subtotal (3½ glands) parathyroidectomy, this technique avoids the risk of devascularization of the parathyroid remnant as well as the significant morbidity associated with neck re-exploration if

TABLE 65–4. Indications for Total Parathyroidectomy and Muscle Autotransplantation

Primary hyperparathyroidism
  Multiple endocrine neoplasia type 1 and type 2
  Familial hyperparathyroidism without associated endocrinopathies
  Four-gland hyperplasia (sporadic)
  Familial hypercalcemic hypocalciuric hyperparathyroidism (FHHH)
  Persistent or recurrent hyperparathyroidism
Secondary and tertiary hyperparathyroidism
Total thyroidectomy*

*Sternocleidomastoid can be used as muscle bed.

recurrent hyperparathyroidism develops. The sternocleidomastoid muscle has also been reported as a suitable bed for parathyroid autograft and is the implantation site of choice in patients with accidental excision of parathyroid gland(s) during thyroid resection. In patients with parathyroid disease secondary to chronic renal failure or four-gland hyperplasia, we prefer to graft the parathyroid tissue in the forearm musculature so that recurrent disease can be easily managed by excision of a portion of the hyperfunctioning graft under local anesthesia. Results of subtotal parathyroidectomy and total parathyroidectomy with autotransplantation in secondary hyperparathyroidism are listed in Table 65–5.

Technique. After removal of the gland that will be autotransplanted and frozen section verification, the parathyroid tissue is placed in a chilled tissue culture medium or in 4°C saline. Once the tissue is firm, it is then sliced into 1×3 mm pieces with a scalpel. While the chilling of the tissue is taking place, a longitudinal incision is made in the lateral aspect of the flexor surface of the nondominant forearm (Fig. 65–7). Fifteen to 20 separate muscle pockets are made, utilizing microsurgical instruments, and the individual pieces of sliced parathyroid tissue are placed into each pocket. Each implantation pocket is then closed with a nonabsorbable suture to provide a marker in case future graft resection is required for recurrent disease and also to avoid extrusion of the implanted graft. Careful attention to hemostasis is important in order to avoid hematomas in the pockets, as hematomas could lead to necrosis of the parathyroid fragment. The total implanted tissue should weigh approximately 100 mg, which is equivalent to the total weight of normal parathyroid glands in the adult. After the implantation of the parathyroid fragments, a portion of the gland is minced and processed for *cryopreservation* (see following section on Cryopreservation).

As a rule, patients who undergo total parathyroidectomy and muscle autotransplantation will have a precipitous decline in the serum calcium level to 6 to 7 mg/100 ml within 48 to 72 hours. Patients with severe renal osteodystrophy are started immediately postoperatively on calcium and vitamin D supplements. Recently, dihydrotachysterol and 1,25-$(OH)_2D_3$ (Rocaltrol) have become commonly used forms of vitamin D replacement in end-stage renal disease patients. If the patients develop hypocalcemic symptoms (perioral or digit tingling, tetany), intravenous calcium should be administered. Once the serum calcium level stabilizes at 8 mg/100 ml or higher, the patient can be discharged from the hospital and followed as an outpatient. As a rule, patients with renal osteodystrophy will require prolonged calcium and vitamin D supplements, sometimes for as long as 6 to 12 months. This is a much longer period of calcium replacement than that required in patients who undergo total parathyroidectomy and muscle autotransplant for primary parathyroid hyperplasia. In 4 to 8 weeks, simultaneous PTH determinations from the grafted arm and the contralateral forearm are obtained, documenting the function of the implanted tissue. Most patients will have a detectable parathormone level gradient between the autotransplanted and the contralateral arm 2 to 6 weeks after implantation. Once a significant gradient is detected, the vitamin D supplement is withdrawn, and if the calcium level remains stable, the calcium supplement is decreased every 2 weeks and is completely withdrawn in 4 to 6 weeks. A PTH gradient between the grafted and nongrafted arms along with maintenance of normal serum calcium attests to the functional viability of the autotransplanted parathyroid tissue. In humans, a gra-

TABLE 65–5. Results of Surgical Treatment of Secondary Hyperparathyroidism

	Total Parathyroidectomy and Autotransplantation			
Author	*Number of Patients*	*Graft-Dependent Hypercalcemia*	*Persistent Hypoparathyroidism*	*Latent Hypoparathyroidism*
Burnett et al., 1977[11]	8	0	0	—
Diethelm et al., 1981[21]	61	0	0	—
Frei et al., 1978[33]	16	0	6	—
Max et al., 1981[53]	16	13%	0	—
Malmaeus et al., 1982[50]	16	13%	31%	—
Mozes et al., 1980[55]	16	6%	25%	19%
Rothmund and Wagner, 1983[61]	46	2%	2%	—
Sicard and Wells, 1983[68]	17	0	12%	6%
Wells et al., 1980, 1977[83, 86]	65	3%	3%	0

	Subtotal Parathyroidectomy			
Author	*Number of Patients*	*Recurrent/Persistent Hyperparathyroidism*	*Persistent Hypoparathyroidism*	*Latent Hypoparathyroidism*
Cordell et al., 1979[19]	36	8.3%	ND*	—
Dubost et al., 1980[23]	10	40%	20%	—
Geis et al., 1973[35]	9	11%	0	—
Lundgren et al., 1977[49]	7	0	43%	—
Malmaeus et al., 1982[50]	30	10%	23%	—
Sicard et al., 1980[70]	14	0	0	—

*Not defined.

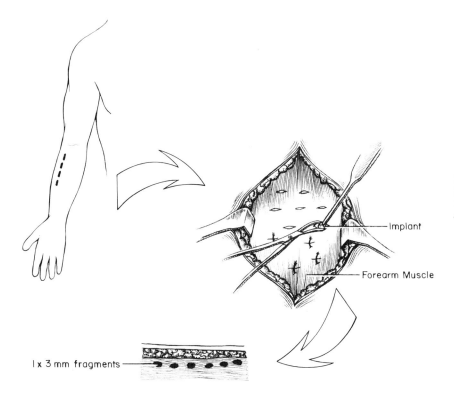

Figure 65–7. In the procedure for forearm muscle autotransplantation, 1 × 3 mm slices of parathyroid tissue are implanted in forearm muscle.

Implant

Forearm Muscle

I x 3 mm fragments

dient of 1.5 to 1 or greater is considered proof of adequate function of the implanted parathyroid tissue.

Cryopreservation. Cryopreservation of parathyroid tissue has gained wide acceptability not only for its investigative applications of parathyroid physiology and mechanisms that control hormone release but also for its potential use in clinical application. Blumenthal and Walsh[5] reported the first histologic documentation of preserved parathyroid glands in cryopreserved thyroid tissue that had been maintained at −70°C. Various investigators attempted the use of various cryoprotective agents and freezing rates of parathyroid tissue with minimal success.[43] Wells and collaborators[82] demonstrated the in vivo function of rat parathyroid glands cryopreserved 3 to 12 months using 10 per cent dimethyl sulfoxide (DMSO) and a slow cooling technique to −80°C, followed by a rapid cooling technique to −196°C. Similarly, Leight and associates[48] successfully cryopreserved dog parathyroid glands for 2 to 9 months utilizing a technique similar to that described by Wells and Christiansen.[82] The function of the autograft was demonstrated by the maintenance of a normal serum calcium and by a PTH gradient between the autografted limb and the contralateral limb. Successful delayed autotransplantation of cryopreserved human parathyroid tissue has been described previously by Wells and associates[84] and Brennan and associates.[7] Wells utilized cryopreserved autograft tissue for 6 weeks and documented the function of the autograft by (1) a PTH gradient in the grafted compared with the nongrafted forearm venous blood, (2) the return from hypocalcemia to normocalcemia, and (3) demonstration of a normal histologic appearance on an autograft biopsy performed 2 years after transplantation. In Brennan's report, suc-

cessful transplantation of the human cryopreserved parathyroid tissue after 18 months of cryopreservation function was documented by both the in vivo stimulation and suppression of PTH release from the autografted arm. The placement of the autograft in the forearm musculature permits the evaluation of function in the autograft compared with the contralateral arm (Fig. 65–8) and also allows the in vivo assessment of the inhibitory and stimulatory effect of various calcium concentrations in the release of PTH by sampling in an antecubital vein.

The tissue utilized for cryopreservation is sliced into 1 × 1 × 3 mm fragments and is placed in a vial containing a chilled solution of 80 per cent tissue culture medium (RPMI 1649) with added glutamine-penicillin-streptomycin, 10 per cent DMSO, and 10 per cent autologous serum. The freezing should start shortly after the addition of the gland to the medium in order to avoid DMSO toxicity, which is commonly seen at room or warm temperatures. The vials are then placed in a freezing chamber,* and freezing is performed at a controlled rate of −1°C/min to −80°C. The vials are then stored in a liquid nitrogen freezer at −196°C. If the cryopreserved tissue is needed for autografting, the tissue is thawed in 37°C bath, and once the crystals have been dissolved, the tissue is immediately washed repetitively with cold saline or cold tissue culture medium in order to eliminate the cytotoxic effect of DMSO at warm temperatures. The tissue is then maintained at 4°C until autografting is performed under sterile conditions.

---

*Linde Biological Freezing Systems, Linde Division, Union Carbide, Indianapolis, Indiana.

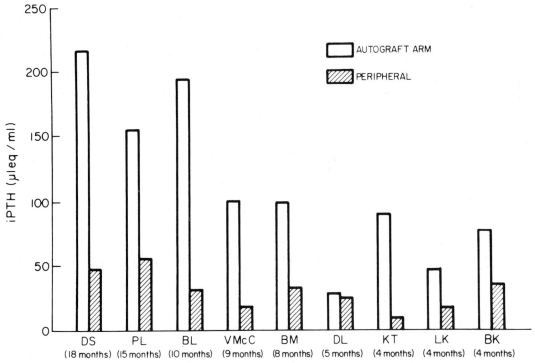

Figure 65–8. Parathormone levels in autograft arm compared with contralateral arm after autotransplantation of parathyroid tissue into forearm muscle in nine patients. The initials in the drawing represent patients' names.

The advantages provided by cryopreserved parathyroid tissue are that it (1) permits delayed autotransplantation of viable tissue if after primary surgery or reoperation no functional parathyroid tissue remains, (2) allows repeated forearm muscle autotransplantation of parathyroid tissue if autografted tissue does not function, and (3) may serve as a possible parathyroid tissue bank for allotransplantation.

Results. Recurrent hyperparathyroidism or latent hypocalcemia is relatively uncommon but should be carefully watched for, making prolonged follow-up necessary for patients who undergo this procedure. The reported incidence of graft-dependent hyperparathyroidism ranges from 0 to 13 per cent (Table 65–5). Fortunately, the placement of the parathyroid autograft in the forearm muscle makes the excision of hyperfunctioning tissue a safer and easier procedure than neck re-exploration, and it can be performed under local anesthesia on an outpatient basis. On the other hand, the reported incidence of persistent hypoparathyroidism ranges from 0 to 31 per cent (Table 65–5). The wide variation in results regarding the incidence of persistent hypoparathyroidism can be explained by the possible loss of autograft function owing to inadequate vascularization of the autograft secondary to hematoma formation in the muscle pockets. If individual pockets are made for each implanted fragment, complications should be lessened, as demonstrated by Wells.[84] Our current practice is not to implant more than two fragments in each pocket and to assure complete hemostasis in the pocket prior to the implantation of the gland.

Tertiary Hyperparathyroidism

After a successful kidney transplant, the renal excretion of phosphorus as well as the active formation of 1,25-dihydroxycholecalciferol [$1,25\text{-}(OH)_2D_3$] normalizes, leading to an increase in the intestinal absorption of calcium and the involution of the hyperplastic parathyroid glands. In most patients the normalization of the serum PTH levels will occur in 1 to 4 months but can take as long as 6 to 18 months. On the other hand, some patients will continue with persistent secondary hyperparathyroidism (tertiary hyperparathyroidism) and progression of bone disease. The persistent hypercalciuria can also lead to significant nephrocalcinosis and irreversible damage of the renal allograft. The incidence of tertiary hyperparathyroidism has been reported to vary from 2 to 41 per cent.[13, 14, 35, 55] Geis and collaborators[35] have reported a 20 per cent incidence of tertiary hyperparathyroidism in their series. Christensen and Nielsen[14] reported marked posttransplant hypercalcemia in 32 (17 per cent) of 188 patients, but only seven of these developed long-term persistent hypercalcemia. In patients with mild hypercalcemia (less than 11 mg/dl) and associated hypophosphatemia, oral phosphates can be used as long as the renal function remains normal. On the other hand, if despite medical management, marked hypercalcemia and hypercalciuria persist, then surgical therapy should be considered.

Subtotal parathyroidectomy has been commonly recommended as the therapy of choice for tertiary hyperparathyroidism. In patients with a long-term well-functioning renal allograft, or in full-matched living related transplant, this may be the procedure of choice. On the other hand, patients with cadaver renal transplants requiring surgical therapy shortly after their renal transplantation, strong consideration should be given to total parathyroidectomy and forearm autotransplantation because the potential for recurrent hyperparathyroidism is considerable if end-stage renal allograft rejection ensues.

REOPERATIVE PARATHYROID SURGERY

Reoperation for recurrent or persistent hyperparathyroidism can be extremely difficult and is associated with a significant morbidity. The true incidence of persistent hyperparathyroidism is unknown and is related to the experience and expertise of the initial operating surgeon. Unfortunately, in the literature the terms "recurrence" and "persistent hyperparathyroidism" have occasionally been used interchangeably, making the true incidence of either very difficult to obtain. Generally, the incidence of recurrent hyperparathyroidism is relatively rare. Clark and collaborators[16] in a literature review found 24 (0.7 per cent) of 3204 patients treated by resection of the enlarged parathyroid gland(s) had recurrent hyperparathyroidism. Identification of patients with the hereditary forms of primary hyperparathyroidism has decreased the incidence of recurrent disease, but even so, the incidence remains considerably high.[83]

Persistent hyperparathyroidism, rather than recurrent hyperparathyroidism, remains the most common indication for reoperation in hyperparathyroidism. Persistent hyperparathyroidism usually results from missing an abnormal gland at the original exploration and rarely from a missed supernumerary gland. The expertise of the surgeon performing the initial exploration, an adequate description (in the operative note) of the location of the glands observed during the original exploration, identification by surgical clips of those glands previously identified, and a thorough evaluation of the patient's family history for other endocrinopathies can help in the preoperative assessment if single- or multiple-gland disease is the cause of the persistent or recurrent disease.

A family history of mild hypercalcemia along with other family members with unsuccessful parathyroid surgery should raise a suspicion of familial hypercalcemic hypocalciuric hyperparathyroidism (FHHH), which has been reported to be present in 9 per cent of patients referred with persistent hypercalcemia.[52] Brennan and collaborators[8] found a higher incidence of multiple-gland disease (37 per cent) in patients referred with persistent or recurrent hypercalcemia than was commonly found in patients at primary operation. Similarly, family history of hypercalcemia or multiple endocrinopathy diseases of other endocrine glands (adrenal, thyroid), the presence of abnormal renal function, and the previous removal of abnormal parathyroid tissue in a setting in which all glands were not identified may indicate the presence of parathyroid hyperplasia. In patients who have been explored by an experienced parathyroid surgeon or who have had more than two unsuccessful neck explorations, the use of localization studies can be very helpful (Table 65–6).

TABLE 65–6. Diagnostic Methods Used in the Localization of Parathyroid Tumors

Noninvasive methods
  Cervical esophagogram
  High-resolution ultrasonography of neck
  Computed tomography (CT) of neck and mediastinum (with and without dye enhancement)
  Thermography

Invasive Methods
  Scanning neck and mediastinum after injection of intravenous [^{75}Se]selenomethionine
  Double isotope scan with ^{125}I and [^{75}Se]selenomethionine
  Scanning after intra-arterial [^{75}Se]selenomethionine injection
  Double isotope scan with ^{99}mTc and ^{201}Th
  Selective arteriography
  Selective venous sampling for parathyroid hormone assay
  Parathyroid hormone assay of aspiration of parathyroid cyst under sonographic or CT guidance
  Ultrasound guided percutaneous fine-needle biopsy of parathyroid gland

Localization Studies

Various noninvasive and invasive techniques have been described in an attempt to localize parathyroid tumors in patients with persistent or recurrent hyperparathyroidism (Table 65–6). Although *esophagography* and *thermography* are simple tests, they have a low localization yield.[64] Most tumors that are detected by barium swallow are extremely large and should be visualized by some other noninvasive technique or easily detected at the time of the operation. Wang[79] found that only 19 (23 per cent) of 83 patients who underwent cervical esophagography had localization by this technique. Brennan and collaborators[8] were able to detect only three (6 per cent) of 51 patients with barium esophagogram abnormalities described as intrinsic defect, and in only two patients (4 per cent) did the defect represent parathyroid tissue. High-resolution real-time *ultrasonography* has been reported to be useful in localizing parathyroid tumors.[26, 63] Unfortunately, in small parathyroid enlargement or parathyroid glands in the superior anterior mediastinum, the results with real-time ultrasonography have been disappointing. The use of [^{75}Se]selenomethionine as a scanning agent for abnormal parathyroid tissue has been described, but the results have been disappointing. The use of a double isotope scanning technique with ^{125}I and [^{75}Se]selenomethionine has been reported to have better results but has not received wide support or evaluation.[29] Recently, the use of a double-tracer scanning technique with subtraction using technetium-99m and thallium-201 has been reported to be extremely successful in detecting parathyroid adenomas in a small series of patients.[32, 90] High-resolution real-time ultrasonography has been reported to be very useful in selected cases of hyperparathyroidism.[71] Similarly, computerized tomography (CT) of the neck and mediastinum is becoming more popular, but its specificity and sensitivity are still under evaluation[22] (Figs. 65–9 to 65–11).

Other more invasive studies have been described to better localize abnormal parathyroid tissue in recurrent

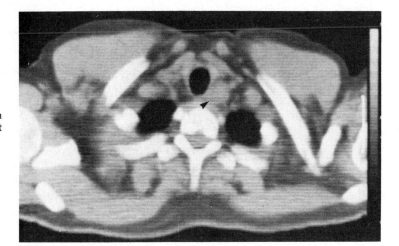

Figure 65–9. CT scan of low neck in patient with persistent hyperparathyroidism. Note large left paratracheal parathyroid (arrow).

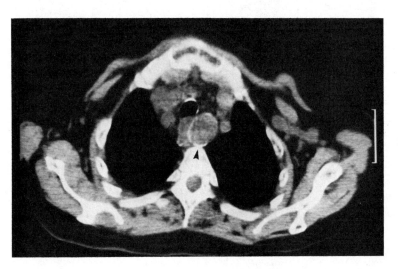

Figure 65–10. CT scan of superior mediastinum from patient with persistent hyperparathyroidism. Note large calcified left paraesophageal mass (arrow). At surgery this was found to be a parathyroid hormone.

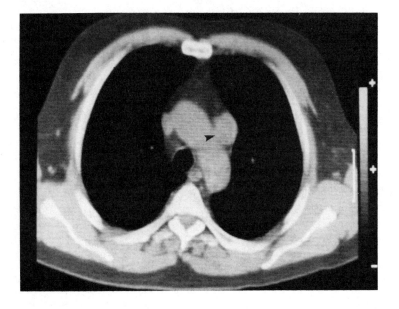

Figure 65–11. CT scan of superior mediastinum from patient with persistent hyperparathyroidism. Note large parathyroid adenoma in superior mediastinum (arrow).

or persistent hyperparathyroidism, some of which have gained widespread acceptance. Intra-arterial [75Se]seleno-methionine scanning has been utilized in patients undergoing localization arteriography and may be useful in the identification of abnormal parathyroid tissue.[74] Unfortunately, this test is not cost-effective and remains of research interest only at the present time.

Selective arteriography and *selective venous sampling* for PTH determination remain the two most successful localization techniques. In an attempt to better localize the abnormal parathyroid gland(s), arteriography should be performed prior to the selective venous sampling for PTH determination (Fig. 65–12). The identification of a parathyroid blush will better guide the radiologist at the time of the venous sampling (Fig. 65–13). In a study of 106 patients undergoing reoperation, Brennan[6] found that in 63 per cent of the cases either the arterial or the venous sampling proved correct in the localization of the abnormal gland. On the other hand, selective arteriography or selective venous sampling alone was correct in only 33 per cent of the cases.

Needle aspiration of parathyroid cysts or glands with PTH determination of aspirate as well as percutaneous needle biopsy guided by high-resolution ultrasound or CT scan has been described, mainly in patients with persistent or recurrent hyperparathyroidism[12, 45] (Fig. 65–14A and B). Except for cases of large parathyroid cysts, this technique should be reserved for unusual cases and

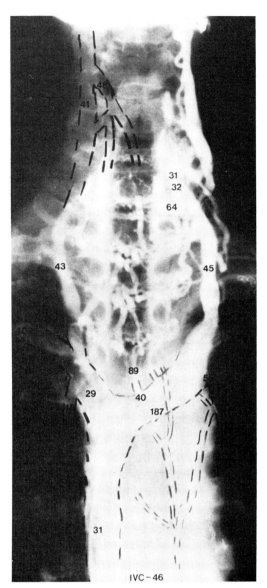

Figure 65–13. Selective venogram with parathyroid hormone (μIEq/ml PTH) values in patient with only three normal parathyroid glands found during original neck exploration. Venous drainage from mediastinum showed high PTH level (187 μIEq/ml). A large adenoma was found in the low superior mediastinum after median sternotomy.

should be performed only by an experienced radiologic group.

The technique of *transcatheter staining* or embolization in the treatment of hyperparathyroidism has proved effective in highly selected cases.[34] In those patients who have mediastinal adenomas with the internal mammary artery as the major vascular supply and who are high operative risks, the technique of transcatheter staining should be considered if it is performed by a highly experienced team.

Operative Technique and Results

Reoperation remains an extremely challenging surgical endeavor and requires an experienced and com-

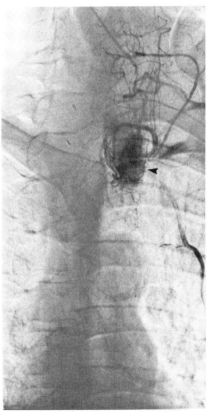

Figure 65–12. Subtraction films of arteriogram of left superior mediastinum. Note increased vascularity (arrow). This was found to be a parathyroid adenoma in a patient with persistent hyperparathyroidism.

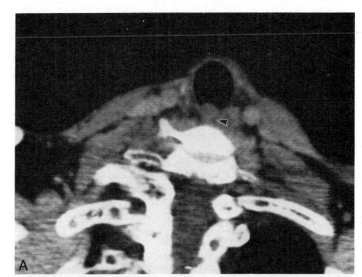

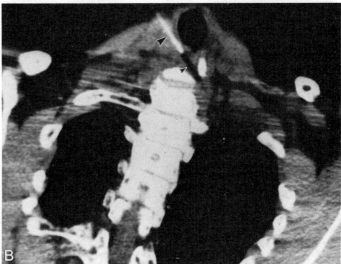

Figure 65–14. Retrotracheal mass. (*A*) This CT scan of the low neck demonstrates a retrotracheal mass (arrow) that proved to be a missed parathyroid gland in a patient with persistent hyperparathyroidism after two explorations. (*B*) Needle aspiration of a retrotracheal mass demonstrated a high parathormone level from the aspirate. At exploration, a large parathyroid adenoma was found.

petent surgeon who is knowledgeable in the anatomy, embryology, and pathology of parathyroid glands. Failure of the surgeon to adequately explore the neck remains the most common cause of unsuccessful primary parathyroid exploration. Another error is the misjudgment of the number of glands that are enlarged, leading to inadequate excision of abnormal tissue. A third common cause of failure in the initial operation is the lack of verification of parathyroid tissue by frozen section, leaving unidentified abnormal tissue behind. However, even when these errors are avoided, a small number (5 per cent or less) of patients still develop recurrent hyperparathyroidism.

One of the most common difficulties in parathyroid reoperation is assessing the total number of glands previously removed. It is not uncommon to find inconsistencies between the surgeon's operative note and the pathology report in reference to the glands removed (for example, inferior versus superior). The strategy and technique used for parathyroid reoperation has been well described by Saxe and Brennan.[65] A small number

of patients may require a mediastinal exploration, for those glands that lie in the anterior superior mediastinum can usually be retrieved through a cervical incision. Edis and collaborators,[27] in a series of reoperative parathyroidectomies, found that 34 (85 per cent) of 40 abnormal glands were retrieved via the neck, and six (15 per cent) of 40 glands required a median sternotomy. Although 21 of the 40 glands were in the mediastinum, only 15 could be retrieved through the cervical incision. Wang[79] reported the experience with reoperation for primary hyperparathyroidism at the Massachusetts General Hospital in 112 patients and found that 89 (81 per cent) of 110 abnormal parathyroid glands were removed through the cervical approach and 21 (19 per cent) of 110 required median sternotomy.

Various techniques have been described to aid in the *intraoperative* localization of abnormal parathyroid tissue. Intravenous use of methylene blue (5 mg/kg of body weight in 500 ml of sodium lactate in Ringer's solution) has gained the most popularity. This technique was originally reported by Dudley[24] and was further popularized by Wheeler and Wade.[87] Devine and collaborators[20] described the use of this technique in patients with persistent or recurrent hyperparathyroidism. In 24 (80 per cent) of 30 patients in which the abnormal parathyroid gland was found, the gland was invariably stained blue. Although it is a potentially useful technique in parathyroid reoperation, its usefulness remains uncertain because the gland must be *visualized* prior to identifying its stain. Other tests, such as the presence or absence of ABO (H) cell surface antigen, determination of deoxyribonucleic acid (DNA), content of parathyroid tissue with flow cytometry, density differences between normal and abnormal parathyroid tissue, intraoperative changes in urinary cylic AMP values, and other intraoperative localization techniques, have been described, but their practicality remains minimal in the clinical setting.[44, 72, 81, 89]

The incidence of permanent hypoparathyroidism remains significant in parathyroid reoperation and has been reported to be as high as 41 per cent.[69] The use of cryopreservation of abnormal parathyroid tissue removed during parathyroid reoperation remains an important adjunct and should help to decrease the incidence of permanent hyperparathyroidism. Delayed autotransplantation of the cryopreserved tissue in those patients who remain hypocalcemic should decrease the incidence of this complication considerably.[66, 67]

Although the need for cryopreservation in the initial operation for single-gland enlargement is not indicated, its use in patients with multiple-gland enlargement should be considered. On the other hand, in parathyroid reoperation the availability of this technique is extremely important because it can considerably decrease the incidence of permanent hypoparathyroidism, which can be very high in this situation. In reoperated patients, when the presence of persistent hypoparathyroidism is documented by very low or absent serum PTH values, delayed autotransplantation of cryopreserved tissue should be performed. Saxe and collaborators[66] described the experience with cryopreserved autografts in 12 patients who underwent autotransplantation of tissue cryopreserved for 2 to 18 months. Seven (58 per cent) of the 12 autografts were functioning, with six of the seven patients requiring no further calcium supplement and the other needing only minimal supplementation. Parathyroid hormone determinations showed that six of the seven patients had a PTH gradient between the grafted and the nongrafted arms of greater than 2:1. The usefulness of this technique has also been reported by other authors.[62, 83, 84]

COMPLICATIONS OF PARATHYROIDECTOMY

Transient hypocalcemia following parathyroidectomy, although common in most cases of single-gland enlargement, usually does not require calcium or vitamin D supplementation. Serum calcium concentration should be checked 12 hours after surgery and every 12 hours thereafter until it stabilizes at 8 mg/dl or higher. Mild or asymptomatic hypocalcemia requires no calcium supplementation. On the other hand, if the patient develops significant circumoral numbness, tingling in the fingers, or a positive Trousseau sign, then immediate calcium supplementation should be started after submitting a blood sample for documentation of the serum calcium level. The presence of a positive Chvostek sign is not a good clinical indicator for calcium supplementation because approximately 25 per cent of normal adults can have a weekly positive response. Prompt institution of calcium supplementation, either orally or intravenously, should avoid the extreme symptoms of hypocalcemia, such as carpopedal spasm or tetany. Untreated severe hypocalcemia can lead to marked laryngeal spasm, stridor, respiratory compromise, and respiratory arrest.

Patients with primary hyperparathyroidism and high serum alkaline phosphatase levels from profound bone disease will commonly have a significant postoperative decrease in the serum calcium level, requiring prolonged calcium and vitamin D supplementation. In these patients, immediate institution of oral calcium at a dose of about 2 to 4 gm of elemental calcium per day as well as vitamin D therapy is important. For short-term therapy of significant hypocalcemia $1,25\text{-}(OH)_2D_3$ should be considered, starting at a dose of 0.25 to 0.50 µg four times a day and adjusting the dosage according to the serum calcium changes. Patients with mild symptomatic persistent hypocalcemia can be treated with oral calcium supplementation (Os-Cal, 500 mg three to four times a day) until the serum calcium remains at a level of 8.0 mg/dl or greater. The patient can then be discharged and the calcium replacement tapered and eventually discontinued over several weeks after normalization of the serum calcium. Nonuremic patients who also require long-term vitamin D supplementation should be started on cholecalciferol, starting at a dose of 100,000 units daily and adjusting this dose as indicated. The advantage of cholecalciferol is that it is relatively inexpensive, but its effect is slow and, once present, remains for 6 to 8 weeks after discontinuation of the drug.[59] New synthetic vitamin D preparations such as dihydrotachysterol (DHT) and $1,25\text{-}(OH)_2D_3$ (Rocaltrol) are faster acting, and their effect ceases shortly after discontinuation. These last two features make it a very useful supplement in patients who require short-term vitamin D supplementation. The disadvantage of these two compounds is their cost, which is much higher than that for cholecalciferol.

Patients who undergo total parathyroidectomy and autotransplantation will have profound hypocalcemia, usually requiring prolonged calcium and vitamin D supplementation. Uremic patients with secondary hyperparathyroidism commonly have profound bone disease and require large amounts of intravenous calcium for various days. We recommend in these patients immediate postoperative institution of Os-Cal, 500 mg four times a day, and Rocaltrol, 0.5 µg four times a day, until a serum calcium level of 8 mg/dl or higher is achieved. Once the patient is discharged from the hospital, frequent monitoring of the serum calcium is important because severe hypercalcemia can occur, requiring the discontinuation or tapering of the Rocaltrol and calcium supplementation. In patients with primary hyperparathyroidism from four-gland hyperplasia who have undergone total parathyroidectomy and autotransplantation, vitamin D and oral calcium replacement therapy is usually maintained for 4 to 8 weeks; then the vitamin D supplement is withdrawn, and if the serum calcium normalizes, the calcium supplement is tapered. On the other hand, patients with secondary hyperparathyroidism from end-stage renal disease commonly require prolonged calcium and vitamin D supplementation, and their persistent osteomalacia may dictate lifelong supplementation despite a functioning autograft.

Hypomagnesemia can occur in patients with primary hyperparathyroidism and can be responsible for persistent and refractory hypocalcemia that is difficult to correct by calcium and vitamin D supplementation. This refractory hypocalcemia associated with magnesium depletion is thought to be secondary to magnesium-sensitive blockade of the peripheral responsiveness to parathyroid hormone or to impaired secretion of parathyroid hormone from the residual parathyroid gland.[39] Parenteral magnesium repletion along with calcium supplementation will allow for the restoration to a normal serum calcium.

Clinically significant injury to the recurrent laryngeal nerve in initial parathyroid surgery remains extremely rare. Nevertheless, the true incidence of this complication is unknown because clinical hoarseness may not be present even in patients who have sustained either paresis or complete transection of the recurrent laryngeal nerve. On the other hand, in parathyroid reoperation the incidence of this complication is higher. Persistent hoarseness postoperatively should be investigated by immediate indirect laryngoscopy. The incidence of significant recurrent laryngeal nerve injury in parathyroid reoperation has been reported to be 1 to 3 per cent.[69] Bilateral recurrent laryngeal nerve injury can be a serious complication, leading to severe respiratory impairment requiring immediate intubation or emergency tracheotomy.

REFERENCES

1. Akerstrom G, Malmaeus J, Bergstrom R: Surgical anatomy of human parathyroid glands. Surgery 95:14, 1984.
2. Albright F, Aub J, Bauer W: Hyperparathyroidism, a common and polymorphic condition illustrated by seventeen proved cases from one clinic. JAMA 102:1276, 1934.
3. Alveryd A: Parathyroid glands in thyroid surgery. ACTA Chir Scand 389:1, 1968.
4. Anderson BJ, Samaan NA, Vassilopoulou-Sellin R, et al: Parathyroid carcinoma: Features and difficulties in diagnosis and management. Surgery 94:906, 1983.
5. Blumenthal HT, Walsh LB: Survival of guinea pig thyroid and parathyroid autotransplants previously subjected to extremely low temperatures. Proc Soc Exp Biol Med 73:62, 1950.
6. Brennan MF: Reoperation for suspected hyperparathyroidism. In Kaplan EL (ed): Clinical Surgery International. Surgery of the Thyroid and Parathyroid Glands. Edinburgh, Churchill Livingstone, 1983.
7. Brennan MF, Brown EM, Sears HF, Aurbach GD: Human parathyroid cryopreservation: In vitro testing of function by parathyroid hormone release. Ann Surg 187:87, 1978.
8. Brennan MF, Marx SJ, Doppman JL, et al: Results of reoperation for persistent and recurrent hyperparathyroidism. Ann Surg 194:671, 1981.
9. Bruining HA: Operative strategy in primary hyperparathyroidism. In Kaplan EL (ed): Surgery of the Thyroid and Parathyroid Glands. Edinburgh, Churchill Livingstone, 1983.
10. Bruining HA, van Houten H, Juffman JR, et al: Results of operative treatment of 615 patients with primary hyperparathyroidism. World J Surg 5:85, 1981.
11. Burnett HF, Thompson BW, Barbour GL: Parathyroid autotransplantation. Arch Surg 112:373, 1977.
12. Charboneau JW, Grant CS, James EM, et al: High resolution-guided percutaneous needle biopsy and intraoperative ultrasonography of a cervical parathyroid adenoma in a patient with persistent hyperparathyroidism. Mayo Clinic Proc 58:497, 1983.
13. Chatterjee SN, Massry SG, Friedler RM, et al: The high incidence of persistent secondary hyperparathyroidism after renal homotransplantation. Surg Gynecol Obstet 143:440, 1976.
14. Christensen MS, Nielsen HE: The clinical significance of hyperparathyroidism after renal transplantation. Scand J Urol Nephrol 42:130, 1977.
15. Churchill ED, Cope O: The surgical treatment of hyperparathyroidism. Ann Surg 104:9, 1936.
16. Clark OH, Way LW, Hunt TK: Recurrent hyperparathyroidism. Ann Surg 184:391, 1976.
17. Cope O: The study of hyperparathyroidism at the Massachusetts General Hospital. N Engl J Med 274:1174, 1966.
18. Cope O, Keynes WM, Roth SI, Castleman B: Primary chief cell hyperplasia of the parathyroid glands. A new entity in the surgery of hyperparathyroidism. Ann Surg 148:375, 1958.
19. Cordell LJ, Maxwell JG, Warden GD: Parathyroidectomy in chronic renal failure. Am J Surg 138:951, 1979.
20. Devine RM, van Heerden JA, Grant CS, Muir JJ: The role of methylene blue infusion in the management of persistent or recurrent hyperparathyroidism. Surgery 94:916, 1983.
21. Diethelm AG, Adams PL, Murad TM, et al: Treatment of secondary hyperparathyroidism in patients with chronic renal failure by total parathyroidectomy and parathyroid autograft. Ann Surg 193:777, 1981.
22. Doppman JL: CT localization of parathyroid glands: It deserves a second look. J Comput Assist Tomogr 6:519, 1982.
23. Dubost C, Drueke T, Jeaneau TL, et al: Secondary hyperparathyroidism: Subtotal parathyroidectomy versus total parathyroidectomy with parathyroid autotransplantation. Nouv Presse Med 9:2709, 1980.
24. Dudley NE: Methylene blue for rapid identification of the parathyroids. Br Med J 3:680, 1971.
25. Edis AJ, Beahrs OH, van Heerden JA, et al: "Conservative" versus "liberal" approach to parathyroid neck exploration. Surgery 82:466, 1977.
26. Edis AJ, Evans TC: High resolution real time ultrasonography in the preoperative location of parathyroid tumors. N Engl J Med 301:532, 1979.
27. Edis AJ, Sheedy PF II, Beahrs OH, van Heerden JA: Results of reoperation for hyperparathyroidism, with evaluation of preoperative localization studies. Surgery 84:384, 1978.
28. Edis AJ, van Heerden JA, Scholz DA: Results of subtotal parathyroidectomy for primary chief cell hyperplasia. Surgery 86:462, 1979.
29. Ell PJ, Pokropek AT, Britton KE: Localization of parathyroid adenomas by computed assisted parathyroid scanning. Br J Surg 62:53, 1975.
30. Esselstyn CB, Levin HS, Eversman JJ, et al: Reappraisal of parathyroid pathology in hyperparathyroidism. Surg Clin North Am 54:443, 1974.
31. Felsenfeld AJ, Harrelson JM, Guttman R, et al: Osteomalacia after parathyroidectomy in patients with uremia. Ann Intern Med 96:34, 1982.
32. Ferlin G, Borsato N, Camerani M, et al: New perspectives in localizing enlarged parathyroids by technetium-thallium subtraction scan. J Nucl Med 24:438, 1983.
33. Frei U, Fassbinder W, Klempa I, et al: Total parathyroidectomy with autograft of parathyroid tissue in treatment of secondary hyperparathyroidism. Proc Eur Dial Transplant Assoc 15:540, 1978.
34. Geelhoed GW, Krundy AG, Doppman JL: Long term follow-up of patients with hyperparathyroidism treated by transcatheter staining with contrast agent. Surgery 94:849, 1983.
35. Geis WP, Popovter MM, Corman JL, et al: The diagnosis and treatment of hyperparathyroidism after renal homotransplantation. Surg Gynecol Obstet 137:997, 1973.
36. Gilmour JR: The gross anatomy of parathyroid glands. J Pathol 46:133, 1938.
37. Glassford DM, Remuers AR, Saues HE, et al: Hyperparathyroidism in the maintenance dialysis patient. Surg Gynecol Obstet 142:328, 1976.
38. Goldman L, Gordan GJ, Roof BS: The parathyroids, progress, problems and practice. Curr Probl Surg (Aug.), 1971, p 1.
39. Habener JF, Potts JT Jr: Parathyroid physiology and primary hyperparathyroidism. In Avioli L (ed): Metabolic Bone Disease. Vol. II. New York, Academic Press, 1978.
40. Haff RC, Ballinger WF: Causes of recurrent hypercalcemia after parathyroidectomy for primary hyperparathyroidism. Ann Surg 173:884, 1971.
41. Heath H, Hodgson SF, Kennedy MA: Primary hyperparathyroidism incidence, morbidity and potential economic impact in a community. N Engl J Med 302:189, 1980.
42. Hoehn JG, Beahrs OH, Woolner LB: Unusual surgical lesions of the parathyroid glands. Am J Surg 118:770, 1969.

43. Huggins CE, Abo S: Preservation of rat parathyroid glands by freezing. *In* Norman JC (ed): Organ Perfusion and Preservation. New York, Appleton-Century-Crofts, 1968.

44. Irving GL, Bagwell CB: Identification of histologically undetectable parathyroid hyperplasia by flow cytometry. Am J Surg *138*:567, 1979.

45. Katz AD, Dunkleman D: Needle aspiration of nonfunctioning parathyroid cysts. Arch Surg *119*:307, 1984.

46. Kelly TR: Primary hyperparathyroidism: A personal experience with 242 cases. Am J Surg *140*:632, 1980.

47. Kuhlback B, Sivula A, Koch B, et al: Secondary hyperparathyroidism and parathyroidectomy in terminal chronic renal failure. Scand J Urol Nephrol *43*:140, 1977.

48. Leight GS, Parker GA, Sears HF, et al: Experimental cryopreservation and autotransplantation of parathyroid glands. Technique and demonstration of function. Ann Surg *188*:16, 1978.

49. Lundgren G, Asaba M, Magnusson G, et al: The role of parathyroidectomy in the treatment of secondary hyperparathyroidism before and after renal transplantation. Scand J Urol Nephrol *42*:149, 1977.

50. Malmaeus J, Akerstrom G, Johansson H, et al: Parathyroid surgery in chronic renal insufficiency. Subtotal parathyroidectomy versus total parathyroidectomy with autotransplantation to the forearm. Acta Chir Scand *148*:229, 1982.

51. Marx SJ, Spiegel AM, Brown EM, et al: Divalent cation metabolism. Familial hypocalciuric hypercalcemia versus typical primary hyperparathyroidism. Am J Med *65*:235, 1978.

52. Marx SJ, Stock JL, Attie MF, et al: Familial hypocalciuric hypercalcemia: Recognition among patients referred after unsuccessful parathyroid exploration. Ann Intern Med *92*:351, 1980.

53. Max MH, Flint LM, Richardson JD, et al: Total parathyroidectomy and parathyroid autotransplantation in patients with chronic renal failure. Surg Gynecol Obstet *153*:177, 1981.

54. McGarity W, Matthews WH, Fulenwider TJ, et al: The surgical management of primary hyperparathyroidism. Ann Surg *193*:794, 1981.

55. Mozes MF, Soper WD, Jonasson D, Lang GR: Total parathyroidectomy and autotransplantation in secondary hyperparathyroidism. Arch Surg *115*:378, 1980.

56. Mundy GR, Cove DH, Fisken R: Primary hyperparathyroidism: Changes in the pattern of clinical presentation. Lancet *1*:1317, 1980.

57. Paloyan E, Lawrence AM, Oslapas R, et al: Subtotal parathyroidectomy for primary hyperparathyroidism. Long term results in 292 patients. Arch Surg *118*:425, 1983.

58. Paloyan E, Paloyan D, Pickleman JR: Hyperparathyroidism today. Surg Clin North Am *53*:211, 1973.

59. Parfitt AM, Frame B: Drug treatment of rickets and osteomalacia. Semin Drug Treatment *2*:83, 1972.

60. Reinhoff WF: The surgical treatment of hyperparathyroidism. Ann Surg *131*:917, 1950.

61. Rothmund M, Wagner PK: Total parathyroidectomy and autotransplantation of parathyroid tissue for renal hyperparathyroidism: A one to six year follow-up. Ann Surg *197*:7, 1983.

62. Rothmund M, Wagner PK, Gunther R: Reoperation bei persistierendem und rezidivierendem hyperparathyreoidismus. Langenbecks Arch Chir *356*:105, 1982.

63. Sample FW, Mitchell SP, Bledsoe RC: Parathyroid ultrasonography. Radiology *127*:485, 1978.

64. Samuels BL, Dowdy AH, Lecky JW: Parathyroid thermography. Radiology *104*:575, 1972.

65. Saxe AW, Brennan MF: Strategy and technique of reoperative parathyroid surgery. Surgery *89*:417, 1981.

66. Saxe AW, Spiegel AM, Marx SJ, Brennan MF: Deferred parathyroid autografts with cryopreserved tissue after reoperative parathyroid surgery. Arch Surg *117*:538, 1982.

67. Scholz DA, Purnell DC: Asymptomatic primary hyperparathyroidism: 10 year prospective study. Mayo Clin Proc *56*:473, 1981.

68. Sicard GA, Wells SA: Surgical treatment of secondary hyperparathyroidism. *In* Kaplan EL (ed): Clinical Surgery International. Surgery of the Thyroid and Parathyroid Glands. Edinburgh, Churchill Livingstone, 1983.

69. Sicard GA, Wells SA: Tumors of the parathyroid gland. *In* Moossa AR (ed): Comprehensive Textbook of Oncology. Baltimore, Williams & Wilkins Co., (in press).

70. Sicard GA, Anderson CB, Hruska KA, et al: Parathormone levels after subtotal and total (autotransplantation) parathyroidectomy for secondary hyperparathyroidism. J Surg Res *29*:541, 1980.

71. Simeone JF, Mueller PR, Ferrucci JT, et al: High-resolution real-time sonography of the parathyroid. Radiology *141*:745, 1981.

72. Spiegel AM, Eastman ST, Attie MF, et al: Utility of rapid measurement of intraoperative urinary cyclic AMP excretion in guiding surgery for primary hyperparathyroidism. N Engl J Med *303*:1457, 1980.

73. Spiegel AM, Marx SJ, Doppman JL, et al: Intrathyroidal parathyroid adenoma or hyperplasia. JAMA *234*:1029, 1975.

74. Stock JL, Krudy AG, Doppman JL, et al: Parathyroid imaging after intra-arterial injection of (^{75}Se) selenomethionine. J Clin Endocrinol Metab *42*:835, 1981.

75. Swanson MR, Beggers JA, Remmers AR, et al: Results of parathyroidectomy for autonomous hyperparathyroidism. Arch Intern Med *139*:989, 1979.

76. Taylor S: Parathyroidectomy: Extent of resection and late results. Br J Surg *64*:153, 1977.

77. van Heerden JA, Kent RB III, Sizemore GW, et al: Primary hyperparathyroidism with multiple endocrine neoplasia syndromes. Arch Surg *118*:533, 1983.

78. Wang CA: The anatomic basis of parathyroid surgery. Ann Surg *183*:271, 1976.

79. Wang CA: Parathyroid re-exploration. A clinical and pathological study of 112 cases. Ann Surg *186*:140, 1977.

80. Wang CA, Castleman B, Cope O: Surgical management of hyperparathyroidism due to primary hyperplasia. A clinical and pathologic study of 104 cases. Ann Surg *195*:384, 1982.

81. Wang CA, Reider SV: A density test for the intraoperative differentiation of parathyroid hyperplasia from neoplasia. Ann Surg *187*:63, 1978.

82. Wells SA, Christiansen C: The transplanted parathyroid gland: Evaluation of cryopreservation and other environmental factors which affect its function. Surgery *75*:49, 1974.

83. Wells SA, Farndon JR, Dale JK, et al: Long term evaluation of patients with primary parathyroid hyperplasia managed by total parathyroidectomy and heterotopic autotransplantation. Ann Surg *192*:451, 1980.

84. Wells SA, Gunnells JC, Gutman RA, et al: The successful transplantation of frozen parathyroid tissue in man. Surgery *81*:86, 1977.

85. Wells SA, Leight GS, Ross AJ: Primary hyperparathyroidism. Curr Probl Surg *17*:397, 1980.

86. Wells SA, Stirman SA, Bolman RM: Parathyroid transplantation. World J Surg *1*:747, 1977.

87. Wheeler MH, Wade JSH: Intraoperative identification of parathyroid glands: Appraisal of methylene blue staining. Am J Surg *143*:713, 1982.

88. Wilson RE, Hanipers CL, Bernstein DS, et al: Subtotal parathyroidectomy in chronic renal failure: A 7 year experience in a dialysis and transplant program. Ann Surg *174*:640, 1971.

89. Woltering EA, Emmott RC, Javadpour N, et al: ABO (H) cell surface antigens in parathyroid adenoma and hyperplasia. Surgery *89*:1, 1981.

90. Young AE, Gaunt JI, Croft DN, et al: Localization of parathyroid adenomas by thallium-201 and technetium-99m subtraction scanning. Br Med J *286*:1384, 1983.

CHAPTER 66

Controversy in the Management of Tumors of the Thyroid and Parathyroid Glands

Oliver H. Beahrs, M.D.

THYROID TUMORS

Many controversies exist regarding the management of thyroid tumors, ranging from the selection of which nodular goiters should be surgically treated to the extent of the surgical procedure when operation is carried out and whether or not additive treatment is indicated following surgery. The various positions have both advocates and opponents. Exactly which position is appropriate is always open to question, but the truth most likely resides somewhere in between. All authors usually express to some extent their bias when reflecting on an issue.

In regard to the issues in this chapter, possibly more questions will be raised than answered. Even though controversies exist in the treatment of thyroid and parathyroid disease, it should be acknowledged that they are infrequently major in magnitude and most often not of consequence to the patient. Actually, in the approach to the problem there is a variance that has little effect on the end result. The physician should use his or her best judgment based on personal knowledge and experience, depending on the laboratory only when necessary, being constantly aware of costs, being conservative, protecting the patient against undue risks, and adequately treating the disease to offer the patient the best chance of cure. This, then, is the art of medicine.

Occurrence

Although nodular goiters are not seen as frequently in clinical practice as during the days when goiters were endemic, the occurrence of nodules in the thyroid gland is not uncommon. Based on necropsy studies, about 50 per cent of thyroid glands contained nodules. In Mortenson's study, 525 glands of 1000 consecutive autopsies had nodules.[9] Primary cancers were present in 5.3 per cent of these nodular goiters, and in 3.4 per cent there were metastatic lesions. Most frequently, these arise from primary cancers in the kidney or breast. The primary lesions in Mortenson's report for the most part were asymptomatic or unknown. These percentages closely approximate earlier figures seen in clinical practice when thyroidectomy was frequently done for any

thyroid nodule. In over 3000 thyroidectomies for exophthalmic goiter, cancer coexisted in 0.5 per cent; in 2229 cases of adenomatous goiter with hyperthyroidism, cancer was present in 1.2 per cent; in 3247 cases of adenomatous goiter without hyperthyroidism when cancer was thought a possibility or unlikely, cancer was seen in 7.4 per cent; and in 3121 cases in which the nodular goiter was symptomatic and not suspected of containing a cancer, it was found in 3.8 per cent.[4] In 605 cases of Hashimoto's thyroiditis operated on, 3 per cent of specimens also contained cancer.[12] These figures reflect the occurrence of cancer in surgical specimens and do not indicate the occurrence of cancer in the general population or in patients with a clinically abnormal thyroid gland.

In 1984, approximately 8000 new cases of cancer of the thyroid were diagnosed, and there were 1000 deaths from the tumor. In frequency, the thyroid ranks about 25th as an anatomic site for cancer. Overall, cancer of the thyroid is not commonly seen and removal of nodular goiter must be done on a selective basis. To remove all nodular goiters (if 50 per cent of adult population has abnormalities) is impractical, unnecessary, and not indicated. Likewise, the occurrence of cancer in nodular goiter is low, and this low risk hardly justifies routine thyroidectomy. At the Mayo Clinic, about 10 per cent of nodular goiters indexed because of clinical findings come to thyroidectomy. Current incidence of cancer in surgical specimens is about 20 per cent.

In the selection of nodular goiter for thyroidectomy, risks other than cancer must be considered. The cosmetic deformity in an exposed part of the anatomy can be a problem for a few patients. Although not seen as frequently as in earlier years, hyperthyroidism is a risk. The magnitude of this risk might be controversial, but it has been variously estimated as being from 10 to 50 per cent, when a nodular goiter is left untreated for years. Lastly, a goiter might enlarge to such a degree as to cause deviation of the trachea or esophagus from the normal anatomic position resulting in embarrassment of the airway or of swallowing. Or the goiter could become impinged in the thoracic inlet or migrate into the mediastinum, causing symptoms due to pressure on vascular structures or other tissue. Decision on the management of a nodular goiter becomes somewhat complex and must be based on multiple factors and not any single one as well as on the overall health of the patient and the projected well-being of the patient over time.

The factors used in decision-making are discussed in the following paragraphs, and the importance of each might be weighed to a different degree by different physicians.

Historical Data

Age. Hayles and associates, in studies of cancer of the thyroid gland in pediatric patients, found that malignant tumors occurred in 50 per cent of those patients having nodular goiters.[8] This high incidence of cancer alone and without other data should support the recommendation for thyroidectomy when a palpable mass is felt in a patient 14 years of age or younger. Assuming that the mass is a discrete, solitary nodule, easily palpated apart from the adjacent thyroid parenchyma in a young patient with many years of life ahead, the most definitive management of the nodular goiter would be thyroidectomy and not prolonged observation or medical management.

Sex. Cancer of the thyroid gland occurs about twice as frequently in women than in men, but nodular goiter itself occurs many times more frequently in women than men. Therefore, a nodule of the thyroid gland in a man should be considered with greater suspicion than one in a woman.

Family History. Although goiter appears to occur in some family groups, it is not considered to be familial in origin. However, the exception is medullary cancer of the thyroid. In about 20 per cent of these cases, the tumor is familial, and in the others it is sporadic.[7] Thus, in a family member with a nodular goiter, with another member having a medullary cancer, there should be no controversy—the nodular goiter should come out. Also, about 20 per cent of medullary cancers function, and this can be determined by the level of plasma calcitonin in the blood. If calcitonin is in the normal range and no lesion is palpable in the thyroid, observation of the patient seems indicated. However, with an elevation of the calcitonin level, regardless of whether an abnormality is felt, thyroid exploration should be considered justified. If surgery is not carried out in a patient without a palpable nodule but with an elevated plasma calcitonin level, very close observation is mandatory.

Personal History. The importance of a history of receiving irradiation to the head and neck area during infancy or early life as an etiologic factor in cancer of the thyroid is of concern. The workshop on this subject at the National Cancer Institute concluded that the risk of cancer of the thyroid in a population group having received irradiation to the head and neck area was four to six times as great as in a population group not having received the irradiation.[2] The magnitude of this risk is most likely overstated, for data from recall studies is highly variable. In the Mayo Clinic recall study, there was no demonstrable increased risk of cancer of the thyroid gland. Nevertheless, patients with a positive history should receive special attention for the development of thyroid disease. The follow-up studies that are indicated in these patients might be somewhat controversial. Most important is periodic evaluation of physical findings, and this is probably all that is necessary. A radioisotope scan might be preferred by some examiners, but as a screening test, it is not justified on a routine basis. A scan will not always correctly identify the correct anatomic location of a small (occult) cancer if one is present. It might be reasonable to consider placing patients at supposed risk on euthyroid doses of suppression therapy, which might have some preventive effect in future formation of nodules or cancer.

Diagnosis

Physical Findings. Certain physical findings are pertinent to decision making. A multinodular goiter, relatively small and asymptomatic and present for many years without significant recent change, hardly warrants thyroidectomy. However, a solitary nodule that has appeared recently and is increasing in size must be considered most likely a surgical problem. Commonly, it is said that a single or solitary or discrete nodule most likely is a cancer, but if the mass is a multinodular gland, the risks of cancer are less. The odds certainly favor a solitary nodule being a cancer, but a multinodular gland can also contain a coexisting cancer at a lesser incidence. Based on surgical experience, what is considered a "single" nodule on clinical examination will prove to be a multinodular gland in 50 per cent of cases.

The physical characteristics of a nodule are important in the decision about management. If it is firm and hard, possibly fixed within the thyroid gland or to adjacent tissues, it more likely is a cancer than if it were soft and cystic. However, it is advisable to remember that about 10 per cent of these cancers have a cystic component.

Coexisting Pathology. As mentioned earlier, cancer, benign nodules, and other disease of the thyroid gland will coexist. Thus, if the patient has a clinical exophthalmic goiter, parenchymatous hypertrophy is present and a cancer may be present as well. Also, in a nodular goiter, one nodule may be an adenoma, yet another may be follicular cancer. Hashimoto's thyroiditis, which may feel like a nodular goiter or a lobular thyroid gland, may be associated with a malignant tumor in about 6 per cent of surgically treated cases.[12] Reidel's struma or fibrous thyroiditis may be confused with a cancer on physical examination, but it is unlikely that a malignant tumor may also be present. De Quervain's or granulomatous thyroiditis is not associated with a cancer. However, in 30 per cent of cases, the process is not painful and will appear as a progressing tumor mass and on these grounds alone may be confused with a cancer.[11] Metastatic cancer will appear in a normal thyroid gland, but other historical and physical facts and diagnoses should make the thyroid diagnosis suspect.

Thyroid Function Tests. Determination of thyroxine levels and other function tests may be of value in diagnosing other thyroid disease but are of no value in confirming a diagnosis of cancer. These tests are frequently done in the overall evaluation of a cancer case, but the results are noncontributory to the diagnosis. To obtain them for diagnosis of cancer is an overutilization of diagnostic capability.

Laboratory Studies. Radioactive isotope (technetium) scans of the thyroid gland are frequently obtained and are of some diagnostic value. The results or the necessity of obtaining the scan may be controversial. One study at the Mayo Clinic showed that in a series of cancers the scan was cold in 61 per cent of cases, neither cold nor hot in 29 per cent, and hot in 10 per cent.[3] In a study by Becker and Southwick, in 63 per cent of scans the nodules that were cold did not correctly identify the anatomic position of an underlying cancer.[5] It is generally recognized that a cold nodule more likely is a cancer than if it is hot or the thyroid is normal. However, it must be remembered that the presence of a normal gland or a hot nodule does not rule out a cancer. A scan is only one parameter to be considered in establishing the clinical diagnosis. But if there are other available data that lead to a management decision, then a scan would be superfluous.

Ultrasonography is of value especially in separating solid from cystic lesions of the thyroid. On the other hand, for many cystic lesions, the physical examination will give comparable information, and it should be remembered in management decisions that about 10 per cent of cancers have a cystic component. If findings by ultrasound or other examination suggests a cystic lesion, then the lesion might first be managed by aspiration. If the lesion disappears and stays away on follow-up, then treatment most likely has been adequate. On the other hand, if the lesion persists totally or in part, then other factors must dictate treatment. Likewise, if a "cystic" lesion reappears after aspiration, surgical treatment must be considered.

Needle and Aspiration Biopsy. Great enthusiasm has been expressed for aspiration by many. In the hands of the expert cytologist, a pretreatment diagnosis (of cancer) can be frequently established. In an environment in which such an expert is available, this approach to diagnosis seems reasonable, but "expert cytologists" are not widely available. Therefore, widespread recommendation for this approach may not be desirable. Also, any false negative reports lead to a delay in the appropriate management in these cases. Data does suggest that the incidence of cancer in cases in which cytologic examination was done is greater than when it has not been used. If this percentage increases too much, it might be reasonable to conclude that cancers in nodular goiter more frequently are being overlooked. Core needle biopsy gives the pathologist more tissue for examination, but it is a more difficult biopsy procedure to perform. Not all pathologists are willing to establish a diagnosis with limited tissue, and the specimen may be inadequate or nonrepresentative. Therefore, open biopsy and removal of the tumor by appropriate thyroidectomy may be the best diagnostic and therapeutic approach. Selection of cases for surgery would be based on the other diagnostic factors that are present. Also, the surgeon would judge the extent of thyroidectomy indicated by the gross findings at operation and also from immediate fresh frozen section diagnosis if the pathologist were willing to make a histologic diagnosis by this technique.

Suppression Therapy. A trial of suppression therapy in the diagnosis of a nodule would be advocated by some doctors. If the lesion disappeared or reduced significantly in size, the trial would be considered fa-vorable for benignancy; if not, cancer would be considered. The value of this approach is controversial because it is uncertain as to what the true underlying disease is. The decreasing lesion might be nodular Hashimoto's thyroiditis, a colloid goiter, or some similar disease. The result of suppression therapy then would be misinterpreted. This author might add that he has not seen what he considered a discrete true nodule tumor of the thyroid gland disappear using this approach to diagnosis.

Treatment

Surgical Experience. The surgical experience within a hospital or institution should hardly be a controversial issue. Nevertheless, if the surgical experience is not extensive and excellent, surgical treatment decisions for nodular goiter must be much more conservative. Today there should be no death associated with thyroid surgery. The morbidity rate should be at an absolute minimum. Iatrogenic injury to the recurrent laryngeal nerve should not occur. Accidental injury resulting in permanent vocal cord paralysis can be prevented by anatomic exposure and preservation of the nerve in the course of an operation. Under certain circumstances, the nerve might be sacrificed to make the operation definitive in the management of the cancer.

Under all circumstances, care must be taken to protect parathyroid tissue. Direct trauma or injury to its immediate blood supply is most damaging to a parathyroid gland. Although it is said that the two superior thyroid and two inferior thyroid arteries should not all be ligated, this is not a contributing factor to parathyroid dysfunction. If the glands are not directly injured, adequate blood supply is obtained from the tracheal and esophageal vessels. Only when a wide-field total thyroidectomy is indicated in the treatment of thyroid disease might parathyroid tissue be in jeopardy. In any case in which parathyroid glands are excised incident to thyroidectomy, they should be implanted or transplanted into the subcutaneous tissue or muscle of the neck or into another anatomic site (forearm). There is documented evidence that parathyroid tissue will function under such circumstances. Permanent tetany is to be prevented if at all possible. In a review of 574 consecutive cases for mortality and morbidity at the Mayo Clinic, there were no deaths, no unexpected vocal cord paralysis, and 3 per cent incidence of tetany. Hemorrhage and infection were rarely encountered.

Management of Benign Tumors. Benign tumors should be treated by conservative thyroidectomy to keep morbidity at a minimum. Upon gross inspection of the thyroid gland on surgical exposure, if the lesions prove to be single and benign, a partial lobectomy would be indicated with excision of the isthmus to expose the trachea just in case airway complication developed, warranting tracheotomy. This approach to such a lesion seems warranted, especially if fresh frozen section diagnosis is immediately available. If it is not and if the surgeon is uncertain of the histologic nature of the tumor, then the best approach would be total lobectomy. But if the lesion proved to be benign, total lobectomy would be overtreatment. Some surgeons might argue always for a total lobectomy. Under any circumstances, the more radical the operation, the greater the risks of morbidity. If multiple lesions are present involving both lobes, then a bilateral subtotal thyroidectomy, double partial resection, and removal of the isthmus is best done. Again, some surgeons would argue for a total thyroidectomy, and even though there are reports that total thyroidectomy can be carried out without morbidity, overall experience does not support this. One could support total lobectomy on one side and partial lobectomy on the other to make a concentrated effort to protect parathyroid tissue. Extending the surgical procedure into the lateral portion of the neck for benign disease is not indicated.

Cancer of the Thyroid Gland

For many years, there was confusion as to the appropriate classification of thyroid cancer, and this led to controversy as to appropriate treatment of any one tumor. The use of many synonyms for similar lesions compounded the confusion. The pathologists of the American Goiter Association (now the American Thyroid Association) met and agreed on four primary types of thyroid cancer. They recommended the classification of (1) papillary adenocarcinoma, (2) follicular adenocarcinoma, (3) medullary adenocarcinoma, and (4) undifferentiated adenocarcinoma of several cellular types. The Association approved the recommendation, and subsequently order has come out of disorder in understanding the biologic behavior of thyroid cancers and appropriate treatment of each type. There is some controversy as to subgroups, such as mixed papillary and follicular and Hürthle cell lesions, but once the behavior of these lesions is studied, it becomes apparent that they fit appropriately into one of the four primary groups. At one time, a cancer of the thyroid was considered as any cancer of the head and neck (most often squamous cell epithelioma). Accordingly, some groups thought radical cancer surgery for the primary lesion was always warranted, meaning total thyroidectomy. Others felt that if lymphadenopathy was present in the lateral neck that a radical neck dissection was indicated. Over the past several decades, the pendulum has come closer to the middle ground, and less controversy exists as to the appropriate surgical procedures. Likewise, the biologic behavior of each type of cancer is better understood; therefore, the operation can be tailored for the particular tumor.

Papillary Adenocarcinoma

Papillary adenocarcinoma is a slow-growing tumor with a good prognosis. Histologically, it is low grade or well differentiated. The lesion is multicentric in the thyroid gland in 20 to 40 per cent of cases. Based on Woolner's study of 1181 cases of cancer of the thyroid, 62 per cent being papillary in type, the most important parameter dictating treatment and prognosis was the extent of the primary lesion in the thyroid gland.[13] This was true even though 40 to 80 per cent of the several subgroups had regional metastatic lymphadenopathy. If the lesion was occult or less than 1.5 cm in diameter, no patient died of papillary cancer in a follow-up of as long as 40 years. Only 3 per cent of the patients died of cancer when the lesion was larger but intrathyroidal, but 16 per cent died when the primary lesion was extrathyroidal involving overlying or underlying tissues adjacent to the thyroid gland. With this favorable outlook, conservative thyroidectomy (total lobectomy, removal of the isthmus, and a partial or subtotal lobectomy on the contralateral side) seems appropriate. This reduces significantly the thyroid parenchyma but permits protection to parathyroid tissue. Also, it would most likely remove multicentric lesions, if present. Practices vary; however, some surgeons would do only a total lobectomy on the side of the lesions and others prefer a total thyroidectomy even though the lesion is single and involves only one lobe. The former seems to be considered undertreatment, and the latter is considered overtreatment.

Because the prognosis of papillary adenocarcinoma is not related to the presence or absence of regional metastasis, radical surgery in the lateral neck does not seem warranted. Some surgeons in the past performed classical radical neck dissection, and others did node "picking" operations. Although these practices persist, a modified neck dissection seems reasonable if metastases are present. A modified neck dissection implies removal of metastatic lymphadenopathy and adjacent node-bearing fascia and fat, thus preserving the sternocleidomastoid muscle for cosmetic reasons and the spinal accessory nerve to preserve function of the trapezius muscle.

Follicular Adenocarcinoma

The prognosis for follicular adenocarcinoma (16 per cent of cases) appears to be related to the presence or absence of blood vessel invasion. This cancer does function and will take up radioactive iodine, more so in the absence of normally functioning thyroid parenchyma. Treatment should then be by total thyroidectomy most often and certainly whenever there is evidence of invasion of blood vessels by the tumor. Resection should be by narrow-field or near-total thyroidectomy, implying a resection that protects parathyroid tissue. Any minimal remaining thyroid tissue could be ablated by a small dose of radioactive iodine, which would not compromise the maximal dose to treat residual cancer or distant metastases.

A contrary view might be to always do a radical total thyroidectomy and have a lesser concern regarding parathyroid tissue. Also, a conservative view would be to do a lobectomy on the side of the lesion, with removal of the isthmus and a part of the contralateral lobe, especially if there is no gross evidence of invasion or none on sampling of the lesion by frozen section. Some surgeons might object to this compromise, but when invasion is absent or minimal, only 3 per cent die of the tumor; when invasion is moderate to severe, 52 per cent die.[13] When distant metastases are present, there would be little controversy that radioactive iodine therapy would be indicated.

Medullary Adenocarcinoma

Medullary adenocarcinoma is a more aggressive cancer, has its origin in the stromal cells of the thyroid C-cells, and is almost always multicentric. The prognosis is related to the presence or absence of regional nodal metastases. The cancer represents 6 per cent of thyroid malignant tumors. There would be little controversy that the primary lesions are best treated by total thyroidectomy. The appropriate management of the regional nodes might be controversial. However, 46 per cent of these patients die of the tumor when nodes are involved, and this supports radical neck dissection as the operation of choice when nodes are thought to be or are known to be metastatic. If a classical radical neck dissection is done, consideration should be given to preservation of the spinal accessory nerve—in so doing there is no functional impairment as a result of the procedure. Difference in opinion exists in the management of the neck in the absence of lymphadenopathy. Observation seems appropriate if the neck is easily and adequately palpated. If not, and there is concern that positive nodes might be present, then an elective (prophylactic) neck dissection might be considered. Six per cent of patients die of the disease even though nodes are negative for metastasis.

Controversy exists regarding appropriate management of cases in which there is an elevated plasma calcitonin in the absence of physical findings indicating a recurrent or primary tumor. For a case not previously operated on, thyroid exploration seems warranted in the presence of an elevation plasma calcitonin. If a patient has had a total thyroidectomy and on follow-up examination has an elevated calcitonin level but no palpable abnormal tissue, the decision is between elective re-exploration of the thyroid area and neck or observation. The decision is difficult to make and has to be arrived at after consideration of all factors in the case.

Anaplastic Adenocarcinoma

These lesions occur in several cellular types, all undifferentiated, that grow rapidly and spread to tissue both adjacent to and distant from the thyroid gland. Most patients die of the disease in 12 months, and almost all die in 36 months. Controversy might exist as to whether or not surgical intervention is justified. Even though surgery is not curative, debulking the tumor might have some value, and freeing up the trachea, protecting the airway, and establishing a tracheostomy if indicated are of real benefit. This might also permit more effective use of radiation treatment of the tumor. Argument might support doing nothing from the surgical standpoint because the outlook is uniformly poor.

Thyroid Replacement Therapy

Euthyroid doses of thyroid medication seem warranted after any type of thyroidectomy for benign or malignant tumors. Myxedema secondary to the extent of thyroid resection or the underlying disease would thus be prevented in all cases. If there is a preventive effect on the further formation of thyroid tumors by the use of exogenous thyroid medication, the patient would benefit in this way. The use of thyroid medication is not critical or expensive, and the medication is taken orally. The controversy concerns whether this should be done in all cases on a routine basis. By practice, it would be better to do it on a selective basis based on the exact pathologic findings and the extent of the thyroidectomy. In other words, if the lesion is small,

well localized, and satisfactorily resected and the remaining thyroid tissue is entirely normal and considered adequate in amount for normal function, then no replacement therapy is justified.

Ablation of Remaining Thyroid Tissue

Real controversy exists in this area. On a selective basis, ablation of remaining normal thyroid tissue is justified, but to routinely do this just because a cancer was present is hardly warranted. Just because the capability to ablate thyroid tissue exists is no reason to do it unless specifically indicated. The cost factor in doing it likewise is not to be ignored. At operation, if it is felt that removal of all thyroid tissue is warranted, the surgeon could do it in the course of the operation. For example, if the lesion is an invasive follicular adenocarcinoma, a total thyroidectomy would have been done. On the other hand, if the lesion was an occult papillary adenocarcinoma with or without nodal involvement and a partial or subtotal thyroidectomy was done, no further treatment of any kind is indicated, and the patient has an excellent prognosis.

Postoperative scans should be done selectively in cases in which residual cancer is thought to be present or distant metastasis exists. If residual thyroid tissue is present in these cases, then ablation of it is justified with the hope that other lesions can be treated with the radioactive isotope.

PARATHYROID TUMORS

From the surgical standpoint there are two areas in which controversies are present in the management of hyperparathyroidism: (1) the use of localizing procedures for the identification of parathyroid glands and (2) the amount of parathyroid tissue that should be resected in the treatment of hyperparathyroidism.

Localization of Parathyroid Glands

A surgeon operating for parathyroid disease must fully appreciate the embryology and anatomy of these glands. It is very clear that the superior parathyroid glands come from the fourth branchial pouch, and they normally descend to positions adjacent to the posterior aspect of the capsule of the upper poles of the thyroid gland. If they overdescend, they do so into the upper posterior mediastinum. Occasionally, they will underdescend and will be in a position above the thyroid pole and adjacent to laryngeal structures. The inferior glands have their origin in the third branchial pouch and normally descend to an area near the lower pole of the thyroid gland. If they overdescend, they may end up in a position in the tracheoesophageal groove or in the anterior mediastinum, not infrequently adjacent to or in the thymus. The normal parathyroid glands weigh 35 to 60 mg; they are well encapsulated, delicate in structure, light to dark chocolate brown in color; and they have a very fine vascular pedicle.

The surgeon who fully appreciates the embryology, anatomy, and gross identification of parathyroid tissue should be able to identify well over 95 per cent of the glands. To use selective venous sampling, arteriography, or CT scans significantly increases the cost of management of the patient's problem. Also, the use of arteriography carries a risk of morbidity. For primary exploration, the use of these sophisticated tests hardly seems indicated or justified. Also, staining techniques are not necessary. In secondary or tertiary operations in which previous exploration was inadequate, CT scans or selective venous sampling might be considered. But even in these cases, a knowledgeable surgeon can find the disease in 75 per cent of cases merely by looking.

Resection of Parathyroid Tissue

There is controversy as to whether solitary parathyroid adenomas exist or whether or not these lesions are merely an expression of diffuse parathyroid hyperplasia. In the experience at the Mayo Clinic, 80 to 90 per cent of cases do prove to be single-gland involvement and require only excision of that abnormal gland and possibly biopsy of a normal gland.[10] An attempt should be made to identify all four glands because in a few cases, adenomas may be present in two or three glands. In following cases for as long as 7 years in which single-gland disease was found, there was only a 1 per cent incidence of possible recurrent hyperparathyroidism. If, in fact, an adenoma was an expression of hyperplasia, a high incidence of recurrence would be expected. Nevertheless, there have been those in the recent past who favored subtotal (3½ gland) resection for "single-gland" disease.

In those cases in which true hyperplasia is present (10 per cent of cases) with involvement to a varying degree of all four glands, then resection of three to three and one-half glands is justified, leaving approximately 100 mg of parathyroid tissue. Controversy does exist as to whether or not the residual tissue should be left in its normal position in situ or transplanted to a new site in the neck or the forearm. To this author, it seems better practice to leave it in situ (from the most accessible gland), describing its location and marking it with a clip or a silk suture. In transplanting the tissue, although function has been well documented, there is the risk of loss.

REFERENCES

1. Beahrs OH: Factors minimizing mortality and morbidity rates in head and neck surgery. Am J Surg 126:443, 1973.
2. Beahrs OH: Irradiation Related Thyroid Cancer. Washington, D.C., U.S. Department of Health, Education and Welfare Public Health Service, DHEW Publications, NO (NIH) 77-1120, 1976.
3. Beahrs OH, Kubista TP: Diagnosis of thyroid cancer. In Cancer Management: A Special Graduate Course on Cancer, sponsored by American Cancer Society, Philadelphia, J. B. Lippincott Co., 1968.
4. Beahrs OH, Pemberton JJ, Black BM: Nodular goiter and malignant lesions of the thyroid gland. J Clin Endocrinol 11:1157, 1951.
5. Becker FO, Economou SG, Southwick HW, Eisenstein R: Adult thyroid cancer after head and neck irradiation in infancy and childhood. Ann Intern Med 83:347, 1975.
6. Cancer Facts and Figures. New York, American Cancer Society, 1984.
7. Chong GC, Beahrs OH, Sizemore GW, Woolner LB: Medullary carcinoma of the thyroid gland. Cancer 35:695, 1975.
8. Hayles AB, Kennedy RLJ, Beahrs OH, Woolner LB: Management of the child with thyroidal carcinoma. JAMA 173:21, 1960.
9. Mortenson JD, Woolner LB, et al: Gross and microscopic findings in clinically normal thyroid glands. J Clin Endocrinol Metab 13:1270, 1955.
10. Purnell DC, Scholz DA, Beahrs OH: Hyperparathyroidism due to single gland enlargement. Arch Surg 112:369, 1977.
11. Woolner LB, McConahey WM, Beahrs OH: Granulomatous thyroiditis (DeQuervain's thyroiditis). J Clin Endocrinol Metab 17:1202, 1957.
12. Woolner LB, McConahey WM, Beahrs OH: Struma lymphomatosa (Hashimoto's thyroiditis) and related disorders. J Clin Endocrinol Metab 19:53, 1959.
13. Woolner LB, Beahrs OH, Black BM, et al: Thyroid Carcinoma: General Considerations and Follow-up Data on 1181 Cases. In Proceedings of the Second Imperial Cancer Research Fund Symposium. Thyroid Neoplasia. London, Academic Press, 1968, pp 51–77, 77–79.

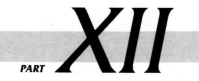

PART XII

Tumors of the Trachea

CHAPTER 67

Management of Tumors of the Trachea

Hermes C. Grillo, M.D.

Primary tracheal tumors are extremely rare, with 2.7 new cases per million estimated to occur per year.[31] Only small series of cases have been accumulated in any single institution. There is even less experience with surgical treatment because techniques that permit adequate resection with primary tracheal reconstruction have been developed only in the last two decades. Thus, 53 primary cancers of the trachea were reported over a 30-year period from the Mayo Clinic,[17] 41 were reported in 33 years from the Memorial Hospital for Cancer and Allied Diseases,[16] 37 were reported from the Toronto General Hospital over 20 years,[28] and 79 cases were gathered from 12 French groups.[7] Perelman and Koroleva[30] reported 76 malignant and 17 benign tumors in 1980. From 1962 to 1981, 110 primary tumors of the trachea were seen at the Massachusetts General Hospital.[15] Another factor that makes it difficult to assess the results of treatment is that one of the two most common types of malignant primary neoplasms in the trachea—adenoid cystic carcinoma—notoriously may have a prolonged course both before diagnosis and after treatment. Few cases have been followed for a sufficient period to be certain that there will be no recurrence. There is an equal paucity of reports of the results of radiotherapy.[31]

Most types of tumors may occur at any level in the trachea, although there are differences in distribution.[11] Adenoid cystic carcinoma often extends far beyond visible disease. Surgical approach to tracheal tumors therefore often involves exposure of the entire trachea. There is little point in arbitrarily dividing the upper and the lower trachea when considering neoplasms of the trachea. The surgeon who undertakes to treat a tumor of the trachea must be prepared either alone or in cooperation with other specialists to view the entire trachea as a single surgical field even if the surgeon should be fortunate enough in an occasional case to deal only with the cervical trachea. Any other approach is likely to do the patient a disservice.

CLASSIFICATION AND CHARACTERISTICS

Squamous cell carcinoma is the most common primary tumor of the trachea (Fig. 67–1). From 1964 through 1982, 43 patients with tracheal squamous cell carcinoma were seen at the Massachusetts General Hospital. There were 33 males and 10 females between 33 and 77 years

of age (mean age, 57.8 years). These excluded patients with extensions into the trachea from squamous cell cancer of larynx, lung, or esophagus. In the same period, 39 patients were seen with adenoid cystic carcinoma (Fig. 67–2). These included 20 males and 19 females who were between 20 and 73 years of age (mean age, 43 years). Adenoid cystic carcinoma was formerly called "cylindroma," which has a deceptively benign sound.

An additional 28 patients were seen with miscellaneous primary tumors. Malignant tumors included the following: one chondrosarcoma (Fig. 67–3), two metastasizing carcinoid tumors, two spindle cell sarcomas, one adenosquamous carcinoma, one malignant fibrous histiocytoma, one sarcoma, two mucoepidermoid carcinomas, and one plexiform neurofibroma. Four additional carcinoid tumors showed no sign of spread (Fig. 67–4). Benign tumors included chondroma, chondroblastoma, squamous papilloma, granular cell tumor (myoblastoma), pleomorphic adenoma, and hemangioma. Small cell undifferentiated carcinoma has been reported as originating in the trachea,[31] but the cases I have seen that appear to be predominantly in the trachea could just as easily have arisen from adjacent lung and invaded the trachea.

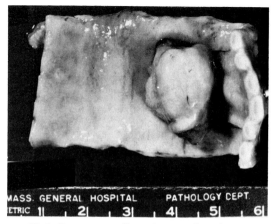

Figure 67–1. Squamous cell carcinoma of trachea, resected surgical specimen. The lesion is exophytic and entirely contained within the trachea. The patient remains alive and well 20 years after resection of the trachea, having meanwhile undergone a right upper lobectomy for squamous cell carcinoma.

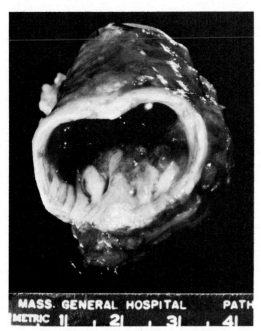

Figure 67–2. Adenoid cystic carcinoma, resected specimen. The infiltrative nature of the tumor is visible here grossly. Additional specimen was resected because of tumor at the margin. The patient was then given postoperative full-dose irradiation. Five years later he developed pulmonary metastases.

Adenoid cystic carcinoma, which is in relative terms common in the trachea, is quite rare in the main bronchi and is even rarer more distally. In contrast, carcinoid tumors are rarely seen in the trachea but are seen quite often in the bronchi.[2] Cartilaginous tumors occur more often in the larynx than in the trachea but are rare even in the larynx.[38]

Like squamous carcinoma of the lung, *squamous carcinoma* of the trachea occurs most commonly in persons in their 50s and 60s. The peak incidence of adenoid cystic carcinoma is about a decade earlier. In children, the most common tumors of the trachea are squamous

cell papilloma, hemangioma, and fibroma. Squamous cell carcinoma of the trachea may appear as an exophytic lesion that is quite circumscribed, or it may spread to involve considerable lengths of the trachea. Several discontinuous foci of squamous carcinoma may be found. Another presentation is as an ulcerative lesion. The tumor may be grossly confined to the trachea or may present with a mass of varying bulk in the mediastinum. Squamous cell carcinoma metastasizes to mediastinal and subcarinal lymph nodes and also directly invades other mediastinal structures, primarily the esophagus. Eighteen of the 43 patients were not surgically explored. In 12 patients the tumor was too extensive for surgical consideration, and in one patient pulmonary metastases were evident. An additional five had had high-dose radiotherapy before being seen. It is not uncommon for a patient with squamous cell cancer of the trachea to have either preceding, concurrent, or subsequent squamous cell carcinoma of the oropharynx or lung.

Adenoid cystic carcinoma is seen as an exophytic lesion, often with poorly defined margins. The lesion may extend circumferentially around the entire trachea. A bulky extratracheal mass may occur. The tumor may displace and compress mediastinal structures such as the pulmonary vessels or aorta without invading them initially. The esophagus may be either displaced or invaded. Adjacent lymph nodes may show metastases, although less commonly than with squamous carcinoma. The most striking characteristic of adenoid cystic carcinoma is its potential for extending long distances submucosally until well beyond what can be seen with the naked eye. It also extends perineurally beyond apparent margins. Frozen section control of the margins of resection is therefore essential. Metastases from adenoid cystic carcinoma frequently extend to the lung. They may enlarge for a prolonged period of time without causing symptoms. Metastases to bone are not uncommon. Brain and other organs may also be involved by the more aggressive tumors. Ten of the 39 patients seen in our series were treated conservatively because of the extent of tumor, the presence of extensive

Figure 67–3. Chondrosarcoma rising in trachea, surgical specimen. This 68-year-old man underwent resection of this bulky tumor, which caused airway obstruction and displacement of upper mediastinal structures, through a curved incision passing over the upper sternum. This allowed for a cervical approach with the addition of an upper sternal division. End-to-end anastomosis was accomplished with cervical flexion.

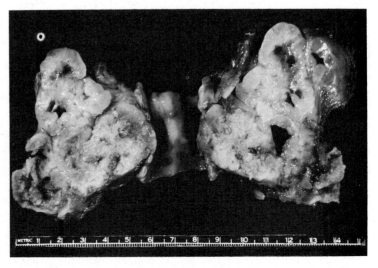

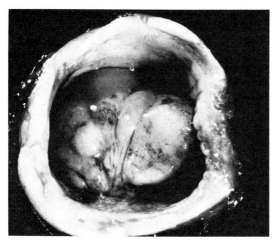

Figure 67–4. Carcinoid tumor of lower trachea, surgical specimen. The patient was 28 years old and suffered from multiple recurrent attacks of bilateral pneumonitis, which responded in each case to antibiotics. A transthoracic sleeve resection was performed.

pulmonary metastases, or prior heavy dose radiation therapy. Three who were explored were found to have tumor too extensive for resection, and in five additional patients it was found impossible to perform primary reconstruction after resection. These were subjected to attempts at staged reconstruction. Adenoid cystic carcinoma may involve the upper trachea and the larynx to such an extent that laryngectomy is also necessary for extirpation. Squamous carcinoma is distributed over all levels of the trachea. Although a wide distribution of adenoid cystic carcinoma is observed, the greatest number occur in the lower trachea and at the carina.

Squamous papillomas may occur in the juvenile in both larynx and trachea but tend to disappear with puberty. In adults, a wide range of squamous papillomas has been observed from solitary lesions to multiple papillomas either in clusters or diffusely spread throughout the tracheobronchial tree. If peripheral, they can cause repetitive instances of bronchial obstruction with sepsis and ultimately may be fatal.

The paucity of experience with the common types of tracheal tumors is accentuated with the uncommon. Scattered observations may be made. Granular cell tumors in the trachea may be accompanied by concomitant granular cell tumors in the bronchi. The growth of benign tumors may be extremely slow. A patient with chondroblastoma had radiologic evidence of the tumor 9½ years prior to diagnosis. During this time he was treated for asthma.

CLINICAL PRESENTATION

Tracheal tumors present in three principal ways: they produce (1) signs and symptoms of upper airway obstruction, (2) hemoptysis, and (3) episodes of pneumonitis or pneumonia. If hemoptysis does not occur, the upper airway obstructive symptoms may be insidious and slow to evolve. In a series of 84 patients with primary tracheal tumors, Weber and Grillo[37] noted the frequency of symptoms to occur in the following order:

dyspnea, hemoptysis, cough, wheezing, dysphagia, change in voice or hoarseness, stridor, and pneumonia.

It is not commonly appreciated that wheezing or stridor, which occurs in 35 per cent of patients with primary tracheal tumors, may be predominant symptoms for some time. Dyspnea on exertion ultimately is present in 54 per cent of the patients. Standard chest x-rays usually show clear lung fields. The assumption is often made that no organic lesion is present, and the patient is often treated for "adult-onset asthma." The signs and symptoms vary with the type of tumor.[26] Hemoptysis is seen prominently in patients with squamous cell carcinoma and therefore leads to earlier diagnosis. Hoarseness as an early symptom may signify advanced disease with recurrent laryngeal nerve involvement. Adenoid cystic carcinoma presents more often with wheezing and stridor as its predominant symptoms, with consequent delay in diagnosis. Only a little over a quarter of the patients with adenoid cystic carcinoma demonstrate hemoptysis early in their course. Dyspnea then becomes the predominant symptom. The mean duration of symptoms prior to diagnosis in patients with squamous cell carcinoma of the trachea was 4 months, but with adenoid cystic carcinoma the mean duration was 18 months. In benign tumors or low-grade malignant tumors, the mean duration of an incorrect diagnosis was 4 years. The mean duration of symptoms with miscellaneous malignant tumors was 11 months. Episodes of obstructive pneumonitis may respond to antibiotics because obstruction is partial.

SECONDARY NEOPLASMS

Carcinoma of the larynx may involve the upper trachea. It may also recur at the tracheal stoma following laryngectomy. Attempts at the radical removal of such extensions or recurrences fail because tumor cells often have permeated the lymphatics all the way to the carina.

Bronchogenic carcinoma that involves the main bronchus may also involve the trachea. Involvement of the carina alone does not make a patient either inoperable or incurable. The patient must be examined carefully for distant disease, and appropriate staging is done at the time of a potential resection. Involvement of mediastinal lymph nodes makes cure unlikely. If nodes are negative, carinal sleeve pneumonectomy or lobectomy may be appropriate.[5, 12, 19] Carcinoma of the esophagus at the middle and upper levels is notorious for invading bronchial or tracheal wall. It is rarely justified to perform concurrent resection of the trachea or carina with the esophageal carcinoma unless it is an unusual lesion that in other respects appears to be favorable and circumscribed.

Cancer of the thyroid—follicular, papillary, mixed follicular and papillary, and poorly differentiated—may involve the trachea. Invasion is usually at isthmic level. Often the patient has had a prior lobectomy, and the surgeon has either knowingly or unknowingly left tumor in or on the trachea. In patients with limited tracheal invasion, even with extension to the lower part of the larynx, palliative resection may be accomplished (Fig. 67–5). If the resection is part of the primary operation, it may conceivably be curative. A relatively small number of patients have been so treated, and it

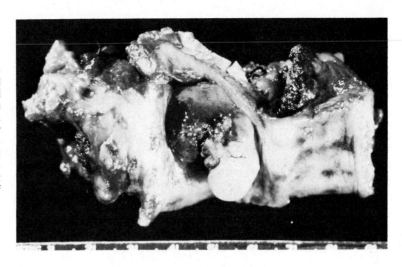

Figure 67–5. Mixed papillary and follicular carcinoma of the thyroid, invading trachea and lower larynx. The patient had undergone total thyroidectomy 6 years before. He presented with a paralyzed vocal cord and airway obstruction. The resected specimen contains recurrent tumor and surrounding cervical tissues, the upper trachea, and an oblique segment of the cricoid cartilage on the involved side. The patient attained excellent palliation with an altered but satisfactory voice for 6 years prior to dying of multiple diffuse bone metastases.

is not possible to be categorical. Resection of the trachea for recurrent or residual thyroid cancer has produced prolonged periods of palliation. Subsequent recurrences have usually been in the bones or other distant sites, justifying such a reconstructive approach.[10, 18] This should not be considered, however, if high-dose irradiation has been given previously.

DIAGNOSTIC STUDIES

Simple radiologic studies, properly performed, will reveal almost all tracheal tumors.[23, 36] Often the tumor can be identified with good radiographic technique in the standard posteroanterior, lateral, and oblique chest x-rays, provided that they are centered high enough to show the trachea well (Fig. 67–6). Overpenetrated, high-kilovolt anteroposterior views utilizing a copper filter in order to obtain greater detail are taken of the entire airway, including the larynx and the carina. A lateral view of the neck in extension shows the larynx and upper trachea. The larynx and trachea are examined fluoroscopically and with selected spot films. The esophagus is opacified with barium. These views usually show the gross extent of the tumor, the presence of mediastinal extension, the extent of trachea that is not involved by the tumor, and the functional state of the glottis. These studies are often amplified with tomography, depending on what additional details need clarification (Fig. 67–7). Intratracheal contrast medium is usually not required.

Computerized tomography has added little to the study of tracheal lesions. It may provide information about mediastinal invasion (Fig. 67–8). In general, transverse sectioning of the airway does not give as good a picture of the critical points about which information is needed: the longitudinal extent of the tumor and the amount of potentially normal trachea available for reconstruction. Xerograms are sometimes helpful because of their precision, but generally they give little more information than do standard roentgenograms. Functional studies of the airway have been of little use but are of interest. On occasion, flow-volume loop changes have led to initial consideration of the presence of an obstructing tracheal lesion.[34] Pulmonary function studies

may inform the surgeon about the patient's tolerance for extended surgical procedures, especially if intrathoracic.

Bronchoscopy and, to a lesser degree, esophagoscopy are essential. If the patient appears to be surgically resectable both from the standpoint of the local lesion and the systemic condition, I often defer the endoscopy to the time of a definitive procedure. Under general anesthesia the patient is examined with a rigid bronchoscope, which provides excellent visualization, using magnifying telescopes. The tumor and the proximal and distal airways are examined. Biopsies may be taken. It is rare for significant bleeding to follow such biopsies, but if it should occur under these circumstances, the surgeon is prepared to proceed as necessary while tamponading the bleeding site with an endotracheal tube or other mechanism. Although massive bleeding has been reported following the biopsy of lesions such as carcinoid tumors, it is rare even in this group. Careful examination of the tumor with a magnifying telescope will give a clue to unusual vascularity. It is essential not to biopsy a hemangioma or hemangiomatous malformation. These lesions are endoscopically apparent. A flexible bronchoscope may be utilized through an endotracheal tube, but in general, the view is not as good. Biopsies are also less satisfactory in size, especially for frozen section diagnosis. Little can be done to control bleeding with such an instrument. The flexible instrument is useful for preliminary observational bronchoscopy if a tumor is suspected from a patient's symptoms. It is preferable to obtain complete radiologic studies beforehand. With an infiltrating tumor, such as adenoid cystic carcinoma, it may be useful to obtain proximal and distal biopsies beyond the obvious gross extension of the tumor. This may well lead to a decision not to proceed with resection if the lesion is too extensive. Esophagoscopy usually adds little.

A rigid bronchoscope is useful for the emergency management of a patient with a tracheal tumor with a high degree of airway obstruction. Under a carefully induced general anesthesia, the bronchoscope may usually be insinuated past the obstructing tumor, and the distal airway is suctioned. An endotracheal tube may be similarly passed if the patient is to have immediate operation. If the extent of the tumor precludes surgery;

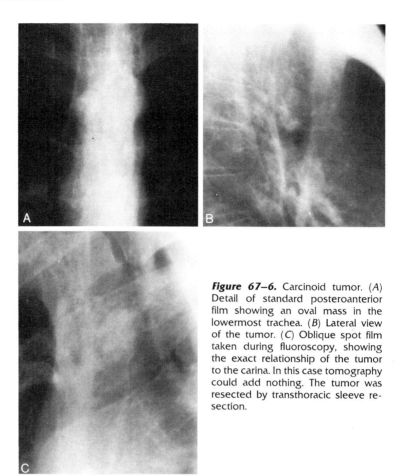

Figure 67–6. Carcinoid tumor. (A) Detail of standard posteroanterior film showing an oval mass in the lowermost trachea. (B) Lateral view of the tumor. (C) Oblique spot film taken during fluoroscopy, showing the exact relationship of the tumor to the carina. In this case tomography could add nothing. The tumor was resected by transthoracic sleeve resection.

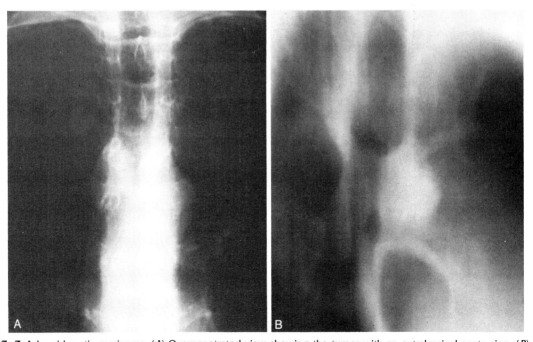

Figure 67–7. Adenoid cystic carcinoma. (A) Overpenetrated view showing the tumor with an extraluminal protrusion. (B) A lateral tomogram, detail. The mass within the lumen may be seen posteriorly extending nearly to the carina. Resection was done transthoracically with the level of division at the carinal spur. Direct end-to-end reconstruction was performed.

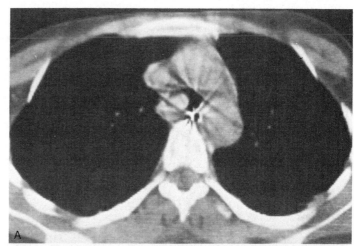

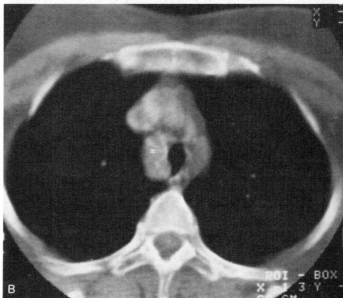

Figure 67–8. Two CT scans of tracheal tumors. (*A*) Carcinoid tumor shown in Figure 67–6. It is intratracheal in extent. (*B*) Adenoid cystic carcinoma shown in Figure 67–7. The compromise of the lumen and the extratracheal extent are clearly seen.

if the patient requires additional workup to determine his or her ability to withstand such surgery, or to exclude the presence of metastases; or if the patient cannot tolerate the surgery, the obstruction may be relieved by removing tumor with biopsy forceps or with the bronchoscope used as a coring instrument. This provides a period of palliation while the patient may be evaluated or radiotherapy commenced. Similar opening of the airway may be achieved with the laser.

SURGICAL ANATOMY

The trachea begins at the lower border of the cricoid cartilage, although the first tracheal cartilage is partly inset beneath the cricoid. The trachea ends at the carinal spur, which represents the midline junction of the right and left main bronchi; those bronchi flair out from the tracheal wall a little more superiorly on the lateral margins. The spur is a useful landmark both radiologically and bronchoscopically. The adult human trachea averages 11 cm in length but varies roughly in proportion to the height of the patient.[14] There are about two cartilaginous rings per centimeter of trachea. There is also 1.5 to 2 cm of subglottic intralaryngeal airway before the lower border of the cricoid cartilage is reached. The cricoid may be identified visually through a bronchoscope with some experience. In a young person with supple tissues, hyperextension of the neck will bring 50 per cent or more of the trachea up into the neck. In an elderly, kyphotic individual, almost no trachea is brought into the neck on attempting to hyperextend the cervical spine. In a young person standing erect, the trachea slopes posteriorly from cricoid to carina but is much more vertical than is the trachea in the elderly. Calcification of cartilages increases with age and with local injury.

The detailed blood supply of the trachea has been described only within relatively recent years.[21, 32] The upper trachea is supplied principally by branches of the inferior thyroid artery, and the lower trachea is supplied by branches of the bronchial arteries with contributions from subclavian, supreme intercostal, internal thoracic, and innominate arteries (Fig. 67–9). The supplying arteries branch anteriorly to the trachea and posteriorly to the esophagus. These vessels arrive at the trachea

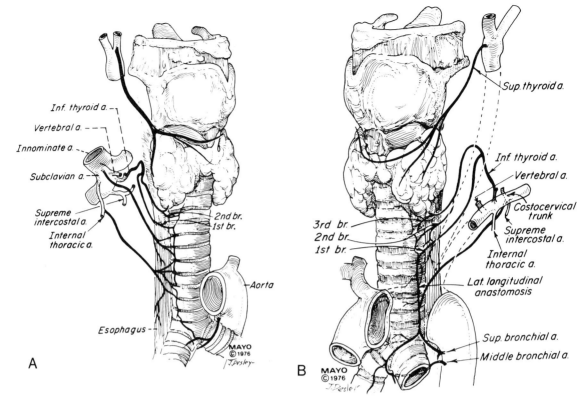

Figure 67–9. Blood supply of the trachea. (A) The lateral longitudinal anastomoses link branches of the inferior thyroid, costocervical trunk, and bronchial arteries. (B) Right anterior view of vessels supplying the trachea. In this specimen the lateral longitudinal anastomoses link branches from the inferior thyroid, the subclavian, the internal thoracic, and the superior bronchial arteries. (From Salassa JR, Pearson BW, Payne WS: Ann Thorac Surg 24:101 and 102, 1977.)

through lateral pedicles of tissue. Longitudinal anastomoses are very fine. Intercartilaginous arteries run transversely, branching into submucosal capillaries. Care must be taken by the surgeon not to destroy the blood supply of the portion of remaining trachea over too great a longitudinal extent, or necrosis will result. These are not theoretical considerations. Such disasters have followed when the surgeon did not take this precaution.

The recurrent laryngeal nerves approach the trachea from both sides, at a sharper angle on the right than on the left. They reach the upper trachea in the groove between trachea and esophagus and then pass medial to the inferior cornu of the thyroid cartilage posterolaterally, entering the larynx at its junction with the cricoid posteriorly.

The thyroid isthmus is intimately adherent to the trachea at the second and third cartilaginous rings. Cancer of the thyroid invades the trachea here. Tumors of the upper trachea may invade the thyroid gland. The posterior surface of the trachea is loosely adherent through areolar tissue to the wall of the esophagus. This becomes fused posterior to the cricoid plate where the esophagus originates just below the arytenoids. Anterior to the trachea at about the midpoint, the innominate artery crosses from the aortic arch to the right side of the mediastinum. The origin of the aorta lies anterior to the carina and arches over the left main bronchus. The recurrent laryngeal nerve at that point lies between the trachea and the aortic arch. The proximity of the major vessels has caused difficulties in the

development of techniques for the reconstruction and especially replacement of the trachea.

Lymph nodes surround the trachea. These nodes are the anterior and posterior subcarinal lymph nodes, and the right tracheobronchial and paratracheal packet, which also has adjacent nodes anterior to the right main bronchus and trachea in its lower portion. The lymph nodes of the left tracheobronchial angle and the right and left upper paratracheal distributions are less prominent. The lymphatic drainage of the trachea has not been as carefully studied as that of the lungs but appears to be generally a regional one to the nodes described. Metastases to both sides of the trachea are not uncommon. Remote metastases from primary tracheal tumors to other lymph nodes in the mediastinum and in the supraclavicular space are not often seen.

SELECTION OF TREATMENT

Data accumulated to date support the approach that both benign and malignant tumors of the trachea are best treated by surgical removal and airway reconstruction.[7, 10, 29, 30] Irradiation is commonly added in treatment of malignant lesions. The application of surgical treatment is guided by two considerations: (1) the potential curability of the disease and (2) the reconstructability of the airway. When there is no evidence of metastatic disease or of extensive local invasion of irremovable structures and when it is clear that the airway can be reconstructed by primary anastomosis, surgical extirpation is in order. There seems to be little point in most situations in exposing the patient to the hazards of extensive tracheal surgery if cure cannot possibly be obtained. A possible exception to this, as proposed by Eschapasse,[7] might be in a patient who has limited pulmonary metastases from adenoid cystic carcinoma in the presence of an otherwise resectable but obstructing tumor of the trachea. The clinical course of such patients may be prolonged over many years. Another exception is palliative resection of thyroid carcinoma in the trachea.

The use of radiotherapy as a primary method of treatment should be reserved for those patients in whom disease is too extensive for cure, who have metastases, or in whom resection would necessitate removal of so much airway that primary reconstruction would not be possible. In general, full-dose radiotherapy will provide the patient with squamous cell carcinoma anywhere from 6 to 18 months before obvious recurrence. Experience is very similar to that in squamous cell carcinoma of the lung. In patients with adenoid cystic carcinoma, the period of relief may be much longer, extending as long as 5 years, although commonly closer to 3 years. Recurrence is most common at the site of the original tumor. Surgical excision is not wise late after full-dose radiotherapy. As will be seen, the group of patients who have undergone surgical excision, usually with postoperative radiotherapy, have the greater number of long-term survivors, possibly with cures, than have those treated by irradiation alone.[7, 10] Preoperative radiotherapy in a more limited dose has been used for adenoid cystic carcinoma,[29] with no clear evidence of improved results.

Early attempts to treat tumors by lateral resection with patching of the defect gave poor results. This was due both to technical failures with leakage and mediastinitis and to early recurrence of the tumor. The concern to leave enough tracheal wall to maintain structural continuity led the surgeon to compromise resection margins. Attempts to replace the trachea with prosthetics have a long and checkered history. Many different materials have been tried. In none have predictably dependable results been obtained.[22, 27, 29] Where initial healing appeared to take place, the patients have later suffered from obstructive granulations or died from erosion of major blood vessels—the innominate artery and aortic arch. Even the currently used intussusceptive prostheses have led to an undue number of deaths from obstructive granulations and arterial hemorrhage. Attempts at staged reconstruction by building interposed cutaneous tubes or other types of tissue replacements have thus far failed more often than not.

Few primary tumors of the trachea, unless they already show metastases or mediastinal invasion, involve such an extensive length of trachea that they cannot be removed and primary reconstruction performed, with the exception of adenoid cystic carcinoma. Squamous lesions involving this length of trachea often have already invaded the mediastinum too extensively to be removed. A truly dependable method of replacement should be evolved for these few but important cases.

When removal is not possible, radiotherapy is the best method of treatment. Chemotherapy has not so far been successful. In an emergency situation, an airway may be established either with a laser or by broncho-

scopic coring, as described earlier. Removal of tumor obstructing the lumen of the trachea, whether by bronchoscopy, cryoprobe, or laser, only serves to crop the obstructing tumor. The tumor remains. Squamous cell carcinoma responds to radiotherapy in much the same pattern as squamous cell carcinoma of the lung. Adenoid cystic carcinoma is more sensitive to radiation in most cases, although this is not universally appreciated. The tumor initially vanishes or all but vanishes. The period of relief may be prolonged, as noted; however, in almost every case it recurs. When tumor recurs following radiotherapy, intraluminal portions may be removed repeatedly for a time by laser. In most cases the tumor will finally also grow extratracheally and push the walls, or what is left of the walls, of the trachea inward. At this point the experienced laser operator recognizes that further removal of tumor will lead to opening into the mediastinum. Additional palliation is obtained in some cases by the insertion of long silicone rubber T tubes, such as those designed by Montgomery.[24] Occasionally, a Y configuration at the lower end may give added time.[39]

A further problem in the management of tracheal tumors is the availability of experienced surgeons. Because of the rarity of these tumors, relatively little experience is gained in training or practice. There is a high potential for complications and death, especially in extensive resections such as those involving the carina.[13]

SURGICAL APPROACH

Anesthesia is usually by inhalation, with halothane preferred, particularly if there is a high degree of obstruction.[8, 40] The surgeon is present with rigid bronchoscopes available so that an emergency airway can be instituted at once if necessary. In most patients with a high degree of obstruction an endotracheal tube above the lesion will permit ventilation past the tumor. If there is insufficient room above the tumor for insertion of such a tube, a rigid bronchoscope can usually be insinuated. In most cases, tumors do not grow circumferentially from the walls of the trachea, and it is possible to pass either a bronchoscope or the endotracheal tube past the tumor along the uninvolved side of the tracheal wall. Ventilation may be easily continued throughout the resection either by a system of tubes across the operative field, which are quite easily managed,[8, 40] or by the use of high-frequency ventilation via catheter.[6] In exceedingly complex resections in which cardiopulmonary bypass might be convenient, the extent of dissection that is required precludes its use because of heparinization. Indeed, in the one patient in whom bypass was used early in our experience because of the complexity of the case, heparinization led to parenchymal bleeding in the two remaining lobes on the operated side; and one remaining lobe on the unoperated side was inadequate to carry the patient. Another experienced tracheal surgeon elsewhere had an identical experience. Bypass is not safe in the few cases in which it might be truly useful.

Positioning of the patient and selection of the incision or potential extensions of the incision are of great importance. In tumors of limited extent, confined to the upper trachea with or without laryngeal involvement, exposure is possible solely by the anterior approach (Fig. 67–10). Adenoid cystic carcinoma extends microscopically for considerable distances beyond where it appears to end grossly. For such patients, even with upper tracheal lesions, it is best to be prepared for intrathoracic extension. For a standard anterior approach, I place the patient supine on the table with an inflatable "thyroid" airbag beneath the shoulders so that the neck is hyperextended reversibly. When there is a possibility of intrathoracic extension of the incision, a support is placed to the right of the midline of the back so that the patient is angled upward on that side. The right arm is then abducted at the shoulder. This will expose the lateral portion of the chest for a thoracotomy extension from a midline incision. The draping frames a surgical field from the chin to a point well below the xiphoid and laterally to the posterior axillary line. A lateral tilt table is used so that the anterior portion of the chest may be horizontal initially.

If the tumor is in the lower trachea or involves the carina, right posterolateral thoracotomy is the optimal incision. Such a tumor may be approached by median sternotomy, between the superior vena cava and the aortic arch, dividing the pericardium anteriorly, and posteriorly retracting innominate artery and pulmonary artery. The exposure, however, is not optimal for an extensive tumor such as one that involves the esophageal wall. Even when the right pleura is open, access to the posterior part of the trachea is inadequate. When posterolateral thoracotomy is used, it is sometimes necessary to have the patient's neck in the operative field so that laryngeal release may be done. In these circumstances no intravenous lines are placed in the right arm,

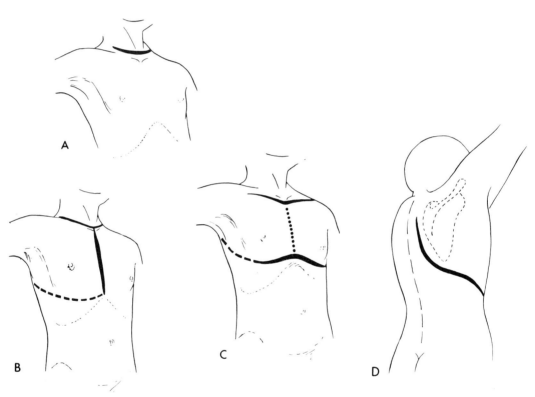

Figure 67–10. Incisions for tracheal resection.

(*A*) Collar incision. The majority of benign strictures of the trachea and neoplastic lesions of the upper trachea are explored initially through a low collar incision. The placement may vary, depending on complexity of the lesion and the existence of open tracheal stomas.

(*B*) Sternotomy extension. After exposure is obtained through the collar incision, an upper sternotomy is sometimes required. Usually this does not extend as far as shown but only past the sternal angle. There is little virtue in a complete sternotomy. The dotted line shows an extension that may be carried through the fourth interspace to provide total exposure of the trachea from cricoid to carina. This incision is now used only for complex cases and has been replaced by posterolateral thoracotomy for lesions of the lower trachea.

(*C*) Occasionally, when it is not clear whether or not a lesion will require a mediastinal tracheostomy, a low horizontal incision is placed so that the anterior cervical skin is intact in case it must be used for first-stage skin reconstruction. A second lower horizontal incision permits raising of a large bipedicled flap. Sternotomy may be done beneath this flap without destroying the integrity of the skin in case mediastinal tracheostomy is required. Extension into the fourth interspace may be used if it is then necessary to expose the carina as well. Occasionally a much lower placed initial horizontal incision will allow for exposure of the neck as well as upper sternotomy with only partial elevation of the flaps and no second incision.

(*D*) Posterolateral thoracotomy. The posterior portion of the incision is carried high because the bed of the fourth rib or the fourth interspace provides the best exposure for major reconstruction of the lower half of the trachea. In complex cases, the skin of the neck is also prepared so that laryngeal devolvement or other maneuvers may be done anteriorly if required.

(From Grillo HC: Surg Gynecol Obstet *129*:347, 1969, with permission.)

and the arm is draped into the field so that it may be turned back and forth for access posteriorly and anteriorly. Right thoracotomy is selected over left because the aortic arch and great vessels make the trachea quite inaccessible from the left. Division of upper intercostal arteries helps little.[1] A rare and special type of carinal problem involving the left main bronchus may be approached from beneath the aortic arch on the left.[13]

TYPES OF SURGICAL APPROACHES

Upper Tracheal Resection

For the anterior approach, a low collar incision is most cosmetic. After initial exploration through the collar incision, additional exposure may be gained by division of the upper sternum to a point 1 or 2 cm below the sternal angle (Fig. 67–11). Partial division of the sternum provides access to the trachea behind the aortic arch and innominate artery down to the carina. Full sternotomy adds nothing. On occasion, a long, curved "smile" incision is placed below the sternal angle. The upper flap may be elevated for the cervical portion of the procedure and yet allow for sternotomy without the vertical incision over the upper chest skin that otherwise is needed.

If access to the entire trachea is required, the incision may be extended by carrying the sternotomy laterally to the right at the fourth interspace to the posterior axillary line. This permits elevation of a trap door of anterior chest wall. The trachea now may be exposed from the cricoid cartilage to the carina behind the innominate artery and vein.

After elevation of the superior flap of skin with platysma, the strap muscles are elevated. If the tumor is invasive, as a thyroid carcinoma may be, the strap muscles are excised with the specimen. A pretracheal plane is established, taking care not to approach its surface too closely where the tumor may lie. Occasionally a lobe of the thyroid is taken with the tracheal specimen if it appears to provide greater margin around a tumor invading the tracheal wall. The pretracheal plane is dissected to the carina to allow for easier sliding of the trachea in the reconstruction. The innominate artery itself is not dissected because leaving its investing tissues over it insures against postoperative hemorrhage from the artery. The amount of peritracheal tissue excised varies with the disease. A compromise may have to be made between leaving behind paratracheal tissue, which may contain positive lymph nodes, and avoiding devascularization of the residual trachea by attempting to do a complete nodal dissection. All lymph nodes adjacent to the segment of the trachea that is to be excised are excised with it. Dissection of that portion of trachea containing the tumor is usually initiated on the side of the trachea away from the tumor. The recurrent nerves are identified and carefully dissected inferior to the tumor. The nerves can then be followed and saved unless directly involved by tumor. This dissection is very different from the approach used for postintubation or other inflammatory lesions. The esophagus is usually left intact, but if the anterolateral wall is involved by tumor, either the muscular wall or full thickness of esophageal wall may be excised with the tumor. The esophagus is reconstructed with two layers of fine, interrupted sutures. Even a markedly narrowed esophagus will serve as a conduit for saliva and liquids. In some cases in which this has been done, the esophagus has later spontaneously dilated sufficiently to function essentially normally even without instrumental dilatations.

The trachea is dissected circumferentially above and below the tumor. If the tumor is in the upper trachea, it is usually simpler to dissect around beneath the tumor initially. Only a small extent of trachea that is to be left in the patient is dissected circumferentially in order to avoid devascularization. If it is impossible to palpate the tumor through the tracheal wall, it may be necessary to rebronchoscope the patient during the operation and mark the limits of the tumor with fine sutures.

Equipment for anesthesia across the operative field is now prepared. Sterile corrugated tubing is passed to the anesthetist at the head of the field, and the distal trachea is intubated with a Tovell armored endotracheal tube. High-frequency ventilation provides a less cumbersome system,[6] although with a little experience the use of endotracheal tubes in the operative field presents little difficulty.[8, 40]

The trachea is opened at a point thought to be below the tumor but on the side of the trachea opposite from the tumor so that tumor will not be transgressed. Inspection is made through the partially divided trachea, and if the incision initially is too close to the tumor, division is done at a greater distance. Prior to division of the trachea, lateral traction sutures of 2–0 vicryl or silk are placed in the lateral wall of the trachea in the midline on either side 1 cm below the expected point of anastomosis. The suture passes through all layers of the trachea so that traction will not tear the endotracheal wall. The divided distal trachea is intubated. The specimen is elevated and dissected away from the esophagus, taking esophageal wall or not, as necessary. The endotracheal tube above is pulled proximally from the operative field. In upper resections a catheter is sutured to the tip of the tube so that it may be replaced through the larynx easily at anastomosis. Proximal transection is completed after proximal traction sutures are placed. An assistant guards the position of the endotracheal tube distally, frequently suctioning to prevent blood from running distally into the lungs, which can occur with the tube cuff inflated.

Biopsies are taken from the residual tracheal ends for frozen microscopic examination to be certain that the margins are clear. It is more conclusive to take these biopsies from the portion of the trachea one expects to leave in the patient than from the specimen that has been excised. If microscopic tumor is present, it may be necessary to excise additional lengths of trachea. However, at some point the presence of microscopic disease must be accepted if further resection would prevent safe primary reconstruction. The possibility of reconstruction may be judged by having the anesthetist flex the patient's neck while the surgeon and assistant each pull upper and lower traction sutures to approximate the trachea. An experienced surgeon can tell whether the tension will be excessive if more trachea is excised. If anastomosis is done under tension, the possibility of separation or stricture increases.[3, 20]

In resection of the upper trachea, additional length may be gained by releasing the larynx. There are two

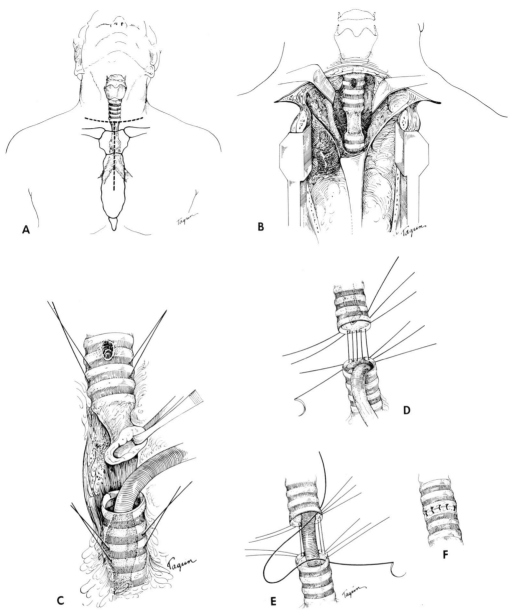

Figure 67–11. Upper tracheal resection.

(*A*) Collar incision and extension for upper sternotomy. Essentially all benign strictures may be most easily resected through this approach, and upper tracheal neoplasms may be resected as well.

(*B*) Dissection is carried anteriorly to the level of the carina. Nothing is gained by dividing the innominate vein. The innominate artery may be gently retracted downward. The pleura is intact.

(*C*) Circumferential dissection has been carried out only immediately beneath the lowermost level of the lesion. Traction sutures are in place, and the patient has been intubated distal to the lesion. The lesion is now being retracted upward to facilitate dissection from the underlying esophagus.

(*D*) Posterior and lateral sutures are placed initially.

(*E*) Anterior sutures are placed after distal endotracheal tube is removed and replaced by proximal tube.

(*F*) Final closure without excessive tension.

(From Grillo HC: Surgery of the Trachea. *In* Ravitch MM et al (eds): Current Problems in Surgery, July, 1970. Copyright © 1970 by Year Book Medical Publishers, Inc., Chicago.)

basic techniques for release. The first is a thyrohyoid release, which divides the thyrohyoid muscles and membrane and the superior cornu of the thyroid cartilage.[4] The superior laryngeal nerves are carefully preserved. Even with preservation of these nerves, a number of these patients develop difficulties with aspiration on deglutition for prolonged periods. I have therefore moved to the use of Montgomery's suprahyoid release.[25] In this procedure the muscles attached to the central part of the superior margin of the hyoid bone are detached. The lesser cornua are divided, and the hyoid is transected on either side anterior to the digastric sling. The stylohyoid tendons are divided. Although this release may not give quite as much length as does the thyrohyoid release, it has a lower incidence of postoperative problems in deglutition. One or 2 cm are gained by this maneuver.

If tumor also involves the larynx, the possibility of partial or complete laryngectomy must be discussed with the patient in advance. This may occur with adenoid cystic or thyroid cancer. It is sometimes possible to obtain a margin around the tumor by beveling the larynx on one side. Margins are checked carefully. Each case must be individualized, so there is no generally describable technique. I partially resect the larynx until a satisfactory margin is obtained. The trachea is beveled inferiorly so that it will fit when mortised to the laryngeal point of division. In such a case the function of one recurrent laryngeal nerve is usually sacrificed if it has not already been paralyzed by the tumor. A nerve stimulator may be helpful in determining whether or not the function of the vocal cord has been preserved in such a high resection. In a case of a granular cell tumor that is benign, it was possible to resect the mucosal and submucosal tissue posteriorly over the cricoid plate where the tumor extended almost to the posterior commissure. The back of the cricoid plate was salvaged, and reconstruction was done by leaving a flap of membranous wall on the distal trachea to cover the cricoid.

Reconstruction is performed with interrupted fine sutures placed so that the knots will be tied outside the lumen. Absorbable synthetic sutures have been free of complications such as granulomas and granulation tissue. I currently use 4–0 vicryl, but other sutures with similar characteristics may function as satisfactorily. Sutures are placed 4 mm from the cut edge of the trachea, usually passing through the cartilage and spaced 4 mm from one another. They are placed serially, posterior to anterior, and are clipped individually to the drapes. They should not cross each other. They will be tied in the opposite order, front to back. Sutures are placed in groups from the midline of the back of the trachea on one side up to the point where the lateral traction sutures will be tied, and they are placed similarly on the other side. The final group of sutures is placed anteriorly so that it will be anterior to the lateral traction sutures on both sides and will not be crossed when these sutures are tied one to the other. After all sutures are placed, the "thyroid" bag is deflated beneath the patient, whose neck is built up into fairly severe flexion by the anesthetist. The proximal endotracheal tube is advanced into the distal trachea. The lateral traction sutures are tied together on both sides simultaneously by the surgeon and the assistant.

This approximates but does not intussuscept the tracheal ends. It is important to avoid excessive tension. Tension greater than 1200 gm in the adult creates a major risk of dehiscence. The child probably tolerates much less tension safely. After initial measurements made years ago using a tensiometer in the operating room, I have depended on surgical judgment for deciding on acceptable tension. This has proved to be dependable.

The decision on whether or not approximation will be possible safely should be made before the resection. If too much trachea has been resected and laryngeal release still has not provided enough relaxation, it may be possible to gain further relaxation by extension of the incision for intrathoracic release of the hilum on the right side. This technique is described later. In general, one does not wish to add a thoracotomy simply for release maneuvers because of the extra hazards involved. Some patients simply cannot tolerate a thoracotomy. Bilateral release would give even more extension, but bilateral thoracotomy is to be avoided because of its great hazards for any patient, even if young and with normal lungs.

The integrity of the suture line is tested under saline with the cuff deflated or placed proximal to the anastomosis. The traction sutures are removed. Second layer closures are not done routinely in the mediastinum. If the thyroid isthmus lies over the anastomosis, it is resutured. If there is special concern about the innominate artery lying adjacent to the anastomosis, a strap muscle may be pedicled between the two.

The incision is closed with drains in the pretracheal and substernal spaces. A heavy suture is placed from a point just beneath the chin to the presternal skin to prevent sudden hyperextension of the neck in the early postoperative period. Most patients are allowed to awaken in the operating room, where they are extubated. Tracheostomy is generally avoided because it can interfere with the healing of the anastomosis and can lead to drying of secretions and to infection.

If intubation is needed, it is better to leave a small endotracheal tube in place. If ventilation is required, the cuff must be placed above or below but not at the anastomosis. If the tube is required only to maintain patency because of glottic edema, a small uncuffed tube is used. If it is thought that a tracheostomy tube will be needed later, it is better to suture tissues over the anastomosis and over the innominate artery and to carefully mark a spot where a tracheostomy tube will later be placed. The actual placement should be deferred, and an endotracheal tube can be used in the meanwhile. This allows time for tissues to seal off the anastomosis and the artery and avoids potential complications from direct placement of a foreign body against either.

Lower Tracheal Resection

In operations for tumors in the lower trachea, a flexible endotracheal tube of extended length is used.[40] The cuff is shorter than the usual endotracheal cuff so that it may be fitted easily within a main bronchus without occluding an upper lobe bronchus or herniating into the trachea. If such a prefabricated tube is not available, one may be fashioned by taking a standard

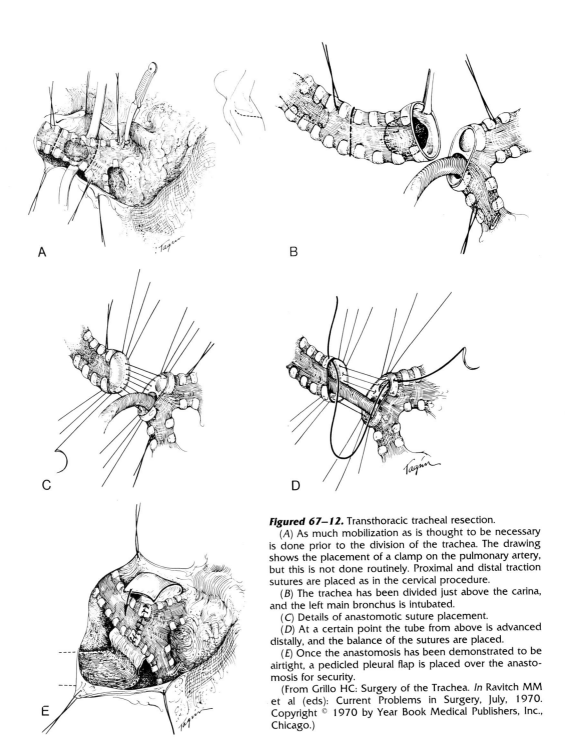

Figured 67–12. Transthoracic tracheal resection.

(A) As much mobilization as is thought to be necessary is done prior to the division of the trachea. The drawing shows the placement of a clamp on the pulmonary artery, but this is not done routinely. Proximal and distal traction sutures are placed as in the cervical procedure.

(B) The trachea has been divided just above the carina, and the left main bronchus is intubated.

(C) Details of anastomotic suture placement.

(D) At a certain point the tube from above is advanced distally, and the balance of the sutures are placed.

(E) Once the anastomosis has been demonstrated to be airtight, a pedicled pleural flap is placed over the anastomosis for security.

(From Grillo HC: Surgery of the Trachea. *In* Ravitch MM et al (eds): Current Problems in Surgery, July, 1970. Copyright © 1970 by Year Book Medical Publishers, Inc., Chicago.)

Tovell tube and connecting it to the proximal end of a cut Rusch tube with a thin-walled metal connecting piece. A double lumen tube is generally too cumbersome for this type of surgery.

The right side of the thorax is entered through the fourth or fifth interspace, the lung is gently compressed, and the mediastinal pleura is opened over the trachea (Fig. 67–12). Adherent pleura is excised with the specimen. The azygos vein is either divided or resected. The tumor and trachea are dissected away from the vena cava anteriorly and from the esophagus posteriorly. Invaded esophagus is excised as part of the specimen. The vagus nerve is sacrificed if it is overlying the tumor, or it is divided to expose the trachea. The right recurrent laryngeal nerve originates high in the thorax beneath the subclavian artery above the point of vagal division. Lymph nodes adjacent to the segment to be removed are left attached to the specimen. Dissection is carried beneath the tumor circumferentially, staying close to the trachea in order not to injure the left recurrent laryngeal nerve, which lies between the trachea and the aortic arch. The anterior surface of trachea is bluntly dissected into the neck. The trachea is transected in the same way as was described for proximal lesions. The tube across the operative field is placed into the left main bronchus in most cases because there is little distal trachea left. This has the added advantage of allowing the right lung to collapse. In low resections, traction sutures are placed in the lateral walls of the right and left main bronchi. After the specimen has been removed and the proximal traction sutures have been placed, anastomosis is accomplished in the same way as was described previously. All anastomotic sutures are placed prior to completion of the anastomosis. The oral endotracheal tube is advanced into the left main bronchus, and the anastomosis is completed. The tube is then pulled proximally, and the integrity of the anastomosis is checked under saline. In thoracic resections a flap of pleura is developed and wrapped around the anastomosis. If there is any question whatsoever about anastomotic security, a pedicled intercostal muscle flap is used. The periosteum must be removed. In one patient in whom periosteum was left intact, it formed a "grommet" of bone around the trachea and required a second operation.

If it is believed that the resection will be of sufficient length to require adjunctive procedures, hilar mobilization is done prior to tracheal division. Mobilization done following resection is more difficult. Sometimes only a portion of the hilar release needs to be done. The inferior pulmonary ligament is divided. A semicircular incision is made in the pericardium inferior to the inferior pulmonary vein. The fibers of attachment that run along the midlateral line of the pericardium to the heart are also divided. This semicircular incision alone may allow sufficient elevation of the right side of the carina so that easier approximation of the anastomosis will be possible. If more relaxation is necessary, the pericardium may be completely circumcised around the hilar vessels front and back. Posteriorly, however, it is done beneath the posterior connective tissue pedicle and lymph nodes that attach to the bronchus. It seems to be important to leave these intact in order to avoid transient lymphatic obstruction postoperatively.

Little can be done from the right to free the left side

of the hilum other than gentle blunt dissection anterior to the left main bronchus. Laryngeal release may be done through the neck, swinging the right arm back, laterally tilting the patient, and gaining access in the semisupine position to the hyoid and cervical regions. However, release of the larynx done in the neck translates very little relaxation to the supracarinal region.

Carinal Resection

Detailed consideration will not be given to the technique of carinal resection and reconstruction because this text is concerned with cancer of the head and neck. Increasing experience has been gained in resection and reconstruction of the carina for primary tumors involving the carina, for bronchogenic tumors involving the carina, and for some cases of secondary tumors.[13] The subject is a complicated one because the exact position of the tumor and its extent in the trachea or in a main bronchus determines what is potentially possible in resection and reconstruction. In some resections no pulmonary tissue has been resected with the carina, and in others concomitant lobectomy, bilobectomy, or pneumonectomy has been done. Reconstructions have varied from the rare reconstitution of a carina in Y fashion to the more common approach in which either the right or left main bronchus is attached to the end of the trachea and the opposite main bronchus is put into a lateral opening on the tracheal wall a centimeter above the anastomosis. In similar fashion, the bronchus intermedius has been elevated also to the side of the trachea in order to preserve middle and lower lobes. As experience has accumulated, a systematic approach has evolved.[13]

Laryngotracheal Resection

In a small number of patients a primary tumor of the trachea or a secondary tumor involving the uppermost trachea will also involve the larynx to such an extent that laryngotrachectomy must be performed. Laryngotracheal resection with pharyngoesophagectomy and concomitant bowel replacement is done for postcricoidal carcinoma of the esophagus. If the tumor does not involve much of the trachea, an end stoma is fashioned in the base of the neck. If a large amount of trachea must also be resected, it is impossible to bring the stoma out of the base of the neck, and mediastinal tracheostomy is required.

Techniques for mediastinal tracheostomy have frequently failed owing to separation of the suture line, too often with subsequent massive hemorrhage from erosion of the innominate artery or the aortic arch. Numerous techniques have been devised to obviate these problems.[9, 35] The technique I favor consists of initial resection through a long transverse incision above the clavicles.[9] A second horizontal incision is made below this, usually at a level above the nipples, although a broad-based bipedicled flap may be made, putting the incision below the nipples and freeing the flap from the chest wall throughout its entire extent. This broad-based flap has excellent vascularity and mobility and can be brought down into the mediastinum to the tracheal end rather than placing tension on the trachea in an attempt to pull it up to the surface. To allow the flap to drop into the mediastinum, the upper portion of the sternum is removed down to the second interspace. The heads of the clavicles on both sides and the cartilages of the first and second ribs on both sides are removed with the sternal plaque. A small circular incision is made in the midline of the flap at an appropriate point, and this is anastomosed with simple sutures to the tracheal margin to form a terminal stoma. The skin incision above is closed to the cervical skin. Inferiorly, there is usually insufficient skin for closure without tension. A skin graft is placed over this defect, which in turn lies over intact chest wall so that the mediastinum will not be exposed if the graft fails. In some cases this relaxing incision is allowed to heal by second intention.

Even with such an approach partial separations and hemorrhage have occurred if the end of the trachea is very distal and lies deeply in the V between the innominate artery and the carotid. In order to avoid these difficulties preoperative carotid and vertebral angiograms are done to determine their patency and the presence of collaterals. Electroencephalographic control is used during surgery as the innominate artery is clamped. If there is no evident change in EEG, the artery is electively divided, and its proximal and distal ends are oversewn with double layers of fine vascular suture material, burying the ends in normal tissues. The omentum is then pedicled from the stomach, using the right gastroepiploic artery as the major blood supply. The omentum is advanced substernally and is placed over the arterial closures described, being interposed between the vascular structures and the trachea and stoma. The upper part of an omental pedicle is brought over the esophageal and pharyngeal closures for added security. It also serves to fill dead space. With these maneuvers (division of the innominate artery and advancement of the omental flap) I have seen no late hemorrhages, even in two patients in whom separation of the skin and tracheal anastomosis occurred because of the need for prolonged ventilation postoperatively. I perform such extensive and destructive surgery only in patients who appear to have a potential for cure.

SURGICAL EXPERIENCE

The length of resection for tumors in the upper trachea varied from 3 to 4.5 cm, in the cervicomediastinal group it ranged from 2 to 6 cm, and in the transthoracic group it ranged from 2 to 7.5 cm. Carinal resections varied in length from 2 to 6 cm. In a group of 32 resections with primary reconstruction five patients had 0 to 2 cm resected, 20 had 2 to 4 cm resected, and seven had 4 to 7.5 cm resected.

Operative procedures varied with extent and type of tumor (Table 67–1). Twenty-nine patients with *adenoid cystic carcinoma* were explored. In three exploration alone was done. Eighteen underwent resection with primary reconstruction, which included 12 carinal resections, four cylindric resections of the trachea with end-to-end anastomosis, and two cylindric resections with partial resection of the larynx. Eight underwent resection without primary reconstruction. There were three laryngotrachectomies. Three carinal and two cylindric resections with staged reconstructions were attempted. The surgical approach in these patients was cervical in four,

TABLE 67–1. Treatment of Primary Tracheal Tumors at the Massachusetts General Hospital, 1962–1982

Procedure	Adenoid Cystic	Squamous	Other
Conservative	10	18	6
Exploration	3	3	1
Resection, Reconstruction	18	19	19
Carinal	(12)	(3)	(5)
Cylindric	(4)	(15)	(12)
With laryngoplasty	(2)	(1)	(2)
Laryngotracheal resection	3	1	1
Staged procedures	5	2	1
Total	39	43	28

cervicomediastinal in three, cervicothoracic in four, transthoracic in 14, plus additional transcervical in four. The lengths of resection ranged between 3 and 8 cm. It is important to note that eight of 19 patients who underwent resection for adenoid cystic carcinoma and survived operation had microscopic tumor found in the margins. Three had histologically positve lymph nodes.

Twenty-five patients with *squamous cell carcinoma* of the trachea were explored. Three underwent exploration alone. Nineteen had primary reconstructions, including three carinal resections, 15 cylindrical resections, and one with partial resection of the larynx. There was one laryngotrachectomy and two attempts at staged reconstruction. The approaches included cervical in two, cervicomediastinal in nine, cervicothoracic in one, transthoracic in 12, and a combination of cervical and transthoracic in one. Lengths of resection ranged between 2.5 and 7 cm.

Twenty-two patients with *miscellaneous tumors*, both benign and malignant, involving the trachea had operations. One was explored only. Nineteen were resected, including five carinal resections, 12 cylindric resections, and two with partial resection of larynx. There was one laryngotrachectomy, and one patient had a cylindric resection with a cutaneous tube reconstruction. The approaches were cervical in seven, cervicomediastinal in three, cervicothoracic in two, and transthoracic in ten. The resections ranged between 2 and 6 cm.

There were 41 patients with secondary lesions (thyroid, lung, esophagus, larynx) subjected to surgical exploration. One with thyroid cancer had exploration only. There were 30 resections with primary reconstruction, including 16 carinal resections, five cylindric, seven cylindric with partial laryngeal resection, and two with wedge resections. The large number of carinal resections reflects primary carcinomas of lung. The large number of partial laryngeal resections reflects involvement by thyroid cancer. There were seven laryngotrachectomies (for cancer of thyroid, esophagus, and larynx) and three attempts at staged reconstruction.

POSTOPERATIVE CARE

The intraoperative course of the patient determines to a great degree what postoperative difficulties may occur. Great attention is given during the operation to preventing secretions and blood from running distally into the lungs. This helps to prevent the need for postoperative ventilation and the sequelae that can follow, including anastomotic separation. The patient is not paralyzed so that he or she will breathe spontaneously at the conclusion of the procedure. Postoperatively, the patient clears the airway by gentle coughing. The patient has been instructed preoperatively in the techniques of chest physiotherapy. If this proves to be inadequate, tracheal suctioning is done gently as often as necessary. A flexible bronchoscope may be used to clear the trachea if other measures fail. It is particularly needed following distal tracheal and carinal resections. The patient is supplied with humidity by face mask. Cervical flexion is maintained with a chin-to-chest suture for 1 week. The suture is then removed, and the patient is advised not to extend the neck vigorously for another week. Feeding is begun cautiously, particularly in patients with laryngeal release, to be sure that there will be no aspiration. Other aspects of postoperative care are routine.

COMPLICATIONS

There are relatively few immediate or early complications of tracheal reconstruction when the operation has been performed precisely without anastomotic tension. Collection of secretions with atelectasis occurs most frequently after carinal resections. Laryngeal edema may occur after procedures that involve the larynx. This may take a week or more to regress. Patients in whom this is feared as a likely possibility because of the nature of the procedure are given racemic epinephrine and inhaled systemic steroids for a few days. All patients are observed for 1 or more days in a respiratory intensive care unit.

Fifty-six patients with primary tumors of the trachea underwent primary reconstruction. Thirty-one of these were cylindric resections with anastomosis, five were cylindric resections and partial laryngeal resections with anastomosis, and 20 were carinal resections. There were four separations of the suture line, which is the most dreaded complication in this type of surgery. Two of these were in complex and extensive carinal resections. In the 36 patients who had cylindric resections with or without partial laryngeal removal, the other major complications were pneumonia in one patient, esophagocutaneous fistula in one, and cord palsies in two. There were six patients with granulations at the suture line, and all were handled bronchoscopically. The majority of the major complications occurred in the smaller group of 20 patients with carinal resection. These included two with respiratory failure, three with partial stenoses of the anastomoses, one with innominate artery hemorrhage, and one with postoperative hypoxemia, which required later removal of a defunctioned lung. There were two with granulations in this group.

Suture line separation or stenosis is most often related to tension on the suture line. If attention is not paid to the blood supply of the airways, necrosis can occur and may cause separation or late stenosis. Minor leakage may seal on conservative treatment.

If tracheal separation occurs in the immediate postoperative phase, a serious technical error must be concluded and prompt reoperation may be considered. Another alternative in the upper trachea is insertion of a T tube or a tracheostomy with corrective surgery to be done months later after regression of inflammation. Resection and reconstruction should not be done in a patient who has had heavy-dose irradiation, which is another cause of separation. Innominate artery hemorrhage should be a rare occurrence after tracheal reconstruction. The danger after mediastinal tracheostomy and in carinal resection or staged reconstructions has been noted. It usually can be prevented in carefully done cylindric resections for benign stenosis or tumor.

The problem of granulations at the suture line has essentially disappeared with the use of absorbable synthetic polymeric sutures. If granulations occur, they can usually be handled bronchoscopically. If stenosis occurs at an anastomotic site it can be managed temporarily by rigid bronchoscopic dilatation. However, if it is a true restenosis, it usually ultimately requires reresection. This should ideally be done no sooner than 4 months following the original resection in order to allow time for regression of inflammation. One anastomotic stenosis occurred in a patient who had suffered partial separation, most probably because he was operated on initially when still on high doses of cortisone for a prior diagnosis of adult-onset asthma. His trachea was later reresected and corrected.

Most deaths following resection with primary reconstruction were in patients who underwent carinal resection. There were four deaths in 23 carinal resections for primary tumors of the trachea. In 37 patients undergoing cylindric resections for primary tumors of the trachea who had primary reconstructions, there was one death. Staged resections are to be avoided.

RESULTS

Because of the long clinical course of patients with adenoid cystic carcinoma it is difficult to speak categorically about the results of current approaches to treatment. Few patients have been followed for the 20-year period that is probably necessary in order to give an accurate statement about cure in adenoid cystic carcinoma. Only relatively small numbers of patients have had contemporary treatment for the other types of primary tumors of the trachea. However, the results attained at the Massachusetts General Hospital are similar to those reported by Perelman and Koroleva[30] for tumors of the trachea in the U.S.S.R.; by Eschapasse,[7] who collected the results of multiple French and Russian groups; and by Pearson and associates,[9] who reported results in a series of adenoid cystic carcinomas from the Toronto General Hospital. The Massachusetts General Hospital results from 1962 through 1982 are as follows: Eighteen patients with *adenoid cystic carcinoma* underwent primary reconstruction after resection. In this group there were three hospital deaths. Thirteen achieved initially good results, and two showed poor results due to stenosis. However, both underwent reresection of their stenosis and achieved good surgical results. As of March, 1983, 11 patients were alive without disease, with a mean follow-up period of 55 months. One was alive with disease at 79 months following resection. Three had died with disease at a mean period of 108 months following resection. It is of note that for seven patients who did not have resection but received radiotherapy the mean survival time was only 45 months.

Of 19 patients who had *squamous cell carcinoma* that was resected primarily and reconstructed, there were two hospital deaths. There were 15 good results and two poor results. These two suffered stenosis and were reresected and achieved good surgical results. In follow-up in 1983 there were eight patients alive without disease at a mean period of 64 months, two alive with metastatic disease, one who had died without disease of other causes, and five who had died with disease in a mean period of 20 months following surgery. In comparison, 18 patients who did not have surgical resection but did receive radiotherapy died in a mean period of 8 months following treatment.

There is not a great deal of meaning to grouping together the wide variety of cases of *other types of tumors*, but the figures are of some general interest. Nineteen patients underwent primary reconstruction after resection, with one hospital death. Sixteen attained good results, and two had poor results. One of these had an anastomotic stenosis and was reresected later with good results. The second one had had a carinal resection with exclusion of the left lung. This caused hypoxemia and tachycardia and later had to be resected to give a good surgical result. Of this group of patients, 15 were alive without disease at a mean period of 67 months. Three had died of disease: one of mucoepidermoid carcinoma, one with spindle cell sarcoma, and one with adeno-squamous carcinoma.

At the present time in the light of these results and the experience of others cited, I recommend that surgical excision be considered the primary mode of treatment for all primary tracheal tumors that can be surgically resected with primary end-to-end anastomosis. In patients with adenoid cystic carcinoma and squamous cell carcinoma who have limited surgical margins, evidence of submucosal or perineural extension, or positive lymph nodes, full-dose postoperative mediastinal radiotherapy should be added. If primary reconstruction does not appear to be feasible, the patient is probably better served at this stage of surgical development by primary treatment with radiotherapy.

Tracheal resection with reconstruction should be considered for selected secondary tumors involving the trachea either when cure appears to be feasible or when long-term palliation is possible, as in resectable carcinoma of the thyroid or in bronchogenic carcinoma with negative mediastinoscopy.

REFERENCES

1. Bjork VO, Rodriguez LE: Reconstruction of the trachea and bifurcation. J Thorac Surg 35:596, 1958.
2. Briselli M, Mark GJ, Grillo HC: Tracheal carcinoids. Cancer 42:2870, 1978.
3. Cantrell JR, Folse JR: The repair of circumferential defects of the trachea by direct anastomosis: Experimental evaluation. J Thorac Cardiovasc Surg 42:589, 1961.
4. Dedo HH, Fishman NH: Laryngeal release and sleeve resection for tracheal stenosis. Ann Otol Rhinol Laryngol 78:285, 1969.
5. Deslauriers J, Beaulieu M, Benazera A, McClish A: Sleeve pneumonectomy for bronchogenic carcinoma. Ann Thorac Surg 28:465, 1979.
6. El-Baz N, Faro RS, Ivankovich AD, et al: One-lung high frequency ventilation for tracheoplasty and bronchoplasty. Ann Thorac Surg 34:516, 1982.
7. Eschapasse H: Les tumeurs tracheales primitives. Traitement chirurgical. Rev Fr Malad Resp 2:425, 1974.
8. Geffin B, Bland J, Grillo HC: Anesthetic management of tracheal resection and reconstruction. Anesth Analg 48:884, 1969.
9. Grillo HC: Terminal or mural tracheostomy in the anterior mediastinum. J Thorac Cardiovasc Surg 51:422, 1966.
10. Grillo HC: Tracheal tumors. Surgical management. Ann Thorac Surg 26:112, 1978.
11. Grillo HC: Tumors of the cervical trachea. In Suen JY, Myers EN (eds): Cancer of the Head and Neck. New York, Churchill Livingstone Publishers, 1981.
12. Grillo HC: Management of tracheal tumors. Am J Surg 143:697, 1982.
13. Grillo HC: Carinal reconstruction. Ann Thorac Surg 34:356, 1982.
14. Grillo HC: Tracheal anatomy and surgical approaches. In Shields TN (ed): Textbook of General Thoracic Surgery. 2nd ed. Philadelphia, Lea & Febiger, 1983.
15. Grillo HC: Tracheal surgery. Scand J Thorac Cardiovasc Surg 17:67, 1983.
16. Hajdu SI, Huvos AG, Goodner JT, et al: Carcinoma of the trachea. Clinicopathologic study of 41 cases. Cancer 25:1448, 1970.
17. Houston HE, Payne WS, Harrison EG Jr, Olsen AM: Primary cancers of the trachea. Arch Surg 99:132, 1969.
18. Ishihara T, Ikeda T, Inoue H, Fukai S: Resection of cancer of lung and carina. J Thorac Cardiovasc Surg 73:936, 1977.
19. Jensik RJ, Faber P, Milloy FJ, Goldin MD: Tracheal sleeve pneumonectomy for advanced carcinoma of the lung. Surg Gynecol Obstet 134:231, 1972.
20. Maeda M, Grillo HC: Effect of tension on tracheal growth after resection and anastomosis in puppies. J Thorac Cardiovasc Surg 65:658, 1973.
21. Miura T, Grillo HC: The contribution of the inferior thyroid artery to the blood supply of the human trachea. Surg Gynecol Obstet 123:99, 1966.
22. Moghissi K: Tracheal reconstruction with a prosthesis of Marlex mesh and pericardium. J Thorac Cardiovasc Surg 69:499, 1975.
23. Momose KJ, MacMillan AS Jr: Roentgenologic investigations of the larynx and trachea. Radiol Clin North Am 16:321, 1978.
24. Montgomery WW: Reconstruction of the cervical trachea. Ann Otol 73:5, 1964.
25. Montgomery WW: Suprahyoid release for tracheal anastomosis. Arch Otol 99:255, 1974.
26. Morgan RJ, Grillo HC: Clinical presentation of primary tracheal tumors—a frequently misdiagnosed entity (unpublished).
27. Neville WE, Bolanowski PJ, Soltanzadeh H: Prosthetic reconstruction of the trachea and carina. J Thorac Cardiovasc Surg 72:525, 1976.
28. Pearson FG: Techniques in the surgery of the trachea. In Smith RE, Williams WG (eds): Surgery of the Lung. The Coventry Conference. Proceedings of a conference held at the Postgraduate Medical Centre, Coventry. London, Butterworths, 1974.
29. Pearson FG, Thompson DW, Weissberg D, et al: Adenoid cystic carcinoma of the trachea. Experience with 16 patients managed by tracheal resection. Ann Thorac Surg 18:16, 1974.
30. Perelman MI, Koroleva N: Surgery of the trachea. World J Surg 4:583, 1980.
31. Rostom AY, Morgan RL: Results of treating primary tumours of the trachea by irradiation. Thorax 33:387, 1978.
32. Salassa JR, Pearson BW, Payne WS: Gross and microscopical blood supply of the trachea. Ann Thorac Surg 24:100, 1977.
33. Sisson GA, Straehley CJ Jr, Johnson NE: Mediastinal dissection for recurrent cancer after laryngectomy. Laryngoscope 72:1064, 1962.
34. Strieder DJ: Case records of the Massachusetts General Hospital, Case 42—1975. N Engl J Med 293:866, 1975.
35. Waddell WR, Cannon B: Technic for surgical excision of the trachea and establishment of sternal tracheostomy. Ann Surg 149:1, 1959.
36. Weber AL, Grillo HC: Tracheal tumor: Radiological, clinical and pathological evaluation. Adv Otol Rhinol Laryngol 24:75, 1977.
37. Weber AL, Grillo HC: Tracheal tumors: A radiological, clinical and pathological evaluation of 84 cases. Radiol Clin North Am 16:227, 1978.
38. Weber AL, Shortsleeve M, Goodman M, et al: Cartilaginous tumors of the larynx and trachea. Radiol Clin North Am 16:261, 1978.
39. Westaby S, Shepherd MP: Palliation of intrathoracic tracheal compression with a silastic tracheobronchial stent. Thorax 38:314, 1983.
40. Wilson RS: Tracheostomy and tracheal reconstruction. In Kaplan JA (ed): Thoracic Anesthesia. New York, Churchill Livingstone Publishers, 1983.

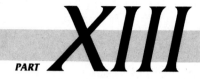

PART *XIII*

Tumors of the Eye, Orbit, and Lacrimal Apparatus

Clinical Evaluation and Pathology of Tumors of the Eye, Orbit, and Lacrimal Apparatus

Jack Rootman, M.D. • Larry H. Allen, M.D.

A detailed description of tumors of the orbit and lacrimal system is beyond the scope of a single chapter. I have therefore chosen to emphasize the broad classification, unique location, clinical features, and methods of investigation as applied to this locale. All tumors exert their effect by virtue of unrestrained or inappropriate growth, infiltration, and metastatic potential. These factors and the unique nature of this location govern the effect of tumors on the sensitive physiology of the visual apparatus. The complex of neurosensory, motor, and secretory structures within the orbit are tightly confined within 30 cm^3, surrounded by bone, nasal sinuses, and the intracranial contents. Disease may originate from or affect any of these spaces independently or conjointly, leading to deterioration of visual or ocular function. The role of the clinical oncologist is to determine the primary site, extent, secondary effects, and the histologic nature of tumors in this location in order to define a rational therapeutic approach.

ANATOMIC CONSIDERATIONS

Bony Anatomy

The orbit is pyramidal in shape with a quadrangular anterior opening with the optic canal and superior orbital fissure at the apex. The roof is made up of the lesser wing of sphenoid and frontal bone and may have a posterior extension of the frontal sinus anteriorly. Apically, the lesser wing contains the optic canal, which is 10 to 12 mm in length and at an axis of 36 degrees to the sagittal plane. Anterolaterally is the lacrimal fossa just above the frontozygomatic suture line.

The lateral wall is made of the greater wing of sphenoid, frontal, and zygomatic bones and is 45 degrees to the medial wall. Posteriorly, it is separated from the roof by the superior orbital fissure and from the floor by the inferior orbital fissures. The medial wall is the thinnest and is made of the maxilla, lacrimal, ethmoid, and lesser wing of sphenoid. The anterior and posterior ethmoid foramina penetrate it and mark the level of the cribriform plate at the frontoethmoid suture line. The ethmoid and frequently the sphenoid (posteriorly) and maxillary (anteriorly) sinuses form the wall.

The floor is shorter, is triangular, and is made up of the maxillary, zygomatic, and palatine bones. It contains the infraorbital sulcus and fissure, which extends forward from the inferior orbital canal opening on the maxilla as the infraorbital foramen. The inferior orbital fissure communicates with the pterygopalatine and infratemporal fossae. Anteromedially is the nasolacrimal fossa and nasolacrimal duct formed by the lacrimal and maxillary bones. It contains the lacrimal sac, which drains into the duct. The duct is 17 to 20 mm long and runs inferolaterally and 15 degrees posteriorly, where it opens under the inferior turbinate. Table 68–1 summarizes the sites and contents of the orbital fissures and canals.

Periorbita and Septa

The periosteum, or periorbita, is generally loosely adherent to the surrounding bones. It is continuous posteriorly with the dura of the optic nerve and that surrounding the superior orbital fissure and anteriorly with the periosteum of the orbital margins. In descriptive terms, the orbit has been divided into the subperiosteal, intraconal spaces (bounded by the rectus muscles and intermuscular fibers), and extraconal spaces. Disease processes may be roughly contained within these spaces, and thus, the concept serves some practical value. Recent work has, however, shown that the intra- and extraconal spaces are highly complex and are divided by radial fibrovascular connective tissue septa.[4] Further, these septa connect to and provide support to all the intraorbital structures, thereby forming complex surgical spaces. These septa invest the orbital fat, which surrounds all the structures as lobules.

Orbital Contents

Extraocular Muscles. There are six extraocular muscles, four recti and two obliques, which control ocular movement. The recti arise from the annulus of Zinn at the apex, where it is continuous with the dural sheath of the optic nerve and periorbita. Thus, apical disease frequently affects all the structures simultaneously. Anteriorly, the recti insert on the globe 5 to 7 mm posterior to the limbus. The superior oblique arises just superior to the annulus and passes forward through the trochlea

TABLE 68–1. Contents of Orbital Fissures and Canals

Structure	Location	Contents
Optic canal	Lesser wing of sphenoid	Optic nerve Meninges Ophthalmic artery Sympathetic fibers
Superior orbital fissure	Lesser and greater wing of sphenoid	Nerves: cranial nerves (superior and inferior division of oculomotor nerve), IV (trochlear nerve), and VI (abducens nerve); sensory root of cranial nerve V (frontal, lacrimal, nasociliary trigeminal branches); sympathetic fibers Vessels: Superior ophthalmic vein, anastomosis of recurrent lacrimal and middle meningeal artery
Inferior orbital fissure	Greater wing of sphenoid, palatine zygomatic and maxillary bones	Nerves: sensory root of cranial nerve V (infraorbital and zygomatic trigeminal branches), parasympathetic branches from pterygopalatine ganglion Vessels: inferior ophthalmic vein and branches to pterygoid plexus
Anterior ethmoid canal	Frontal and ethmoid	Nerve: anterior ethmoid becomes dorsal nasal Vessel: anterior ethmoid artery
Posterior ethmoid canal	Frontal and ethmoid	Nerve: posterior ethmoid Vessel: posterior ethmoid artery
Nasolacrimal fossa	Lacrimal and maxillary bones	Nasolacrimal sac and duct

(4 mm posterior to the orbital margin just medial to the supraorbital notch), whence it extends posterolaterally to insert on the superior aspect of the globe. The inferior oblique arises from the bone just lateral to the nasolacrimal fossa and passes posterolaterally, where it inserts on the inferolateral aspect of the eye. The superior oblique is innervated by the trochlear, the lateral rectus by the abducens, and the remaining muscles by the oculomotor nerves. The levator palpebrae (oculomotor innervation) originates from the annulus and inserts on the upper lid. It is attached anteriorly to Müller's muscle, a sympathetically innervated smooth muscle. Disease affecting either may alter the lid position or function.

Optic Nerve. The optic nerve is a nerve fiber tract, 4.5 to 5 cm long (intracranial, 1 cm; intracanalicular, 10 to 12 mm; and intraorbital, 3 cm), extending from the globe to the chiasm. The subarachnoid space and meningeal linings sheath the nerve and extend from the canal forward to the globe. The ophthalmic artery is covered in dura in the canal where it lies inferolateral to the nerve. At the orbital end of the canal, it loses the dural coat and crosses medially in the intraconal space.

Peripheral Nerves. The major sensory supply of the orbit is the ophthalmic division of the trigeminal nerve with the maxillary (via the infraorbital and zygomatic branches) supplying the inferior orbital, cheek, and temporal regions. The frontal and lacrimal branches of the ophthalmic nerve run forward between the periorbita and the levator complex to supply the forehead and lacrimal gland. The nasociliary branch is intraconal, crosses medially over the optic nerve, and terminates as the ethmoidal and infratrochlear nerves. The trochlear nerve extends forward in the same space as the frontal and lacrimal. The oculomotor nerve enters the cone as a superior division (supplying the levator and superior rectus) and an inferior division (supplying the medial and inferior rectus and inferior oblique). Just temporal to the optic nerve 1 cm anterior to the apex is the ciliary ganglion containing the major parasympa-

thetic supply to the eye. The sympathetic supply accompanies the orbital vessels, and the secretory fibers to the lacrimal gland (postganglionic from the sphenopalatine) arrive via the zygomatic and lacrimal nerves.

Vascular Supply. The major vascular supply of the orbit is via the branches of the ophthalmic artery, including the central retinal, choroidal, recurrent branch to the middle meningeal, muscular, ethmoidal and supraorbital arteries. The orbital veins are valveless, the superior ophthalmic draining to the cavernous sinus via the superior orbital fissure and the inferior to the pterygoid plexus.

Lacrimal System. The lacrimal gland weights 78 gm, measures 20 × 12 × 5 mm, and is divided into a palpebral and orbital part by the levator aponeurosis. The ducts (10 to 12) pass through the palpebral lobe into the superolateral conjunctival fornix. The gland is tubuloracemose, resembling the parotid. Tears flow across the eye and are drained into the lacrimal sac through the canaliculi of the upper and lower lid via a pump system initiated by blinking.

The lacrimal sac fills the lacrimal fossa and is enveloped by the periorbita and the medial canthal tendon anteriorly. It drains via the nasolacrimal duct beneath the inferior turbinate.

Anatomic Patterns of Disease

The effect of any disease in the orbit is governed not only by the primary nature of the process but also by the anatomic pattern of involvement. Location within the tight confines of the orbit has profound effect on the clinical presentation of the disease. For instance, a small tumor in the orbital apex may produce a profound early effect on the function of the second, third, fourth, fifth, and sixth nerves, as in a case of a small hemangiopericytoma that presented with the sole feature of rapid loss of vision (Fig. 68–1A and B). In simple terms, most disease can be viewed as having either functional or mass effect. Functional effects lead to interference

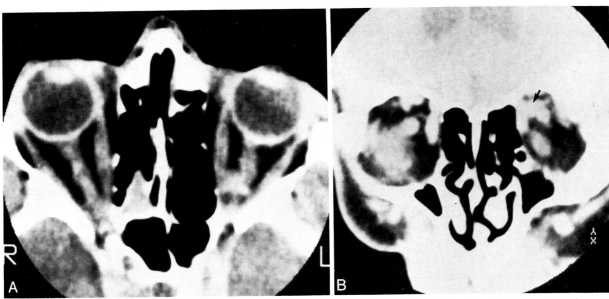

Figure 68–1. (*A*) CT scan, axial view, showing a small, apically located, smooth orbital mass causing displacement of the optic nerve. Clinically, this was associated with decreased vision as a result of compressive optic neuropathy. (*B*) Coronal scan of same patient with contrast medium. Note smooth perineural hemangiopericytoma showing enhancement (arrow).

with the motor or sensory physiology of adjacent structures. Mass effect shifts orbital structures by occupying or increasing space or by cicatrization. For instance, an ethmoidal mass causes lateral displacement, whereas destruction of the orbital floor (Fig. 68–2) leads to enophthalmos and downward displacement.

The pattern of anatomic involvement can generally be divided into anterior, diffuse, myopathic, lacrimal, perineural (apical),[8] periocular, intraconal, periorbital, and lacrimal drainage system. Anterior lesions cause greater direct ocular effects owing to immediate relationship to the globe, whereas diffuse disease involves motor and sensory structures of the entire orbit that may lead to fixation of the globe or sensory deficits (pain, paresthesia, or loss of visual function). Apical disease tends to affect the optic, motor, and sensory nerves earlier, as in a case of minimal apical infiltration by squamous carcinoma of the maxillary sinus with profound early motor (ptosis and limitation of movement), sensory (infraorbital paresthesia), and visual loss without much evidence of mass effect (proptosis) (Fig. 68–3). Lacrimal disease is dominated by functional and structural alterations of the gland (tearing or drying), lacrimal fossa, and the outer third of the upper lid. A tumor here may cause displacement of the globe down and in, sensory effect on the frontotemporal and frontozygomatic nerves, and an S-shaped deformity of the lid (Fig. 68–4). Myopathic disease such as thyroid ophthalmopathy leads to restriction of ocular movement due to either mass effect, scarring, or neuromotor dysfunction (Fig. 68–5). Ocular diseases have symptomatic functional change (visual loss, floaters, photopsia, pain, photophobia) affecting primarily vision and are usually readily accessible to clinical examination of the globe. Processes within the tight periorbital space can cause a profound and even sudden effect, such as an abscess (Fig. 68–6), with the displacement governed by the site of involvement. A mass in the ethmoids leads to lateral

displacement, one in the roof leads to downward displacement, and one in the floor leads to upward displacement. Disease of the lacrimal drainage system is usually characterized by obstruction leading to tearing with or without infection.

PATHOLOGIC PROCESS AS APPLIED TO THE ORBIT

Although the emphasis here is on neoplasia, it is important to have a broad conceptual framework in approaching orbital diagnosis because tumors can in a pathophysiologic sense overlap, combine with, or mimic other diseases. As a simplification, there are five disease processes seen in the orbit: inflammation, neoplasia, structural abnormality, vascular, and degeneration and deposition. These are not mutually exclusive, but in our experience the incidence of these as primary orbital processes is summarized in Table 68–2. A breakdown of specific types of orbital and lacrimal lesions is noted in Tables 68–3 and 68–4.

Inflammation

The underlying pathophysiologic substrate determines the nature of the clinical presentation and development of inflammatory disease. This substrate ranges in character from acute inflammatory cells and their pharmacologic intermediates to delayed infiltration in the case of misdirected immune responses and granulomatous disorders. The character and location of the infiltrate affects the clinical pattern, which may be acute (dominated by pain, injection, systemic malaise, and loss of function) to chronic (dominated by entrapment or mass effect). In short, the clinical patterns of inflammation are acute, subacute, and chronic and either infiltrative or noninfiltrative.

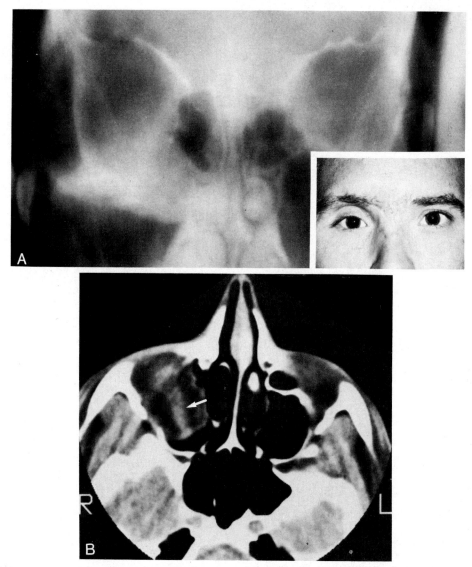

Figure 68–2. (A) *Inset:* Patient shows downward displacement of the right eye following a blow to the orbit. Note deepened superior sulcus. X-ray tomogram shows disruption of the orbital floor with downward displacement of soft tissues. (B) Axial CT scan of same patient showing inferior rectus muscle (arrow) surrounded by fat displaced downard into maxillary sinus.

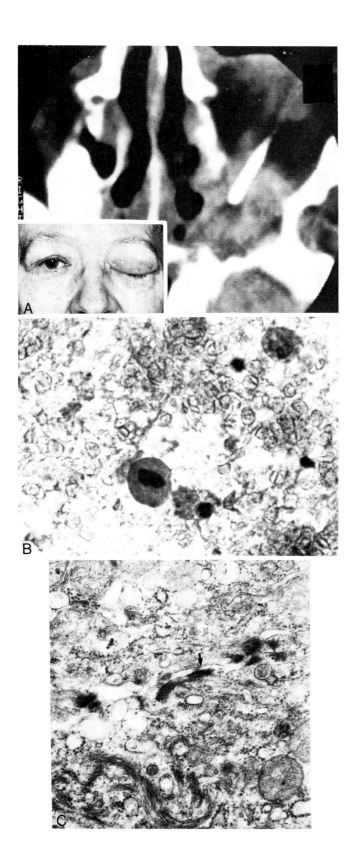

Figure 68–3. (*A*) *Inset:* This patient presented with a 3-month history of slow onset of complete ptosis, restriction of ocular movements, and decreased vision. The CT scan shows aspiration needle placed in apical infiltrating orbital mass arising from the underlying sinus and leading to destruction of bony margins. (*B*) Histopathologic photograph of cytologic specimen obtained from aspirate of tumor shown in *A*. Note large squamoid cells. (H & E, × 100.) (*C*) Electron micrograph of aspirate from tumor from *A* shows desmosomes (arrow) and subcellular organelles consistent with squamous cell origin.

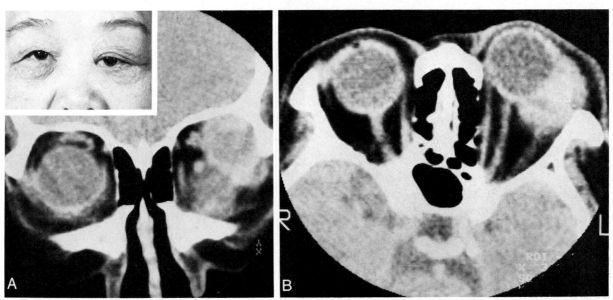

Figure 68–4. (A) *Inset:* patient with long-standing history of slowly developing downward and inward displacement of the left eye. Axial CT scan shows a smooth, well-contained mass with focal excavation of bone. (B) Axial CT scan of patient shown in A. Well-contained mass in lateral orbit leads to inward displacement and axial proptosis.

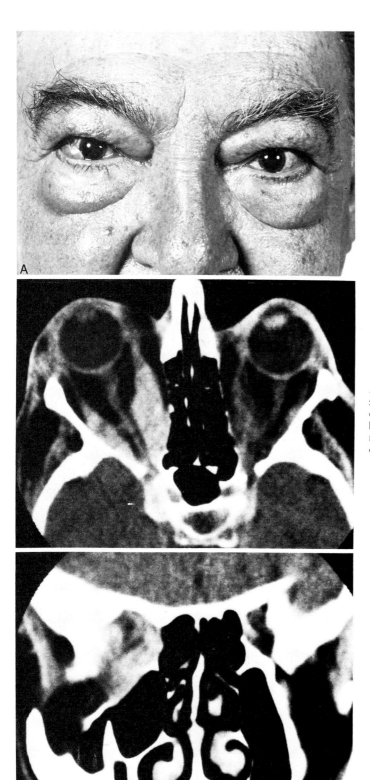

Figure 68–5. (*A*) Patient with thyroid ophthalmopathy shows bilateral infiltrative disease with chemosis and lid edema. (*B*) Composite CT scan showing marked enlargement of extraocular muscles, particularly on the right side. Coronal and axial scan shows marked apical crowding, which accounts for an optic neuropathy.

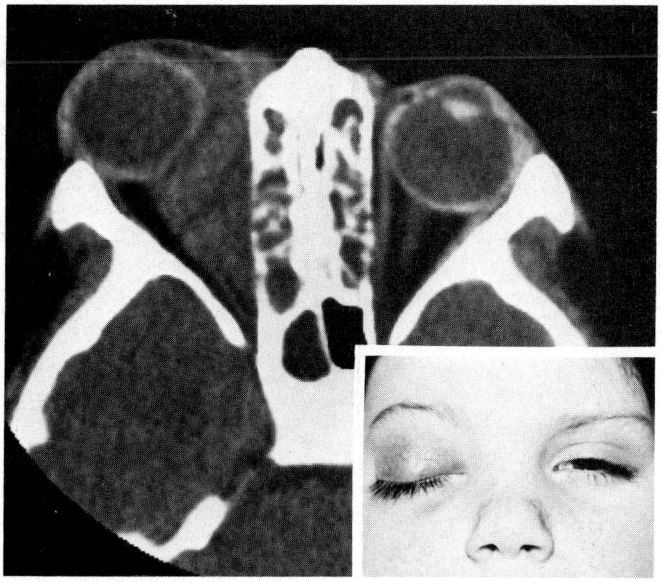

Figure 68–6. Inset: This 10-year-old child presented with a 2-day history of sudden onset of ptosis, infection of right lid, decreased vision, and marked limitation of ocular movement owing to a subperiosteal abscess shown in CT scan arising from an ethmoid sinusitis.

Infective cellulitis is the model for acute inflammation and is characterized by rapid onset (days to weeks) of proptosis, pain, injection, edema, and functional damage to orbital structures. The majority of disorders in this category are sinal in origin, especially in children, but may be ocular (Fig. 68–6), pyemic, or secondary to wound infection. The practical differential diagnosis of acute inflammation consists of about six disorders: infective cellulitis, acute idiopathic orbital inflammation (pseudotumor), ocular inflammation (keratitis, conjunctivitis, iritis, as in Fig. 68–7), fulminant neoplasia (rhabdomyosarcoma, lymphoma, or metastasis), acute myositis, and a sudden event in a pre-existing lesion (such as a hemorrhage in a varix or tumor, as in Fig. 68–8).

Subacute inflammation generally presents with two patterns—either a slower onset of inflammatory signs or a remitting pattern with progressive signs and symptoms. Infiltrative thyroid ophthalmopathy is the most common example of subacute inflammatory disease of the orbit (Fig. 68–5), but adult sinus disease may produce subacute inflammation as a result either of incomplete or inappropriate treatment of the sinus infection (or the sinus obstruction) or as the result of fistula formation with intermittent drainage. The simple differential diagnosis of subacute inflammation includes idiopathic orbital inflammation (pseudotumor), thyroid ophthalmopathy, infective cellulitis, primary ocular inflammation (scleritis, uveitis), collagen vascular disease, and neoplasia (Fig. 68–9).

TABLE 68–2. Summary of Diseases of the Orbital Processes, University of British Columbia, 1975–1983

Type of Disease	Incidence
Inflammation	
Thyroid ophthalmopathy	52%
Other	12.2%
Neoplasia	17.7%
Structural	13.3%
Vascular	3.5%
Degeneration and deposition	1.3%

TABLE 68–3. Incidence of Various Orbital Lesions, University of British Columbia Orbital Clinic, 1975–1983

Type of Lesion	Number*
Inflammatory (64.2% of total)	
Thyroid ophthalmopathy	456
Cellulitis	36
Pseudotumor	46
Miscellaneous: sarcoid, Wegener's granulomatosis, granulomatous inflammations, etc.	25
Neoplastic (17.7% of total)	
Hemangioma	25
Meningioma: sphenoid wing (17), optic nerve (4)	21
Metastatic	21
Lymphoma	17
Neurofibroma	16
Contiguous or secondary invasion	13
Schwannoma	9
Lacrimal epithelial	8
Fibrous dysplasia	5
Glioma	4
Lymphangioma	4
Miscellaneous	12
Structural (13.3% of total)	
Trauma	60
Cystic: dermoid (25), mucocele (20), lacrimal cyst (6)	51
Asymmetry	6
Vascular (3.5% of total)	
Varix	16
AV fistula	11
Hematic cyst	2
Vein thrombosis	2
Degenerative and deposition (1.3% of total)	
Socket contraction	4
Myopia	3
Fat prolapse	2
Scleroderma	1
Amyloid	1

*Total number of lesions = 877.

TABLE 68–4. Incidence of Lacrimal Gland Lesions

Type of Lesion	Number*
Neoplasic	
Carcinoma	8
Benign mixed tumor (2)	
Mucoepidermoid (2)	
Adenoid cystic (2)	
Basaloid carcinoma (1)	
Spindle cell carcinoma (1)	
Lymphoma	8
Inflammatory	9
Pseudotumors (7)	
Sarcoid (1)	
Sjögren's syndrome (1)	
Structural	9
Lacrimal cysts (6)	
Dermoid cysts (3)	

*Total number of lesions = 34.

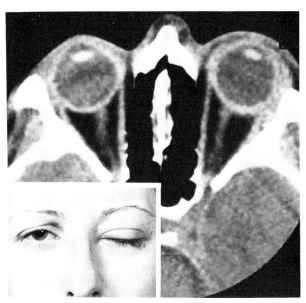

Chronic orbital inflammation is dominated by a silent progressive pattern of displacement with or without evidence of entrapment or interference with orbital function. A classical chronic infiltrative pattern may be seen in the progressive idiopathic sclerosing inflammation (pseudotumor). The misdirected immune infiltrate stimulates a desmoplastic response that leads to fixation of structures. The differential diagnosis for chronic infiltrative inflammation includes lymphoproliferative disease, idiopathic sclerosing inflammation (pseudotumor), thyroid ophthalmopathy, primary and secondary neoplasia, collagen vascular disease, and rare disorders such as orbital amyloidosis. On the other hand, chronic inflammation may simply produce a mass effect. The location of the mass will affect the clinical presentation.

Figure 68–7. *Inset:* This patient developed lid edema, chemosis, ptosis, and superficial ocular inflammation associated with mild proptosis. The CT scan shows thickened ocular coats on the left side in particular, consistent with ocular inflammation ultimately associated with hearing loss and corneal infiltrates and a diagnosis of Cogan's syndrome. Note enhancement of scleral coats on left side.

For example, a mucocele of the ethmoid will cause lateral displacement, and one of the frontal sinus will cause downward displacement (Fig. 68–10). The simple differential diagnosis of chronic inflammatory disease with mass effect is any tumor, either primary or secondary.

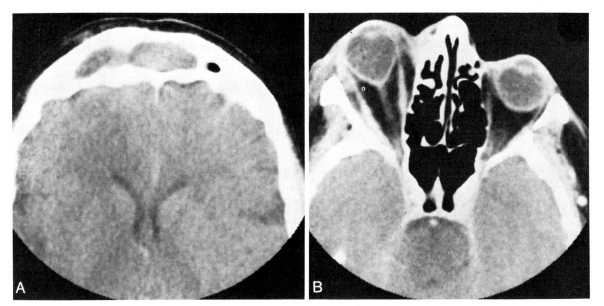

Figure 68–8. (*A*) CT scan of frontal sinus of a patient presenting with an explosive onset of severe proptosis and loss of vision as a result of an abscess in the sinus. The abscess penetrated into the superior subperiosteal space of the orbit, leading to massive and sudden proptosis (*B*). The marked posterior tenting of the globe is a result of extensive orbital pressure and forward displacement of the globe from the abscess.

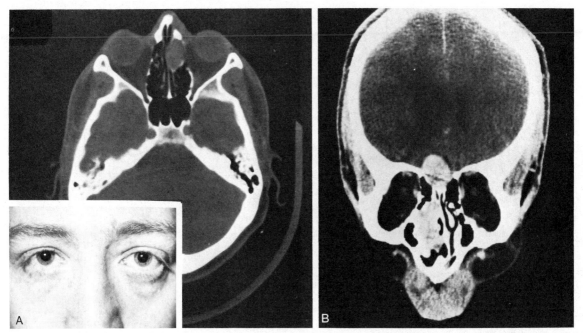

Figure 68–9. (A) Inset: This 23-year-old man presented with mild periorbital swelling, proptosis, and displacement of the left eye as a result of the presence of a mass in the ethmoid sinus shown on CT scan. Surgically, this was associated with an accumulation of mucopurulent material and underlying tumor mass, which proved to be histologically a schwannoma. (B) Coronal CT scan of the same patient shown in A taken 3 years later, showing extension of residual mass into anterior cranial fossa and nasopharynx.

Neoplasia

Neoplasia accounts for one fifth of our orbital cases and is an important aspect of differential diagnosis in disease of the orbit. The specific list of neoplasms affecting the orbit is extensive, but from a practical point of view, they can be defined on the basis of biologic behavior. In effect, tumors within the orbit, both benign and malignant, are either infiltrative or noninfiltrative in behavior.

Noninfiltrative neoplasms exert simple mass effect and generally lead to functional damage late unless they are critically located. The adult cavernous hemangioma is a good example of a benign lesion that is noninfiltrative and well defined and simply leads to proptosis and indentation of the globe (Fig. 68–11). Another benign growth that is frequently noninvasive and exerts mass effect is fibrous dysplasia of bone. On the other hand, benign locally infiltrative neoplasia such as fibrous histiocytoma and hemangiopericytoma are both conditions with orbital propensity and may have locally invasive behavior.

Malignant lesions can, in fact, show similar patterns of behavior. For example, the patient demonstrated in Figure 68–4 had a history of downward and inward displacement of the globe without functional deficit, either motor or sensory. She had a well-contained lacrimal gland lesion without bone destruction, but excavation was shown on CT scan and x-ray, suggesting a noninfiltrative longstanding mass. At surgery, it was an encapsulated tumor, which was histologically a well-differentiated mucoepidermoid carcinoma. On the other hand, malignant tumors are more frequently infiltrative and lead to both functional deficit and mass effect (Fig. 68–12). In particular, tumors secondarily invading the orbit such as this nasopharyngeal carcinoma (Fig. 68–12) have devastating effects by virtue of their infiltrative and destructive behavior.

Structural Abnormalities

Structural abnormalities include congenital bony deformities such as Crouzon's disease or maxillary hypoplasia, as shown in Figure 68–13. The acquired structural abnormalities are post-traumatic lesions, the trauma including all types of physical damage. Enophthalmos secondary to a traumatic blow-out fracture (Fig. 68–2) is an example.

Vascular Disease

Four per cent of the cases seen in our clinic were vascular in character and constituted the fourth most common process. Pathologically, there are many lesions in this category, but pathophysiologically, there are fundamental patterns based on blood flow. In effect, lesions of this kind are either nonobstructive, low flow or high flow, or they are obstructive, and they may be arterial, venous, or both.

An example of arterial high flow lesion may be seen in some infantile hemangiomas, as in a child with an intraconal hemangioma that presented with proptosis and pulsating exophthalmos and a rapid arterial blush on angiography (Fig. 68–14). In contrast, the adult cavernous hemangioma on arteriography shows minimal arterial blood flow, suggesting a low flow lesion (see Fig. 68–11). Arteriovenous lesions may also demonstrate high or low flow characteristics, depending on the size of the shunt. The larger the shunt, the more profound the orbital findings.

Text continued on page 1718

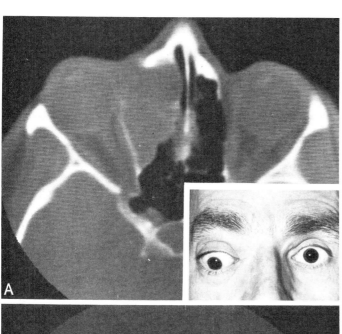

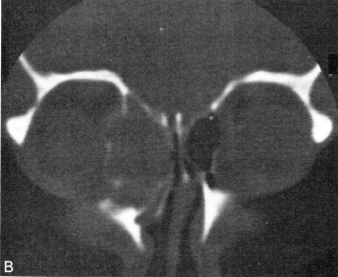

Figure 68–10. *Inset:* A 48-year-old man shows downward and outward displacement of his right globe as a result of the presence of a frontal ethmoid mucocele shown on CT scan in axial (*A*) and coronal (*B*) views. Note evidence of both bony erosion and expansion. This lesion was not enhanced on contrast scan.

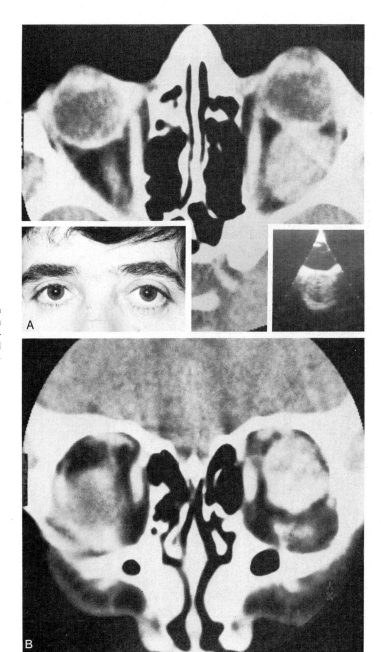

Figure 68–11. (A) *Left inset*: A 35-year-old woman shows left axial proptosis as a result of a smooth contrast-enhancing intraconal hemangioma. *Right inset*: B-scan ultrasound showing smooth margins and internal echos consistent with hemangioma. (B) Coronal CT scan showing enhancing intraconal lesion.

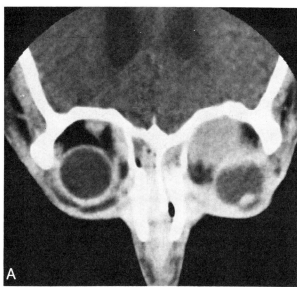

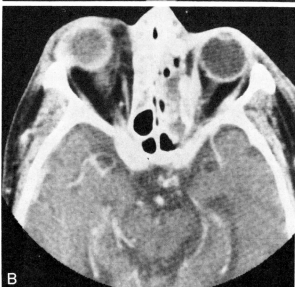

Figure 68–12. (A) Coronal CT scan showing infiltrating orbital mass arising from adjacent sinus and nasopharynx. This was histologically a malignant, poorly differentiated squamous cell carcinoma. (B) Same mass in axial view with evidence of compression of the optic nerve.

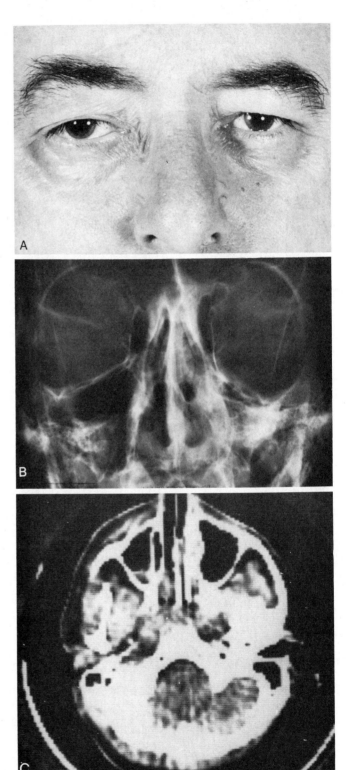

Figure 68–13. (*A*) This patient presented with apparent right proptosis, but in fact had left enophthalmos, which was the result of maxillary hypoplasia, shown on routine x-ray (*B*) and on CT scan (*C*).

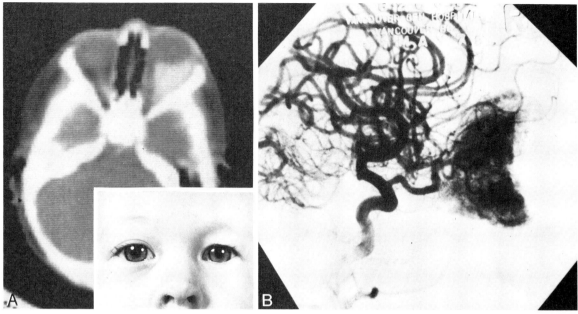

Figure 68–14. (A) Inset: Infant with right pulsating exopthalmos, the result of the presence of a capillary hemangioma within the muscle cone shown enhancing on CT scan (A) and as extensive tumor blush on angiography (B).

On the venous side of the circulation, there are a number of lesions that may also show high or low flow characteristics. The orbital varix is frequently low flow and simply manifests recurrent episodes of hemorrhage. On the other hand, if it is high flow, the patient may show profound alterations of proptosis depending on jugular venous pressure (Fig. 68–15).

Some of the foregoing lesions have obstructive elements, but both arterial and venous obstruction may occur independently as either primary or secondary features of orbital disease. For example, venous thrombosis may occur secondary to cavernous sinus inflammation, as was seen in a case of sphenoid sinusitis that also led to middle cerebral artery obstruction (Fig. 68–16).

Degeneration and Deposition

Degenerations include processes of atrophy, deposition, and cicatrization, the commonest being senile fat atrophy of the orbit. Localized amyloidosis is an example of deposition that may occur in the orbit, leading to functional and structural change. Myopia is a common degenerative process that may present as pseudoproptosis owing to the large size of the globe (Fig. 68–17).

INCIDENCE OF SINUS, NASOPHARYNGEAL, AND ORBITAL DISEASE

Overall, 12.8 per cent (112 cases) of our orbital series (877 cases) were in the category of lesions occurring in the orbit, sinus, or nasopharynx (Table 68–5). In relative terms, the incidence within this group was (1) structural, 52.7 per cent; (2) inflammatory, 24.1 per cent; and (3) neoplastic, 23.2 per cent.

The 26 neoplastic lesions of this group represented 16.7 per cent of all orbital neoplasms and 3 per cent of orbital lesions in our series. It is difficult to compare

TABLE 68–5. Orbital, Sinus, Nasopharyngeal Lesions, University of British Columbia Orbital Clinic, 1976–1983

Type of Lesion	Number*	Total (%)
Structural		59 (52.7%)
Cystic		23 (20.5%)
Mucocele	16	
With cellulitis	2	
With enophthalmos	2	
Dermoid cyst	2	
Rathke pouch cyst	1	
Trauma		36 (32.2%)
Orbital sinus	33	
Foreign body	2	
Congenital hypoplasia	1	
Inflammatory		27 (24.1%)
Orbital cellulitis with sinusitis	16	
Subperiosteal abscess	4	
Wegener's granulomatosis	3	
Aneurysmal bone cyst	1	
Sinus polyposis	1	
Sclerosing pseudotumor	1	
Cavernous sinus thrombosis with sinusitis	1	
Neoplastic		26 (23.2%)
Carcinoma	13	
Squamous cell (5)		
Transitional (3)		
Adenocarcinoma (1)		
Adenoid cystic (2)		
Basal cell (1)		
Neuroendocrine (1)		
Fibrous dysplasia	4	
Chondrosarcoma	2	
Osteoma	2	
Ewing's sarcoma	1	
Myeloma	1	
Lymphoma	1	
Neurofibroma	1	
Schwannoma	1	

*Total number of lesions = 112.

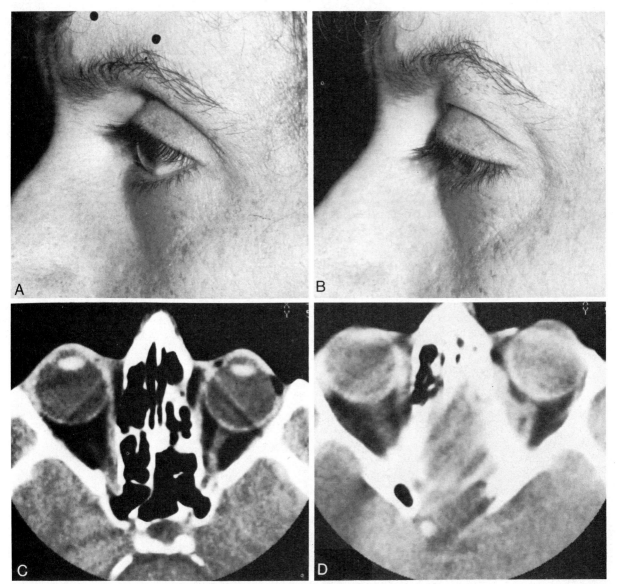

Figure 68–15. (*A*) Lateral view of patient with left enophthalmos and a clinical history of intermittent exophthalmos. (*B*) Same patient during Valsalva maneuver. Note increasing fullness of upper and lower lids and axial proptosis during Valsalva maneuver. (*C*) Axial CT scan of the same patient. Note normally enophthalmic position. (*D*) Contrast-enhanced scan of same patient with a dependent position of her head, showing expanded medial orbital varix.

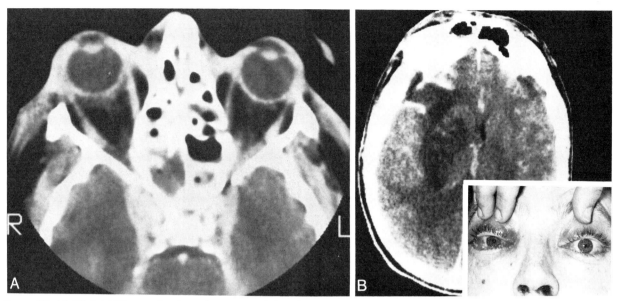

Figure 68–16. (*A*) Axial CT scan of patient who presented clinically with catastrophic onset of bilateral proptosis, chemosis, limitation of ocular movement, and lid edema. (*B*) *Inset:* Patient at presentation. Note opacification of sphenoid sinus and enlargement of the cavernous sinus. The CT scan shows a large infarct of the right hemisphere due to obstruction of middle cerebral artery.

these figures to other series because the reports of sinus nasopharyngeal orbital lesions are frequently not clearly delineated, and figures vary as to means of ascertainment and the nature of the center studying them. From pooled series Reese shows 6 per cent of orbital lesions are from the sinus and 2 per cent are neoplastic.[6] In Moss's clinical series he identifies 3 per cent mucoceles but does not specifically identify the neoplasms in terms of origin from these sites.[5] Ingall's text indicates 7 per cent of his series of biopsy-proved orbital tumors were

extensions from the nasal sinuses.[3] Henderson in his most recent text on orbital disease indicates 7.9 per cent (60 of 774) were epithelial neoplasms from the sinus or nasopharynx, and 8.5 per cent (65 of 774) were mucoceles.[15] It is difficult to determine how many of the other neoplasms in his large series were in these sites, as they are defined histologically rather than by location. As a summation, the incidence of neoplasia bounding these areas varies from about 3 to 8 per cent, depending on the series studied.

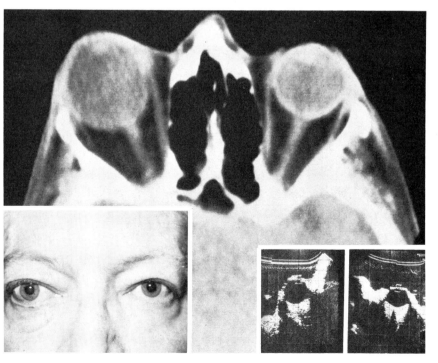

Figure 68–17. *Left inset:* This patient presented with apparent right proptosis, which was the result of a degenerative myopia leading to a large right globe, shown both on CT scan and ultrasound (*right inset*).

CLINICAL EVALUATION

The clinical evaluation of patients is the most important method of assessing orbital disease and sets the stage for diagnostic investigation.[7] In simple terms, the history and physical examination should be directed toward answering two questions:

1. Where is the disease located?
2. How has the disease affected the orbital structures—that is, what dynamic alteration has occurred? Synthesis of the answers allows formulation of a rational investigation.

Location of Disease

The question of location is usually the easier to answer because it reflects the shifting of orbital structures induced by disease. When a process occupies space, it tends to push structures away from it, having a positive effect (Fig. 68–18). On the other hand, disease that draws structures toward it through cicatrization or excavation exerts a negative effect (Fig. 68–19). For example, a mass from the ethmoid sinus with positive effect displaces orbital structures laterally. Whereas, in a case of cicatrizing metastatic carcinoma, the orbital structures are drawn toward the lesion, producing enophthalmos and fixation (Fig. 68–20). In rare instances both a positive and negative effect may occur in different circumstances, as in the previously demonstrated patient with an orbital varix (Fig. 68–15). In normal circumstances the patient is enophthalmic; however, she showed increasing axial proptosis and fullness of the lid with a Valsalva maneuver or when bending over.

The physical examination should provide information on the degree and direction of displacement of the affected orbital structures and can be measured in the following manner:

1. Measure horizontal displacement by recording the distance at the level of the canthi from the center of the nose to the medial edge of the limbus with the patient looking in the axial direction (Fig. 68–21A).
2. Measure vertical displacement by recording the position of the globe above or below the level of the canthi (Fig. 68–21B).
3. Measure proptosis with an exophthalmometer, one eye at a time, with the patient regarding an object

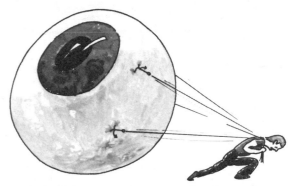

Figure 68–19. Diagrammatic representation of a negative process pulling the eye, or displacing the eye toward the lesion.

(preferably your eye) along the central visual axis (Fig. 68–21C).

Dynamic Alteration

Dynamic alteration is more difficult to assess and involves an analysis of two clinical features of disease: temporal change and the abnormal process.

TEMPORAL CHANGE

The character of temporal change is extracted from the patient's history with emphasis on diurnal variation, time of onset, rapidity of development, or intermittent nature. For example, a patient with thyroid ophthalmopathy frequently has more proptosis, lid edema, and diplopia in the morning secondary to orbital swelling accentuated by lying prone at night. Both the time and rapidity of the onset may provide a clue to the nature of the disease. A catastrophic change suggests either hemorrhage in a pre-existing lesion or fulminant inflammation. For example, a patient with an aneurysmal bone cyst affecting the frontal sinus and orbit presented with a catastrophic onset of proptosis secondary to bleeding within the mass (Fig. 68–22).

Changes that occur at a regular but rapid rate (weeks to a few months) suggest either an inflammatory process (Fig. 68–5) or a fulminant neoplasm (see Fig. 68–12), whereas insidious change implies low-grade inflammation or infiltrative neoplasm. Finally, intermittent change, such as pulsation or alteration with Valsalva maneuver, suggest either a bony defect of the wall of the orbit or a relationship to the vascular system (Figs. 68–14 and 68–15).

ABNORMAL PROCESS

The abnormal pathophysiology can be divided into three basic categories that are not necessarily independent but provide a working framework for characterization of a particular orbital problem. One tends to associate certain clinical signs with each of these processes:

1. *Inflammation.* Inflammation is characterized by signs and symptoms of pain, warmth, loss of function, and mass effect. The degree to which the clinician characterizes the process as either acute or chronic is related to the severity of signs and the rapidity of onset. For instance, in acute infective cellulitis there is a sudden

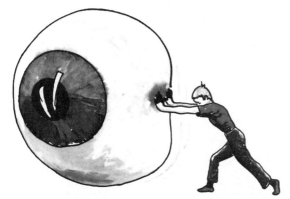

Figure 68–18. Diagrammatic representation of a positive orbital process leading to displacement of the globe away from a mass lesion.

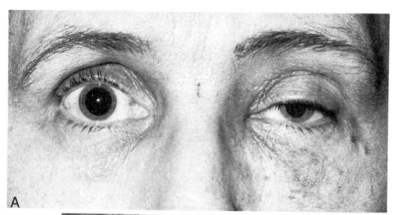

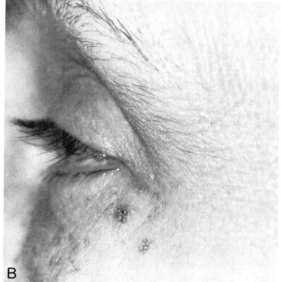

Figure 68–20. (*A*) This patient presented with insidious onset of restricted left ocular movement, ptosis, and enophthalmos (*B*), the result of a cicatrizing metastatic breast carcinoma.

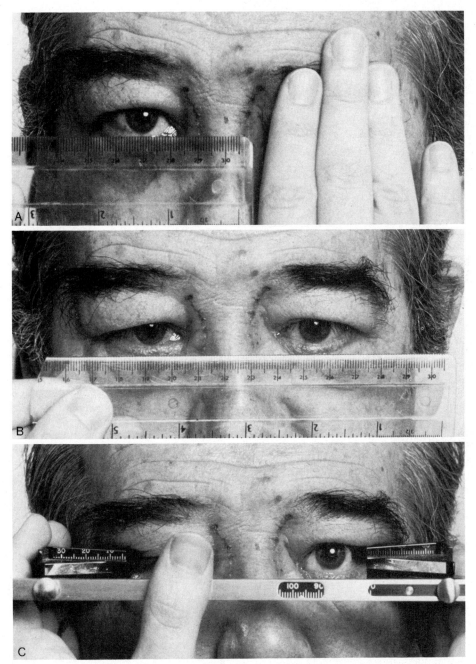

Figure 68–21. (A) Method of measurement of lateral displacement of the globe. Note central marking on the nose. Measurement is taken from this marking to the inner canthus with the patient looking in the axial direction. (B) The horizontal ruler should be aligned with the outer canthi to demonstrate any vertical displacement of the globe. (C) Exophthalmometer shows measurement of axial proptosis. Note that the opposite eye is occluded and that the patient looks in the central axial direction.

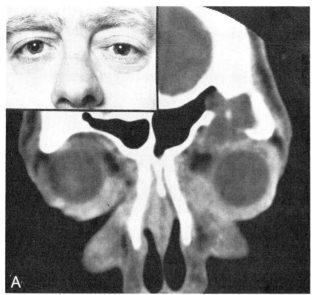

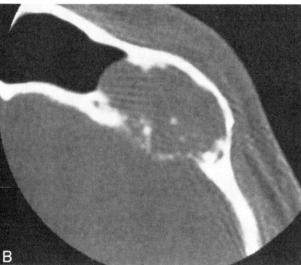

Figure 68–22. (A) *Inset*: A 42-year-old man presented with a sudden (occurring over a 1-week period) onset of downward displacement and proptosis of the left globe, the result of a hemorrhage within a pre-existing aneurysmal bone cyst, which is shown on CT scan both in coronal (A) and axial (B) planes. Note erosion of bone and involvement of frontal sinus.

development of inflammation with marked limitation of movement, proptosis, injection, and pain (Fig. 68–6). In contrast, more insidious diseases such as some idiopathic sclerosing conditions (pseudotumor) are characterized by more subtle features of inflammation.

2. *Mass effect*. Mass effect leads to displacement with or without signs of involvement of sentient or neuromuscular structures and as stated helps to localize disease.

3. *Infiltration*. Infiltration causes entrapment and damage to orbital structures as previously demonstrated in a case of metastatic cicatrizing carcinoma with a slow but progressive course (Fig. 68–20). On the other hand, infiltration may occur more rapidly in tumors with more aggressive biologic behavior.

To make a clinical diagnosis of orbital disease one should bring together information from the history and physical examination that identifies displacement, characterizes temporal development, and defines the disease process. Virtually every combination of location and dynamic alteration may occur, and the clinical definition of the specifics prepares for a rational investigative formulation.

INVESTIGATION

The purpose of investigation is to define the nature, location, size, and effect of disease on the visual and ocular apparatus. Therapeutic decisions are made on the basis of these investigations and the clinical findings. The basic categories of investigation are orbital imaging, ocular and visual function assessment, and pathologic study.

Orbital Imaging

Recent advances in the imaging process allow for increasing specificity in terms of defining the nature, progress, and position of lesions. Radiologic and ultrasound procedures can assess lesions for evidence of infiltration, capsular definition, tissue characteristics, and relationship to the vascular system and adjacent structures. In addition, change in a lesion with time can aid in diagnosis or in assessment of treatment.

For example, in the diagnosis and differential diagnosis of the patient with axial proptosis, computed tomographic (CT) scanning localized the disease to the intraconal space in the case of a hemangioma (Fig. 68–11) and to the orbital apex and medial wall in a case of chondrosarcoma of the sinus (Fig. 68–23). On the other hand, both CT and ultrasound scans helped to define the difference between an infiltrative and noninfiltrative medial orbital mass in cases of carcinoma (Figs. 68–12,

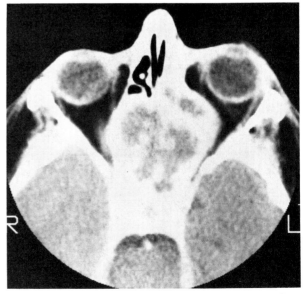

Figure 68–23. Axial CT scan showing right proptosis resulting from a medial orbital mass arising in the nasopharynx and sinus. Histologically, this was proved to be a chondrosarcoma.

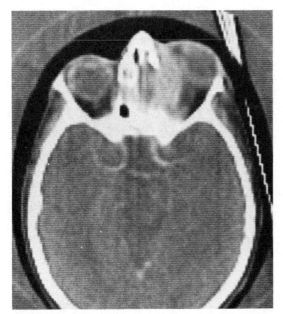

Figure 68–24. Axial CT scan showing erosion of the right medial orbital wall by an infiltrating nasopharyngeal carcinoma, which resulted in proptosis, limitation of ocular movement, and visual deficit.

68–24, and 68–26) and mucocele in this location (Figs. 68–10 and 68–25). Localization of tumors preoperatively or for ancillary diagnostic procedures, such as aspiration needle biopsy (Fig. 68–3), can be effectively achieved with modern imaging devices. Finally, disease progress or the effect of treatment can be monitored as shown in a patient with Ewing's sarcoma of the orbit and nasopharynx treated with radiotherapy and systemic chemotherapy (Fig. 68–26).

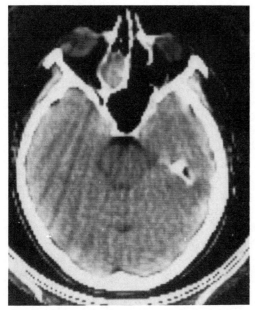

Figure 68–25. Axial CT scan showing posterior ethmoid mucocele that has led to expansion of the adjacent bony orbital wall.

Computed Tomography. High-resolution CT scanning permits a detailed assessment of the orbit and surrounding structures. We routinely do 3 mm axial and coronal cuts with selected 1.5 mm sections for sites of special interest. The angle of the gantry may be changed to study particular structures such as the optic canal, where the angle is at 10 degrees from the orbitomeatal line. The resolution is approximately 1 mm, allowing detailed visualization of the globe, optic nerve, muscles, larger vessels, and adjacent structures.

In disease processes the scanner can define the margins as smooth (Figs. 68–1, 68–4, 68–9, and 68–11), infiltrative (Figs. 68–3, 68–12, and 68–31), or nodular (Figs. 68–15, 68–27, and 68–28). Contrast enhancement may show rim enhancement in the case of a hematic cyst (Fig. 68–27), tumor blush in the case of a hemangioma (Figs. 68–11 and 68–14) or nonenhancement in the case of a mucocele or some solid tumors of the sinus (Fig. 68–10). The density of masses can be assessed, allowing differentiation between fat-containing (Fig. 68–29), calcium-containing (Fig. 68–30), and homogeneous structures. Site of origin and degree of extension can be defined in the case of combined orbital-nasopharyngeal-intracranial lesions (Figs. 68–9, 68–15, and 68–31). Bony erosion in destructive lesions (Figs. 68–23 and 68–26) and excavation (Fig. 68–25) in expanding masses can be identified. Erosion suggests an aggressive disease process, whereas excavation and expansion implies long-standing noninfiltrative disease. In some instances features of both processes may be noted (Figs. 68–10 and 68–22). Generalized expansion of the orbit is frequently a feature of masses in childhood (Fig. 68–28). In trauma, the site, extent, and degree of fracture as well as the presence of a foreign body may be assessed (Figs. 68–2 and 68–32). In addition, the structural effects of trauma on tissues can be delineated. More sophisticated contrast techniques, such as intrathecal metrizamide injection, may rarely be used to assess continuity or lack of continuity to the subarachnoid space. Contrast enhancement combined with dependent positioning or Valsalva maneuver may show varices, allowing preoperative localization of an essentially intermittent lesion (Fig. 68–15).

Routine Radiographic Methods. Routine and tomographic x-ray studies are an important part of orbital assessment, particularly in terms of the effect on bony structures. Plain film studies are done in the Caldwell view (for an unobstructed assessment of the bony margins, ethmoid sinuses, sphenoid wing, posterior orbital floor, superior orbital fissure, and lacrimal fossa), Waters view (for sinuses, orbital roof and floor), lateral views (roof, floor, and ethmoid sinuses), and base views (lateral and medial walls, sphenoid wings and sinus, pterygoid fossa, optic canal, and lacrimal fossa). Tomography provides thin cuts and thus finer resolution of the bony structures.

Dense tumors such as osteomas may be clearly defined and separated from soft-tissue components of disease (Fig. 68–33). Generalized expansion of the orbit in childhood masses and localized expansion in long-standing adult lesions may be studied. Bony erosion in the case of destructive lesions and site, extent, and degree of fractures can be identified (Fig. 68–2).

Vascular Studies. Vascular studies, both arterial and venous, are particularly useful in assessing selected

Text continued on page 1731

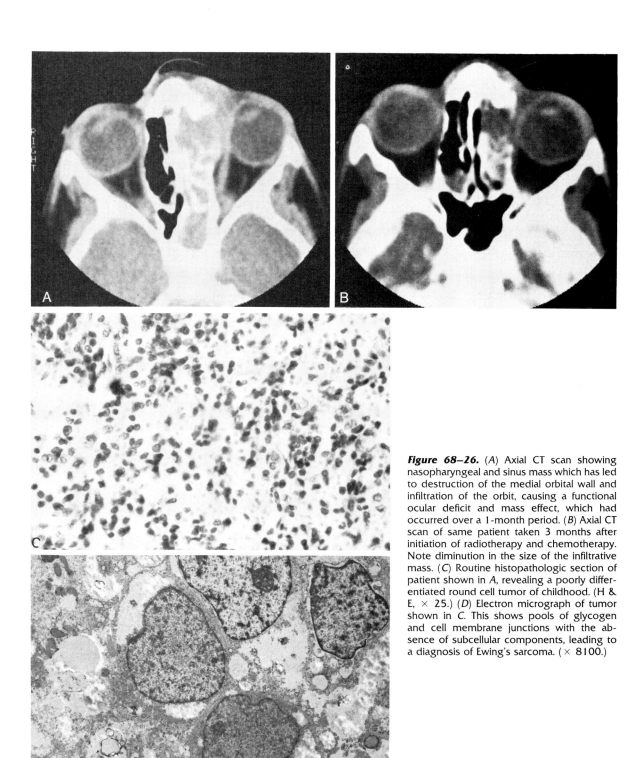

Figure 68–26. (*A*) Axial CT scan showing nasopharyngeal and sinus mass which has led to destruction of the medial orbital wall and infiltration of the orbit, causing a functional ocular deficit and mass effect, which had occurred over a 1-month period. (*B*) Axial CT scan of same patient taken 3 months after initiation of radiotherapy and chemotherapy. Note diminution in the size of the infiltrative mass. (*C*) Routine histopathologic section of patient shown in *A*, revealing a poorly differentiated round cell tumor of childhood. (H & E, × 25.) (*D*) Electron micrograph of tumor shown in *C*. This shows pools of glycogen and cell membrane junctions with the absence of subcellular components, leading to a diagnosis of Ewing's sarcoma. (× 8100.)

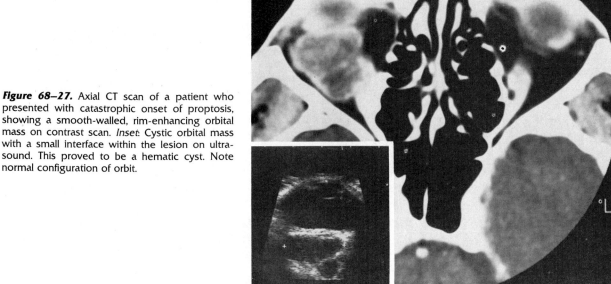

Figure 68–27. Axial CT scan of a patient who presented with catastrophic onset of proptosis, showing a smooth-walled, rim-enhancing orbital mass on contrast scan. *Inset*: Cystic orbital mass with a small interface within the lesion on ultrasound. This proved to be a hematic cyst. Note normal configuration of orbit.

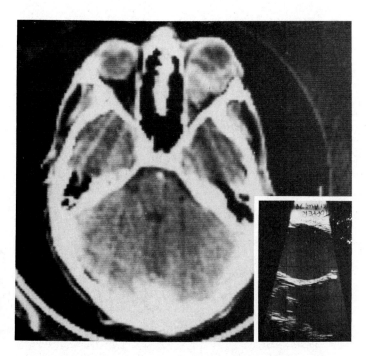

Figure 68–28. Axial CT scan of a left orbital mass that occurred in a patient who presented with a catastrophic onset of proptosis that had occurred on several previous occasions. Note the multilobular borders and evidence of loculation shown in ultrasound (*inset*). This proved to be due to a hemorrhage in a pre-existing orbital varix. Note also evidence on an enlarged orbit, suggesting chronic raised intraorbital pressure.

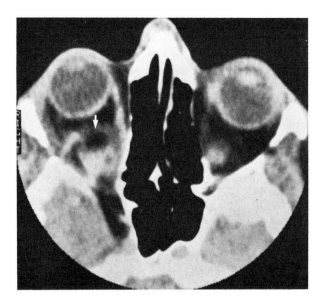

Figure 68–29. Axial CT scan of an intraconal apical orbital mass showing an anterior area of decreased density due to the presence of fat (arrow) in this orbital dermoid cyst.

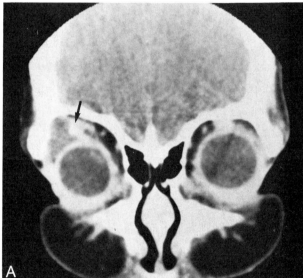

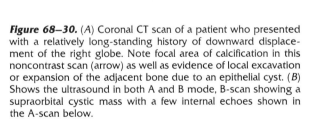

Figure 68–30. (A) Coronal CT scan of a patient who presented with a relatively long-standing history of downward displacement of the right globe. Note focal area of calcification in this noncontrast scan (arrow) as well as evidence of local excavation or expansion of the adjacent bone due to an epithelial cyst. (B) Shows the ultrasound in both A and B mode, B-scan showing a supraorbital cystic mass with a few internal echoes shown in the A-scan below.

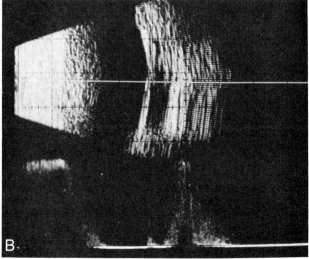

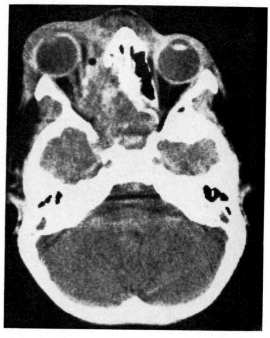

Figure 68–31. Axial CT scan of a patient who presented with a rapid, regular onset of proptosis on the right side due to the presence of giant cell reparative granuloma that had led to destruction of the sinuses, nasopharynx, and adjacent wall of middle cranial fossa.

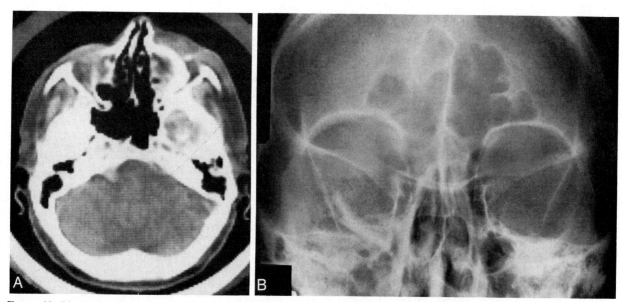

Figure 68–32. (*A*) Axial CT scan of a patient presenting with a right infraorbital laceration due to a large fragment of glass that lodged within both the maxillary sinus and right orbit. (*B*) Routine x-ray of patient in *A* showing two large shards of glass.

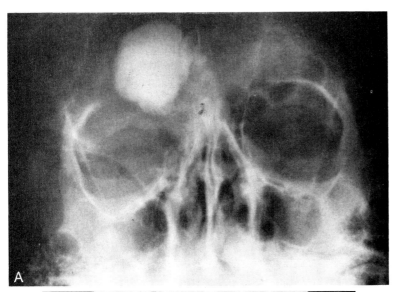

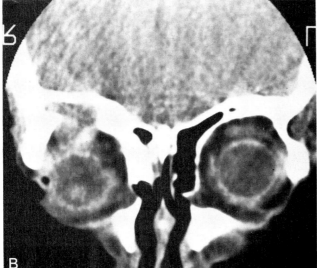

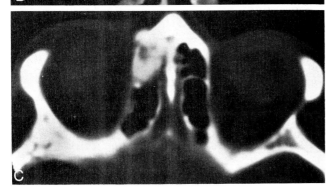

Figure 68–33. (A) Routine x-ray of a patient presenting with slow onset of downward displacement of the right orbit, showing a dense, ossified mass within his frontal sinus. (B) Coronal CT scan of patient shown in A, revealing a soft-tissue mass in the lateral part of the right frontal sinus. The mass led to destruction of the orbital roof and extension of this mucocele, which had resulted from the obstruction produced by what proved to be an osteoma on axial CT scan (C).

aspects of orbital tumors and vascular lesions. Detailed magnified and subtracted views of the arterial supply can aid in defining the location and the character of the blood supply of tumors preoperatively (Figs. 68–34 to 68–36). Indeed, therapy of highly vascular tumors and fistulas can now be achieved via selected arterial embolization and occlusion (Fig. 68–37). Phlebography is rarely indicated in the study of orbital disease except for varices in which a specific localization or definition may be possible. Orbital venograms are routinely done via the angular tributaries but may also be studied via retrograde jugular venous supply in selected circumstances. The recent introduction of digital subtraction methods may circumvent the need for direct and complicated intra-arterial injection studies in selected instances.

Lacrimal Drainage System.[2, 10] The lacrimal drainage system can be assessed by tomographic and CT studies. In the case of obstruction, contrast medium injected into the drainage system can help to outline intraluminal masses or sites of the obstruction secondary to extraluminal pressure. This may be particularly useful in combined nasopharyngeal and orbital lesions. The method involves intubation of the canaliculi and injection of radiopaque dyes (Fig. 68–38*B*, arrow).

Echography.[1] Orbital echography is a noninvasive ultrasound technique that provides useful information regarding the size, shape, location, tissue characteristics, and vascular features of orbital disease. The technique of standardized echography combines information obtained from A scan, B scan, and Doppler echography. The A scan uses a small probe that emits sound waves, the reflections of which can be displayed on an oscilloscope. These reflections, when studied, can help to differentiate the reflectivity, structure, sound attenuation, location, shape, size, borders, mobility, and compressibility of lesions (Figs. 68–30, 68–39, and 68–40*D*). With the added two-dimensional modality of B

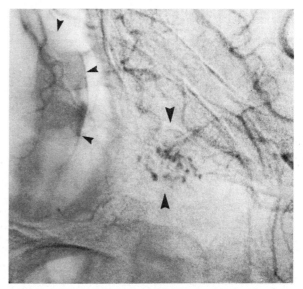

Figure 68–34. Coned-down subtraction view of a mass in the orbit following carotid injection. Note a focal area of minor pools of dye between large arrows. Small arrows show the choroidal crescent. This proved to be a hemangioma.

scan, location and size can be graphically demonstrated (Figs. 68–17, 68–27, 68–28, 68–30, 68–39, and 68–40). Doppler echography provides information concerning vascularity. The overall technique should involve a combination of these methods, depending on the type of lesion being studied.

New Techniques. There are several innovative technologic developments becoming available that may provide special functional and structural information in orbital disease. In particular, positron emission tomography and nuclear magnetic resonance promise to pro-

Text continued on page 1738

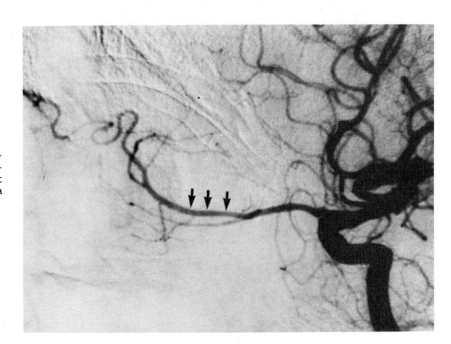

Figure 68–35. Subtraction view of internal carotid injection showing downward displacement of the ophthalmic artery as a result of the presence of a non-enhancing orbital mass (arrows).

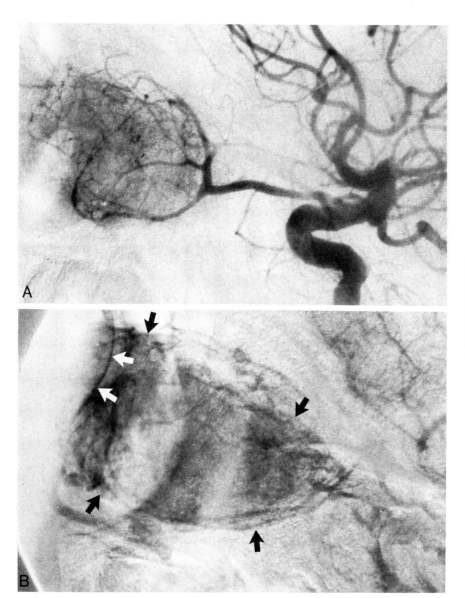

Figure 68–36. (A) Early arterial phase injection showing a rapid tumor blush, which persisted into the late phase (B). Black arrows show extent of tumor, and white arrows show choroidal crescent. This proved to be a tumor blush associated with a meningioma of the optic nerve.

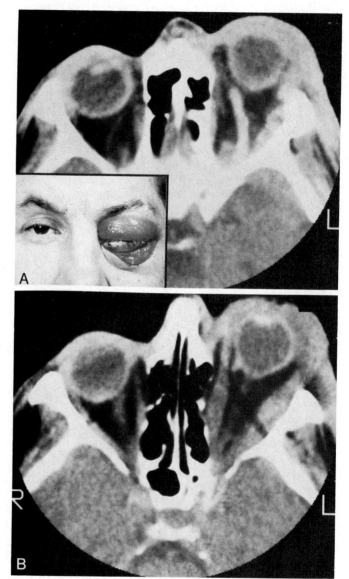

Figure 68–37. (*A*) *Inset*: This patient presented with persistent exophthalmos, chemosis, ptosis, lack of ocular movement, and loss of vision as a result of facial trauma received several weeks earlier. Clinically, there was evidence of pulsation. The adjacent axial contrast CT scan shows a large superior ophthalmic vein and marked proptosis. (*B*) An axial scan of the same patient shows tenting of the globe caused by the extreme proptosis and enlargement of the extraocular muscles.

Illustration continued on following page

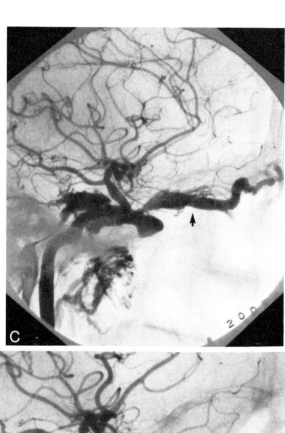

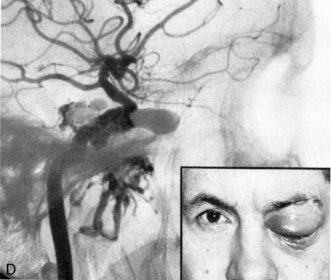

Figure 68–37 *Continued.* (*C*) Angiogram of same patient showing a carotid cavernous fistula with extensive filling of the superior ophthalmic vein (arrow). (*D*) Angiogram shows placement of balloons, which have obstructed the shunt and lead to marked improvement, as shown in inset. This was taken 1 week after balloon catheterization.

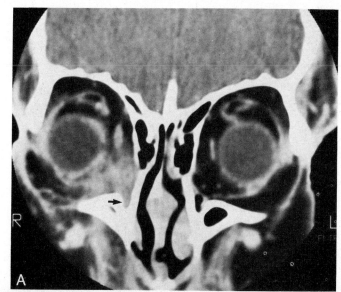

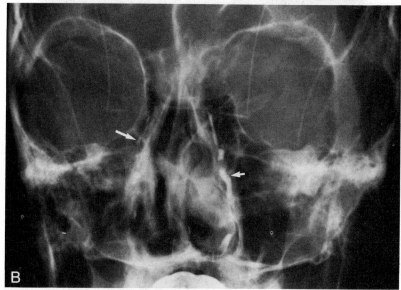

Figure 68–38. (*A*) Coronal CT scan shows an infiltrative right inferior orbital mass, which has led to outward and upward displacement of the globe and extends into the lacrimal duct (arrow). (*B*) Contrast dacryocystogram of same patient shows normal filling of the left lacrimal system (small arrow), as opposed to marked decrease in filling of the right system (large arrow) resulting from extraluminal pressure arising from what proved to be an idiopathic sclerosing inflammation (pseudotumor) of the orbit.

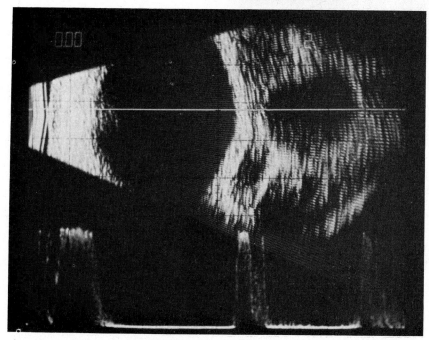

Figure 68–39. A- and B-scan ultrasound of a retrobulbar multilocular cystic mass caused by a hemorrhage in an orbital varix.

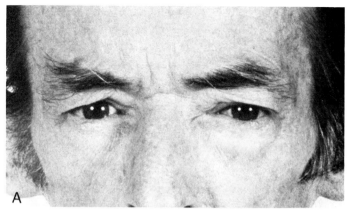

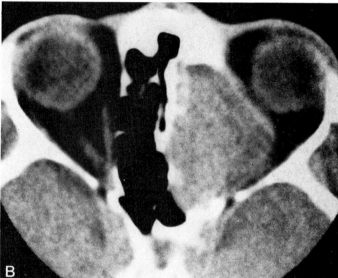

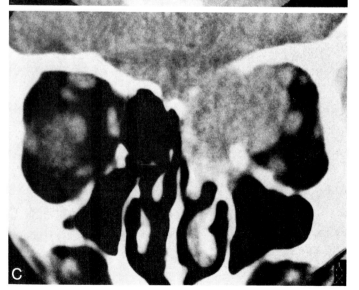

Figure 68–40. (A) This patient presented with an outward and axial displacement of the left globe owing to the presence of a mass within the sinus and nasopharynx shown on axial CT scan (B) and on coronal CT scan (C). Note bone destruction and infiltration.

Illustration continued on opposite page

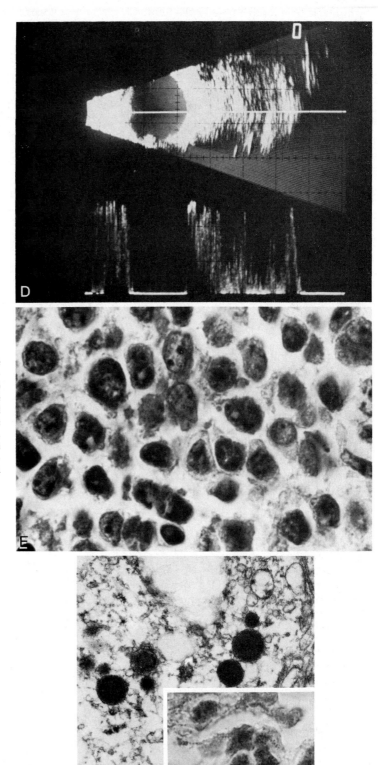

Figure 68–40 *Continued.* (*D*) An A- and B-mode ultrasound of the same lesion shows multiple interfaces characteristic of an infiltrating orbital mass. (*E*) High-power photomicrograph of a biopsy of the lesion, showing a poorly differentiated round cell tumor of the nasopharynx. (H & E, × 100.) (*F*) *Inset:* Grimelius stain was positive for argyrophil granules. (Grimelius, × 100.) The larger picture is an electron micrograph of the same lesion and shows membrane-bound neuroendocrine granules, confirming a diagnosis of neuroendocrine carcinoma.

vide added physiologic information regarding the effect of disease. These are currently being studied and will be available on a routine basis in the future.

Visual Function

It is important to assess the effect of disease on the ocular and orbital structures. There is a vast array of sophisticated methods available to study ocular motility, psychovisual function, ocular vascularity, tear production, and drainage. In particular, the effect of disease on the optic nerve may be delineated early in the course by study of color vision, visual fields, electroretinography, and visually evoked response. This kind of assessment allows for definition of need for, and effect of, therapeutic intervention as well as the effect of the primary disease itself. Evidence of dysfunction of the muscles or neuromuscular apparatus can also be detected early and assessed on a temporal basis for similar reasons. Tear production, or absence, as well as drainage can be assessed by both simple and sophisticated (scintillography) technology.[10]

Technology of Pathology

It is important to realize the fullest diagnostic potential from any specimen, and this is especially true in the case of orbital disease. Frequently, lesions here are not easily accessible and require considerable technical expertise to obtain both for biopsy and on extirpation. Once the specimen is obtained, it is important to have a clear plan as to the disposition of the specimen. The technology of pathology[9] has undergone an explosive change in the last decade, and the specificity of diagnosis is becoming increasingly important because effective therapy, particularly in cancer, is also becoming specific in orientation. There are four major areas of advances in pathologic assessment: cytology, histochemistry, immunohistochemistry, and electron microscopy.

Cytologic methods and ancillary technology, including *histochemistry* and *electron microscopy*, are routinely available. In the orbit, as in other areas, this has facilitated fine needle aspiration, which is particularly useful in secondary invasions in which it avoids open biopsy. For instance, the previously demonstrated aspiration of a progressive infiltrative lesion of the orbit arising from the maxillary antrum yielded an aspirate that proved to be a squamous cell carcinoma on routine histologic and electron microscopic examination (Fig. 68–3).

The introduction of *immunohistochemical techniques,* particularly the immunoperoxidase method, has allowed for an ever-increasing range of specificity in tissue diagnosis. Identification of component antigens for immunoprotein, muscle, keratin, glial protein, prostatic antigen, endocrine granules, and many others are becoming routinely available. For example, the nasopharyngeal carcinoma shown in Figure 68–40 appeared on routine histologic tests to be a poorly differentiated malignancy with a wide-ranging differential diagnosis. Immunoperoxidase stain ruled out immunoglobulin, myoglobulin, and glial fiber protein. Routine histochemical staining for argyrophil granules was strongly posi-

tive, suggesting a carcinoma with neuroendocrine features. Immunohistochemistry is most successful with fresh frozen tissue or tissue briefly fixed in acetone or Bouin's or Carnoy's solution. In use of these procedures, proper management of the tissues is important in order to obtain accurate results.

Ultrastructural methods are particularly useful in distinguishing tissue types, as demonstrated in our previous example who showed membrane-bound neuroendocrine granules (Fig. 68–40F). In another case of a poorly differentiated round cell tumor of the nasopharynx seen in childhood, the electron microscopic appearance showed pools of glycogen and the presence of cell membrane junctions with the absence of other subcellular components, leading to a diagnosis of Ewing's sarcoma (Fig. 68–26C and D). This method is particularly valuable in the study of small round cell tumors of childhood and the adult. Once again, it is important to get appropriate fixation (glutaraldehyde) and rapid transportation to the laboratory for maximal results.

The best way of handling biopsy tissues is to alert pathologists in advance, discuss the differential diagnosis, and ask for guidance in the handling of tissue. This informed multidisciplinary approach to biopsy will assure maximum diagnostic information.

REFERENCES

GENERAL

1. Bryne SF, Glaser JS: Orbital tissue differentiation with standard echography. Ophthalmology 90:1071, 1983.
2. Hurwitz JJ, Welham RAN, Lloyd GAS: The role of intubation macrodacryocystography in the management of problems of the lacrimal system. Can J Ophthalmol 10:361, 1975.
3. Ingalls RG: Tumors of the Orbit and Allied Pseudotumors. Springfield, Ill., Thomas, 1953.
4. Koorneff L: New insights in the human orbital connective tissue. Arch Ophthalmol 95:1269, 1977.
5. Moss HM: Expanding lesions of the orbit, a clinical study of 230 consecutive cases. Am J Ophthalmol 54:761, 1962.
6. Reese AB: Expanding lesions of the orbit. Trans Ophthalmol Soc UK 91:85, 1971.
7. Rootman J: An approach to diagnosis of orbital disease. Can J Ophthalmol 18:102, 1983.
8. Rootman J, Nugent R: The classification and management of acute orbital pseudotumors. Ophthalmology 84:1040, 1982.
9. Rootman J, Quenville N, Owen D: Recent advances in pathology as applied to orbital biopsy—practical considerations. Ophthalmology 91:708, 1984.
10. Rosenstock T, Hurwitz JJ: Functional obstruction of the lacrimal drainage passages. Can J Ophthalmol 17:249, 1982.

ANATOMY

11. Duane TD (ed): Biomedical Foundations of Ophthalmology. Vol. I. New York, Harper & Row, 1982.
12. Elder D: System of Ophthalmology, Vol. II. Anatomy of the Visual System. London, Henry Kimpton, 1961.
13. Last RJ: Anatomy of the Eye and Orbit. Philadelphia, W. B. Saunders Co., 1968.

ORBITAL DISEASE

14. Elder D: System of Ophthalmology. Vol. XIII. London, Henry Kimpton, 1974.
15. Henderson JW: Orbital Tumors. 2nd ed. New York, Decker/Thieme-Stratton, 1980.
16. Jakobiec FA (ed): Ocular and Adnexal Tumors. Birmingham, Ala., Aesculapius, 1978.
17. Jones IS, Jakobiec FA: Diseases of the Orbit. New York, Harper & Row, 1979.

CHAPTER 69

Treatment of Tumors of the Eye, Orbit, and Lacrimal Apparatus

Jonathan J. Dutton, M.D., Ph.D. • *Richard L. Anderson, M.D.*

The eyes, eyelids, and ocular adnexa are common sites for malignancy. A large number of primary tumors may occur here, and secondary lesions frequently invade periocular tissues from adjacent paranasal sinuses or the intracranial vault. In the Third National Cancer Survey (1975), tumors of the eye itself and orbit constituted 0.3 per cent of all malignancies in the United States, with an age-adjusted incidence of 0.8 per 100,000 for Caucasians and 0.4 per 100,000 for blacks. An estimated 1700 new cases of malignant eye cancers were diagnosed in 1975.

Preservation of visual function depends upon early diagnosis and definitive therapy with minimal destruction of adjacent normal tissues. This is usually very difficult to achieve for malignant processes because of the crowded juxtaposition of so many vital structures within the eye and orbit. Compounding the problem is the relationship of orbital structures to the intracranial contents through bony foramina, allowing spread of tumors backward into the central nervous system.

The recognition and diagnosis of ophthalmic malignancies can be a challenging task. External tumors of the eyelids exhibit variable presentations, often masquerading as benign processes, such as blepharitis, chalazion, or papilloma. Orbital lesions usually manifest with proptosis, with or without associated visual loss or motility disturbance. New diagnostic modalities, as discussed in the previous chapter, may narrow down the possible etiologies but, for the most part, are no substitute for tissue diagnosis. However, obtaining such biopsy material may require major orbital surgery.

Intraocular malignancies may go unrecognized until rather advanced stages of visual loss have occurred or, in children, until leukokoria or strabismus is noticed by the parents. Diagnosis may be even more difficult than with orbital lesions because histologic confirmation is usually impossible before definitive treatment is rendered. Yet, nowhere is accurate diagnosis more important, as therapy frequently involves loss of useful vision in the involved eye.

Numerous therapeutic modalities for ophthalmic malignancies have been advocated in an attempt to preserve vision. In some cases less extensive and more cosmetically acceptable procedures have replaced older treatments without worsening the long-term prognosis. The appropriate management of ophthalmic malignancies varies with the specific lesion, its precise location,

and the philosophy of the surgeon. We will discuss the more common malignant tumors of the eyelid, eye, and orbit and the various treatments in current practice.

SURGICAL ANATOMY

Eyelids

The eyelids, along with the orbital rims and brows, serve to protect the exposed anterior surfaces of the eye. Their unique anatomic structure, physiology, and constant reflex and voluntary movements provide defensive and protective mechanisms against glare, foreign matter, desiccation, trauma, and infection.

The eyelids form the thin outer covering of the orbit. They extend from the brow above to the cheek below, and from the medial to the lateral orbital rims. Between the lids is the interpalpebral fissure, which measures from 25 to 28 mm horizontally and from 7 to 11 mm vertically. Movements of the lids are complex and allow intimate contact between the conjunctival surfaces of both eyelids with the underlying cornea in all positions of gaze. Lying medially between the plica and medial canthus is the caruncle, a fleshy mass that measures 4 to 5 mm vertically by 3 mm horizontally.

The eyelid margins are formed from modified skin anteriorly and conjunctiva posteriorly, with a mucocutaneous junction separating them. On the anterior edge of the lid margins are several rows of cilia, which serve to protect the eye from wind-blown particles. In the posterior half of the lid, margins are the openings of the meibomian glands. These are large sebaceous glands lying within the tarsal plates, numbering about 25 in the upper lid and 20 in the lower lid, and they supply the lipid component to the precorneal tear film.

Glands of Zeis are microscopic sebaceous glands associated with each eyelash follicle. Moll's glands are modified sweat glands that empty onto the lid margins between the cilia. Unlike the meibomian glands and Zeis glands, which are holocrine glands, Moll's glands are apocrine glands.

The main portion of the eyelid is a thin structure composed of several laminae (Fig. 69–1). At a level 3 mm proximal to the lid margin these laminae are, from anterior to posterior, (1) skin, (2) subcutaneous areolar tissue, (3) pretarsal orbicularis muscle, (4) postorbicular

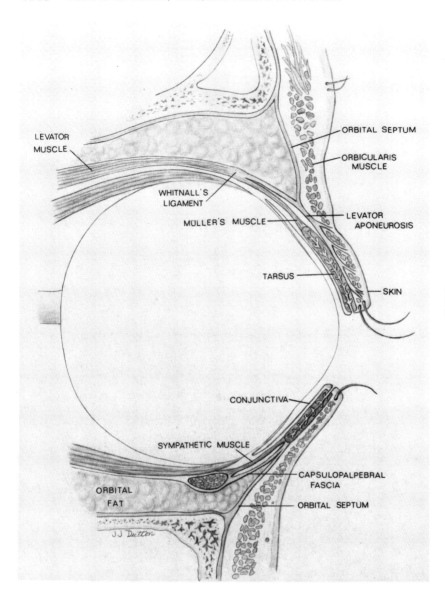

Figure 69–1. Cross section of the anterior orbit showing lamellar structure of the upper and lower eyelids.

areolar tissue, (5) tarsal plate, and (6) conjunctiva. At a level 15 mm above the upper lid margin, the laminae are as follows: (1) skin, (2) subcutaneous areolar tissue, (3) preseptal orbicularis muscle, (4) postorbicular areolar tissue, (5) orbital septum, (6) preaponeurotic fat pad, (7) levator aponeurosis, (8) Müller's sympathetic muscle, and (9) conjunctiva.

The skin of the eyelids is exceptionally thin and is loosely attached to underlying tissues except in the pretarsal portions of the eyelids and at the canthi. This accounts for a number of conditions such as stretched redundant skin (dermatochalasis) in older patients and the easy accumulation of preseptal subcutaneous edema and hemorrhage.

Beneath the subcutaneous areolar tissue the orbicularis oculi fibers run parallel to the lid margins. The orbicularis muscle is divided anatomically into several portions. The orbital portion arises from the medial orbital rim, fans out above, and passes around the periphery of the eyelids to insert near its site of origin at the medial orbital rim. The palpebral portion is confined to the mobile portion of the lids. It arises from the medial canthal tendon, arcs superiorly and inferiorly, and inserts along the lateral horizontal raphe and lateral canthal tendon. It is further subdivided into a pretarsal portion, overlying the anterior surface of the tarsal plates, and a preseptal portion, which overlies the orbital septum proximal to the tarsal plates. Along the lid margins and forming a delicate band of striated fibers is the muscle of Riolan. The main pretarsal orbicularis fibers pass laterally into the lateral canthal tendon, which inserts into the periosteum at the lateral orbital tubercle, and medially into the medial canthal tendon, which inserts into the periosteum on the frontal process of the maxillary bone. Small slips of orbicularis, Horner's muscle, pass from the deep medial portion of the pretarsal fibers and from the muscle of Riolan and insert into the periosteum of the posterior lacrimal crest.

They contribute to functioning of the lacrimal pump system by shortening the canaliculus. The orbicularis muscle is innervated by branches of the seventh cranial nerve. The postorbicular areolar plane is composed of loose connective tissue and contains the seventh cranial nerve fibers that supply the orbicularis muscle.

The orbital septum originates from the arcus marginalis formed by the junction of periorbita and periosteum around the periphery of the orbital rim. In the upper lid the septum blends distally into the fibers of the underlying levator aponeurosis about 4 to 6 mm above the tarsal plate. In the lower lid the septum extends from the arcus marginalis at the lower orbital rim to the lower border of the tarsal plate, where it joins the lower lid retractors. Medially, the orbital septum of both lids pass behind the lacrimal sac, blending with fibers of the posterior crus of the medial canthal tendon, to insert onto the posterior lacrimal crest. Laterally, the septum fuses to and forms the posterior layer of the lateral palpebral raphe. Weak and thin areas in the septum permit herniation of orbital fat into the lids; this is especially prominent in the elderly. The orbital septum acts as a barrier to the spread of infection and hemorrhage.

Between the orbital septum and the levator aponeurosis in the upper lid is the preaponeurotic fat pad, which is a forward extension of orbital fat. It is an important surgical landmark, and its prolapse into weak areas of the septum is a major cause of baggy eyelids.

The levator palpebrae superioris muscle, which elevates the lid, takes origin from the lesser wing of the sphenoid bone just above the optic foramen and annulus of Zinn. It travels forward in close approximation to the underlying superior rectus muscle. As it crosses the equator of the globe, the muscle fibers pass into a fibrous aponeurosis that fans out horizontally to occupy the entire orbital width. A thickened condensation of fibrous tissue, the superior suspensory ligament of Whitnall, extends across the orbit within this tendon, just at its junction with the muscular portion of the levator. Whitnall's ligament is attached to the orbital wall medially at the trochlea and laterally to the capsule of the lacrimal gland and periosteum of the orbital wall. This ligament serves to support the levator and to change its vector force from horizontal in the orbit to vertical in the lid. As the aponeurosis passes forward into the upper lid, it fans out to occupy the entire orbital width. It fuses with the distal fibers of the orbital septum about 4 to 6 mm above the tarsal plate and sends fibrous slips that interdigitate between fibers of the orbicularis to insert into the intermuscular septa, forming a prominent lid crease. The aponeurosis attaches to the anterior aspect of the tarsal plate. Medial and lateral extensions of the aponeurosis, forming the "horns," insert into the medial and lateral canthal tendons, respectively. The levator muscle derives its innervation from the superior division of the third cranial nerve.

Müller's muscle is supplied by sympathetic fibers and lies just behind the levator aponeurosis. It originates from the distal fibers of the levator muscle and inserts onto the proximal border of the tarsal plate. In the lower lid, analogous but less developed fibers take origin from the fascia of the inferior rectus muscle and pass to the lower border of the tarsus. Lockwood's ligament, or the inferior suspensory ligament, is a condensation of the capsules of the inferior oblique and inferior rectus muscles and spans the inferior orbit, helping to support the orbital contents. A fascial expansion from Lockwood's ligament and the inferior rectus sheath, the capsulopalpebral fascia, passes upward to insert into the inferior surface of the tarsus, forming an analogue of the levator aponeurosis.

The tarsal plates are flat, dense, fibrous structures that give support to the eyelids. About 20 to 30 meibomian glands lie within the plates in each lid and provide the important lipid component to the tear film.

Lining the posterior surface of both lids is the conjunctiva, a highly vascular mucous membrane that contains numerous mucus-secreting goblet cells as well as small accessory lacrimal glands of Krause and Wolfring. From the eyelids the palpebral conjunctiva passes into the fornices and is continuous with the bulbar conjunctiva covering the globe.

The vascular supply of the eyelids is extensive. Arterial blood derives mainly from the ophthalmic artery via the medial superior and inferior palpebral arteries that penetrate the orbital septum nasally. These run laterally as three arcades: the marginal arcades near the lid margins in the upper and lower lids and the superior peripheral arcade that runs near the upper border of the tarsus in the upper lid. An inferior peripheral arcade may be present but is generally poorly defined. These arcades anastomose temporally with the lateral superior and lateral inferior palpebral arteries derived from the lacrimal artery. Further anastomotic branches join the external carotid system via the transverse facial and superficial temporal arteries laterally and the dorsal nasal and angular arteries medially.

Venous drainage anterior to the tarsal plate is into the angular and superficial temporal veins. A deeper system, draining posterior to the tarsus, empties into tributaries of the ophthalmic veins.

Lymphatic vessels in the lateral two thirds of the upper lid and the lateral one third of the lower lid enter the preauricular lymph nodes. The medial third of the upper lid and medial two thirds of the lower lid drain into the submaxillary nodes.

The sensory nerve supply to the lids is from the fifth cranial nerve. The supraorbital and supratrochlear branches of the ophthalmic division supply the upper lid, with some branches of the infratrochlear and lacrimal nerve also contributing. The lower lid is supplied principally from infraorbital branches of the maxillary division of the trigeminal nerve, along with some contribution from the infratrochlear nerve.

The Orbit

The bony orbit has the approximate shape of a pear, with the stem directed toward the optic canal. Vertically, its widest portion lies about 1.5 cm behind the rims. The lateral rim is formed by the frontal process of the zygomatic bone and the zygomatic process of the frontal bone. The lateral wall behind the rim is formed from the orbital plates of the zygomatic and greater wing of the sphenoid bones. Superiorly, crossing the lateral rim, is the frontozygomatic suture. About 1 cm above this suture begins the anterior cranial fossa. This relationship is important to keep in mind when performing a lateral orbitotomy. Inferiorly, the lateral rim passes into the zygomatic arch. During orbital surgery, the lateral wall is usually removed to the superior border of the arch. Rarely, the zygomatic arch may be removed for greater exposure, but care must be taken not to injure structures in the inferior orbital fissure, which lies immediately medial to it. As the orbital plate of the greater wing of the sphenoid passes back toward the apex, it is joined by the main body of the wing to form the anterior surface of the middle cranial fossa. In removing the more posterior portion of this wall during a lateral orbitotomy, the appearance of thick cancellous bone marks this junction. Bleeding from this bone is occasionally brisk but is easily controlled with bone wax. Low on the lateral wall, near the anterior end of the inferior orbital fissure, are the zygomaticotemporal and zygomaticofacial foramina, transmitting branches of the zygomatic nerve and vessels to the face and temporal fossa. These may be disrupted while elevating periorbita from the lateral wall, but this is of little consequence. More posteriorly is Hyrtl's canal, a foramen in the greater wing of the sphenoid near its suture with the frontal bone, which transmits a branch of the middle meningeal artery into the orbit. Excessive posterior dissection of periorbita may transect this vessel with subsequent bleeding.

Immediately inside periorbita, along the middle of the lateral wall, is the lateral rectus muscle and, above it, the lacrimal artery and nerve. Damage to these structures may result from tearing periorbita during orbitotomy or during the surgical opening of it.

The lateral orbital tubercle is a small elevation on the orbital surface of the zygomatic bone just inside the rim. It is located 10 to 12 mm below the frontozygomatic suture. Attached to the tubercle are the lateral canthal tendon, the lateral horn of the levator aponeurosis, and tendinous attachments to the medial rectus muscle sheath. These are dissected off with periorbita during lateral orbital approaches. Careful reapproximation of periorbita and periosteum over the lateral rim will maintain the anatomic relationships of these structures.

The orbital roof is formed by the orbital plate of the frontal bone with a small posterior contribution by the lesser wing of the sphenoid bone. The roof is very thin, and in elderly patients, there may be areas of bony dehiscence through which dura and periorbita are in contact. During surgery in this region or during exenteration, dissection of periorbita from the roof with instruments or even with the fingers can fracture this bone. If a dural tear occurs, a cerebrospinal fluid leak will result.

Immediately beneath periorbita in the middle of the roof is the frontal nerve, and in the anterior half of the orbit, it is accompanied by the supraorbital artery. More medially, the supratrochlear nerve also lies just beneath periorbita. Tears in the periorbita during surgery along the roof may damage these structures.

Superolaterally and anteriorly on the roof, and extending onto the upper portion of the lateral wall, is the lacrimal fossa, a slight indentation on the zygomatic process of the frontal bone. Just within periorbita in the region of the fossa is the lacrimal gland and its associated vascular and nerve supply, as well as orbital fat, with which the gland might be confused.

Superomedially, the cartilaginous trochlea and adjacent periorbita are firmly attached to the orbital roof about 4 mm behind the orbital rim. This may be dissected off for exposure of the roof during anteromedial orbital surgery but must be carefully repositioned, with periorbita sutured to periosteum, to avoid superior oblique muscle imbalance.

The supraorbital notch is a separation in the superior orbital rim at the junction of its lateral two thirds and medial one third and is easily palpated. It transmits the supraorbital vessels and nerve out of the orbit. These structures are easily damaged during superomedial surgery.

The medial orbital wall lies parallel to the midsagittal plane. It is formed from front to back by the frontal process of the maxillary bone, the lacrimal bone, the lamina papyracea of the ethmoid bone, and the body of the sphenoid bone. The paper-thin ethmoid bone makes up the largest portion of the medial wall and separates the orbit from the ethmoidal air cells. This wall can be easily penetrated by probing instruments and even by the surgeon's finger. Anteriorly, between maxillary and lacrimal bones, is the nasolacrimal fossa and canal. It is bounded by the anterior and posterior lacrimal crests, and within the fossa lies the lacrimal sac. Just in front of the sac, the medial canthal tendon attaches to the frontal process of the maxillary bone, and behind, posterior fibers of the orbicularis muscle (Horner's muscle) and the orbital septum attach to the posterior lacrimal crest. During medial orbital surgery the lacrimal sac may inadvertently be damaged.

Perforating the medial wall within the frontoethmoid suture are the anterior and posterior ethmoidal foramina, which transmit branches of the ophthalmic artery with the same names. Surgery along the medial wall may transect these arteries, resulting in profuse bleeding.

Just behind the ethmoid bone, at the level of the frontoethmoid suture in the anterior half of the orbit, lies the lamina cribrosa, forming the roof of the nasal cavity. Removal of the medial wall above this level may involve this structure, with the possibility of a cerebrospinal fluid leak.

Just beneath periorbita along the medial wall is the medial rectus muscle and just above it is the infratrochlear nerve. The superior oblique muscle lies in the angle between the medial wall and roof.

The floor of the orbit is composed principally of the orbital plate of the maxillary bone, with small contributions from the zygomatic bone laterally and the palatine bone posteriorly. Running in the floor from back to front is the infraorbital groove, which becomes bridged over at its midportion to continue forward as the infraorbital canal. This transmits the infraorbital nerve and vessels. Surgery on the orbital floor may damage these structures.

Below the floor is the maxillary sinus, which extends from the maxilloethmoid suture to just lateral to the infraorbital canal and back to the posterior portion of the orbit, ending just in front of the superior orbital fissure. The floor is separated from the lateral wall by the inferior orbital fissure, which transmits the maxillary nerve and its zygomatic branch, ascending branches from the sphenopalatine ganglion, and the infraorbital vessels. Separating the orbital floor from the roof is the apex, containing the optic canal and superior orbital fissure. These latter two openings are separated from each other by a bony bar, the optic strut. Within the apex is the tight juxtaposition of all the major vascular and neural elements entering the orbit from the middle cranial fossa. These are not generally encountered in routine orbital procedures, but their relationships become exceedingly important in surgery at the apex for tumors or for canal decompressions, either through a transcranial or transorbital approach.

Just beneath periorbita in the middle of the floor lies the inferior rectus muscle. The inferior oblique muscle lies transversely in the anterior orbit between periorbita and the inferior rectus. It is very easily injured during surgery along the orbital floor.

On the inferior orbital rim, about 4 to 5 mm below the margin, is the infraorbital foramen, which carries the infraorbital nerve and vessels. Incision of periosteum along the rim in inferior orbital approaches should be made above this level to avoid transecting these structures.

Within the bony orbit, four surgical spaces may be defined. Most peripherally is a potential subperiosteal space bounded externally by the bony walls and internally by periorbita. Anteriorly, this space is closed by the orbital septum and globe. The second, or peripheral orbital space, lies between periorbita and the muscle cone. It contains intraorbital fat; lacrimal gland; supraorbital, supratrochlear, lacrimal, and frontal nerves; and supraorbital and supratrochlear arteries and their branches. The third, or central surgical space, lies within the muscle cone. It is bounded anteriorly by Tenon's capsule and contains many vital structures, including the extraocular muscles and their nerves, the ophthalmic artery and superior ophthalmic vein and their branches, the ciliary ganglion and posterior ciliary nerves, the nasociliary nerve, and the optic nerve. The fourth space lies between Tenon's capsule and the globe.

MALIGNANT TUMORS OF THE EYELIDS AND CONJUNCTIVA

Types of Tumors

Eyelid tumors are very common, but only about 20 per cent of such lesions are malignant. Of the latter, greater than 90 per cent are basal cell carcinomas. Squamous cell carcinomas constitute the majority of remaining malignant lesions, with sebaceous cell carcinomas and malignant melanomas being relatively uncommon. Carcinoma of sweat gland origin is exceedingly rare in the eyelids. Although malignant lymphomas and metastatic lesions may occur in the eyelids, these most frequently involve the orbit with contiguous spread to the lids.

Clinically, most eyelid lesions are easily visible and noticed by the patient. Certain features, such as loss of eyelashes, bleeding and ulceration, and rapid growth, are more suggestive of a malignant process. Physical examination must include palpation of subcutaneous tissues. Both skin and conjunctival surfaces of the lid and the fornices must be examined to determine the extent of the lesion and to note the presence of multicentric tumors. Regional lymph nodes should be palpated when malignancies other than basal cell carcinoma are suspected. If potentially metastasizing tumors are suspected, a systemic examination as well as appropriate laboratory studies will be required. With large tumors that extend into the orbit, appropriate radiographic and echographic studies are indicated to determine the dimensions of the mass and involvement of orbital tissues, bones, and adjacent structures, such as paranasal sinuses or intracranial vault.

Basal Cell Carcinoma

Basal cell carcinomas are the most common skin malignancies occurring on the face and represent more than 90 per cent of all cancers of the eyelids.[75, 111, 147] They typically are slow-growing tumors that metastasize with exceptional rarity. Local invasion of the underlying dermis is usual, and larger lesions may involve the adjacent orbit or, rarely, even the eye itself.[74, 149] In the past, 2 to 22 per cent of patients with basal cell carcinoma of the eyelid required enucleation or exenteration, and the ultimate mortality rate has been as high as 11 per cent with conventional modes of therapy.[16, 113, 133, 155]

Basal cell carcinomas occur most commonly in middle-aged to elderly individuals who are predisposed by chronic sunlight exposure, chronic irritation, or mechanical or chemical injury. Light-skinned individuals are particularly susceptible to this tumor. The lesions are found most commonly on the lower eyelid, followed by the medial canthus, upper lid, and lateral canthus, in decreasing order of frequency.[75]

Clinically, basal cell carcinomas may present in numerous forms. The nodular-ulcerative type frequently begins as a small, elevated, waxy nodule with telangiectatic surface vessels. It slowly enlarges and undergoes central ulceration. The ulcer crater is usually surrounded by a rolled, pearly border (Fig. 69–2). Variable amounts of pigmentation and even cystic changes may be present. Growth may be atypical, resembling a benign papilloma. The morpheaform or sclerosing form of basal cell carcinoma appears as a firm, slightly elevated plaque with ill-defined borders. The tumor margins

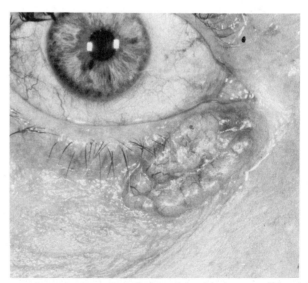

Figure 69–2. Basal cell carcinoma of the right lower eyelid and medial canthus. Note the typical pearly, raised borders and the depressed center resulting from necrosis.

frequently extend well beyond the clinically definable edges of the lesion. Such tumors not uncommonly extend deep into lid and orbital structures.

Left untreated, basal cell carcinomas grow slowly with progressive involvement of orbit, bones, paranasal sinuses, sclera, and even brain. Recurrent lesions after incomplete treatment tend to be more extensive and more widely invasive. This is particularly true of medial canthal tumors, in which inadequate excision is common owing to reluctance on the part of the surgeon to damage canthal and lacrimal drainage structures.

Squamous Cell Carcinoma

Squamous cell carcinomas involve the eyelids far less frequently than do basal cell carcinomas. They tend to occur on exposed areas of skin damaged by sunlight, or can arise in pre-existing lesions such as senile keratoses, chronic ulcers, burn scars, or areas of chronic inflammation. These tumors are far more common on the conjunctiva, where they have a predilection for the limbus. They may be indolent, but in general grow rapidly, with contiguous spread into adjacent structures, including the orbit, sclera,[74, 122] and even corneal epithelium.[24, 74] These tumors show a tendency toward local recurrences after any form of treatment, and there does not appear to be a clear relationship between invasiveness through the basement membrane and later recurrence.[79] The incidence of metastasis has been reported at 0.5 to 5.0 per cent,[6, 96] and metastasis occurs primarily via regional lymphatics.

Clinically this tumor begins as an elevated keratinized area, often with an ulcerated center (Fig. 69–3). It may resemble a basal cell carcinoma, or occasionally may form a fungating, verrucous mass (Fig. 69–4). Because of the tumor's invasiveness and potential for metastasis, early recognition is important. The clinician must be aware of the various pre-existing lesions that may give rise to squamous cell carcinomas, and any suspicious lesions must be biopsied.

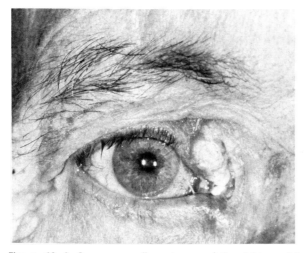

Figure 69–3. Squamous cell carcinoma of the right medial canthus with areas of necrosis. This lesion extended into the underlying periosteum and back into the orbit, requiring radical exenteration for treatment.

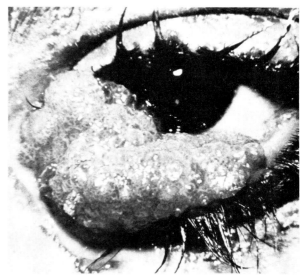

Figure 69–4. Squamous cell carcinoma of the palpebral conjunctiva of the left lower eyelid.

Sebaceous Cell Carcinoma

Sebaceous cell adenocarcinoma is a malignant tumor that may arise in the meibomian and sebaceous glands of the eyelids. It represents between 0.2 and 5.3 per cent of all eyelid tumors.[22, 25, 148] This lesion tends to occur in older individuals in the sixth and seventh decades and appears to be somewhat more common in females.[126]

Sebaceous carcinomas around the eye occur most frequently in the eyelids, with about 7 per cent of lesions arising in the caruncle. The upper eyelid is involved in about 60 per cent of cases, and the lower eyelid is involved in about 20 per cent. The remainder occur in the canthal region or eyebrows. Multicentric origin has been reported.[25] These tumors spread by direct extension. Seventeen to 19 per cent have been reported to involve the orbit.[18, 120] Metastatic spread is by regional lymphatics and is seen in up to 28 per cent of patients.[64]

Clinically, this tumor appears as a small, firm nodule near the lid margin, without ulceration. It may present a rather benign and indolent appearance and may be mistaken for a chalazion that is unresponsive to treatment in up to 40 per cent of cases, thus delaying diagnosis and definitive therapy.[18] A more diffuse growth pattern with conjunctival changes may simulate a chronic blepharoconjunctivitis or trachoma. Eventually, the lid margin becomes distorted with loss of lashes, and a large fungating mass may result.

The ultimate prognosis depends upon several factors. In their review of 95 cases of sebaceous carcinoma, Rao and associates[120] found a 43 per cent mortality rate for patients in whom symptoms were present for more than 6 months, compared with 13 per cent for those with symptoms of shorter duration. Histologic differentiation showed a marked relationship with prognosis, from a 7 per cent mortality rate for well-differentiated tumors to a 60 per cent mortality rate for poorly differentiated lesions. Similarly, those lesions with a high degree of infiltration carried four times the mortality rate (40 per cent) than those with minimal infiltrations.

It is clear that early diagnosis and aggressive treatment is essential in the management of sebaceous carcinoma.[68] Any patient with a chalazion-like lesion that is unresponsive to medical therapy or recurrent despite repeated curettage requires biopsy, as does any persistent unilateral blepharoconjunctivitis. Wet biopsy tissue must be submitted for fat stains, which are crucial to the diagnosis. Treatment should consist of exenteration if there is any involvement of orbital tissues.

Sweat Gland Carcinoma

These are rare malignancies that have been reported to occur on the eyelids.[85, 109] They are slow-growing tumors and frequently are neglected by patients for many years. They tend to recur locally, may be aggressively invasive, and have a high potential for metastasis.[135] Three cases of orbital and sinus involvement have been reported.[67, 85, 140] There is no characteristic clinical appearance, and histologic examination is in general the only means of diagnosis.

Malignant Melanoma

Periocular malignant melanoma is a rare tumor that usually arises from pre-existing pigmented lesions, such as junctional or compound nevi, or acquired melanosis. They may also arise from dermal melanoblasts associated with oculodermal melanocytosis. Malignant melanomas are highly aggressive tumors that are frequently misdiagnosed.

Clinically, malignant melanomas appear as a gradually enlarging mass that may look quite benign (Figs. 69–5 and 69–6). The surface may show some bleeding or frank ulceration. Pigmentation is variable and occasionally may be absent. Metastases usually occur via lymphatics to the regional lymph nodes and later by a hematogenous route to the liver, lungs, and skin.

Periocular and conjunctival melanomas may occur as focal nodular lesions arising as isolated tumors or as

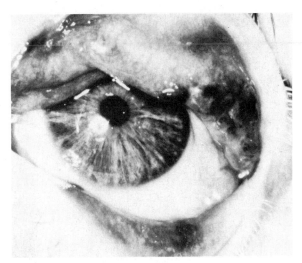

Figure 69–6. Acquired melanosis of the palpebral conjunctiva with nodules of malignant melanoma.

diffuse intraepithelial growths with extensive radial proliferation.[81] The latter seems to be more aggressive, with many patients ultimately requiring enucleation or exenteration.[93]

Management Modalities

The eyelids perform a vital function in protecting the eye from foreign bodies and desiccation. Without eyelids or an adequate substitute, useful vision is not possible. Because of this, treatment of malignant lesions in the lids is fraught with difficulty. Neoplastic tissue must be completely eliminated while at the same time preserving as much normal structure as possible for eyelid reconstruction. We feel that adequate removal of eyelid tumors can be done only by surgical excision with histologic confirmation of margins. We favor the *Mohs technique of microsurgical excision followed by immediate reconstruction.*[10, 23, 106] In the largest series of patients with eyelid malignancies treated with this method, only four recurrences in 250 patients (1.6 per cent) were reported after 2 to 5 years of follow-up, and all four had invasion of orbital tissues at the time of initial excision.[11] This contrasts with recurrence rates of 3.5 to 18.5 per cent with uncontrolled surgery.[1, 14, 113, 119]

The originally described Mohs technique utilized zinc chloride paste to fix tissues in situ prior to excision of each tissue layer, followed by mapping, staining, and microscopic examination of all margins for residual tumor.[105] The technique allowed controlled excision of tumor extensions beyond the clinically visible borders. A modification of this method utilizing fresh-frozen tissue instead of the more destructive procedure of chemical fixation[143] has proved to be more acceptable for excision of eyelid and orbital tumors.

Following microsurgically controlled excision of eyelid malignancies, the eyelids are restored by any of a number of plastic reconstructive techniques (Fig. 69–7). Medial canthal lesions present the greatest challenge because of the frequent involvement of the lacrimal drainage apparatus. When portions of the eyelids are missing, excessive laxity in elderly patients may permit direct closure of the defect and suturing of the remaining

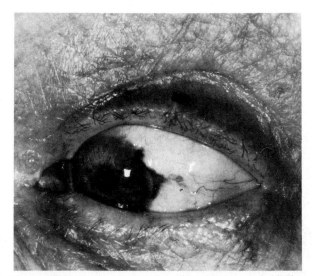

Figure 69–5. Conjunctival malignant melanoma at the limbus of the left eye. At surgery the lesion was found to be invasive into the corneal stroma and underlying sclera.

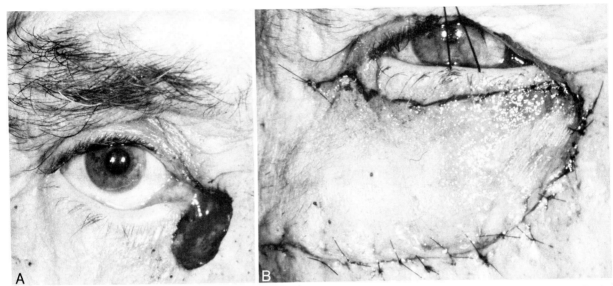

Figure 69–7. (*A*) Final defect resulting form a Mohs microsurgical excision of a medial canthal basal cell carcinoma. (*B*) Following reconstruction by a sliding myocutaneous flap.

tarsus to periosteum on the orbital process of the maxillary bone. If periosteum has not been preserved, a transnasal or canthal wire through bone will permit reconstruction of the medial canthus. If additional eyelid length is needed, this may be achieved with a free tarsal-conjunctival graft from the opposite eye to either upper or lower lid, periosteal flaps, sliding tarsal-conjunctival flaps from upper to lower lid, or with nasal cartilage-mucosal grafts. Skin defects can be closed with sliding or rotational myocutaneous flaps or with thin skin grafts. Occasionally, small defects may be left to granulate with acceptable cosmetic results.

The major complications encountered in reconstructions of the eyelids are instability of the lids or poor lid contour with resultant corneal exposure and abrasion. Lower lid ectropion is caused by vertical shortening of skin, laxity of the lid, and inadequate fixation at the canthi. Sufficient vertical height is achieved with the use of free skin grafts or generous flaps and the use of tarsorrhaphy (Frost) sutures for 1 week postoperatively to counteract cicatricial forces. Lid laxity is prevented by use of advancement flaps that are not excessively large for the defect. It is best to leave these tissues with some degree of tension. Lateral and medial canthal fixation should be done with permanent sutures to periosteum. The lateral canthus should create an upward vector to support the lateral lower lid and prevent postoperative sag. Meticulous attention to closure of

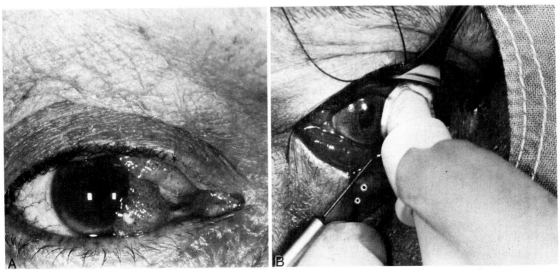

Figure 69–8. (*A*) Squamous cell carcinoma of the conjunctiva, invasive into underlying sclera. (*B*) Cryotherapy to the dissection bed following local excision of the tumor.

central lid defects will avoid eyelid notching, which can result in corneal irritation. Finally, in any plastic reconstructive procedure, complete hemostasis is a must, especially if free skin grafts are used. Thick grafts are to be avoided because they will tend to mask tumor recurrences. When the lacrimal drainage system has been sacrificed, its reconstruction is delayed for several years to avoid spread of possible recurrences into the nasopharynx.

Cryosurgery has been advocated for the treatment of basal cell carcinomas[38, 144, 154] and has been used extensively for bovine ocular squamous cell carcinomas.[39, 57] Clinical response has been reported to be excellent,[15, 39, 56–58, 101, 154] with clinical recurrence rates of 2 to 8 per cent. However, one study found biopsy-proved residual tumor in 20 per cent of cases following cryosurgery alone.[63] Combined localized surgery plus cryotherapy to the residual bed has been used for intraepithelial melanoma of the conjunctiva, and although some of these patients had recurrences, none developed extensive invasive disease or metastases.[80] In three patients with scleral invasion of a basal cell carcinoma, squamous cell carcinoma, and malignant melanoma, in whom radical surgery could not be done, we performed a similar combined limited local excision with cryotherapy for clinical eradication of tumor and found no recurrences in a 32- to 40-month follow-up period (Fig. 69–8).

Radiotherapy has had limited success in the treatment of basal cell and squamous cell carcinomas. Ocular complications, including damage to the lens and cornea, and secondary orbital malignancies are a potential hazard. Recurrence rates of 2 to 9 per cent have been reported.[28, 44, 91] Radiotherapy must be delivered in fractionated doses over several weeks and if recurrences develop, this mode cannot be repeated. It suffers from the same limitation of all noncontrolled modalities, that is, inability to monitor adequacy of treatment at the tumor margins.

Radiotherapy has been recommended as a primary treatment for sebaceous carcinoma of the eyelid.[72, 77] However, recurrence rates appear to be high, and this modality cannot be recommended as the initial treatment of this potentially lethal malignancy.[110]

Photoradiation therapy is a new method of treating malignancies that utilizes a photosensitizing pigment, hematoporphyrin derivative (HpD), which is selectively retained in neoplastic tissues. Exposure of these tissues containing HpD to a laser-generated red light at a frequency of 630 nm initiates the formation of a highly reactive state of oxygen that results in selective cytotoxicity of the tumor cells. This method has shown promising preliminary results against a number of solid human malignancies.[29, 34, 49, 90, 146] Its use in the treatment of basal cell carcinomas of the eyelids and face in nevoid basal cell carcinoma syndrome has given results comparable to other noncontrolled modalities (D. Tse, personal communication). The use of the CO_2 laser for the treatment of skin cancers has been reported,[8] but this method frequently leaves residual tumor, and recurrence rates have been as high as 50 per cent.

In summary, management of malignant lesions of the eyelids is best performed with excision by the Mohs microsurgical technique. Other modalities, although useful in selected patients, do not achieve the cure rates obtainable with this method.

INTRAOCULAR MALIGNANCIES

Types of Intraocular Tumors

Malignant tumors that occur within the eye present unique problems in both diagnosis and therapy. Because of the functional integrity of the eye, such lesions are not amenable to biopsy, and diagnosis must frequently rely on clinical history and ophthalmoscopic appearance alone. In the past a high percentage of eyes suspected of having malignant tumors have had benign lesions instead.[132] Therapeutic options are varied and depend in large part on the specific tumor diagnosis and location of the lesion, as well as visual status of the affected and fellow eye, age and health of the patient, and previous treatments given. Some tumors are best managed by surgery, others by less radical modalities, and still others by periodic observation.

Retinoblastoma

Retinoblastoma is a highly malignant tumor that arises from the retina (Fig. 69–9). It is the most common intraocular malignancy of childhood, occurring in one out of 18,000 live births in the United States.[35] Retinoblastoma ranks second after malignant melanoma as the most frequently encountered primary intraocular cancer in any age group.[125] The average age of patients at diagnosis is approximately 18 months, and the vast majority of cases present prior to 3 years of age. About 70 per cent of retinoblastoma cases are unilateral, and 25 to 30 per cent are bilateral.

Retinoblastoma is the only cancer known to be genetically determined. The gene behaves as an autosomal dominant with incomplete penetrance.[136] Approximately 5 per cent of affected patients will have a positive family history for this malignancy. In the remaining 95 per cent of cases, the tumor arises as a spontaneous mutation, of which about 80 per cent are believed to be of

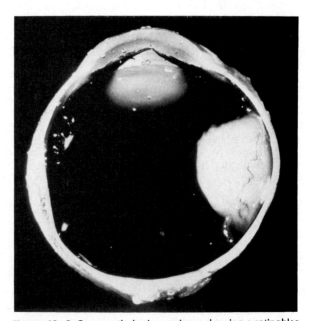

Figure 69–9. Gross pathologic specimen showing a retinoblastoma in the equatorial region.

somatic origin, with 20 per cent of germinal origin. Only the latter have hereditary implications.

There is an unusually high incidence of second primary tumors in retinoblastoma survivors, mostly osteogenic sarcoma. This is seen in about 10 to 15 per cent of bilateral cases.[5]

The clinical manifestations of retinoblastoma vary with the severity of the disease at the time of presentation. Two thirds of patients present with leukokoria, which is a white pupillary reflex due to moderately advanced tumor size. One fourth will show motility disturbances resulting from macular involvement and inability to fixate. About half of retinoblastoma children have rubeosis of the iris, which may cause spontaneous hyphema. In advanced lesions the tumor may invade the optic nerve and subarachnoid space, with subsequent dissemination to the brain. It may penetrate the globe to involve the orbit directly or may metastasize to regional lymph nodes, bones, or visceral organs. About 1 per cent of retinoblastomas will regress spontaneously.[122]

Because of its hereditary potential, an important aspect in the management of retinoblastoma is genetic counseling. The treating physician must be familiar with the mode and risk of transmission of the gene to subsequent generations for this particular patient.

The *management of retinoblastoma* is complex and depends in large part on staging of the disease. Prior to the advent of chemotherapy in 1953, the survival rate of children with this tumor was less than 50 per cent. Since then, with combined modality therapy, overall survival rates have risen to 90 per cent or more.[7, 92] Concomitant with longer survivals, the incidence of heritable cases has risen significantly.

Pretreatment staging has been recommended as a basis for therapy selection in most cases, and has been associated with excellent survival rates.[76] However, ophthalmoscopic evaluation does not always correlate with the extent of extraretinal extension. High risk of recurrence and poor prognosis are associated with invasion of tumor into the choroid or emissary veins, into the optic nerve, or through the sclera into the orbit. The presence of extracranial metastases correlates with a high mortality rate.

Photocoagulation of small lesions in the posterior pole has had some success.[130] Such lesions must be away from the optic disk and fovea to preserve vision, and the technique is ineffective if any vitreous seeding is present.

Cryotherapy has also proved of value for small peripherally located tumors near the ora serrata.[141] Limited vitreous seeding over the tumor may also be destroyed with this method.

The use of *radiotherapy* in the management of retinoblastoma has been widely accepted. The tumor is quite radiosensitive, and results have been encouraging.[37] Treatment may be applied by cobalt plaque application[129] or by external beam irradiation.[3] The use of scleral plaques is limited to small tumors 6 to 15 mm in diameter and not closer than 3 mm to the optic disk or fovea. External beam radiation may be used in cases with multifocal lesions of larger size, including those in the fovea or over the optic disk. It is advocated in unilateral cases in which less than half the retina is involved and vision is salvageable and in bilateral cases in which one eye has been enucleated or both eyes harbor small lesions. Radiation of the orbit is indicated in cases in which tumor is found extending beyond the cut section of optic nerve following enucleation.

Enucleation is the procedure of choice in unilateral cases with extensive tumors occupying more than half the retinal surface and in eyes with massive vitreous seeding. Some authors advocate enucleation for all unilateral cases. However, for smaller lesions other modalities may be appropriate, although the risk of metastasis is greater.[129] In bilateral cases, one eye is generally far advanced. Enucleation of this eye should be performed, with alternative treatment of the fellow eye depending upon degree of tumor involvement. Massive bilateral tumors with loss of useful vision are best treated with bilateral enucleations. Simultaneous irradiation of advanced bilateral retinoblastomas has been reported with unsatisfactory long-term results.[2] In cases in which extraocular extension has occurred, enucleation plus adjunctive radiotherapy is indicated.

Chemotherapy has been advocated for all cases in which tumor has extended beyond the retina into the choroid, emissary vessels, or through the sclera. Cases with demonstrated tumor beyond the cut edge of the optic nerve following enucleation and those with distant metastases are also treated with chemotherapy.[152] In bilateral cases in which radiation therapy is utilized, adjunctive chemotherapy may be beneficial. Any case of orbital recurrence following enucleation should be treated with chemotherapy in addition to radiation. More recently, adjunctive chemotherapy has also been recommended whenever extraretinal extension cannot be determined, that is, in eyes treated by modalities other than enucleation.[76]

After any method of treatment periodic follow-up examinations are essential for the remaining eye at regular intervals until the child is at least 5 years old. Genetic counseling is a vital part of any management program.

Malignant Melanoma

Malignant melanoma is an aggressive tumor that may arise from epidermal melanocytes, nevus cells, or dermal melanoblasts. More than 90 per cent of melanomas within the eye occur as primary tumors of the choroid, but they may also be seen in the ciliary body or iris. Melanoma is the second most common intraocular malignancy in adults after metastatic lesions, with an incidence of five to seven per million population per year.[127, 150] The lesion is extremely rare in nonwhites. The incidence of malignant melanoma is higher in patients with ocular melanosis affecting the uveal tract, oculodermal melanocytosis (nevus of Ota), and neurofibromatosis.[127]

For small choroidal lesions the rate of metastasis is about 4 per cent overall, and about 11 per cent for tumors that show documented growth.[61] For larger tumors the rate of metastasis is higher, and mortality rates as high as 50 to 65 per cent after 10 years have been reported.[83, 157] Metastatic spread occurs via hematogenous routes, primary sites being liver, lung, and bone. Choroidal and ciliary body melanomas metastasize much more frequently than do those of the iris.

Uveal melanomas are diagnosed most frequently in

patients between 50 and 60 years of age, but because of their slow growth, the age of onset is difficult to assess. Males and females are affected equally.

Iris melanomas are easily visible and exhibit a wide variety of clinical appearances (Fig. 69–10). They tend to occur in younger patients (40 to 50 years of age), and are most frequently seen in the inferior half of the iris. These tumors may be circumscribed, elevated, and irregular with variable pigmentation or may be diffuse, flat infiltrating lesions that cover a large part of the iris and adjacent angle structures. Secondary glaucoma and spontaneous hyphema may be seen as the initial clinical feature. Cytologically, most iris melanomas are composed of low-grade spindle-B or rarely mixed spindle-B and epithelioid cells. The prognosis for preservation of vision is excellent, and long-term survival rates are better than 95 per cent.[12]

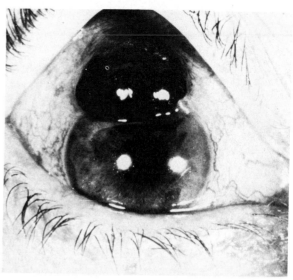

Figure 69–11. Malignant melanoma arising from the ciliary body and extending through the overlying sclera.

Melanomas of the ciliary body are hidden behind the iris and may attain a large size before diagnosis (Fig. 69–11). The patient frequently presents with blurring of vision or field loss due to distortion or dislocation of the lens, cataract encroachment on the pupillary aperture, or associated retinal effusion or detachment. As with iris lesions, the growth pattern may be nodular or diffuse. Pigmentation varies from heavily melanotic to amelanotic. Tortuous and dilated episcleral vessels may be seen overlying the ciliary body tumor, and extension through the scleral wall may be seen.

Choroidal melanomas often remain asymptomatic for long periods, depending upon their size and location (Figs. 69–12 and 69–13). In the posterior pole they frequently produce field loss, floaters, and decreased vision resulting from overlying retinal detachment. Pain is not a common feature. Characteristically, choroidal melanomas assume a nodular growth, which may break

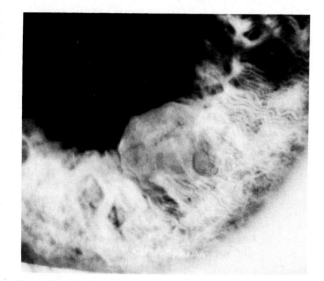

Figure 69–10. Nodular malignant melanoma of the iris involving the pupillary border, but not extending to the base. Note disturbance of iris stromal architecture and the prominent vasculature.

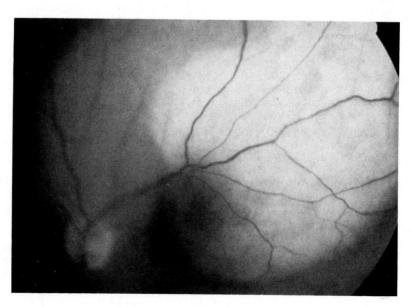

Figure 69–12. Choroidal malignant melanoma as seen with indirect ophthalmoscopy.

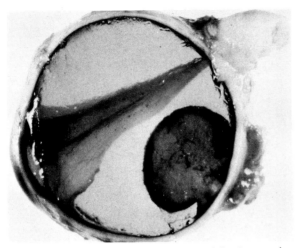

Figure 69–13. Gross pathologic specimen following enucleation for a large choroidal malignant melanoma. The specimen has extended through Bruch's membrane and demonstrates the classic mushroom-shaped configuration.

through Bruch's membrane to produce the familiar mushroom-shaped lesion. The tumor may extend through the sclera into the orbit.

The *management of melanomas* of the choroid is the subject of much controversy. In the past, enucleation was considered the procedure of choice for intraocular melanomas. However, up to 20 per cent of eyes enucleated for suspected melanoma had been benign lesions instead.[40, 132] Many tumors with spindle-A cell histologic appearance, previously considered a low-grade malignant melanoma treated by enucleation, are now classified as benign spindle cell nevi without malignant potential.[98] Also, clinical studies have shown that many small pigmented choroidal lesions followed over long periods do not grow or metastasize.[61] Recently, it has been suggested that manipulation of the eye during enucleation for malignant melanoma may hasten metastatic spread.[137, 156]

Numerous treatment modalities have been advocated for intraocular melanomas. For any given patient and lesion, several methods of therapy might be appropriate, and the selection will depend upon the specific tumor site, experience of the surgeon, and the willingness of the patient to accept certain procedures.

Periodic observation of small melanomas that show little tendency to grow has been advocated in recent years.[31, 61, 156] Those lesions that do show demonstrable growth during this period should receive definitive treatment. At present there is no firm evidence that observation of such small lesions increases a patient's risk for metastasis.

Observation may be indicated for small stable lesions less than 10 mm in diameter and 3 mm in thickness, for small or medium-sized lesions in elderly or debilitated patients, and in one-eyed individuals.[129] Examination every 3 months with fundus photographs and periodic fluorescein angiography and echography is appropriate.

The indications for *enucleation* in the treatment of intraocular melanomas will depend upon the philosophy of the surgeon. In general, any tumor judged too large for local resection or nonsurgical modalities, tumors that have resulted in severe visual loss, or cases with evidence of optic nerve extension should be managed with enucleation. The "no-touch" techniques have been devised to minimize manipulation and subsequent increased intraocular pressure that might facilitate metastatic spread.[55, 89, 97, 151] Although theoretically of great value, the long-term survival benefits of such techniques remain unproved, and metastases following such procedures have been seen.[129] The 5-year mortality rate from metastatic disease following standard enucleation remains in the range of 30 to 45 per cent.[128]

Exenteration is a radical procedure for removal of all orbital contents. It is reserved for cases with evidence of nonencapsulated extrascleral extension into the orbit, or in which orbital recurrence follows primary enucleation or some other treatment modality. The procedure offers only palliative value in cases with demonstrable metastases. The benefits of extenteration in prolonging survival remain controversial.[9]

The feasibility of full-thickness eye wall resection for choroidal tumors has been under investigation for many years, but only recently has some success been achieved.[116] The method is applicable to tumors less than 10 mm in basal diameter and not closer than 4.5 mm from the optic disk. Ocular media must be clear enough to permit visualization, and there should be no evidence of metastases. The number of reported cases treated so far is small, and preservation of useful vision has not been impressive.

Anteriorly situated melanomas of the iris or ciliary body may be resected en bloc by techniques that preserve the eye and useful vision. Indications for iridocyclectomy include small lesions not over four clock hours (120 degrees) in circumferential extent, and involving the iris and pars plicata of the ciliary body. Preservation of the globe has been achieved in 75 to 85 per cent of cases, and useful vision has been preserved in 50 per cent of cases.[51, 107] Deaths from metastatic spread following surgery have been no greater than with enucleation, despite a high incidence of incomplete resections with this technique.

The use of *photocoagulation* to treat intraocular melanomas was introduced in 1952 and has proved useful in selected cases.[103, 128] The technique requires clear ocular media. Indications for its use include small lesions sufficiently posterior to allow placement of burns around the entire tumor. Tumors beneath the fovea or closer than 3 mm from the optic disk cannot be treated without loss of vision. In addition, accepted criteria for treatment include a size not exceeding 10 mm in diameter and 2 mm in elevation and no retinal detachment overlying the tumor.[53] Recurrences and mortality rates have been comparable to other methods of treatment. Deviation from treatment criteria is associated with very high failure rates.[36] Close follow-up is essential, and enucleation is indicated for any recurrences.

Cryotherapy has had only limited use for intraocular melanomas. The technique requires small, anteriorly situated lesions and appears capable of controlling such tumors in selected cases.[4] However, long-term efficacy is unknown.

Malignant melanomas are not especially radiosensitive, but *radiation therapy* has proved of value, and its use is increasing. Indications include small to medium-sized tumors in eyes with useful or salvageable vision where photocoagulation cannot be applied, and tumors of any size in monocular patients. Radiation may be applied by cobalt-60 plaques,[131] iodine-125 seeds,[112] or rhodium/rubidium applicators,[95] external proton beam irradiation,[65] and helium ion irradiation.[26] In general, long-term survival rates appear to be comparable to or perhaps slightly better than with enucleation,[129] but with preservation of vision in a large number of cases.

Metastatic Intraocular Malignancies

Metastatic neoplasms to the eye represent the most common intraocular malignancies in adults. They reach the uvea by hematogenous dissemination. Most of these lesions occur in the choroid of the posterior pole of the eye, which has the greatest blood flow. Sarcomas rarely metastasize to the eye, and most secondary choroidal tumors are carcinomas. Breast carcinoma is the most frequent primary site, representing 40 to 65 per cent of metastases to the choroid.[42, 129] Lung carcinoma is the next most frequent primary site (6 to 30 per cent), with metastases from other sites such as kidney, pancreas, prostate, and gastrointestinal tract occurring considerably less commonly. Despite extensive search, the primary origin for intraocular metastases remains unknown in about 9 to 18 per cent of cases.

Metastatic malignancies to the uveal tract occur most commonly in patients aged 40 to 70 years. There is frequently a history of previous extraocular cancer, particularly of the breast, although ocular involvement may be the presenting manifestation of systemic carcinoma, especially lung cancer.[129]

Metastases to the iris and ciliary body are exceedingly rare, representing less than 12 per cent of all metastases to the eye and orbit.[43] Clinical features of anterior segment metastases include decreased vision, visible mass, redness of the eye, pain, secondary glaucoma, iridocyclitis, and recurrent hyphema. Iridocyclitis is a common intraocular disorder but is ordinarily not associated with hyphema. Therefore, any patient with iridocyclitis and hyphema should be suspected of having an occult tumor or mestastasis to the anterior segment.

Choroidal metastases most frequently present with decreased vision and ocular pain. Proptosis, retinal detachment, uveitis, and secondary glaucoma are much less common. Ophthalmoscopically, these lesions appear as a slightly elevated yellowish mass in the posterior pole. A serous detachment of the retina overlying the tumor is seen in about 75 per cent of cases.

Once intraocular metastases develop, the prognosis for survival is grave. In the largest series of such patients studied, Ferry and Font[43] found an overall mortality rate of 93 per cent from systemic metastatic disease, with a median survival of 7.4 months.

Management of metastatic intraocular malignancies depends upon the site of the primary tumor, degree of systemic involvement, and the patient's health.[138] In general, treatment is not indicated if the eye remains pain-free and the tumor is controlled with chemotherapy. For decreased vision, local control of the tumor may be achieved with radiotherapy to the posterior pole for choroidal lesions using fractionated external beam irradiation of 2500 to 3000 rads tumor dose. Dramatic reduction in the size of such lesions and improvement in vision can often be achieved.[27, 99] Cobalt plaque application may also be used for peripherally located choroidal lesions.[129] For those cases in which the choroidal tumor cannot be controlled, or in which intraocular pain from secondary glaucoma is present, enucleation may be necessary.

Specific Management Methods

The choice of a particular therapeutic approach to intraocular malignancies depends upon the type of tumor, its location within the eye, the visual status of the fellow eye, and the age and medical status of the patient. The rationale for selecting procedures has been discussed previously. Here, we briefly discuss these treatment modalities and the complications associated with each.

Cryotherapy

Cryotherapy involves the use of a cryoprobe utilizing nitrous oxide. It is applicable for peripherally located lesions that can be reached with this device. Freezing is performed trans-sclerally, with the probe used as a scleral depressor over the tumor and with visualization of the ice ball using indirect ophthalmoscopy.

Treatment consists of a double or triple freeze-thaw-refreeze cycle to -60 to $-70°C$. Maximum tissue destruction follows the second or subsequent freezes from disruption of intracellular organelles, pH changes, dehydration, and ischemia.[108] For larger lesions the probe is moved to an adjacent area, and the cycle is repeated. Retrobulbar or topical anesthesia is required. The treatment may have to be repeated after 3 to 4 weeks.

Complications of ocular cryotherapy include subconjunctival hemorrhage at the site of treatment. Chemosis may on occasion be so severe that conjunctiva protrudes through the eyelid's fissure. An antibiotic and steroid combination applied four times daily will hasten resolution. Minimal iritis is not uncommon and generally does not require specific treatment. With extensive peripheral cryotherapy, damage to the ciliary nerves to iris and ciliary body may result in pupillary and accommodation abnormalities that may last for many months. Choroidal detachment with associated narrowing of the anterior chamber and increased intraocular pressure may result from extensive cryotherapy.

Cryotherapy has been used successfully in the treatment of small peripheral retinoblastomas,[131] malignant melanomas, and metastatic choroidal lesions.[94] Its use in the management of conjunctival pigmented lesions[81] and for scleral invasion of malignant conjunctival tumors has shown promising preliminary results.

Photocoagulation

During the past several years photocoagulation has become increasingly important in the treatment of selected intraocular tumors.[103] This is especially true for small lesions that may be treated prior to attaining a size requiring enucleation. Photocoagulation utilizes visible light to destroy tumors by thermal effect. The light source may be generated from a xenon arc white light photocoagulator or a monochromatic laser, either argon or krypton. Treatment is delivered by a transcorneal approach. The technique requires clear ocular media for visualization, and the tumor must be located sufficiently posterior to allow placement of a ring of burns around its base. Lesions beneath the fovea cannot be treated with photocoagulation without permanent loss of central vision.

Retrobulbar anesthesia is used for xenon photocoagulation. With the laser, topical anesthetic is usually sufficient. Therapy is delivered in several treatment sessions. First, a double row of confluent burns is placed around the tumor base. After about 3 to 4 weeks this procedure is repeated to obliterate the tumor's vascular supply.[129] For retinal tumors, only enough power to close retinal vessels is required. For choroidal lesions, heavier burns and multiple treatment sessions will be needed. Subsequent treatment sessions at 3- to 5-week intervals are directed at the tumor surface and are repeated until adequate tumor destruction has been achieved.

Complications of photocoagulation include retinal and vitreous hemorrhage from rupture of superficial vessels, branch retinal vascular obstructions, vitreoretinal traction and macular pucker, cystoid macular edema, and retinal detachment.[129] If large branches of the central retinal vessels are obliterated, neovascularization may develop at the edge of the treated area. Such complications occur less frequently with argon laser, and their incidence can be reduced by careful technique.

Radiotherapy

Radiation therapy may be applied to intraocular tumors by external beam irradiation or with the use of plaques applied to the scleral surface. Successful treatment has been obtained for metastatic lesions, melanomas, and retinoblastoma.[142]

Radioactive applicators utilizing cobalt-60 or other sources of radiation[95, 112, 131] may be used for small lesions in the posterior pole that are not beneath the fovea or adjacent to the optic nerve head. The tumor is localized by transillumination or indirect ophthalmoscopy, and surface diathermy is used to mark the sclera, delineating the area to be treated. The active plaque is sutured to the sclera over the lesion, the dose having been carefully planned in advance. Typical doses are 3500 to 4500 rad to the tumor apex for retinoblastomas, and 8000 to 10,000 rad for choroidal melanomas.[129] Following appropriate dose delivery, the plaque is removed under local anesthesia.

Complications of plaque applications have been few. These include radiation retinopathy,[20] radiation optic neuropathy,[19] vitreous hemorrhage, cataract, keratoconjunctivitis, and pupillary abnormalities. Vitreous hemorrhage will generally clear with time, and cataracts, if significant, will require extraction. Results in the treatment of more than 300 patients with posterior uveal melanomas have so far been encouraging.[131]

External beam radiotherapy may utilize cobalt beam, ortho- or supervoltage techniques, helium ion, or proton beam irradiation.[26, 65, 66] The latter two techniques have shown some success in the management of melanomas. External beam radiotherapy can be used for tumors beneath the fovea or adjacent to the optic disk.

For retinoblastomas, treatment is delivered through an anterior, temporal, or combined port in a dose of 3500 to 4000 rad in divided doses over a 3-week period. A shield is used to protect the lens, and the beam is angled to avoid the opposite eye and the pituitary gland.[3]

Metastatic tumors to the choroid are treated through an anterior or lateral port with orthovoltage dosages of 3000 to 4000 rad over 3 to 4 weeks, or with supervoltage techniques at 10 MeV through the lateral or nasal field to avoid the lens.[27]

Complications of external beam irradiation are similar to those for plaques and include cataract, radiation retinopathy, and optic neuropathy. Damage to small retinal and optic disk vasculature may result in neovascularization and optic atrophy. Atrophy of orbital fat may cause enophthalmos. Secondary tumors such as orbital sarcomas in the treatment field are an important long-term complication of radiotherapy.[124]

Iridectomy and Iridocyclectomy

En bloc removal of the ciliary body and iris is required for the management of small anterior segment tumors. Malignant melanomas restricted to the iris and showing evidence of growth can be managed with a sector iridectomy. Iris lesions extending onto the trabecular meshwork, but not involving the ciliary body, and producing uncontrolled glaucoma or documented evidence of growth should be removed by iridotrabeculectomy. Iridocyclectomy is used for malignancies extending into the ciliary body. This procedure is usually limited to lesions less than four clock hours (120 degrees) in circumferential extent.

Iridectomy involves removing a sector of iris only. It is performed through a limbal corneoscleral incision of about 180 degrees adjacent to the tumor. Radial incisions are made in the iris to either side of the lesion from the base to the pupil, and the involved iris segment is torn from or cut across at its root. The corneoscleral wound is closed with multiple sutures to achieve a watertight closure.

Iridocyclectomy is the en bloc resection of iris, trabecular mesh and ciliary body. It is performed by reflecting a fornix-based conjunctival flap and securing the globe with a Flieringa ring sutured to episclera. Margins of the tumor are carefully located by transillumination. A lamellar scleral flap is fashioned over the tumor, allowing at least 3 mm overlap around it. The flap is reflected toward the cornea, and diathermy is applied to the margins of the dissection bed. The anterior chamber is entered along the limbus, and a sector iridectomy is cut as for an iridectomy. These radial incisions are extended across the ciliary body through the diathermy burns, and the iris-ciliary body segment is removed en bloc. The scleral flap is sutured into place, and the conjunctiva is pulled over it. Alternatively, it has been argued that all scleral layers should be removed over the tumor with repair of the defect using a scleral patch.[107]

Complications include significant bleeding from the ciliary body, but this usually stops spontaneously. Vitreous loss is a potential complication that can be minimized by softening the eye preoperatively and avoiding undue pressure during the procedure. Local opacities in the lens may develop adjacent to the site of resection.

Enucleation

Although in recent years less radical methods of treating intraocular tumors have become more common, enucleation is still indicated for many malignancies. It is recommended for large tumors not easily treated by other means, and for eyes with pain from tumor-induced uncontrolled glaucoma.

The procedure is performed under local or general anesthesia. A 360-degree limbal conjunctival peritomy incision is made. Tenon's capsule is separated from underlying sclera by blunt dissection between the rectus muscles. The muscles are individually hooked. If a movable implant is to be used, a suture is passed through the muscle insertions and tied prior to disinserting them at the sclera. Alternatively, the muscles may be cut from the sclera and allowed to retract free. The superior and inferior oblique muscles are hooked, clamped, and cut. A hemostat or silk traction suture is placed on the stump of the medial rectus muscle, gentle forward traction is applied, and a curved clamp is passed around the globe between Tenon's capsule and sclera. The optic nerve is identified by strumming it, and the clamp is applied as far posteriorly as possible. This is left in position for 3 to 5 minutes. The clamp is removed, and an enucleation scissors is used to transect the optic nerve. After removal of the globe, the orbital contents are compressed with gauze packing or an orbital compressor for 5 minutes until hemostatis is adequate. A careful examination of the enucleated globe is made to rule out any extrascleral extension. An orbital implant is placed in Tenon's capsule, and the latter is closed in layers over it with interrupted absorbable sutures. Conjunctiva is closed separately. Antibiotic ointment is applied, and a conformer is placed beneath the lids. A pressure dressing is applied for 48 hours.

If there is any evidence of orbital extension of tumor, more extensive dissection of soft tissues may be required.

In recent years a "no-touch" cryoring technique has been advocated in order to minimize intraoperative dissemination of tumor cells.[55] In this procedure the rectus muscles are cut without hooking them to avoid elevation of intraocular pressure. A specially designed cryoring is placed on the sclera around the tumor base. When a satisfactory ice ball is formed, the optic nerve is cut and the globe is removed.

Complications of enucleation may occur early or late. Bleeding at the time of surgery is usually easily controlled with pressure. Most late complications involve extrusion of the orbital implant. This can be decreased by proper selection of an appropriately sized implant, and meticulous closure of Tenon's capsule.

LACRIMAL GLAND TUMORS

Clinical Features

Epithelial tumors of the lacrimal gland represent about 5 to 7 per cent of all expanding mass lesions of the orbit.[69, 122] Of these, about half are malignant neoplasms. In contrast to salivary gland malignancies, adenoid cystic carcinoma is by far the most common epithelial cancer of the lacrimal gland, with adenocarcinomas being less common, and malignant mixed and muco-epidermoid carcinomas being relatively rare.

Lacrimal gland malignancies may occur in any age group, although they are exceptionally rare in children under 10 years old.[32] Adenoid cystic carcinoma is seen more frequently in the fourth decade and is more common in females, whereas adenocarcinomas are more prevalent in the sixth decade and are more common in males.

Clinical symptoms include proptosis and inferonasal displacement of the globe (Fig. 69–14). A palpable mass in the superotemporal quadrant is usually present. Diplopia and ptosis are variable features.

Pain is a common feature of malignant lacrimal tumors and is usually not present with benign tumors. It probably results from perineural invasion by neoplastic cells and from bone destruction. Duration of symptoms tends to be shorter with malignant tumors, generally 6 months to a year.

With any method of treatment recurrence rates are very high, being 70 per cent in the largest reported series.[46] Half of these recurrences are confined to the orbital soft tissues, but the orbital bones, paranasal sinuses, and intracranial cavity may also be involved.

The 5-year survival rate for all malignant epithelial tumors of the lacrimal gland is 57 per cent.[46] Prognosis appears to be significantly improved for cancers arising in benign mixed tumors. For de novo adenoid cystic and adenocarcinomas, however, the 5-year survival rate is less than 40 per cent. For adenoid cystic tumors, histologic structure has been shown to correlate with prognosis, with a basaloid pattern associated with significantly reduced survival rates.[60]

Malignant mixed tumors arise from persistent or recurrent benign mixed tumors with a frequency estimated at 10 per cent after 20 years.[46] These are aggressive tumors with a variable but generally lethal course.[71, 119]

The differential diagnosis of a lacrimal gland mass includes inflammatory and granulomatous disease, lymphoma, benign parenchymal tumors of the lacrimal gland, dermoids, and histiocytic lesions of the histiocytosis X group.

Management Modalities

The aggressive nature of lacrimal gland malignancies and their generally poor prognosis have led to some controversy regarding appropriate management. Unless there is evidence of extraorbital extension or metastases, surgical excision is the treatment of choice.

Part of the controversy surrounds the justification for biopsy prior to surgery. In the case of a benign mixed tumor, which may not always be distinguishable from a malignancy, it has been clearly demonstrated that pre-excisional biopsy carries a recurrence rate 10 times higher than excision within an intact capsule.[46] For primary epithelial malignancies Font and Gamel reported a 29 per cent 5-year survival rate for patients undergoing biopsy prior to excision, in contrast to a 70 per cent survival rate for those having excision with the capsule left intact.[46] The routes of biopsy were not given, and it must be assumed that some of these were via a lateral orbitotomy, which has a greater risk of orbital

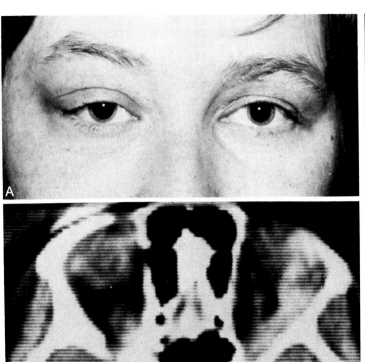

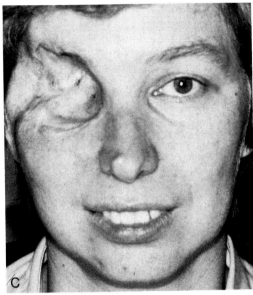

Figure 69–14. Lacrimal gland tumor. (*A*) Patient with painful proptosis of the right eye of several months' duration. (*B*) Early generation orbital CT scan showing a large adenoid cystic carcinoma of the lacrimal gland (right side of figure). (*C*) Patient after a radical exenteration with resection of bone.

contamination. Nevertheless, these authors recommended en bloc excision of suspected malignancies without prior biopsy.

When preoperative evaluation suggests a circumscribed or encapsulated tumor, every effort should be made to remove it intact. For more infiltrative lesions, we prefer biopsy and histologic confirmation of malignancy prior to definitive surgery. When this is deemed desirable, biopsy should always be performed via an anterior transseptal orbitotomy approach. The entire biopsy tract can thus be excised in any further extirpative procedure. With modern high-resolution CT scanners, and a careful evaluation of the patient's clinical history, a more accurate preoperative diagnosis is possible, even obviating the need for biopsy in many cases.[82, 139]

The *surgical approach* to lacrimal gland malignancies must attempt complete excision of the tumor without contamination of adjacent tissues. The emphasis on resection of adjacent bone was made by Reese and Jones in 1964,[123] and most subsequent authors have agreed with this approach. The dissemination of tumor cells through periorbita and into the haversian canals of orbital bones may occur early in the growth of such lesions and may account for the high recurrence rates when bone is not resected.[71]

In 1976 Henderson and Neault recommended the en bloc removal of the lacrimal gland tumor and adjacent adnexa, its periorbital base, and surrounding bone.[72] This is performed as a one-stage procedure in which

biopsy of the lesion, if necessary, is done after its partial isolation from the orbital contents but prior to complete removal. This technique allows removal of the tumor with preservation of the eye.[46, 71] The technique may also be used following a translid biopsy.[114] For this procedure an S-shaped lateral orbitotomy incision is made, beginning beneath the lateral brow and extending laterally in a laugh line. Subcutaneous tissues are separated from underlying periosteum and orbital septum along the entire lateral orbital rim. The orbital septum is opened, and the tumor is isolated, separating it from orbital structures as needed, but without disturbing its base along the lacrimal fossa. The periosteum is incised along the lateral rim and is elevated into the temporalis fossa, displacing temporalis muscle laterally. A Stryker saw is used to cut the orbital rim above and below the tumor, and the bone is fractured outward along the zygomaticosphenoid suture. Periorbita is then cut posterior to attachment of the tumor. The tumor, its attached bone, and periorbita are removed en bloc. The temporalis muscle is displaced into the lateral defect and the fascia is fastened to the remaining orbital rim. Subcutaneous tissue and skin are closed in the usual manner.

A more radical approach has been advocated by some workers because of the dismal long-term survival even following en bloc resection. Here a translid biopsy is performed, and if positive for malignancy, it is followed by *radical exenteration* including all orbital contents, eyelids, and both the lateral and superolateral orbital walls.[139, 153] A specific admonition against a transcranial approach has been made because of the risk of intracranial spread.[46] More recently, however, a radical combined intra- and extracranial en bloc resection has been recommended on the grounds that it provides better assessment of resectability, protects the dura and underlying cortex during resection, and allows frozen-section evaluation of tumor spread along cranial nerve routes.[100]

Radiotherapy, either alone or in combination with surgery, has not proved to be of any additional value in the treatment of lacrimal gland malignancies.[21, 46]

ORBITAL TUMORS

Types of Orbital Tumors

Orbital malignancies present a difficult and challenging diagnostic problem. Limited approaches to diagnosis include routine radiography, computerized tomographic scanning, and standardized echography. Fine needle aspiration biopsy under CT control is a new procedure that will significantly improve our diagnostic capabilities in the future. Nuclear magnetic resonance scanners are only just coming into use, and their potential contribution to the evaluation of orbital disease seems promising.

Excluding lacrimal gland lesions, malignant neoplasms represent approximately 25 per cent of all orbital tumors.[69, 121] In children, the figure may be as high as 35 per cent.[117] The unique anatomy of the orbit allows for early detection of such lesions, and thus a greater potential for cure. The bony confines of the orbital space result in proptosis as an early sign, often bringing the patient to medical attention while the lesion is still quite small. The lack of lymphatics within the orbit limits the routes of metastatic spread.

Although numerous malignant lesions have been seen in the orbit, most are quite rare in that location. In adults lymphomas, invasive tumor from adjacent lids or sinuses and metastatic lesions represent the majority of orbital cancers. In children, rhabdomyosarcoma alone accounts for 50 to 75 per cent of all malignant tumors,[78, 117] with metastatic neuroblastoma, lymphoid tumors, and extraocular retinoblastomas making up most of the remainder.

The philosophy in managing some of these tumors has changed drastically in recent years and for the most part requires a multispecialty approach, including an orbital surgeon, often with the collaboration of the otolaryngologist and neurosurgeon, as well as the radiation and medical oncologist.

Lymphoid Tumors

Orbital neoplasms of the lymphoreticular systems are often confusing to both the ophthalmologist and the pathologist. Lymphomas represent approximately 8 per cent of all orbital tumors, and lymphoid infiltrations account for about 15 per cent.[50, 69, 121, 134] It is only recently that some clarification of the cytogenetics, histopathology, and immunology of these lesions has been gained, resulting in better correlation with their natural history.[87] Malignant lymphomas are, in some cases, not readily distinguishable from some lymphoid hyperplasias.

These latter have been referred to as atypical lymphoid hyperplasia composed of an admixture of small, mature-looking lymphocytes and larger lymphoid cells of questionable maturity.[87] They lack characteristic features of both benign pseudolymphomas and malignant lymphomas.[86] Immunologic studies have demonstrated that lymphoid infiltrates can be further divided into polyclonal proliferations, which show benign histologic features, and monoclonal B-cell proliferations, which show malignant characteristics.[87] This finding is rapidly altering our approach to the diagnosis of orbital lymphoid lesions, although recent evidence suggests that this distinction may not be absolute.

In the orbit, malignant lymphomas outnumber benign lymphoid infiltrates 2:1. This contrasts to similar tumors in the conjunctiva, where benign proliferations outnumber lymphomas 5:1. The most common cytologic type is the lymphocytic lymphoma. In their review of 400 ocular adnexal lymphoid tumors, Knowles and Jakobiec[87] found 15 per cent of the lesions classified as inflammatory pseudotumor or benign lymphoid hyperplasia to disseminate. Of those lesions classified as lymphocytic lymphomas, 60 per cent overall were eventually associated with systemic disease. Of the latter, 58 per cent had concurrent orbital and systemic lesions at the time of diagnosis, and 42 per cent developed systemic involvement within 5 years of the orbital tumor. Further, they found a correlation between histology and prognosis. Only 25 per cent of patients characterized with diffuse, well-differentiated lymphocytic lymphomas ultimately acquired disseminated disease, whereas 60 per cent of those with nodular, poorly differentiated lymphomas developed extraorbital lesions.

Orbital lymphoma is a disease almost exclusively of adults in the fifth and sixth decades of life. Patients generally present with a palpable mass (Fig. 69–15). Other less frequent symptoms include ptosis, pain, and diplopia. The disease may be bilateral in 5 per cent of cases.[87]

Lymphomas are radiosensitive, and irradiation is the treatment of choice for localized disease or for treatment of symptomatic orbital lesions in disseminated cases. Surgical intervention is limited to biopsy, generally through an anterior orbitotomy approach. Treatment consists of 3000 rad delivered by anterior and lateral ports, with appropriate shielding of the lens.[52] For reticulum cell sarcoma, a higher dose, 3500 to 4000 rad over 3 to 4 weeks, is given. Complications may be seen in 30 per cent of cases and include conjunctivitis and cataracts.[54] Corneal erosions and marked cutaneous erythema and edema may also be seen. For systemic disease, chemotherapy is indicated.

Rhabdomyosarcoma

Rhabdomyosarcoma is the most common primary orbital malignancy in childhood. Without treatment, it is rapidly fatal. In recent years understanding of this lesion has changed the accepted therapeutic modalities so that improved survival is now obtainable without the mutilating surgery once deemed necessary.

Rhabdomyosarcoma represents about 10 per cent of all malignant solid neoplasms in the orbit. It arises from mesenchymal cell rests, having the potential to differentiate toward striated muscle.

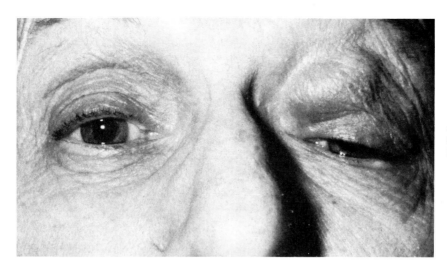

Figure 69–15. Orbital lymphoma presenting as a palpable mass in the superior anterior orbit.

The tumor occurs predominantly in children under 10 years of age, with a mean age of 7.8 years.[13, 59, 84, 118] The disease occurs more frequently in males, having a male-female ratio of 5:3.[88]

The most common clinical presentation is proptosis evolving rapidly over days to weeks (Fig. 69–16). In some cases a palpable mass may be seen in the lid or beneath the conjunctiva, or ptosis may be seen early in the course. Orbital pain and headache are not prominent features until late in the disease process. Decreased vision and motility disturbances may also be seen. Diagnosis is based on routine radiographic studies, which frequently show bone destruction, standardized echography, and computerized tomography in both axial and coronal planes, along with the clinical history. Tissue diagnosis is essential and should be obtained immediately upon suspecting the lesion. It is not uncommon for these tumors to double their size in a matter of days, and any delay in diagnosis and treatment may have disastrous consequences.

Rhabdomyosarcoma is an aggressive tumor locally, with a propensity to recur and invade adjacent sinuses and intracranial cavity. Metastases are predominantly to the lungs and bones.[118] Regional lymph node involvement occurs when the tumor gains access to the lids where lymphatics are present.

The major histologic types are pleomorphic, embryonal, alveolar, and botryoid rhabdomyosarcoma.[88] Orbital lesions are predominantly of the embryonal type, in which the infrequency of cross striations makes the diagnosis more difficult.

Rarely, a rhabdomyosarcoma may present as a small, well-circumscribed lesion that can be removed completely at surgery (Fig. 69–17). Until recently, radical surgery was considered the treatment of choice for larger orbital rhabdomyosarcomas.[84, 88] This usually consisted of immediate orbital exenteration. Even so, the best survival rates were about 30 to 40 per cent after 3 years.[13, 59, 84, 118] Until the advent of chemotherapy for this disease in the late 1960s, the presence of metastases was uniformly fatal. In 1972, the Intergroup Rhabdomyosarcoma Study was established to preoperatively evaluate newer treatment modalities.[102] Based on their findings, current therapy consists of staging patients into four groups as follows: Group I, completely resected without residual tumor; Group II, resected with

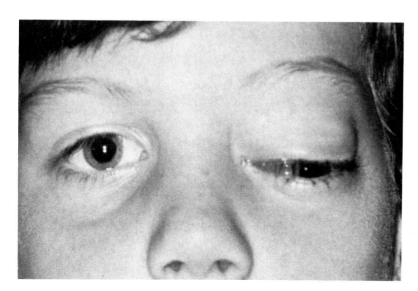

Figure 69–16. Rhabdomyosarcoma of the left orbit with proptosis and downward displacement of the globe.

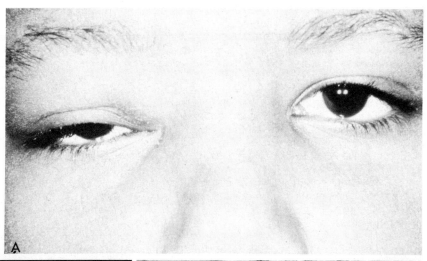

Figure 69–17. Rhabdomyosarcoma. (*A*) Anterior orbital mass with downward displacement of the right globe in a child. (*B*) Orbital CT scan showing a well-circumscribed rhabdomyosarcoma in the anterior medial orbit (left side of figure). (*C*) At surgery by anterior orbitotomy, the lesion was removed in toto.

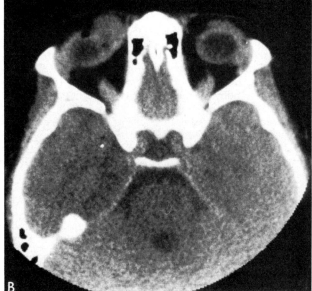

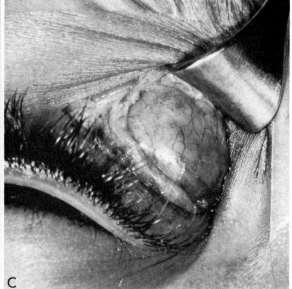

histologic evidence of microscopic residual tumor; Group III, gross residual tumor; and Group IV, documented metastatic disease. Except for Group I, chemotherapy consisting of vincristine, cyclophosphamide, and dactinomycin, along with radiotherapy, is given in various combinations according to a strict protocol. For Group IV patients, adriamycin may be added to the regimen. With such combined therapy, prognosis was dramatically improved during the past decades, with overall survival rates in the 70 per cent range being reported. Patients with metastases have the worst prognosis.

Current recommendations are for immediate biopsy followed by radiotherapy consisting of 4500 rad over 6 weeks. Adjuvant chemotherapy is given in an 84-day cycle and may be coincident with the radiation or may follow it. Complications of radiotherapy include orbital growth retardation in young children, conjunctivitis, keratitis, and cataract formation. Chemotherapy is associated with some toxicity in up to 70 to 80 per cent of cases. The more severe complications include leuko-

penia, thrombocytopenia, infections, and with adriamycin, cardiac toxicity.

Metastatic Orbital Malignancies

Malignant tumors metastatic to the orbit represent about 3 to 5 per cent of all solid orbital mass lesions[69, 121, 134] and about 15 per cent of malignant tumors in that site. Orbital metastases are far less common than those to the choroid and account for only about 12 per cent of metastases to the eye and orbital region.[45] In 4 to 7 per cent of cases, there is bilateral orbital involvement.

The primary site for orbital metastases is similar to that for secondary choroidal tumors. In adults about 29 per cent overall were breast carcinomas (62 per cent of female patients), and 14 per cent were lung cancers (20 per cent of male patients).[45] Less common sites included kidney, testis, prostate, pancreas, and ileum. In about one third of cases, the primary site cannot be determined. The vast majority of orbital metastases are carcinomas. In children metastatic neuroblastoma may involve the orbit and is bilateral in 50 per cent of cases. Neuroblastoma represents about 1.5 per cent of all orbital tumors in childhood, and about 4 per cent of malignant orbital tumors in that age group.[117] In most cases, however, evidence of abdominal or thoracic primary disease precedes the orbital lesion.

Clinically, the most common presenting symptom of orbital metastasis is proptosis, seen in 75 per cent of cases (Fig. 69–18). Pain, decreased vision, periorbital swelling, palpable mass, and motility disturbance all occur frequently. Enophthalmos may be seen with metastatic scirrhous carcinomas of the breast.[45] In about 60 per cent of cases orbital and ocular symptoms will precede detection of the primary neoplasm.[41] Diagnosis is based on radiographic, CT, and echographic studies and tissue biopsy.

Management of orbital metastases is quite variable. In most cases evidence of systemic disease argues against radical surgery. Nevertheless, survival rates for many cancers are improving, and treatment should be aimed at achieving maximum visual potential and minimal disability. Local resection or exenteration of the orbit is generally not indicated but may be considered for control of intractable pain. With rare exceptions, such surgical therapy will not prolong life in cases of metastatic disease. In patients with breast or prostatic metastases, hormonal therapy may be used effectively, usually in conjunction with radiotherapy or chemotherapy. In such instances, treatment is directed at systemic metastases, not just the orbital lesions. Specific chemotherapy is generally indicated and is dependent upon the primary site of involvement. In most patients with orbital metastases, radiotherapy remains the treatment of choice for reduction in tumor size and improvement in symptoms and vision.

Despite treatment, the prognosis for patients with metastatic carcinoma to the orbit is poor. Font and Ferry[45] reported a 79 per cent mortality rate for their series, with a median survival period of 15.6 months.

Other Orbital Malignant Tumors

Extensions of malignant tumors from adjacent paranasal sinuses and eyelids account for about 15 to 20 per cent of orbital cancers. Squamous cell carcinomas compose the majority of these lesions, followed by basal cell carcinomas and, rarely, sebaceous cell carcinomas. Treatment consists of radical surgery with or without adjunctive local radiotherapy or cryotherapy.

Malignant optic nerve gliomas are rare tumors, occurring almost exclusively in adults, although they may be seen in children as well.[69] We have treated a young child with atypical glioma felt to be of low-grade malignancy (Fig. 69–19). Optic sheath meningiomas may occur as a rare malignant neoplasm in children. In both cases, excision of the optic nerve with adjunctive radiotherapy is indicated. Rarely, a small anteriorly situated meningioma may be removed from the optic nerve with preservation of vision. For intracranial extension, a transfrontal approach is required.

Extension of intraocular retinoblastomas and malignant melanomas account for about 15 per cent of orbital malignant disease (Fig. 69–20). Because this is a local process, orbital exenteration, usually with adjunctive radiotherapy and chemotherapy, is generally indicated as discussed in previous sections.

Hemangiopericytomas are vascular tumors characterized by prominent vascular spaces with small solid areas of cellular proliferation resembling pericytes. These are slowly growing mass lesions, producing proptosis and less commonly a palpable mass. Diplopia and visual loss are seen infrequently. Pain may be a feature in up to one third of patients. In more than three fourths of cases the tumor is located in the superior orbit. A clear-cut distinction between benign and malignant hemangiopericytoma is difficult to establish, and the clinical behavior of these lesions is not always predictable from histologic features.[30]

The treatment of choice is surgical excision.[30, 70] The tumor is generally circumscribed, and sometimes encapsulated, facilitating complete removal in most cases. Incomplete or piecemeal removal is associated with a significant increase in recurrence rate. The lateral orbitotomy approach is preferred, and the transfrontal route should be avoided to prevent possible intracranial spread. This tumor is generally considered to be radio-resistant, although some response has been reported.[104] For metastatic disease, chemotherapy may be effective.

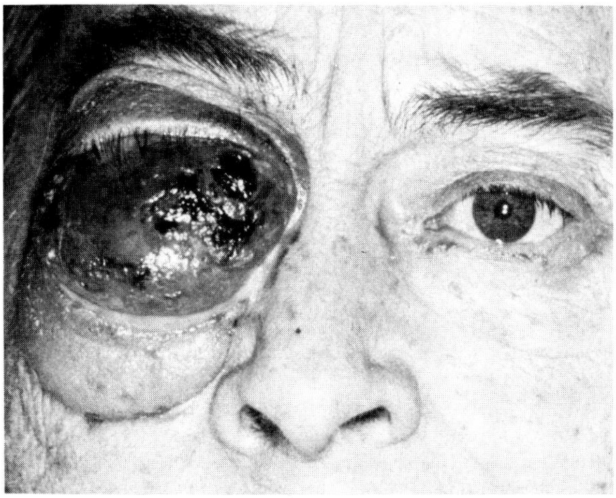

Figure 69–18. Large orbital mass in a patient with a history of breast cancer. Biopsy revealed the presence of metastatic breast carcinoma.

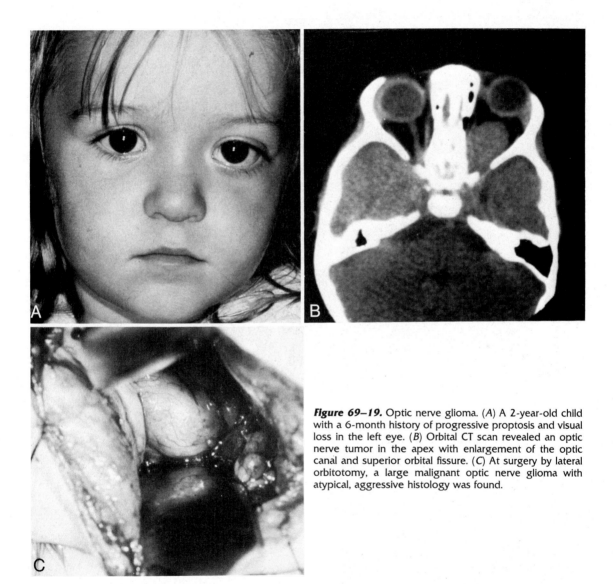

Figure 69–19. Optic nerve glioma. (*A*) A 2-year-old child with a 6-month history of progressive proptosis and visual loss in the left eye. (*B*) Orbital CT scan revealed an optic nerve tumor in the apex with enlargement of the optic canal and superior orbital fissure. (*C*) At surgery by lateral orbitotomy, a large malignant optic nerve glioma with atypical, aggressive histology was found.

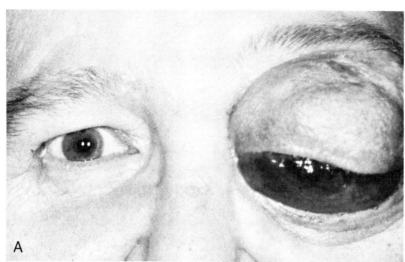

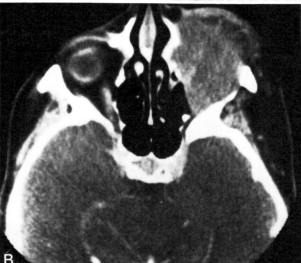

Figure 69–20. Orbital melanoma. (*A*) This patient presented with a large pigmented orbital mass ipsilateral to cutaneous pigmentation in the distribution of the trigeminal nerve consistent with oculodermal melanocytosis (nevus of Ota). Biopsy revealed a malignant melanoma. (*B*) CT scan showing the mass to completely fill the left orbit with erosion of the lateral wall. Treatment consisted of radical exenteration, with excision of bone, and adjunctive cryotherapy.

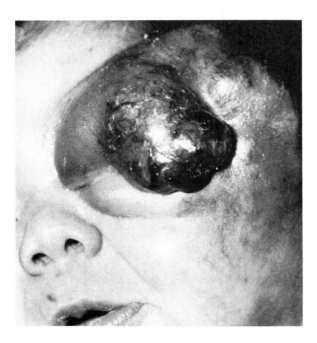

Figure 69–21. Four-week-old infant with a rapidly growing undifferentiated carcinoma of the left orbit and eyelids, progressing to death within four weeks.

Primary orbital malignant melanoma is rare, but has been reported in association with oculodermal melanocytosis. Numerous other rare malignancies have been reported in the orbit (Fig. 69–21). Rare occurrences of lesions such as alveolar soft-tissue carcinoma,[48] malignant fibrous histiocytoma,[47] malignant schwannoma, fibrosarcoma, leiomyosarcoma, liposarcoma, chondrosarcoma, and osteogenic sarcoma have been reported.[69, 121, 122] Local excision or exenteration, with or without adjuvant therapy, is indicated, depending upon the size, location, and invasiveness of the lesions.

Surgical Management Methods

The surgical procedure utilized for any specific lesion will depend upon its location, size, and suspected histopathology. If a malignant tumor is the working diagnosis, a lateral orbitotomy is necessary for removal in toto. A small, well-circumscribed palpable lesion may be excised through an anterior route. A transcranial approach, which may be required for a posteriorly situated optic nerve or apical lesion, would not usually be considered for a malignant tumor confined to the orbit because of the potential for intracranial contamination.

Transseptal Anterior Orbitotomy

In this approach the skin incisions are made through the eyelids over the palpable tumor mass. Entrance into the orbit is made through the orbital septum, giving access directly to the peripheral orbital space outside the muscle cone. This route leaves both periorbita and the intermuscular septum intact and is useful for lesions such as anteriorly situated lymphomas and for biopsy of some anterior tumors in which contamination of adjacent orbital spaces should be avoided.

In exploration of the superolateral orbit, care must be taken to identify the lacrimal gland. This is frequently displaced forward by expanding orbital lesions, and biopsy of suspected tumors in this region not uncommonly shows only normal lacrimal tissue.

The orbital septum need not be closed separately, and attempts at doing so inferiorly frequently result in foreshortening of the lower eyelid, with subsequent cosmetic deformity.

Transconjunctival Anterior Orbitotomy

For this approach, the initial incision is made in the conjunctival fornix. In the lower lid, the peripheral orbital space, between the muscle cone and periorbita, may be entered by incising the lower lid retractors. In both lower and upper lids the intraconal central space is entered by opening Tenon's capsule between insertions of the rectus muscles, or by removing these muscles at their insertions. Exposure is generally poor by this approach, and damage to extraocular muscles with resultant motility disturbance is a potential complication. The transconjunctival route is useful only for small, anteriorly placed lesions, but for deeper tumors it rarely has any advantage over other procedures. It may be combined with a lateral orbitotomy to provide greater visualization medially for access to the optic nerve or optic canal.

Lateral Orbitotomy

The lateral approach gives better visualization to the retrobulbar space than any of the anterior routes. It is preferred for any posterior lesion and for more anteriorly placed tumors that extend back behind the equator of the globe.

Numerous variations in detail have been advocated since the procedure was first introduced by Krönlein. Of the various skin incisions proposed, the S-shaped opening of Stallard, extending from beneath the lateral brow, along the lateral orbital rim, and laterally in a laugh line, gives excellent exposure and avoids having to repair the lateral canthal tendon and angle (Fig. 69–22). The initial incision is carried down to, but not through, periosteum. Periosteum is incised with a scalpel blade about 2 mm lateral to the orbital rim and is elevated from underlying bone. Once the dissection is carried into the temporalis fossa, periosteum and muscle will be firmly adherent to bone. Separation is facilitated by forcing a gauze sponge into the dissection plane with a periosteal elevator to just behind the sphenozygomatic suture. This will result in a clean bony surface. The periosteum is dissected from the orbital rim, where it is firmly adherent. However, once within the orbital space, periorbita is easily separated from bone.

Removal of the lateral wall requires two saw cuts, the exact placement of which depends in part upon the size and position of the anticipated lesion and the exposure required. For routine orbitotomies, the lower cut is made with a Stryker saw at the level of the upper border of the zygomatic arch. A higher incision will significantly reduce exposure. The upper cut should be at or up to 5 mm above the frontozygomatic suture. Protection of the orbital contents with a broad malleable band retractor is essential during this maneuver. Once the bone incisions are made, the lateral wall is fractured outward, using a double-action rongeur. It is not necessary to leave the fragment attached to a muscle flap, and better visualization is obtained by removing the bone completely and storing it in saline until replacement. Exposure of the orbital space may be significantly enhanced by further removal of bone along the lateral wall with rongeurs until cancellous bone of the greater wing of the sphenoid is encountered.

Access to the peripheral and intraconal spaces is achieved by opening the periorbita. This is best performed with an anteroposterior cut made just above or below the lateral rectus muscle. This may be extended by a perpendicular cut anteriorly to form a T-shaped opening. After the lesion has been identified, the remaining procedure will depend upon the nature of the disease and the involvement of adjacent structures. If well defined or encapsulated, complete removal should be attempted. This is greatly facilitated with the use of a cryoprobe for bloodless traction on the lesion and a Freer elevator for blunt dissection. More infiltrative lesions cannot be removed in toto without radical exenteration. Biopsy with frozen sections will help in planning further therapy.

When lesions are encountered that are better treated by means other than surgery, such as lymphoma or metastatic carcinoma, the orbitotomy should be closed without further disruption of orbital contents. In some cases, however, debulking of the tumor may make subsequent treatment more effective. However, because

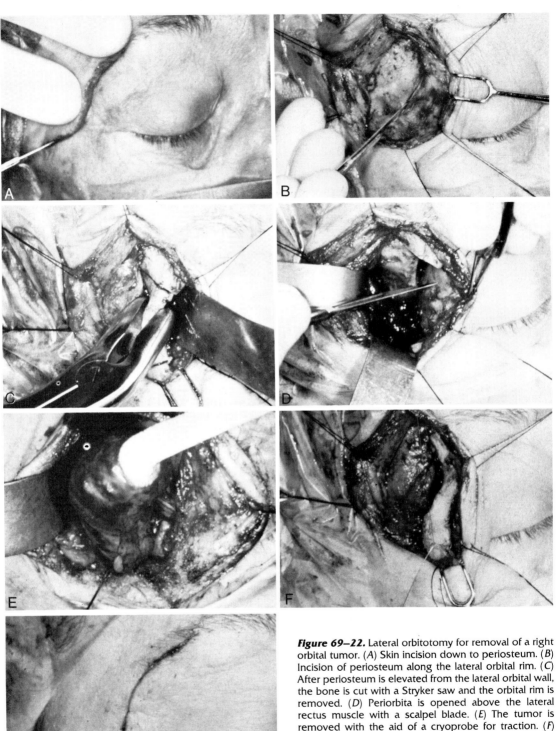

Figure 69–22. Lateral orbitotomy for removal of a right orbital tumor. (*A*) Skin incision down to periosteum. (*B*) Incision of periosteum along the lateral orbital rim. (*C*) After periosteum is elevated from the lateral orbital wall, the bone is cut with a Stryker saw and the orbital rim is removed. (*D*) Periorbita is opened above the lateral rectus muscle with a scalpel blade. (*E*) The tumor is removed with the aid of a cryoprobe for traction. (*F*) The lateral orbital rim is replaced and wired into position. (*G*) The subcutaneous tissues are closed, followed by skin sutures.

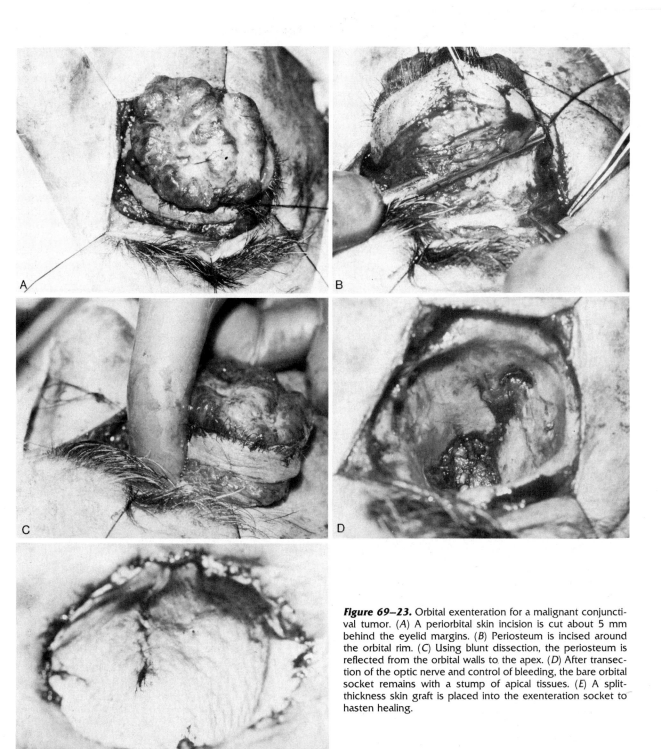

Figure 69–23. Orbital exenteration for a malignant conjunctival tumor. (*A*) A periorbital skin incision is cut about 5 mm behind the eyelid margins. (*B*) Periosteum is incised around the orbital rim. (*C*) Using blunt dissection, the periosteum is reflected from the orbital walls to the apex. (*D*) After transection of the optic nerve and control of bleeding, the bare orbital socket remains with a stump of apical tissues. (*E*) A split-thickness skin graft is placed into the exenteration socket to hasten healing.

these lesions are amenable to less invasive means of treatment, orbital structures should not be further compromised during attempted resection.

Periorbita should be left open to allow decompression of orbital blood and edema into the temporalis fossa. The orbital rim may be replaced and wired into position. Periosteum is tightly closed to provide nourishment to the bony rim and to reposition the lateral canthal tendon. Muscle and skin layers are closed separately.

Postoperatively, a light pressure dressing is applied for 24 hours. The use of a tight headroll may only contribute to increased intraocular pressure and is never a substitute for meticulous hemostasis. Drains are pulled 1 day after surgery, and sutures are removed after 7 days. If any significant trauma to the optic nerve was sustained, systemic steroids for several days are indicated. If entrance into the paranasal sinuses was performed, coverage with antibiotics for several days might be considered.

The most common postoperative complications are ptosis and lid edema, both generally transient. Weakness of the lateral rectus muscle is avoided by minimizing its manipulation. When present, however, it is usually transient. If persistent, 6 months should be allowed before considering intervention.

Transfrontal Approach

The transcranial approach to the orbit allows wide access to the apex and optic canal that would not be possible through a lateral orbitotomy. It is the procedure of choice for deep optic nerve and apical lesions that involve both the orbital and intracranial compartments. In 1941 Dandy suggested that all orbital surgery be performed by this route because in his series nearly 75 per cent of orbital tumors showed some intracranial extension.[33] With modern diagnostic techniques, however, the transcranial approach can be limited to those lesions that can be documented to be inoperable by other routes.

The procedure requires the collaboration of a neurosurgeon to provide access to the orbital roof. A curved scalp incision extends from the ear to the midline, then forward to the forehead. The skin and galea are reflected from the periosteum, and the latter is elevated. Bur holes are drilled, and the dura is separated from the overlying bone between the holes. The frontal bone is then cut with a wire saw. Radiographs in both frontal and lateral projections are necessary to determine the size and position of the frontal sinus prior to making these cuts. Dura is opened and the frontal lobe is reflected up to expose the orbital roof. A dural flap is fashioned, the roof is opened at its thinnest point, and this opening is enlarged with rongeurs. The periorbita is opened. Care must be exercised at this point not to injure the frontal artery and nerve, the trochlear nerve, and the levator-superior rectus complex, all of which lie immediately beneath periorbita.

Complications with this approach include cerebrospinal fluid rhinorrhea if the paranasal sinuses are inadvertently entered. Meningitis is a severe potential risk. Damage to the vascular supply in the area of the chiasm may lead to serious bleeding, and injury to the internal carotid artery would be disastrous. At the close of the procedure, dura is closed over the orbit. Pulsating

exophthalmos, a possible long-term complication, is usually not a problem.

Orbital Exenteration

Exenteration may be necessary when a malignant tumor cannot be completely excised by more conservative procedures. The technique involves removal of all orbital contents within an intact periorbita. If possible, the eyelid skin may be saved by placing skin incisions just behind the lid margins and separating skin from underlying muscle to the level of the orbital rims (Fig. 69–23). If the eyelids are involved with tumor, the skin incision is made directly over the orbital rim down to the level of periosteum. Periosteum is incised around the orbit and is gently dissected from bone to the orbital apex. An enucleation scissors is used to cut the optic nerve as close as possible to the apex, and the specimen is removed en bloc. Bleeding from the ophthalmic artery is controlled with cautery. The orbital cavity is allowed to heal by granulation, or a split-thickness skin graft may be placed. If adjacent orbital bones are involved with tumor, the exenteration must be combined with more radical excision of orbital walls or adjacent sinuses.

REFERENCES

1. Abraham JC, Jaboley ME, Hoopes JE: Basal cell carcinoma of the medial canthal region. Am J Surg 126:492, 1973.
2. Abramson DH, Ellsworth RM, Tretter P, et al: Simultaneous bilateral radiation for advanced bilateral retinoblastoma. Arch Ophthalmol 99:1763, 1981.
3. Abramson DH, Jereb B, Ellsworth RM: External beam radiation for retinoblastoma. Bull NY Acad Med 57:787, 1981.
4. Abramson DH, Lisman RD: Cryopexy of a choroidal melanoma. Ann Ophthalmol 11:1418, 1979.
5. Abramson DH, Ronner HT, Ellsworth RM: Second tumors in non-irradiated bilateral retinoblastoma. Am J Ophthalmol 87:624, 1979.
6. Ackerman LV, de Regato JA: Cancer. 2nd ed. St. Louis, The C. V. Mosby Co., 1954.
7. Acquaviva A, Barberi L, Bernardini C, et al: Medical therapy of retinoblastoma in children. J Neurosurg Sci 26:49, 1982.
8. Adams EL, Price NM: Treatment of basal cell carcinoma with a carbon dioxide laser. J Dermatol Surg Oncol 5:803, 1979.
9. Affeldt JC, Minckler DS, Azen SP, Yeh L: Prognosis in uveal melanoma with extrascleral extension. Arch Ophthalmol 98:1975, 1979.
10. Anderson RL: Oculoplastic updates. Cryosurgery of the ocular adnexa. *In* Symposium on Diseases and Surgery of the Lids, Lacrimal Apparatus, and Orbit. Trans New Orleans Acad Ophthalmol, St. Louis, The C. V. Mosby Co., 1982.
11. Anderson RL, Ceilley RJ: A multispecialty approach to the excision and reconstruction of eyelid tumors. Ophthalmology 85:1150, 1978.
12. Orentesen TJ, Green WR: Melanoma of the uvea: Report of 72 cases treated surgically. Ophthalmic Surg 6:23, 1975.
13. Ashton N, Morgan G: Embryonal sarcoma and embryonal rhabdomyosarcoma of the orbit. J Clin Pathol 18:599, 1965.
14. Aurora AL, Blodi FC: Reappraisal of basal cell carcinoma of the eyelids. Am J Ophthalmol 70:329, 1970.
15. Beard C, Sullivan JH: Cryosurgery of eyelid disorders including malignant tumors. *In* Zacarian SA (ed): Cryosurgical Advances in Dermatology and Tumors of the Head and Neck. Springfield, Charles C Thomas, 1977.
16. Birge HL: Cancer of the eyelids. I. Basal cell and mixed basal cell and squamous cell epitheliomas. Arch Ophthalmol 19:700, 1938.
17. Bloch RS, Gartner S: The incidence of ocular metastatic carcinoma. Arch Ophthalmol 85:673, 1971.
18. Boniuk M, Zimmerman LE: Sebaceous carcinoma of the eyelids, eyebrows, caruncle and orbit. Trans Am Acad Opthalmol Otol 72:619, 1968.
19. Brown GC, Shields JA, Sanborn G, et al: Radiation optic neuropathy. Ophthalmology 89:1489, 1982.

20. Brown GC, Shields JA, Sanborn G, et al: Radiation retinopathy. Ophthalmology 89:1494, 1982.
21. Byers R, Berkeley RG, Luna M, Jesse RH: Combined therapeutic approach to malignant lacrimal gland tumors. Am J Ophthalmol 79:53, 1975.
22. Callahan M, Callahan A: Sebaceous gland carcinoma. In Jakobiec FA (ed): Ocular and Adnexal Tumors. Birmingham, Ala., Aesculapius Publishing Co., 1978.
23. Callahan A, Monheit GD, Callahan MA: Cancer excision from eyelids and ocular adnexa: The Mohs fresh tissue technique and reconstruction. CA 32:322, 1982.
24. Carroll JM, Kuwabara T: A classification of limbal epitheliomas. Arch Ophthalmol 73:545, 1965.
25. Cavanagh HD, Green WR, Goldberg HV: Multicentric sebaceous adenocarcinoma of the meibomian gland. Am J Ophthalmol 77:326, 1974.
26. Char DH, Castro JR, Quivey JM, et al: Helium ion charged particle therapy for choroidal melanoma. Ophthalmology 87:565, 1980.
27. Chu FCH, Huh SH, Nisce LZ, Simpson LD: Radiation therapy of choroidal metastases from breast cancer. Int J Radiat Oncol Biol Phys 2:273, 1977.
28. Cobb GM, Thompson GH, Allt WEC: Treatment of basal cell carcinoma of the eyelids by radiotherapy. Can Med Assoc J 91:743, 1964.
29. Cortese DA, Kinsey JH: Endoscopic management of lung cancer with hematoporphyrin derivative phototherapy. Mayo Clin Proc 57:542, 1982.
30. Croxatto JO, Font RL: Hemangiopericytoma of the orbit: A clinicopathologic study of 30 cases. Hum Pathol 13:210, 1982.
31. Curtin VT, Cavender JC: Natural course of selected malignant melanomas of the choroid and ciliary body. Mod Probl Ophthalmol 12:523, 1974.
32. Dagher G, Anderson RL, Ossoinig KC, Baker JD: Adenoid cystic carcinoma of the lacrimal gland in a child. Arch Opthalmol 98:1098, 1980.
33. Dandy WE: Results following the transcranial operative attack on orbital tumors; Arch Ophthalmol 25:191, 1941.
34. Daugherty TJ, Kaufman JE, Goldfarb A, et al: Photoradiation therapy for the treatment of malignant tumors. Cancer Res 38:2628, 1978.
35. Devesa SS: The incidence of retinoblastoma. Am J Ophthalmol 80:263, 1975.
36. Duvall J, Lucas DR: Argon laser and xenon arc coagulation of malignant choroidal melanomata: Histologic findings in six cases. Br J Ophthalmol 65:464, 1981.
37. Ellsworth RM: The practical management of retinoblastoma. Trans Am Ophthalmol Soc 67:462, 1969.
38. Elton RF: Cryosurgery of advanced cancer of the skin. In Zacarian SA (ed): Cryosurgical Advances in Dermatology and Tumors of the Head and Neck. Springfield, Ill., Charles C Thomas, 1972.
39. Farris HE: Cryosurgical treatment of bovine ocular squamous cell carcinoma. Vet Clin North Am [Small Anim Pract] 10:861, 1980.
40. Ferry AP: Lesions mistaken for malignant melanoma of the posterior uvea. Arch Ophthalmol 72:463, 1964.
41. Ferry AP: Tumors metastatic to the eye and ocular adnexa. In Jakobiec FA (ed): Ocular and Adnexal Tumors. Birmingham, Aesculapius Publishing Co., 1978.
42. Ferry AP, Font RL: Carcinoma metastatic to the eye and orbit. I. A clinicopathologic study of 227 cases. Arch Ophthalmol 92:276, 1974.
43. Ferry AP, Font RL: Carcinoma metastatic to the eye and orbit. II. A clinicopathologic study of 26 patients with carcinoma metastatic to the anterior segment of the eye. Arch Ophthalmol 93:472, 1975.
44. Fitzpatrick PJ, Jamiesan DM, Thompson GH, Allt WEC: Tumors of the eyelids and their treatment by radiotherapy. Radiology 104:661, 1972.
45. Font RL, Ferry AP: Carcinoma metastatic to the eye and orbit. III. A clinicopathologic study of 28 cases metastatic to the orbit. Cancer 38:1326, 1976.
46. Font RL, Gamel JW: Epithelial tumors of the lacrimal gland: An analysis of 265 cases. In Jakobiec FA (ed): Ocular and Adnexal Tumors. Birmingham, Ala., Aesculapius Publishing Co., 1978.
47. Font RL, Hidayat AA: Fibrous histiocytoma of the orbit: A clinicopathologic study of 150 cases. Hum Pathol 13:199, 1982.
48. Font RL, Jurico S III, Zimmerman LE: Alveolar soft-part sarcoma of the orbit: A clinicopathologic analysis of seventeen cases and a review of the literature. Hum Pathol 13:569, 1982.
49. Forbes IJ, Cowled PA, Leong ASY, et al: Phototherapy of human tumors using hematoporphyrin derivative. Med J Aust 2:489, 1980.
50. Forrest AW: Intraorbital tumors. Arch Ophthalmol 41:198, 1949.
51. Forrest AW: Iridocyclectomy for ciliary body tumors: Pathologic criteria for operative success. In Jakobiec FA (ed): Ocular and Adnexal Tumors. Birmingham, Ala., Aesculapius Publishing Co., 1978.
52. Foster SC, Wilson CS, Tretter PK: Radiotherapy of primary lymphoma of the orbit. Am J Roentgenol 111:343, 1971.
53. Francois J: Treatment of malignant choroidal melanomas by photocoagulation. Ophthalmologica 184:121, 1982.
54. Franklin CV: Primary lymphoreticular tumors in the orbit. Clin Radiol 26:137, 1975.
55. Fraunfelder FT, Boozman FW III, Wilson RS, Thomas AH: No-touch technique for intraocular malignant melanomas. Arch Ophthalmol 95:1616, 1977.
56. Fraunfelder FT, Chappell CW: External ocular and periocular diseases. In Ablin RJ (ed): Handbook of Cryosurgery. New York, Marcel Dekker, Inc., 1980.
57. Fraunfelder FT, Wallace TR, Farris HE, et al: The role of cryosurgery in external ocular and periocular disease. Trans Am Acad Ophthalmol Otol 83:713, 1977.
58. Fraunfelder FT, Zacarian SA, Limmer BL, Wingfield D: Cryosurgery for malignancies of the eyelid. Ophthalmology 87:461, 1980.
59. Frayer WC, Enterline HT: Embryonal rhabdomyosarcoma of the orbit in children and young adults. Arch Ophthalmol 62:203, 1959.
60. Gamel JW, Font RL: Adenoid cystic carcinoma of the lacrimal gland: The clinical significance of a basaloid histologic pattern. Hum Pathol 13:219, 1982.
61. Gass JDM: Problems in the differential diagnosis of choroidal nevi and malignant melanomas. Am J Ophthalmol 83:299, 1977.
62. Gass JDM: Observation of suspected choroidal and ciliary body melanomas for evidence of growth prior to enucleation. Ophthalmology 87:523, 1980.
63. Gill EG, Harris RB: Bowen's disease (intraepithelial epithelioma). Am J Ophthalmol 43:111, 1957.
64. Ginsberg J: Present status of meibomian gland carcinoma. Arch Ophthalmol 73:271, 1965.
65. Gragoudas ES: The Bragg Peak of proton beams for treatment of uveal melanoma. Int Ophthalmol Clin 20:123, 1980.
66. Grant GD, Shields JA, Brady LW: The radiotherapy of ocular disease. In Brady LW, Perez CA (eds): Basic and Clinical Practice of Radiation Oncology. New York, John Wiley and Sons, 1979.
67. Grizzard WS, Torczynski E, Edwards WC: Adenocarcinoma of eccrine sweat gland. Arch Ophthalmol 94:2119, 1976.
68. Harvey JT, Anderson RL: The management of meibomian gland carcinoma. Ophthalmic Surg 13:56, 1982.
69. Henderson JW: Orbital Tumors. 2nd ed. New York, Brian C. Decker, 1980.
70. Henderson JW, Farrow GM: Primary hemangiopericytoma: An aggressive and potentially malignant neoplasm. Arch Ophthalmol 96:666, 1978.
71. Henderson JW, Farrow GM: Primary malignant mixed tumors of the lacrimal gland. Report of 10 cases. Ophthalmology 87:466, 1980.
72. Henderson JW, Neault RW: En bloc removal of intrinsic neoplasms of the lacrimal gland. Am J Ophthalmol 82:905, 1976.
73. Hendley RL, Rieser JC, Cavanaugh HD, et al: Primary radiation therapy for meibomian gland carcinoma. Am J Ophthalmol 87:206, 1979.
74. Hogan MJ, Zimmerman LE: Ophthalmic Pathology. An Atlas and Textbook. 2nd ed. Philadelphia, W. B. Saunders Co., 1962.
75. Hollander L, Krugh FJ: Cancer of the eyelids. Am J Ophthalmol 27:244, 1944.
76. Howarth C, Meyer D, Omar Huster H, et al: Stage-related combined modality treatment of retinoblastoma. Cancer 45:851, 1980.
77. Ide CH, Ridings GR, Yamashita T, Buesseler JA: Radiotherapy of a recurrent adenocarcinoma of the meibomian gland. Arch Ophthalmol 79:540, 1968.
78. Iliff WJ, Green WR: Orbital tumors in children. In Jakobiec FA (ed): Ocular and Adnexal Tumors. Birmingham, Ala., Aesculapius Publishing Co., 1978.
79. Irvine AR Jr: Dyskeratotic epibulbar tumors. Trans Am Ophthalmol Soc 61:246, 1963.
80. Jakobiec FA, Brownstein S, Albert W, et al: The role of cryotherapy in the management of conjunctival melanoma. Ophthalmology 89:503, 1982.
81. Jakobiec FA, Brownstein S, Wilkinson RD, et al: Combined surgery and cryotherapy for diffuse malignant melanoma of the conjunctiva. Arch Ophthalmol 98:1390, 1980.
82. Jakobiec FA, Yeo JH, Trokel SL, et al: Combined clinical and computed tomographic diagnosis of primary lacrimal fossa lesions. Am J Ophthalmol 94:785, 1982.
83. Jensen OA: Malignant melanomas of the human uvea: 25-year

follow-up of cases in Denmark, 1943-1952. Acta Ophthalmol 60:161, 1982.

84. Jones IS, Reese AB, Kraut J: Orbital rhabdomyosarcoma: An analysis of 62 cases. Am J Ophthalmol 61:721, 1966.

85. Khalil M, Brownstein S, Codère F, Nicolle D: Eccrine sweat gland carcinoma of the eyelid with orbital involvement. Arch Ophthalmol 98:2110, 1980.

86. Knowles DM II, Jakobiec FA: Orbital lymphoid neoplasms. A clinicopathologic study of 60 patients. Cancer 46:576, 1980.

87. Knowles DM II, Jakobiec FA: Ocular adnexal lymphoid neoplasms: Clinical, histopathologic, electron microscopic and immunologic characteristics. Hum Pathol 13:148, 1982.

88. Knowles DM II, Jakobiec FA, Potter GD, Jones IS: The diagnosis and treatment of rhabdomyosarcoma of the orbit. In Jakobiec FA (ed): Ocular and Adnexal Tumors. Birmingham, Ala., Aesculapius Publishing, Co., 1978.

89. Kramer KK, LaPiana FG, Whitmore PV: Enucleation with stabilization of intraocular pressure in the treatment of uveal melanomas. Ophthalmic Surg 11:39, 1980.

90. Laws ER Jr, Cortese DA, Kinsey JH, et al: Photoradiation therapy in the treatment of malignant brain tumors. A phase I (feasibility) study. Neurosurgery 9:672, 1981.

91. Lederman M: Discussion. In Boniuk M (ed): Ocular and Adnexal Tumors: New and Controversial Aspects. St. Louis, The C. V. Mosby Co., 1964.

92. Lennox EL, Draper GJ, Sanders BM: Retinoblastoma. A study of natural history and prognosis of 268 cases. Br Med J 3:731, 1975.

93. Liesegang TJ, Cambell RJ: Mayo Clinic experience with conjunctival melanomas. Arch Ophthalmol 98:1385, 1980.

94. Lincoff H, McLean J, Lang R: The cryosurgical treatment of intraocular tumors. Am J Ophthalmol 63:389, 1967.

95. Lommatzsch PK: Experiences in the treatment of malignant melanoma of the choroid with ^{106}Ru/^{106} Rh beta ray applicators. Trans Ophthalmol Soc UK 93:119, 1973.

96. Lund HZ: How often does squamous cell carcinoma of the skin metastasize? Arch Dermatol 92:635, 1965.

97. McCubbin JA, Spratt JS: The value of no-touch isolation technique for resection of cancer. The eye as a model. Arch Surg 115:224, 1980.

98. McLean IW, Zimmerman LE, Evans RM: Reappraisal of Callender's spindle-A type of malignant melanomas of the choroid and ciliary body. Am J Ophthalmol 86:557, 1978.

99. Maor M, Chan RC, Young SE: Radiotherapy of choroidal metastases. Breast cancer as primary site. Cancer 40:2081, 1977.

100. Marsh JL, Wise DM, Smith M, Schwartz H: Lacrimal gland adenoid cystic carcinoma: Intracranial and extracranial en bloc resection. Plast Reconstr Surg 68:577, 1981.

101. Matthaus W, Lang G, Roitzch E: Die Kryotherapie von Lid- und Bindehauttumoren. Ophthalmologica 173:53, 1976.

102. Maurer HM, Moon T, Donaldson M, et al: The intergroup rhabdomyosarcoma study. A preliminary report. Cancer 40:2015, 1977.

103. Meyer-Schwickerath G, Vogel MH: Malignant melanoma of the choroid treated with photocoagulation. A 10-year follow-up. Mod Probl Ophthalmol 12:544, 1973.

104. Mira HG, Chu FCH, Fortner JG: The role of radiotherapy in the management of malignant hemangiopericytoma: Report of 11 new cases and review of the literature. Cancer 29:1254, 1977.

105. Mohs FE: Chemosurgery: Microscopically controlled method of cancer excision. Arch Surg 42:279, 1941.

106. Mohs FE: Chemosurgery for skin cancer. Arch Dermatol 112:211, 1976.

107. Naumann GOH, Volker HE, Gackle D: The block excision of malignant melanomas of the ciliary body and the peripheral choroid. Doc Ophthalmol 50:43, 1980.

108. Neel HB III, Ketchan AS, Hammond WG: Requisites for successful cryogenic surgery of cancer. Arch Surg 102:45, 1971.

109. Ni C, Dryja TP, Albert DM: Sweat gland tumors in the eyelids. A clinicopathologic analysis of 55 cases. In Ni C, Albert DM (eds): Tumors of the Eyelids and Orbit: A Chinese-American Collaborative Study. Int Ophthalmol Clin 22:1, 1982.

110. Nunery WR, Welsh MG, McCord CD: Recurrence of sebaceous carcinoma of the eyelid after radiation therapy. Am J Ophthalmol 86:10, 1983.

111. Owen M: Basal cell carcinoma—A study of 836 cases. Arch Pathol 10:386, 1930.

112. Packer S, Rotman M: Radiotherapy of choroidal melanoma with iodine-125. Ophthalmology 87:582, 1980.

113. Payne JW, Duke JR, Butner R, Eifrig DE: Basal cell carcinoma of the eyelids. A long-term follow-up study. Arch Ophthalmol 81:553, 1969.

114. Perzin KH, Jakobiec FA, Livolsi VA, Desjardins L: Lacrimal gland malignant mixed tumors (carcinomas arising in benign mixed tumors). A clinicopathologic study. Cancer 45:2593, 1980.

115. Peyman GH, Axelrod AJ, Graham RO: Full-thickness eyewall resection. Arch Ophthalmol 91:219, 1974.

116. Peyman GA, Raichand M: Resection of choroidal melanoma. In Jakobiec FA (ed): Ocular and Adnexal Tumors. Birmingham, Aesculapius Publishing Co., 1978.

117. Porterfield JT: Orbital tumors in children: A report on 214 cases. Int Ophthalmol Clin 2:319, 1962.

118. Porterfield JT, Zimmerman LE: Rhabdomyosarcoma of the orbit: A clinicopathologic study of 55 cases. Virchows Arch [Pathol Anat] 335:329, 1962.

119. Rakofsky SI: The adequacy of the surgical excision of basal cell carcinoma. Ann Ophthalmol 5:596, 1973.

120. Rao NA, McLean IW, Zimmerman LE: Sebaceous carcinoma of eyelids and caruncle. Correlation of clinicopathologic features with prognosis. In Jakobiec FA (ed): Ocular and Adnexal Tumors. Birmingham, Aesculapius Publishing Co., 1978.

121. Reese AB: Expanding lesions of the orbit (Bowman Lecture). Trans Ophthalmol Soc UK 91:85, 1971.

122. Reese AB: Tumors of the Eye. 3rd ed. New York, Harper & Row, 1976.

123. Reese AB, Jones IS: Bone resection in the excision of epithelial tumors of the lacrimal gland. Arch Ophthalmol 71:382, 1964.

124. Sagerman RH, Cassady JR, Tretter P, Ellsworth RM: Radiation induced neoplasia following external beam therapy for children with retinoblastoma. Am J Roentgenol 105:529, 1969.

125. Sang DN, Albert DM: Retinoblastoma: Clinical and histopathologic features. Hum Pathol 13:133, 1982.

126. Scheie HG, Yanoff M, Frayer WC: Carcinoma of sebaceous glands of the eyelids. Arch Ophthalmol 72:800, 1964.

127. Shammas HF, Watzke RC: Bilateral choroidal melanomas: Case report and incidence. Arch Ophthalmol 95:617, 1977.

128. Shields JA: Current approaches to the diagnosis and management of choroidal melanomas. Surg Ophthalmol 21:443, 1977.

129. Shields JA: Diagnosis and Management of Intraocular Tumors. St. Louis, The C. V. Mosby Co., 1983.

130. Shields JA, Augsburger JJ: Current approaches to the diagnosis and management of retinoblastoma. Surv Ophthalmol 25:347, 1981.

131. Shields JA, Augsburger JJ, Brady LW, Day JL: Cobalt plaque therapy for posterior uveal melanomas. Ophthalmology 89:1201, 1982.

132. Shields JA, Zimmerman LE: Lesions simulating malignant melanomas of the posterior uvea. Arch Ophthalmol 89:466, 1973.

133. Shulman J: Treatment of malignant tumors of the eyelids by plastic surgery. Br J Plast Surg 15:37, 1962.

134. Silva D: Orbital tumors. Am J Ophthalmol 65:318, 1968.

135. Smith CK: Metastasizing carcinoma of the sweat gland. Br J Surg 43:80, 1955.

136. Sorsby A: Bilateral retinoblastoma: A dominantly inherited affliction. Br Med J 2:580, 1972.

137. Stanford GB, Reese AB: Malignant cells in the blood of eye patients. Trans Am Acad Ophthalmol Otol 75:102, 1971.

138. Stephens RF, Shields JA: Diagnosis and management of cancer metastatic to the uvea: A study of 70 cases. Ophthalmology 86:1336, 1979.

139. Stewart WB, Krohel GB, Wright JE: Lacrimal gland and fossa lesions: An approach to diagnosis and management. Ophthalmology 86:886, 1979.

140. Stout AP, Cooley SGE: Carcinoma of sweat glands. Cancer 4:521, 1951.

141. Tolentino FI, Tablante RT: Cryotherapy of retinoblastoma. Arch Ophthalmol 87:52, 1972.

142. Tretter P: Radiotherapy of ocular and orbital tumors. In Reese AB (ed): Tumors of the Eye. New York, Harper & Row, 1976.

143. Tromovitch TA, Stegman SJ: Microscopically controlled excision of skin tumors: Chemosurgery (Mohs): Fresh tissue technique. Arch Dermatol 110:231, 1974.

144. Vered IY, Rosen G: Cryosurgery for basal cell carcinoma of the head and neck. S Afr Med J 56:26, 1979.

145. Wagoner MD, Beyer CK, Gonder JR, Albert DM: Common presentations of sebaceous gland carcinoma of the eyelid. Ann Ophthalmol 14:159, 1982.

146. Ward BG, Forbes IJ, Cowled PA, et al: The treatment of vaginal recurrences of gynecologic malignancy with phototherapy following hematoporphyrin derivative pretreatment. Am J Obstet Gynecol 142:356, 1982.

147. Ward GE, Hendrick JW: Tumors of the Head and Neck. Baltimore, Williams & Wilkins Co., 1950.

148. Welch RB, Duke JR: Lesions of lids. Statistical note. Am J Ophthalmol 45:415, 1958.
149. Wiggs EO: Morpheaform basal cell carcinoma of the canthi. Trans Am Acad Ophthalmol Otol 79:649, 1975.
150. Wilkes SR, Robertson DM, Kurland LT, Cambell JR: Incidence of uveal malignant melanoma in the resident population of Rochester and Olmstead County, Minnesota. Am J Ophthalmol 87:639, 1979.
151. Wilson RS, Fraunfelder FT: No-touch cryosurgical enucleation: A minimal trauma technique for eyes harboring intraocular malignancy. Ophthalmology 85:1170, 1978.
152. Wolff JA: Chemotherapy of retinoblastoma. *In* Jakobiec FA (ed): Ocular and Adnexal Tumors. Birmingham, Ala., Aesculapius Publishing Co., 1978.

153. Wright JE, Stewart WB, Krohel GB: Clinical presentation and management of lacrimal gland tumors. Br J Ophthalmol 63:600, 1979.
154. Zacarian SA: Cryosurgery in dermatology. Int Surg 47:528, 1967.
155. Zacarian SA: Cryosurgical Advances in Dermatology and Tumors of the Head and Neck. Springifield, Ill., Charles C Thomas, 1977.
156. Zimmerman LE, McLean IW, Foster WP: Does enucleation of an eye containing a malignant melanoma prevent or accelerate the dissemination of tumor cells? Br J Ophthalmol 62:420, 1978.
157. Zimmerman LE, McLean IW, Foster WD: Statistical analysis of follow-up data concerning uveal melanomas and the influence of enucleation. Ophthalmology 87:557, 1980.

XIV

Special Topics

CHAPTER 70

Tumors of the Head and Neck in Children

Robin T. Cotton, M.D., F.A.C.S., F.R.C.S.(C) • **Edgar T. Ballard, M.D.**
Jacquelyn A. Going, M.D. • **Charles M. Myer III, M.D.** • **Richard B. Towbin, M.D.**
Kwan Y. Wong, M.B.B.S.

The major forms of cancer in children are leukemia, central nervous system tumors, lymphoma, neuroblastoma, and soft-tissue tumors (Fig. 70–1). The frequency of leukemia and neuroblastoma decreases after age 5 years, whereas lymphoma and thyroid tumors have peak frequencies in later childhood (Figs. 70–2 and 70–3). Approximately 40 per cent of pediatric malignancies occur in children under 5 years old.[1]

Primary malignant neoplasms of the head and neck in children are not common,[123] accounting for about 5 per cent of neoplasms occurring in childhood (Fig. 70–4). Malignant lymphomas and soft-tissue sarcomas, mainly rhabdomyosarcomas, are the most common tumors seen.[110, 123, 200] Other neoplasms seen less frequently in the head and neck of children include nasopharyngeal carcinoma, neuroblastoma, salivary gland carcinoma, and thyroid carcinoma.

We reviewed the records of children presenting with malignancies of the head and neck at Children's Hospital Medical Center, Cincinnati, Ohio, from January, 1971 to December 31, 1982. Intracranial tumors, orbital tumors except for rhabdomyosarcoma, odontogenic tumors, and tumors metastatic to the head and neck were excluded (Table 70–1). The two most common malignancies were lymphomas (43 per cent) and rhabdomyosarcoma (21 per cent), and a variety of tumors composed the remainder.

The most common presentation of a tumor in the head and neck area is the appearance of a mass, which is often painless. It may be difficult to differentiate a tumor from infection, and the decision to perform a biopsy depends on the experience of the examiner. As shown in Table 70–1, lymphoid malignancy is the most common tumor in the head and neck region in children. Infection is by far the commonest cause of cervical lymphadenopathy in children. Biopsy should be considered for a significantly enlarged lymph node still present or enlarging 6 weeks after a 2-week course of antibiotics. If the node shows decrease in size at this time, biopsy should be deferred. Other factors that may dictate an earlier biopsy include multiple palpable nodes in other areas of the body, an abnormal blood count or smear, palpable liver or spleen, or evidence of mediastinal lymphadenopathy on chest x-ray.

Other symptoms of tumors in the head and neck area

are secondary to mass effect on adjacent tissue. Prolonged nasal obstruction and recurrent epistaxis deserve a thorough ear, nose, and throat examination. If facial nerve palsy complicates an otitis media, the middle ear should be carefully examined for tumor. Horner's syndrome can be associated with a cervical or upper mediastinal neuroblastoma. Facial plethora and engorgement of neck veins signify compression of the superior vena cava, usually by non-Hodgkin's lymphoma.

When a malignant process is suspected, certain laboratory tests are helpful to determine the extent of involvement and the planning of treatment. Complete blood count may show a mild anemia with changes in the blood smear indicating bone marrow involvement. These changes include the presence of teardrop red blood cells, nucleated red blood cells, young myeloid cells, or young platelets. The erythrocyte sedimentation rate is elevated in both infection and malignancy and is not a helpful test. Bone marrow examination is mandatory if there is an abnormal blood count or if lym-

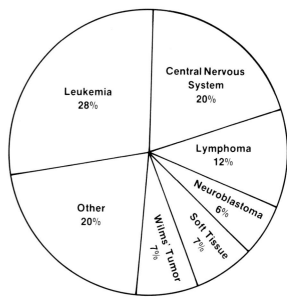

Figure 70–1. Major forms of cancer in children.

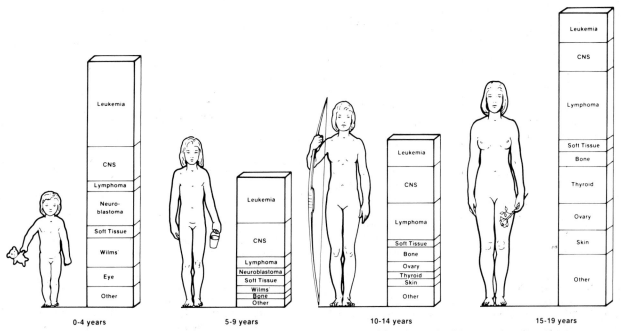

Figure 70–2. Relative proportions of major malignancies in four age groups of females under 20 years old. (Modified from Altman AJ, Schwartz AD: Malignant Diseases of Infancy, Childhood, and Adolescence. 2nd ed. Philadelphia, W. B. Saunders Co., 1983.)

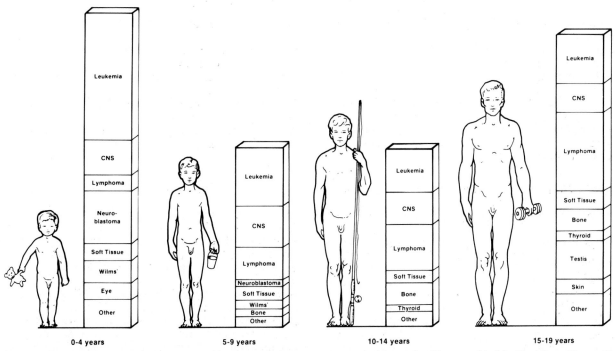

Figure 70–3. Relative proportion of major malignancies in four age groups of males under 20 years old. (Modified from Altman AJ, Schwartz AD: Malignant Diseases of Infancy, Childhood, and Adolescence. 2nd ed. Philadelphia, W. B. Saunders Co., 1983.)

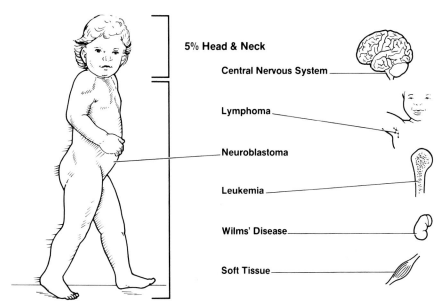

Figure 70–4. Types of primary malignant neoplasms.

phoma is suspected. The finding of blast cells in the bone marrow enables the diagnosis of lymphoma or granulocytic sarcoma (chloroma) without biopsy of the lymph node or mass.

The radiographic evaluation of diseases involving the head and neck has traditionally centered around plain radiographs, contrast examination of the oropharynx and nasopharynx, and occasionally angiography. However, these modalities have not been able to demonstrate fully the extent of disease and the relationship to surrounding structures. With the introduction and application of ultrasound and particularly computed tomography (CT), a more thorough and accurate diagnostic evaluation can be achieved.

A common site for metastasis in childhood malignancy is the lung. When the suspicion of malignancy is high, tomography or computed tomography (CT) of the chest is indicated prior to any surgical procedure. After anesthesia there could be areas of atelectasis in the lungs, and this would make the interpretation of the CT scan difficult.

Bone metastases are also common in childhood malignancies. Radionuclide imaging is more sensitive than radiographic examination of the skeleton, with the exception of purely osteolytic lesions.

The staging system in childhood malignancy is different from the TNM system that is commonly used for adult carcinomas. Histologic subtypes have been shown to have prognostic significance and must be considered in treatment planning.

Adjuvant chemotherapy after complete resection of tumor is often necessary to treat micrometastasis to prevent recurrence of the tumor.[111] Radiation therapy can provide tumor control locally at the primary site. With good tumor control using a combination of radiation therapy and chemotherapy, radical resection of tumor such as orbital exenteration for rhabdomyosarcoma, is seldom necessary. Extirpation of tumor may also be possible at a later date after a course of radiotherapy or chemotherapy. Thus, a diagnostic biopsy is a common surgical procedure for head and neck tumors in childhood.

RHABDOMYOSARCOMA

Soft-tissue sarcomas account for about 7 per cent of all malignant neoplasms in children under 15 years of age in the United States; over half of these are rhabdomyosarcomas.[273] The annual incidence of rhabdomyosarcoma is 4.4 per million in white children and 1.3 per million in black children under 15 years of age. In frequency of location for primary tumors, 38 per cent are in the head and neck region, 21 per cent are in the genitourinary tract, 18 per cent are in the extremities, 7 per cent are in the trunk, 7 per cent are in the retroperitoneum, and 9 per cent are at other sites[169] (Fig. 70–5). Head and neck primary tumors are most commonly found in the orbit, followed by the pharynx and soft tissue of the face and neck[17, 221, 247] (Table 70–2) (Fig. 70–6). The peak incidence of rhabdomyosarcoma is around 5 years of age,[247, 248] with a slight predominance in males.[169]

TABLE 70–1. Types of Head and Neck Malignancies in Children

Type of Malignancy	Children's Hospital Medical Center, 1971–1982	Jaffe and Jaffe[123]	Sutow[246]
Malignant lymphoma	26	97	53
Hodgkin's disease	16	46	31
Non-Hodgkin's disease	10	51	22
Rhabdomyosarcoma	13	20	35
Other soft-tissue sarcomas	2	15	11
Osteogenic sarcoma	2	2	1
Ewing's sarcoma	1	3	4
Parotid malignancies	1	2	3
Thyroid malignancies	1	9	15
Squamous cell carcinoma	5	7	7*
Malignant histiocytosis	1		
Neuroblastoma	1	9	3
Histiocytosis X	8		
Malignant melanoma		4	3
Malignant teratoma		1	2

*Includes three basal cell carcinomas.

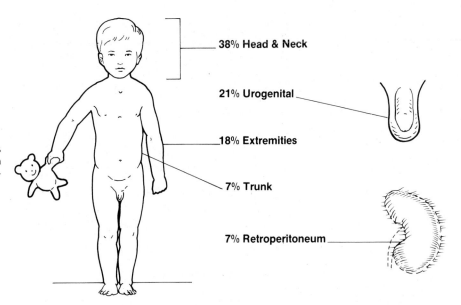

Figure 70–5. Relative frequencies of rhabdomyosarcoma based on sites of origin in the pediatric patient.

- 38% Head & Neck
- 21% Urogenital
- 18% Extremities
- 7% Trunk
- 7% Retroperitoneum

Pathology

Rhabdomyosarcomas include a heterogeneous group of neoplasms, which were originally classified by Horn and Enterline[118] into embryonal, botryoid, alveolar, and pleomorphic. Certain undifferentiated tumors and tumors of uncertain histogenesis are also grouped in this category for convenience. Although there is considerable histologic overlap between the various groups, certain characteristic features can be identified.[97]

Embryonal rhabdomyosarcomas account for the majority of head and neck rhabdomyosarcomas in childhood. These are densely cellular tumors, composed of lymphocyte-sized cells with hyperchromatic round to oval nuclei and stellate or bipolar cell processes (Fig. 70–7). The tumor cells exhibit a variable arrangement of syncytial or interlacing bands of cells and at times a myxoid-appearing background. Rhabdomyoblastic differentiation may be evident as sarcoplasm-like eosinophilic striated or granular cytoplasm or cross striations in single nucleated or multinucleated "strap" cells. The botryoid variety is generally considered a subcategory of the embryonal and occurs when the tumor arises beneath a mucous membrane surface, producing a polypoid configuration. A unique feature of the latter type is the condensed cambial layer immediately beneath the mucosa (Fig. 70–8).

The alveolar rhabdomyosarcomas are characterized by cells of moderate size (15 to 30 μm) separated into alveolar groupings by fibrous septa (Fig. 70–9). Within the alveolar groupings peripherally placed cells appear to have an orientation to the fibrous septa. Centrally, there is lack of cellular cohesiveness and degenerative change. There are blunt, grooved nuclei, which may be lobulated or reniform. Multinucleation is common, and evidence of rhabdomyoblastic differentiation may be evident as cross striations or the presence of variable cell forms with eosinophilic cytoplasm, including strap cells, racquet cells, or multinucleated cells with a wreath of peripherally placed nuclei, so-called spider cells.

The pleomorphic type is composed of large bizarre pleomorphic tumor cells that have differentiating features of skeletal muscle and appear to arise in mature skeletal muscle in contrast to the previous groups, which are tumors of embryonic tissue. Pleomorphic rhabdomyosarcomas are for practical purposes seen only in adults.

In addition to the classically described types of rhabdomyosarcoma, a number of tumors of uncertain histogenesis are generally classified with the rhabdomyosarcomas. One of these is the group of soft-tissue tumors that histologically resemble Ewing's sarcoma of bone. The remainder are undifferentiated tumors without clear rhabdomyoblastic differentiation and generally are referred to as undifferentiated, small, round-cell mesenchymal sarcomas, type undetermined. Of the established subtypes, the alveolar rhabdomyosarcoma, which occurs predominantly in older children and young adults, has the worst prognosis. The Intergroup

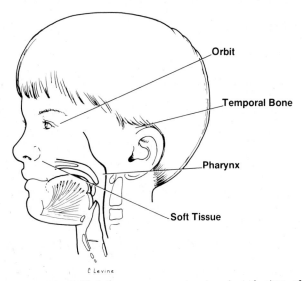

- Orbit
- Temporal Bone
- Pharynx
- Soft Tissue

C Levine

Figure 70–6. Rhabdomyosarcoma—head and neck sites of origin.

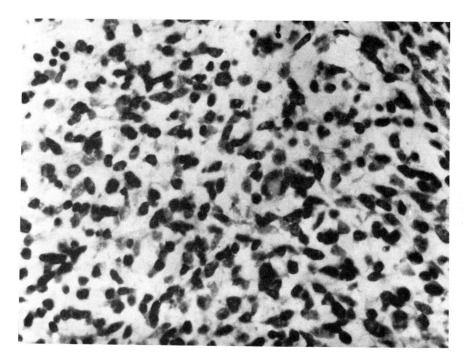

Figure 70–7. Embryonal rhabdomyosarcoma. There is a diffuse infiltration of embryonal rhabdomyoblasts. Note the stellate appearance of tumor cells, occasional multinucleated cells, and myxoid appearance. (× 760)

Rhabdomyosarcoma Study (IRS) is currently evaluating whether additional histologic features have prognostic significance.

Although the majority of rhabdomyosarcomas can be diagnosed by routine histologic examination, in only 23 to 33 per cent of cases will definite cross striations or other evidence of striated muscle differentiation be demonstrable by light microscopy. The use of immunohistologic and electron microscopic examination may be helpful in identifying rhabdomyoblastic differentiation in a greater percentage of cases than is possible by light microscopy alone. Kahn and associates[130] have shown that the use of immunoperoxidase staining for myoglobin and the MM isoenzyme of creatine kinase identifies definite evidence of rhabdomyoblastic differentiation in a greater percentage of cases than indicated by light microscopy. Electron microscopy of rhabdomyosarcomas reveals a pattern of cellular differentiation that is similar to normal embryonic myogenesis.[176] A minimal ultrastructural criterion is the presence of specific thick and thin cytoplasmic myofilaments or Z-band material.

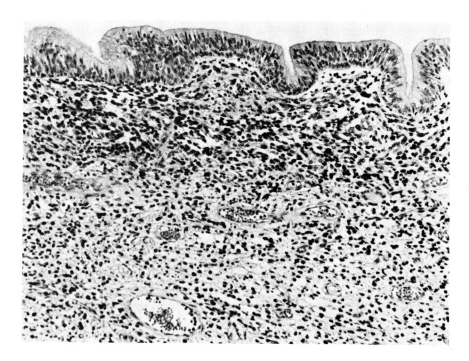

Figure 70–8. Botryoid rhabdomyosarcoma. The compressed cambial layer of tumor cells immediately beneath the mucosa is a unique feature of this tumor. (× 570)

TABLE 70–2. Rhabdomyosarcoma—Frequency of Head and Neck Primary Tumors by Site

Site	Batsakis[17]	Schuller et al.[221]	Sutow[246]	Children's Hospital Medical Center, 1971–1982	Total	Percentage of All Rhabdomyosarcomas
Orbit	54	8	52	5	119	29%
Soft tissue					82	20%
Neck	18	5	19		42	
Head	22	4	13	1	40	
Pharynx					99	24%
Nasopharynx	16	3	39	3	61	15%
Oropharynx	15	5	11	2	33	8%
Hypopharynx	3	2			5	1%
Oral cavity	15	3			18	4%
Nasal cavity			3		3	0.7%
Infratemporal fossa			13	1	14	3.5%
Paranasal sinus	3	2	20		25	6%
Temporal bone	12	2	18	1	33	8%
Larynx		1	1		2	0.5%
Parotid gland			11		11	2.7%
Total	158	35	200	13	406	

Clinical Manifestations

The clinical presentation varies with the anatomic site. In the orbit, there is usually a rapidly developing proptosis due to the small confines of the orbit, and early diagnosis is usually possible. Tumor in the soft tissue of the head and neck usually presents as a painless, enlarging mass. Symptoms related to tumors in the nasopharynx or middle ear are often initially ascribed to an intercurrent upper respiratory tract infection. Otorrhea, nasal speech, epistaxis, serous otitis media, earache, and sinusitis may be present. As the disease advances, a polypoid mass may be seen in the nasopharynx or middle ear. Lower motor neuron paralysis of the seventh cranial nerve may also be present. When there is a delay in the resolution of an upper respiratory tract infection or otitis media, a careful ear, nose, and throat examination is warranted.

Based on the extent of disease at the outset of treatment, patients can be categorized into four clinical groups[169] (Table 70–3). Twenty per cent of patients have evidence of metastases at the time of diagnosis.[169] In the head and neck the largest number of patients are in group III. This is due to the fact that radiation and chemotherapy have been shown to be relatively effective, and, therefore, there is a natural reluctance of the surgeon to perform mutilating surgery. An excessive

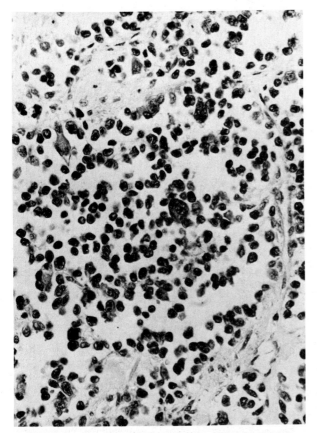

Figure 70–9. Alveolar rhabdomyosarcoma. This subtype is characterized by alveolar groupings of cells enclosed by delicated fibrous septa. (× 500)

TABLE 70–3. IRS Staging in Rhabdomyosarcoma

Stage	Description
Group I	Localized disease confined to organ of origin or with contiguous involvement (not including regional nodes) completely resected
Group II	Grossly resected tumor with microscopic residual disease Regional disease (regional nodal involvement or extension to adjacent organ) completely resected Regional disease with nodal involvement grossly resected with microscopic residual disease
Group III	Incomplete resection or biopsy only with gross residual tumor
Group IV	Metastatic disease present at onset

Source: Adapted from Maurer HM, Moon T, et al: Cancer 40:2015, 1977.

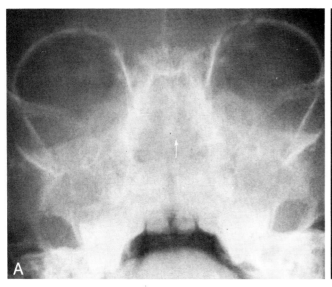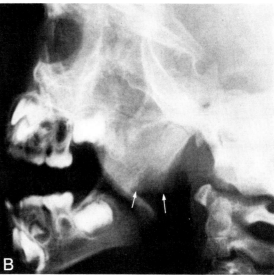

Figure 70–10. Waters' (*A*) and lateral (*B*) radiographs show a large, noncalcified nasopharyngeal soft-tissue mass (arrows) invading and destroying the nasal septum (arrows), nares, and posterior antra. The antra are opacified secondary to extrinsic obstruction and tumor invasion. (Figures reprinted with permission from Radiographics vol. 2, no. 2, May 1982.)

number of patients with parameningeal primary tumors had group III or group IV disease.[247] Of special note is that the incidence of metastatic disease is extremely low in patients with orbital rhabdomyosarcoma (4 per cent in IRS-I).[247] In IRS-I, 35 per cent of patients with parameningeal primary lesions (nasopharynx, paranasal sinuses, and middle ear) had evidence of direct extension to the meninges and had a 90 per cent mortality rate.[251] About 14 per cent of patients with parameningeal lesions already had distant metastases at diagnosis.[247] The common sites of metastasis are the lungs, lymph nodes, skeletal system, bone marrow, liver, brain, and breast.[234]

Diagnostic Studies

Careful evaluation of the extent of tumor involvement is necessary to determine the type of surgical approach or to define the field of radiation treatment. The roentgen evaluation of patients with rhabdomyosarcoma involving the head and neck depends to a great extent on the location of the primary tumor mass. In the past, skull and sinus series, laminagraphy, and angiography were the mainstay of diagnostic radiographic evelution. However, CT is now the preferred imaging modality for both diagnostic evaluation and therapeutic planning. Computed tomography has largely replaced laminagraphy and angiography and is the best method to delineate tumor location, tumor extent, and response to therapy.[277]

Computerized tomography is performed in axial projection prior to and after bolus injection of 2 to 3 ml per kg of body weight (maximum of 100 ml) of contrast material. If possible, postcontrast direct coronal images are also obtained. Five- or 10-mm thick contiguous or overlapping images are obtained, depending on patient size and ability to cooperate. Sagittal re-formated images are routinely made.

Radiographic features are not specific for rhabdomyosarcoma. In nasopharyngeal rhabdomyosarcoma, plain radiography usually demonstrates a noncalcified, exo-phytic nasopharyngeal mass projecting into the air space (Fig. 70–10). Associated destruction of the skull base with contiguous or distant spread is often noted. Computed tomography usually demonstrates a noncalcified, enhancing, exophytic nasopharyngeal mass, which often invades and destroys adjacent structures, including the paranasal sinuses, nasal cavity, skull base, orbit, and temporal bone. Direct intracranial extension into the middle cranial fossa may also occur.

When the petrous bone is primarily involved, plain radiography and laminagraphy will document opacified or destroyed mastoid air cells (Fig. 70–11). The degree of bone destruction is often out of proportion to the patient's clinical symptoms. Computed tomography has replaced laminagraphy because it better demonstrates the extent of bone destruction, soft-tissue mass, and intracranial extension (Fig. 70–12).[42, 84] Computed tomography appears to be the most sensitive method and provides the best anatomic display of tumor spread.[60, 223, 277]

Chest radiograph should be evaluated for metastatic lesions. Chest CT is more sensitive than conventional chest radiography. Preferably, CT should be done prior to general anesthesia because postanesthetic atelectasis may mask some metastatic lesions. Bone metastasis can be evaluated by radionuclide bone scan. Liver scan should also be considered.

Cytologic or cytocentrifugation smear from cerebrospinal fluid should be examined if the tumor arises from parameningeal areas. Bone marrow should be examined for tumor cells by an aspiration sample and either a concentrated (buffy coat) specimen from the aspirate or a bone marrow biopsy. Ideally, bone marrow samples from two different sites should be examined.

Principles of Therapy

Local control of tumor is usually achieved by resection of the tumor followed by radiation treatment to the tumor bed. However, wide surgical resection of tumors

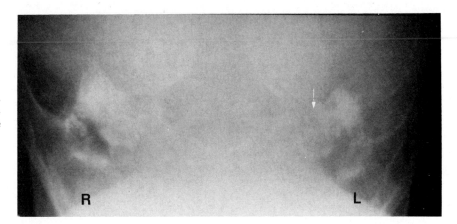

Figure 70–11. Opacification and destruction of left temporal bone (arrow). However, extent of disease cannot be determined.

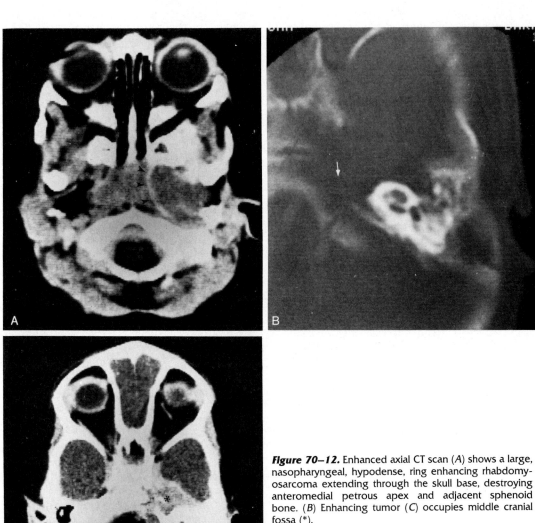

Figure 70–12. Enhanced axial CT scan (A) shows a large, nasopharyngeal, hypodense, ring enhancing rhabdomyosarcoma extending through the skull base, destroying anteromedial petrous apex and adjacent sphenoid bone. (B) Enhancing tumor (C) occupies middle cranial fossa (*).

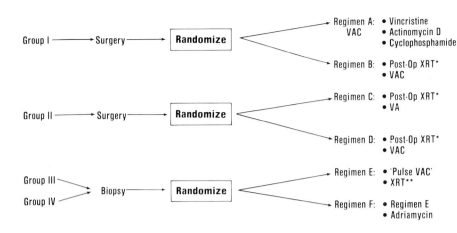

Figure 70–13. Intergroup rhabdomyosarcoma Study (IRS-I) protocol. Therapeutic regimen: XRT* = Radiotherapy given for 42 days before chemotherapy; XRT** = radiotherapy given after 6 weeks of chemotherapy.

in the head and neck area is often impossible or achieved only with unacceptably disfiguring results. Moreover, the concept of the presence of micrometastases at diagnosis is supported by the lower rate of recurrence or metastasis in those patients who received chemotherapy in addition to complete surgical resection and local radiotherapy.[111] In IRS-I protocol, there was no difference in the disease-free survival rate between group I and group II patients (Fig. 70–13). Thus, wide surgical margins do not appear to be necessary to assure local control. The initial surgical approach for the patient with suspected rhabdomyosarcoma should be an incisional biopsy. If complete resection is not possible after careful evaluation, chemotherapy and radiation treatment should be given first to reduce the size of the tumor. A second surgery is then planned to remove the tumor if necessary.

Radiation treatment in the range of 4000 to 6000 rad is effective in local control of the tumor. Results from IRS-I protocol indicate that radiation treatment is not necessary in those patients with complete resection of the tumor[169] and that local control is as effective with 4000 to 4500 rad and combined chemotherapy as with higher doses if the tumor is less than 5 cm in diameter.[252] Thus, in IRS-II protocol, dosages between 4000 and 4500 rad with a 5 cm margin are currently recommended for all ages with group II tumors and for children under 6

years of age with group III tumors less than 5 cm in diameter. In children older than 6 years, 4500 to 5000 rad will be delivered if the tumor is less than 5 cm, and 5000 to 5500 rad are given if the tumor is greater than 5 cm in diameter[168] (Fig. 70–14).

Effective chemotherapeutic agents used singly include vincristine (59 per cent response rate), actinomycin D (24 per cent), cyclophosphamide (54 per cent), doxorubicin (31 per cent), dacarbazine (DTIC) (11 per cent), and mitomycin C (36 per cent).[99] A combination of vincristine, actinomycin D, and cyclophosphamide (VAC) appears to be most successful and is most commonly used. The duration of chemotherapy is usually 18 to 24 months. In IRS-II protocol, the question of shorter duration of treatment for group I patients will be answered by a randomized study.[168] More aggressive approach or refinement in the chemotherapy regimens is needed for patients with metastatic disease.

Prognosis

With the current multimodal therapy for rhabdomyosarcoma, the prognosis is closely related to the initial extent of disease. The overall 2-year survival rate for clinical group I patients is 92 per cent, with a disease-free survival of 83 per cent. For group II patients the figures are 78 per cent and 72 per cent, respectively.

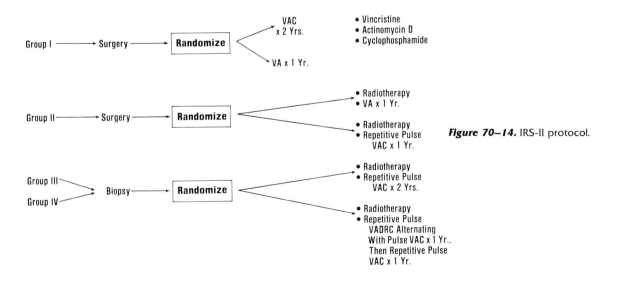

Figure 70–14. IRS-II protocol.

TABLE 70–4. Survival of Patients with Head and Neck Rhabdomyosarcoma

	Group I			Group II			Group III			Group IV		
	Total No.	Failures	2 Yr. (%)	Total No.	Failures	2 Yr. (%)	Total No.	Failures	2 Yr. (%)	Total No.	Failures	2 Yr. (%)
Disease-free survival (I, II) or length of time on study (III, IV)												
Head and neck	0			29	5	82	97	49	53	21	18	10
Orbit	0			15	1	93	36	9	68	0		
Survival												
Head and neck	0			30	3	88	97	41	58	21	14	27
Orbit	0			15	1	93	36	4	83	0		
Survival (all sites)	73	5	92	130	27	78	238	83	64	113	68	35

Source: Adapted from Gehan EA, Glover FN, Maurer HM, et al: Natl Cancer Inst Monogr 56:83–92, 1981.

The 2-year survival rate for group III is 64 per cent, and for Group IV it is 35 per cent[202] (Table 70–4).

Management and Diagnosis of Special Sites

The distribution of rhabdomyosarcoma in the head and neck area is shown in Table 70–2. The majority of the tumors are of the embryonal or botryoid types. The alveolar type occurs in 6 per cent of the orbital lesions and 10 per cent of tumors from other sites in the head and neck.[247] Most of the patients had group III disease (62 per cent) and metastatic disease occurred in 11 per cent of the patients.[247]

The prognosis of localized disease (groups I, II and III) is related to the site of the primary tumor: 3-year disease-free survival for orbital lesions is 91 per cent, for parameningeal lesions it is 45 per cent, and for other head and neck sites it is 75 per cent. The same survival rate for patients with metastatic disease is only 18 per cent.[95, 247]

With the high mortality rate in patients with meningeal extension of tumor from parameningeal sites,[251] treatment to the central nervous system is given in addition to intensive chemotherapy and radiation treatment to the tumor area.[168] Cranial radiation is given to those patients with intracranial extension, erosion of skull base, or cranial nerve palsy. Chemotherapy with methotrexate, cytosine arabinoside, and hydrocortisone is also given intrathecally. Those patients with tumor cells in the cerebrospinal fluid or cord compression due to tumor received additional spinal axis radiation. The preliminary results are encouraging.[202]

Rhabdomyosarcoma of the ear occurred in 28 (4 per cent) patients in the IRS-I protocol, 26 involving the middle ear and two involving the external ear.[201] All the tumors were embryonal or botryoid type. The common clinical presentation includes bloody or purulent ear discharge, refractory otitis media, presence of a mass in the auditory canal, and cranial nerve palsy, especially of the facial nerve.[56, 155, 201]

Surgical resection appeared possible only in those patients with primary tumor in the external ear,[5, 56, 155, 201] and the prognosis has been good. The majority of the patients had group III disease after biopsy or mastoidectomy. Only 37.5 per cent of these patients were free of tumor from 2.2 to 5.7 years (median, 4 years)

after beginning therapy.[201] About 20 per cent of the patients had metastatic disease at diagnosis, and none of them were alive.[201] The survival rate of these children appears to have improved with the addition of cranial irradiation and intrathecal chemotherapy.[202]

SOFT-PART SARCOMA

Besides rhabdomyosarcoma, other malignant soft-part sarcomas in the head and neck include fibrosarcoma, synovial sarcoma, liposarcoma, malignant fibrous histiocytoma, alveolar soft-part sarcoma, hemangiopericytoma, and neurogenic sarcoma.[76, 80] Although these tumors are generally found in the extremities and the trunk, primary tumors of the head and neck occasionally occur. Local recurrence rate is high with soft-tissue sarcoma and may occur late with evidence of metastasis. Tumors that tend to recur locally and rarely metastasize include liposarcoma, well-differentiated fibrosarcoma, and superficial malignant fibrous histiocytoma.[76] Tumors with tendency to long-delayed metastases include synovial sarcoma, alveolar soft-part sarcoma, and fibrosarcoma.[76] Radiation treatment and chemotherapy are probably indicated for some of these tumors.

Fibrosarcoma

Fibrosarcoma is rare in children, but the diagnostic criteria are the same as for adults. Briefly, these tumors are composed of a proliferation of anaplastic spindle cells arranged in a herringbone pattern (Fig. 70–15). The degree of anaplasia, cellularity, differentiation, and mitotic activity are used in determining histologic grade. The prognosis for these tumors in children, however, is much better than for adults. In the study by Soule and Pritchard,[235] children less than 5 years of age had a 7.3 per cent chance of developing metastatic spread, compared with a 50 per cent incidence of metastasis in children 10 years or older. However, few of these cases involved the head and neck area, and extrapolation of these data to tumors of the paranasal area would be ill advised.

The major source of diagnostic confusion is with the heterogeneous group of fibroblastic proliferations known collectively as fibromatosis.[211] The etiology is

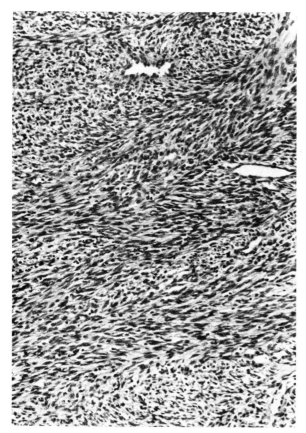

Figure 70–15. Infantile fibrosarcoma. This lesion is composed of parallel bundles of fibroblasts that exhibit an interlacing or "herringbone" pattern. Histologically, the differentiation of this lesion from aggressive fibromatosis in children or from the more malignant fibrosarcomas of older patients is difficult. (× 208)

unknown, and the lesions are composed of a mixture of fibroblasts and collagen. The histologic subtypes encompass a spectrum of cellularity and aggressive features that range from bland scar-like lesions, such as sternomastoid tumor, to aggressive fibromatosis. These conditions, depending on the histologic subtype, have the potential for local invasion and recurrence following excision or for spontaneous regression, but they do not metastasize. Aggressive fibromatosis, an uncommon lesion, is the most controversial of these lesions, for there is considerable overlap with low-grade fibrosarcomas in both clinical behavior and microscopic appearance of these lesions. A conservative approach to therapy is urged for all these lesions because of a low potential for distant spread.

Fibrosarcoma can originate from either bone or soft tissue but, regardless of origin, has no specific radiographic features. When bone is the primary site of origin, there may be geographic or permeative bone destruction, associated soft-tissue mass, and dystrophic calcification (Fig. 70–16).[205]

Unfortunately, it has not been possible to predict which tumors are capable of metastasis on the basis of microscopic study.[52, 241] Wide local excision is the treatment of choice for both primary and recurrent tumors. Radiation treatment in doses over 6000 rad may offer some tumor control, although this type of tumor is not particularly radiosensitive.[243] Chemotherapy is indicated for metastatic disease, and occasional success is seen with the use of vincristine, actinomycin D, cyclophosphamide, doxorubicin, and 5-fluorouracil in various combination regimens.

Synovial Sarcoma

Synovial sarcoma is a slow-growing tumor that does not originate within joints or bursal surfaces. The tumor arises in or near tendons and tendon sheaths. Synovial sarcomas tend to be solitary, well-circumscribed lesions.[77] The cut surface is soft, moist, glistening, and yellowish gray. Microscopically, synovial sarcomas of the neck are similar to those in other sites. There may be the characteristic biphasic pattern of epithelioid cells forming gland-like spaces or clefts surrounded by fibrosarcoma-like areas. Other tumors are predominantly fibrosarcoma with little synovial differentiation.

In the head and neck it may be found in the retropharynx.[216] Local recurrence rate is high, and metastasis to lungs usually occurs within 2 years.[40, 106] Treatment is wide local excision. If complete removal is not possible, postoperative radiation treatment and chemotherapy should be given in a manner similar to that of treatment of rhabdomyosarcoma.

Lipoblastoma

Lipoblastoma and liposarcoma are found in infants and adolescents.[51] Lipoblastomas (localized form) and lipoblastomatosis (diffuse form) are benign tumors that occur in infancy and early childhood, predominantly on the extremities. They are composed of lobules of immature fat cells surrounded by myxoid connective tissue. The latter results in a resemblance to a myxoid liposarcoma. Liposarcomas, however, are rare in children, but when they occur, they tend to be of the myxoid variety.[227] Treatment should be local excision. Radiation treatment and chemotherapy may be considered for recurrent tumors.

Malignant Fibrous Histiocytoma

Malignant fibrous histiocytoma is composed of spindle cells arranged in a storiform pattern with frequent neoplastic histiocyte cells that may be multinucleated.[233, 258] Only one third of the patients failed to have recurrence of tumor after surgical resection.[258] Chemotherapy for recurrent or metastatic disease with actinomycin D, cyclophosphamide, DTIC, and doxorubicin was only partially effective.[152]

Alveolar Soft-Part Sarcoma

Alveolar soft-part sarcoma is a rare tumor of uncertain histogenesis; it occurs predominantly in adolescents and young adults. The tumors grossly are well circumscribed and highly vascular. Microscopically, they are characterized by a strikingly uniform pseudoalveolar pattern of polygonal cells that may contain characteristic cytoplasmic crystalline structures. In the head and neck, it may be found in the orbital area.[88] Metastases of this tumor can occur more than 10 years after primary therapy,[157] and this makes evaluation of the treatment of the primary tumor extremely difficult.

Hemangiopericytoma

Hemangiopericytoma is a neoplasm of vascular origin. Histologically, the tumor consists of spindle-shaped cells (pericytes) grouped about capillaries. Mitoses are common. The tumor can be benign or malignant.[135] In the head and neck, it may be found in the orbit.[113, 124, 132] Treatment is wide excision. Radiation treatment and chemotherapy are of doubtful value.

LYMPHOMA

Lymphoma is the second most common malignant solid tumor in children[273] and is the most common malignancy in the head and neck. Hodgkin's disease frequently presents with cervical lymph node enlargement. Non-Hodgkin's lymphoma, on the other hand, tends to be widespread at diagnosis, and enlargement of neck nodes is only part of the clinical picture rather than the presenting chief complaint. In rare instances, myelogenous leukemia may present as a soft-tissue mass or lymph node enlargement, termed granulocytic sarcoma or chloroma. The common site for granulocytic sarcoma is the orbit,[128] followed by intracranial location[122] and other head and neck areas.[31, 33] Biopsy material from these masses may be interpreted as non-Hodgkin's lymphoma if the esterase stain is not used in the evaluation. Granulocytic sarcoma may precede the leukemia picture by months to over a year.[260]

Cervical lymph node enlargement is a common occurrence in children. Frequently, it has an infectious etiology. Lymphoid hyperplasia in response to infection is much more common in children than adults. However, persistent lymphadenopathy often poses a diagnostic and therapeutic problem, particularly in timing of a biopsy. A common practice is to treat the child with lymphadenopathy with an adequate course of antibiotics, and if there is no response, biopsy is indicated. This

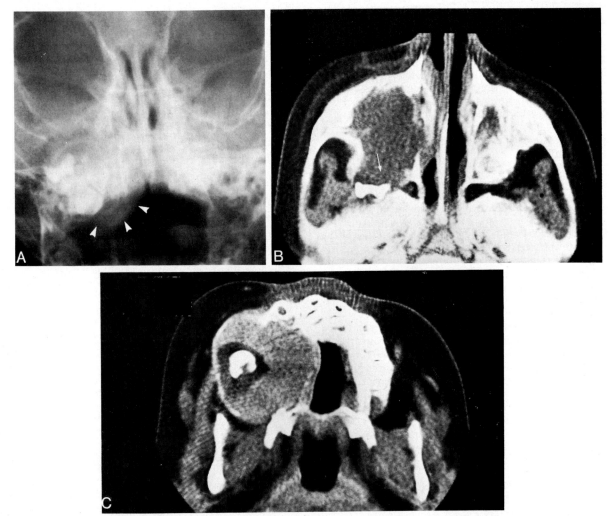

Figure 70–16. One-year-old male with a rapidly growing palatal fibrosarcoma. Anteroposterior view of face (*A*) reveals a soft-tissue mass originating within the right maxilla and projecting into the oropharynx (arrows). (*B*) Subtle destruction of the maxilla (arrow) is present. (*C*) Contrast-enhanced CT scan shows a large destructive mass (approximately 43 mm in diameter) involving the maxilla and extending into, enlarging, and destroying the maxillary antrum. The mass contours a cystic and hypovascular component and floating tooth.

is an oversimplified statement. Some viral infection may be associated with prolonged lymphadenopathy, such as mononucleosis syndrome. Besides infectious causes, diphenylhydantoin (Dilantin) hypersensitivity, rheumatoid arthritis, and systemic lupus erythematosus can produce enlargement of lymph nodes, mimicking lymphoma.[71] Thus, the decision to perform a biopsy should be made by an experienced specialist. Lymph node biopsies should include central areas of tumor to avoid the diagnostic difficulty frequently encountered in small specimens taken at the periphery of a tumor mass. Initial biopsies early in disease may be nondiagnostic or may reveal only atypical hyperplasia, necessitating further follow-up and repeat biopsy.

Hodgkin's Disease

The incidence of Hodgkin's disease is about 5.8 per million. Studies have shown a bimodal age peak incidence: the first peak occurs in teenage children and young adults, and the disease has a fairly good prognosis; the second peak occurs in patients over 40 years of age, and the prognosis is less optimistic.[162] It is rare in children under 5 years of age. There is a male predominance in the preteen years (3:1 ratio). The incidence in the female increases with age, and in the older age group the incidence in both sexes appears similar.

Hodgkin's disease is generally recognized as a malignancy of the lymphoreticular system. The tumor histologically consists of a polymorphous infiltration of malignant cells (Reed-Sternberg cells and their mononuclear variants) and morphologically normal reactive cells (lymphocytes, plasma cells, and eosinophils). The diagnostic Reed-Sternberg cells are large cells with multiple nuclei, which are often mirror image in configuration. Each nucleus has a single prominent eosinophilic nucleolus. Condensation of the nuclear chromatin beneath the nuclear membrane results in a perinucleolar halo. The cytoplasm is moderately abundant and stains variably, although it is usually slightly eosinophilic. The current classification is the Rye modification of the Lukes Butler classification[159, 160, 164] (Table 70–5), which divides Hodgkin's disease into lymphocytic predominance, mixed cellularity, lymphocyte depletion, and nodular sclerosis.

Lymphocyte depletion, mixed cellularity, and lymphocyte predominance are distinguished primarily by the relative proportions of Reed-Sternberg cells and non-neoplastic cells, mostly lymphocytes. Lymphocyte predominance is characterized by either partial or complete effacement of nodal architecture and occasional paracortical infiltration with sparing of lymphoid follicles. Reed-Sternberg cells are rare, and patients usually have a more favorable prognosis. Lymphocyte depletion Hodgkin's disease is characterized by predominance of

TABLE 70–5. Histologic Subtypes of Hodgkin's Disease

Lymphocyte predominance
Nodular sclerosis
Mixed cellularity
Lymphocyte depletion

Reed-Sternberg cells and variants, necrosis, fibrosis, and a paucity of lymphocytes and other reactive cells. Mixed cellularity Hodgkin's disease is intermediate between the previous two types in relative proportions of the neoplastic Reed-Sternberg cells and non-neoplastic lymphocytes. In addition, there is often a heterogeneous mixture of eosinophils, plasma cells, lymphocytes, and non-neoplastic histiocytes.

The nodular sclerosis variety of Hodgkin's disease is somewhat variable but has distinct clinical and histologic features. This disease occurs more frequently in adolescents and young adults in lower cervical, supraclavicular, and mediastinal lymph nodes and has a more favorable prognosis. Two features serve to distinguish this variety histologically: (1) a thickened capsule with thick bands of birefringent collagen dividing the tumor into descrete lobules and (2) the presence of a variant of the Reed-Sternberg cell, the lacunar cell. These cells have abundant pale eosinophilic cytoplasm, unusually delicate nuclear chromatin with small nucleoli, and an unusual degree of nuclear hyperlobation. In formalin-fixed material the cell cytoplasm tends to retract, resulting in a "lacunar"-like appearance.

The relative frequency of these four histologic subtypes in children is as follows: lymphocyte predominant, 23.0 per cent; nodular sclerosis, 38.8 per cent; mixed cellularity, 33.5 per cent; and lymphocyte depleted, 4.7 per cent.[199] The lymphocyte predominant and mixed cellularity types display a marked male predominance (3.9:1 and 5.2:1, respectively), whereas the nodular sclerosis and lymphocyte depletion types show a lower male-female ratio of about 2:1.[199]

Clinical Picture and Staging

Clinically, the majority of patients present with painless adenopathy, with 80 to 90 per cent involving cervical lymph nodes. The disease usually progresses by direct lymphatic spread. Thus, left supraclavicular node involvement is often associated with abdominal disease, and right supraclavicular node involvement is associated with mediastinal disease.

Some patients may have associated systemic symptoms, which include fever, night sweats, and weight loss. The fever pattern is a recurrent or relapsing type, with a body temperature of 39 to 40°C, mainly in the afternoon and evening (Pel-Ebstein fever). Significant weight loss is defined as more than 10 per cent reduction in body weight in the 6 months prior to diagnosis. Pruritus is seen in 10 to 15 per cent of adults and rarely in children.[255] The prognostic significance of this symptom has been questioned, and currently, pruritus is not considered to be a specific symptom of Hodgkin's disease. However, severe pruritus associated with multiple excoriations and resistant to antipruritics may be associated with a poor prognosis.[83, 96]

The Ann Arbor staging system[44] is used universally to describe the extent of disease involvement (Table 70–6). Each stage is subdivided into A or B, the former being asymptomatic and the latter associated with weight loss, fever, or night sweats. The majority of children present with early-stage disease: stage I, 27 per cent; stage II, 44 per cent; stage III, 21 per cent; and stage IV, 8 per cent.[188]

TABLE 70—6. Staging in Hodgkin's Disease (Ann Arbor)

Stage	Description
Stage I	Involvement of a single lymph node region
IE	Involvement of a single extralymphatic organ
Stage II	Involvement of two or more lymph node regions on the same side of the diaphragm
IIE	Localized involvement of extralymphatic organ or site and of one or more lymph node regions on the same side of the diaphragm
Stage III	Involvement of lymph node regions on both sides of the diaphragm
IIIE	Involvement of lymph node regions on both sides of diaphragm with localized involvement of extralymphatic organ or site
IIIS	As in III, with involvement of spleen
IIISE	As in III, with involvement of spleen and extralymphatic organ or site
Stage IV	Diffuse or disseminated involvement of one or more extralymphatic organs or tissues, with or without associated lymph node enlargement

Evaluation

Laboratory evaluation should include a complete blood count, erythrocyte sedimentation rate, liver chemistry, and serum copper level. There may be mild anemia and leukocytosis with eosinophilia and relative lymphopenia. The erythrocyte sedimentation rate and serum copper level[119] are elevated during active disease and are useful parameters for follow-up evaluation. The yield of bone marrow examination is low and is recommended for patients with systemic symptoms.[212] A skeletal survey and bone scan will detect bone involvement with Hodgkin's disease. Liver and spleen scan is not particularly helpful, and abdominal CT will provide information on the size of these organs as well as the remainder of the abdominal contents. Percutaneous liver biopsy is indicated if the liver function tests are abnormal or if the liver is enlarged.[10]

To evaluate lymph nodes in the abdomen, lymphangiography and CT have their advantages and disadvantages. The lymphangiogram does not delineate celiac, mesenteric, perisplenic, and perihepatic nodes; CT is helpful in such areas. On the other hand, lymphangiography is capable of demonstrating abnormality within the node before it is enlarged. Gallium scan is of limited value for abdominal disease.[45]

The role of staging laparotomy and splenectomy has to be carefully evaluated. The clinical staging may be altered in 20 to 30 per cent of children after the procedure.[29, 70] Fifty per cent of palpably enlarged spleens and 25 per cent of clinically normal spleens are infiltrated by Hodgkin's disease.[109, 213] The incidence of post-splenectomy sepsis in children with Hodgkin's disease is about 10 per cent with a 50 per cent mortality.[50] Partial splenectomy has been proposed, but splenic involve-ment may be limited to a few localized nodules without visible subcapsular lesions and could be missed by partial splenectomy.[64] Thus, staging laparotomy and splenectomy should be performed in those patients without definite clinical evidence of abdominal involvement, and the therapeutic approach will be influenced by the information derived from the procedure. Splenectomy is not indicated for patients under 5 years of age.

Treatment

The role of surgery in the treatment of Hodgkin's disease has changed. Although complete resection of stage I disease is possible, radical node dissection can be mutilating and is followed by a high local recurrence rate. The effective control of disease with radiation treatment has limited the initial surgical procedure to a diagnostic biopsy. The important role of surgery is to provide an accurate staging of the disease to help in treatment planning. In staging laparotomy, the abnormal lymph nodes identified by preoperative lymphangiogram must be biopsied. In addition, celiac, portal, para-aortic, iliac, and mesenteric lymph nodes are sampled. The spleen and splenic nodes are totally removed. A large wedge biopsy and two deep needle biopsies from the liver should be taken. Oophoropexy is performed if radiation treatment has to be delivered to the pelvic nodes. If liver involvement is strongly suspected from clinical evaluation, laparoscopy is a simpler procedure than laparotomy. It allows direct visualization of the surfaces of the liver and biopsy of any suspicious areas. Lymph nodes can be inspected and biopsies done, except those in the retroperitoneal area. The overall mortality rate for staging laparotomy is less than 1 per cent.[148]

Selected patients may not need staging laparotomy. Patients with high cervical nodes, lymphocyte-predominant, or nodular sclerosis histologic appearance and clinical stage IA may be treated with extended-field radiotherapy alone with excellent chance of cure.[92] On the other hand, patients with mixed cellularity or lymphocyte depletion histologic appearance, ''B'' symptoms, bulky mediastinal or abdominal disease, or clinical stage IV should be treated with combined radiotherapy and chemotherapy, and staging laparotomy is not necessary.

The use of laparotomy to document a complete remission after treatment has been proposed in order to identify persistent disease early or false positive clinical evaluation.[98, 245] In general, residual disease is rarely found in patients with normal clinical evaluation, and patients with abnormal clinical tests frequently have residual disease. Thus, the value of this procedure is questionable.

There is a clear dose-response relationship in radiotherapy for Hodgkin's disease.[131] When an adequate dose, such as 3500 to 4500 rad, is delivered, local recurrence is uncommon. Radiation treatment can be directed to the areas with known disease (involved field, IF) or can include additional sites adjacent to the involved area or the next lymph node groups (extended field, EF). For stage III disease, total nodal irradiation can be given. The overall survival for patients with stage

I and II disease is excellent with different modes of radiotherapy. Relapse of Hodgkin's disease can be effectively treated with chemotherapy. Thus, the goal of treatment is directed at maximizing relapse-free survival. The 10-year survival rate for stage IA and IIA patients treated with extended field radiotherapy is 95 per cent; the relapse-free survival rate is 80 per cent.[112] In one study, there was no difference in the survival or relapse-free survival between local and extended field radiotherapy.[105] However, in the Intergroup Hodgkin's Disease study, extended field was better than local radiotherapy in preventing recurrence.[244]

Most of the stage I and II patients have disease above the diaphragm. If the disease is limited to the mediastinum, the prognosis is good, with an 85 per cent relapse-free survival and a 100 per cent overall survival at 8 years.[167] However, if there is large mediastinal lymphadenopathy (mediastinum-thorax ratio greater than 1:3), recurrence within mediastinum or regional areas is common with radiotherapy alone.[105, 150, 166, 167, 215] The 5-year relapse-free survival is only about 60 per cent.

In general, treatment of stage III disease is total nodal irradiation. The 10-year survival rate is about 70 per cent, and the relapse-free survival rate is 40 to 57 per cent.[112, 117] Patients with upper abdominal involvement appear to have superior survival rates compared with patients with lower abdominal involvement.[239] Symptomatic patients also fare less well. Although the addition of chemotherapy to these patients did not change the overall survival rate, the relapse-free survival has been improved.[112, 117, 129, 239]

Chemotherapy for Hodgkin's disease was pioneered by De Vita and colleagues using a drug combination commonly known as MOPP (nitrogen mustard, vincristine, procarbazine, and prednisone) (Table 70–7). Long-term follow-up of advanced-stage patients treated with MOPP indicated that 55 per cent of all patients remained in their first remission for at least 5 years.[68] A high complete response rate to MOPP is also seen in patients who relapse from primary radiation treatment. Modification of MOPP by substitution, deletion, or addition of drugs has not been shown to be superior to MOPP itself.[43] A totally different drug combination (Table 70–7) commonly known as ABVD (Adriamycin, bleomycin, vinblastine, and DTIC) is as effective as MOPP in treating patients with advanced disease[27] as well as patients resistant to MOPP.[219] Because there is no cross resistance between MOPP and ABVD, treatment regimens with MOPP alternating with ABVD are currently being tested.

Late complications from intensive treatment of Hodgkin's disease include infertility, immunosuppression, psychosocial problems, and development of a second malignancy. Infertility is definitely a problem in young men who have received MOPP chemotherapy.[47, 54, 259] A

TABLE 70–7. Chemotherapy Regimens for Hodgkin's Disease

MOPP	ABVD
Nitrogen Mustard	Adriamycin
Oncovin	Bleomycin
Procarbazine	Vinblastine
Prednisone	DTIC

second malignancy is seen more frequently in patients treated with combined radiotherapy and chemotherapy than with either treatment modality alone. The most common type of second malignancy is acute nonlymphoblastic leukemia, with an incidence ranging from 0 to 4.65 per cent.[104] The Stanford experience indicates that the actuarial risk of leukemia at 5 and 7 years is 1.5 per cent and 2.0 per cent, respectively, for all patients, and 2.9 and 3.9 per cent for those treated with combined radiotherapy and chemotherapy.[54] The Copenhagen experience estimates a risk of about 4 per cent at 5 years and 10 per cent at 9 years.[194] Bonadonna and associates[27] found a 1.5 per cent incidence of leukemia in patients initially treated with radiotherapy and MOPP and a 6.1 per cent incidence in patients who had primary radiotherapy and subsequent salvage chemotherapy.[256] However, leukemia was not seen in any of the 84 patients treated with ABVD and radiotherapy.[256] It appears that leukemia is related to the use of an alkylating agent with or without radiotherapy.

With the long-term effects of treatment in mind, the goal of the current investigation is to maximize relapse-free survival and to minimize complications by combining chemotherapy with reduced radiotherapy as initial treatment of all stages of Hodgkin's disease. Radiation treatment can be IF, low-dose EF, or low-dose IF to areas of bulky disease only.[105, 126, 244, 272] Staging laparotomy and splenectomy may be omitted if chemotherapy is used.[126] The preliminary results are encouraging while awaiting long-term follow-up results.

Non-Hodgkin's Lymphoma

Non-Hodgkin's lymphoma in children differs from the disease in adults in that the nodular histologic pattern is rare in children. The majority of children with lymphoma have widespread disease at diagnosis, and bone marrow involvement is common. Histologically, cytologically, and immunologically, the tumor cells in lymphoma and acute lymphoblastic leukemia share common properties. It may be difficult to distinguish one disease from the other. Clinically, patients with leukemia may have massive enlargement of the lymph nodes; and patients with lymphoma may have bone marrow infiltration. Arbitrarily, if more than 25 per cent of the cells in the bone marrow are lymphoblasts, it is defined as leukemia. The term "leukemia-lymphoma" syndrome appears to be more appropriate for this type of clinical presentation.

In contrast to a peak incidence of acute lymphoblastic leukemia at 2 to 5 years of age, non-Hodgkin's lymphoma tends to occur in older children between 7 to 11 years. It is more common in boys, with a male-female ratio of 3:1.

For practical purposes a modified histologic classification of non-Hodgkin's lymphoma is used for childhood lymphomas because of the rarity of both nodular lymphomas and well-differentiated lymphomas in children.[41, 57, 139] Also uncommon in children are those tumors associated with a monoclonal gammopathy. Because of the frequency in children of conditions that cause follicular lymphoid hyperplasia, strict diagnostic criteria must be applied before a diagnosis of follicular lymphoma is made.[91] The nodular lymphomas in children, except for the rare instance when a Burkitt lymphoma may have a nodular pattern, appear to be distinguished by a better prognosis than that of their counterparts in adults or the more common childhood lymphomas.

A useful and practical classification of childhood lymphomas divides the most commonly encountered types into three histologic types: (1) malignant lymphoma, lymphoblastic type (30 to 35 per cent of cases); (2) malignant lymphoma, undifferentiated (Burkitt's lymphoma and non-Burkitt's lymphoma) (40 to 50 per cent of cases); and (3) large cell lymphomas (15 to 20 per cent of cases).

Although widespread dissemination of disease is common at diagnosis, there is some correlation of the histologic subtype with the anatomic sites of the tumor. Lymphoblastic lymphoma is common above the diaphragm, frequently associated with a mediastinal mass, but rarely involving Waldeyer's ring. Undifferentiated lymphomas, both Burkitt and non-Burkitt types, have a high predilection for the gastrointestinal tract, abdominal cavity, and Waldeyer's ring. Although the American Burkitt lymphoma is characteristically an abdominal tumor, it may occur in the head and neck area, as is so typical of the African variety. Extranodal primary tumors, such as those in bones, are histiocytic lymphomas.

Malignant lymphomas of the lymphoblastic type are similar morphologically to acute lymphoblastic leukemia. Although immunologically heterogeneous, a majority have T-cell markers, suggesting they are of thymic origin. Histologically, they are characterized by a diffuse uniform infiltrate of cells with scant cytoplasm and rounded or convoluted nuclei with a finely stippled chromatin pattern and rare nucleoli (Fig. 70–17). A starry sky pattern of reactive histiocytes may be present.

A paracortical pattern of infiltration of lymph nodes with sparing of non-neoplastic germinal centers may be seen. In imprints the cells resemble L-1 lymphoblasts of the FAB classification. Useful histochemical markers include glycogen and terminal deoxynucleotidyl transferase (TdT).

Malignant lymphoma, undifferentiated (small noncleaved cell type) includes both Burkitt lymphoma and in some classifications a subgroup, the non-Burkitt pleomorphic type. Burkitt lymphomas are characterized by monotonous proliferation of primitive cells 10 to 25 μm in diameter with round to oval nuclei and two to five nucleoli (Fig. 70–18). There is frequently a starry sky pattern of phagocytic histiocytes, and the tumor cell nuclei are approximately the same size as the histiocyte nuclei. There is a high mitotic index. Histochemically, the cells are characterized by cytoplasmic pyroninophilia and frequent cytoplasmic lipid vacuoles. There is no cytoplasmic glycogen. Monoclonal surface immunoglobins of the IgM class can usually be demonstrated, suggesting a B-cell origin. The non-Burkitt type is primarily characterized by greater nuclear pleomorphism and a wider age span, being much less common in children, and may be difficult to distinguish as a separate entity.

Malignant lymphomas of the diffuse large cell and immunoblastic types represent a heterogeneous group of tumors that traditionally were termed "histiocytic" lymphomas.[9] The majority of these tumors are lymphoid rather than true histiocytic. The classification of tumors in this category is similar for children and adults.

The staging system for Hodgkin's disease may be applied to non-Hodgkin's lymphoma (Table 70–6). However, non-Hodgkin's lymphoma usually progresses rapidly in children, and treatment should be started without too much delay in the staging procedure. It would suffice to classify patients into localized disease and nonlocalized disease for treatment purposes.[3] Localized disease is defined as a tumor limited anatomically either to a single extranodal site, with or without positive regional nodes, or to lymph nodes in one or two adjacent lymphatic regions. Grossly, a gastrointestinal tract tumor that can be completely excised is

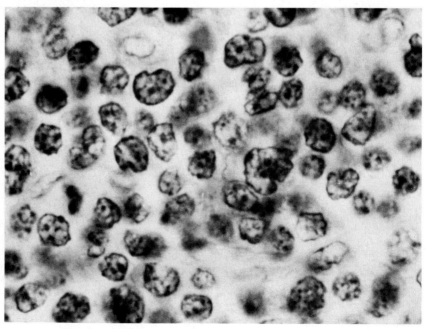

Figure 70–17. Lymphoblastic lymphoma. In this example the nuclei exhibit prominent nuclear convolutions and inconspicuous nucleoli. (× 2500)

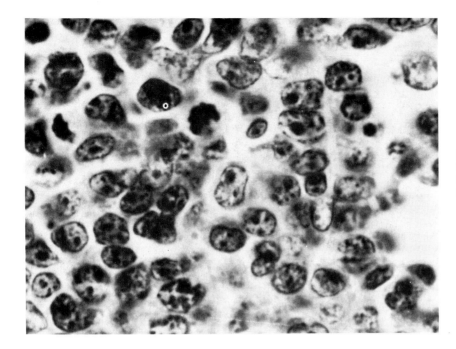

Figure 70–18. Burkitt's lymphoma. Nuclei are uniformly round to slightly oval and have multiple prominent nucleoli. (× 2500)

classified as localized disease. All other tumors, including any mediastinal mass, are considered to be nonlocalized.

About 15 per cent of non-Hodgkin's lymphomas arise in the head and neck area.[183] Besides the presence of tumor mass, symptoms related to pressure on vital structures by the tumor are common, such as tracheal compression or superior vena cava compression syndrome. Primary tumors arising from Waldeyer's ring may present with middle ear effusion or nasal obstruc-

tion. Burkitt lymphoma may present as large tumor in the jaw, thyroid gland, or parotid gland.

Hodgkin's and non-Hodgkin's lymphoma involving the head and neck cannot be differentiated from one another radiographically. In addition, there are no specific roentgen features that distinguish malignant lymphoma from other nasopharyngeal malignant processes (Fig. 70–19). Nevertheless, when the radiographic distribution of disease is coupled with the history, physical examination, and pertinent laboratory data, the correct

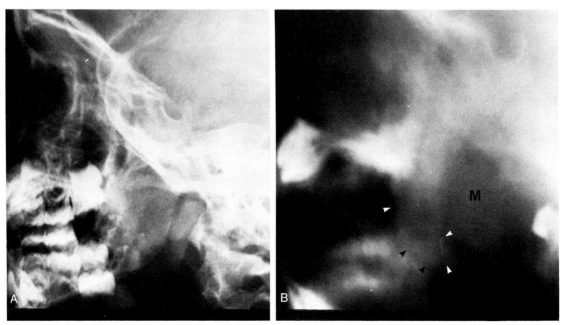

Figure 70–19. Four-year-old male with non-Hodgkin's lymphoma presenting with difficulty in breathing. Lateral view of nasopharynx (A) and midline laminagram (B) demonstrate a bulky, noncalcified mass (M) obstructing the nasopharynx and displacing the soft palate and uvula inferiorly (arrowheads).

diagnosis may be suspected. However, biopsy remains the ultimate diagnostic tool.

The radiographic appearance of malignant lymphoma depends upon the site of origin and the presence of distant metastases. In the head and neck, lymphoma may present as a discrete mass involving any portion of the upper airway, tonsils, base of tongue, lingual surface of epiglottis, paranasal sinuses, or nose. The nasopharynx is the most common site of origin, with tumor most frequently arising from the fossa of Rosenmüller or the lymphatic tissue about the torus tubarius. This results in a lateral nasopharyngeal mass. Tumor arising from the nasopharyngeal roof or superoposterior wall is also common. Rarely, tumor will be found on the nasopharyngeal surface of the soft palate, producing an anterior mass.

Diagnostic evaluation of nasopharyngeal disease has included radiographs in anteroposterior, lateral, and often submentovertex projections. Complex motion laminagraphy in two or more positions and nasopharyngography have been utilized in selected cases. However, with these modalities intracranial extension can only be inferred when skull base destruction is identified. Angiography was then performed to define the location and extent of intracranial disease. Computed tomography is now the single best imaging modality for examining the nasopharynx and has replaced laminagraphy and angiography in most instances. The CT scan better defines the anatomic location and extent of disease and aids in pre- and postoperative therapeutic planning. It can accurately image nasopharyngeal mucosal contour, the superficial and deep anatomic planes, and intracranial spread of tumor. Although CT findings are not pathognomonic, they can help differentiate benign from aggressive disease processes. In aggressive benign processes and malignancies, the pharyngobasilar fascia is penetrated, and deep structures are invaded. With normal variants, such as hypertrophied adenoids and benign processes, the nasopharynx remains supple, the superficial planes are maintained, and the paranasopharyngeal spaces are always visualized. In patients with nasopharyngeal lymphoma, CT most commonly demonstrates an isodense or slightly hyperdense, non-enhancing mass that grows in a bulky, circumferential manner (Fig. 70–20). Associated adenopathy, skull base destruction, or contiguous spread may be identified.

Diagnostic evaluation would be quite limited with rapidly progressive tumor. A careful physical examination, complete blood count, chest radiograph, bone marrow examination, and cerebrospinal fluid examination will assess the extent of disease involvement. Liver and spleen scans, gallium scan, sonography, and CT of abdomen are of limited value. Laparotomy is not necessary except for abdominal primary tumors. More important, evaluation of blood chemistry should include liver function, renal function, serum uric acid, calcium, and phosphorus because of the rapid cell turnover and the possibility of acute tumor lysis syndrome[53] when treatment is initiated.

Current research in cytogenetics has identified marker chromosomes in certain human cancers. The 14q+ marker chromosome is seen in Burkitt lymphoma and other forms of non-Hodgkin's lymphoma.[165, 179] Another important area of research is the characterization of immunologic markers of the tumor cells in order to understand the biology of cancer.[89, 210] It would be a significant contribution to cancer research if every effort is made to ensure that fresh biopsy materials are studied cytogenetically and immunologically.

Because of the general tendency for rapid dissemi-

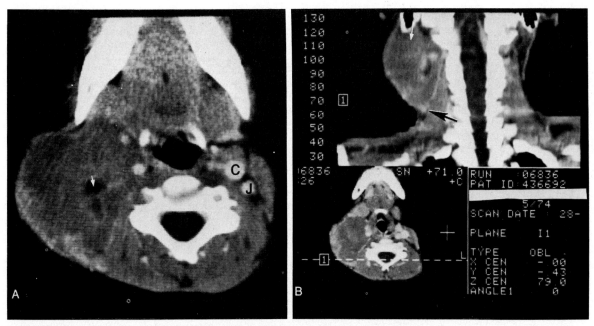

Figure 70–20. Nine-year-old male with non-Hodgkin's lymphoma presenting with enlarging neck mass and tonsil. (*A*) Contrast-enhanced CT scan shows a large hypodense, inhomogeneous enhancing mass with central necrosis (arrow) in the posterior cervical triangle. (*B*) Mass extends from mastoid tip (white arrow) to neck base (black arrow), anteriorly displaces the carotid artery, and involves the parotid gland. The right jugular vein is thrombosed. C is the opposite normal carotid artery, and J is the normal jugular vein.

nation of disease with non-Hodgkin's lymphoma, surgical resection is seldom performed except for gastrointestinal tumors, Burkitt lymphoma, or perhaps some instances of localized disease. The prognosis of Burkitt lymphoma is directly proportional to the volume of the tumor, and surgical reduction of tumor bulk should be considered.[163] Radiation treatment is indicated for immediate symptomatic relief of pressure symptoms such as tracheal compression or superior vena cava syndrome. A single dose of 500 to 600 rad will be sufficient. Radiation treatment is also indicated for gastrointestinal tumors after surgical resection. The role of radiotherapy to bulky disease areas in addition to chemotherapy remains to be determined.

In the past, most children with non-Hodgkin's lymphoma relapsed within a year despite treatment, and long-term survival was rare. Wollner and her colleagues treated 39 patients with a ten-drug program, LSA_2-L_2 (Table 70–8), using several combinations of drugs in cycles and radiation to areas with bulky disease.[264, 265] A long-term disease-free survival rate of 73 per cent was reported. The results of a randomized study by Children's Cancer Study Group indicated that the type of treatment program can be determined by the extent of disease at diagnosis and the histologic type.[3] A four-drug combination (COMP: cyclophosphamide, vincristine, methotrexate, and prednisone) was compared with a 10-drug combination (modified LSA_2-L_2). There was no difference in the treatment results with either treatment regimen for localized disease, with 84 per cent disease-free survival at 2 years (Fig. 70–21). Less treatment toxicity was observed with COMP than with LSA_2-L_2. No relapse was observed after the first year of treatment. With nonlocalized disease, LSA_2-L_2 produced superior treatment results in patients with a lymphoblastic histologic appearance, and COMP was more effective for patients with nonlymphoblastic histologic subtypes (Figs. 70–22 and 70–23). The 2-year relapse-free survival rate was 76 per cent for lymphoblastic lymphoma and 57 per cent for nonlymphoblastic lymphoma in this study.[3]

Systemic chemotherapy is the treatment of choice for Burkitt lymphoma. The initial chemotherapy should be adequate, for patients who fail to respond to initial treatment invariably die within several months. High doses of cyclophosphamide (1000 mg per m² or 40 mg per kg) or drug combinations such as COMP, including high doses of cyclophosphamide, are effective regimens.[38, 275, 276] Patients with bone marrow involvement, head and neck tumors, paraspinal tumors, or large,

TABLE 70–8. Chemotherapy Regimens for Non-Hodgkin's Lymphoma

COMP
Cyclophosphamide
Oncovin
Methotrexate
Prednisone

LSA₂—L₂	
Cyclophosphamide	Cytarabine
Vincristine	Thioguanine
Methotrexate	Asparaginase
Daunomycin	Carmustine
Prednisone	Hydroxyurea

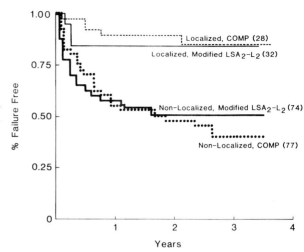

Figure 70–21. Survival data for non-Hodgkin's lymphoma: Localized and nonlocalized diseases treated with two different drug combinations. Figures in parentheses indicate numbers of patients. (Reproduced with permission from Anderson JR et al: N Engl J Med *308*:559, 1983.)

disseminated abdominal tumors are at high risk of tumor involvement of the central nervous system. The use of cranial irradiation, intrathecal chemotherapy, or infusion of high-dose methotrexate should be considered in these patients.

During treatment of lymphoma with radiotherapy or chemotherapy, it is important to monitor renal function and serum chemistry because of the high uric acid load on the kidneys. Allopurinol should be given to promote urinary excretion of uric acid. In addition, hydration with intravenous fluid and alkalinization of the urine are wise measures.

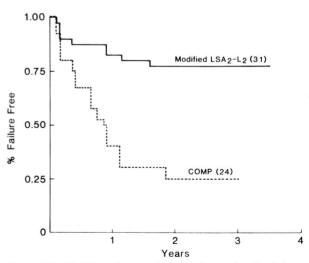

Figure 70–22. Failure-free survival data for nonlocalized, lymphoblastic lymphoma treated with COMP and LSA_2-L_2. Figures in parentheses indicate numbers of patients. (Reproduced with permission from Anderson JR et al: N Engl J Med *308*:559, 1983.)

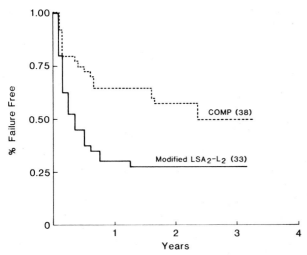

Figure 70–23. Failure-free survival data for nonlocalized, non-lymphoblastic lymphoma treated with COMP and LSA_2-L_2. Figures in parentheses indicate numbers of patients. (Reproduced with permission from Andersen JR et al: N Engl J Med *308*:559, 1983.)

Dialysis may be necessary in patients with renal failure secondary to uric acid nephropathy. Hyperkalemia, hyperphosphatemia, and hypocalcemia can occur as a result of tumor destruction.[53] Good supportive care is crucial in the initial phase of treatment of non-Hodgkin's lymphoma.

HISTIOCYTOSIS X

Histiocytosis X is a group of syndromes of unknown etiology characterized by a proliferation of histiocytes. The benign end of this disease spectrum is the solitary eosinophilic granuloma of bone. The most malignant course is represented by Letterer-Siwe disease in which multiple organ systems are involved, such as liver, spleen, lung, bone, lymph node, hematopoietic system, and skin. These patients quite often are seen by the otolaryngologist because of chronic otitis media and otorrhea. Hand-Schüller-Christian disease describes a triad of clinical findings: defects in membranous bones, exophthalmos, and diabetes insipidus.[108] This term is being used loosely to describe all the conditions with varying extent of bone or organ involvement other than eosinophilic granuloma and Letterer-Siwe disease. It seems appropriate for Lichtenstein to introduce the term histiocytosis X to integrate these disease entities because of the similar basic histologic features.[156]

Histiocytosis X is characterized histologically by the infiltration of Langerhans' histiocytes (Fig. 70–24).[81] The cells average 12 μm in diameter and have abundant finely granular eosinophilic cytoplasm and distinct cell margins. The nuclei have an open chromatin pattern and are often folded, lobulated, or bean-shaped. The cells are rarely phagocytic. Multinucleated giant cells are often seen, particularly in the solitary lesions. Although the Langerhans' histiocyte is the pathognomic cell, the variable presence of numerous eosinophils and

lymphocytes is also characteristic. Definitive identification of the Langherhans' cell is most easily made by ultrastructural examination for the presence of typical Langherhans' cell granules (Fig. 70–25).

The solitary eosinophilic granuloma and multifocal and systemic forms of the disease may exhibit varying histologic patterns. Bone lesions, whether solitary or multiple, generally have syncytial sheets of Langerhans' cells with indistinct cell membranes and frequently have eosinophils, giant cells, and necrosis. In the skin and visceral lesions the cells show little cohesion and necrosis, and giant cells are less common.

Newton and Hamoudi[186] have subclassified these lesions histologically into "benign" type II lesions, corresponding roughly to the solitary eosinophilic granuloma, and "malignant" type I lesions, which are characterized by less cohesiveness of the cells and infrequent giant cells, necrosis, and eosinophils. Although these histologic types do not clearly predict behavior, there is some correlation with clinical staging.

There are similarities between severe combined immunodeficiency and histiocytosis X.[46, 190] Osband and associates demonstrated a deficiency of suppressor T-lymphocytes, and they treated these patients with thymic extract.[192] However, a recent study by Children's Cancer Study Group failed to document a primary immunodeficiency disease in any of the patients with histiocytosis X.[146]

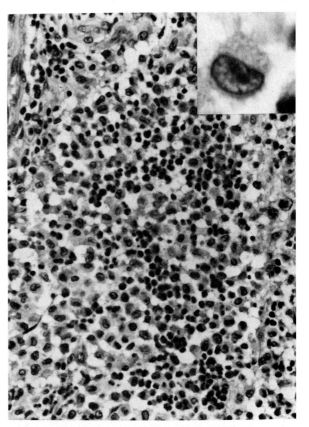

Figure 70–24. Histiocytosis X. There is a diffuse infiltration of Langerhans' histiocytes (inset, × 3000) and eosinophils in a skull lesion. Note the abundant cytoplasm resulting in the ameboid appearance of the cell, the bean-shaped nucleus, and the lack of phagocytosis. (× 5000)

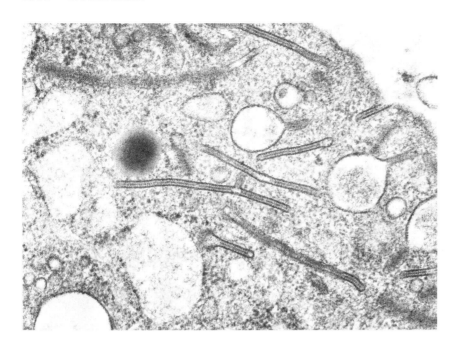

Figure 70–25. Langerhans' cell granules. The characteristic cells of histocytosis X contain "zipper"-shaped tubular inclusions that often end in a spherical cytoplasmic vesicle (× 64,000)

The clinical presentation is usually a soft-tissue mass with the typical well-circumscribed lytic lesion in the underlying bone. Skull bones are frequently involved. Other findings include seborrhea-like dermatitis, lymph node enlargement, ear discharge, mobile or "floating" teeth, hepatomegaly, anemia, diabetes insipidus, exophthalmos, and abnormal chest radiograph. Involvement of the head and neck area accounts for 15 per cent of all patients with histiocytosis X,[170] but the incidence can be as high as 80 per cent if the head and neck finding is associated with other presenting complaints.[220] Rarely, eosinophilic granuloma can present as solitary lymph node enlargement, and in such cases cervical lymph nodes are commonly involved.[182]

Eosinophilic granuloma is a benign process usually involving the skeleton with the skull, mandible, spine, ribs, and long bones most often affected. Although solitary bone lesions predominate, multiple bone lesions also occur.[74] In the skull, the destructive process originates within the diploic space and destroys both inner and outer tables. The outer table tends to be more severely affected and is responsible for the typical "beveled edge" appearance on skull radiographs (Fig. 70–26A).[74] The bone margins are usually sharp but not sclerotic, and a central "button sequestrum" may be noted.[180] The CT scan may be helpful in atypical or difficult cases and best demonstrates the adjacent enhancing soft-tissue mass and button sequestrum (Fig. 70–26B and C).[174, 180] The hard and soft tissues of the oral cavity may also be involved, with the mandible more frequently involved than the maxilla. The bone lesions tend to affect the alveolar bone and do not extend downward to the inferior border of the mandible. The lytic lesions tend to be periapical and undermine the tooth stability, creating the "floating teeth" sign radiographically.[236]

The mastoid and temporal bones are another frequent site of involvement. Otologic manifestations have been reported in 15 to 61 per cent of cases. Radiographically, lytic destruction with or without a soft-tissue mass may

be identified.[170] Computed tomography is probably the diagnostic method of choice at this time. Unusual sites of involvement such as the orbit,[12] sinuses, and nasal cavity[187] have been reported.

The roentgen characteristics of Hand-Schüller-Christian and Letterer-Siwe diseases are similar to eosinophilic granuloma in that skeletal lesions predominate. In Hand-Schüller-Christian disease the roentgen findings may be limited to the skeletal lesion. However, thickening of the pituitary stalk and destruction of the sella turcica may be present. Letterer-Siwe disease is characterized by systemic involvement; however, no distinct radiographic features are found.

The differential diagnosis of solitary or multiple lytic skull lesions would include osteomyelitis, localized fibrous dysplasia, epidermoid tumor, hemangioma, and intradiploic neural heterotopia. Osteomyelitis is the most difficult to differentiate from histiocytosis X because it also begins within the diploic space and can destroy both bony tables. However, it usually does not produce a beveled-edge lesion. Instead, it causes geographic destruction and frequently is adjacent to a paranasal sinus or is the result of a fracture or previous surgery. Localized fibrous dysplasia often has a lobulated margin and expands the outer bony table and may have a ground-glass appearance. Epidermoid tumors generally appear round and are surrounded by dense peripheral sclerosis. Calvarial hemangiomas are lucent lesions with sclerotic margins and dense internal trabeculation. Intradiploic neural heterotopia is a rare lesion, and it presents with a well-circumscribed margin with or without sclerosis.[136]

The treatment for a solitary lesion is curettage or low-dose radiotherapy. For multifocal disease, chemotherapy is indicated. The use of single drugs or combination of drugs yields about the same results.[145, 237, 238] The drugs that are commonly used include steroids, vinblastine, vincristine, cyclophosphamide, methotrexate, and chlorambucil. Local radiation to special sites, such as lesions in the spine, may be necessary in addition to

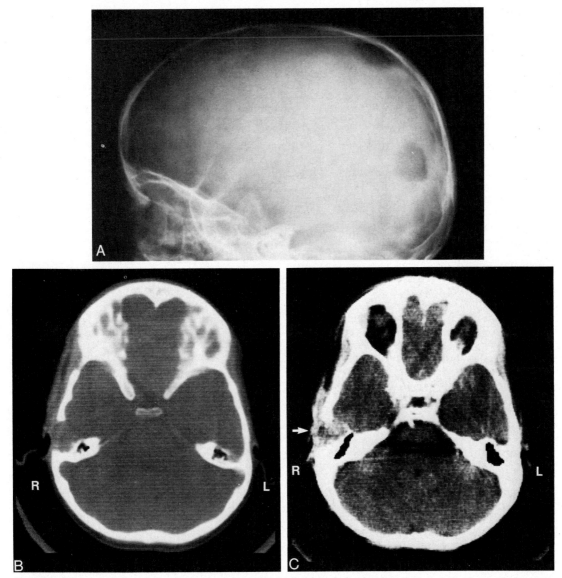

Figure 70–26. (*A*) Lateral skull radiograph demonstrates two typical beveled edge lytic lesions with sharp margins but without peripheral sclerosis. A CT scan in a different patient without contrast (*B*) and with contrast (*C*) material demonstrates an isodense, enhancing lytic lesion (arrow) of the right temporal bone with adjacent small soft-tissue mass.

chemotherapy.[61] Hormonal replacement is necessary if there is diabetes insipidus or growth failure.

The prognosis of histiocytosis X depends on the age of onset, the extent of disease, histologic features and presence or absence of dysfunction of certain organ systems.[141, 144, 146, 147] Patients under 2 or 3 years of age do not respond well to treatment, and in general, the younger the patient, the poorer the prognosis. They also tend to have more organ system involvement. Letterer-Siwe disease is common in infancy. A scoring system was devised on the basis of the number of organ systems involved clinically or radiographically.[147] The organ systems are skin, bone, liver, spleen, lung, pituitary gland, and the hematopoietic system. The prognosis is poor if there are more than two organ systems involved. However, this scoring system is not as valu-

able as the presence or absence of dysfunction of certain crucial organs such as liver, lung, and hematopoietic system.[144]

Lung dysfunction is considered if the patient experiences tachypnea, dyspnea, cyanosis, pneumothorax, or pleural effusion attributable to the disease rather than infection.[144]

Hematopoietic dysfunction is considered when there is anemia (less than 10 gm per ml hemoglobin), leukopenia (less than 4000 white blood cells per mm³), neutropenia (neutrophil count less than 1500 cells per mm³), or thrombocytopenia (less than 100,000 thrombocyctes per mm³). Excessive number of histiocytes in the bone marrow without cytopenia is not an evidence of dysfunction.[144]

Of 50 patients without organ dysfunction, 66 per cent

TABLE 70–9. Prognostic Groups in Histiocytosis X

Group	Organ Dysfunction	Age
Good risk	None	≥2
Intermediate risk	None	<2
Poor risk	Yes	All

Source: Adapted from Komp DM, Herson J, et al: A staging system for Histiocytosis X; A Southwest Oncology Group Study. Cancer 47:798, 1981.

responded to therapy with only a 4 per cent mortality rate. In contrast, only 33 per cent of patients with organ dysfunction responded to treatment, with a mortality rate of 66 per cent.[144]

With consideration of age and organ dysfunction, patients can be classified into three groups: those given a good prognosis are over 2 years of age, without organ dysfunction; those given an intermediate prognosis are under 2 years of age, with organ dysfunction; and those considered to have a poor prognosis may be any age, with organ dysfunction (Table 70–9).[141] The 5-year survival rates are about 90, 65, and 45 per cent, respectively, for these three groups (Fig. 70–27).

There are long-term sequelae of histiocytosis X besides the need for permanent hormonal replacement therapy. There may be cirrhosis of the liver or pulmonary fibrosis as a result of healing. Psychoneurologic complications such as delayed motor development, learning difficulties, ataxia, and behavioral changes may occur. The development of a second neoplasm has been reported.[140]

NEUROBLASTOMA

Neuroblastoma is a malignant tumor arising from the sympathetic nervous system. The most common site of primary tumor is the adrenal gland and retroperitoneal area (Fig. 70–28); however, primary cervical and skull

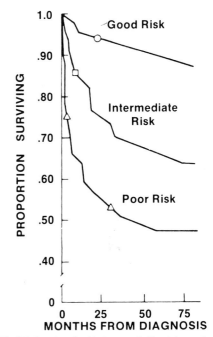

Figure 70–27. Staging for histiocytosis X—risk survival curves.

olfactory origin occurs in approximately 5 and 2 per cent of cases, respectively (Table 70–10).[34, 66, 101, 138, 249, 274] Primary cervical neuroblastoma tends to occur within the first 6 months of life.[58]

The pathologic classification of tumors of the sympathetic nervous system is based upon the degree of cellular differentiation within the tumor. Neuroblastomas are densely cellular neoplasms composed of lymphocyte-sized oval or fusiform cells with round or oval nuclei that resemble embryonic neuroblasts. The formation of pseudorosettes or a delicate neurofibrillary stroma is a variable but diagnostic feature. The presence

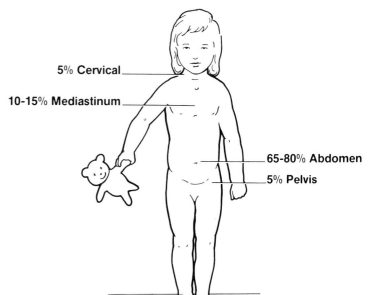

Figure 70–28. Incidence of primary sites for neuroblastoma.

TABLE 70–10. Cervical Neuroblastomas, Series Comparison

Series	Cervical/Total Neuroblastomas	Survival (%)
deLorimier[66]	5/512 (2.0)	2/5 (40)
Young[274]	3/35 (8.5)	2/3 (67)
Swank[249]	5/125 (4.0)	4/5 (80)
Brown[34]	4/105 (3.8)	0/4 (0)
Grosfeld[101]	3/160 (1.8)	3/3 (100)

TABLE 70–11. Staging System for Neuroblastoma

Stage	Description
Stage I	Tumors confined to the organ or structure of origin.
Stage II	Tumors extending in continuity beyond the organ or structure of origin but not crossing the midline. Regional lymph nodes on the homolateral side may be involved.
Stage III	Tumors extending in continuity beyond the midline. Regional lymph nodes bilaterally may be involved.
Stage IV	Remote disease involving skeleton, parenchymatous organs, soft tissues or distant lymph node groups (see IVS).
IVS	Patients who would otherwise be stage I or II, but who have remote disease confined to only one or more of the following sites: liver, skin, or bone marrow (without radiographic evidence of bone metastases on complete skeletal survey).

Source: Evans AE, et al: Cancer 27:374, 1971.

of prominent vascular connective tissue septa produces a trabecular architecture. A spectrum of maturational changes from the most immature neuroblastoma to benign ganglioneuroma is seen. In the latter, mature tumor ganglion cells and neural tissue compose the tumor. Partial differentiation may be seen in otherwise pure neuroblastomas, but this has little implication for prognosis. The only form that has a prognosis intermediate between neuroblastoma and ganglioneuroma is the composite ganglioneuroblastoma in which a mixture of neuroblastoma and mature ganglioneuroma is seen.[30] Electron microscopy is not usually essential for diagnosis but the identification of neurosecretory granules and microtubules in neuritic tumor cell processes may be helpful in differentiating undifferentiated neuroblastomas from other small cell sarcomas.[55, 209, 250]

Olfactory neuroblastomas (esthesioneuroblastoma) are similar microscopically and ultrastructurally to the neuroblastomas of the sympathetic system, and on the basis of biochemical and ultrastructural studies appear to be of neural crest origin, arising from neuroepithelial cells of the olfactory mucosa.[49] In contrast to other neuroblastomas, they occur at a later age and have a more insidious clinical course. Because of their rarity, differentiation from more common tumors in this area is a major problem.

The staging system by Evans and associates[78] is commonly used (Table 70–11). Cervical neuroblastoma is frequently localized, thus being stage I or stage II. When there is extension of the tumor through a spinal foramen to the extradural space, it is not considered as stage II, although literally it crosses the midline. The prognosis for this type of tumor is similar to that of stages I and II.

Primary cervical neuroblastoma presents with a painless mass, sometimes associated with Horner's syndrome and heterochromia of the iris. Pressure symptoms may include hoarseness of voice, stridor, dysphagia, and respiratory difficulty. Metastatic neuroblastoma may present with findings in the head and neck area, and careful examination will reveal the location of the primary tumor elsewhere. Proptosis with periorbital ecchymosis is a common sign of metastatic neuroblastoma. Bone metastases may manifest as masses over the skull and mandible. Subcutaneous metastatic nodules may be another manifestation, and they have a bluish color.

Diagnostic evaluation should include chest radiograph and ultrasound examination of the abdomen and pelvis for evidence of other tumor masses besides the cervical mass. Multiple primary tumors can occur with neuroblastoma, especially in young infants.[48, 149, 266] Radionuclide bone scan, liver scan, and bone marrow

examination are necessary, as the common sites of metastases are bone, bone marrow, and liver.

With osseous metastases, involvement of the calvarium, epidural space, orbit, ribs, and long bone are most common; however, any bone can be involved (Fig. 70–29). Neuroblastoma may originate within the cervical sympathetic ganglia and result in a variably sized prevertebral soft-tissue mass that displaces and distorts the adjacent laryngopharynx. Stippled or amorphous calcification may be present (Fig. 70–30).[274] Tumor can extend into the spinal extradural space via the neural foramina. Metastatic spread to the cervical lymph nodes or vertebrae can also occur and may result in a retropharyngeal mass. Occasionally, direct extension from a posterior mediastinal primary site can lead to a cervical mass.[6] Regardless of the etiology of neck involvement, this area is best evaluated using plain radiographs of the neck and chest followed by CT (Fig. 70–31). Currently, CT better demonstrates the extent of disease, the relationship between the tumor mass and adjacent structures, and the presence or absence of calcification or intracranial extension and is useful for therapeutic planning.[6, 138, 177]

Olfactory neuroblastoma is a rare, neurogenic tumor arising from the olfactory mucosa within the nasal cavity. It is most often recognized within the second to third decade of life. In the past, radiographic evaluation has included sinus series, examination of the nasopharynx with anteroposterior, lateral, and submental views; hypocycloidal laminagraphy; and occasionally angiography.[214] Today, after preliminary radiographs, CT is the imaging modality of choice and usually replaces all other forms of examination.[37, 214] The most common roentgen features include a noncalcified, unilateral mass involving the nasal cavity and ethmoid sinus and bone destruction involving the nasal septum, cribriform plate, lamina papyracea, and nasomaxillary wall. Orbital extension occurs in approximately 17 per cent, intracranial

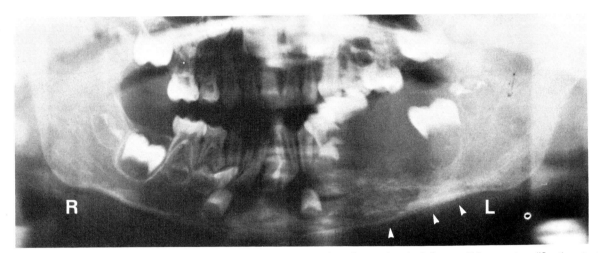

Figure 70–29. Neuroblastoma. Orthopantomogram shows permeative destruction in left mandible, causing "floating teeth" appearance. The upper cortex has been destroyed, and inferiorly, there is periosteal new bone formation (arrowheads).

spread in 15 per cent, and distant metastases in 20 per cent.[37]

The majority of patients with neuroblastoma excrete large quantities of catecholamines in the urine. This biochemical marker is useful in the follow-up evaluation, as the values will return to normal levels when the patients have a complete remission.

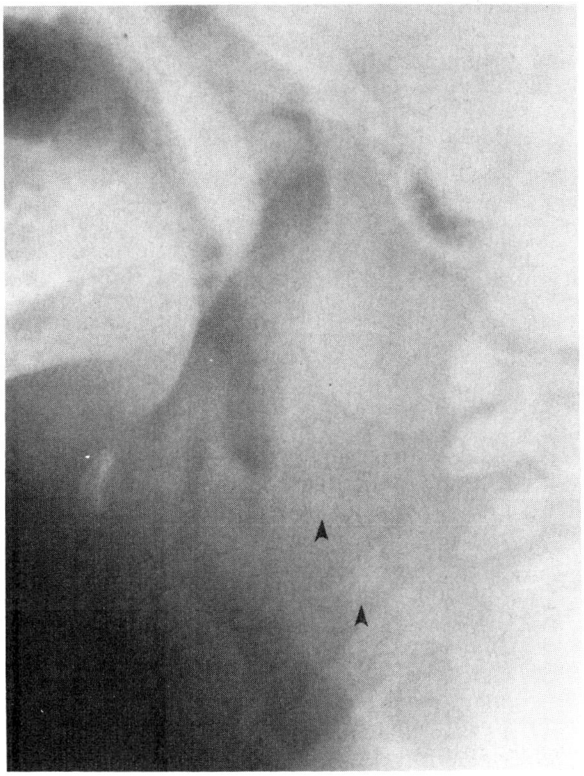

The prognosis of neuroblastoma is related to age at diagnosis and stage of the disease.[32] Children under 1 year of age have the best prognosis. Stages I, II, and IVS have favorable rates.

Total removal of localized tumors (stages I and II) offers the best chance of cure. For large tumors, a course of chemotherapy or radiotherapy may be able to reduce the bulk of the tumor, and resection becomes possible. Both treatment modalities can be used for residual tumor after incomplete resection. The commonly used therapeutic agents for neuroblastoma are vincristine and cyclophosphamide. Cervical neuroblastoma tends to have a favorable prognosis and usually occurs in young infants. It is preferred to omit radiation treatment in these patients to avoid growth retardation and late complications.[58]

Figure 70–30. Lateral neck radiograph in a 2-month-old with neuroblastoma. A retropharyngeal mass containing faintly seen amorphous calcification (arrows). The hypopharynx and proximal trachea are anteriorly displaced. There is no bone destruction.

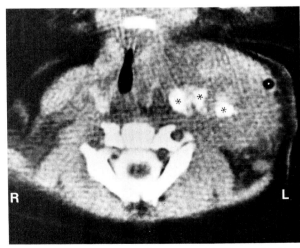

Figure 70–31. Cervical neuroblastoma, axial CT scan. Metrizamide opacifies subarachnoid space. No extradural mass is present. Amorphous calcifications (asterisks) are identifed in the left prevertebral tissue, causing mild compression and rightward displacement of the hypopharynx. Gas in soft tissue is from recent biopsy.

NASOPHARYNGEAL CARCINOMA

Nasopharyngeal carcinoma is rare in children, accounting for less than 1 per cent of all childhood malignancies.[273] However, there is an increase in incidence in blacks, especially among the teenage group.[11, 25, 67, 73, 86, 100, 125, 127, 158, 197, 231, 273]

The classification of nasopharyngeal carcinoma has not been uniform in the literature, and a variety of terms have been used synonymously, including transitional carcinoma, undifferentiated carcinoma, and lymphoepithelioma.[271] The latter designation refers to a subgroup of tumors composed of transitional or undifferentiated tumor cells in which there is a prominent lymphoid cell infiltrate and does not imply a lymphoid neoplasm. The term transitional cell carcinoma has been used by various authors to indicate tumors that arise from intermediate cells of squamous mucosa or tumors arising from nonkeratinizing mucous membranes such as bladder, trachea, nasal passages, and cervical canal. In the nasopharyngeal area these tumors are composed of small uniform undifferentiated cells that fail to show squamous characteristics. The transitional tumors differ from classically described lymphoepithelioma by the lack of lymphocytic infiltration but share the tendency to be radiosensitive. The majority of nasopharyngeal carcinomas are epidermoid tumors rather than adenocarcinoma or sarcoma. A variety of cell patterns may be seen in addition to typical squamous cell carcinoma, including transitional cell, spindle cell, clear cell, and polyhedral cell patterns. These patterns have formed the basis of various classifications, but by usual criteria, the majority of such tumors, regardless of subclassification, are undifferentiated. Therefore, a simplified approach to classification is that adopted by the United Nations World Health Organization (WHO)[226] in which three types are proposed: (1) keratinizing squamous cell carcinoma, (2) nonkeratinizing squamous cell carcinoma, and (3) undifferentiated carcinoma. The undifferentiated tumors may exhibit ultrastructural features of squamous cell differentiation such as desmosomes and tonofilaments.

The most common presenting sign is the presence of cervical adenopathy, which reflects regional lymph node involvement by the tumor. Quite often the node is tender and is treated for infection. There may be a history of nasal obstruction, epistaxis, or pain referred to the ear, neck, or throat. Erosion of the base of the skull and cranial nerve paresis occur with extensive tumors. Distant metastasis appears to be uncommon at diagnosis.

The extent of tumor involvement at diagnosis can be best described with the TNM system of The American Joint Committee for Cancer Staging and End-Results Reporting (Table 70–12).[2] The most common site of the primary tumor in the nasopharynx is the lateral wall, followed by the posterosuperior wall, posterior wall, and anterior wall.[22]

The radiologic evaluation of patients with nasopharyngeal carcinoma should include chest roentgenogram, skeletal survey, or bone scan as the most common sites of metastases are the bone and the lungs. Previously, the primary site and disease extent were examined by skull series, including submentovertex view, and conventional tomography. Angiography was occasionally performed, especially if juvenile angiofibroma was suspected, diagnostic difficulties were encountered, or the operating surgeon requested it. There are no pathognomonic radiographic features of nasopharyngeal carcinoma; however, the combination of a nasopharyngeal mass with destruction of the skull base raises this diagnostic possibility (Fig. 70–32). Currently, the diagnostic examination of choice is CT, for it better evaluates tumor location and extent.

The differential diagnosis to consider in a child with nasopharyngeal mass and skull base destruction centers around malignant and aggressive benign processes. The most common malignant tumors are lymphoma, rhabdomyosarcoma, neuroblastoma, and nasopharyngeal carcinoma.[121] Occasionally, juvenile angiofibroma and inflammatory processes destroy bone and only rarely will there be diagnostic confusion with these benign processes.

The association of Epstein-Barr virus (EBV) with nasopharyngeal carcinoma has been correlated with the histologic types. In the differentiated tumor, EBV-genome copies could be found in the cells, whereas the undifferentiated tumors tended to be EBV-DNA negative.[4] High titers of antibody against the viral capsid antigen and the diffuse (D) component of the early antigen complex have been demonstrated in patients with the undifferentiated nasopharyngeal carcinoma.[4, 22, 184] These titers decrease to undetectable levels within 12 to 30 months in patients who have responded to treatment; and a subsequent increase in the antibody titers may precede clinical recognition of recurrent tumors by 1 to 6 months.[184]

A high response rate can be achieved with radiation to the tumor area, with doses of 5000 to 6500 rad. Local recurrence may occur and can be further treated with radiotherapy.[125] The 5-year relapse-free survival rate varied from 19 to 60 per cent,[11, 25, 67, 86, 125, 127, 158, 197, 231] and patients with T1 and T2 tumors had a significantly better survival rate.[158] The extent of cervical node involvement did not seem to influence the final outcome.[158] Adjuvant chemotherapy with cyclophosphamide has been suggested[25, 67, 86, 127, 184, 197]; however, it did not reduce the incidence of relapse in another study.[158] Moreover, the majority of the patients who developed metastases died despite chemotherapy.

THYROID CARCINOMA

Thyroid carcinoma is relatively uncommon in childhood and occurs mainly in children 10 years of age or older.[107, 229] It is more common in females.[36]

There is a relationship between thyroid carcinoma and radiation therapy to the head and neck in infancy and childhood given for benign diseases such as thymic "enlargement," tonsillar and adenoidal hypertrophy, hemangiomas, and cystic hygroma. Popularity for radiation treatment to such benign conditions reached a peak in the 1940s. Winship and Rosvoll obtained a history of prior irradiation in 80 per cent of patients in whom an attempt was made to obtain this in a history.[261] The average dose was 512 rad, and the average interval from irradiation to diagnosis of thyroid carcinoma was 8.5 years.[262] Most of the reported carcinomas are differentiated papillary or follicular.[82] With the realization of

1796 · SPECIAL TOPICS

TABLE 70–12. TNM Classification for Nasopharyngeal Carcinoma

Stage	Description
Primary tumor (T)	
TX	Tumor that cannot be assessed by rules
T0	No evidence of primary tumor
Nasopharynx	
TIS	Carcinoma in situ
T1	Tumor confined to one site of nasopharynx or no tumor visible (positive biopsy only)
T2	Tumor involving two sites (both posterosuperior and lateral walls)
T3	Extension of tumor into nasal cavity or oropharynx
T4	Tumor invasion of skull or cranial nerve involvement, or both
Oropharynx	
TIS	Carcinoma in situ
T1	Tumor 2 cm or less in greatest diameter
T2	Tumor more than 2 cm but not more than 4 cm in greatest diameter
T3	Tumor more than 4 cm in greatest diameter
T4	Massive tumor more than 4 cm in diameter with invasion of bone, soft tissues of neck, or root (deep musculature) of tongue
Hypopharynx	
TIS	Carcinoma in situ
T1	Tumor confined to the site of origin
T2	Extension of tumor to adjacent region or site without fixation of hemilarynx
T3	Extension of tumor to adjacent region or site with fixation of hemilarynx
T4	Massive tumor invading bone or soft tissue of neck
Nodal involvement (N)	
NX	Nodes cannot be assessed
N0	No clinically positive node
N1	Single clinically positive homolateral node 3 cm or less in diameter
N2	Single clinically positive homolateral node more than 3 cm but not more than 6 cm in diameter or multiple clinically positive homolateral nodes none more than 6 cm in diameter
N2a	Single clinically positive homolateral node more than 3 cm but not more than 6 cm in diameter
N2b	Multiple clinically positive homolateral nodes none more than 6 cm in diameter
N3	Massive homolateral node(s), bilateral or contralateral node(s)
N3a	Clinically positive homolateral node(s), one more than 6 cm in diameter
N3b	Bilateral clinically positive nodes (in this situation, each side of the neck should be staged separately, that is, N3b: right, N2a: left, N1)
N3c	Contralateral clinically positive node(s) only
Distant metastasis (M)	
MX	Not assessed
M0	No (known) distant metastasis
M1	Distant metastasis present

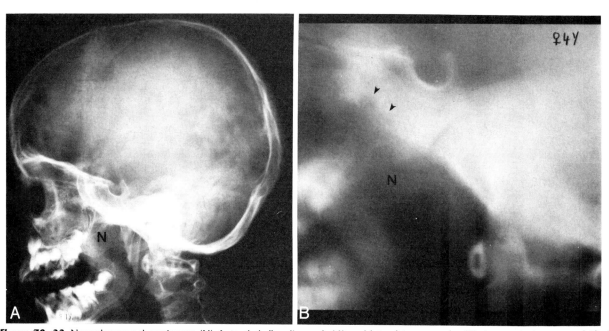

Figure 70–32. Nasopharyngeal carcinoma (N). Lateral skull radiograph (A) and lateral tomography (B) demonstrate a noncalcified nasopharyngeal mass that destroys the sphenoid bone anteriorly (arrowheads).

this association in the 1950s, use of radiation therapy for benign disease declined. The emphasis on increased incidence due to irradiation has shifted to the adult population.[204, 222] However thyroid carcinoma has been reported in three cases, 8, 10, and 12 years after mantle irradiation for Hodgkin's disease[173] so that in long-term survivors following combined therapy for head and neck malignancies thyroid carcinoma may become a problem.

Long-term TSH stimulation may produce hyperplasia or nodule formation with possible malignant changes that may be relevant in children with enzymatic defects in thyroxine synthesis.[1, 36]

Medullary carcinoma of the thyroid (MCT) can occur in a familial form in about 10 to 20 per cent of cases.[134] It is transmitted in an autosomal dominant form[1] and may occur in multiple endocrine neoplasia, type 2b (MEN2b) and MEN2a. It is worst in MEN2b.

Carcinoma of the thyroid is generally divided into four groups: papillary, follicular, medullary, and undifferentiated or anaplastic. Papillary adenocarcinoma is the most common type seen in children.[262] It is a well-differentiated tumor with epithelium, usually containing a single layer of cuboidal cells arranged on fibrovascular stalks that project into cystic spaces. Squamous metaplasia, psammoma bodies, oxyphilic change, and lymphatic invasion are frequent findings in these tumors.[175]

Follicular adenocarcinoma is the second most common type and constitutes about 18 per cent of thyroid carcinomas in children.[36, 262] Microscopically, these tumors exhibit a variable pattern of solid and follicular growth, some closely resembling normal thyroid. Malignancy is judged primarily by demonstration of invasiveness.[36] Psammoma bodies may be present but not as commonly as in papillary carcinoma. Blood vessel invasion, pulmonary metastases, and osseous metastases are more common than with papillary carcinoma.[1, 262] Many tumors have both papillary and follicular elements and are termed mixed papillary and follicular carcinoma. Meissner and Warren recommend that they be classified according to the predominant pattern.[175]

Medullary carcinoma accounts for between 5 and 10 per cent of all thyroid carcinomas.[175] These tumors originate from neural crest cells, which migrate to the thyroid during embryogenesis, the parafollicular or C cells. In general, medullary carcinoma is composed of clusters of round or polyhedral cells with granular eosinophilic cytoplasm and a dense, often amyloid-containing stroma, although considerable histologic variability is possible. Lymph node metastases occur early and are seen in about 50 per cent of patients.[134] Widespread metastases to other nodal groups, lung, liver, and bone may occur. In the familial forms of the disease a spectrum of C-cell hyperplasia or occult medullary carcinoma may be seen in patients whose only clinical finding is elevated calcitonin.[65]

Anaplastic or undifferentiated carcinoma occurs mainly in older age groups but constitutes approximately 9 per cent of thyroid carcinomas in children.[261] Histologically, there are two major subcategories—small cell carcinoma and giant cell carcinoma—or there may be a mixture of patterns.[175] These tumors are aggressive and are associated with widespread metastases.

There is no staging system in general use for thyroid carcinomas. The more differentiated carcinomas (papillary and follicular) most frequently present as cervical lymphadenopathy or a thyroid nodule.[79, 261] In Winship

and Rosvoll's series, 76 per cent had cervical nodules at presentation, as opposed to 23 per cent with thyroid nodules only.[261] One per cent presented with pulmonary metastases only. Other series have also reported a high incidence of cervical metastasis, ranging from 43 to 87 per cent.[79] Anaplastic carcinoma may present as a bulky, rapidly growing mass in the thyroid fixed to surrounding neck structures with symptoms of hoarseness, respiratory distress, and dysphagia.[36] With medullary carcinoma there may be stigmata associated with MEN-2 syndromes such as mucosal neuromas, marfanoid habitus, acromegalic facies, or hypertension. The patient may have a history of diarrhea. Exposure to ionizing radiation and goitrogens should be ascertained, as well as a family history of such tumors as pheochromocytoma.

Laboratory evaluations should include T_3, T_4, and TSH, although most patients with carcinoma are euthyroid.[120, 222] Plasma immunoreactive calcitonin (iCT), a humoral marker for MCT, should be measured if MCT is suspected from the history and physical examination. Examination of a case of MCT discovered with calcitonin (CT) assay in an 18-month-old infant whose mother had MCT has been described,[240] and periodic screening by calcitonin immunoassay after stimulation with calcium or pentagastrin is advised for those at risk, from an early age until age 30.[93, 222, 240] In a study of 123 patients by the Mayo Clinic, 29 had MEN2a.[217] A significant relationship was shown between the method of diagnosis of MCT and the pathologic stage of disease. Among the 29 patients with clinical disease, the tumor had metastasized to cervical lymph nodes in 12 (41 per cent); of 14 patients whose diagnosis was made solely on the basis of an elevated concentration of basal iCT, 12 (86 per cent) had tumor confined to the thyroid and only two (14 per cent) had nodal metastasis. All 14 (100 per cent) patients who had normal concentrations of basal iCT and who underwent operation because of elevated concentrations of iCT after stimulation had disease restricted to the thyroid, without incidence of nodal spread. These findings emphasize the advisability of screening members of MEN2 families, with the resultant finding of less advanced disease.

A soft-tissue x-ray of the neck may be useful, as the more differentiated tumors may contain calcifications. A chest x-ray should be obtained in view of the incidence of pulmonary metastasis. Thyroid scanning is important because malignancy is more likely with a "cold" nodule (Table 70–13). However, this does not always hold true, and malignancy has been reported in 14.3 per cent[120] to 40 per cent[137] of solitary nodules, not all of which were cold on scanning. Consideration should be given to excision of all solitary nodules in children.[120, 137] Scanning is also important to rule out congenital anomalies such as hemiagenesis or faulty thyroid anlage migration.[120, 222] The common radioisotopes used are ^{131}I and technetium pertechnetate. [131]I may be used but delivers more radiation to the gland. Ochi and associates have described scanning with thallium [Tl[201]] chloride, in which a delayed scan shows a malignant nodule to remain "hot" in 94.6 per cent of cases but shows no remaining activity with benign thyroid enlargement in 89.7 per cent of cases.[189]

Surgery is the mainstay of treatment for thyroid carcinomas. Current recommendations for papillary and follicular carcinoma range from lobectomy and isthmu-

TABLE 70–13. Solitary Thyroid Nodules in Children

Study	Malignant Nodules/ Total (%)	Histologic Type	Age Range (years)	Metastasis at Presentation Cervical	Lung
Kirkland[137]	12/30 (40%)	Papillary Follicular Mixed	2–15	8	1
Scott and Crawford[222]	6/36 (17%)	Papillary Follicular	6–19	6	1
Silverman[229]	5/14 (35%)	Papillary Mixed	7–18	3	
Hung[120]	5/35 (14.3%)	Papillary Mixed One undifferentiated	3–15	NA	0

sectomy only[263] for localized disease to subtotal or total thyroidectomy.[23, 107] There seems to be general agreement that with clinically involved nodes a modified radical neck dissection with preservation of the sternocleidomastoid muscle and spinal accessory nerve,[263] and in some instances the internal jugular vein,[222] be performed. Patients with pulmonary metastases who will receive radioactive iodine need a total thyroidectomy, which enhances the uptake of iodine by the metastases.[23, 107, 263]

Medullary carcinoma, especially the familial form, tends to be multicentric, and total thyroidectomy is indicated.[23, 217] In addition, central compartment (delphian, subisthmic, tracheoesophageal, and superior mediastinal nodes) nodal dissection bilaterally has been recommended, along with sampling of midjugular nodes. If positive, a modified neck dissection is recommended.[217] Radioactive iodine is not useful for metastases.

With anaplastic carcinoma total surgical removal should be attempted. External radiation as well as chemotherapy has been used, but the prognosis remains poor. Exogenous thyroid is recommended following surgery for thyroid carcinoma.[263]

The more differentiated thyroid carcinomas follow an indolent course, and 5- or even 10-year follow-up is not enough. In a series of 20 patients with papillary or follicular carcinoma there were two deaths from recurrence at 12- and 20-year follow-up.[263] In Winship and Rosvoll's 20-year study, there was an overall mortality rate of 17 per cent. The best survival was with papillary carcinoma (86.3 per cent), followed by follicular (85.3 per cent), medullary (44 per cent), and undifferentiated (19 per cent) types. In 75 per cent of patients the immediate cause of death was infection, obstruction, and asphyxia caused by tumor in the neck, mediastinum, or lungs.[262]

BENIGN NEOPLASMS

Almost all benign neoplasms of the head and neck region in adults may be found in the pediatric patient. A review of such entities is both impractical and unnecessary in a text of this nature. Rather, this section will focus selectively on a limited number of conditions that have their major impact on patients before adulthood.

Fibro-osseous Lesions

Fibro-osseous lesions are a heterogenous mixture of conditions that share similar histologic features as their common denominator (benign cellular fibrous tissue containing variable amounts of mineralized material) and are usually grouped with neoplasms of the head and neck.[14] In these lesions, the normal bony architecture is replaced by tissue composed of collagen, fibroblasts, and various amounts of osteoid and calcified tissue. Diagnosis is often impossible under the microscope alone and requires clinical and radiographic correlation. There are three general types, all differing in their treatment: (1) osseous dysplasia (cementoma), (2) fibrous dysplasia, and (3) ossifying fibroma (cementifying fibroma).

Bony dysplasias of the facial bones are separated into their different categories based upon their histopathologic features and clinical behavior. Microscopic features of the various lesions overlap, and certain aspects of the different lesions may even coexist in the same specimen. Because of this, it is the predominant pathologic process identified histologically in combination with the clinical presentation that determines the label placed on the disease entity.

A brief review of the normal ossification process of the maxilla is necessary before describing the various fibro-osseous lesions. In the development of the normal membranous bone of the maxilla, mesenchymal cells assume an orderly linear arrangement. The cells begin enzymatic function and are subsequently transformed into osteoblasts. Collagen fibrils are produced and are then laid into the matrix of mucopolysaccharides (osteoid). New osteoblasts are continually formed in a trabecular pattern. This constitutes formation of cancellous or spongy bone. Stress becomes a factor with aging, and the osteoblasts lay down rings of bone between the trabecula so that compact bone is formed.[208]

Osseous Dysplasia

Osseous dysplasia is a reactive lesion that occurs predominantly in black females over age 20 years. It most commonly occurs in the periapical alveolar bone of the anterior mandibular teeth. The patients are generally asymptomatic. The early lesions appear radiographically as either a periapical lucency or as multiple lucencies that resemble periapical granulomas or cysts but with the involved tooth always appearing vital. The late lesions exhibit calcification and become opaque with a thin lucent rim. The lesions themselves may be either multiple or single but always surround tooth roots unless the teeth have been extracted. One subtype of osseous dysplasia is florid osseous dysplasia. This is an extensive lesion, which is present in multiple quadrants of the mouth and is associated with expansion, dull pain, and traumatic bone cysts. Therapy required is simple excision.

Fibrous Dysplasia

Fibrous dysplasia is a developmental lesion that usually presents in the first or second decade of life. It generally presents as a diffuse, painless, bony swelling with subsequent facial deformity, especially when there is hemorrhage into an area of cystic degeneration. The intraoral mucosa and dentition appear normal. The lesions do not cross the midline, and their growth rate appears to decline as the patient reaches adulthood. Females are more commonly afflicted with fibrous dysplasia than are males, and there is thought to be a slightly higher incidence of the disease in blacks than in whites. In addition, the maxilla is more commonly affected than the mandible.[208]

Most investigators consider fibrous dysplasia to be a developmental lesion, although there is a school of thought that attributes it to a traumatic etiology. Regardless, the origin of fibrous dysplasia is based upon osseous metaplasia of medullary bone. Identification of oxytalan fiber when examined with the polarization microscope helps distinguish fibrous dysplasia from the other fibro-osseous lesions.[14] Grossly, the lesion has a variable consistency, depending on the amount of bone being present. When there is a large amount of bone present, the lesion has a gritty texture. Microscopically, one sees highly cellular fibrous tissue with strands of immature bone. There are no lamellae seen, nor are osteoblasts visualized.[208, 218] The connective tissue may appear active, quiescent, or inactive. Radiographs of facial bones that are involved with fibrous dysplasia often show a ground-glass appearance (Fig. 70–33). Of the facial bones, the maxilla is most frequently affected. There is often a fusiform narrowing of the maxillary sinus with indistinct margins. There can be involvement of the lamina dura and cortical bone as well. The x-ray appearance varies, depending on the degree of mineralization of the abnormal bone. Therefore, sclerotic, mixed, and lytic variants may be found. The sclerotic type predominates in the skull with involvement of the skull base and sphenoid wings most often found. When the lytic type predominates, there may be local or widespread expansion of the diploic space. In the skull this expansion occurs mainly at the expense of the outer table. In the monostotic form the skull is affected in 10 to 25 per cent of patients, and with the polyostotic variety the calvarium is involved in approximately 50 per cent.[69, 114, 185]

Plain radiographs are often sufficient to diagnose long bone involvement. Radionuclide bone scan is nonspecific. However, it can demonstrate the extent of disease.[114, 185] The CT scan appears to be the most useful modality in craniofacial disease because it (1) defines the magnitude of bone involvement, (2) demonstrates

the degree of proptosis, (3) detects orbital lesions and possible encroachment upon the optic canal, basal foramina, sinuses, and nasal cavity, (4) aids in surgical planning, (5) establishes diagnosis when plain films are equivocal, (6) helps evaluate patients with possible malignant degeneration, and (7) assists in the determination of the biopsy site.[59, 114, 171] Computed tomography can also establish the diagnosis of pseudotumoral fibrous dysplasia of the maxillary sinus. This is characterized by a rapid progression of clinical symptoms, raising the possibility of malignancy. Radiographically, there is opacification and poor definition of sinus walls. Histologically, there may be difficulty in establishing the diagnosis of fibrous dysplasia. The CT scan will demonstrate an intact and possibly thickened sinus wall, which suggests a benign process. Bone scanning may also be helpful.[257]

Several groupings of fibrous dysplasia have been identified, all of which have similar histologic features. In the monostotic variety, only one bone is affected. In the polyostotic variety, more than one bone is affected. The facial bones are usually spared in the polyostotic variety. The latter type may be associated with Albright's syndrome in which the patients present with precocious puberty and abnormal pigmentation, especially, café au lait spots.[85] A third type of fibrous dysplasia is the juvenile aggressive form, in which rapidly growing lesions cause marked deformity of the maxilla and destruction of tooth buds. It is generally refractory to treatment.[14]

Though fibrous dysplasia is usually associated with a good prognosis in the long term, its short-term course is marked by alternating periods of rapid and slow growth and multiple recurrences. Biopsy of the lesion may be necessary to differentiate it from malignant sarcomatous changes. Therapy should always be individualized. When symptoms are minimal, no therapy is necessary. Conservative surgical therapy is mandatory when the patient complains of cosmetic deformity, pain, or a functional abnormality. Surgical treatment generally involves the removal of excess tissue through either a Caldwell-Luc approach or a lateral rhinotomy. Radiation therapy should never be used in the treatment of fibrous dysplasia.[208]

Ossifying Fibroma

The ossifying fibroma is a benign neoplasm arising from periodontal fibrous connective tissue and is felt by some to be a variant of fibrous dysplasia.[14] Like fibrous dysplasia, the lesion may present as a small asymptomatic growth or as an extensive lesion with gross facial deformity. The mass generally presents, however, as a painless swelling in the cortex of bone with displacement of teeth. It may occur in any age group or location, but is most commonly seen in the mandible in female patients under the age of 20.[208]

The lesion is visualized as a well-demarcated lucency on x-ray with no, scant, or dense opacification, depending on the amount of maturation and mineralization present. Divergence of tooth roots is commonly seen. Although ossifying fibromas may be more locally aggressive than fibrous dysplasia, the tumor may often be removed much more easily. Microscopically, one sees a fibrous stroma with spicules of bone surrounded by osteoblasts and osteoclasts. A closely related entity is

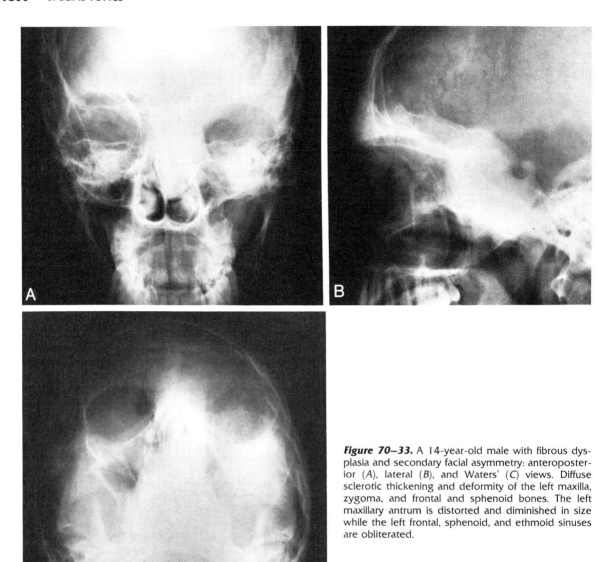

Figure 70–33. A 14-year-old male with fibrous dysplasia and secondary facial asymmetry: anteroposterior (A), lateral (B), and Waters' (C) views. Diffuse sclerotic thickening and deformity of the left maxilla, zygoma, and frontal and sphenoid bones. The left maxillary antrum is distorted and diminished in size while the left frontal, sphenoid, and ethmoid sinuses are obliterated.

the juvenile active ossifying fibroma. This neoplasm grows to enormous proportions and may cause death by encroachment of vital structures. It is found primarily in children and adolescents and appears as a large expansile lesion on x-ray.[14]

Giant Cell Lesions

Giant cell lesions in the head and neck most commonly involve the maxillary sinus. They generally present with signs and symptoms of an expanding mass with evidence of bone destruction.[208] One of the more common giant cell lesions is the *reparative granuloma*, a mass of proliferating fibroblastic granulation tissue. Its etiology is uncertain, although trauma appears to be the most likely explanation. It is often seen following tooth removal when there is injury to the periodontal membrane or odontogenic mesenchyme. Two basic types of reparative granulomas are found: the more common peripheral type and a less commonly occurring central type. The peripheral type presents as a sessile or pedunculated mucosa-covered mass that is reddish or blue in color. It arises from the gingiva or alveolar mucosa and is found most commonly in the anterior mandible. The central type, on the other hand, is an endosteal lesion, and is usually found in the mandible anterior to the first molar. Although peripheral lesions are found more commonly in female patients over the age of 20 years, central lesions are usually seen in male patients during the second decade of life. Radiographically, the lesion appears as a lytic, expansile, unilocular cavity with well-demarcated, nonsclerotic margins, which may cross the midline (Fig. 70–34). However, multiple lytic foci with ill-defined margins can also occur. The bony cortex is usually thinned but intact. Both displacement of teeth and root resorption are often noted.[161, 206, 268] If the lesion is circumscribed, simple excision is the only therapy necessary.[14] When the lesion is more diffuse, thorough curettage may be necessary.[208]

Reparative granuloma should be distinguished from the true giant cell tumor, which is a lesion usually seen in an older age group and is rarely found in the head and neck. Two other lesions that must be considered in the differential diagnosis of reparative granuloma are the brown tumor of hyperparathyroidism and Paget's disease. The former lesion is associated with serum chemical abnormalities, including calcium, phosphorus, alkaline phosphatase, and parathormone. Once the primary disease process of hyperparathyroidism is brought under control, the bone lesions usually regress.[208]

Cherubism

Cherubism is a familial condition in which there is proliferation of fibrous tissue and giant cells in the jaws. Although the true etiology is unknown, it does appear to be a developmental disturbance of the "bone-forming" mesenchyme. Its inheritance is autosomal dominant, with 100 per cent penetrance in males and 50 to 70 per cent penetrance in females. Not all patients appear the same, however, as there is variable expressivity. Although uncommon, there have been some spontaneous mutations reported. Several investigators

have questioned whether the condition is actually a form of hereditary fibrous dysplasia. Although up to 33 per cent of the patients may have some sort of pigmentation abnormalities, the bony components found in fibrous dysplasia are generally lacking. Its histologic appearance is, in fact, essentially the same as that seen in the giant cell reparative granuloma.

Although the patients appear normal at birth, they begin to manifest symmetric fullness of the cheeks, especially at the angle of the mandible, by age 3 years. The angle of the mandible is the most common location of the tumor, but the maxilla may be involved in up to 67 per cent of the cases. Extensive involvement of this structure can produce a narrow V-shaped palatal vault. The patients commonly lose their deciduous teeth at an early age and have delayed eruption of their permanent teeth. The lesions exhibit rapid growth for the first several years after their discovery before entering a slow growth phase for the next 5 years. Involution of the lesion usually begins by age 10 and is most often complete by puberty. The patients generally function normally, and the lesions are usually associated with minimal or no pain. Cervical adenopathy is frequently associated with cherubism and usually regresses at the same time as the jaw lesions.

Radiographic features associated with this condition include multilocular lucencies with sharply defined margins and thinning of the overlying cortex. If longstanding, the affected facial bones may be deformed with radiographic evidence of sclerosis or a diffuse ground-glass appearance. Capillary hemorrhage often occurs in this condition with the production of new tissue and jaw growth. Giant cells are characteristically absent. Bone formation can occur, most often in response to inflammation. When regression is not complete, curettage may be necessary in order to obtain ideal cosmetic results. Radiotherapy should never be used in the treatment of cherubism.[14]

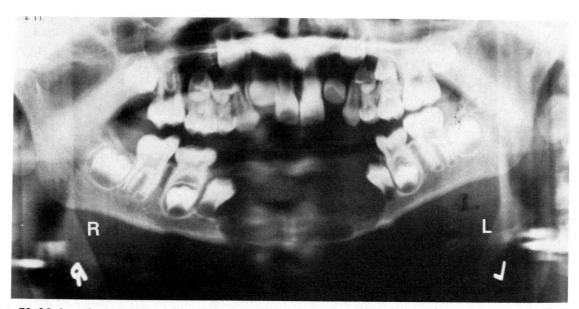

Figure 70–34. An orthopantomogram of a 9-year-old girl with a large reparative granuloma occupying the mid-mandible. No internal architecture is apparent; however, the cortical thinning and endosteal scalloping of the lower mandibular margin and absent teeth are noted.

Myxoma

Another type of benign tumor commonly seen in young patients is the myxoma. It is a lesion limited almost exclusively to the mandible and maxilla and whose origin is postulated to be either odontogenic, osteogenic, or some combination of the two. Some investigators argue that the tumor arises from nonodontogenic mesenchyme. It is seen most commonly in young patients, with 67 per cent of the patients being between ages 10 and 29 years. Males and females have a similar incidence. The mandible is more commonly involved than the maxilla, although the symphysis is not usually affected. Bilateral mandibular involvement is also quite rare. In the maxilla, involvement of the zygomatic process with invasion of the maxillary sinus is commonly seen.

Myxomas of the jaws are slowly progressive and commonly present with swelling of the facial features. The teeth are often loosened and pushed aside. The mucosa is bulging but intact. If left untreated, the lesions will eventually erode bone and grow into the overlying soft tissue. Pain may or may not be present with these lesions. They appear radiographically as multilocular cysts surrounded by a dense margin. Although the growths appear grossly encapsulated, this is in fact a pseudocapsule, thus explaining the high incidence of recurrence after excision. Therapy generally consists of either curettage or wide local excision with or without chemical or electrical cautery. For larger lesions, mandibular resection or partial maxillectomy may be necessary. Again, radiotherapy is not employed for the treatment of this type of fibro-osseous lesion.[14]

TUMORS OF THE PERIPHERAL NERVOUS SYSTEM

Neurogenic tumors of the head and neck in children are uncommon. The specific tumors encountered in the pediatric population are not unique to this age group, and they present similar problems in terms of diagnosis and management to those found in the adult population. One difference between the age groups, however, appears to be the propensity of the pediatric patients with neurogenic tumors to develop systemic disease, compared with adult patients, who more commonly develop isolated neural sheath tumors. The tumors may be either superficial or deep-seated, the latter more often being associated with a delay in recognition and subsequent management. Neurogenic tumors may be solitary or may be part of the clinical presentation of von Recklinghausen's disease. When solitary, about 25 per cent of the tumors arise along the course of a cervical or cranial nerve. Several basic types of benign neurogenic tumors in the head and neck have been identified, including neurofibromas and solitary schwannomas.[206]

It is generally agreed that neurogenic tumors arise from the neural sheath cells and not from the nerve cells themselves. A nerve is normally surrounded by both Schwann cells and endoneurial fibroblasts. A thin connective tissue sheet, the neurilemma, surrounds both of these cells. Controversy exists as to whether the Schwann cell or the endoneurial fibroblast is the parent cell of the nerve sheath tumors. In spite of questions concerning their cell of origin, schwannomas and neurofibromas, the most common tumors of the peripheral nerves, are distinct entities whose clinical differences demand separate categorization.[19]

The tumors arise from multiple sites within the head and neck. A progressive peripheral facial palsy is the usual presenting complaint when a tumor arises from the seventh cranial nerve. Any portion of the seventh cranial nerve may be involved—intracranial, intratemporal, or extratemporal. A tumor presenting in the neck may arise from any of the multiple motor or sensory cervical nerves or from the brachial plexus itself. Within the oral cavity, the tongue is the site most commonly involved, but the gingiva, buccal mucosa, and floor of mouth may also be involved. Surgical removal of these tumors is necessary to prevent chronic oral irritation and harmful effects on dentition. Neurogenic tumors in the nasal cavity or paranasal sinus region are distinctly unusual in children. Although the exact site of origin may not be known, it is certain that the tumors do not arise from the olfactory nerve because this structure does not have Schwann cells. Intraosseous tumors have been reported, with schwannomas being the most frequently occurring. These generally involve the mandible, especially the body and ascending ramus. Other possible sites of neurogenic tumors include the parapharyngeal space (vagus nerve and cervical sympathetic chain), larynx, and salivary gland.[19]

Schwannomas are solitary encapsulated lesions that arise from peripheral nerve sheaths. If the nerve of origin can be identified, nerve fibers are seen to be attached to and compressed by the tumor. Microscopically, solitary schwannomas are composed of two types of tissue: cellular Antoni type A and less cellular Antoni type B tissue. In the cellular areas the tumor is composed of compact spindle cells in parallel orientation. Often, nuclei are oriented in rows, resulting in a palisading pattern. When these palisading areas are oriented around parallel bundles of fibers, Verocay bodies are formed. The Antoni type B tissue is characterized by abundant acellular matrix containing collagen and a more random orientation of nerve fibers. These tumors rarely undergo malignant transformation and are not associated with *von Recklinghausen's neurofibromatosis.*

Neurofibromas may occur sporadically as solitary lesions or in association with von Recklinghausen's neurofibromatosis, in which case they are usually multiple and have a plexiform configuration. The solitary lesions are well circumscribed. The plexiform lesions occur as poorly defined or multinodular masses. Microscopically, neurofibromas are composed of bundles of Schwann cells and collagen in a mucinous matrix. Some plexiform neurofibromas diffusely invade the nerve of origin. This is in contrast to solitary schwannomas. Normal nerve elements are often found within the neurofibroma in a distorted, sometimes proliferating, fashion. Mast cells are not infrequently found in these lesions. Nuclear atypia may be quite prominent but are less reliable criteria of aggressive behavior than are mitotic rate, overall cellularity and loss of the nerve fiber pattern.

Neurofibromas may be either multiple or solitary. Several types of solitary neurofibromas are found in children, including cutaneous and subcutaneous, plexiform, elephantiasis neuromatosa, and molluscum fibrosum.[269] The cutaneous and subcutaneous lesions arise in the vicinity of the termination of small cutaneous nerves. The lesions present as soft, elevated, nodular, pedunculated masses with the overlying skin exhibiting increased melanin production. Plexiform neurofibromas, on the other hand, are more deeply seated and arise from major nerve trunks. It is thought by some to be seen only in von Recklinghausen's disease.[19]

Multiple neurofibromatosis is a syndrome marked by multiple neurofibromas, abnormal skin pigmentation, and certain bony abnormalities.[269] Von Recklinghausen's disease is the most common type of multiple neurofibromatosis and is inherited in an autosomal dominant pattern with variable penetrance. There is a high mutation rate, and only 50 per cent of cases have a positive family history. It occurs in approximately one out of 3000 live births. The signs and symptoms of the disease manifest themselves at an early age and include the appearance of café au lait spots as well as the tumors themselves. Half of the patients with von Recklinghausen's disease are identified at birth, and 67 per cent may be identified as a result of their distinctive features by the age of 1 year. Café au lait spots do not have to be present for the diagnosis to be made; 25 to 90 per cent of patients with von Recklinghausen's disease will have café au lait spots.[19] The café au lait spots seen in von Recklinghausen's disease have a smoother border than those found in the McCune-Albright syndrome. If patients do have more than six spots of at least 1.5 cm diameter, then von Recklinghausen's disease can be diagnosed. There is usually a truncal distribution of these pigmentary abnormalities, with pigment ranging from light brown to dark brown. One may see areas of vitiligo as well. Up to 30 per cent of patients have axillary freckling.[269] Multiple congenital anomalies may be seen in patients with von Recklinghausen's disease. These patients often have associated gliomas, meningiomas, acoustic neuromas, spina bifida, syndactyly, hemangiomas, retinal abnormalities, visceral abnormalities, pheochromocytoma, and medullary thyroid carcinoma.[19] Many bony abnormalities have been identified in patients with von Recklinghausen's disease. These include macroencephaly, macrocranium, cervical kyphosis,[269] bowing of the lower limbs, pressure erosion, and bone growth disorders. Osseous disturbance results from mesodermal dysplasia usually in the absence of adjacent neurofibromatous tissue. These dysplastic bony changes can affect any portion of the skeleton, but alteration of the facial bones, dental structures, and distortion of the sphenoid and petrous bones are well known.[116] The syndrome itself is marked by a persistent, slow increase in both the size and number of the neurofibromas. The condition has an associated mortality secondary to the multiple anomalies found in a large number of patients with von Recklinghausen's disease and the possibility of malignant degeneration of tumors in up to 16 per cent of patients.[19]

Orbitofacial disfigurement and proptosis may result from one or more processes: plexiform neurofibroma, orbital osseous dysplasia, orbital neoplasia, and congenital glaucoma. Plexiform neurofibromas may occur in any motor or sensory nerve within the head and neck (Fig. 70–35) and can remain local or become extensive in distribution. Plain radiographs of affected areas are often adequate to suggest the diagnosis (Fig. 70–36). However, CT is the imaging technique of choice, for it better demonstrates the location and extent of the lesion(s). Plexiform neurofibromas generally are irregular,

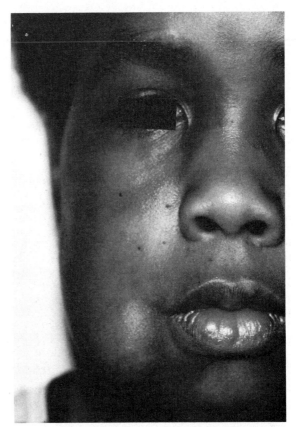

Figure 70–35. Adolescent male with large facial plexiform neurofibroma causing obvious cosmetic distortion.

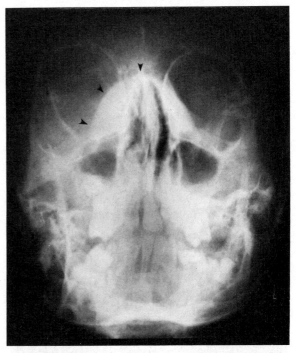

Figure 70–36. Eleven-year-old girl with perinasal soft-tissue thickening (arrowheads) but no osseous change owing to plexiform neurofibroma. A CT scan (not shown) confirmed the radiographic findings.

contrast-enhancing masses that enlarge and distort both superficial and deep anatomic planes (Fig. 70–37).[278] However, a plexiform neurofibroma may be inhomogeneous and may contain nonenhancing components (Fig. 70–38). Bony dysplasia involving the facial and orbital structures is also easily examined.

In children with neurofibromatosis, 75 per cent of optic gliomas develop before age 12. Holt[116] and others[62] believe that either unilateral or bilateral disease is indicative of neurofibromatosis. The CT scan best demonstrates the optic nerve enlargement and potential intracranial extent.

Otologic involvement is manifested by widening of the external auditory canal or internal auditory canal, which can be the result of dysplastic osseous change or the development of acoustic neuromas, respectively. Acoustic neuromas have a well-recognized association with neurofibromatosis, and when they are bilateral, the diagnosis of neurofibromatosis is suggested. However, acoustic neuromas are rare in childhood. Large acoustic neuromas are easily recognized by petrous CT, which demonstrates a rounded, isodense enhancing mass in the cerebellopontine angle with associated widening and foreshortening of the internal auditory canal (Fig. 70–39). Small lesions within the cerebellopontine angle or intracanalicular lesions can be difficult to diagnose, and air-CT cisternography may be necessary.[143]

The treatment for schwannomas as well as for neurofibromas is surgical excision. Depending on the size of the lesion, staged excision may be necessary for diagnosis.[143] The prognosis is excellent for solitary neurofibromas or for schwannomas that are completely excised. Although incomplete excision of these masses may result in tumor recurrence, the overall prognosis is still good. When dealing with schwannomas, one should always attempt enucleation with preservation of the nerve of origin. When dealing with neurofibromas, the nerve of origin must generally be sacrificed. In those situations, primary grafting is recommended. In von Recklinghausen's disease, surgical removal of all tumors may be impractical. When the mass causes a significant cosmetic or functional impairment, excision is required.[19]

LYMPHANGIOMA

Lymphangiomas (cystic hygromas) are soft, painless, compressible masses that represent areas of regional lymphatic dilatation. The majority of cervical tumors are thought to arise from sequestration of tissue adjacent to the primative jugular lymphatic sac. Lymphangiomas have been divided arbitrarily into three histologic groupings, depending on the size of the lymph channels present. These histologic patterns—simple (capillary), cavernous, and cystic—may coexist in the same lesion.[133] Little clinical significance can be attached to such a histologic classification. Hemorrhage into a lesion may result in the appearance of a hemangioma or may cause difficulty in distinguishing between the two.

The rarity of lymphangiomas is well documented. The tumors are most commonly seen shortly after birth. Approximately 50 to 60 per cent of the tumors present before the age of 1 year, and about 90 per cent of the lesions occur prior to the end of the second year of life. They may be seen, however, as late as the fourth or fifth decade.[203] The reason these lesions remain dormant for such a lengthy period of time is unknown, but it is speculated that local infection may precipitate the rapid growth of a previously unrecognized lesion.[151]

The clinical presentation of cystic hygromas is referable to their site of origin. The diagnosis of cystic hygroma can be made in utero, when a sonogram shows thin-walled, multiseptated, fluid-filled cysts. When this finding is associated with tubular serpiginous or multiloculate intradermal fluid collections within the subcu-

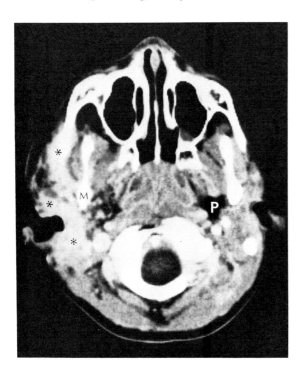

Figure 70–37. Eleven-year-old male with a predominantly superficial, homogeneously enhancing lesion that infiltrates and deforms the right cheek and periauricular tissue (*). There is posteromedial displacement of the jugular vein and infiltration of the infratemporal fat. The mandible (M) is dysplastic. Parapharyngeal space fat (P) is seen on the uninvolved side. Notice the distortion of the tumor side.

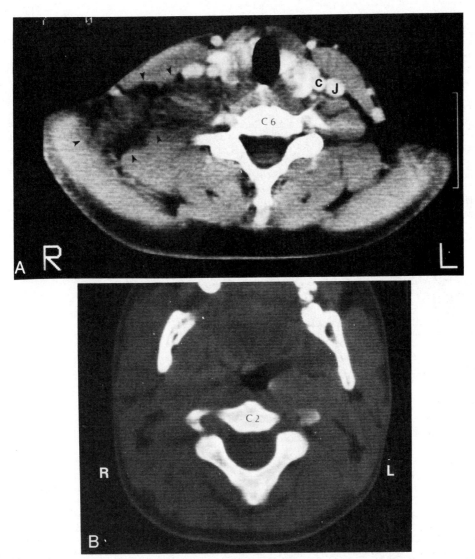

Figure 70–38. Fourteen-year-old male with a hypodense, minimally enhancing plexiform neurofibroma (*A*). The superficial and deep structures of the right cervicothoracic region (arrows) are involved. At C6, muscular and fascial planes are infiltrated and distorted while the jugular vein and carotid artery are anteriorly displaced. C indicates the normal carotid artery; J shows the normal jugular vein. (*B*) The right C2 neural foramen is widened by neurofibromatous tissue.

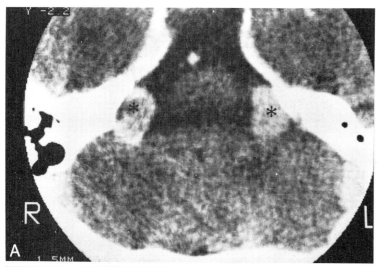

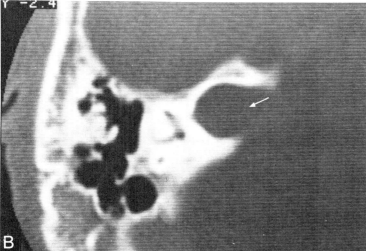

Figure 70–39. Fifteen-year-old female with neurofibromatosis. (*A*) Petrous CT scan demonstrates bilateral enhancing masses (*) occupying the internal auditory canals and cerebellopontine angles. (*B*) Bone window shows a dysplastic, widened, and foreshortened internal auditory canal (arrow).

taneous tissue of the thorax or abdomen, Phillips and associates[196] believe it is pathognomonic of cystic hygroma.

Except for the obvious cosmetic deformity (Fig. 70–40), most cervical lymphangiomas do not cause symptoms. They must be differentiated from branchial cleft cysts, thyroglossal duct cysts, lymphomas, and true neoplasms. The most common location is the posterior triangle of the neck. When the anterior triangle of the neck is involved, intraoral extension with pharyngeal compression and airway compromise may result. Children with head and neck involvement are best evaluated by anteroposterior and lateral neck radiographs, chest radiograph, and neck ultrasound (Fig. 70–41). CT can occasionally be helpful, especially if there is extensive mediastinal or bony involvement.[178, 198, 228] Lymphangiography is rarely performed. The most common radiographic finding is a noncalcified neck mass of variable size, which may extend into the mediastinum in approximately 5 per cent of patients. If large, the mass can displace and compress adjacent structures.[153, 198] Neck sonography is helpful in the evaluation of childhood neck masses, for it aids in determining the character and extent of the mass and its relationship to

surrounding structures. The most common sonographic finding in a patient with a cervical cystic hygroma is a thin-walled, multiseptated cyst. However, solid or mixed echogenicity patterns can also occur, adding difficulty to differential diagnosis.[153, 196, 198] Cystic hygroma may also involve other areas including the epiglottis (Fig. 70–42*A*), trachea (Fig. 70–42*B*), orbit, and face. The laryngeal involvement may be either primary or secondary to extension of a cervical lymphangioma.[203]

Surgical excision is the only acceptable mode of therapy for cystic hygromas. Although complete excision should always be the goal, the surgeon must remember that he is dealing with a benign tumor. Normal structures should not be sacrificed in order to obtain total extirpation of the tumor. If all macroscopic disease has been resected, recurrence is uncommon. If, on the other hand, gross tumor is left behind, a 15 per cent recurrence rate has been quoted.[133] Laryngeal lesions should be approached through a standard cervical incision as employed for other laryngeal tumors. Endoscopy may prove quite beneficial in dealing with persistent cystic hygromas in the larynx. Unless laryngeal lesions are recognized early, tracheotomy is almost always required for airway maintenance.[203]

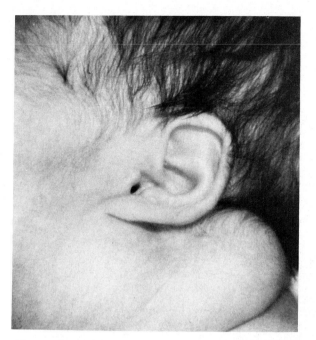

Figure 70–40. This large cervical lymphangioma exhibited growth in the neonatal period.

HEMANGIOMA

Hemangiomas are the single most common head and neck neoplasm in children. They are predominantly located on cutaneous surfaces, but they may be found on mucosal surfaces as well. The scalp is the most frequently involved region, followed by the neck and face. Females are more frequently affected than males, and the tumors are more often solitary than multifocal.[20]

Hemangiomas can be defined as benign nonreactive processes in which there is an increase in the number of normal- and abnormal-appearing blood vessels. Several different types have been described. *Capillary hemangiomas* are composed of nests of capillary vascular channels lined by endothelial cells and surrounded by pericytes. The endothelial cells of early lesions may be quite plump, obscuring the lumen of the capillaries, and the vascular nature of the lesion may not be immediately apparent. The cutaneous birthmark (nevus flammeus) is a capillary hemangioma located in the dermis. The strawberry nevus is a subcutaneous mass and is actually a hypertrophic type of capillary hemangioma. This tumor is marked by a period of slow evolution, which is then followed by a rapid growth phase and then, possibly, involution.[94]

Cavernous hemangiomas are composed of tortuous large vascular spaces lined by endothelial cells. They are larger, more frequently involve deep structures than do capillary hemangiomas, and are unlikely to regress spontaneously. There is frequently adventitial fibrosis. Phleboliths may develop as a result of dystrophic calcification in the thrombi.[94] Cavernous hemangiomas can be found in skin or in deeper tissues. These lesions are often permanent, especially if they are not present at birth. Those that are present at birth tend to involute spontaneously.

Arteriovenous hemangiomas occur in deep soft tissue and are referred to by some as arteriovenous malformations. The clinical findings of a pulsatile mass and the physiologic manifestations of an anteriovenous shunt are as important diagnostically as the histopathologic findings. Histologically, many features of a capillary or cavernous hemangioma may be present. Diagnosis can be made by the finding of intimal thickening in veins or by demonstration of diverse arteriovenous connections in serial sections.[94]

Hemangiomas are lesions of infancy; less than one third of these lesions are present at birth. They typically are noted in the first month of life, grow during the first year, and involute in approximately 90 per cent of cases without treatment. Angiographically, hemangiomas are well-circumscribed lobular masses that have a persistent dense tissue stain and are supplied by multiple slightly enlarged arteries. The proximal artery surrounds the lesion, and smaller arteries enter the hemangioma at right angles. Arteriovenous shunting can be noted but is usually not present. In contrast to vascular neoplasms, vascular malformations are always present at birth, although not always identified, grow proportional to the child, and do not involute. The angiographic appearance depends on the type of vessels involved Capillary venous malformations have dilated, ectatic spaces that fill during the venous phase and demonstrate prolonged contrast pooling. Arterial-venous—lymphatic vascular malformations are high-flow communications with enlarged and more numerous vessels.[39]

Mucosal hemangiomas may appear anywhere in the upper aerodigestive tract, especially in the oral cavity and nose. Nasal hemangiomas are most commonly found in older adolescent patients. A great deal of controversy exists as to their etiologic basis. They are found most commonly arising from the anterior nasal septum in Little's area. They are usually isolated lesions and are generally not part of a systemic disorder with multiple angiomatous lesions.[193] Nasal hemangiomas are most likely the result of local irritation. Little evidence exists that they are present congenitally. Likewise, there seems to be little to support the concept that these lesions are hamartomas, that is, local accentuations of blood vessels normally present. Rather, their development appears to be the result of post-traumatic proliferation of a local group of blood vessels with an associated increase in regional hydrostatic pressure.[8]

Hemangiomas in the nares must be differentiated from exuberant granulation tissue, which also occurs secondary to local trauma.[20] Nasal hemangiomas most commonly present as polypoid or sessile masses and can usually be diagnosed on gross clinical examination. Their size ranges from several millimeters to more than 2 cm in diameter.[193] The tumor is generally confined to the nasal passages but may extend into the nasal skeleton and surrounding structures. There seems to be no sex predilection, and most patients present with epistaxis and nasal obstruction, generally of less than 6 months' duration.

In spite of its apparent traumatic etiology, the growth behaves clinically as a true neoplasm. This concept is based upon the tumor's distinctive morphology and its propensity for local recurrence when inadequately excised.[8] Radiographs of the facial bones and paranasal

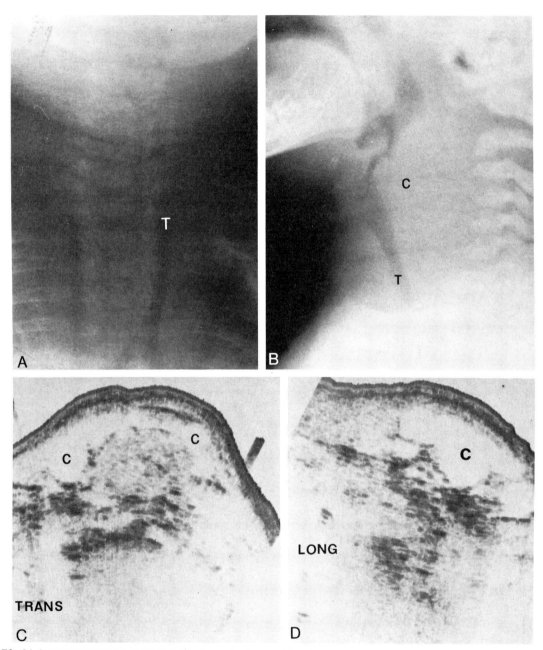

Figure 70–41. Anteroposterior (*A*) and lateral (*B*) views of a 4-year-old male with a cystic hygroma (C). The hypopharynx is distorted by a large retropharyngeal tumor. The trachea is bowed anteriorly and leftward by the large cervical-mediastinal mass. Transverse (*C*) and longitudinal (*D*) ultrasound images show a hypoechogenic neck mass (M) in a different patient with rare internal echoes typical of cystic hygroma.

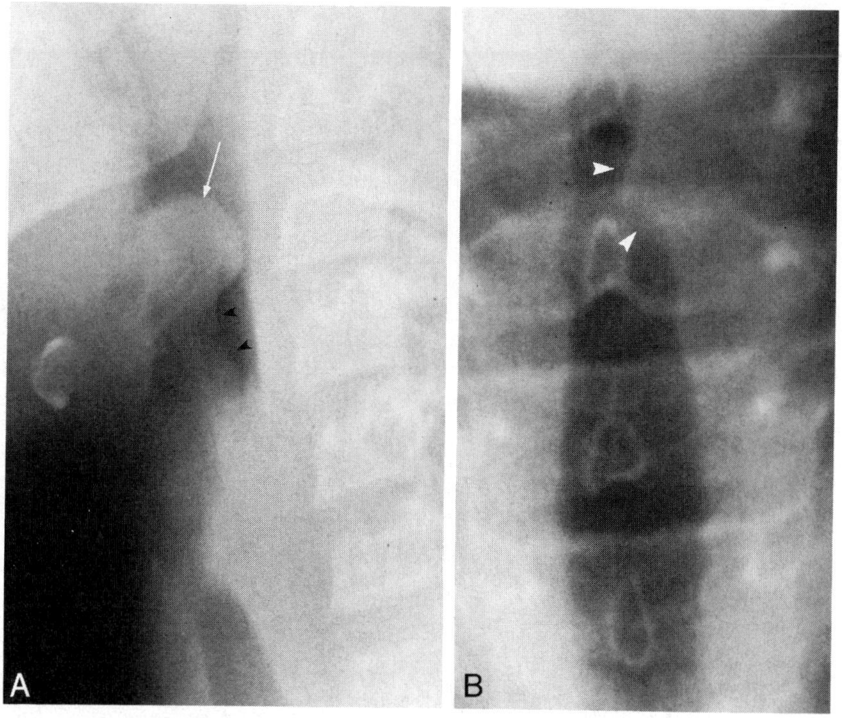

Figure 70–42. Epiglottic lymphangioma causing rounded enlargement of the epiglottis (white arrow). The aryepiglottic folds (black arrowheads) are normal (A). A second lymphangioma bulges the left proximal tracheal wall (B).

sinuses are the only investigative procedures that are obtained routinely. Arteriography may be of benefit in those rare lesions that are quite extensive and must be differentiated from nasopharyngeal angiofibromas.[154] The majority of congenital hemangiomas involute spontaneously, but those arising on the nasal septum generally require some form of definitive therapy. Radiotherapy, injection of a sclerosing agent, conservative excision, and radical excision have all been proposed as possible treatment modalities for these lesions. In general, however, the best method of treatment appears to be wide resection of the mass together with a cuff of underlying mucosa and perichondrium. Minimal bleeding occurs. Failure to include the perichondrium is associated with a high rate of recurrence. The exposed cartilaginous septum may be left to granulate. Obviously, therapy must be individualized, and locally infiltrative tumors may require radical surgery.[20]

Hemangiomas may be located anywhere in the oral cavity in children, with the lips, cheek, and tongue most commonly affected. The lesions may be either superficial or deeply invasive with subsequent deformity of oral structures. The superficial lesions are usually reddish blue and are easily compressible. They may appear partially submerged. The deep lesions are usually firm, diffuse, and less circumscribed. The patients are usually less than 5 years of age. Most oral hemangiomas are solitary, but they can be multicentric with clustering.[20]

Although most cutaneous and mucosal hemangiomas do not appear circumscribed, they are usually not invasive in spite of their histologic appearance. Hemangiomas located in deep subcutaneous tissues, fascia, and muscles tend to be infiltrating and difficult to treat. The lesions do not undergo malignant degeneration or metastasize, but local control is difficult and is often not achieved. Children are more frequently affected than

adults. An example of an invasive lesion is the intramuscular hemangioma, which is most commonly found in the masseter and trapezius muscles. It usually presents as a localized mass with a rubbery consistency and distinct margins. It is mobile and not associated with a bruit, thrill, or pulsation. Cutaneous involvement is not uncommon, nor is functional impairment of the involved muscle. Patients may complain of pain due to compression. Capillary hemangiomas are the most common type of intramuscular hemangioma and are associated with a 20 per cent recurrence rate after appropriate therapy. Cavernous intramuscular hemangiomas are the second most common type seen, and they are associated with a 9 per cent recurrence rate. Mixed types are uncommonly found but are associated with a 25 per cent recurrence rate. Therapy for these intramuscular hemangiomas requires ligation of the feeding vessels and excision of the mass. The surgeon must remember that these are benign lesions, and care must be taken to save all vital structures.[20]

Conservative therapy is the rule for most hemangiomas. The majority of congenital lesions involute spontaneously. One must constantly reassure both the child and parent that involution is expected. When the tumors show unusually rapid growth, biopsy is indicated, and some form of definitive therapy may be indicated. This must be individualized based on several factors, including patient age, site of lesion, size of lesion, depth of extension, and the general characteristics of the mass. The use of steroids, radiotherapy, and sclerosing agents has been proposed both as alternatives and as adjuncts to surgical excision. Oral mucosal lesions may be treated in a fashion similar to that for cutaneous hemangiomas with conservative local excision when conditions warrant.[20] Vascular malformations present a more difficult problem and often require embolization or surgery (Fig. 70–43). Embolization may

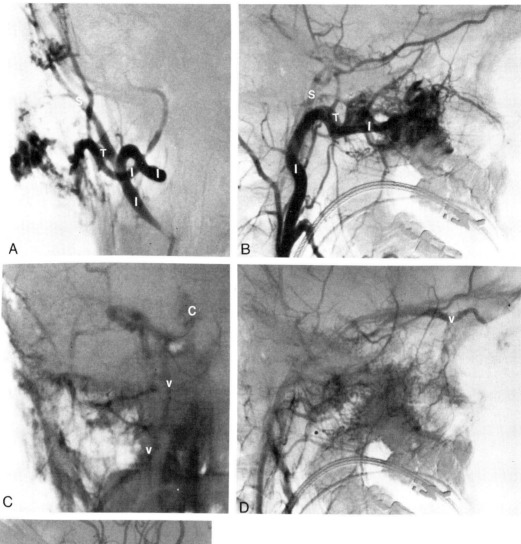

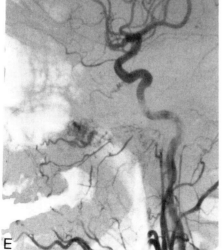

Figure 70–43. Nine-year-old female with a pulsatile right facial vascular malformation. In arterial phase right external carotid arteriogram, anteroposterior (*A*) and lateral (*B*) views demonstrate enlarged internal maxillary (I) and transverse facial (TF) arteries supplying a hypervascular malformation. Venous phase: anteroposterior (*C*) and lateral (*D*) views reveal early venous drainage via enlarged superficial facial (F) and angular (A) veins, which drain into the cavernous sinus (C). (*E*) Seven weeks later: lateral common carotid arteriogram after Ivalon embolization. The large vascular malformation has been reduced considerably. Only minimal residual supply from the ascending pharyngeal artery and palatal collaterals.

be used either as a primary treatment or to reduce blood flow preoperatively. For successful embolic obliteration of vascular malformation, detailed superselective angiography followed by infusion of particulate matter, glues, coils, or other materials[267] can be performed by an experienced angiographer.

Hemangiomas of specific sites deserve special mention, especially those found in the parotid gland and in the larynx.[18] Before the age of 1 year, capillary hemangiomas make up greater than 50 per cent of all salivary gland tumors. It is usually detected before 6 months of age because the maximum growth stage occurs during this time period. Females are affected more frequently than males, and the parotid gland is the most frequently involved salivary gland (Fig. 70–44). The diagnosis can usually be made without a tissue examination.

Hemangiomas are the most common cause of parotid swelling in infants. There are often overlying skin hemangiomas or telangiectasias, and bluish skin discoloration may result from the underlying neoplasm. Crying is associated with an increase in the size of the mass. It has a cystic feel and usually can be compressed. The most common location for parotid hemangiomas is at the angle of the mandible with extension anteriorly and superiorly along the ascending ramus.

Hemangiomas can cause the parotid gland to increase up to five times its normal size. There is an increase in the number of individual lobules, and the gland assumes a spongy consistency. It is purple to red in color. The histopathologic appearance is characteristic; the general lobular architecture of the gland is preserved, but the parenchyma is characterized by endothelial proliferation with vascular differentiation. The changes are multifocal, and related abnormalities are seen in the periparotid soft tissues and interlobular septa. Nuclear

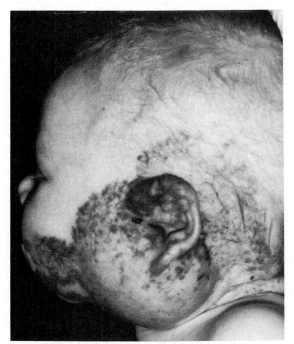

Figure 70–44. Large parotid hemangioma with extensive cervical involvement, which necessitated a tracheostomy.

pleomorphism and atypia are absent, but mitoses may be present.

The best therapy for parotid hemangiomas is observation while waiting for the lesions to regress spontaneously. As with hemangiomas elsewhere, one may be forced to operate when there is infection, hemorrhage, ulceration, or a failure to involute. Should involution occur in other cutaneous lesions, involution of a hemangioma of the parotid gland will most likely occur. When surgery is performed, recurrence is unusual unless the child is less than 4 months old. The seventh cranial nerve should always be preserved.[18]

Hemangiomas of the larynx have been separated into adult and infantile types. The adult type is usually a glottic or a supraglottic hemangioma and consists of circumscribed reddish blue lesions that present with signs and symptoms of hoarseness and occasionally airway distress. The true incidence of infantile hemangiomas of the larynx is unknown, but they are certainly not rare lesions. Females are more frequently affected than males, and infants are usually asymptomatic at birth but develop increasing stridor during their first 3 to 6 months of life. The stridor is usually inspiratory but sometimes becomes biphasic. The condition is not usually associated with hoarseness or change in cry, and the infants often present with respiratory distress, which increases with excitement or infection. It is generally felt that an increase in venous pressure causes an increase in symptoms.

Infantile hemangiomas of the larynx are most commonly found in the subglottic region. Because about 50 per cent of children with subglottic hemangiomas have other associated cutaneous hemangiomas, the finding of such a cutaneous lesion in a child with stridor and dyspnea suggests the diagnosis of subglottic hemangioma. The lesion can usually be recognized endoscopically as a unilateral, sessile, compressible mass arising between the undersurface of the true vocal cord and lower border of the cricoid ring. The mass may have some discoloration. Radiographs of the airway characteristically show an asymmetric subglottic narrowing due to the posterolateral subglottic mass (Fig. 70–45).

The treatment of *subglottic hemangiomas* is dependent upon the infant's clinical condition. When the infant presents with acute airway distress, a tracheotomy must be performed. This should be placed lower than normal to ensure that the tumor is not entered. When there is no immediate airway danger, diagnosis is confirmed endoscopically. Controversy exists with respect to the advisability of biopsy. Our preference is to avoid biopsy because of the danger of hemorrhage. Therapy most often consists of observation because the majority of lesions regress spontaneously within 6 months after diagnosis. If this is not the case, laser excision or steroids may be employed to avoid a tracheotomy.[13] If a tracheotomy has been performed, one should wait for the tumor to regress rather than employ additional therapeutic maneuvers, which may involve risk to the larynx.

JUVENILE NASOPHARYNGEAL ANGIOFIBROMA

The juvenile nasopharyngeal angiofibroma (JNA) is the most commonly encountered vascular mass found

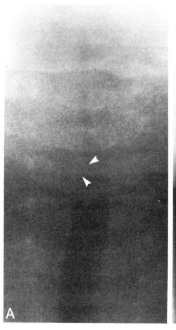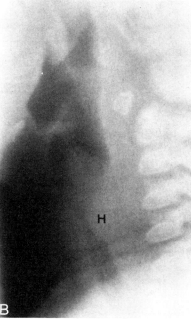

Figure 70–45. Subglottic hemangioma (H). Anteroposterior (*A*) and lateral (*B*) views of airway radiographs demonstrating asymmetric subglottic narrowing (arrowheads) due to a posterolateral mass.

in the nasal cavity. Its name reflects the fact that the tumor's primary manifestations occur during adolescence. The patients' ages range from 7 through 21 years, with a peak between 14 and 18 years of age. Only rarely have females been diagnosed with this lesion; when this does occur, one must seriously question the diagnosis or perform chromosome analysis on the patient.[20]

Although the etiology is uncertain, the tumor appears to arise from the characteristic fibrovascular stroma normally seen in the nasopharynx. The tumor is broad-based and generally arises on the posterolateral wall of the nasal cavity at the sphenopalatine foramen. From this description, it is easy to understand how the tumor can spread to involve the sphenoid sinus and the pterygomaxillary fossa. Orbital and intracranial spread can also occur.[20] Histologically, the tumor is composed of stellate or spindle fibrocytes in a varying amount of connective tissue stroma with many wide, thin-walled vessels (Fig. 70–46).

The clinical signs and symptoms associated with the JNA are certainly characteristic but are by no means diagnostic. Nasal obstruction and recurrent severe epistaxis are most commonly reported. Purulent rhinorrhea occurs when there is a secondary infection of the surrounding paranasal sinuses. The locally invasive nature of the tumor can lead to gross facial deformity with involvement of the palate, midface, and pharynx. Hyponasal speech is a common finding in these patients, and they frequently complain of anosmia. Rarely, signs of intracranial mass effect may be encountered from intracranial extension of the tumor.[20]

Imaging is extremely important in the diagnosis and management of juvenile angiofibroma. Prior to the introduction of CT, the diagnostic evaluation of a pubescent male with a nasopharyngeal mass consisted of skull and sinus series, complex motion laminagraphy, and angiography. However, CT has now replaced laminagraphy, and our current recommendations include skull and sinus series, CT, angiography, and preoperative embolization.

Radiographic evaluation usually begins with skull and sinus series. A nasopharyngeal mass is usually evident on lateral, open mouth Waters', or submentovertex views without evidence of gross bony destruction (Fig.

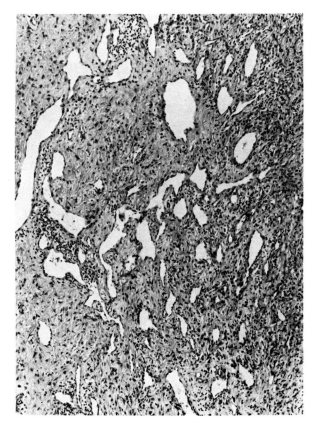

Figure 70–46. Juvenile nasal angiofibroma. The lesion is composed of slit-like vascular spaces separated by a fibrous or fibromyxoid stroma and occasionally a nonspecific inflammatory infiltrate. (× 130)

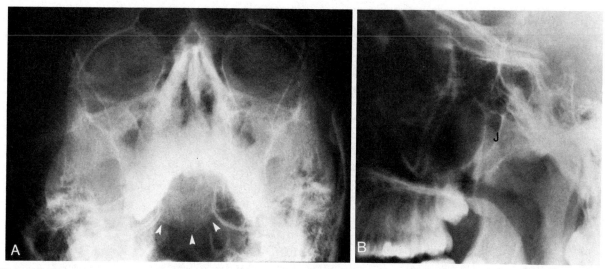

Figure 70–47. Juvenile nasal angiofibroma. Open-mouth Waters' projection (A) demonstrates mucosal thickening of both maxillary antra and a large mass (arrowheads). Lateral projection (B) localizes the mass (J) to the nasopharynx.

70–47). The tumor is slow growing and extends along and through the natural fissures and foramina of the skull base, pushing rather than destroying bone. Typically, there is widening of the sphenopalatine foramina[224] and anterior bowing of the posterior maxillary wall (Holman-Miller sign) (Fig. 70–48).[115] The maxillary, ethmoid, and frontal sinuses may also be involved. If tumor extends superiorly, it can cause obstruction of the sphenoid sinus ostium or fill the sinus cavity. Occasionally, erosion of the anterior sphenoid wall occurs, resulting in a lytic lesion with sclerotic margins. Extension may also occur through the superior orbital fissure and may be accompanied by erosion of the inferomedial sphenoid wing.

Laterally, the tumor may extend into the infratem-

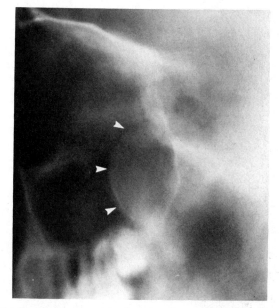

Figure 70–48. Lateral laminagram shows anterior bowing of the posterior maxillary wall (arrowheads) by a large nasopharyngeal juvenile angiofibroma.

poral fossa but rarely erodes the zygomatic arch. This soft-tissue involvement is difficult to appreciate with conventional radiography alone. Anteriorly, extension into the nasal fossa can produce erosion and displacement of nasal septum;[225] CT demonstrates these changes quite well. Although the numerous bony changes may be better delineated by laminagraphy, this technique does not accurately predict the soft-tissue extent of the tumor, especially in the region of the infratemporal fossa and intracranially.[253]

Computed tomography is now the method of choice in the preoperative evaluation and follow-up of these patients. Bryan and colleagues[35] have recommended pre- and postcontrast axial and direct coronal images (Figs. 70–49 and 70–50). However, in order to reduce radiation exposure, we currently are scanning these patients in the axial and coronal planes only after the addition of contrast material and reformatting images in the sagittal plane as needed. We find this method to be highly diagnostic, as it demonstrates accurately the characteristics and extent of the tumor. To date, all untreated tumors have been enhanced to a greater degree than adjacent muscle and have been easy to recognize.

Computed tomography is extremely important in preoperative planning. Because there are multiple potential routes for tumor extension, no single therapeutic approach is possible. Sessions and associates[224] have proposed a staging classification based on CT:

Stage I
A Disease represents tumor limited to the posterior naris or nasopharyngeal bulbs. No paranasal sinus extension.
B Same as 1A with extension into one or more paranasal sinuses.

Stage II
A Minimal lateral extension through the sphenopalatine foramina, into and including a minimal part of the medialmost part of the pterygomaxillary foramina.
B Full occupation of the pterygomaxillary foramina, displacing the posterior wall of the maxillary antrum anteriorly. Lateral or anterior displacement

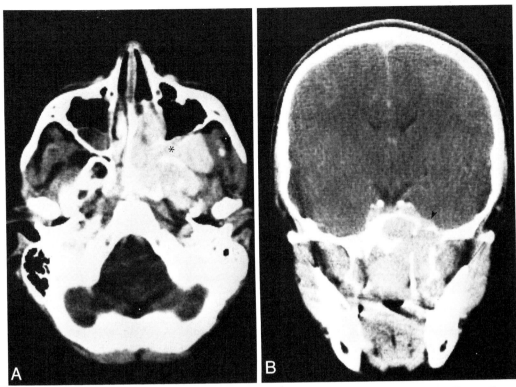

Figure 70–49. Post-contrast axial (*A*) and direct coronal (*B*) images in this 11-year-old male with stage III juvenile angiofibroma. Densely enhancing tumor widens the pterygomaxillary foramina (*) with medial extension into the nasopharynx, lateral spread into infratemporal fossa, and superior extension into the sphenoid sinus and middle cranial fossa with adjacent bone erosion (arrow).

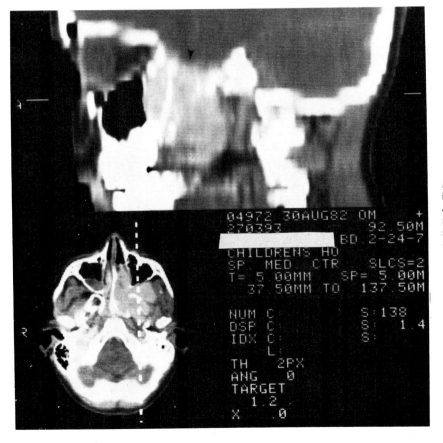

Figure 70–50. Sagittal re-formated image: tumor in pterygomaxillary foramina with anterior bowing of posterior maxillary wall and skull base erosion (arrowhead) with intracranial extension identified.

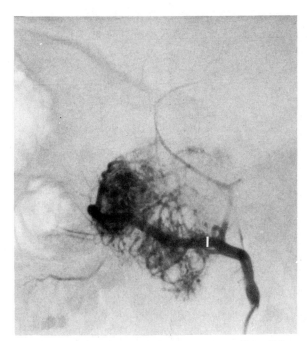

Figure 70–51. Pre-embolization selective internal maxillary artery injection. Lateral subtraction view. Enlarged internal maxillary artery (I) with hypervascular tumor blush.

of branches of the maxillary artery. Superior extension may occur, eroding the orbital bones.

C Extension through the pterygomaxillary foramina into the cheek and temporal fossa.

Stage III Intracranial extension.

This staging classification is important because treatment regimens can be based on the various stages.

Angiography remains an important modality in evaluation of JNA. It no longer is performed to define tumor extent because CT is more accurate. The main value of angiography is defining the tumor's vascular supply and for preoperative embolization. Bilateral internal and external carotid artery and left vertebral artery injections are made to document completely the vascular supply. Magnification and subtraction techniques are utilized. Typically, the JNA is supplied by the internal maxillary and ascending pharyngeal arteries, both originating from the external carotid artery (Fig. 70–51). Contralateral supply is occasionally present, particularly in larger tumors. The angiographic features are consistent and include hypertrophy and increased numbers of small arterial branches without beading, segmental narrowing, dilatation, or aneurysm formation. The circulation through the tumor is rapid, with early venous opacification and a persistent dense capillary stain.[207]

In the past, we performed diagnostic angiography and preoperative embolization at separate examinations. However, because of the small total contrast dose and increased familiarity with the procedure, we now will perform both components during a single examination. We prefer to embolize the angiofibroma 18 to 24 hours prior to surgical removal. This procedure is usually performed under general anesthesia, although it may occasionally be accomplished using heavy sedation. A 5 French catheter is positioned within the internal maxillary artery, and Gelfoam pledgets suspended in dilute contrast material are injected. Embolization is continued until blood flow is reduced (Fig. 70–52). The procedure is repeated in all vessels that provide a significant vascular supply to the neoplasm.

Certain precautions are necessary to avoid complications. Congenital vascular variations such as ophthalmic artery origin from the middle meningeal artery, communication between the posterior division of the ascending pharyngeal and vertebral artery, and internal carotid and vertebral (pro-atlantial) artery communication at the level of the posterior arch of C1 must be excluded. After embolization, the patient may develop a low-grade fever, scalp pain lasting 1 to 3 days, or pain referred to the region of the tumor bed. If pain is severe, narcotic analgesia may be necessary. We prefer Gelfoam because of its ease of use, low cost, and short occlusive

Figure 70–52. Postembolization, lateral view. Embolization with gelatin sponge (Gelfoam) pledgets has successfully obliterated tumor hypervascularity.

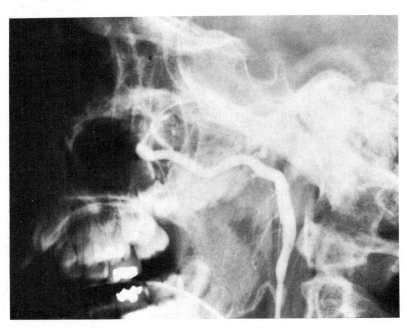

life. However, other materials such as Ivalon, latex spheres, Gianturco coils, and tissue adhesives can be used singly or in combination. In our experience and that of others[35, 207] embolization has been effective in diminishing intraoperative blood loss from approximately 2500 ml to 800 ml. In addition, total tumor volume is reduced.

The differential diagnosis of a nasopharyngeal mass without bone destruction, presenting in a pubescent male, is extensive. Some abnormalities to consider include congenital nasal or sphenoid encephalocele; persistent, enlarged adenoid tissue; and malignant tumors in their early stages, which would include lymphoma, rhabdomyosarcoma, nasopharyngeal carcinoma, and olfactory neuroblastoma. Benign neoplasms such as antrochoanal[254] and angiomatous polyps[232] also need to be considered. CT and angiography can help in differentiating many of these entities. Malignancies usually are associated with bone destruction and penetrate the pharyngobasilar fascia. This is unusual in JNA. The main entity causing difficulty in differential diagnosis is the *angiomatous polyp*. These patients present with similar symptoms; however, they tend to present at a slightly older age, during the third decade, and the CT and angiographic appearances allow differentiation. On CT, the angiomatous polyp expands the nasal vault and extends into the nasopharynx but does not invade the pterygopalatine fossa or sphenoid sinus. The mass is either hypovascular or avascular and is supplied predominantly by ethmoid branches of the internal carotid artery. Surgery is the treatment of choice, and preoperative embolization is not necessary because intraoperative bleeding is not a problem.[232]

The natural history of the JNA is usually one of slowly progressive enlargement. Only rarely has a reduction in tumor size been documented as the patient has passed out of adolescence. With this in mind, it is imperative that a treatment plan be developed. Careful observation of the tumor does not constitute one of these therapeutic alternatives.[20]

Various surgical approaches have been developed, depending on the exact site of the tumor. The transpalatal approach is indicated when the tumor is confined to the nasopharynx, but the majority of tumors require a wide lateral rhinotomy approach.[26]

Various adjuncts to surgical therapy have also been suggested, including estrogen therapy, cryotherapy, and the previously described arterial embolization. Although histologic studies do show involution of blood vessels after estrogen therapy, their efficacy in diminishing surgical blood loss in the treatment of the JNA has not been proved. Cryotherapy has a limited use in the surgical treatment of these lesions. Its major advantage is in controlling bleeding from small tumors.[87] An alternative treatment modality is radiotherapy with about 3500 rad. Approximately 20 per cent of patients will require a surgical procedure to remove significant residual tumor.[87]

The long-term prognosis of patients with JNA is good. Batsakis[20] reports a recurrence rate of about 50 per cent but a mortality rate of only 3 per cent. Recurrence usually occurs within the first 12 months after therapy and is unusual after 24 months. Several factors predispose these patients to recurrent tumors. The multilob-

ular nature of this tumor accounts for its ability to irregularly invade the adjacent sinuses and fascial spaces. In addition, the anatomic irregularity of the nasopharynx itself makes complete tumor extirpation difficult. Lack of aggressiveness on the part of the surgeon may further compromise tumor removal.

INFANTILE HEMANGIOPERICYTOMA

Infantile hemangiopericytomas are multilobulated subcutaneous lesions occurring in the first year of life. Despite the occurrence of endovascular proliferation, increased mitotic activity, and focal necrosis, which are all changes indicative of malignancy in adult tumors, these tumors follow a benign clinical course.

TERATOMA

True teratomas contain tissue elements derived from all three germinal layers. The cells found in the lesion may be in any stage of differentiation, and when cells are quite immature, malignancy is suggested. This, however, is probably quite rare and most likely reflects only the immaturity of the tissue.

Cervical Teratomas

Cervical teratomas are sometimes referred to as teratomas of the thyroid. They are encapsulated and usually partially cystic, having a variegated appearance on cut section. Microscopically, cervical teratomas are composed of a mixture of mature elements derived from ectoderm, mesoderm, and endoderm and of immature or embryonic tissue, mostly embryonic neuroectoderm (Fig. 70–53). Consequently, most are embryonal teratomas. Malignancy is determined by the presence of a malignant neoplastic component such as embryonal carcinoma or yolk sac tumor. One case in our experience at Children's Hospital Medical Center, Cincinnati, Ohio, recurred at age 23 months as a yolk sac tumor (Fig. 70–54) in the nasopharynx after local excision of an embryonal teratoma of the face at 5 days of age.[63]

Cervical teratoma presents as a mass in the neck and is usually discovered at birth. It may be seen in stillborn children and rarely presents after the age of 1 year. The diagnosis can be made in utero ultrasonically by demonstration of a cervical mass that is of mixed echogenicity and displaces the trachea posteriorly. Calcification may be detected. In the past, amniocentesis and amniography have also been performed. Cystic hygroma can cause diagnostic confusion but is typically a multilocular, noncalcified cystic mass.[103]

Symptoms are caused from pressure, resulting in upper airway compression and obstruction that leads to stridor and possible apnea. The patients may present with cyanosis. Dysphagia from esophageal compression is also seen. Neck radiographs document a soft-tissue mass that contains speckled calcification in approximately 50 per cent of cases; the mass displaces the trachea and esophagus posteriorly and may be associated with pulmonary atelectasis and collapse. Ultrasonically, a teratoma is generally of mixed echogenicity and then develop over time. The patients do not seem to have an increased incidence of other congenital anomalies, but maternal hydramnios has been incriminated as a predisposing factor.

The differential diagnosis of these cervical lesions is quite broad. Cystic hygromas usually can be differentiated because of their more cystic appearance and ill-defined margins. The cystic hygroma is also capable of transillumination. Branchial cleft cysts are distinguished on the basis of their size, location, and fluctuance. Other things that must be considered are the cavernous hemangioma, thyroglossal duct cyst, laryngocele, goiter, desmoid tumor, and lipoma.[63]

Once the diagnosis of a cervical teratoma is made, immediate surgical excision is necessary to prevent pulmonary problems. Without this intervention, all such patients die. Even in those patients who do survive long enough to undergo surgery, there is a mortality rate associated with the condition.[21]

Nasopharyngeal Teratomas

Besides the cervical region, another common location for teratomas in the head and neck is the nasopharynx. The tumors arise from the superior or lateral walls of the nasopharynx and often present at birth. Females are affected more commonly than males.[102] Many authors consider the nasopharyngeal teratoma to be any nasopharyngeal neoplasm that consists of multiple types of tissue extrinsic to its site of origin. When this broad definition is applied, dermoid cysts, teratoid tumors, epignathi, and true teratomas are all classified together.

In the nasopharynx, the dermoid cyst is the most common teratoma. The patients usually present with a "hairy polyp" filling the nasal cavity or oral cavity. This is actually a dermoid covered by hairy skin that arises from the nasopharynx or the palate. The tumors may extend intracranially. When examined histologically, fibroadipose tissue, bone, cartilage, and skeletal muscle all can be identified. Neural tissue may also be seen.

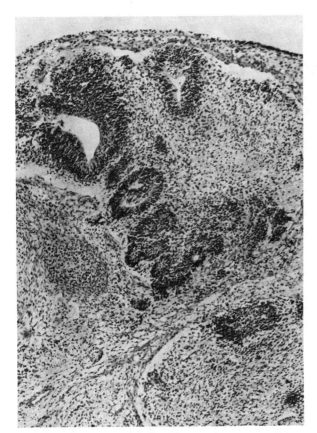

Figure 70–53. Embryonal teratoma. The presence of embryonic tissue—in this case, embryonic neuroectoderm—determines whether a teratoma is embryonal. (× 130)

can usually be differentiated from a cystic hygroma, which typically appears as a multilocular cyst and may extend into the mediastinum, and from a congenital goiter, which appears solid.[90] Symptoms are usually present at birth, but they may be absent initially and

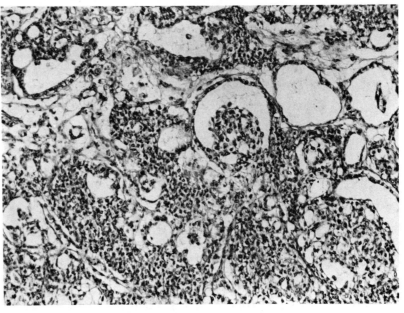

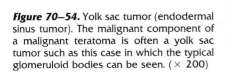

Figure 70–54. Yolk sac tumor (endodermal sinus tumor). The malignant component of a malignant teratoma is often a yolk sac tumor such as this case in which the typical glomeruloid bodies can be seen. (× 200)

Signs and symptoms depend on the site of origin. A long pedicle may cause intermittent symptoms due to excessive mobility of the mass.[16] Radiographs of the nasopharynx alone or combined with contrast injection can assist in diagnosis.[90] The patients present with varying degrees of nasal obstruction and, possibly, difficulty with mouth breathing, depending on the amount of prolapse of the mass. If the symptoms are mild, diagnosis may be delayed or even missed.

Treatment involves surgical excision. When the lesion is pedunculated, a snare may be used. Forceps are usually required for sessile masses. Unless intracranial involvement is present, a good prognosis can be expected. Before treating any nasopharyngeal teratoma, the surgeon must ensure that the mass is not an extension of an orbital teratoma.[16] Computerized tomography is a valuable tool in making this distinction. An ophthalmologist should be consulted to assist in the removal of such a lesion.

RECURRENT RESPIRATORY PAPILLOMATOSIS

Squamous cell papillomas of the oral cavity, sinonasal tract, and larynx are commonly seen in children. Laryngeal papillomas are, in fact, the most common tumor of the larynx in infants and children. Although the condition has been known historically as juvenile laryngeal papillomatosis, this is probably a poor choice of terms. Most patients do present before age 15, but 36 per cent present after the adolescent period. Papillomatosis may not be confined to the larynx. It can be seen in any upper aerodigestive site as well as the lungs. Papillomas in the upper aerodigestive tract are similar histologically in all age groups. In addition, these papillomas have a histologic appearance similar to squamous papillomas elsewhere in the body.[242] Microscopically, there are papillary growths with a vascular connective tissue core covered by stratified squamous epithelium showing a normal pattern of maturation. Mild variability in nuclear size may be seen, but there is no atypia and mitoses are rarely present.[15]

Two broad classifications of recurrent respiratory papillomatosis have arbitrarily evolved. In the "juvenile" type, children are the most frequently involved portion of the population. The growths are almost always multiple and recurrent in spite of therapy. Spontaneous resolution can occur, often at puberty. When this does not happen, papillomatosis can become a lifelong problem. All regions of the upper aerodigestive tract can be affected.[15]

In the "senile" type of respiratory papillomatosis, an older age group of patients is usually affected. Papillomas are usually single, and recurrence is rare after their removal. In spite of their histologic appearance being the same as that of the "juvenile" type, these papillomas are more friable when manipulated.[15]

The true etiology of recurrent respiratory papillomatosis is unknown, but the papova virus has been incriminated. The lesions are not thought to represent true neoplasms but are actually thought to be an abnormal tissue response to an initiating factor. There is some thought that affected patients have an immune disorder that may predispose them to the development of this condition. The parents of patients with recurrent respiratory papillomatosis frequently are found to have venereal condyloma acuminatum.[242]

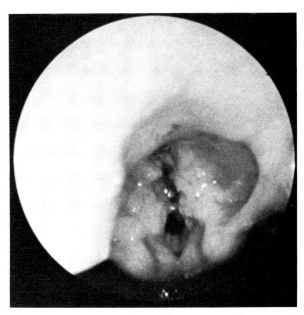

Figure 70–55. Endoscopic view of recurrent respiratory papillomas partially obstructing laryngeal introitus.

The growths appear as pinkish red glistening nodules that are quite friable and bleed easily. The signs and symptoms depend on the site or origin. When the larynx is involved, the patients present with respiratory obstruction (Fig. 70–55). Growth is usually insidious, but the obstruction may be sudden and may require urgent tracheotomy. Hoarseness, or even aphonia, is a frequent presenting complaint.[15]

Roentgen examination of patients with papillomatosis should include frontal and lateral radiographs of the upper airway and chest. CT scans can be used for more detailed pulmonary examination when pulmonary spread is suspected. The hallmark for recognition of laryngeal involvement is enlargement and deformity of the glottis by variably sized nodular masses (Fig. 70–56).[72] Tracheal and pulmonary involvement is unusual but most often occurs in patients who have had surgical manipulation for removal of papillomas or have had a tracheotomy. The tracheobronchial tree is affected in approximately 2 per cent of cases.[230] Pulmonary involvement generally is manifested by either bronchial obstruction or parenchymal disease and can be recognized up to 25 years after discovery of laryngeal disease. When bronchial obstruction occurs, the large bronchi are usually affected, resulting in segmental collapse. Superimposed infection and bronchiectasis form a common sequela. Interestingly, one case of bronchial papilloma without laryngeal disease has been reported.[75] Parenchymal disease is more frequently seen and can present with gradually expanding thin- or thick-walled cavities (Fig. 70–57) or pulmonary nodules without cavities. Rarely, the esophagus can be involved (Fig. 70–58).

Many different forms of therapy have been proposed over the years. These have included antibiotics, hormones, electrocoagulation, cryotherapy, radiotherapy,

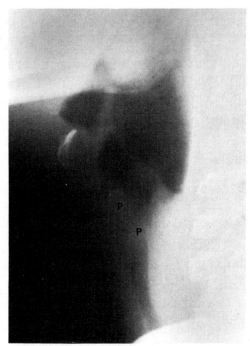

Figure 70–56. Lateral view of the upper airway. Rounded nodular masses of glottis (P) are due to recurrent respiratory papillomas with secondary obstructive distention of hypopharynx and collapse of proximal trachea.

transfer factor, surgical excision, laser excision, autogenous vaccine, mumps vaccine, and interferon. Whatever one does, it should be conservative. The mortality rate of 15 per cent, which is often quoted for recurrent respiratory papillomatosis, is more likely to reflect the

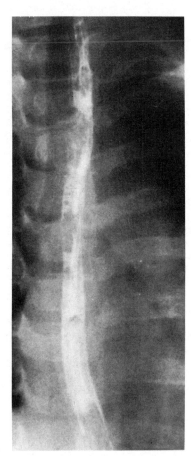

Figure 70–58. Esophagogram. Recurrent respiratory papillomatosis with spread to esophagus: multiple small intraluminal filling defects of the esophagus.

therapy than the disease itself.[15] Spontaneous remission can and does take place, but the true incidence of this occurrence is unknown. If it is going to occur, it usually occurs before age 10 or after age 40. It rarely happens during adolescence. Unfortunately, even when patients have a spontaneous remission, there may be late recurrence years after the initial remission.[242] Microlaryngoscopy with laser excision of papillomas is the preferred treatment at this time for laryngeal papillomatosis. A biopsy should always be obtained to ensure that malignant degeneration has not taken place. This method allows precise ablation of the abnormal tissue while preserving vital underlying structures.[15] Tracheotomy should be avoided if at all possible because of the increased risk of distal spread. It is thought that the tracheotomy results in abrasion and drying of the mucosa, with subsequent seeding of papillomas. The goal of treatment, then, should be to maintain normal function until spontaneous remission occurs. The patient should be monitored frequently and papillomas removed as often as necessary. In addition, the patients and their families need a great deal of psychologic support because of the recurrent nature of the illness and the financial burden associated with repeated hospitalizations and surgical procedures. Radiotherapy should never be utilized in the treatment of these patients for fear of inducing malignant change.[242]

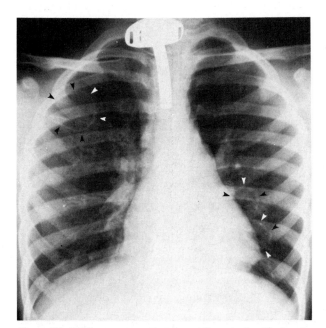

Figure 70–57. Recurrent respiratory papillomatosis with alveolar spread. Anteroposterior chest x-ray shows large, thin-walled cyst within right upper (arrowheads); several smaller cysts are within the left lower lobe (arrowheads).

MISCELLANEOUS TUMORS

Calcifying Epithelioma of Malherbe

An unusual cutaneous lesion is the calcifying epithelioma of Malherbe. The lesion is also known as pilomatrixoma and is a benign tumor of skin seen almost exclusively in whites.[7] Over half of these tumors present in the head and neck region,[191] where they arise from hair follicles.[181] They are found most frequently on the brow, lid, and cheek.[195] The tumors have been identified in neonates,[181] and 40 per cent of patients are seen in the first decade of life. An additional 20 per cent of patients present before age 20. Tumors are most commonly solitary,[181, 195] but they may be multiple in up to 6 per cent of cases.[181]

Pilomatrixomas present clinically as solid or cystic freely movable nodules covered by normal skin. A reddish or bluish discoloration can develop in the overlying skin.[191] The tumors range in size up to 3 cm in diameter. Growth of the tumors is usually quite slow, and they are often asymptomatic. Pain may result from pressure or when the growths become secondarily infected with subsequent bleeding and ulceration.[181] Although the tumor is quite distinct histologically, it must be differentiated clinically from squamous cell carcinomas, skin cysts, and subcutaneous cysts.[191] Most authors recommend total excision of these tumors,[7, 191, 195] but there are proponents of incision and curettage.[181] Recurrence is unusual after adequate surgical excision.[195]

Granular Cell Tumor

A multitude of names have been used to identify the granular cell tumor. These have included Abrikossoff's tumor, congenital epulis, nonchromaffin paraganglioma, granular cell myoblastoma, granular cell neurofibroma, myoblastic myoma, uniform myoblastoma, and embryonal myoblastoma. The controversial nature of the tumor's histogenesis is reflected in the large number of names assigned to it. Both myogenic and neurogenic tissues have been proposed as possible sources for the development of the granular cell tumor. In addition, both histiocytes and fibroblasts have been implicated as potential sources of tumor development. Regardless of its origin, the granular cell tumor is recognized as a benign lesion most commonly found in the upper aerodigestive tract.

Two distinct types of granular cell tumors have been identified in humans. Although there are minor histologic differences between them, they may be divided for practical purposes on the basis of their locale and age at presentation. The *congenital epulis* presents a distinct submucosal mass along the crest of the alveolar ridge in the incisor region of newborns. The maxilla is more commonly involved than the mandible, but both jaws may be involved simultaneously. The tumor is found eight times more frequently in females than males.[19] Simple excision has been recommended as the treatment of choice,[270] but no therapy is probably necessary because the lesion will most likely undergo spontaneous regression.[19] Recurrence is uncommon following surgical removal.[270]

The second type of granular cell tumor is primarily *a lesion of young adults*. The lesions are found more frequently in female patients, and there is a higher incidence in blacks than in whites. The most frequent locations for the tumor are the tongue (33 to 50 per cent of cases) and subcutaneous regions (33 per cent of cases), but any submucosal site in the upper respiratory tract may be involved, including the larynx and bronchus. The growths appear as well-circumscribed nodules with a variable diameter. Up to 10 per cent of patients may have multiple lesions in various regions of the body. Wide local excision is the treatment of choice for these benign tumors. Recurrence is uncommon unless inadequate surgery has been performed.[19]

Melanotic Neuroectodermal Tumor of Infancy

The melanotic neuroectodermal tumor of infancy is an infrequently seen lesion known by a plethora of terms. It has been called congenital melanocarcinoma, melanotic progonoma, pigmented or melanotic ameloblastoma, pigmented epulis, retinal anlage tumor, and melanotic neuroectodermal tissue of infancy. This large number of names no doubt reflects the uncertainties surrounding the tumor's histogenesis. Although the possibility of neural crest origin seems the most likely, other plausible theories of origin include congenital melanoma, odontogenic origin, retinal anlage origin, neurectodermal development, and keratoma.[28, 172]

In spite of its infiltrative appearance, the melanotic neuroectodermal tumor of infancy is considered to be a benign lesion. It is most commonly found in infants under 1 year of age. Its most frequent site of presentation is the anterior maxilla unilaterally. Other reported locations are the anterior mandible, anterior fontanelle, shoulder, epididymis, cerebellum, and mediastinum.[142] Local excision is the recommended mode of therapy for these lesions; chemotherapy and radiotherapy should not be used. Recurrences can be treated with further conservative surgery. Treatment of intraoral tumors can result in dental deformities, but the overall prognosis is good.[172]

REFERENCES

1. Altman AJ, Schwartz AD: Malignant Diseases of Infancy, Childhood, and Adolescence. 2nd ed. Philadelphia, W. B. Saunders Co., 1983.
2. American Joint Committee for Cancer Staging and End-Results Reporting: Manual for Staging of Cancer. American Joint Committee, 1978.
3. Anderson JR, Wilson JF, Jenkin DT, et al: Childhood non-Hodgkin's lymphoma. The results of a randomized therapeutic trial comparing a 4-drug regimen (COMP) with a 10-drug regimen (LSA$_2$–L$_2$). N Engl J Med 308:559, 1983.
4. Andersson-Anvret M, Forsby N, Klein G, et al: Relationship between the Epstein-Barr virus and undifferentiated nasopharyngeal carcinoma: Correlated nucleic acid hybridization and histopathological examination. Int J Cancer 20:486, 1977.
5. Angervall L, Dahl I, Ekedahl C: Embryonal rhabdomyosarcoma in the external ear. Acta Otolaryngol 73:513, 1972.
6. Armstrong EA, Harwood-Nash DC, Fitz CR, et al: CT of neuroblastomas and ganglioneuromas in children. AJR 139:571, 1982.
7. Arole G, Mosadomi A, Arain AH: Calcifying epithelioma of Malherbe (pilomatrixoma) of the cheek. J Oral Maxillofac Surg 41:121, 1983.
8. Ash JE, Old JW: Hemangiomas of the nasal septum. Trans Am Acad Ophthalmol 54:350, 1950.
9. Azar HA, Jaffe ES, Berard CW, et al: Diffuse large cell lymphomas (reticulum cell sarcomas, histiocytic lymphomas). Cancer 46:1428, 1980.

10. Bagley CM Jr, Roth JA, Thomas LB, et al: Liver biopsy in Hodgkin's disease. Clinicopathologic correlations in 127 patients. Ann Intern Med 76:219, 1972.
11. Baker SR, McClatchey KD: Carcinoma of the nasopharynx in childhood. Otolaryngol Head Neck Surg 89:555, 1981.
12. Bass RM: Eosinophilic granuloma in the head and neck. J Otolaryngol 9:250, 1980.
13. Batsakis JG: Neoplasms of the larynx. In Batsakis JG (ed): Tumors of the Head and Neck: Clinical and Pathological Considerations. 2nd ed. Baltimore, Williams & Wilkins Co., 1979.
14. Batsakis JG: Non-odontogenic tumors of the jaws. In Batsakis JG (ed): Tumors of the Head and Neck: Clinical and Pathological Considerations. 2nd ed. Baltimore, Williams & Wilkins Co., 1979.
15. Batsakis JG: Squamous cell "papillomas" of the oral cavity, sinonasal tract and larynx. In Batsakis JG (ed): Tumors of the Head and Neck: Clinical and Pathological Considerations. 2nd ed. Baltimore, Williams & Wilkins Co., 1979.
16. Batsakis JG: Teratomas of the head and neck. In Batsakis JG (ed): Tumors of the Head and Neck: Clinical and Pathological Considerations. 2nd ed. Baltimore, Williams & Wilkins Co., 1979.
17. Batsakis JG (ed): Tumors of the Head and Neck: Clinical and Pathological Considerations. 2nd ed. Baltimore, Williams & Wilkins Co., 1979.
18. Batsakis JG: Tumors of the major salivary glands. In Batsakis JG (ed): Tumors of the Head and Neck: Clinical and Pathological Considerations. 2nd ed. Baltimore, Williams & Wilkins Co., 1979.
19. Batsakis JG: Tumors of the peripheral nervous system. In Batsakis JG (ed): Tumors of the Head and Neck: Clinical and Pathological Considerations. 2nd ed. Baltimore, Williams & Wilkins Co., 1979.
20. Batsakis JG: Vasoformative tumors. In Batsakis JG (ed): Tumors of the Head and Neck: Clinical and Pathological Considerations. 2nd ed. Baltimore, Williams & Wilkins Co., 1979.
21. Batsakis JG, Littler ER, Oberman HA: Teratomas of the neck: A clinicopathological appraisal. Arch Otolaryngol 79:619, 1964.
22. Batsakis JG, Solomon AR, Rice DH: The pathology of head and neck tumors: Carcinoma of the nasopharynx, Part 11. Head Neck Surg 3:511, 1981.
23. Bell MJ, Bower RJ, Ternberg JL: Selected topics in pediatric surgery. Current concepts of diagnosis and management. Mo Med 78:403, 1981.
24. Berenstein A, Kricheff II: Catheter and material selection for transarterial embolization: Technical considerations. II. Materials. Radiology 132:631, 1979.
25. Berry MP, Smith CR, et al: Nasopharyngeal carcinoma in the young. Int J Radiat Oncol Biol Phys 6:415, 1980.
26. Biller HF, Sessions DG, Ogura JH: Angiofibroma: A treatment approach. Laryngoscope 84:695, 1974.
27. Bonadonna G, Zucali R, et al: Combination chemotherapy of Hodgkin's disease with adriamycin, bleomycin, vinblastine, and imidazole carboxamide versus MOPP. Cancer 36:252, 1975.
28. Borello ED, Gorlin RJ: Melanotic neuroectodermal tumor of infancy: A neoplasm of neural crest origin. Cancer 19:196, 1966.
29. Botnick LE, Goodman R, Jaffe N, et al: Stages I–III Hodgkin's disease in children. Results of staging and treatment. Cancer 39:599, 1977.
30. Bove KE, McAdams AJ: Composite ganglioneuroblastoma. An assessment of the significance of histological maturation in neuroblastoma diagnosed beyond infancy. Arch Pathol Lab Med 105:325, 1981.
31. Brama I, Goldfarb A, et al: Tumour of the nose as a presenting feature of leukaemia. J Laryngol Otol 96:83, 1982.
32. Breslow N, McCann B: Statistical estimation of prognosis for children with neuroblastoma. Cancer Res 31:2098, 1971.
33. Brooks HW, Evans AE, Glass RM III, Glass RM, et al: Chloromas of the head and neck in childhood. The initial manifestation of myeloid leukemia in three patients. Arch Otolaryngol 100:306, 1974.
34. Brown RJ, Szymula NJ, Lore JM Jr: Neuroblastoma of the head and neck. Arch Otolaryngol 104:395, 1978.
35. Bryan RN, Sessions RB, Horowitz BL: Radiographic management of juvenile angiofibroma. AJNR 2:157, 1981.
36. Bumsted RM: Thyroid disease: A guide for the head and neck surgeon. Ann Otol Rhinol Laryngol (Suppl) 89:1, 1980.
37. Burke DP, Gabrielsen TO, Knake JE, et al: Radiology of olfactory neuroblastoma. Radiology 137:367, 1980.
38. Burkitt D: Long-term remissions following one and two-dose chemotherapy for African lymphoma. Cancer 20:756, 1967.
39. Burrows PE, Mulliken JB, Fellows KE, et al: Childhood hemangiomas and vascular malformation: Angiographic differentiation. AJR 141:483, 1983.
40. Cadman NL, Soule EH, Kelly PJ: Synovial sarcoma: An analysis of 134 cases. Cancer 18:613, 1965.
41. Callihan TR, Berard CW: Childhood non-Hodgkin's lymphomas in current histologic perspective. In Rosenberg HS, Berstein J (eds): Perspectives in Pediatric Pathology, Vol. 7. New York, Raven Press, 1982.
42. Canalis RF, Gussen R: Temporal bone findings in rhabdomyosarcoma with predominantly petrous involvement. Arch Otolaryngol 106:290, 1980.
43. Canellos GP, Come SE, Skarin AT: Chemotherapy in the treatment of Hodgkin's disease. Semin Hematol 20:1, 1983.
44. Carbone PP, Kaplan HS, Musshoff K, et al: Report of the Committee on Hodgkin's Disease Staging Classification. Cancer Res 31:1860, 1971.
45. Castellino RA: Imaging techniques for staging abdominal Hodgkin's disease. Cancer Treat Rep 66:697, 1982.
46. Cederbaum DS, Niwayama G, et al: Combined immunodeficiency presenting as the Letterer-Siwe syndrome. J Pediatr 85:466, 1974.
47. Chapman RM, Sutcliffe SB, Malpas JS: Male gonadal dysfunction in Hodgkin's disease. A prospective study. JAMA 245:1323, 1981.
48. Chatten J, Voorhess ML: Familial neuroblastoma. Report of a kindred with multiple disorders, including neuroblastomas in four siblings. N Engl J Med 277:1230, 1967.
49. Chaudhry AP, Haar JG, Koul A, et al: Olfactory neuroblastoma (esthesioneuroblastoma): A light and ultrastructural study of two cases. Cancer 44:564, 1979.
50. Chilcote RR, Baehner RL, Hammond D: Septicemia and meningitis in children splenectomized for Hodgkin's disease. N Engl J Med 295:798, 1976.
51. Chung EB, Enzinger FM: Benign lipoblastomatosis. Analysis of 35 cases. Cancer 32:482, 1973.
52. Chung EB, Enzinger FM: Infantile fibrosarcoma. Cancer 38:729, 1976.
53. Cohen LF, Balow JE, et al: Acute tumor lysis syndrome. Am J Med 68:486, 1980.
54. Coleman CN, Williams CJ, Flint A, et al: Hematologic neoplasia in patients treated for Hodgkin's disease. N Engl J Med 297:1249, 1977.
55. Conde E, Lafarga M, Bureo E, et al: Unusual ultrastructural findings in neuroblastoma. Cancer 50:1115, 1982.
56. Conte PJ, Sagerman RH: Embryonal rhabdomyosarcoma of the middle ear with long-term survival. N Engl J Med 284:92, 1971.
57. Crist WM, Kelly DR, Ragab AJ, et al: Predictive ability of Lukes-Collins classification for immunologic phenotypes of childhood non-Hodgkin's lymphoma: An institutional series and literature review. Cancer 48:2070, 1981.
58. Cushing BA, Slovis TL, et al: A rational approach to cervical neuroblastoma. Cancer 50:785, 1982.
59. Daffner RH, Kirks DR, Gehweiler JA Jr, et al: Computed tomography of fibrous dysplasia. AJR 139:943, 1982.
60. Danziger J, Handel SF, Jing BS, et al: Computerized tomography in rhabdomyosarcoma of the head and neck. Cancer 44:463, 1979.
61. Dargeon HW: Considerations in the treatment of reticuloendotheliosis. AJR 93:521, 1965.
62. David FA: Primary tumors of the optic nerve (a phenomenon of Recklinghausen's disease). A clinical and pathologic study with a report of five cases and a review of the literature. Arch Ophthalmol 23:735, 1940.
63. Day LH, Arnold GE: Rare tumors of the ear, nose and throat: Second series: Uncommon benign tumors of the head and neck. Laryngoscope 81:1138, 1971.
64. Dearth JC, Gilchrist GS, Telander RL, et al: Partial splenectomy for staging Hodgkin's disease: Risk of false-negative results. N Engl J Med 299:345, 1978.
65. De Lellis RA, Wolfe HJ: The pathobiology of the human calcitonin (C) cell: A review. Pathol Annu 16:22, 1981.
66. deLorimier AA, Bragg KU, Linden G: Neuroblastoma in childhood. Am J Dis Child 118:441, 1969.
67. Deutsch M, Mercado R Jr, Parsons JA: Cancer of the nasopharynx in children. Cancer 41:1128, 1978.
68. De Vita V Jr, Simon RM, et al: Curability of advanced Hodgkin's disease with chemotherapy. Long-term follow-up of MOPP-treated patients at the National Cancer Institute. Ann Intern Med 92:587, 1980.
69. Dodd GD, Jing B: Radiology of the Nose, Paranasal Sinuses and Nasopharynx. Baltimore, Williams & Wilkins Co., 1977.
70. Donaldson SS, Glatstein E, Rosenberg S, et al: Pediatric Hodgkin's disease. II. Results of therapy. Cancer 37:2436, 1976.
71. Dorfman RF, Warnke R: Lymphadenopathy simulating the malignant lymphomas. Hum Pathol 5:519, 1974.

72. Dunbar JS: Upper respiratory tract obstruction in infants and children. AJR 109:227, 1977.
73. Easton JM, Levine PH, Hyams VJ: Nasopharyngeal carcinoma in the United States. A pathologic study of 177 U.S. and 30 foreign cases. Arch Otolaryngol 106:88, 1980.
74. Edeiken J, Hodes PJ: Roentgen Diagnosis of Diseases of Bone. 2nd ed. Baltimore, Williams & Wilkins Co., 1973.
75. Elliott CB, Belkin A, Donald WA: Cystic bronchial papillomatosis. Clin Radiol 13:62, 1962.
76. Enterline HT: Histopathology of sarcoma. Semin Oncol 8:133, 1981.
77. Enzinger FM, Weiss SW: Soft Tissue Tumors. St. Louis, The C. V. Mosby Co., 1983.
78. Evans AE, D'Angio GJ, Randolph J: A proposed staging for children with neuroblastoma. Children's cancer study group A. Cancer 27:374, 1971.
79. Exelby PE, Frazell EL: Carcinoma of the thyroid in children. Surg Clin North Am 49:249, 1969.
80. Farr HW: Soft part sarcomas of the head and neck. Semin Oncol 8:185, 1981.
81. Favara BE: The pathology of "histiocytosis." Am J Pediat Hemat Oncol 3:45, 1981.
82. Favus MJ, Schneider AB, et al: Thyroid cancer occurring as a late consequence of head-and-neck irradiation. Evaluation of 1056 patients. N Engl J Med 294:1019, 1976.
83. Feiner AS, Mahmood T, Wallner SF: Prognostic importance of pruritus in Hodgkin's disease. JAMA 240:2738, 1978.
84. Feldman BA: Rhabdomyosarcoma of the head and neck. Laryngoscope 92:424, 1982.
85. Feldman F: Tuberous sclerosis, neurofibromatosis, and fibrous dysplasia. In Resnick D, Niwayama G (eds): Diagnosis of Bone and Joint Disorders. Philadelphia, W. B. Saunders Co., 1981.
86. Fernandez CH, Cangir A, Samaan NA, et al: Nasopharyngeal carcinoma in children. Cancer 37:2782, 1976.
87. Fitzpatrick PJ, Briant TD, Berman JM: The nasopharyngeal angiofibroma. Arch Otolaryngol 106:234, 1980.
88. Font RL, Jurco S III, Zimmerman LE: Alveolar soft-part sarcoma of the orbit: A clinicopathologic analysis of seventeen cases and a review of the literature. Hum Pathol 13:569, 1982.
89. Foon KA, Schroff RW, Gale RP: Surface markers on leukemia and lymphoma cells: Recent advances. Blood 60:1, 1982.
90. Frech RS, McAlister WH: Teratoma of the nasopharynx producing depression of the posterior hard palate. J Can Assoc Radiol 20:204, 1969.
91. Frizzera G, Murphy SB: Follicular (nodular) lymphoma in childhood. A rare clinical-pathological entity. Report of eight cases from four cancer centers. Cancer 44:2218, 1979.
92. Fuller LM, Hutchison GB: Collaborative clinical trial for Stage I and II Hodgkin's disease: Significance of mediastinal and nonmediastinal disease in laparotomy and non-laparotomy-staged patients. Cancer Treat Rep 66:775, 1982.
93. Gagel RF, Jackson CE, Block MA, et al: Age-related probability of development of hereditary medullary thyroid carcinoma. J Pediatr 101:941, 1982.
94. Garfinkle TJ, Handler SD: Hemangiomas of the head and neck in children—a guide to management. J Otolaryngol 9:439, 1980.
95. Gehan EA, Glover FN, et al: Prognostic factors in children with rhabdomyosarcoma. Natl Cancer Inst Monogr 56:83, 1981.
96. Gobbi PG, Attardo-Parrinello G, Lattanzio G, et al: Severe pruritus should be a B-symptom in Hodgkin's disease. Cancer 51:1934, 1983.
97. Gonzalez-Crussi F, Black-Schaffer S: Rhabdomyosarcoma of infancy and childhood, problems of morphologic classification. Am J Surg Pathol 3:157, 1979.
98. Goodman GE, Jones SE, et al: Surgical restaging of Hodgkin's disease. Cancer Treat Rep 66:751, 1982.
99. Green DM, Jaffe N: Progress and controversy in the treatment of childhood rhabdomyosarcoma. Cancer Treat Rep 5:7, 1978.
100. Greene MH, Fraumeni JF, Hoover R: Nasopharyngeal cancer among young people in the United States: Racial variations by cell type. J Natl Cancer Inst 58:1267, 1977.
101. Grosfeld JL, Baehner RL: Neuroblastoma: An analysis of 160 cases. World J Surg 4:29, 1980.
102. Grosfeld JL, Ballantine TVN, Lowe D, Baehner RL: Benign and malignant teratomas in children: Analysis of 85 patients. Surgery 80:297, 1976.
103. Gundry SR, Wesley JR, Klein MD, et al: Cervical teratomas in the newborn. J Pediatr Surg 18:382, 1983.
104. Grunwald HW, Rosner F: Acute myeloid leukemia following treatment of Hodgkin's disease: A review. Cancer 50:676, 1982.

105. Hagemeister FB, Fuller LM, et al: Stage I and II Hodgkin's disease: Involved-field radiotherapy versus extended-field radiotherapy versus involved-field radiotherapy followed by six cycles of MOPP. Cancer Treat Rep 66:789, 1982.
106. Hajdu SI, Shiu MH, Fortner JG: Tendosynovial sarcoma: A clinicopathological study of 136 cases. Cancer 39:1201, 1977.
107. Halpern S: Thyroid carcinoma in childhood. Med Pediatr Oncol 9:143, 1981.
108. Hand A: Defects of membranous bones, exophthalmos and polyuria in childhood; is it dyspituitarism? Am J Med Sci 162:509, 1921.
109. Hays DM, Karon M, et al: Hodgkin's disease. Technique and results of staging laparotomy in childhood. Arch Surg 106:507, 1973.
110. Healy GB: Malignant tumors of the head and neck in children: Diagnosis and treatment. Otolaryngol Clin North Am 13:483, 1980.
111. Heyn RM, Holland R, Newton WA Jr, et al: The role of combined chemotherapy in the treatment of rhabdomyosarcoma in children. Cancer 34:2128, 1974.
112. Hellman S, Mauch P: Role of radiation therapy in the treatment of Hodgkin's disease. Cancer Treat Rep 66:915, 1982.
113. Henderson JW, Farrow GM: Primary orbital hemangiopericytoma. An aggressive and potentially malignant neoplasm. Arch Ophthalmol 96:666, 1978.
114. Higashi T, Iguchi M, Shimura A, et al: Computed tomography and bone scintigraphy in polyostotic fibrous dysplasia. Report of a case. Oral Surg 50:580, 1980.
115. Holman CB, Miller WE: Juvenile nasopharyngeal fibroma. AJR 94:292, 1965.
116. Holt JF: Neurofibromatosis in children. AJR 130:615, 1978.
117. Hoppe RT, Cox RS, et al: Prognostic factors in pathologic stage III Hodgkin's disease. Cancer Treat Rep 66:743, 1982.
118. Horn RC Jr, Enterline HT: Rhabdomyosarcoma: A clinicopathological study and classification of 39 cases. Cancer 11:181, 1958.
119. Hrgovcic M, Tessmer CF, et al: Serum copper levels in lymphoma and leukemia. Special reference to Hodgkin's disease. Cancer 21:743, 1968.
120. Hung W, August GP, Randolph JG, et al: Solitary thyroid nodules in children and adolescents. J Pediatr Surg 17:225, 1982.
121. Hunter DW, L'Heureux PR, Latchaw RE: Malignant facial tumors in children: Radiologic evaluation. Stressing value of conventional and computerized tomography. Pediatr Radiol 10:2, 1980.
122. Infante AJ, Miller RH, et al: Intracranial granulocytic sarcoma complicating childhood acute myelomonocytic leukemia. Am J Pediatr Hematol Oncol 3:173, 1981.
123. Jaffe BF, Jaffe N: Diagnosis and treatment: Head and neck tumors in children. Pediatrics 51:731, 1973.
124. Jakobiec FA, Howard GM, et al: Hemangiopericytoma of the orbit. Am J Ophthalmol 78:816, 1974.
125. Jenkin RD, Anderson JR, et al: Nasopharyngeal carcinoma—a retrospective review of patients less than thirty years of age: A report of Children's Cancer Study Group. Cancer 47:360, 1981.
126. Jenkin D, Chan H, et al: Hodgkin's disease in children: Treatment results with MOPP and low-dose, extended-field irradiation. Cancer Treat Rep 66:949, 1982.
127. Jereb B, Huvos AG, et al: Nasopharyngeal carcinoma in children: Review of 16 cases. Int J Radiat Oncol Biol Phys 6:487, 1980.
128. Jha BK, Lamba PA: Proptosis as a manifestation of acute myeloid leukemia. Br J Ophthalmol 55:844, 1971.
129. Jones SE, Coltman CA Jr, et al: Conclusions from clinical trials of the Southwest Oncology Group. Cancer Treat Rep 66:847, 1982.
130. Kahn HJ, Herman Y, et al: Immunohistochemical and electron microscopic assessment of childhood rhabdomyosarcoma, increased frequency of diagnosis over routine histologic methods. Cancer 51:1897, 1983.
131. Kaplan HS: Evidence for tumoricidal dose level in the radiotherapy of Hodgkin's disease. Cancer Res 26:1221, 1966.
132. Kapoor S, Kapoor MS, et al: Orbital hemangiopericytoma: A report of a three-year-old child. J Pediatr Ophthalmol Strabismus 15:40, 1978.
133. Karmody CS, Fortson JK, Calcaterra VE: Lymphangiomas of the head and neck in adults. Otolaryngol Head Neck Surg 90:283, 1982.
134. Kaufman FR, Roe TF, Isaacs H Jr: Metastatic medullary thyroid carcinoma in young children with mucosal neuroma syndrome. Pediatrics 70:263, 1982.
135. Kauffman SL, Stout AP: Hemangiopericytoma in children. Cancer 13:695, 1960.
136. Kim KS, Rogers LF, Weinberg PE: Intradiploic neural heterotopia. Rare calvarial defect. Radiology 125:425, 1977.

137. Kirkland RT, Kirkland JL, et al: Solitary thyroid nodules in 30 children and report of a child with a thyroid abscess. Pediatrics 51:85, 1973.
138. Kirks DR: Practical Pediatric Imaging; Diagnostic Radiology of Infants and Children. Boston, Little, Brown and Company, 1984.
139. Kjeldsberg CR, Wilson JF, Berard CW: Non-Hodgkin's lymphoma in children. Hum Pathol 14:612, 1983.
140. Komp DM: Long-term sequelae of histiocytosis X. Am J Pediatr Hematol Oncol 3:165, 1981.
141. Komp DM, Herson J, Starling KA, et al: A staging system for histiocytosis X: A Southwest Oncology Group Study. Cancer 47:798, 1981.
142. Koudstaal J, Oldhoff J, Panders AK, Hardank MJ: Melanotic neuroectodermal tumor of infancy. Cancer 22:151, 1968.
143. Kricheff II, Pinto RS, et al: Air-CT cisternography and canalography for small acoustic neuromas. AJNR 1:57, 1980.
144. Lahey ME: Histiocytosis X—analysis of prognostic factor. J Pediatr 87:184, 1975.
145. Lahey ME: Histiocytosis X—comparison of three treatment regimens. J Pediatr 87:179, 1975.
146. Lahey ME: Prognostic factors in histiocytosis X. Am J Pediatr Hematol Oncol 3:57, 1981.
147. Lahey ME: Prognosis in reticuloendotheliosis in children. J Pediatr 60:664, 1962.
148. Larson RA, Ultmann JE: The strategic role of laparotomy in staging Hodgkin's disease. Cancer Treat Rep 66:767, 1982.
149. Leape LL, Lowman JT, Loveland GC: Multifocal nondisseminated neuroblastoma. Report of two cases in siblings. J Pediatr 92:75, 1978.
150. Lee CK, Bloomfield DC, Goldman AI, et al: Prognostic significance of mediastinal involvement in Hodgkin's disease treated with curative radiotherapy. Cancer 46:2403, 1980.
151. Leipzig B, Rabuzzi DD: Recurrent massive cystic lymphangioma. Otolaryngology 86:758, 1978.
152. Leite C, Goodwin JW, Sinkovics JG, et al: Chemotherapy of malignant fibrous histiocytoma: A Southwest Oncology Group report. Cancer 40:2010, 1977.
153. Leonida JC, Brill PW, Bhan I, et al: Cystic retroperitoneal lymphangioma in infants and children. Radiology 127:203, 1978.
154. Levey M: Hemangioma of the nasal septum. Int Surg 61:344, 1976.
155. Leviton A, Davidson R, Gilles F: Neurologic manifestations of embryonal rhabdomyosarcoma of the middle ear cleft. J Pediatr 80:596, 1972.
156. Lichtenstein L: Histiocytosis X; integration of eosinophilic granuloma of bone, Letterer-Siwe disease, and Schüller-Christian disease as related manifestations of a single nosologic entity. Arch Pathol 56:84, 1953.
157. Lieberman PH, Foote FW Jr, et al: Alveolar soft-part sarcoma. JAMA 198:1047, 1966.
158. Lombardi F, Gasparini M, Gianni C, et al: Nasopharyngeal carcinoma in childhood. Med Pediatr Oncol 10:243, 1982.
159. Lukes RJ, Butler JJ: The pathology and nomenclature of Hodgkin's disease. Cancer Res 26:1063, 1966.
160. Lukes RJ, Craver LF, Hall TC, et al: Report of the nomenclature committee. Cancer Res 26:1311, 1966.
161. Lund BA: Nonodontogenic tumors of the jawbones. In Stafne EC, Gibilisco JA (eds): Oral Roentgenographic Diagnosis. 4th ed. Philadelphia, W. B. Saunders Co., 1975.
162. MacMahon B: Epidemiology of Hodgkin's disease. Cancer Res 26:1189, 1966.
163. Magrath I, Lee YJ, et al: Prognostic factors in Burkitt's lymphoma: Importance of total tumor burden. Cancer 45:1507, 1980.
164. Mann RB, Jaffe ES, Berard CW: Malignant lymphomas—a conceptual understanding of morphologic diversity. A review. Am J Pathol 94:105, 1979.
165. Manolov G, Manolova Y: Marker band in one chromosome 14 from Burkitt lymphomas. Nature 237:33, 1972.
166. Mauch P, Goodman R, Hellman S: The significance of mediastinal involvement in early stage Hodgkin's disease. Cancer 42:1039, 1978.
167. Mauch P, Gorshein D, et al: Influence of mediastinal adenopathy on site and frequency of relapse in patients with Hodgkin's disease. Cancer Treat Rep 66:809, 1982.
168. Maurer HM: The Intergroup Rhabdomyosarcoma Study II: Objectives and study design. J Pediatr Surg 15:371, 1980.
169. Maurer HM: The intergroup rhabdomyosarcoma study: update, November 1978. Natl Cancer Inst Monogr 56:61, 1981.
170. McCaffrey TV, McDonald TJ: Histiocytosis X of the ear and temporal bone: Review of 22 cases. Laryngoscope 89:1735, 1979.
171. McCormick CC: Computed tomography of the maxillary antra and

adjacent regions. Normal anatomy and its alteration by pathological processes. Australas Radiol 24:7, 1980.
172. McCormick MV, Hogg DS, Chrystal V, Cook MRB: Melanotic neuro-ectodermal tumour of infancy: A case report. J Laryngol Otol 97:755, 1983.
173. McDougall IR, Coleman CN, et al: Thyroid carcinoma after high-dose external radiotherapy for Hodgkin's disease. Report of three cases. Cancer 45:2056, 1980.
174. McGahan JP, Osborn RA, Dublin AB, et al: CT of eosinophilic granuloma of the skull with sonographic correlation. Am J Neurol 1:576, 1980.
175. Meissner WA, Warren S: Tumors of the Thyroid Gland. Atlas of Tumor Pathology. Armed Forces Institute of Pathology, Washington, D.C., 1969.
176. Mierau GW, Favara BE: Rhabdomyosarcoma in children: Ultrastructural study of 31 cases. Cancer 46:2035, 1980.
177. Miller EM, Norman D: Role of computed tomography in the evaluation of neck masses. Radiology 133:145, 1979.
178. Miller EM, Norman D: The role of computed tomography in the evaluation of neck masses. Radiology 133:145, 1979.
179. Mitelman F: Marker chromosome 14q+ in human cancer and leukemia. Adv Cancer Res 34:141, 1981.
180. Mitnick JS, Pinto RS: Computed tomography in the diagnosis of eosinophilic granuloma. J Comput Assist Tomogr 4:791, 1980.
181. Morales A, McGoey J: Pilomatrixoma: Treatment by incision and curettement. J Am Acad Dermatol 2:44, 1980.
182. Motoi M, Helbron D, Kaiserling E, et al: Eosinophilic granuloma of lymph nodes—a variant of histiocytosis X. Histopathology 4:585, 1980.
183. Murphy SB: Classification, staging and end results of treatment of childhood non-Hodgkin's lymphomas: Dissimilarities from lymphomas in adults. Semin Oncol 7:332, 1980.
184. Naegele RF, Champion J, Murphy S: Nasopharyngeal carcinoma in American children: Epstein-Barr virus—specific antibody titers and prognosis. Int J Cancer 29:209, 1982.
185. Nance FL, Fonseca RJ, Burkes EJ Jr: Technetium bone imaging as an adjunct in the management of fibrous dysplasia. Oral Surg 50:199, 1980.
186. Newton WA Jr, Hamoudi AB: Histiocytosis; a histologic classification with clinical correlation. In Rosenberg AS, Bolande RP (eds): Perspectives in Pediatric Pathology. Vol 1. Chicago, Year Book Medical Publishers, 1973.
187. Nirodi NS, Gowrinath K, Onuora CA: Histiocytosis X of the nose. J Laryngol Otol 93:193, 1979.
188. Norris DG, Burgert EO Jr, Cooper HA, et al: Hodgkin's disease in children. Blood 40:974, 1972.
189. Ochi H, Sawa H, Fukuda T, et al: Thallium-201 chloride thyroid scintigraphy to evaluate benign and/or malignant nodules: usefulness of the delayed scan. Cancer 50:236, 1982.
190. Ochs HD, Davis SD, et al: Combined immunodeficiency and reticuloendotheliosis with eosinophilia. J Pediatr 85:463, 1974.
191. O'Grady RB, Spoerl G: Pilomatrixoma (benign calcifying epithelioma of Malherbe). Ophthalmology (Rochester) 88:1196, 1981.
192. Osband ME, Lipton JM, et al: Histiocytosis X. Demonstration of abnormal immunity, T-cell histamine H2-receptor deficiency, and successful treatment with thymic extract. N Engl J Med 304:146, 1981.
193. Osborn DA: Haemangiomas of the nose. J Laryngol Otol 73:174, 1959.
194. Pedersen-Bjergaard J, Larsen SO: Incidence of acute nonlymphocytic leukemia, preleukemia and acute myeloproliferative syndrome up to 10 years after treatment of Hodgkin's disease. N Engl J Med 307:965, 1982.
195. Perez RC, Nicholson DH: Malherbe's calcifying epithelioma (pilomatrixoma) of the eyelid. Clinical features (clinical conference). Arch Ophthalmol 97:314, 1979.
196. Phillips HE, McGahan JP: Intrauterine fetal cystic hygromas; sonographic detection. AJR 136:799, 1981.
197. Pick T, Maurer HM, McWilliams NB: Lymphoepithelioma in childhood. J Pediatr 84:96, 1974.
198. Pilla TJ, Wolverson MK, Sundaram M, et al: CT evaluation of cystic lymphangiomas of the mediastinum. Radiology 144:841, 1982.
199. Poppema S, Lennert K: Hodgkin's disease in childhood. Histopathologic classification in relation to age and sex. Cancer 45:1443, 1980.
200. Raney RB Jr, Handler SD: Management of neoplasms of the head and neck in children. II. Malignant tumors. Head Neck Surg 3:500, 1981.
201. Raney RB Jr, Lawrence W Jr, et al: Rhabdomyosarcoma of the ear

in childhood. A report from the Intergroup Rhabdomyosarcoma Study—I. Cancer 51:2356, 1983.

202. Raney RB Jr, Tefft M, et al: Results of intensive treatment of children with cranial parameningeal sarcoma: A report from the Intergroup Rhabdomyosarcoma Study (IRS). Proc Am Assoc Cancer Res 23:120, 1983.

203. Ravitch MM, Rush BF: Cystic hygroma. In Ravitch MM, Welch KJ, Benson CD, et al (eds): Pediatric Surgery. 3rd ed. Chicago, Year Book Medical Publishers, 1979.

204. Reiter EO, Root AW, Rettig K, et al: Childhood thyromegaly: Recent developments. J Pediatr 99:507, 1981.

205. Resnick D, Niwayama G: Diagnosis of Bone and Joint Disorders: With Emphasis on Articular Abnormalities. Philadelphia, W. B. Saunders Co., 1981.

206. Rice DH, Coulthard SW: Neurogenic tumors of the head and neck in children. Ann Plastic Surg 2:441, 1978.

207. Roberson GH, Price AC, Davis JM: Therapeutic embolization of juvenile angiofibroma. AJR 133:657, 1979.

208. Rogers JH, Fredrickson JM, Noyek AM: Management of cysts, benign tumors, and bony dysplasia of the maxillary sinus. Otolaryngol Clin North Am 9:233, 1976.

209. Romansky SG, Crocker DW, Shaw KN: Ultrastructural studies on neuroblastoma: Evaluation of cytodifferentiation and correlation of morphology and biochemical and survival data. Cancer 42:2392, 1978.

210. Roper M, Crist WM, Metzgar R, et al: Monoclonal antibody characterization of surface antigens in childhood T-cell lymphoid malignancies. Blood 61:830, 1983.

211. Rosenberg HS, Stenback WA, Spjut HJ: The fibromatoses of infancy and childhood. Perspect Pediatr Pathol 4:269, 1978.

212. Rosenberg SA: Hodgkin's disease of the bone marrow. Cancer Res 31:1733, 1971.

213. Rosenberg SA: Place of splenectomy in evaluation and management. JAMA 222:1296, 1972.

214. Rosengren JE, Jing BS, Wallace S, et al: Radiographic features of olfactory neuroblastoma. AJR 132:945, 1979.

215. Roskos RR, Evans RC, et al: Prognostic significance of mediastinal mass in childhood Hodgkin's disease. Cancer Treat Rep 66:961, 1982.

216. Roth JA, Enzinger FM, Tannenbaum R: Synovial sarcoma of the neck; a follow up study of 24 cases. Cancer 35:1243, 1975.

217. Russell CF, Van Heerden JA, Sizemore GW, et al: The surgical management of medullary thyroid carcinoma. Ann Surg 197:42, 1983.

218. Samuel E, Lloyd G: Clinical Radiology of the Ear, Nose and Throat. 2nd ed. Philadelphia, W. B. Saunders Co., 1978.

219. Santoro A, Bonfante V, Bonadonna G: Salvage chemotherapy with ABVD in MOPP-resistant Hodgkin's disease. Ann Intern Med 96:139, 1982.

220. Schloss MD, Klein A, Black MJ: Histiocytosis X of the head and neck. J Otolaryngol 10:189, 1981.

221. Schuller DE, Lawrence TL, Newton WA Jr: Childhood rhabdomyosarcomas of the head and neck. Arch Otolaryngol 105:689, 1979.

222. Scott MD, Crawford JD: Solitary thyroid nodules in childhood: Is the incidence of thyroid carcinoma declining? Pediatrics 58:521, 1976.

223. Scotti G, Harwood-Nash DC: Computed tomography of rhabdomyosarcomas of the skull base in children. J Comput Assist Tomogr 6:33, 1982.

224. Sessions RB, Bryan RN, Naclerio RM, et al: Radiographic staging of juvenile angiofibroma. Head Neck Surg 3:279, 1981.

225. Sessions RB, Wills PI, Alford BR, et al: Juvenile nasopharyngeal angiofibroma: Radiographic aspects. Laryngoscope 86:2, 1976.

226. Shanmugaratnam K, et al: Histopathology of nasopharyngeal carcinoma correlations with epidemiology, survival rates and other biological characteristics. Cancer 44:1029, 1979.

227. Shmookler BM, Enzinger FM: Liposarcoma occurring in children. An analysis of seventeen cases and review of the literature. Cancer 52:567, 1983.

228. Silverman PM, Korobkin M, Moore AV: CT diagnosis of cystic hygroma of the neck. J Comput Assist Tomogr 7:519, 1983.

229. Silverman SH, Nussbaum M, Rausen AR: Thyroid nodules in children: A ten year experience at one institution. Mt Sinai J Med (NY) 46:460, 1979.

230. Smith L, Gooding CA: Pulmonary involvement in laryngeal papillomatosis. Pediatr Radiol 2:161, 1974.

231. Snow JB Jr: Carcinoma of the nasopharynx in children. Ann Otol Rhinol Laryngol 84:817, 1975.

232. Som PM, Cohen BA, Sacher M, et al: The angiomatous polyp and the angiofibroma: Two different lesions. Radiology 144:329, 1982.

233. Soule EH, Enriquez P: Atypical fibrous histiocytoma, malignant fibrous histiocytoma, malignant histiocytoma, and epithelioid sarcoma. Cancer 30:128, 1972.

234. Soule EH, Mahour GH, Mills SD, et al: Soft-tissue sarcomas of infants and children: A clinicopathologic study of 135 cases. Mayo Clin Proc 43:313, 1968.

235. Soule EH, Pritchard DJ: Fibrosarcoma in infants and children: A review of 110 cases. Cancer 40:1711, 1977.

236. Stafne EC, Gibilisco JA: Oral Roentgenographic Diagnosis. 4th ed. Philadelphia, W. B. Saunders Co., 1975.

237. Starling KA, Donaldson MH, et al: Therapy of histiocytosis X with vincristine, vinblastine, and cyclophosphamide. The Southwest Cancer Chemotherapy Study Group. Am J Dis Child 123:105, 1972.

238. Starling KA, Iyer R, et al: Chlorambucil in histiocytosis X: A Southwest Oncology Group study. J Pediatr 96:266, 1980.

239. Stein RS, Golomb HM, Wiernik PH, et al: Anatomic substages of stage IIIA Hodgkin's disease: Follow-up of a collaborative study. Cancer Treat Rep 66:733, 1982.

240. Stjernholm MR, Freudenbourg JC, et al: Medullary carcinoma of the thyroid before age 2 years. J Clin Endocrinol Metab 51:252, 1980.

241. Stout AP: Fibrosarcoma in infants and children. Cancer 15:1028, 1962.

242. Strong MS, Vaughn CW, Healy GB: Recurrent respiratory papillomatosis. In Healy GB, McGill TJ (eds): Laryngo-tracheal Problems in the Pediatric Patient. Springfield, Charles C Thomas, Publisher, 1979.

243. Suit HD, Russell WO, Martin RG: Sarcoma of soft tissue: Clinical and histopathologic parameters and response to treatment. Cancer 35:1478, 1975.

244. Sullivan MP, Fuller LM, et al: Intergroup Hodgkin's disease in children study of Stages I and II: A preliminary report. Cancer Treat Rep 66:937, 1982.

245. Sutcliffe SB, Wrigley PF, et al: Posttreatment laparotomy as a guide to management in patients with Hodgkin's disease. Cancer Treat Rep 66:759, 1982.

246. Sutow WW: Cancer of the head and neck in children. JAMA 190:414, 1964.

247. Sutow WW, Lindberg RD, Gehan EA, et al: Three-year relapse-free survival rates in childhood rhabdomyosarcoma of the head and neck: Report from the Intergroup Rhabdomyosarcoma Study. Cancer 49:2217, 1982.

248. Sutow WW, Sullivan MP, Ried HL, et al: Prognosis in childhood rhabdomyosarcoma. Cancer 25:1384, 1970.

249. Swank RL, Fetterman GE, et al: Prognostic factors in neuroblastoma. Ann Surg 174:428, 1971.

250. Tannenbaum M: Ultrastructural pathology of adrenal medullary tumors. Pathol Annu 5:145, 1970.

251. Tefft M, Fernandez C, Donaldson M, et al: Incidence of meningeal involvement by rhabdomyosarcoma of the head and neck in children: A report of the Intergroup Rhabdomyosarcoma Study (IRS). Cancer 42:253, 1978.

252. Tefft M, Lindberg RD, et al: Radiation therapy combined with systemic chemotherapy of rhabdomyosarcoma in children: Local control in patients enrolled in the Intergroup Rhabdomyosarcoma Study. Natl Cancer Inst Monogr 56:75, 1981.

253. Thomas RL: Computed tomography in the assessment of patients with juvenile post-nasal angiofibroma. J Otolaryngol 9:334, 1980.

254. Towbin R, Bove K, Dunbar JS: Antrochoanal polyps. AJR 132:27, 1979.

255. Ultmann JE, Cunningham JK, Gellhorn A: The clinical picture of Hodgkin's disease. Cancer Res 26:1047, 1966.

256. Valagussa P, Santoro A, Bellani F, et al: Absence of treatment-induced second neoplasms after ABVD in Hodgkin's disease. Blood 59:488, 1982.

257. Vanel D, Couanet D, Micheau C, et al: Pseudotumoral fibrous dysplasia of the maxilla: Radiological studies and computed tomography contribution. Skeletal Radiol 5:99, 1980.

258. Weiss SW, Enzinger FM: Malignant fibrous histiocytoma: An analysis of 200 cases. Cancer 41:2250, 1978.

259. Whitehead E, Shalet SM, Blackledge G, et al: The effects of Hodgkin's disease and combination chemotherapy on gonadal function in the adult male. Cancer 49:418, 1982.

260. Wiernik PH, Serpick AA: Granulocytic sarcoma (chloroma). Blood 35:361, 1970.

261. Winship T, Rosvoll RV: Childhood thyroid carcinoma. Cancer 14:734, 1961.

262. Winship T, Rosvoll RV: Thyroid carcinoma in childhood: Final report on a 20 year study. Clinical Proceedings of the Children's Hospital of Washington, D.C. *26*:327, 1970.

263. Withers EH, Rosenfeld L, et al: Long-term experience with childhood thyroid carcinoma. J Pediatr Surg *14*:332, 1979.

264. Wollner N, Exelby PR, Lieberman PH: Non-Hodgkin's lymphoma in children. A progress report on the original patients treated with the LSA$_2$-L$_2$ protocol. Cancer *44*:1990, 1979.

265. Wolner N, Burchenal JH, et al: Non-Hodgkin's lymphoma in children. A comparative study of two modalities of therapy. Cancer *37*:123, 1976.

266. Wong KY, Hanenson IB, Lampkin BC: Familial neuroblastoma. Am J Dis Child *121*:415, 1971.

267. Work WP: Hemangiomas of the head and neck. Ann Otol Rhinol Laryngol *87*:633, 1978.

268. Worth HM: Principles and Practice of Oral Radiologic Interpretation. Chicago, Year Book Medical Publishers, 1963.

269. Wright BA, Jackson D: Neural tumors of the oral cavity. A review of the spectrum of benign and malignant oral tumors of the oral cavity and jaws. Oral Surg *49*:509, 1980.

270. Yarrington CT Jr: Tumors and cysts of the oral cavity. *In* Paparella MM, Shumrick DA (eds): Otolaryngology. 2nd ed. Philadelphia, W. B. Saunders Co., 1980.

271. Yeh S: A histological classification of carcinomas of the nasopharynx with a critical review as to the existence of lymphoepitheliomas. Cancer *15*:895, 1962.

272. Young CW, Straus DJ, Myers J, et al: Multidisciplinary treatment of advanced Hodgkin's disease by an alternating chemotherapeutic regimen of MOPP/ABVD and low-dose radiation therapy restricted to originally bulky disease. Cancer Treat Rep *66*:907, 1982.

273. Young JL Jr, Miller RW: Incidence of malignant tumors in U.S. in children. J Pediatr *86*:254, 1975.

274. Young LW, Rubin P, Hanson RE: The extra-adrenal neuroblastoma; high radiocurability and diagnostic accuracy. AJR *108*:75, 1970.

275. Ziegler JL: Burkitt's lymphoma. N Engl J Med *305*:735, 1981.

276. Ziegler JL: Treatment results of 54 American patients with Burkitt's lymphoma are similar to the African experience. N Engl J Med *297*:75, 1977.

277. Zimmerman RA, Bilaniuk LT, Littman P: Computed tomography of pediatric craniofacial sarcoma. CT *2*:113, 1978.

278. Zimmerman RA, Bilaniuk LT, Metzger RA, et al: Computer tomography of orbital facial neurofibromatosis. Radiology *146*:113 1983.

CHAPTER 71

Lymphoreticular Disorders of the Head and Neck

PATHOLOGY OF LYMPHORETICULAR DISORDERS

Kenneth D. McClatchey, D.D.S., M.D. • Bertram Schnitzer, M.D.

A discussion of lymphoreticular disorders of the head and neck region centers on three areas: (1) reactive lesions, (2) non-Hodgkin's lymphomas, and (3) Hodgkin's disease. This discussion also requires a thorough understanding of lymph node anatomy, including such areas as afferent and efferent lymphatics, subcapsular sinus, radiating sinus, interfollicular areas, follicular mantle, and follicular center. Individual cells within these anatomic areas are characterized according to size, immunologic markers (T cell, B cell), cellular enzymes, electron microscopy, and even cytogenetic studies. The combination of pattern and cellular characteristics has been the foundation of morphologic diagnosis of lymphoreticular disorders.

REACTIVE LYMPHORETICULAR DISORDERS

Nonspecific Follicular Hyperplasia

Lymph node enlargement in children and adolescents is most often due to follicular hyperplasia associated with an unknown immune stimulus. The histomorphologic picture consists of a variable number of enlarged follicles throughout the lymph node with or without sinus histiocytosis. The enlargement and even coalescence of the follicles is associated with increased numbers of follicle center cells, which include cleaved and noncleaved (transformed) lymphocytes, tingible body macrophages, and even occasional plasma cells. An often important feature of reactive follicles seen at low-magnification microscopy is the sharp demarcation of the follicle center from the surrounding mantle of small lymphocytes (Fig. 71–1). These histologic features are associated with two diseases in adults: (1) rheumatoid arthritis and (2) syphilis.

Giant Lymph Node Hyperplasia

Castleman first described giant lymph node hyperplasia as a lesion of the mediastinum.[7] Other solitary anatomic locations since described for this lesion include cervical and axillary regions, skeletal muscle, pulmonary parenchyma, abdomen, and retroperitoneum.[24] We have recently seen a case of giant lymph node hyperplasia in the pelvis of a young woman. Multiple lymph node sites as well as lesions of the spleen have been reported.[14, 15] In all reported cases, there has been no sex preference or specific age group affected.

Two histomorphologic types of giant lymph node hyperplasia are recognized:

1. The *hyaline vascular type* (80 per cent) has numerous small follicular centers, which have variable numbers of small hyalinized capillaries, radially arranged, penetrating the follicles. The interfollicular areas contain numerous prominent capillaries. Most of the cells in the interfollicular region are lymphocytes. A few plasma cells and eosinophils are found. The vast majority of the patients are asymptomatic except for compression or other symptoms associated with the mass.

2. The *plasma cell type* (20 per cent) has large hyperplastic follicle centers (not unlike those seen in follicular hyperplasia associated with rheumatoid arthritis) associated with sheets of plasma cells in the interfollicle zone.

The plasma cell type, in contrast to the hyaline vascular type, is often associated with clinical symptoms other than just the mass effect. Half of the patients will have hematologic abnormalities, including a syndrome of fever, anemia, and hypergammaglobulinemia.

Sinus Histiocytosis

Sinus histiocytosis is a common finding in lymph node biopsies associated with or without follicular hyperplasias. It is characterized by dilated subcapsular and trabecular sinuses partially or completely filled with histiocytes (macrophages). The histiocytes originate from sinus-lining cells. Sinus histiocytosis is often seen in lymph nodes draining inflammatory lesions or carcinoma.

Histomorphologically, the lesion is characterized by the presence of intrasinusoidal histiocytes with abundant cytoplasm and round to oval indented nuclei with a delicate chromatin pattern and an inconspicuous nucleolus. In addition, the histiocytes may contain phagocytized pigment such as carbon, tattoo pigment, and hemosiderin drained to the lymph node from adjacent areas.

Rosai and Dorfman described sinus histiocytosis with massive lymphodenopathy of unknown etiology.[39, 40] The disease is seen in young blacks (first and second decades) with a prolonged course, even years, and spontaneous regression. Laboratory findings include elevated erythrocyte sedimentation rate, polyclonal hypergammaglobulinemia, and neutrophilic leukocytosis.

Dermatopathic Lymphadenopathy

General exfoliative dermatitis is classically associated with lymph node enlargement histomorphologically characterized by paracortical expansion caused by a proliferation of large histiocytes (macrophages).[8, 19] The paracortical expansion may be so extreme as to compress follicles beneath the capsule. Because the lymph nodes affected are ones that drain the skin, lipid and melanin are often found in the histiocytes. The descriptive term "lipomelanotic reticulosis" has been used to define the process.[19]

Toxoplasmosis Lymphadenitis

Toxoplasmosis lymphadenitis exhibits itself as cervical lymph node enlargement, especially of the posterior triangle; it occurs usually on only one side. The patient often has a history of ingestion of raw or undercooked meat or contamination by cat feces. The striking histomorphologic features are (1) marked reactive follicular hyperplasia and (2) multiple small aggregates of epithelioid histiocytes within interfollicular areas (Fig. 71–2).[44]

In addition, the enlarged follicles contain abundant mitotic figures and a striking number of tingible body macrophages. The subcapsular and trabecular sinuses may be filled with atypical monocytoid cells.[10, 44] The parasites or "parasitic cysts" are rarely seen in the enlarged lymph nodes. The specific diagnosis is made by serologic assays, such as the IgM immunofluorescent antibody test. The differential diagnosis associated with toxoplasmosis includes sarcoidosis, mycobacterial infections, primary and secondary syphilis, Lennert's lymphoma, and even Hodgkin's disease.

Cat-Scratch Disease

Cat-scratch disease involves axillary or cervical lymph nodes and occurs 3 to 50 days (usually about 2 weeks) after a person is scratched by a cat or, less frequently, a dog. The characteristic histomorphologic picture includes centrally suppurative granulomas in the paracortex of the lymph node. These suppurative granulomas consist of irregular branching stellate abscesses surrounded by palisading histiocytes and fibroblasts.[51] Definitive diagnosis requires a clinical history, skin testing, and the presence of accompanying characteristic granulomas.

HODGKIN'S DISEASE

The lymphoma most commonly presenting as a painless cervical mass is Hodgkin's disease. The disease was first described in 1843 by Thomas Hodgkin.[17] Although persons of all ages can be affected, the disease has a bimodal age distribution, with an early cluster of patients in the 15- to 34-year age group and a second cluster of patients older than 55 years. Males are affected more often than females.

Rarely, extranodal involvement can be a presenting symptom. Typical sites for such involvement include the liver, spleen, bone marrow, and, very rarely, skin and intestines.

The histologic manifestations of Hodgkin's disease include a diverse admixture of neoplastic and non-neoplastic inflammatory cells characterized by malig-

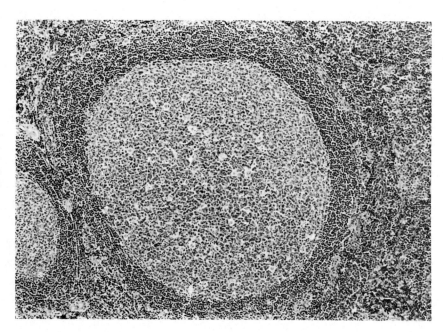

Figure 71–1. Reactive follicular hyperplasia showing a follicle center surrounded by a mantle of small lymphocytes. A "starry sky" appearance is evident in the follicle center. (H&E, ×20)

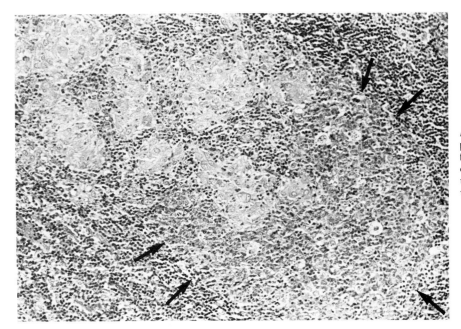

Figure 71–2. Toxoplasmosis lymphadenitis. A poorly demarcated follicle center (arrows) contains clusters of epithelioid histiocytes that are also present adjacent to the follicle. (H&E, ×20)

nant lymphoid cells and non-neoplastic inflammatory cells, such as lymphocytes, histiocytes, eosinophils, and plasma cells.

The Reed-Sternberg cell must be present for the diagnosis of Hodgkin's disease to be made. This classic cell is identified as a large cell with a bilobate nucleus, each lobe containing a large inclusion-like nucleolus. There also may be two nuclei, each containing a large nucleolus (Fig. 71–3). In either instance, fine strands of chromatin can be seen emanating from the nucleolus and condensed at the periphery beneath the nuclear membrane. It is important to note that the diagnosis of Hodgkin's disease should not be made unless bilobate, binucleate, or multinucleate Reed-Sternberg cells are

present (Fig. 71–4). Reed-Sternberg cells *alone* are not pathognomonic for Hodgkin's disease because similar cells can be seen in viral disorders, especially in infectious mononucleosis, in immunoblastic proliferations, in peripheral or node-base T-cell lymphomas, and in a variety of non-Hodgkin's lymphoma following therapy.[33, 43, 45, 52] A monoclonal antibody, Leu M1, is useful in identifying true Reed-Sternberg cells.[18]

The Rye modification of the Lukes and Butler classification of 1966 condensed the descriptive morphologic scheme into four prognostically significant types of Hodgkin's disease: (1) lymphocyte predominance, (2) nodular sclerosis, (3) mixed cellularity, and (4) lymphocyte depletion.[30, 32, 41] The most favorable prognosis is

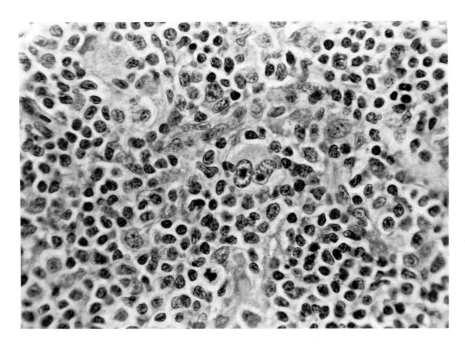

Figure 71–3. Hodgkin's disease showing binucleate Reed-Sternberg cell containing prominent nucleoli. (H&E, ×500)

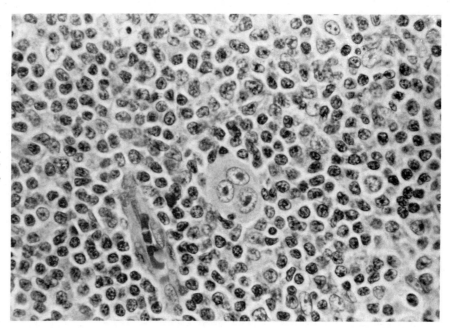

Figure 71—4. Trinucleate Reed-Sternberg cell, each nucleus containing a prominent nucleosis. (H&E, ×500)

associated with the lymphocyte-predominant type, and the least favorable prognosis is associated with the lymphocyte-depleted histologic form.

In lymphocyte-predominant Hodgkin's disease, the predominant cell is a small, mature-appearing lymphocyte. Admixed with the numerous lymphocytes are scattered histiocytes, some arranged in clusters. The malignant cell, the Reed-Sternberg cell, is rare. In addition, eosinophils and plasma cells are rarely present. This type of Hodgkin's disease may be confused histologically with well-differentiated lymphocytic lymphoma (chronic lymphocytic lymphoma), Lennert's lymphoma, and toxoplasmosis lymphadenopathy.

Nodular sclerosis Hodgkin's disease is the most frequent type of Hodgkin's disease in both adults and children. It is also the most common type seen in females. Histologically, there is an admixture of bands of collagen extending from the capsule into the lymph node and islands of abnormal lymphoreticular tissue containing numerous variants of Reed-Sternberg cells called lacunar cells. The lacunar cells are surrounded by clear spaces or lacunae, which are the result of fixation artifact.

As the name implies, mixed cellularity Hodgkin's disease is composed of a mixture of lymphocytes, eosinophils, plasma cells, neutrophils, and benign-appearing histiocytes. Reed-Sternberg cells and malignant-appearing mononuclear cells with cytologic features of Reed-Sternberg cells are easily found. Foci of necrosis and fibrosis are found, yet collagen bands are absent.

Mixed cellularity Hodgkin's disease must be differentiated from angioimmunoblastic lymphadenopathy and T-cell lymphomas, which may contain cells morphologically identical to Reed-Sternberg cells.

There are two types of lymphocyte depletion Hodgkin's disease: diffuse fibrosis and reticular. The diffuse fibrosis type is characterized by disorderly fibrosis, and the reticular pattern is characterized by a proliferation of malignant large cells ("histiocytes"). The malignant "histiocytes" are large, often bizarre, with prominent nucleoli. Reed-Sternberg cells are easily found. In addition to a depletion of lymphocytes in both the diffuse fibrosis or reticular pattern, areas of necrosis are often found. Many cases, which in the past have been diagnosed as lymphocyte depletion, are in fact non-Hodgkin's T-cell lymphomas. Immunologic studies are needed to make this differential diagnosis.

The clinicopathologic staging of Hodgkin's disease is most important in determining prognosis. Clinical staging includes initial biopsy, history, physical examination, laboratory tests, radiographic studies, and staging laparotomy.

NON-HODGKIN'S LYMPHOMA

It is commonly known that non-Hodgkin's lymphoma occurs in nodal and extranodal forms. In the head and neck region, extranodal presentation has an increased incidence owing to the presence of abundant lymphoid tissue, particularly in Waldeyer's ring.[11a] Supraclavicular manifestations of more generalized lymphomas in 1269 cases were noted by Rosenberg and associates to occur in 8.9 per cent of their cases.[42]

General anatomic locations and incidence are the most straightforward components of any discussion of non-Hodgkin's lymphoma; the more difficult component is the terminology of classifications and the derivation of the neoplastic cells.

The anatomic distribution of extranodal non-Hodgkin's lymphoma in the head and neck is as follows[42]:

1. Anterior nasal cavity and paranasal sinuses, 49 to 52 per cent.
2. Submandibular gland, 0 to 16 per cent.
3. Parotid gland, 10 to 23 per cent.
4. Thyroid gland, 0 to 8 per cent.
5. Orbit, 0 to 8 per cent.
6. Palate, 0 to 8 per cent.
7. Lip, 0 to 8 per cent.
8. Postauricular area, 0 to 8 per cent.

Most extranodal non-Hodgkin's lymphomas of the head and neck are histomorphologically defined as diffuse large-cell (histiocytic) lymphoma or diffuse, follicular, cleaved small-cell, poorly differentiated lymphocytic lymphoma.[48]

The staging of extranodal non-Hodgkin's lymphoma of the head and neck has shown that most cases at presentation are clinical stage IE or IIE. The actual staging of extranodal non-Hodgkin's lymphoma is as follows:

Stage IE: Single extranodal site.
Stage IIE: Localized involvement of an extranodal site and its contiguous lymph node.
Stage IIIE: Localized involvement of an extranodal site and involvement of lymph node regions on both sides of diaphragm.
Stage IV: Diffuse or disseminated involvement of more than one extranodal region with or without associated lymph node enlargement.

The 5-year survival for extranodal non-Hodgkin's lymphoma ranges from 60 to 70 per cent after regional radiotherapy. The disease-free survival after irradiation is less than 50 per cent for patients with stage IIE disease. Death in treatment failures is preceded by visceral (lungs, gastrointestinal tract) involvement.[12, 22]

In a recent publication on malignant lymphomas, Tindle states:

"Classification of tumors, in order to be useful, must have relevance in the clinical approach to the patient's treatment, must be easily reproducible among various diagnosticians to allow for universal acceptance and use of the terminology and should be scientifically correct as relates to current concepts of pathogenesis and etiology."[49]

Non-Hodgkin's lymphomas have undergone an evolution of classifications based on the continued increase in knowledge of the pathogenesis of lymphoreticular disease. As Tindle has noted, lymphocyte populations are now being identified cytologically as well as by immunologic and cytochemical methods, thus giving credibility to attempts to classify lymphomas on a functional basis.[50]

There are two classic cell lines in a discussion of lymphomas: (1) T cells, involved in cell-mediated immune mechanisms; and (2) B cells, involved in humoral immune mechanisms (antibody production). Both cell lines are derived from stem cells in the bone marrow. T-cell differentiation comes under the influence of the thymus, and B-cell differentiation comes under the influence of the bursa equivalent.

Not long ago, the pathologist's interpretation of well-prepared tissue was the only means of lymphoma classification. In the last 15 years or so, there has been a steady evolution of laboratory methods to ascertain specific monoclonicity.[34]

In the past, B-cell abnormalities have been defined using antiglobulin to cell surface immunoglobulins. Specific testing involves, first, polyvalent immunoglobulin antiserum, and if an abnormality is found, this is followed by antisera specific for the kappa and lambda light chains. Both immunofluorescence and immunoperoxidase methodologies can be used in detecting surface immunoglobulins, with the immunoperoxidase technique having the advantage of availability for use on paraffin-embedded tissue. Classically, in the past, T-cell abnormalities have been identified by the E rosette method, a technique in which sheep red blood cells rosette around human T lymphocytes in response to a poorly defined membrane marker system.

Electron microscopy has continued to be useful in defining poorly differentiated lymphoreticular disorders, especially subtle cytoplasmic or surface membrane abnormalities.

Nuclear enzymes, such as the enzyme terminal deoxynucleotidyl transferase (TdT), have been used to identify lymphoreticular "blast" forms or cells best identified as stem cells.[5] The enzyme TdT is especially useful in confirming a diagnosis of an aggressive thymus-derived lymphoblastic lymphoma.[5]

In the last several years, the advent of certain developments has brought on a rapid redefinition of lymphoreticular abnormalities, both benign and malignant[29]: (1) better defined immunoperoxidase techniques, (2) specific monoclonal antibodies to T-cell and B-cell subsets, as well as to myeloid and monocytic cells, and (3) reliable clinical flow cytometry equipment.

Using all these diagnostic techniques, then, lymphoma diagnosis still begins with an anatomic and histomorphologic tissue examination. In contrast to the classification of Hodgkin's disease, which is universally accepted, there remains considerable controversy and confusion about the histologic classifications of non-Hodgkin's lymphomas. The classification of Rappaport is familiar to most pathologists, surgeons specializing in the head and neck, and oncologists.[37] This classification was reproducible by pathologists and was of considerable clinical relevance as far as choosing appropriate therapeutic regimens and predicting prognoses was concerned. Since the institution of the Rappaport classification, our knowledge about the function and immunology of cells of the lymphoreticular system, which is the anatomic arm of the functional immune system, has been vastly expanded. The increased knowledge of the biology of lymphoid cells resulted in a rash of new classification schemes in the mid-1970s.[4, 9, 16, 28, 31] Clinicians and pathologists became alarmed and confused by the number of new classifications and by the many different and often strange terms applied to various subgroups in the new schemes. The National Cancer Institute, therefore, sponsored and organized a large-scale, international, multi-institutional clinicopathologic study of 1175 cases of non-Hodgkin's lymphomas to evaluate the various new classification schemes and to attempt to develop a unifying scheme.[35] The results of this study resulted in a "Working Formulation for Clinical Usage." This formulation was not proposed as yet another new classification but as a means of translating the terms of the other classifications so that reports of case studies and clinical trials from medical centers throughout the world could be compared with each other.[27] This new formulation is illustrated in the following discussion.

Histomorphologic Classification of Lymphomas

In contrast to previous classification systems, the new formulation is divided into three distinct, prognostically significant subgroups: (1) low grade, (2) intermediate grade, and (3) high grade. Lymphomas of low grade are generally associated with a relatively good prog-

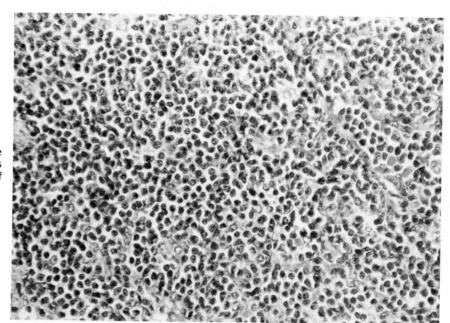

Figure 71–5. Diffuse lymphoma. The architecture of the lymph node is effaced by a diffuse proliferation of neoplastic cells. (H&E, ×200)

nosis, those of high grade have a poor outlook, and those of the intermediate group are associated with a survival rate between the two. There are ten major subtypes within the three groups, and there is also a miscellaneous group within groups 1 and 2: the lymphomas have either a diffuse (Fig. 71–5) or a follicular (Fig. 71–6) pattern.

Low-Grade Lymphomas

Malignant lymphoma, small lymphocytic (lymphocytic, well-differentiated[37]; small lymphocytic, plasmacytoid[31]): Of 1175 cases, 41 (3.6 per cent) had the histologic features of this type of lymphoma. The median age of

the patients was 60.5 years. Median survival was 5.8 years, and the 5-year survival rate was 59 per cent. Histologically, the pattern is diffuse, and the lymph node architecture is effaced by small lymphocytes with round to oval nuclei with clumped chromatin and absent or inconspicuous nucleoli (Fig. 71–7). Mitotic figures are few or absent. These histologic features are identical to those seen in tissue involved by chronic lymphocytic leukemia. Immunologically, the vast majority of these cells are B-cell neoplasms.

In a variant of the small lymphocytic type, varying numbers of cells have plasmacytoid features (lymphoid plasma cells). The nuclei are eccentrically placed in amphophilic cytoplasm (Fig. 71–8), and these cells may

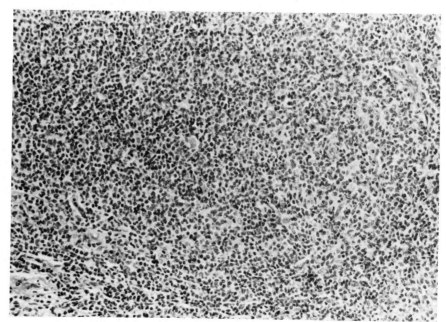

Figure 71–6. Follicular (nodular) lymphoma. The neoplastic small cleaved cells are arranged in a follicular pattern. (H&E, ×200)

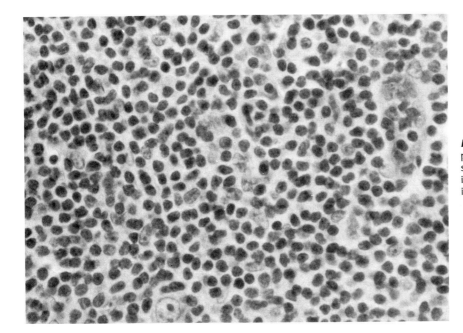

Figure 71–7. Diffuse small-cell lymphocytic lymphoma characterized by small cells with round nuclei containing aggregated chromatin and invisible nucleoli. (H&E, ×800)

have intranuclear or cytoplasmic inclusions (Dutcher bodies and Russell bodies). The patients may have monoclonal immunoglobulinemia.

Malignant lymphoma, follicular, predominantly small-cell, cleaved (nodular, poorly differentiated lymphocytic;[37] small-cell, cleaved, follicular center, follicular or follicular and diffuse[31]): This was the most common histologic type, found in 259 cases (22.5 per cent). The median age of the patients was 54.3 years, the median survival was 7.2 years, and the 5-year survival was 70 per cent. Either the histologic pattern was completely follicular (nodular), or both follicular and diffuse areas were present. The follicles are generally fairly uniform in size and shape, and most are surrounded by a mantle of

lymphocytes. The neoplastic cells are slightly larger than those of normal lymphocytes, and their nuclei are irregular and have varying numbers of clefts (Fig. 71–6). The chromatin is clumped, and nucleoli are inconspicuous. Mitoses are few. As all follicular lymphomas arise from follicle centers, which are B-cell areas, these neoplasms are always composed of B cells.

Malignant lymphoma, follicular, mixed small-cell cleaved and large-cell (nodular, mixed lymphocytic-histiocytic;[37] small-cell, cleaved, follicle center, follicular or large-cell, cleaved follicle center[31]): Eighty-nine cases (7.7 per cent) had this histologic appearance. The median age of the patients was 56.1 years. The median survival was 5.1 years, and the 5-year survival was 50 per cent. In this

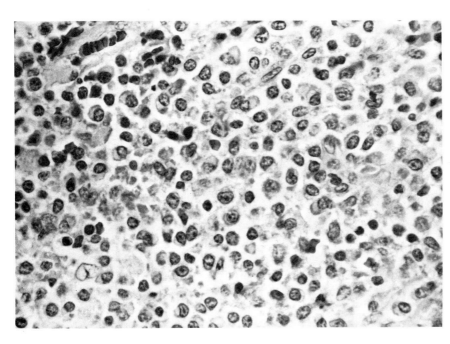

Figure 71–8. Diffuse small lymphocytic lymphoma with plasmacytoid features. (H&E, ×800)

category, the neoplastic follicles contain both small cleaved lymphocytes and large cleaved and noncleaved cells. There is no clear preponderance of either cell type. The large lymphocytes have vesicular nuclei, with one to three nucleoli often adjacent to the nuclear membrane; the small cells have cleaved nuclei. Diffuse areas may be present.

Intermediate-Grade Lymphomas

Malignant lymphoma, follicular, predominantly large-cell (nodular histiocytic;[37] large-cell or noncleaved follicular center, follicular[31]): Forty-four (3.8 per cent) cases had this histologic picture. The median age of these patients was 55.4 years. The median survival was 45 per cent. Most of the cells within the neoplastic follicles are large with either cleaved or noncleaved nuclei. In most cases, the nuclei are predominantly noncleaved. In many cases, diffuse areas are present. Mitotic figures are often numerous. Thin bands of fibrous tissue (sclerosis) resulting in compartmentalization of tumor cells are not unusual, especially in the diffuse areas.

Malignant lymphoma, diffuse small-cell cleaved (diffuse lymphocytic, poorly differentiated[37]; small-cell, cleaved follicular center, diffuse[31]): Seventy-nine cases (6.9 per cent) were of this histologic type. The median age of these patients was 57.9 years. Median survival was 3.4 years, and 5-year survival was 33 per cent. This lymphoma is most likely the diffuse counterpart of the follicular, small-cell cleaved type. Cytologically, the cells are identical (Fig. 71–9). The mitotic rate may be higher than that seen in the follicular type. The majority of these lymphomas are B-cell neoplasms. Occasional cases are T-cell lymphomas.

Malignant lymphoma, diffuse, mixed small- and large-cell (diffuse, mixed lymphocytic-histiocytic[37]; small-cell cleaved, large-cell cleaved, or large-cell noncleaved, follicle center, diffuse[31]): Fifty-seven patients (6.7 per cent of cases) had this histologic appearance. Median age was 58 years. The median survival was 2.7 years,

and the 5-year survival was 28 per cent. Some of these cases represent the diffuse counterpart of the follicular type of mixed small-cell cleaved and large-cell types (Fig. 71–10). Others, however, have been found to be T-cell lymphomas and are, therefore, not the same as those B-cell mixed lymphomas arising from the follicles, which are B-cell regions. The small lymphocytes of the T-cell lymphomas have nuclei with irregular contours rather than cleaved nuclei characteristic of B lymphocytes. The nuclei of the large cells of the T-cell lymphomas may be either irregular or round. When numerous clusters of epithelioid histiocytes are found among the neoplastic cells, the lymphoma is called Lennert's lymphoma (Fig. 71–11).[6, 25] Immunophenotyping of the neoplastic cells must be carried out to distinguish between the B-cell and T-cell types with certainty.

Malignant lymphoma, diffuse, large-cell (diffuse histiocytic[37]; large-cell cleaved or noncleaved, follicle center, diffuse[31]): There were 277 cases (19.7 per cent) with this histologic picture. The median age of these patients was 56.8 years. The median survival was 1.5 years, and the 5-year survival was 35 per cent. The cells of the lymphoma may be large cleaved or noncleaved or both (Fig. 71–12). In most cases, however, the noncleaved cells predominate. Small cleaved cells may be noted among the large cells, but they make up the minority of the cell population. Fine sclerotic bands may subdivide groups of cells, resulting in compartmentalization. The majority of these lymphomas are B-cell neoplasms.

High-Grade Lymphomas

Malignant lymphoma, large-cell, immunoblastic (diffuse histiocytic[37]; immunoblastic sarcoma B-cell or T-cell type[31]): Ninety-one cases (7.9 per cent) were diagnosed as this type of lymphoma. The median age of the patients was 51.3 years. The median survival was 1.3 years, and the 5-year survival was 32 per cent. This lymphoma is subdivided into plasmacytoid, clear-cell, and polymorphous types. The plasmacytoid type, which

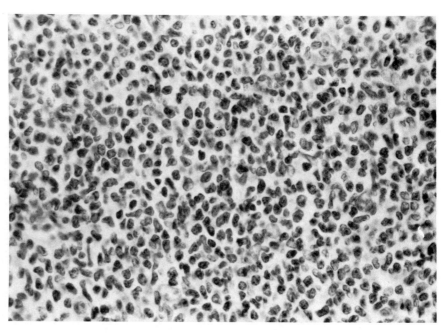

Figure 71–9. Diffuse small-cell cleaved lymphoma. Most of the cells have cleaved nuclei with inconspicuous nucleoli. Scattered large cells with prominent nucleoli are also present. (H&E, ×500)

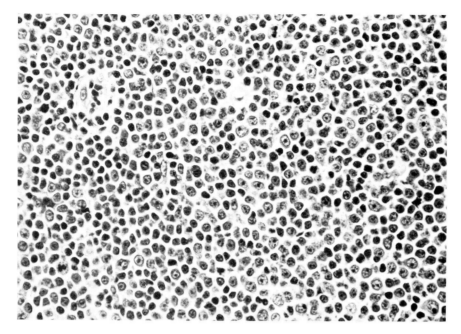

Figure 71–10. Diffuse mixed cleaved small- and large-cell lymphoma. A mixture of small and large cells is evident. (H&E, ×500)

usually is a B-cell neoplasm, is characterized cytologically by large vesicular nuclei with a single or several prominent centrally placed nucleoli. As in plasma cells, the nuclei are eccentrically located in the amphophilic, strongly pyroninophilic cytoplasm (Fig. 71–13). The clear-cell type has a large amount of pale-staining, weakly pyroninophilic cytoplasm, and the nucleus is usually centrally placed. Immunologically, this is usually a T-cell neoplasm and corresponds to the T-cell immunoblastic sarcoma in the Lukes-Collins classification. The polymorphous variant is also a T-cell lymphoma. A mixture of cells ranging in size from small to large is noted. The small cells have irregular nuclear contours, and the large cells often have abundant, clear-

staining cytoplasm. The latter cells may be multilobated, and muitinucleated giant cells resembling Reed-Sternberg cells may be present. Clusters of plasma cells as well as epithelioid histiocytes may be seen. When the latter cells are prominent, the neoplasm is called lymphoepithelioid cell lymphoma, or Lennert's lymphoma.[6, 25] Although the B- or T-cell nature of the neoplastic cells may be suspected on cytologic grounds, surface or cytoplasmic marker studies are needed to establish this definitively.

Malignant lymphoma, lymphoblastic (lymphoblastic, convoluted or nonconvoluted[37]; convoluted T cell[31]): Forty-nine patients (4.2 per cent were diagnosed as having lymphoblastic lymphoma. The median age of the pa-

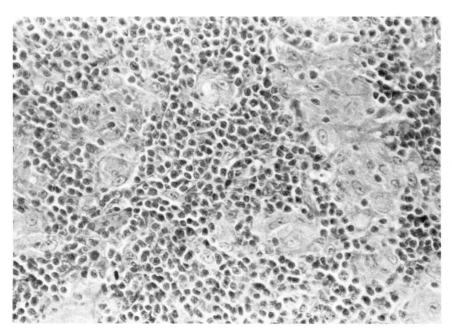

Figure 71–11. Diffuse mixed small- and large-cell lymphoma with numerous clusters of epithelioid histiocytes. (H&E, ×300)

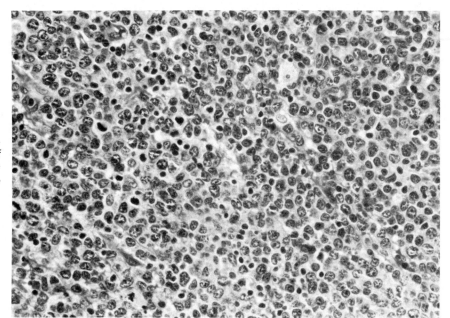

Figure 71–12. Diffuse large-cell noncleaved lymphomas composed of cells with round or oval nuclei containing one or more nucleoli. (H&E, ×25)

tients was 16.9 years. The median survival was 2.0 years, and the 5-year survival was 28 per cent. This lymphoma always has a diffuse pattern. A "starry sky" pattern similar to that seen in Burkitt's lymphoma may be present. The convoluted cells are characterized by deep nuclear subdivisions, giving the nuclei a convoluted appearance (Fig. 71–14). In other cases, the cells have round nuclei (Fig. 71–15). In both types, the nuclei have finely dispersed chromatin with a single, inconspicuous nucleus and scanty cytoplasm. The mitotic rate is high. Immunologically, this is a T-cell lymphoma, and it is the only lymphoma that is TdT positive. The TdT positivity is useful in confirming a diagnosis of lymphoblastic lymphoma.

Malignant lymphoma, small-cell, noncleaved (undifferentiated, Burkitt's and non-Burkitt's[37]; small-cell noncleaved, follicular center[31]): Fifty-eight cases (5 per cent) were diagnosed as small-cell, cleaved type. The median age of the patients was 29.8 years. The median survival was 0.7 years, and the 5-year survival was 23 per cent. This lymphoma includes both undifferentiated Burkitt's and non-Burkitt's types. A starry sky pattern is usually evident and often is prominent. This histologic picture is due to the presence of benign macrophages among the neoplastic cells. The latter cells have nuclei that are round or oval, are uniform in size and shape, and contain two to five small nucleoli (Fig. 71–16). The sizes of the nucleoli are approximately the same as those of

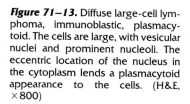

Figure 71–13. Diffuse large-cell lymphoma, immunoblastic, plasmacytoid. The cells are large, with vesicular nuclei and prominent nucleoli. The eccentric location of the nucleus in the cytoplasm lends a plasmacytoid appearance to the cells. (H&E, ×800)

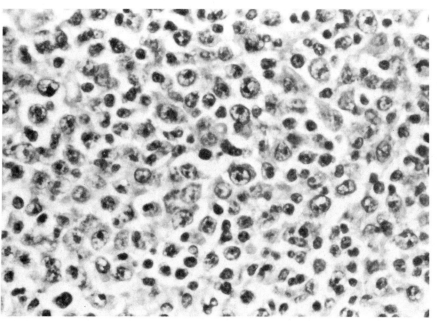

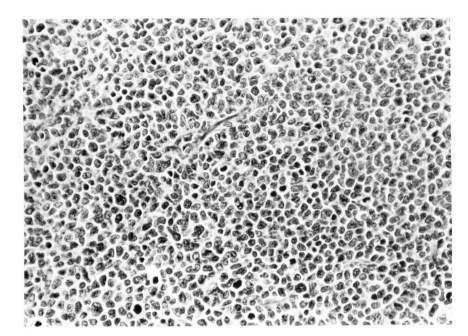

Figure 71–14. Lymphoblastic lymphoma, convoluted type. The neoplastic cells have convoluted nuclei, inconspicuous nucleoli, and little cytoplasm. (H&E, ×500)

the starry sky macrophages. Lymphomas with similar cytologic features but greater nuclear pleomorphism are characteristic of undifferentiated non-Burkitt's type. The nuclei of other cells tend to have single nucleoli that are larger than those in Burkitt's type, and occasional neoplastic giant cells may be present. These lymphomas are always B-cell malignancies.

Flow Cytometric Diagnosis of Lymphomas

The morphologic classification of lymphomas discussed in the preceding sections is not entirely satisfactory because of the subjectivity involved in the interpretation of lymphoid neoplasms and in differentiating them from benign lesions that may mimic lymphomas both morphologically and clinically. This subjectivity is eliminated by the application of new automated analytical immunologic techniques to normal lymphoid populations as well as to lymphomas and leukemias. This new technology is known as automated cytometry or, as applied to lymphoid lesions, flow cytometry.[29] With the use of a battery of monoclonal antibodies that are highly specific for surface antigens of benign and neoplastic cells, lymphomas and leukemias can be immunophenotyped into B- or T-cell subgroups, and thus, they can be categorized immunologically into prognostically significant subgroups. Immunophenotyping of lymphoid cells in this manner, together with histomorphologic description of lymphoid malignancies, has resulted in immunomorphologic classifications of lym-

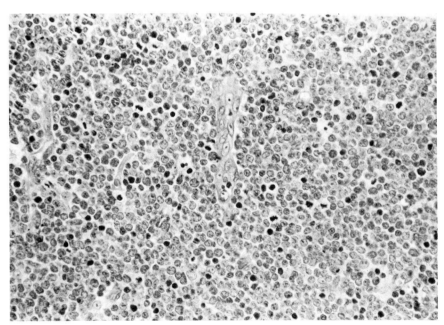

Figure 71–15. Lymphoblastic lymphoma, nonconvoluted. The neoplastic cells have little cytoplasm, round nuclei containing finely dispersed chromatin, and inconspicuous nucleoli. A high mitotic rate is evident. (H&E, ×25; inset, H&E, ×500)

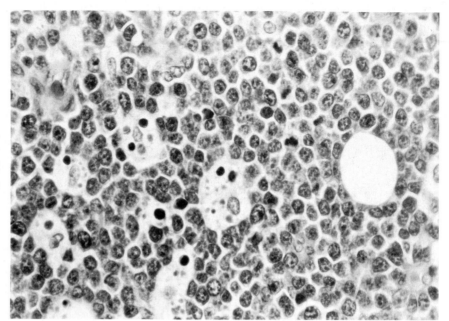

Figure 71–16. Diffuse small-cell non-cleaved (Burkitt's) lymphoma characterized by uniform cells with round, noncleaved nuclei containing one or more nucleoli. A starry sky pattern is evident. (H&E, ×800)

phomas and leukemias which will, in the future, supplant the less precise and heterogeneous purely morphologic classification schemes. Precise immunophenotyping of cells will be necessary in the future when specific immunotherapy is more widely used in the treatment of lymphomas and leukemias. In addition, DNA analysis by flow cytometry offers the possibility of rapidly recognizing aneuploid populations of cells. Not only is aneuploidy the most reliable and constant marker of malignancy, which may aid in differentiating benign from neoplastic lymphoproliferations, but cell cycle analysis by flow cytometry may prove to be another important predictor of prognosis in lymphomas and leukemias.

Miscellaneous Lymphomas

Composite lymphoma has been defined as two distinctly demarcated types of non-Hodgkin's lymphoma or both Hodgkin's disease and non-Hodgkin's lymphoma within the same organ or tissue. The prognosis of a composite lymphoma depends upon the one which is of higher grade.

Mycosis fungoides and *Sézary syndrome,* which is the leukemic phase of mycosis fungoides, are included among the cutaneous T-cell lymphomas. These neoplasms are characterized by irregular or convoluted nuclei. In the blood, these cells have a "cerebriform" appearance. *Extramedullary plasmacytomas* are often found in the upper respiratory tract. They may eventually spread to and involve the bone marrow. Lymphomas of *"true histiocytes"* (macrophages) are rare and can be diagnosed only with the aid of cytochemistry, immunologic markers, flow cytometry, or electron microscopy.

Lymphomas of the Head and Neck

In a review of non-Hodgkin's lymphomas of the head and neck seen and treated at the Institute of Laryngol-

ogy and Otology, in London, during the years 1962 to 1980, Evans noted 58 cases.[11] The majority of the cases (54) were extranodal (Table 71–1).

A discussion of lymphomas occurring in selected specific head and neck sites is worthy of consideration. In Freeman's study, in 1972, 417 patients (28 per cent) of a total of 1467 patients with non-Hodgkin's lymphoma were noted to have their disease in specific head and neck sites (Table 71–2).[12]

It is interesting to note that one third of head and neck non-Hodgkin's lymphomas will demonstrate remote disease at the time of diagnosis. In 40 per cent of cases cervical lymph nodes are palpable at the time of diagnosis.[12]

Non-Hodgkin's Lymphoma of Larynx

Primary non-Hodgkin's lymphoma of the larynx must probably develop in the lymphoid collections of the supraglottic lamina propria and laryngeal ventricles. In

TABLE 71–1. Distribution of Head and Neck non-Hodgkin's Lymphoma

Site	Number of Lesions
Ear	1
Ethmoid and orbit	1
Uvula and epiglottis	1
Larynx, primary	2
Larynx, secondary	2
Antroethmoidal	4
Nasal passages	5
Lung and neck	10
Waldeyer's ring	
Tonsil and palate	21
Tongue and floor of mouth	5
Posterior nasal space	6
Total	58

Source: Modified from Evans C: Clin Oncol 7:23, 1981.[11]

TABLE 71–2. Head and Neck Sites of Presentation of non-Hodgkin's Lymphoma

Site	Number of Lesions
Tonsil	162
Adenoid	37
Salivary gland	69
Thyroid	36
Nose	33
Orbit	32
Larynx	8
Oral cavity	40
TOTAL	417

Source: Modified from Freeman C, Berg JW, Cutler SJ: Cancer 29:252, 1972.[12]

a review[18] of non-Hodgkin's lymphoma cases limited to the larynx Swerdlow and associates[46] noted that the single most frequent presenting sign was hoarseness (eight cases). The patients ranged in age from 14 to 81 years (mean age, 57.1 years). The male-female ratio was 1:1.6. It was noted that if localized laryngeal disease is confirmed, radiotherapy appeared to be the curative treatment of choice.

Lymphoma of the larynx is an unusual lesion accounting for less than 1 per cent of laryngeal neoplasms. A study from the Mayo Clinic from 1952 to 1968 by DeSanto and Weisland reported nine patients with lymphoma of the larynx. This accounted for less than 0.2 per cent of a total of 5319 patients seen with malignant lymphoma.[9a] Similar statistics have been reported by Anderson[1a] and associates.

The majority of laryngeal lymphomas have presented as supraglottic masses.[1a] All the reported laryngeal lymphomas have been of the lymphocytic type. The majority of extranodal lymphomas of the larynx have or will soon develop extralaryngeal disease. Initial treatment should be irradiation; however, chemotherapy may be required for control of widespread disease.

Non-Hodgkin's Lymphoma of Salivary Glands

Non-Hodgkin's lymphomas of major or minor salivary glands are rare. Batsakis and Regezi noted that at the University of Michigan Medical Center in a 25-year period two primary non-Hodgkin's lymphomas were diagnosed.[3] The two non-Hodgkin's lymphomas were found among 580 primary parotid tumors diagnosed during that 25-year period. In another study, Nime and associates only found one case of major salivary gland (parotid gland) non-Hodgkin's lymphoma of 2636 cases of lymphoma.[36]

Even though non-Hodgkin's lymphoma is rare in all salivary glands, the parotid salivary gland is the most common site. The apparent "predilection" for the parotid gland is probably associated with the incidence of lymphoid tissue or lymph nodes in the parotid gland. Interestingly, as reported by Thompson and Bryant, lymph nodes or encapsulated lymphoid aggregates are absent in the embryonic and adult submandibular and sublingual glands.[48]

Criteria are established for defining primary non-Hodgkin's lymphoma[3]:

1. No known extrasalivary lymphoma.

2. Absolute histologic proof that the lymphoma involves salivary gland parenchyma.

3. Absolute confirmation of the malignant nature of the lymphoreticular infiltrate.

The association of benign lymphoepithelial lesions (including Sjögren's syndrome) and neoplasia, both epithelial malignancies and lymphoreticular malignancies, has been documented.[20] Batsakis has recently suggested the term "carcinoma ex lymphoepithelial lesion" to describe the epithelial malignancy.[1,2] Lymphoreticular abnormalities associated with benign lymphoepithelial lesions and Sjögren's syndrome include pseudolymphomas, macroglobulinemias, hyperglobulinemias, and malignant lymphoma.[26] It is important to note that "pseudolymphoma" is the most common and is suspected to be a precursor form to lymphoma.[1,20] Although the rare non-Hodgkin's lymphoma that develops in the major salivary gland of a person with a benign lymphoepithelial lesion may be more often than not solitary, the lymphoma that develops in a patient with Sjögren's syndrome is a manifestation of generalized lymphoma. Malignant lymphomas develop in up to 5 per cent of patients with Sjögren's syndrome. The relative risk in this group of patients is estimated to be 44 times that of the normal population. The lymphomas arising in patients with Sjögren's syndrome have all been non-Hodgkin's type and have also been almost exclusively extrasalivary. In addition, non-Hodgkin's lymphomas that develop in patients with Sjögren's syndrome (and its associated autoimmune abnormalities) are often rapidly fatal, with many patients surviving less than 3 years after diagnosis.

Non-Hodgkin's Lymphoma of the Nose and Paranasal Sinuses

Non-Hodgkin's lymphoma of the nose and paranasal sinuses is the most common nonepithelial malignancy in the area. The sites most often affected, in order of decreasing frequency, are the maxillary antrum, nasal cavity, and ethmoid sinus.[13,50] Interestingly, a point often overlooked by clinicians and pathologists alike is that non-Hodgkin's lymphomas have the propensity to destroy bone and invade adjacent soft tissue, just as the other small, round-cell malignancies that occur in the area, such as anaplastic carcinoma, melanoma, affecting neuroblastoma, Ewing's sarcoma, embryonal rhabdomyosarcoma, plasmacytoma, and chloroma.[13,26] As noted by Kapidia and associates, there are also some benign lesions that occur in the area and must be differentiated from non-Hodgkin's lymphoma, such as polymorphic reticulosis, Wegener's granulomatosis, and pseudolymphoma.[23]

As noted by Frierson and associates, the most common presenting symptoms were nasal obstruction and unilateral focal swelling.[13] The most common histologic form of non-Hodgkin's lymphoma in their study was diffuse large cell immunoblastic. The mean survival time for patients with non-Hodgkin's lymphoma in this study was 6.4 months.

Lymphomas of the Facial Bones

Lymphoma involving the facial bones is unusual and may be considered either a primary lesion or a secondary lesion in a patient with regional or diffuse lymphoma. The diagnosis of primary lymphoma should meet several criteria, as established by Topolnicki[49a] and associates:

1. The lesion should originate in a single bone.
2. Secondary involvement should be ruled out.
3. Histologic appearance should be the same as lymphomas seen in other tissues.
4. A long history of the disease should exist.
5. Metastatic lesions should be limited to regional lymph nodes.
6. The lesion should be radiosensitive.[49a]

Reimer and associates[38] suggest that lymphomas presenting in bone account for approximately 5 per cent of all extranodal lymphomas. In the region of the paranasal sinuses, it is often difficult to differentiate those lesions originating in bone from those originating in the paranasal sinuses. In those lesions presenting in the maxillary sinus, presenting symptoms include nasal obstruction, facial swelling, and proptosis. Excluding the maxillary antrum, the mandible is the most common site for facial bone involvement with lymphoma.

Patients are often males in the fifth to seventh decades, and the average duration of symptoms is 10 to 11 months. The radiographic picture is nonspecific and demonstrates osteolytic destruction. The majority of these lesions are pathologically classified as "mixed lymphomas," indicating that histiocytic cells, lymphoblasts, and lymphocytes are all variably present. Reimer and associates[38] have stated that histiocytic lymphoma is the most common type, with diffuse poorly differentiated lymphocytic, diffuse lymphocytic histiocytic, and undifferentiated lymphomas occurring in decreasing order of frequency. At the time of presentation, 86 per cent of patients with primary lymphoma of bone had stage IV disease. Yet the prognosis in lymphoma of bone does appear to be better than that for other malignancies of bone. The 5-year survival approaches 25 per cent. These tumors are generally considered to be radiosensitive, and radiation therapy is the primary mode of treatment.

REFERENCES

1a. Anderson HA, Maisel RH, Cantrell RW: Isolated laryngeal lymphoma. Laryngoscope 86:1251, 1976.
1. Batsakis JG: Carcinoma ex lymphoepithelial lesion. Ann Otol Rhinol Laryngol 92:567, 1983.
2. Batsakis JG: The pathology of head and neck tumors: The lymphoepithelial lesion and Sjögren's syndrome. Head Neck Surg 5:150, 1982.
3. Batsakis JG, Regezi JA: Selected controversial lesion of salivary tissues. Otolaryngol Clin North Am 10:309, 1977.
4. Bennett MH, et al: Classification of non-Hodgkin's lymphoma. Lancet 2:405, 1974.
5. Brazielle RM, Keneklis T, Donlon JA, et al: Terminal deoxynucleotidyl transferase in non-Hodgkin's lymphoma. Am J Clin Pathol 80:655, 1983.
6. Burke JS, Butler JJ: Malignant lymphoma with a high content of epithelioid histiocytes (Lennert's lymphoma). Am J Clin Pathol 66:1, 1976.
7. Castleman B, Iverson I, Menendez VP: Localized mediastinal lymph node hyperplasia resembling thymoma. Cancer 9:822, 1956.
8. Cooper RA, Dawson PJ, Rambo OM: Dermatopathic lymphadenopathy: A clinicopathologic analysis of lymph node biopsy over a 15-year period. Colo Med 106:170, 1967.
9a. DeSanto LW, Weiland LH: Malignant lymphoma of the larynx. Laryngoscope 80:966, 1970.
9. Dorfman RF: Classification of non-Hodgkin's lymphoma. Lancet 1:1295, 1974.
10. Dorfman RF, Remington JS: Value of lymph node biopsy in the diagnosis of acute acquired toxoplasmosis. N Engl J Med 289:878, 1973.
11. Evans C: A review of non-Hodgkin's lymphomata of the head and neck. Clin Oncol 7:23, 1981.
11a. Fierstein JT, Thawley SE: Lymphoma of the head and neck. Laryngoscope 88:582, 1978.
12. Freeman C, Berg JW, Cutler SJ: Occurrence and prognosis of extranodal lymphomas. Cancer 29:252, 1972.
13. Frierson HF, Mills SE, Innes DJ: Non-Hodgkin's lymphomas of the sinonasal region: Histologic subtypes and their clinicopathologic features. Am J Clin Pathol 81:721, 1984.
14. Frizzera G, Masarelli G, Banks PM, Rosai J: A systemic lymphoproliferative disorder with morphologic features of Castleman's disease: Pathologic findings in 15 patients. Am J Surg Pathol 7:211, 1983.
15. Gaba AR, Stein RS, Sweet DL, Variakojis D: Multicentric giant lymph node hyperplasia. Am J Clin Pathol 69:86, 1978.
16. Gerard-Marchant R, et al: Classification of non-Hodgkin's lymphomas. Lancet 2:406, 1974.
17. Hodgkin T: On some morbid appearances of the absorbent glands and spleen. Med Chir Trans 17:68, 1832.
18. Hsu SM, Jaffe ES: Leu M1 and peanut agglutination stain the neoplastic cells of Hodgkin's disease. Am J Clin Pathol 82:29, 1984.
19. Hurwitt E: Dermatopathic lymphadenitis: Focal granulomatous lymphadenitis associated with chromic generalized skin disorders. J Invest Dermatol 3:197, 1942.
20. Hyman GA, Wolff M: Malignant lymphomas of the salivary glands: Review of the literature and report of 33 new cases, including four cases associated with the lymphoepithelial lesion. Am J Clin Pathol 65:421, 1976.
21. Ivins JC, Dahlin DC: Malignant lymphoma (reticular cell sarcoma) in bone. Proc Mayo Clin 38:375, 1963.
22. Jones SE: Non-Hodgkin lymphoma. JAMA 234:633, 1975.
23. Kapadia SB, Barnes L, Deutsch M: Non-Hodgkin's lymphoma of the nose and paranasal sinuses: A study of 17 cases. Head Neck Surg 3:490, 1981.
24. Keller AR, Hochholzer L, Castleman B: Hyaline-vascular and plasma-cell types of giant lymph node hyperplasia of mediastinum and other locations. Cancer 29:670, 1972.
25. Kim H, et al: Malignant lymphoma with a high content of epithelioid histiocytes. A distinct clinicopathologic entity and a form of so-called "Lennert's lymphoma." Cancer 41:620, 1978.
26. Kim YH, Fayos JV, Schnitzer B: Extranodal head and neck lymphomas; result of radiation therapy. Int J Radiat Oncol Biol Phys 4:789, 1978.
27. Krueger GRF, et al: A new working formulation of non-Hodgkin's lymphomas. A retrospective study of the new NCI classification proposal in comparison to the Rappaport and Kiel classifications. Cancer 52:833, 1983.
28. Lennert K, Mohri N, Stein H, et al: The histopathology of malignant lymphoma. Br J Haematol (Suppl) 31:193, 1975.
29. Lovett EJ, et al: Application of flow cytometry to diagnostic pathology. Lab Invest 50:115, 1984.
30. Lukes RJ, Butler JJ: The pathology and nomenclature of Hodgkin's disease. Cancer Res 26:1063, 1966.
31. Lukes RJ, Collins RD: Immunopathologic characterization of human malignant lymphomas. Cancer 34:1488, 1974.
32. Lukes RJ, Craver LL, Hall TC, et al: Hodgkin's disease: Report of nomenclature committee. Cancer Res 26:1311, 1966.
33. Lukes RJ, Tindle BH, Parker JW: Reed-Sternberg-like cells in infectious mononucleosis. Lancet 2:1003, 1969.
34. Mann RB, Jaffe ES, Berard CW: Malignant lymphomas—A conceptual understanding of morphologic diversity. A review. Am J Pathol 94:105, 1979.
35. National Cancer Institute sponsored study of the classification of non-Hodgkin's lymphomas: Summary and description of a working formulation for clinical usage. Cancer 49:2112, 1982.
36. Nime FA, Cooper HS, Eggleston JC: Primary malignant lymphomas of the salivary glands. Cancer 37:906, 1976.
37. Rappaport H: Tumors of the hematopoietic system. In Atlas of Tumor Pathology, section 3, fasc 8. Washington, D.C., Armed Forces Institute of Pathology, 1966.
38. Reimer DR, Chabner BA, Young RC, et al: Lymphomas presenting in bone: Results of histopathology, staging and therapy. Ann Intern Med 87:50, 1977.
39. Rosai J, Dorfman RF: Sinus histiocytosis with massive lymphadenopathy: A newly recognized benign clinicopathologic entity. Arch Pathol 87:63, 1969.

40. Rosai J, Dorfman RF: Sinus histiocytosis with massive lymphad-enopathy—a pseudolymphomatous benign disorder: Analysis of 34 cases. Cancer 30:1174, 1972.
41. Rosenberg SA: Report of the committee on staging of Hodgkin's disease. Cancer Res 26:1310, 1966.
42. Rosenberg SA, Diamond HD, Jaskowitz B, Grover LF. Lympho-sarcoma: A review of 1269 cases. Medicine 40:31, 1961.
43. Schnitzer B: Reed-Sternberg–like cells in lymphocytic lymphoma and chronic lymphocytic leukemia. Lancet 1:1399, 1970.
44. Stanfield AG: The histological diagnosis of toxoplasmic lymphad-enitis. J Clin Pathol 14:565, 1961.
45. Strum SB, Park JK, Rappaport H: Observation of cells resembling Sternberg-Reed cells in conditions other than Hodgkin's disease. Cancer 26:176, 1970.
46. Swerdlow JB, et al: Non-Hodgkin's lymphoma limited to the larynx. Cancer 53:2546, 1984.
47. The non-Hodgkin's lymphoma pathologic classification project.

National Cancer Institute sponsored study of the classification of non-Hodgkin's lymphomas: Summary and description of a work-ing formulation for clinical usage. Cancer 49:2112, 1982.
48. Thompson AS, Bryant HC Jr: Histogenesis of papillary cystad-enoma lymphomatosum (Warthin's tumors) of the parotid sali-vary glands. Am J Pathol 26:807, 1950.
49. Tindle BH: Malignant lymphomas. Am J Pathol 116:119, 1984.
49a. Topolnicki W, White RJ: Primary reticulum cell sarcoma of the skull: Response to irradiation. Cancer 24:569, 1969.
50. Wilder WH, Harner SG, Banks PM: Lymphoma of the nose and paranasal sinuses. Arch Otolaryngol 109:310, 1983.
51. Winship T: Pathologic changes in so-called cat scratch fever: Review of findings in lymph nodes of 29 patients and cutaneous lesions in 2 patients. Am J Clin Pathol 23:1012, 1953.
52. Wright DH: Reed-Sternberg–like cells in recurrent Burkitt lym-phoma. Lancet 1:1052, 1970.

DIAGNOSIS AND TREATMENT OF LYMPHOMAS

Jay Marion, M.D.

NON-HODGKIN'S LYMPHOMA

The head and neck surgeon is often the first physician to evaluate the patient with a lymphoma. Such patients often present with cervical, occipital, or tonsillar ade-nopathy. The non-Hodgkin's lymphomas represent sev-eral clinical disorders of malignant lymphocytes. These disorders are often placed in categories that are defined by their clinical differences and similarities. There has been much diversity in the various classification systems used, and there is still ongoing controversy regarding the optimal classification. This diversity in classification systems is in part responsible for the confusion faced by the clinician who treats the patient with a non-Hodgkin's lymphoma. A working formulation classifi-cation has recently been introduced, and it is hoped that it will decrease this confusion and aid in patient management.[27]

Incidence, Etiology, and Epidemiology

The estimated incidence of the non-Hodgkin's lym-phomas is approximately 15,000 new cases per year in the United States. This represents about 2 per cent of all malignancies. The etiology of these disorders is not well defined. Possible etiologic factors include exposure to drugs,[9] infectious agents,[15] ionizing radiation,[18] and immunosuppression.[21] Because the non-Hodgkin's lym-phomas represent a heterogeneous group of clinical entities, it is no surprise that a clear etiology has not been identified.

There is a steady increase in the incidence of the non-Hodgkin's lymphomas from childhood through late adulthood in the United States. The incidence rates for the non-Hodgkin's lymphomas vary from country to country. For example, in Africa and New Guinea, Bur-kitt's lymphoma is very common, whereas it is rare in the United States. Similarly, the frequency of non-Hodgkin's lymphomas in younger age groups is higher in Egypt than in the United States.

Lymphomas have been reported with increasing fre-quency in patients with the acquired immunodeficiency syndrome (AIDS).[32] This disorder is caused by a human T lymphocyte–tropic retrovirus. The agent has been termed "human T-cell lymphotropic virus (HTLV)-III by Gallo and colleagues.[4a] Data from the Centers for Dis-ease Control on seropositivity in apparently healthy homosexual males indicates widespread dissemination of the virus.[26] The number of patients with clinically definable disease will continue to increase, since reports have indicated that up to 10 per cent of persons who are seropositive for HTLV-III may develop disease over a 2-year follow-up period.[17a] Most homosexual men with chronic lymphadenopathy, however, will not be diag-nosed as having lymphoma. Burns studied 69 homosex-ual men with chronic lymphadenopathy who all under-went lymph node biopsies. Only ten of these patients were diagnosed as having malignant lymphoma. The most common histologic pattern noted in these 69 patients was florid reactive follicular hyperplasia (43 cases).[2a] Since homosexual males with chronic lymph-adenopathy may have lymphoma as well as opportun-istic infection, it is important that lymph node biopsies be performed for histologic evaluation and culture.

Classification and Staging

The Rappaport system of classification is presently in widest use, even though it suffers from major faults and limitations. It has the advantage of being fairly reproducible among pathologists. It cross-classifies lym-phomas by nodal architecture—nodular (N) or diffuse (D)—and by cellular histologic features—well-differentiated lymphocytic (WDL), poorly differentiated lymphocytic (PDL), mixed lymphocytic-histiocytic (M), histiocytic (H), and undifferentiated (U). Because the majority of clinical studies have used this classification, there is prognostic and therapeutic importance in gaining familiarity with it. There are, however, several major weaknesses in this system. For example, it suffers from inexact terminology. The so-called "histiocytic" lymphoma is rarely (< 5 per cent) a disorder of histiocytes. It is most commonly a disease of transformed B-lymphocytes. Similarly, the Rappaport classification suffers from overly simplistic grouping. We now know that the category of diffuse histiocytic lymphoma (DHL) comprises a heterogeneous mixture of neoplasms with different natural histories. Most of them arise from B-lymphocytes, some from T-lymphocytes, and only a few from true histiocytes.[20] Because the biologic behavior of these subsets is different, adhering to the Rappaport classification alone may obscure important prognostic and therapeutic information. However, most of the published studies to date are based upon the Rappaport classification; thus, it will be used throughout this section.

The Ann Arbor staging system, which was developed for Hodgkin's disease, is also commonly used for the non-Hodgkin's lymphomas (Table 71–3). There are, however, limitations that become apparent, as this system is applied to the non-Hodgkin's lymphomas. Hodgkin's disease usually spreads in a contiguous and thus predictable fashion. This is rarely the case for many of the non-Hodgkin's lymphomas. For example, approximately 60 per cent of patients with poorly differentiated lymphocytic lymphoma, nodular type (PDLL-N), will have bone marrow involvement at presentation; this suggests that hematogenous spread may occur early in the course of the disease.[28] Furthermore, the Ann Arbor system does not address an important prognostic factor in some of the non-Hodgkin's lymphomas—bulk of disease. A patient with diffuse histiocytic lymphoma (DHL) who has bilateral cervical disease with the largest node being 2 to 3 cm in diameter has stage II disease. Similarly, a patient with DHL who has massive retroperitoneal and abdominal adenopathy, with nodes being larger than 7 to 10 cm in diameter, also has stage II disease. The ultimate prognosis for these two patients, however, is not the same.[19] The patient with bulky infradiaphragmatic disease will do less well than the patient with minimal cervical disease. Within the literature, however, these two patients might well be lumped together as stage II patients.

Natural History

As mentioned earlier, the non-Hodgkin's lymphomas are a heterogeneous group of malignant disorders. The aggressiveness of the various subtypes of lymphomas varies considerably. The median survival ranges from months to several years, even in untreated patients. Despite the problems with the Rappaport classification, this system has produced information that allows some prognostication when a patient is diagnosed as having a non-Hodgkin's lymphoma. Two major clinical groups of patients with non-Hodgkin's lymphomas can be identified within the Rappaport classification: those with histologically "favorable" lymphomas and those with histologically "unfavorable" lymphomas.

Histologically "Favorable" Lymphomas

This category of lymphomas includes well-differentiated lymphocytic diffuse (WDLL-D), poorly differentiated lymphocytic nodular (PDLL-N), and nodular mixed lymphocytic-histiocytic (NM). The histologically favorable lymphomas tend to be widely disseminated at the time of diagnosis and are characterized by an indolent growth. Despite high complete response rates to chemotherapy, these lymphomas tend to be incurable, and the patient remains at continuous risk for relapse. The median age at the time of diagnosis is approximately 55 years. The usual presenting complaint is that of slowly progressive lymphadenopathy. Systemic symptoms may be present in approximately 10 to 20 per cent of patients. Coombs' positive hemolytic anemia or immunogenic thrombocytopenia may complicate these disorders.[10]

TABLE 71–3. AJCC Modification of the Ann Arbor Staging Classification for Hodgkin's Disease

Stage I   Involvement of a single lymph node region (1) or of a single extralymphatic organ or site (I_E).

Stage II   Involvement of two or more lymph node regions (number to be stated) on the same side of the diaphragm (II), or localized involvement of an extralymphatic organ or site and of one or more lymph node regions on the same side of the diaphragm (II_E).

Stage III Involvement of lymph node regions on both sides of the diaphragm (III), which may also be accompanied by localized involvement of extralymphatic organ site (III_E) or by involvement of the spleen (III_S) or both (III_{ES}).

Stage IV Diffuse or disseminated involvement of one or more extralymphatic organs or tissues with or without associated lymph node enlargement. The reason for classifying the patient as stage IV is identified further by specifying sites according to the following notation:

Pulmonary—PUL	Bone marrow—MAR
Osseous—OSS	Pleura—PLE
Hepatic—HEP	Skin—SKI
Brain—BRA	Eye—EYE
Lymph nodes—LYM	Other—OTH

Systemic symptoms:
  A Asymptomatic
  B Unexplained weight loss of more than 10 per cent of body weight in the 6 months before admission
    Unexplained fever with temperature above 38°C
    Night sweats

*From Beahrs OH, Myers MH (eds): American Joint Committee on Cancer: Manual for Staging of Cancer, 2nd ed. Philadelphia, J. B. Lippincott Co., 1983, p. 227.

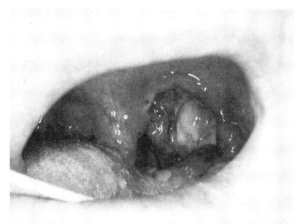

Figure 71–17. Lymphoma of Waldeyer's ring involving the tonsil.

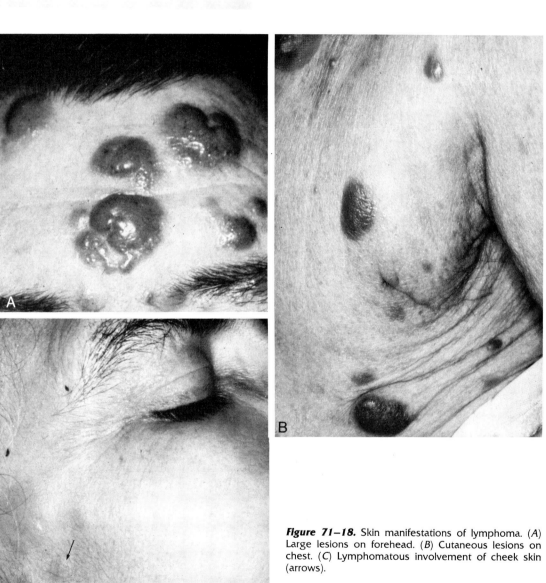

Figure 71–18. Skin manifestations of lymphoma. (*A*) Large lesions on forehead. (*B*) Cutaneous lesions on chest. (*C*) Lymphomatous involvement of cheek skin (arrows).

Histologically "Unfavorable" Lymphomas

This category includes the histiocytic lymphomas with diffuse or nodular architecture (DHL, NHL), poorly differentiated lymphocytic diffuse (PDLL-D), and mixed lymphocytic-histiocytic diffuse (DM). DHL is the most common subtype, composing approximately 30 per cent of the non-Hodgkin's lymphomas. The median age at diagnosis is approximately 50 years. Patients usually present with rapidly progressive lymphadenopathy. Extranodal disease is frequently found in such sites as Waldeyer's ring (Fig. 71–17), the gastrointestinal tract, the meninges, skin, and lung (Fig. 71–18). Approximately 25 per cent of patients with DHL will present with localized disease (stage I or II). Systemic symptoms may be present and usually correlate with the extent of disease. These lymphomas tend to run an aggressive course and result in early death unless a complete remission can be obtained. Once a complete remission is obtained, however, it may remain durable in certain subtypes and the patient may be cured. Nearly 50 per cent of patients with DHL will be cured with aggressive therapy.[23]

Patient Evaluation

Once the diagnosis of a non-Hodgkin's lymphoma is achieved, further studies are often indicated to assess the "stage" of the disease. Exhaustive staging studies should not be undertaken in all patients as a matter of routine. As a general rule, staging studies should be performed only in patients in whom a change in stage would result in a change in initial therapy. For example, the initial therapy for a patient with a clinical stage I diffuse histiocytic lymphoma would depend upon the true, or pathologic, stage of disease. If such a patient were found during staging studies to have more advanced disease, systemic chemotherapy would most likely be recommended. If, however, localized disease was confirmed after the staging evaluation, radiation therapy would probably be recommended. However, in the patient with a histologically favorable lymphoma, such as a nodular, poorly differentiated lymphocytic lymphoma, the treatment strategy is rarely altered by the true stage of disease. Because the histologically favorable lymphomas are generally incurable at presentation, therapy is usually reserved for the palliation of associated symptoms, regardless of stage.[24]

Staging studies are thus carried out until enough information is obtained to allow for the initiation of an individualized treatment plan for the given patient. In some instances, however, there is a second purpose for staging patients with non-Hodgkin's lymphomas. An adequate "base line" is sometimes desired so that the response to cytotoxic therapy can be monitored. For example, in a patient with a curable lymphoma, one would want to be sure that all measurable disease had been eradicated prior to stopping cytotoxic therapy. This obviously requires knowing the extent of disease prior to initiating therapy.

The following procedures are useful in staging the patient with a non-Hodgkin's lymphoma:

1. *History.* When obtaining a history from a patient with newly diagnosed lymphoma, it is important to investigate for the presence of constitutional symptoms. Unexplained fevers, weight loss, and night sweats may provide prognostic information in some of the lymphomas. Patients who have such symptoms have the suffix "B" added to their numerical stage.

2. *Complete physical examination.* All node-bearing areas must be examined carefully, and the size of all nodes should be recorded (Fig. 71–19). Areas of extranodal lymphoid tissue, such as Waldeyer's ring (Fig. 71–20), should also be evaluated carefully. Virtually any mass in the head and neck area should be suspect for lymphoma (Figs. 17–21 and 17–22). The liver and spleen should be examined, and there should be a search for bone tenderness.

3. *Laboratory studies.* Complete blood counts, including a differential and platelet count, should be obtained in all patients with newly diagnosed lymphoma. Liver function and renal function studies should also be obtained. If available, cell surface phenotyping studies should be obtained in difficult histologic diagnoses. These studies can often classify lymphomas as either B-cell or T-cell neoplasms.

4. *Radiographic studies.* Chest x-rays and abdominal CT scans (Fig. 71–23) are often obtained routinely in the patient with a newly diagnosed non-Hodgkin's lymphoma. Other studies such as lymphangiography, liver-spleen scans, and bone scans are less often ordered routinely but are occasionally helpful in certain settings. Because approximately 10 per cent of patients with Waldeyer's ring lymphoma have gastrointestinal tract involvement, barium studies are indicated in these patients to rule out occult abdominal disease (Fig. 71–24).[2] Sinus CT scans can document the extent of initial disease and show the response to therapy (Figs. 71–25 and 71–26).

5. *Invasive staging studies.* A bone marrow biopsy is often performed during the staging of a patient with a non-Hodgkin's lymphoma to promptly rule in or rule out stage IV disease. A formal staging laparotomy is rarely indicated as part of the evaluation of a patient with a non-Hodgkin's lymphoma.

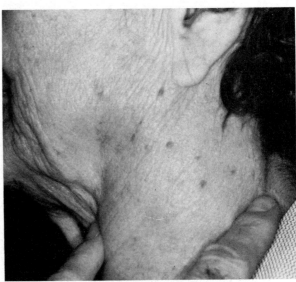

Figure 71–19. Extensive cervical lymphadenopathy from lymphoma.

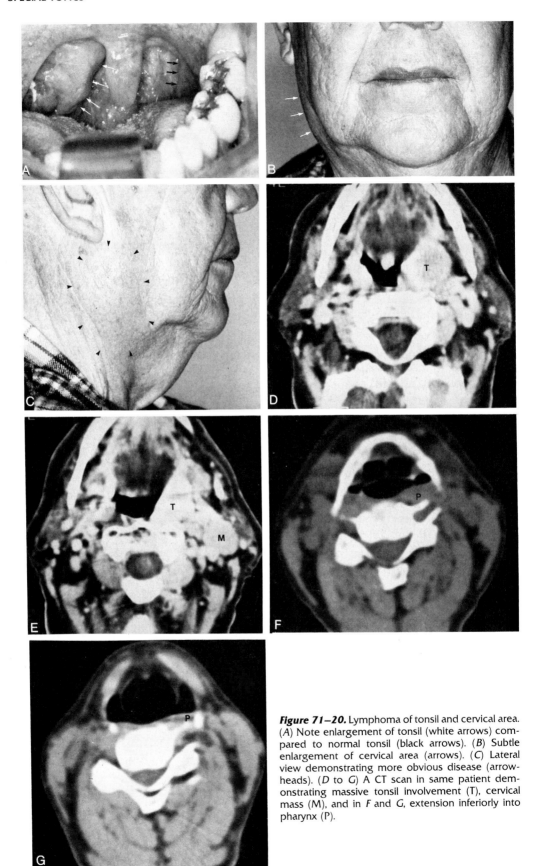

Figure 71–20. Lymphoma of tonsil and cervical area. (*A*) Note enlargement of tonsil (white arrows) compared to normal tonsil (black arrows). (*B*) Subtle enlargement of cervical area (arrows). (*C*) Lateral view demonstrating more obvious disease (arrowheads). (*D* to *G*) A CT scan in same patient demonstrating massive tonsil involvement (T), cervical mass (M), and in *F* and *G*, extension inferiorly into pharynx (P).

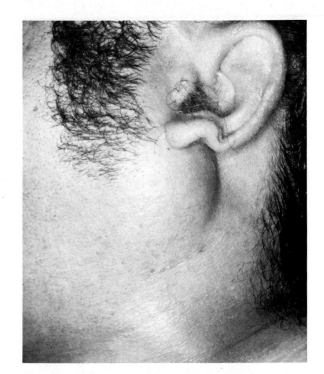

Figure 71–21. Parotid mass from lymphoma involvement of parotid lymphoid tissue.

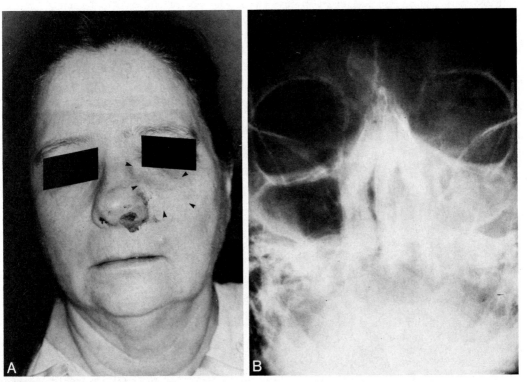

Figure 71–22. (A) Mass of cheek (arrowheads) from lymphoma of maxillary sinus. (B) Sinus radiograph demonstrates opacification of the left maxillary sinus secondary to lymphoma.

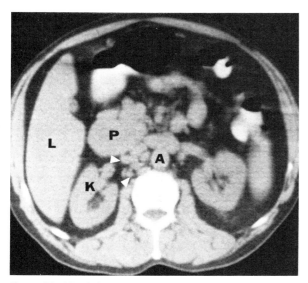

Figure 71–23. Abdominal lymphoma. Peripancreatic lymphadenopathy (P) and enlarged retroperitoneal lymph nodes (arrowheads). Areas labeled are liver (L), kidney (K), and aorta (A).

Treatment

There are two major indications for treating a patient with a non-Hodgkin's lymphoma. Some patients will have a curable neoplasm and should be treated early with curative intent. Others will have an incurable disease, and treatment will be reserved for the control of symptoms. Prior to initiating any therapy, the physician should define the goal of treatment as cure or palliation.

Histologically Indolent ("Favorable") Lymphomas

In general, the histologically "favorable" lymphomas, such as PDLL-N and WDLL-D, are incurable but "indolent" neoplasms. They are often associated with long symptom-free periods, and thus, no initial systemic therapy is usually recommended.[24] Treatment is usually initiated when the disease becomes rapidly progressive or when systemic symptoms develop. Local symptomatic disease is often treated effectively with local radiotherapy. Similarly, the rare patient who presents with stage I disease may benefit from involved-field radiotherapy. The survival of patients with clinical stage I PDLL-N who are treated with regional radiotherapy is 100 per cent at 5 years, with 60 per cent being relapse-free.[7]

Ultimately, most patients with histologically "favorable" lymphomas will develop systemic signs or symptoms that will warrant the institution of systemic chemotherapy. Progressive anemia, thrombocytopenia, neutropenia, weight loss, night sweats, fevers, and bulky adenopathy are all indications for systemic chemotherapy. Initial systemic treatment often consists of single-agent alkylator therapy. Cyclophosphamide and chlorambucil can both be given by the oral route to induce and maintain clinical remissions. Disease that demonstrates rapid progression despite single-agent therapy is best managed with combination chemother-

apy. Combinations such as CVP (cyclophosphamide, vincristine, and prednisone) can induce clinical remissions in the majority of treated patients (Fig. 71–27). Unfortunately, relapse occurs at a rate of approximately 10 to 15 per cent per year, with less than 30 per cent of patients remaining disease-free at 10 years.

Histologically Aggressive ("Unfavorable") Lymphomas

In contrast to the histologically "favorable" lymphomas, the "unfavorable" lymphomas are frequently curable. Thus, curative therapy is offered to the patient at the time of diagnosis, regardless of the presence or absence of systemic symptoms. Patients with clinical stage I disease are often treated for cure with radiotherapy. Five-year disease-free survivals of approximately 40 per cent are reported for patients with clinical stage I DHL who are treated with radiotherapy alone.[3] Patients who are found to have pathologic stage I disease, after undergoing a staging laparotomy, enjoy an approximate 90 per cent disease-free survival.[30]

Patients with more advanced disease (stages II, III, and IV) are generally treated initially with combination chemotherapy. Curative potential has been demonstrated for many such combinations (Table 71–4).

All the regimens listed in Table 71–4 have greatly improved the prognosis of the "unfavorable" lymphomas. Greater than 40 to 50 per cent of aggressively treated patients with diffuse histiocytic lymphoma can expect to be cured. However, because approximately 50 per cent of patients still fail primary therapy, newer induction regimens for untreated patients and better salvage regimens for previously treated patients need to be developed.

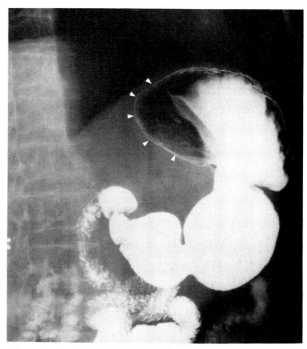

Figure 71–24. Barium film demonstrating gastric lymphoma.

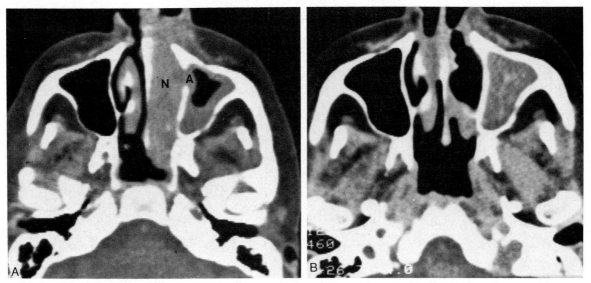

Figure 71–25. Nasal and maxillary sinus lymphoma. (*A*) Initial lesion with extensive involvement of nasal cavity (N), turbinates, and thickening maxillary sinus mucosa. Surgical nasoantral window for drainage purposes (A). (*B*) Same area 9 months later following irradiation. Note almost complete resolution of nasal disease. Opacification of maxillary sinus was residual sinusitis, which cleared following repeat drainage procedure.

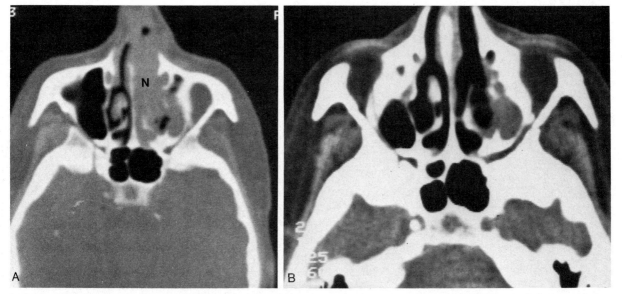

Figure 71–26. (*A*) Initial nasal sinus lymphoma with complete obstruction of nose (N). (*B*) Resolution of lesion following radiation.

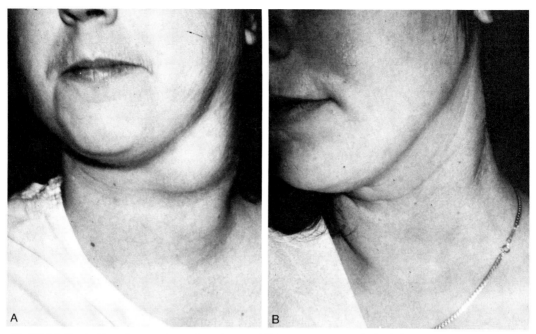

Figure 71–27. (*A*) Cervical lymphoma prior to drug therapy. (*B*) Same patient 6 months following combination drug therapy.

Future Directions in Management

As mentioned, newer induction and salvage chemo-therapeutic regimens are being evaluated in the non-Hodgkin's lymphomas. In some selected patients, bone marrow transplantation is being used for poor-risk patients.[1, 22] Monoclonal antibodies directed against malignant lymphocytes are being evaluated for therapeutic potential with encouraging preliminary results.[25] Similarly, the various interferons are being studied for their therapeutic potential in the non-Hodgkin's lymphomas. Objective responses have been reported.[29]

TABLE 71–4. Treatment Programs for Diffuse Aggressive Lymphomas

Regimen	Complete Remissions (%)	Long-term Survivors (%)
C-MOPP	45	37
BACOP	46	37
CHOP	58	<30
COMLA	55	48
M-BACOD	72	59
ProMACE-MOPP	74	65

Key:
MOPP = mechlorethamine, vincristine, procarbazine, prednisone.
C-MOPF = cyclophosphamide + MOPP.
BACOP = bleomycin, adriamycin, cyclophosphamide, vincristine, prednisone.
CHOP = cyclophosphamide, adriamycin, vincristine, prednisone.
COMLA = cyclophosphamide, vincristine, methotrexate, leucovorin rescue, cytarabine.
M-BACOD = high-dose methotrexate, leucovorin rescue, bleomycin, adriamycin, cyclophosphamide, vincristine, dexamethasone.
ProMACE-MOPP = cyclophosphamide, adriamycin, VP-16-213, high-dose methotrexate, mechlorethamine, vincristine, procarbazine, prednisone.
Source: Pinedo H, Chabner B: Cancer Chemotherapy, Annual 5. New York, Elsevier Publishing Co., 1983.

HODGKIN'S LYMPHOMA

Hodgkin's disease is a lymphoreticular malignancy that usually presents as painless lymphadenopathy. At the time of diagnosis, the patient may also be aware of systemic symptoms such as unexplained weight loss, fevers, or night sweats. As in patients with non-Hodgkin's lymphomas, the head and neck surgeon is often the first physician to evaluate the patient with Hodgkin's disease.

Incidence, Etiology, and Epidemiology

Hodgkin's disease is a relatively rare disease, accounting for only 1 per cent of new cancers in the United States. There appears to be a bimodal age-incidence curve. In the United States, incidence rates begin to rise sharply after age 10, peak in the late 20s, and then decline to age 45. After age 50, the incidence rises steadily with advancing age. There has been much concern voiced that Hodgkin's disease might be a contagious illness. Gutensohn and associates noted the similarities between the epidemiology of Hodgkin's disease and paralytic poliomyelitis.[6] The peak age of incidence for both diseases is delayed as living conditions improve. Risk is also increased for both diseases with small family size and increasing social class. These authors have thus suggested that Hodgkin's disease, like paralytic poliomyelitis, may be a rare manifestation of a common infection with the probability of developing clinical illness increasing as the patient's age at the time of infection increases. To date, though, no etiologic agent has been discovered, and most studies do not suggest that Hodgkin's disease is a contagious illness. Certainly, it is no more prevalent in physicians than it is within the general population.[5]

Classification and Staging

In 1965, an International Symposium was held in Rye, New York, and a classification scheme was agreed upon. The Rye classification has generally been accepted by clinicians because of its simplicity and ability to allow for prognostication. Within this classification, Hodgkin's disease is subclassified into four subtypes (Table 71–5).[26]

The subclassification of cases into the four histologic types is mostly subjective. There are no clear-cut guidelines that exist for unequivocal subtyping. Despite this, the Rye classification has both clinical and prognostic value. Except for nodular sclerosis, Hodgkin's disease may evolve from one subtype to another. Specifically, a lymphocyte-predominant neoplasm may evolve into mixed cellularity or lymphocyte-depleted Hodgkin's disease. It is not known why the nodular sclerosis subtype does not demonstrate such evolutionary progression.

The cellular population in a Hodgkin's node is not composed, for the most part, by malignant cells. Instead, there is a heterogeneous population of lymphocytes, histiocytes, plasma cells, eosinophils, mononuclear cells and Reed-Sternberg (R-S) cells. A histopathologic diagnosis of Hodgkin's disease requires the presence of the giant Reed-Sternberg cells in a characteristic pleomorphic background. Despite the malignant appearance of the Reed-Sternberg cell, it does not appear capable of replication. Instead, it appears to be derived from a "putative" neoplastic cell, which may be a malignant macrophage.[11, 14]

The anatomic staging system, which had been developed at the Ann Arbor Conference in 1971, is widely accepted by clinicians treating Hodgkin's disease. It was updated in 1977 by the American Joint Committee for Cancer Staging and is shown in Table 71–3.[17] This system has more utility when applied to Hodgkin's disease than when applied to the non-Hodgkin's lymphomas. Whereas the pattern of spread in the non-Hodgkin's lymphomas is often random, the usual mode of spread in Hodgkin's disease is more predictable and nonrandom. There is usually an orderly spread via lymphatic channels to contiguous lymph node chains and lymphatic structures. Similarly, in Hodgkin's disease, there is an axial or central proclivity for involved nodes (cervical, mediastinal, para-aortic). Mesenteric, epitrochlear, and popliteal nodes are rarely involved. The liver is almost never involved unless there is disease within the spleen.[13] Fewer than 1 per cent of patients with Hodgkin's disease will have involvement of the tonsils and Waldeyer's ring.

Various constitutional symptoms may occur with Hodgkin's disease. Generalized malaise, fatigue, anorexia, weakness, fever, weight loss, night sweats, pruritus, and pain in nodal areas of involvement after alcohol ingestion are all commonly seen in patients with Hodgkin's disease. Three of these symptoms have been associated with a reduction in survival and thus have been included in the Ann Arbor staging system.[16, 31] These have been titled B symptoms and include:

1. Night sweats.
2. Unexplained weight loss of more than 10 per cent of the body weight in 6 months.
3. Unexplained fevers above 38°C.

It is essential to document the presence or absence of B symptoms and to include the appropriate suffix to the numerical stage when discussing a patient with Hodgkin's disease.

Patient Evaluation

After the diagnosis of Hodgkin's disease is made, further studies are usually indicated to allow for the appropriate "staging" of the patient. As in the non-Hodgkin's lymphomas, exhaustive staging studies should not be undertaken in all patients as a matter of routine. Staging studies should be performed only in patients in whom a change in stage would result in a change in initial therapy. The clinical stage (CS) is determined by the information gathered from the history, physical examination, laboratory studies, radiographic studies, and radioisotopic procedures. The pathologic stage (PS) is determined by the information obtained from biopsies of specific tissues. As mentioned previously, not all patients should be subjected to pathologic staging. There remains much controversy regarding the role of aggressive staging in various patient subsets. It is beyond the scope of this chapter to delve into this controversy.

The following procedures are useful in staging the patient with Hodgkin's disease:

1. *History.* As discussed previously, it is essential to investigate for the presence of unexplained fevers, weight loss, and night sweats. Patients who have such symptoms have the suffix B added to their numerical stage. The presence of a B symptom has prognostic implications and occasionally necessitates a more aggressive therapeutic approach.

2. *Complete physical examination.* All node-bearing areas must be examined carefully, and the size of all nodes should be recorded (Figs. 71–28 and 71–29). The liver and spleen should be examined for evidence of enlargement or tenderness.

3. *Laboratory studies.* Complete blood counts, liver function studies, and renal function tests should be obtained in all patients with newly diagnosed Hodgkin's disease. Erythrocyte sedimentation rates and serum copper levels are sometimes obtained as base-line studies.

4. *Radiographic studies.* Chest x-rays and abdominal CT scans are routinely obtained in the patient with newly diagnosed Hodgkin's disease. Cervical CT scans may also be helpful (Fig. 71–30). Thoracic CT scans are often obtained if the chest x-ray is abnormal (Fig. 71–31). Lymphangiography (Fig. 71–32) is occasionally useful in detecting lymphomatous involvement of normal-sized lower retroperitoneal nodes. Bone scans rarely add useful information in the setting of a normal alkaline phosphatase in an asymptomatic patient. A liver-spleen

TABLE 71–5. The Rye Classification of Hodgkin's Disease

Subtype	Relative Frequency (%)
Lymphocyte Predominance (LP)	10–12
Nodular Sclerosis (NS)	45–55
Mixed Cellularity (MC)	30–35
Lymphocyte Depletion (LD)	8–10

Source: Rosenberg SA: Report of the committee on the staging of Hodgkin's disease. Cancer Res 26:1310, 1966.

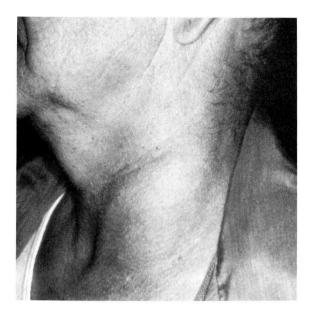

Figure 71–28. Hodgkin's lymphoma of cervical area.

scan is usually obtained unless the abdominal CT scan reveals evidence for involvement of those organs.

5. *Invasive staging studies.* Bilateral posterior iliac crest core biopsies are often obtained early to demonstrate occult marrow involvement. Such demonstration allows for the designation of pathologic stage IV disease and may obviate the need for other staging studies.

Staging laparotomies are performed in selected patients in whom the information obtained would result in a change in initial therapy. For example, a patient with clinical stage IIIB mixed cellularity Hodgkin's disease is likely to be treated with aggressive chemotherapy regardless of the results of a staging laparotomy. The presence of B symptoms and the mixed cellularity subtype place the patient in a poor prognostic group. Most physicians would treat such a patient with systemic chemotherapy whether the pathologic stage were IIB, IIIB, or IVB. Thus, it is unlikely that the information obtained during a staging laparotomy would result in a change of therapy for the patient. Conversely, in a patient with clinical stage IIA mixed cellularity disease, the results of a staging laparotomy might well alter the initial therapy. If the patient were found to have pathologic stage IIA disease, treatment would likely be extended field radiotherapy. If, however, the patient were found to have pathologic stage IIIA or IVA disease,

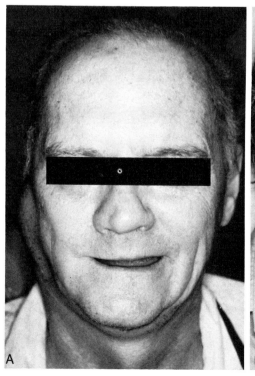
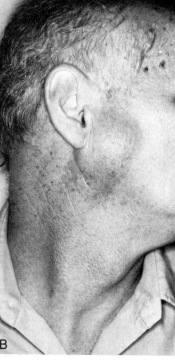

Figure 71–29. (A and B) Hodgkin's lymphoma of parotid node.

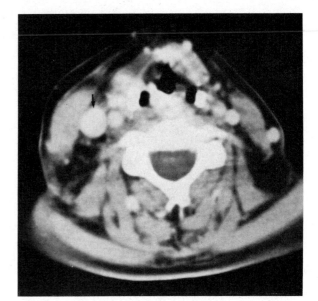

Figure 71–30. Cervical CT scan demonstrating enlarged node (arrow).

treatment would more likely be multiagent chemotherapy. The risks associated with a staging laparotomy could thus be justified in this patient.

If performed, a staging laparotomy should include the following:

1. Careful inspection and exploration of the abdominal contents.

2. Wedge and needle biopsies of both hepatic lobes.

3. Splenectomy.

4. Biopsy of para-aortic, iliac mesenteric, celiac, hepatic portal, and splenic hilar lymph nodes.

5. Biopsy of any lymph nodes that appeared abnormal on the lymphangiogram.

6. An open iliac crest bone marrow biopsy.

7. Placement of radiopaque markers at the sites of node biopsies, the splenic pedicle, and at the margins of tumor masses.

8. Oophoropexy in women of childbearing age to remove the ovaries from potential radiation ports.

Treatment

Approximately 70 per cent of all patients with Hodgkin's disease can be cured. Radiation therapy has curative potential in early stage disease, and combination chemotherapy is similarly effective in advanced stage disease. Because choice of the initial therapy is often dependent upon the stage of disease, outcome is affected by the accuracy of the staging process.

Radiation Therapy

Radiotherapy has demonstrated curative potential in patients with stage IA and IIA disease.[8] Similarly, some

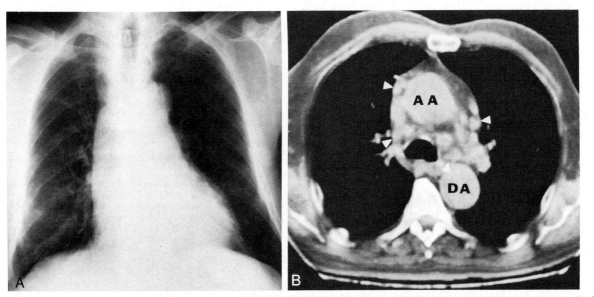

Figure 71–31. (A) Chest radiograph demonstrating mediastinal widening. (B) CT scan in the same patient demonstrates multiple enlarged mediastinal lymph nodes (arrowheads), ascending aorta (AA), and descending aorta (DA).

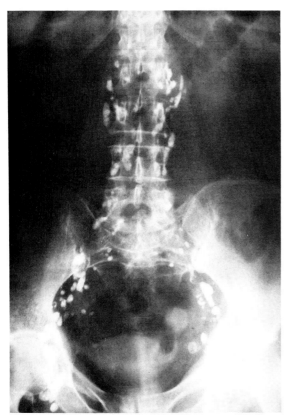

Figure 71–32. Lymphangiogram demonstrating visualization of abdominal nodes.

subsets of patients with stage IIIA disease are also curable with appropriately delivered radiotherapy. However, the use of radiation alone for patients with stage IB, IIB, and IIIB disease is controversial. The usual technique prescribed consists of an extended-field port that includes the areas of known disease and the contiguous lymph node chains. Radiation delivered to a total dose of 4000 rad, in 200-rad daily fractions, will result in an in-field failure rate of less than 5 per cent.[12] Treatment-related complications may include radiation pneumonitis, chronic pericarditis, hypothyroidism, myelosuppression, and infertility (if the gonads are not shielded).

Chemotherapy

Multiagent systemic chemotherapy is the treatment of choice for patients with stage IIIB, IVA, and IVB disease. Selected patients with stage IIB and IIIA disease are also best treated initially with chemotherapy. Several multiagent regimens have been, and are being, tested in advanced disease. To date, none has demonstrated consistent superiority to the MOPP regimen (nitrogen mustard, vincristine, prednisone, and procarbazine). Approximately 80 per cent of all patients with stage IIIB or IV disease will obtain a complete remission after six monthly cycles of MOPP. Unfortunately, not all remissions are durable, and thus, the cure rate in advanced disease is only approximately 50 per cent.[4] Frequent toxicities associated with the MOPP regimen include,

nausea, vomiting, myelosuppression, neuropathy, infertility, and mood swings.

Future Directions in Management

Presently, multiple clinical trials are ongoing to evaluate new drug combinations in advanced stage Hodgkin's disease. Similarly, there are trials under way to evaluate various combinations of radiotherapy and chemotherapy in selected patients. Salvage regimens are being evaluated in patients who fail primary therapy or who relapse after an initial remission. Finally, study is ongoing into the etiology and pathogenesis of Hodgkin's disease so that preventive therapies can be designed.

REFERENCES

1. Appelbaum FR, et al: Treatment of non-Hodgkin's lymphoma with marrow transplantation in identical twins. Blood 58:509, 1981.
2. Banfi A, et al: Malignant lymphomas of Waldeyer's ring: Natural history and survival after radiotherapy. Br Med J 3:140, 1972.
2a. Burns BF, Wood GS, Dorfman RF: The varied histopathology of lymphadenopathy in the homosexual male. Am J Surg Pathol 9:287, 1985.
2b. Centers For Disease Control: Antibodies to a retrovirus etiologically associated with acquired immunodeficiency syndrome (AIDS) in populations with increased incidences of the syndrome. MMWR. 33:377, 1984.
3. Chen MG, et al: Results of radiotherapy in control of stage I and II non-Hodgkin's lymphoma. Cancer 43:1245, 1979.
4. DeVita VT, et al: Curability of advanced Hodgkin's disease with chemotherapy. Ann Intern Med 92:587, 1980.
4a. Gallo RC, Salahuddin SZ, Popovic M, et al. Frequent detection and isolation of cytopathic retroviruses (HTLV-III) from patients with AIDS and at risk for AIDS. Science 224:500, 1984.
5. Grufferman S: Clustering and aggregation of exposures in Hodgkin's disease. Cancer 39:1829, 1977.
6. Gutensohn N, et al: Epidemiology of Hodgkin's disease in the young. Int J Cancer 19:595, 1977.
7. Hellman S, et al: The place of radiation therapy in the treatment of non-Hodgkin's lymphomas. Cancer 39:843, 1977.
8. Hellman S, et al: The place of radiation therapy in the treatment of Hodgkin's disease. Cancer 42:971, 1978.
9. Hyman GA, et al: The development of Hodgkin's disease and lymphoma during anticonvulsant therapy. Blood 28:416, 1966.
10. Jones SE: Autoimmune disorders and malignant lymphoma. Cancer 31:1092, 1973.
11. Kadin ME, et al: Exogenous immunoglobulin and the macrophage origin of Reed-Sternberg cells in Hodgkin's disease. N Engl J Med 229:1208, 1978.
12. Kaplan HS: Evidence of a tumoricidal dose level in the radiotherapy of Hodgkin's disease. Cancer Res 26:1221, 1966.
13. Kaplan HS: Contiguity and progression in Hodgkin's disease. Cancer 31:1811, 1971.
14. Kaplan HS, et al: "Sternberg-Reed" giant cells of Hodgkin's disease: Cultivation in vitro, heterotransplantation, and characterization as neoplastic macrophages. Int J Cancer 19:511, 1977.
15. Kaplan HS, et al: Biology and virology of the human malignant lymphomas. Cancer 43:1, 1979.
16. Lobell M, et al: The clinical significance of fever in Hodgkin's disease. Arch Intern Med 117:335, 1966.
17. Manual for Staging of Cancer 1978. Chicago, American Joint Committee for Cancer Staging and End-Results Reporting, 1978.
17a. Melbye M, Biggar R, Ebbesen P, et al: Seroepidemiology of HTLV-III antibody in Danish homosexual men: Prevalence, transmission, and disease outcome. Br Med J 289:573, 1984.
18. Miller RW: Delayed radiation effects in atomic bomb survivors. Science 166:569, 1969.
19. Monyak D, et al: The cure of low stage large cell lymphomas treated by radiotherapy alone. (Submitted for publication.)
20. Nathwani BN: A critical analysis of the classifications of non-Hodgkin's lymphomas. Cancer 44:347, 1979.
21. Penn I: The incidence of malignancies in transplant recipients. Transplant Proc 7:323, 1975.

22. Philips GL, et al: Treatment of resistant malignant lymphoma with cyclophosphamide, total body irradiation, and transplantation of cryopreserved autologous marrow. N Engl J Med 310:1557, 1984.
23. Pinedo H, Chabner B: Cancer Chemotherapy, Annual 5. New York, Elsevier Publishing Co., 1983, p 258.
24. Portlock CS, et al: No initial therapy for stage III and IV non-Hodgkin's lymphomas of favorable histologic types. Ann Intern Med 90:10, 1979.
25. Ritz J, et al: Utilization of monoclonal antibodies in the treatment of leukemia and lymphoma. Blood 59:1, 1982.
26. Rosenberg SA: Report of the committee on the staging of Hodgkin's disease. Cancer Res 26:1310, 1966.
27. Rosenberg SA, et al: National Cancer Institute sponsored study of classifications of non-Hodgkin's lymphomas; summary and descrip-

28. Stein RS, et al: Bone marrow involvement in non-Hodgkin's lymphoma. Implications for staging and therapy. Cancer 37:629, 1976.
29. Stiehm ER, et al: Interferon: Immunobiology and clinical significance. Ann Intern Med 96:80, 1982.
30. Sweet DL, et al: Survival of patients with localized diffuse histiocytic lymphoma. Blood 58:1218, 1981.
31. Tubiana M, et al: Prognostic factors in 454 cases of Hodgkin's disease. Cancer Res 31:1801, 1971.
32. Ziegler JL, Levine AM, Metroka CE, et al: Non-Hodgkin's lymphoma in 90 homosexual men: Relationship to generalized lymphadenopathy and acquired immunodeficiency syndrome (AIDS). N Engl J Med 311:565, 1984.

tion of a working formulation for clinical usage. Cancer 49:2112, 1982.

LYMPHORETICULAR AND GRANULOMATOUS DISORDERS OF THE HEAD AND NECK

Joseph H. Graboyes, M.D.

Some of the lymphoreticular and granulomatous disorders of the head and neck may present with a head and neck manifestation that initially may be construed as a tumor. Some of the more common and confusing disorders are discussed in this chapter to help the clinician accurately diagnose and treat these lesions.

SINUS HISTIOCYTOSIS WITH MASSIVE LYMPHADENOPATHY

Sinus histiocystosis with massive lymphadenopathy (SHML) is a benign pseudolymphomatous disorder. It was first described in 1969 by Rosai and Dorfman in four patients. In the next decade, approximately 120 patients were described, making this a very uncommon disorder yet one that may present initially to the head and neck specialist. Most patients with SHML are children or young adults with massive painless lymphadenopathy. Diagnosis is made when a specific histopathologic pattern seen on lymph node biopsy is associated with a chronic benign clinical course. The typical patient is a male younger than 20 years of age. Although ages have ranged from 7 months to 45 years, very few cases present in persons over 20 years of age. Blacks are affected more commonly than whites.

The most prominent manifestation of SHML is cervical lymphadenopathy. These painless, often bilateral, lymph nodes persist for days to years before the patient seeks consultation, with an average interval being 3 to 9 months. All lymph node groups of the neck may be involved. When only one node or nodal group is involved, the submandibular area is the most common. The nodes begin as mobile discrete masses before becoming adherent, producing a large multinodular mass. Cervical lymph node involvement occurs more fre-

quently than axillary or inguinal lymphadenopathy. The lymph nodes persist from 6 months to several years before final resolution occurs in the majority of cases. Lymphadenopathy may rarely persist as long as 11 years after diagnosis. A few cases may show intermittent recurring lymphadenopathy.

Although the lymphadenopathy is protracted, the patient's general condition is benign during the several years it takes lymphadenopathy to regress. The only symptom that usually accompanies lymphadenopathy is fever. This may be present in 75 per cent of patients and ranges from 37.8 to 38.9°C. Patients are otherwise in excellent condition, with malaise and weight loss occurring rarely. Other unusual manifestations of SHML include tonsillitis, orbital mass, otitis media, conjunctivitis, eyelid swelling, nasal obstruction, testicular enlargement, skin nodules, cellulitis of the leg, paraplegia secondary to spinal epidural involvement, and upper airway obstruction.

Although cervical lymphadenopathy is a major manifestation of SHML, about 25 to 30 per cent of patients demonstrate extranodal involvement; occasionally, this may be the most prominent clinical manifestation. The most common location of extranodal involvement with SHML is the nasal cavity. The presence of diffuse inflammation or nasal polyps, often bilateral, results in partial or complete nasal obstruction. Epistaxis and rhinitis also occasionally occur. The salivary gland is the next most common location of extranodal involvement. This is occasionally mistaken for a tumor or a lymph node preoperatively. Other areas of involvement include the larynx, paranasal sinuses, tonsils, and trachea. Up to one half of these patients may demonstrate extranodal involvement at multiple sites. Two thirds of the patients with ear, nose, or throat involvement have SHML occurring at a second nonlymphoid location.

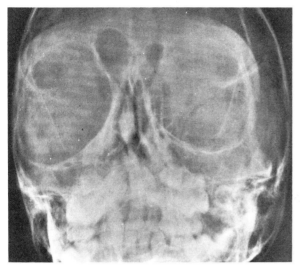

Figure 71–33. Bilateral orbital enlargement from sinus histiocytosis with massive lymphadenopathy.

Eye disease is an early manifestation in 5 per cent of patients. In another 5 per cent, ocular involvement will develop up to 20 years following initial presentation of the disease. Commonly, patients with ocular SHML will have significant peripheral lymphadenopathy. In addition, over half of the patients with ocular disease will demonstrate an additional site of extranodal involvement. The most frequent location of eye disease in SHML occurs in orbital soft tissue as firm, rubbery, nontender masses. Lacrimal gland and eyelid involvement occurs. Resultant exophthalmos may be bilateral (Fig. 71–33). Eyelid involvement, although usually asymptomatic, has been reported to cause blepharoptosis.

Bony lesions of SHML occur in approximately 4 per cent of patients. The long bones are most commonly involved, although other affected bones include the skull, vertebral bodies, ribs, metacarpals, phalanges, and pelvis. Radiographically, the lesions appear lytic with ill-defined margins. The lesions usually are medullary, but cortical defects may be present with no surrounding periosteal reaction. Serial roentgenograms show a gradual resolution of lytic lesions.

Occasionally, massive lymphadenopathy may result in compression of adjacent structures. Up to one fifth of these patients have dysphagia secondary to pharyngeal or esophageal compression. Retropharyngeal masses have resulted in stridor, with the need for an emergency tracheotomy.

Radiographically, SHML is indistinguishable from many other conditions that cause lymphadenopathy in children. Routine chest roentgenograms demonstrate perihilar or mediastinal masses in half of the patients. Perihilar involvement is unilateral in half of these patients and bilateral in the other half. Focal pulmonary infiltrates can occur. Retroperitoneal lymphangiography shows involvement of inguinal, iliac, and para-aortic lymph nodes with a reticular pattern or interruption in the marginal sinuses suggesting lymphoma.

To exclude the presence of lymphoma, it is best to perform a lymph node biopsy. Light microscopy reveals a proliferation of sinus histiocytes that completely replaces normal nodal architecture. The presence of lymphocytes and occasionally other hematopoietic cells within the cytoplasm of histiocytes is a constant feature. These intracellular inclusions are not unique to SHML and may be seen in salmonellosis, rhinoscleroma, and histoplasmosis.

Extranodal biopsy tissue from the nasal cavity, paranasal sinuses, and pharynx have cell populations identical to those seen in lymph nodes with histiocytes, lymphocytes, and plasma cells containing Russell bodies. The epithelium overlying the infiltrate is intact. In some cases, the aggregation of cells creates the illusion of sinuses. In all cases, typical histiocytes are present. Salivary gland infiltrates are similar in cell type to that in lymph nodes. In some cases, a correct diagnosis of SHML can be made from extranodal tissue; however, in others, study of an involved lymph node will be needed.

Routine laboratory studies generally are not helpful. The most common finding is that of an elevated erythrocyte sedimentation rate and hypergammaglobulinemia. Each of these is present in over 75 per cent of cases. Leukocytosis and neutrophilia are other common manifestations in this disease.

Multiple causes of lymphadenopathy in children must be entertained in the differential diagnosis of this disorder. Following biopsy, the histopathologic differential diagnosis of this disorder can be difficult, for several lymphoreticular malignant neoplasms including lymphoma, Hodgkin's lymphoma, malignant histiocytosis, and monocytic leukemia may partially resemble SHML. In contrast to the benign appearance of histiocytes in SHML, the cytologic atypia present in the aforementioned malignancies may assist in the proper diagnosis.

Attempts to document an infectious etiology of SHML have been unsuccessful despite microscopic examinations, cultures, and serologic testing. Defects in host immunity have been inconsistently identified. The etiology of SHML, therefore, remains unknown.

Because the cause of this disorder has yet to be determined, treatment is largely empiric. Antibiotics have been used, but are currently thought to have no effect. The use of steroids has resulted in the disappearance of fever, but lymphadenopathy persists. There is no consistent response of lymphadenopathy to steroids, radiation, or chemotherapy. Surgical excision of affected lymph nodes has resulted in complete cure in some patients. Others, however, have had local recurrences at the site of excision. These local recurrences may develop as late as 6 years following the initial surgery. Given the relatively benign nature and rarity of this disorder, no clear conclusions may be made concerning efforts to influence its clinical course. Fortunately, sinus histiocytosis with massive lymphadenopathy, a newly recognized, distinct, pseudolymphomatous disorder with characteristic microscopic features, is a rare, chronic, benign disease.

ANGIOIMMUNOBLASTIC LYMPHADENOPATHY WITH DYSPROTEINEMIA

There are a number of non-neoplastic lymphadenopathies that simulate malignant lymphoma. Within the last decade, a lymphadenopathy associated with the immunologic abnormalities of polyclonal gammopathy, hemolytic anemia, or both has received special attention. While reviewing cases of Hodgkin's disease that lacked diagnostic Reed-Sternberg cells and exhibited consistent clinical and laboratory features,[11] Frizzera, Moran, and Rappaport discovered this entity, which they called angioimmunoblastic lymphadenopathy with dysproteinemia (AILD).

Patients affected with this disease have signs similar to those of malignant lymphoma. Peripheral lymphadenopathy, hepatosplenomegaly, skin rash, and systemic manifestations occur. Changes may also occur in bone marrow and lung. The group of patients affected with this disease is nonhomogeneous, with variable states of immunologic abnormalities. Some patients experience a benign reversible process with a temporary immunologic deficiency; others follow a progressively fulminant course with a nearly complete breakdown of immunologic defenses.

The prevalence of AILD is uncertain. Males and females are equally affected. The average age of presentation is in the fifth and sixth decades.

The clinical manifestations of AILD are suggestive of Hodgkin's disease. There is a rapid onset of lymphadenopathy. In approximately one fourth of patients, this follows a drug ingestion and is interpreted as drug sensitivity. On retrospective analysis, commonly implicated therapeutic agents include penicillin, sulfonamide, aspirin, halothane, and primidone.

The nodes average 2 to 3 cm in size and are soft, mobile, nonmatted, and only occasionally tender. The lymphadenopathy is generalized in 80 per cent, but involves only regional nodes in 20 per cent of cases. There is a predisposition of lymph nodes to localize in the head and neck. Approximately half of these patients will have cervical lymphadenopathy; supraclavicular nodes will be involved in 15 per cent, and postauricular and submandibular nodes each may be involved in approximately 5 per cent of cases. Accompanying the lymphadenopathy will be hepatomegaly and splenomegaly, each involving over 50 per cent of patients.

Systemic manifestations also frequently occur. Fever and weight loss will be present in over half of the patients. A maculopapular rash and pruritus will each occur in approximately one third of patients. Pneumonia, with radiologic evidence of bilateral infiltrates and pleural effusion, may resolve with appropriate therapy, leaving the patient with an unknown source for the febrile episodes. Alternatively, these pulmonary infiltrates and effusion may reflect a primary involvement of the lung with AILD. In this situation, pleural biopsy will demonstrate an infiltrate of immunoblasts, plasma cells, and lymphocytes. Nonetheless, pneumonia remains the primary consideration in these patients, for it occurs in many patients with AILD.

Routine laboratory data demonstrate dysproteinemias and a Coombs-positive hemolytic anemia. The Coombs-positive anemia will be present in approximately 50 per cent of patients and may be direct or indirect. Some patients will demonstrate changes consistent with hemolytic anemia on peripheral blood smears. Non–Coombs-positive anemia also occurs. Polyclonal hyperglobulinemia is another characteristic finding. Approximately 85 per cent of patients with AILD will have

hyperglobulinemia. There may be diffuse involvement of all categories or selective involvement of IgG and IgM. Leukocytosis and leukopenia may occur, and eosinophilia is present in at least 20 per cent of patients. Thrombocytopenia may also occur. Thus, a constellation of laboratory findings with characteristic hemolytic anemia and polyclonal hyperglobulinemia characterizes patients with AILD.

Radiologic studies of these patients mistakenly thought to have lymphoma demonstrate classical findings on lymphangiogram and liver spleen scans. There is an increase in iliac and para-aortic lymph nodes. They have a foamy appearance with filling defects demonstrable on lymphangiograms. Liver-spleen scans show enlargement of the liver and spleen with a slight decrease in radioactive uptake and no specific filling defects. Chest roentgenograms may show mediastinal and hilar lymphadenopathy. An occasional pleural effusion occurs. The combination of characteristic radiologic and laboratory findings is insufficient to exclude the diagnosis of malignant lymphoma. Most patients, therefore, present for lymph node biopsy before the correct diagnosis can be confirmed.

The nodes are similar to those of other lymphoproliferative disorders, being large, pale, and rubbery. Necrosis and "fish flesh" consistency and appearance rarely occur. Lymph nodes of the head and neck are both commonly present and are easily accessible for biopsy. Skin lesions may also be present for biopsy. Needle biopsies of the liver and bone marrow biopsies will demonstrate nonspecific changes consistent with AILD, but these extranodal specimens lack the diagnostic specificity present only in lymph nodes.

The histopathologic picture demonstrates a diffuse disruption of nodal architecture by a mixed cellular proliferation of immunoblasts, vascular proliferation and arborization, and acidophilic interstitial material. Biopsy of extranodal sites is insufficient to make the diagnosis of AILD, but characteristic changes are noted. Liver biopsies demonstrate normal hepatocytes with lymphocyte and plasma cell infiltrates of portal triads. Bone marrow biopsy in patients with hemolytic anemia will show only hyperplastic changes. Biopsy of involved skin areas shows focal cellular infiltrates in the upper and lower dermis with epidermal sparing. Immunoblasts are present, as is an increase in the number of capillaries. All these extranodal surgical specimens lack the diagnostic specificity present in lymph nodes. Thus, biopsy of the lymph node remains the only source of material permitting the diagnosis of AILD.

One of the major problems facing pathologists is the distinction between reactive proliferation of lymphoreticular tissue and malignant neoplasms. This differential diagnosis is complicated by the fact that lymphoid tissue may react intensely to a variety of infectious and other antigenic stimuli, and the resulting proliferative process may simulate that of a malignant neoplasm. Furthermore, the finding of changes consistent with AILD within a portion of a single lymph node does not exclude the diagnosis of malignant lymphoma. Further sectioning within a single node may show areas consistent with malignant lymphoma. The principal differential diagnosis after lymph node biopsy includes reactive lesions that may occur with Hodgkin's disease, immunoblastic lymphoma, postvaccinal lymphadenopathies, and viral lymphadenopathies including herpes simplex, herpes zoster, and infectious mononucleosis. In most viral lymphadenopathies, however, nodal architecture is usually preserved.

The clinical course with AILD is variable. It ranges from prolonged survival in the absence of therapy to a rapid, more fulminant progression than that seen in patients treated for malignant lymphoma. In addition to those patients who die of AILD, despite therapy, one third of the patients with AILD will ultimately develop malignant lymphoma.

Both radiation therapy and chemotherapy have been used alone or in combination to treat AILD. Chemotherapeutic agents used have included glucocorticoids, cyclophosphamide, vincristine, bleomycin, and nitrogen mustard. On the basis of limited nonprospective data, corticosteroids are the best therapeutic agent. Results of therapy with prednisone have varied. Approximately two thirds of those patients treated with oral prednisone, at 20 to 120 mg per day, will have a complete remission. Approximately half of the patients treated with oral prednisone will undergo a complete remission and remain asymptomatic after stopping all therapy. Two thirds of those treated with oral prednisone will be alive 12 to 57 months after diagnosis, and the median survival for the entire group will be approximately 32 months. Results for patients treated with combination or single-drug chemotherapy are similar. Thus, the spectrum of survival in AILD includes those few patients who have a spontaneous remission without any therapy, those patients who have a long disease-free survival after chemotherapy, and those patients who rapidly die of their disease despite chemotherapy.

In addition, some patients with AILD will later develop immunoblastic lymphoma. This subset of patients has a much poorer response to either prednisone or chemotherapy than do the patients with AILD who do not progress to immunoblastic lymphoma. Given the nonhomogeneity of patients with AILD, and the great variability in the natural course of this disease, recommendations for specific therapeutic regimens, based on previous nonprospective trials, must be limited to the observation that corticosteroids appear to be as beneficial as more toxic chemotherapeutic agents in the control of AILD.

With the rapidly progressive course in AILD, cytotoxic agents indeed may enhance the patient's susceptibility to overwhelming infection, which may be the terminal event. The various mycotic and opportunistic infections, together with gastrointestinal ulcerations, massive hepatic necrosis, acute pancreatitis, and acute renal failure, are common causes of patients dying of AILD.

The etiology of this condition is unknown, and its classification is indefinite. Lukes and Tindle suggest that AILD is a form of reticuloendothelial proliferation.[13] As in other disorders such as Sjögren's syndrome and systemic lupus erythematosus, malignant lymphoma may occur following AILD. Noting that one fourth of cases of AILD were temporally related to a drug reaction, a reactive mechanism as a possible etiology of AILD exists. There are also similarities between AILD and graft-versus-host reactions. Cell surface markers indicate that although plasma cells are present within nodal lesions, most cells in the abnormal lymph node are of T-cell lineage, with B cells accounting for only 25

per cent. AILD therefore may result from an abnormal T-cell response to unknown antigenic agents.

Our understanding of the lymphadenopathies associated with abnormal immunologic reaction is still incomplete. Perhaps AILD and immunoblastic lymphoma, with clinical and morphologic similarities, are identical entities. Alternatively, they may constitute distinct disorders sharing abnormal immune reactions. The diagnosis of a new entity, angioimmunoblastic lymphadenopathy with dysproteinemia, appears justified based upon a distinctive histopathologic pattern, immunologic features such as polyclonal gammopathy and hemolytic anemia, common clinical features, and a distinctive, albeit variable, clinical course that often progresses to lymphoma.

HISTIOCYTOSIS X

Histiocytosis X is a disorder of the reticuloendothelial system that is characterized by the proliferation of cytologically benign histiocytes. Histiocytosis X, a term coined in 1953 by Lichtenstein, relates three disease complexes of unknown etiology and variable clinical expression to a common histologic lesion. The three clinical expressions of the disease, in increasing degree of severity, are eosinophilic granuloma, Hand-Schüller-Christian disease, and Letterer-Siwe disease. The overlapping manifestations of the disease complexes, the unpredictable evolution, and the multiple modalities of therapy result in clinical confusion concerning histiocytosis X. A comparison of these three types is presented in Table 71–6.

There is an important difference between histiocytosis X and true malignant neoplasms. The course of histiocytosis X is characterized by spontaneous remissions and exacerbations, whereas the course of true cancer is unrelentingly progressive. The lesions of true neoplasms are usually pathologically homogeneous, whereas those of histiocytosis X are generally heterogeneous. Moreover, histiocytosis X has similarities to various immunologic disorders including severe combined immunodeficiency disease and graft-versus-host reactions.

There are those who support the concept of a single all-encompassing nosologic entity and those who dispute that concept. Most workers now use the term Hand-Schüller-Christian (HSC) syndrome to describe a disseminated or multifocal eosinophilic granuloma. Indeed, the classic triad of exophthalmos, diabetes insipidus, and bony defects occurs in only 10 per cent of cases with HSC syndrome. When described in this manner, solitary or multifocal eosinophilic granulomas each appear to be a single disease process.

More than 75 per cent of patients have one or more head and neck manifestation of histiocytosis X at the time of presentation. The most frequent complaint is local pain and a low-grade fever. Although localized forms of the disease usually have a favorable outcome, disseminated forms of histiocytosis X vary greatly in severity and prognosis.

Eosinophilic granuloma, the mildest form of the disease, was first described in 1940 by Jaffe and Lichtenstein. This benign condition may occur at any age and is seen predominantly in children over 5 years of age and in young adults. Typically, the disease is restricted to bone. The skull, long bones, ribs, and vertebrae are usually affected, with pain and local tenderness being the presenting symptoms. It is associated with a high degree of spontaneous tumor resolution. Eosinophilic granuloma may be considered the unifocal manifestation of disease, and HSC syndrome is the multifocal manifestation of disease.

Hand-Schüller-Christian syndrome is used to designate widespread eosinophilic granuloma of the bone as well as histiocytic infiltrates of the liver, lung, spleen, skin, and brain. This moderately favorable syndrome has slow tumor growth and occasional spontaneous resolution. It occurs in children less than 5 years old and rarely occurs in adults. Males are affected twice as frequently as females.

Letterer-Siwe (LS) syndrome almost invariably occurs in infants less than 3 years of age and rarely occurs in adults. This most severe form of histiocytosis X is characterized by multiple organ involvement and dysfunction. Patients usually lack bony involvement but suffer from anemia, thrombocytopenia, jaundice, respiratory insufficiency, lymphadenopathy, and skin infiltration. LS syndrome has a rapidly progressive downhill course, with death occurring within 1 to 2 years after the onset of disease.

The unifying feature in histiocytosis X is the pathologic lesion. In an attempt to correlate the pathologic appearance with the clinical course of histiocytosis X, two separate subtypes of lesions have been described. The type 1 (malignant) lesion is characterized by a diffuse monomorphous infiltration of the reticuloendothelial system and other tissues by histiocytes. There is a definite absence of multinucleated giant cells, eosinophils, necrosis, and fibrosis. The type 2 (benign) disease is characterized by variegated lesions infiltrated by histiocytes mixed with eosinophils, multinucleated giant cells, and foci of necrosis. Patients with type 2 disease have a more benign protracted form of the disorder. Type 2 disease includes HSC syndrome and eosinophilic granuloma. The type 1 form of disease occurs mainly in LS syndrome. It has a short course and a poor prognosis. Some investigators note patients with type 2 disease who present with a picture identical to LS syndrome have a better prognosis than patients with type 1 histologic and clinical picture. Nonetheless, the histologic appearance of histiocytosis X appears to be highly variable. It depends upon the tissue selected for biopsy and upon the time of the biopsy in the course of the disease. Simultaneous biopsies of a cutaneous lesion and a bony lesion in the same patient may confirm the histologic pleomorphism of histiocytosis X and therefore the limited prognostic value of histologic subtyping.

The etiology and origin of histiocytosis X remain unclear. Although males are involved twice as often as females, mortality rates are approximately equal. Thus, a more severe form appears to affect females. There is no apparent racial predisposition.

Disseminated histiocytosis X (DHX) includes the entities of Hand-Schüller-Christian syndrome and Letterer-Siwe syndrome. Studies needed to define the extent of disease include a complete blood count with a peripheral smear, erythrocyte sedimentation rate, serum calcium and phosphate levels, liver function tests, and measurements of hypothalamic and pituitary function (growth hormone, ACTH, TSH, plasma osmolality, and ADH). Roentgenographic studies include chest and skeletal surveys and both liver and spleen radionuclide scans.

Disseminated histiocytosis X has a variable clinical course. In some patients the disease is rapidly progressive, with death occurring within 2 years. In others, the active phase lasts a minimum of 2 years, and disease may reappear after a period of stabilization. Following termination of drug therapy, there may be sudden phases of disease activity. During these periods cutaneous lesions and visceral lesions, particularly of liver and spleen, increase in size. The reappearance of skin and pulmonary lesions signifies a poor prognosis, and if skin lesions are evident after 2 years, the patient rarely survives. Those patients with DHX who survive have numerous and variable sequelae. Most frequently, diabetes insipidus develops. Growth stunting caused by spinal lesions, pituitary insufficiency, or prolonged corticosteroid therapy is another common result. Intellectual retardation is usually the result of blindness or deafness.

Histiocytosis X can affect almost any organ in the body. Skin is a frequently involved tissue. Skin lesions are initially present in 40 per cent of patients and ultimately occur in 80 to 100 per cent of patients with DHX. Skin lesions are most commonly found on the scalp and hair line areas and vary from resistant dandruff to weeping dermatitis. Scalp lesions are often misdiagnosed as eczema and may be an early sign of dissemination. In severe cases, the skin is scaly, yellow-brown, and greasy, with a purpuric or hemorrhagic rash resembling scald burns (Fig. 71–34). There are protein and fluid losses and secondary infection. Because the skin is almost invariably involved, the prognostic value of skin involvement at presentation is minimal.

Bone lesions are also common manifestations of histiocytosis X. The flat bones of the skull, pelvis, scapula, and ribs are more frequently involved than the long bones. Bone lesions with pain or functional impairment are presenting symptoms in 20 per cent of patients. A dull pain with adjacent soft-tissue swelling is the typical presentation, although asymptomatic lesions may be incidental findings. Ultimately, 80 per cent or more of

TABLE 71–6. A Comparison of Three Clinical Forms of Histiocytosis X

Feature	Eosinophilic Granuloma	Hand-Schüller-Christian Disease	Letterer-Siwe Disease
Age	Over 5 years	Under 5 years	Under 3 years
Bone involvement	+	+	−
Other organ involvement	−	+	+
Course	Possible spontaneous remission	Longer than 1–2 years	Fatal in 1–2 years

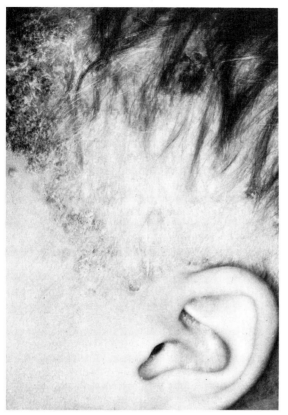

Figure 71–34. Skin manifestations of histiocytosis X with scaling, erythema, and purpura.

these patients develop bony involvement. Many lesions appear as the disease progresses, and single lesions may later progress to multiple sites. Spontaneous resolution has been observed, and if lesions remain unchanged for 12 or more months, then progression is unlikely. The disease replaces both endochondral and membranous bone. Sites affected in order of decreasing incidence include the skull (most frequently the temporal bone), ribs, scapula, and femur. Half of the patients with solitary bony lesions are children younger than 10 years of age, although adults are not immune. Bony lesions do not adversely affect the prognosis.

The roentgenographic appearance of bony lesions is distinctive but not pathognomonic. Frank bone defects are the most common changes. In the calvarium, greater destruction of the outer table gives a beveled edge to the lucencies and a scalloped margin. Cyst-like lesions progress into multiloculated, irregularly marginated defects with a map-like design, giving rise to the term "geographic skull" (Fig. 71–35). Sclerosis rarely occurs in the skull or in flat bones. Erosion of the cortical layer may stimulate periosteal reaction. These lesions radiologically simulate osteomyelitis, Ewing's sarcoma, or metastatic tumor. Exophthalmos, usually bilateral, results from involvement of bony orbital walls. Spinal infiltration by histiocytes results in vertebral collapse with subsequent widening of the disk space. Vertebral body collapse may be uniform, or an incomplete wedge-shaped deformity may occur anteriorly. A return to normal dimensions rarely occurs following therapy.

Oral involvement is nonspecific and occurs in conjunction with maxillofacial involvement. Osseous lesions may occur on the palate, maxilla, or mandible. Posterior mandible or alveolar ridge involvement is the most common intraoral location. Symptoms include swelling and pain when soft tissue becomes involved. Histiocytic infiltration of the alveolar bone and mucosa simulates periodontal disease and periapical infection. Loosening of teeth and exfoliation of teeth may be found with a characteristic radiologic picture of "floating teeth." Primary histiocytic infiltration of the mucosa is less common.

The reported incidence of otologic involvement in histiocytosis X ranges from 15 to 60 per cent. This variability results from the method of patient evaluation as well as the definition of otologic involvement. Involvement occurs more frequently in patients with systemic involvement than in those with localized osseous involvement. It is most often observed in the first decade of life and generally in patients less than 4 years of age. Among those patients with otologic involvement, one third will present with otologic symptoms as the initial manifestation of histiocytosis X. The most frequent symptoms are aural discharge and swelling over the temporal area. When otologic involvement is the sole manifestation of histiocytosis X, the otolaryngologist may suspect the diagnosis only after antibiotics fail to control otitis externa or when chronic otitis media and mastoid destruction lead to a mastoidectomy.

Histiocytosis X may originate in the temporal bone. Initially, the lesions are asymptomatic. Erosion of any portion of the temporal bone can occur, including the labyrinthine capsule or cochlea. Destruction of the tegmen may allow tumor invasion of the middle or posterior cranial fossa. Granulation tissue in the external auditory canal with a fistula through the bony canal into the mastoid cavity may occur. Involvement of the facial canal can produce facial paralysis. Facial nerve paralysis occurs in less than 5 per cent of patients with temporal bone destruction even when the nerve traverses the area of active disease. Facial paralysis is more common when multifocal disease occurs.

Suppurative otitis media is the most common clinical manifestation of otologic involvement, although bloody otorrhea is rare. It is indistinguishable from common suppurative otitis media. Otitis externa also commonly occurs. A swollen and inflamed ear canal, similar to that seen in diffuse bacterial otitis externa, may yield characteristic findings when biopsied. Perforations of the tympanic membrane usually result from infection rather than from histiocytic infiltration. Conductive hearing loss is commonly present, with sensorineural hearing loss and vertigo being unusual findings that are indicative of labyrinthine involvement.

Temporal bone lesions are punched-out radiolucent defects without reactive sclerosis. Because of its indolent nature, eosinophilic granuloma of the temporal bone may be confused with neoplasms, granulomatous disorders, chronic infections, and surgical or traumatic defects. Disease entities to be excluded include radiation necrosis, cystic osteomyelitis, tuberculosis, syphilis, cholesteatoma, solitary bone cysts, giant cell tumor of bone, plasmacytoma, multiple myeloma, benign bone cysts, fibrous dysplasia, osteitis fibrosa cystica, Ewing's sarcoma, sinus histiocytosis with massive lymphadenopathy, meningioma, neuroblastoma, lymphoma, sarcoma, and metastatic tumors.

Grossly, the intraosseous lesion in the temporal bone is a demarcated area of soft gray or reddish brown granular material with areas of necrosis, cysts, and hemorrhage. Secondary infection of the temporal bone often occurs; thus, suppuration may be present.

Current management of temporal bone involvement includes surgery, radiation therapy, or chemotherapy. A useful management strategy includes conservative mastoid surgery to allow exteriorization of the disease with preservation of vital structures and retention of useful hearing. Low-dose radiation is given separately or in combination with surgery in doses of 600 to 1000 rad. Chemotherapy is unjustified in the management of new unifocal disease but is essential for recurrent or multifocal disease. When disease is confined to the mastoid, mastoidectomy alone or in combination with radiation therapy is effective in controlling the disease.

A long-term sequela of chronic DHX is diabetes insipidus. Diabetes insipidus may be present in 6 per cent of patients at presentation and will eventually occur in half of all patients with chronic DHX. Thought to result from a lesion of the hypothalamus or pituitary, the lesion responds poorly to local radiation therapy. The diabetes insipidus appears to be permanent but is easily treated. It is interesting that the presence of diabetes insipidus is a prognostically favorable finding. When an inadequate level of somatotropin occurs, impaired sexual development and stunted growth result. A lack of other hormones is rarely found. Other central nervous system lesions result from compressive effects or extension of osseous skull lesions. Blindness may occur. Sensory deficits of hearing loss and blindness often lead to mental retardation.

Lymphadenopathy is a frequent finding in DHX. In 5 per cent of patients, lymph node enlargement is the first manifestation of histiocytosis X, although ultimately, half of these patients will develop lymphadenopathy. It most commonly manifests itself as regional node involvement with accompanying lytic bone lesions or cutaneous manifestations. Less frequently, histiocy-

tosis X presents as lymphadenopathy without extranodal involvement and remains localized. There is a slight predilection for the anterior cervical chain, although any group may be affected. Lymphadenopathy may be generalized or localized and intermittently recurrent over a period of 1 to 6 years in untreated patients. The patients with recurrent intermittent lymphadenopathy are asymptomatic between episodes but develop systemic symptoms of fever, malaise, and night sweats with the lymphadenopathy. The systemic symptoms are notably transient, appearing and resolving over a period of weeks. With isolated lymphadenopathy a simple excision of the involved nodes is curative, but patients must be re-examined periodically for recurrence or progression of disease.

Pulmonary lesions are rarely the initial site of localization of histiocytosis X and may occur in generalized disease or as a primary isolated lesion in young adults. Bilateral diffuse infiltrates can be found in both generalized and localized involvement (Fig. 71–36). A honeycomb-like pattern on chest roentgenograms results when fibrosis leads to multiple cystic lesions. There is often no correlation between pulmonary symptoms and roentgenographic findings. Symptoms of dry cough, dyspnea, shortness of breath, respiratory insufficiency, and cor pulmonale all carry a poor prognosis. Asymptomatic pulmonary involvement is of no prognostic significance.

Involvement of the gastrointestinal tract may occur. Moderate enlargement of the liver and spleen with normal organ function is not unusual. With aggressive disease, extreme enlargement and evidence of organ dysfunction indicates a poor prognosis. When jaundice or clinical signs of hepatic insufficiency develop, the disease is almost inevitably fatal. Although splenectomy is dangerous, reports of benefit following this procedure may justify the risk.

Hematologic manifestations of histiocytosis X are frequently observed in disseminated cases. Anemia, leukocytosis, thrombocytopenia, and an elevated erythrocyte sedimentation rate all occur. Cases of spontaneous thrombocytopenia and severe anemia are almost always

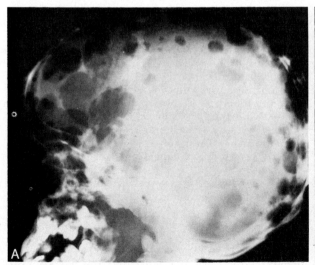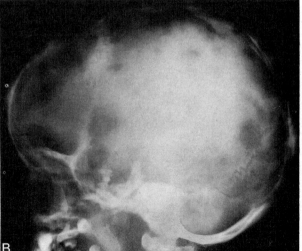

Figure 71–35. Multiloculated cyst-like lesions of the skull are characteristic of histiocytosis X. (*A*) Before treatment. (*B*) After treatment. Note improvement in skull lesions.

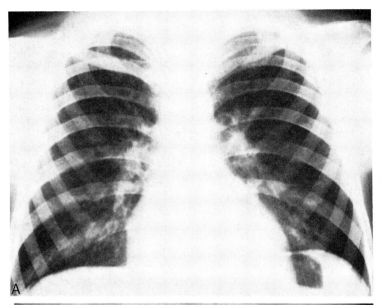

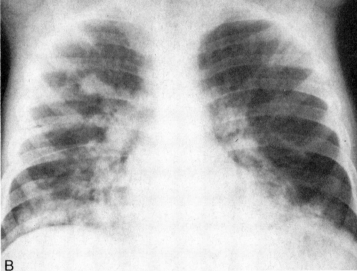

Figure 71-36. (*A*) Pulmonary infiltrate from histiocytosis X. (*B*) Same patient 8 months later. This disease progressed in spite of therapy. It is interesting to note that the skull lesions improved while the lung lesions worsened.

fatal. Pancytopenia indicates either iatrogenic suppression of bone marrow or bone marrow replacement by disease. Anemia, thrombocytopenia, and splenomegaly may be seen despite a nearly normal bone marrow examination.

The prognosis of histiocytosis X is based on a variety of factors. Patients older than 2 years of age without organ dysfunction generally have a good prognosis. Patients younger than 2 years of age without organ dysfunction have a fair prognosis, but those younger than 2 years of age with organ dysfunction have a poor prognosis. The peak occurrence of disseminated histiocytosis X is during the first 6 months of life. Those patients who develop DHX after 2 years of age have an 80 per cent survival rate with treatment, compared with a 33 per cent survival rate for patients presenting under 2 years of age. Nonetheless, the extensiveness of the lesion, rather than the age of the patient at which it occurs, is most critical. Lahey devised a system to evaluate the prognosis of DHX. When one point is given for each of the nine changes of cutaneous eruption, hepatic insufficiency, splenomegaly, impaired respiratory function, bone localization, pituitary involvement, anemia, leukopenia, and thrombocytopenia, then the mortality rate is linearly related to the number of involved localities. There is a 25 per cent mortality rate when two organs are involved, a 33 per cent mortality when three or four organ are involved, a 72 per cent mortality when five or six organs are involved, and a 100 per cent mortality when more than six organs are involved.

HSC syndrome is a chronic illness with an active phase lasting a minimum of 2 years. Relapses occur, but these are rare after 3 years of quiescence. Sequelae are frequent and include stunting of growth, mental retardation, blindness, deafness, and diabetes insipidus. In fatal cases, death occurs within 2 years from cutaneous, pulmonary, or bone marrow involvement. Deaths from bone marrow aplasia, septicemia, or opportunistic infection are common. Severe cachexia is present, regardless of the cause of death. In those patients dying of histiocytosis X, the course is rapid, with death usually occurring within 2 years. Rare delayed deaths occurring after 2 years have been noted in patients with bone marrow aplasia.

Conservative treatment of localized lesions by limited surgery or curettage in combination with low-dose radiation, from 300 to 1000 rad, is effective. Higher doses of radiation up to 4000 rad have been used in inaccessible areas or in sites associated with a high morbidity. Spontaneous remissions have occurred. With aggressive disseminated disease many publications advocate the use of specific therapeutic protocols of chemotherapy. A variety of chemotherapeutic drugs have been tried, including vincristine, vinblastine, methotrexate, chlorambucil, and various drug combinations. Because of a lack of well-controlled trials, it is difficult to assess the efficacy of these regimens. Deaths due to aggressive chemotherapy have been reported with bone marrow aplasia and drug-induced immunosuppression. As both the illness and the treatment are complex, it is not possible to make value judgments about specific therapies. Nonetheless, the prognosis for untreated Letterer-Siwe syndrome is grave, although modification through chemotherapy has been possible.

A recent recognition of immunologic abnormality associated in over half of patients with histiocytosis X has attracted much interest. Over 50 per cent of patients with histiocytosis X lack suppressor T-cells. When treated daily with intramuscular injections of thymic extract, clinical remission occurred coincident with an increase in suppressor T-cell populations. A response rate of 60 per cent is similar to that seen in patients treated with chemotherapy. The time from the onset of treatment until remission is shorter with thymic extract treatment than it is with chemotherapy, and the duration of remission is longer after thymic extract treatment than after chemotherapy. Additional clinical trials are needed to verify this finding.

The prognosis and treatment of patients should be based upon the staging and extent of disease. Localized disease should be treated conservatively, recognizing that spontaneous resolution may occur. Similarly, localized disease may progress to diffuse systemic disease. Continued clinical observation is therefore necessary. Low-dose radiation therapy is efficacious in treating localized nonsurgically accessible lesions. Randomized treatment protocols are necessary to clarify the value of chemotherapy and immunotherapy in patients with aggressive disseminated disease.

SARCOIDOSIS

The word "sarcoid" was coined by Boeck in 1899 to describe skin eruptions of multiple, small, discrete infiltrations that he considered to be paravascular sarcomatoid tissue. Schaumann and other authors later noted the occurrence of systemic manifestations beyond the skin.

Because no agent or factor that causes sarcoidosis has yet been discovered, sarcoidosis cannot be etiologically defined. Sarcoidosis is a disease characterized by noncaseating epithelioid cell granulomas in several organs and tissues. Because a variety of infectious and malignant diseases as well as local foreign body reactions can cause localized noncaseating granulomas, the diagnosis of sarcoidosis must indicate that a widespread granulomatosis is present. The complete lack of necrosis and failure to histologically demonstrate infectious agents are compatible with the diagnosis, but the absence of a known cause for granulomatous change is required for a definitive diagnosis.

Sarcoidosis can be a self-limiting benign disease that requires no therapy or minimal therapy. The natural history of the disease includes an insidious onset and progression over the years, with an occasional variation wherein a patient has an acute onset. Some patients experience a chronic progressive course with resultant severe illness.

Although generally involving the reticuloendothelial system, sarcoidosis also affects almost every other structure and organ in the body. The otolaryngologist will encounter this disease because of the frequency of lesions involving the head and neck, including the nose, tonsils, salivary glands, larynx, and cervical lymph nodes. Furthermore, the otolaryngologist will encounter multiple lesions that are easily accessible for biopsy.

Sarcoidosis has its most common onset in the third decade with the earliest age of presentation being 7 years and the latest age being roughly 75 years. The peak incidence occurs in the third decade, in which 40 per cent of the cases present. Sarcoidosis is 11 times more prevalent in blacks than in Caucasians. In nonmilitary series white males and females are equally affected. Negro females, however, are affected with twice the frequency of Negro males. In military personnel, a higher incidence of sarcoidosis among men born in the southern United States has been reported. Others note no differences between sarcoidosis patients and control patients with regard to place of birth, residence, vacations, or trips to the South.

Symptoms in a patient presenting with sarcoidosis can be divided into two groups: those of a general nature and those of specific organ involvement. Approximately 85 per cent of patients have some symptoms, indicating that the disease is not usually an incidental finding. Approximately 43 per cent of patients note vague complaints such as fatigue, malaise, and weakness. Next in frequency are respiratory symptoms such as cough and dyspnea, followed by ocular and cutaneous lesions. About a quarter of patients note weight loss, and a slightly smaller percentage will present with fever. Nonetheless, there is a noticeable frequency of asymptomatic organ involvement. There is a striking contrast between minimal symptoms and the degree of involvement present. Local symptoms may not become manifest until after extensive organ involvement has occurred. The disease is generally benign, although the outcome may be poor in 15 to 20 per cent of patients. Those patients dying of disease do so as a result of cardiac, pulmonary, or central nervous system lesions.

The typical histologic picture is insufficient to make the diagnosis of sarcoidosis. Typically, the presence of numerous similar granulomas composed mainly of epithelioid cells with an occasional giant cell, and with the absence of caseation is seen. The granulomas may appear fresh for months or years with little evidence of scarring. They may ultimately resolve completely, leaving no residual change, or alternatively, the granulomas may undergo hyaline fibrosis. The factors that influence progression toward resolution or fibrosis remain unknown. The presence of extensive areas of central or intragranulomatous eosinophilic necrosis of collagen may make histologic differentiation from caseating tuberculosis difficult. Granular necrosis may closely resemble caseation.

The differential diagnosis of sarcoidosis depends both upon the location of the lesion and the findings obtained on biopsy. When patients have caseating tuberculosis, the possibility of sarcoidosis remains and will cause difficulty in clinical diagnosis. Granulomatous changes may also be found in patients having some forms of autoimmune deficiency disease. Epithelioid granulomas can be seen in lymph nodes of patients with malignant lymphadenopathy and may obscure the underlying malignancy. When biopsies show a local granulomatous reaction, or fail to show a characteristic granuloma but rather display poorly formed collections of inflammatory cells or necrotic granulomas, a problem arises. Equally problematic is the patient who refuses biopsy. It is unreasonable to specify a single set of diagnostic criteria applicable to the many clinical manifestations of sarcoidosis. When cases conform to a well-recognized pattern and lack discordant features, then a confirmatory histologic picture from an affected tissue is sufficient. Alternatively, consistent biopsies from multiple sites may still leave room for doubt, with the need to follow a patient's clinical course. Physicians now have two alternatives to establishing or supporting the diagnosis of sarcoidosis.

The Kveim-Siltzbach test may assist in the diagnosis of sarcoidosis. A positive test combined with a clinical picture suggesting sarcoidosis increases the probability of the disease. A negative test diminishes the probability to a degree, varying with the apparent stage of the disease. With the Kveim-Siltzbach test, a saline suspension of human sarcoidal spleen or lymph node tissue from a patient with sarcoidosis is injected intracutaneously into another patient with suspected sarcoidosis. In 2 to 6 weeks a palpable purple nodule arises at the site of injection. Biopsy of this nodule in a positive Kveim-Siltzbach test will show a caseating granulomatous reaction. A classic case with bilateral hilar lymphadenopathy and erythema nodosum may have a 10 to 15 per cent false negative test; here a negative test is almost noncontributory. Given bilateral hilar lymphadenopathy with constitutional symptoms, a positive Kveim-Siltzbach test makes these other diagnoses very unlikely. When granulomatous involvement is found in only a single organ, without clinical or radiologic evidence of granulomatosis elsewhere, a positive Kveim-Siltzbach test response can be the equivalent of finding granulomas at a second location, thereby strongly supporting the diagnosis of sarcoidosis.

Two difficulties diminish the utility of this test. First, the test may be falsely positive in cases with certain other diseases, notably Crohn's disease, infectious mononucleosis, chronic lymphocytic leukemia, and nonspecific lymphadenopathy. Usually, clinical or histopathologic information can exclude these diagnoses. A more serious difficulty arises because of the limited availability of potent validated antigen for this test.

The second test of utility to the clinician in diagnosing and following a patient with suspected sarcoidosis involves measurement of blood levels of serum angiotensin-converting enzyme (ACE). This enzyme is elevated in patients with active sarcoidosis. The percentage of substantially elevated levels has varied in different studies, ranging from 35 to 80 per cent in patients with known sarcoidosis. Patients with stage 0 and 1 disease have elevated angiotensin-converting enzyme levels in approximately 30 per cent of cases. Patients with stage 2 disease, characterized by bilateral hilar adenopathy together with pulmonary infiltration on chest roentgenograms, have the highest incidence of ACE elevation; 77 per cent of these patients will have elevated enzyme levels. Patients with resolved sarcoidosis will have normal levels. Similarly, patients treated with steroids will have a rapid fall of their ACE levels within 2 to 3 weeks. Thus, levels correlate with the activity of clinical disease and are useful in judging a patient's progression despite a paucity of symptoms. ACE levels may be increased in a number of diseases such as leprosy, Gaucher's disease, primary biliary cirrhosis, silicosis, miliary tuberculosis, lymphoma, extrinsic allergic alveolitis, talc granulomatosis, asbestosis, fibrosing alveolitis, chronic lymphocytic pneumonitis, and berylliosis. Many of these disease states can be clinically or histologically distinguished from sarcoidosis, thereby increasing the utility of this test. Positive immunohistologic staining for angiotensin-converting enzyme was found in 38 of 39 cases of sarcoidosis, but it was not present in any of 37 cases with granulomas of known etiology of normal lymph nodes or of normal control subjects. Because the pathologic diagnosis of sarcoidosis is basically one of exclusion, this test may have great utility. At present, angiotensin-converting enzyme histochemical analysis is not available at all major medical centers.

Pulmonary involvement is the most common presentation for patients with sarcoidosis. Thirty per cent of patients will complain of cough, and one third of them will have a productive cough. Thirty per cent will complain of shortness of breath, and 15 per cent will complain of chest pain, perhaps secondary to the cough or to marked hilar involvement. Chest roentgenographic abnormalities will be present in 90 per cent or more of patients during their period of observation. Radiologic examination will show bilateral, diffuse, localized, or patchy interstitial infiltration followed later by fibrosis. Radiologic assessment of pulmonary involvement can be divided into four stages: stage 0 shows no evidence of disease, stage 1 patients have bilateral hilar lymphadenopathy (Fig. 71–37), stage 2 patients have bilateral hilar lymphadenopathy and pulmonary infiltration (Fig. 71–38), and stage 3 patients have parenchymal infiltration or fibrosis without bilateral hilar lymphadenopathy (Fig. 71–39).

Skin lesions occur in one third of patients with sarcoidosis. The most common lesions are maculopapular (Fig. 71–40) and are often missed because they are small. These lesions are commonly located about the mouth, nose, eyes, ears, and nape of neck, thus being convenient for biopsy. These maculopapular eruptions may be transient. Other skin lesions include erythema nodosum, lupus pernio, skin plaques, and scars. Although erythema nodosum is commonly seen in Great Britain, it occurs less frequently in the United States. The lesions in erythema nodosum are bright red or pink, rounded,

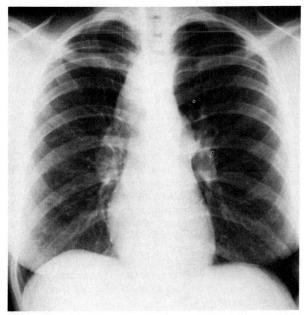

Figure 71–37. Sarcoidosis, stage I, with bilateral hilar adenopathy.

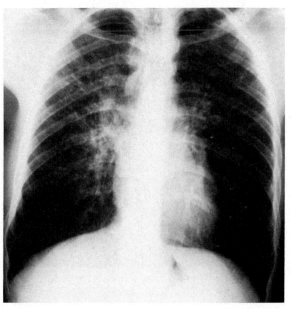

Figure 71–39. Sarcoidosis, stage III, parenchymal infiltration without bilateral adenopathy.

slightly raised, tender nodules in the skin or subcutaneous tissue. Constitutional symptoms often accompany these lesions. Reversible bilateral hilar lymphadenopathy occurs in two thirds of patients with erythema nodosum. Skin plaques are large, purple, elevated, nontender patches commonly occurring on the limbs, buttocks, and abdominal wall. Subcutaneous nodules are painless and, on biopsy, reveal noncaseating granulomas. The lesions of lupus pernio, skin plaques, and scars are associated with a chronic persistent course of sarcoidosis.

The incidence of sarcoidosis in the head and neck is difficult to ascertain. Some series note an incidence of 2

to 10 per cent, but often the lesions are small and readily overlooked. Sarcoidosis in the upper respiratory tract has a significant predilection for women, with a female-male ratio of approximately 6 to 1, unlike the balanced sex ratio with disease involvement noted in other locations. The nose is most frequently involved, and the tonsils are probably the second most frequent site of involvement in the head and neck excluding lymphadenopathy. In a series at the Mayo Clinic, 1 per cent of

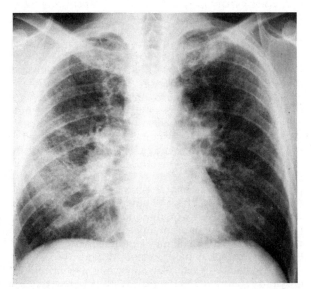

Figure 71–38. Sarcoidosis, stage II, pulmonary infiltration and bilateral hilar adenopathy.

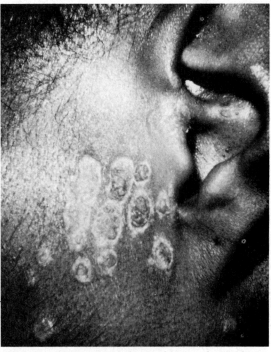

Figure 71–40. Maculopapular skin lesions of sarcoidosis.

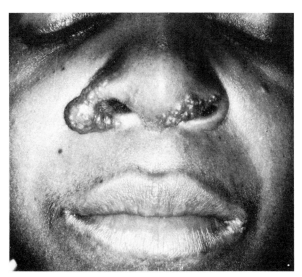

Figure 71–41. Sarcoid lesions of the nose.

the patients had nasal lesions.[36] Nasal lesions occur mainly on the septum and inferior turbinates. Disseminated nodules, 1 to 4 mm in diameter, are gray-white with a hyperemic border. They are firm, arise in the submucosa, and later reach the mucosal surface forming a yellow plaque. The symptoms include nasal obstruction in 82 per cent, with epistaxis occurring in 25 per cent and anosmia in 6 per cent. Rhinitis with turgescence and serosanguineous or mucopurulent discharge occurs. Nasal mucosa is dry and friable, and crusting occurs in two thirds of patients. Ulceration occurs occasionally. Hypertrophy and fibrosis with polypoid mucosal changes occur in the end stage, with resultant thickening of the septum and turbinates resulting in nasal obstruction. Perforation of the cartilaginous septum has been reported. Lesions of the external nose are rare (Fig. 71–41).

The tonsils are probably the second most frequent site of involvement in the head and neck following the nose. Except for hypertrophy, clinical evidence of sarcoidosis is usually lacking. Being part of the lymphatic system, tonsillar tissue is a preferred site for sarcoidosis. The symptoms of tonsillar sarcoidosis include systemic manifestations, such as malaise, low-grade fever, and fatigue. A sense of fullness, dysphagia, and odynophagia may occur with tonsillar enlargement, mimicking chronic infective tonsillitis. Involvement of the oral cavity, paranasal sinuses, and nasopharyngeal lymphatic tissue is uncommon.

Laryngeal involvement is also rare in sarcoidosis, occurring in approximately 1 per cent of patients. Unlike lesions of the nose and oral cavity, which are often poorly examined by nonotolaryngologists, the reported incidence of laryngeal involvement may reflect its true incidence, for many patients undergo bronchoscopy. Two forms of laryngeal sarcoidosis occur. In one type a discrete sarcoid nodule forms, and in the other a diffuse fibrotic involvement is seen (Fig. 71–42). Symptoms pertaining to the larynx may precede, coincide, or follow other manifestations of the disease. In the absence of extralaryngeal disease, the diagnosis is difficult to document.

When the combination of chronic fibrotic laryngeal disease, described as pseudoedema or thickening, occurs in the absence of extralaryngeal manifestations of sarcoidosis, then malignant neoplasms, cartilaginous tumors, granulomatous infections such as syphilis, histoplasmosis, coccidioidomycosis, blastomycosis, actinomycosis, as well as amyloidosis must be excluded. Metabolic diseases such as myxedema and collagen vascular diseases must likewise be considered. Sarcoidosis in the larynx most frequently involves the epiglottis. Most patients are symptomatic, with hoarseness, dysphagia, and dyspnea frequently being seen. The true vocal cords are unaffected, and the subglottis is rarely affected. In the epiglottis, brown-white nodules coalesce to form a turban-shaped epiglottis. This appearance is strikingly characteristic and, indeed, near pathognomonic. The supraglottic larynx is pale pink and is diffusely enlarged, with the epiglottic rim full, rounded, and thickened. At times in the supraglottic larynx, reddened or granular areas are seen. When subglottic involvement occurs, these reddened, granular changes are the only changes seen. Biopsy usually yields noncaseating granuloma.

The natural history of laryngeal sarcoidosis is one of slow, progressive growth and fibrosis. Some patients will require a tracheotomy, although a proportion of these are subsequently decannulated following therapy. It is difficult to recommend any specific therapy because sarcoidosis has frequent spontaneous remissions and exacerbations. The efficacy of systemic steroids in treatment of laryngeal involvement is controversial. Certainly, impending laryngeal obstruction is an indication for therapy. In a small series of patients treated with local steroid injections, some patients improved and others showed no change. Both systemic and local steroid therapy have shown some success in treating this disease.

Abnormal peripheral lymph nodes that are enlarged are clinically firm. At times, a careful search is required to locate these nodes. Most patients have asymptomatic lymphadenopathy.

A wide variety of neurologic involvement, both central and peripheral, occurs in 5 to 15 per cent of the patients with sarcoidosis. Approximately 50 per cent of the neurologic disease involves the central nervous system. In a retrospective analysis of patients with neurologic sarcoidosis, three fourths of the patients had a neurologic symptom as the first sign of the disease. This, however, was unrecognized at the time of presentation. Facial palsy is the most common clinical neurologic disorder. Involvement of the facial nerve appears secondary to direct granulomatous infiltration and is invariably of the lower motor neuron rather than the upper motor neuron. One third to one half of facial palsies are bilateral. Most series report that cranial peripheral neuropathies are transitory, but central nervous system lesions have a slow and often incomplete recovery. Diabetes insipidus and peripheral neuropathies are other common manifestations of sarcoid neurologic involvement. Basal leptomeningitis with acquired hydrocephalus occurs not infrequently.

The frequency of olfactory abnormality in sarcoidosis is approximately 1.5 per cent. This rarity may reflect a failure to perform relevant history taking and physical examination. The symptoms of anosmia or hyposmia are rarely a presenting complaint. The etiology is secondary to basal meningitis with compression and infiltration of the olfactory bulbs and tract by granuloma. Patients with anosmia have a high incidence of other neurologic disorders, with about 75 per cent having facial nerve involvement, 40 per cent with optic nerve involvement, and about 30 per cent having diabetes insipidus.

Neurosensory hearing loss occurs in approximately 5 per cent of cases of neurologic sarcoidosis. A majority of these patients also have diminished responses to caloric testing. Temporal bone studies have been notably infrequently done. Those which exist indicate a posterior fossa granulomatous meningitis as the etiology. The finding of other neurologic signs in association with acousticovestibular symptoms is a more common occurrence than the finding of isolated acousticovestibular changes. Sudden hearing loss has been reported and fluctuating neurosensory hearing loss also occurs. Neurologic problems are generally more chronic than other manifestations of sarcoidosis. Treatment with steroids may yield complete recovery; alternatively, it may result in no improvement. Acoustic losses may similarly be temporary, with complete recovery, or permanent. Vestibular losses are more often permanent.

Ocular involvement, present in 20 per cent of patients, is worrisome because of the possibility of progression to blindness. In addition to uveitis, abnormalities can occur in conjunctiva, sclera, cornea, lens, retina and lacrimal glands. The uveal tract is the most common site of involvement. Slit-lamp examination will reveal conjunctival granulomas in a majority of patients. Palpebral conjunctival biopsy is one tissue source for making the diagnosis of sarcoidosis.

Involvement of salivary glands is found in a small percentage of patients. Parotid enlargement is the most commonly recognized. Splenomegaly occurs in over 20 per cent of patients and can rarely cause hypersplenism. Liver involvement, determined by papability, occurs in approximately 25 per cent of patients and is usually asymptomatic. Biopsy, however, will show involvement in a majority of patients. Renal damage occurs in 5 to 10 per cent of patients as a result of either renal infiltration or hypercalcemia. Joint involvement also occurs in some patients, with a fleeting polyarthritis being the most common finding.

Routine laboratory studies are nondiagnostic and are used mainly to exclude entities in the differential diagnosis of sarcoidosis. Anemia is present in 3 to 20 per cent of patients and may reflect the patient's underlying nutritional status. Leukopenia occurs in 30 per cent, and eosinophilia is seen in 25 per cent. Thrombocytopenia occurs in approximately 2 per cent and may reflect splenic involvement. The erythrocyte sedimentation rate is increased in 45 to 70 per cent of patients, and total serum proteins are increased with inversion of the albumin-globulin ratios. Hyperglobulinemia occurs in 25 to 50 per cent of patients. Liver function tests may demonstrate an elevation of serum alkaline phosphatase; however, normal levels can coexist with extensive liver disease.

The diagnosis of sarcoidosis is dependent upon demonstration of an appropriate pathologic picture. Visible skin lesions, oral lesions, and enlarged peripheral lymph nodes, when present, provide readily accessible biopsy sites. Organs that appear normal clinically may show noncaseating granulomas on random biopsies, for many clinically uninvolved tissues contain sarcoid changes. Transbronchial lung biopsies with a fiberoptic bronchoscope are often the initial procedure. If six or eight

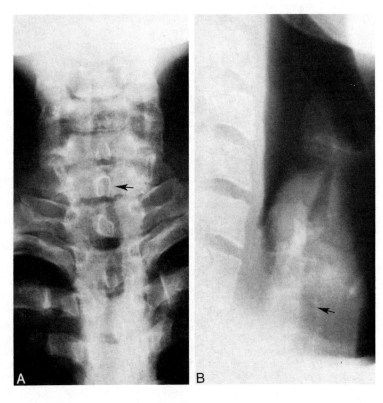

Figure 71–42. Sarcoid fibrosis of the subglottic area with narrowed subglottic airway (arrow). (*A*) Anterior view. (*B*) Lateral view of same patient; narrowed subglottic airway (arrow).

random biopsies are done, the chance of obtaining noncaseating granulomas from lung parenchyma is good despite apparently normal chest roentgenograms. Positive biopsies will be obtained in approximately 70 per cent of patients with stage 1 sarcoidosis, and 85 per cent of patients in stages 2 or 3 of sarcoidosis will be positive when six or eight random transbronchial biopsies are done. Random percutaneous liver biopsy will yield positive results in two thirds to three quarters of patients. Conjunctival biopsies will be positive in 30 to 50 per cent of cases, and skin biopsies will be positive in 30 per cent of patients. In a prospective study 50 per cent of random lower lip biopsies of minor salivary glands in patients with sarcoidosis yielded findings compatible with sarcoidosis. This compares favorably with skin or conjunctival biopsy results and is minimally morbid. Biopsy of minor salivary glands of the lower lip is useful as an initial outpatient procedure because it provides means of demonstrating involvement of several organ systems, namely, skin, salivary gland, and possibly lymph node. Other sites of easy accessibility to the otolaryngologist include tonsillar biopsy and nasal mucosa biopsy.

Patients with sarcoidosis have defective cell-mediated immunity with a tendency for a weak or absent tuberculin skin test response. Despite the decreasing prevalence of tuberculosis in the general population, the proportion of patients with chronic sarcoidosis who show a high degree of tuberculin sensitivity exceeds that of the general population, at 4 to 5 per cent. Thus, skin reactivity to a small dose of tuberculin does not exclude the diagnosis of sarcoidosis. A positive skin test reflects previous mycobacterial infection; it does not indicate acutely active tuberculosis. When the patient with sarcoidosis develops caseating tuberculosis, skin tests often will convert from negative to positive. Alternatively, in some patients with the clinical picture associated with sarcoidosis, mycobacterial tuberculosis can be isolated despite a nonreactive skin test. Similar impairment of cutaneous delayed cell-mediated immunity may occur with the mumps, *Candida albicans,* and *Trichophyton* skin tests. The reappearance of normal cell-mediated immunity in patients who have recovered from sarcoidosis is variable but usually does not occur. Cell-mediated immunity is sufficient for one third of those vaccinated with bacillus Calmette-Guérin (BCG) to become tuberculin-positive. Skin homographs in sarcoidosis patients with tuberculin anergy are rejected normally despite the anergy. Antibody formation does not appear abnormal in sarcoidosis, and B-lymphocyte activity is enhanced.

At the present time, no factor exists that can be corrected or eliminated as part of the therapy of sarcoidosis. It is not surprising, therefore, that no specific treatment as yet exists. Symptoms of the early inflammatory changes can be controlled by anti-inflammatory steroidal or nonsteroidal drugs. It is doubtful, however, whether these agents influence the end results except for a few manifestations such as uveitis and hypercalcemia. Symptomless bilateral pulmonary lymphadenopathy needs no therapy. Patients with hilar lymphadenopathy with erythema nodosum and febrile arthropathy usually respond to aspirin and nearly always respond to phenylbutazone or indomethacin. Pulmonary sarcoidosis is treated primarily for the relief of symptoms rather than to improve radiographic findings. Dyspnea on exertion is the commonest and most important pulmonary symptom. Large doses of steroids are used until maximal improvement in pulmonary testing has occurred. The dosage is then slowly reduced until the smallest dose that maintains this improvement is reached. This dosage is then continued for 6 to 12 months and finally is tapered. If symptoms resume upon tapering, then the suppressive dose is reinstituted. Short-term corticosteroid therapy will improve the condition of patients with pulmonary sarcoidosis. Long-term prognosis, however, may not be altered by steroid therapy.

Radiologic abnormalities cannot be used to infer that all decreases in diffusing capacity are permanent. That is, some patients will show improvement despite prolonged radiographic changes. Hypercalcemia and hypercalciuria occur in a few cases of sarcoidosis. This requires control to prevent renal damage. Initial attempts to control the calcium level involve dietary modification to limit ingestion of calcium and vitamin D as well as avoidance of strong sunlight to decrease vitamin D formation. If these measures do not suffice, low-dosage corticosteroid therapy is required. Alternatively, inorganic phosphate and sodium phytate can be useful in reducing serum and urinary calcium by decreasing the calcium absorption from the gastrointestinal tract.

Absolute indications for steroid therapy include hypercalcemia, ocular lesions, cardiac involvement, and central nervous system lesions. Some unsightly disfiguring skin lesions should also be treated for cosmetic reasons. Oral prednisone, 20 to 40 mg daily, can be used as the initial treatment. Alternatively, skin lesions may be treated solely by local injection of triamcinolone acetonide directly into the lesion at a concentration of 2 to 5 mg per milliliter diluted with 1 per cent chloroquine and repeated at 1- to 2-week intervals.

Chloroquine is also useful in the management of lupus pernio. The dosage is 250 mg daily for 3 months. Simultaneous usage of chloroquine allows reduction of the steroid dosage. Chloroquine, however, may lead to irreversible retinopathy, and careful ophthalmologic observation is mandatory with treatment. Nasal symptoms of sarcoidosis can be treated with topical beclomethasone inhalant. In addition, nasal irrigation with normal saline can relieve discomfort from nasal crusting. Local depot steroid injection will offer relief of tonsillar symptoms.

Although sarcoidosis is primarily a benign disease of long duration, some 3 to 6 per cent of patients will die directly or indirectly as a result of sarcoidosis. Causes of death have commonly been cardiopulmonary from prolonged pulmonary fibrosis, adrenal insufficiency from adrenal involvement, and direct cardiac involvement.

WEGENER'S GRANULOMATOSIS

Wegener's granulomatosis is an uncommon cause of granulomatous disease involving the head and neck. In 1936 Friederich Wegener described the syndrome in three patients who died of sepsis. These patients had necrotizing granulomas of the upper and lower respiratory tracts, a generalized arteritis, and renal changes similar to those of toxic glomerulonephritis. Reviews by Goodman and Churg in 1954 resulted in the establishment of definitive criteria for the diagnosis of the disease. They described the pathologic changes of disseminated necrotizing vasculitis involving both small arteries and veins of the upper and lower respiratory system together with a glomerulonephritis. Carrington and Liebow in 1966 identified a localized form of Wegener's granulomatosis limited to the upper and lower respiratory tracts.[46] In the majority of patients, however, there is generalized rather than localized disease.

The clinical incidence of Wegener's granulomatosis is difficult to determine. Although it is a relatively uncommon disorder, sufficient reports of small series of patients have been published to indicate that many cases probably are no longer reported. Cases of Wegener's granulomatosis in general have a slight male predominance. With an average patient age of 40 years, the disease may occur in an age range of 15 to 75 years.

Prior to the development of effective chemotherapy, Wegener's granulomatosis was a rapidly fatal disease. The mean survival was 5 months, and 80 per cent of patients died within 1 year, with 95 per cent of patients dying within 2 years. Over 85 per cent of deaths were secondary to renal failure, and the rest of the deaths were secondary to pneumonia. Spontaneous remission without x-ray, laboratory, or clinical evidence of disease occurred less frequently than did prolonged survival.

Although the disease entity can be clearly defined pathologically, the clinical features of Wegener's granulomatosis may create significant difficulty in establishing a correct diagnosis. In the past, a major problem has been its confusion with numerous other pathologic entities. Currently, the diagnosis of typical Wegener's granulomatosis is easily made when it is considered and the appropriate diagnostic tests are ordered. Nevertheless, other disease processes must be considered in the differential diagnosis of Wegener's granulomatosis. These other disorders include infectious granulomatous diseases, disorders that have a vasculitic or granulomatous component, and other diseases affecting the kidney and lung. The differential diagnosis of vasculitic diseases includes periarteritis nodosa, hypersensitivity angiitis, systemic lupus erythematosus, scleroderma, dermatomyositis, Sjögren's syndrome, Henoch-Schönlein purpura, giant cell arteritis, and rheumatoid arthritis. Biopsy in these diseases may show a vasculitis but no granulomas will be present. Disease entities that are predominantly granulomatous include sarcoidosis, berylliosis, and polymorphic reticulosis. These entities are notable for a lack of vasculitic lesions on biopsy. Mixed granulomatous and vasculitic disease occurs in allergic granulomatosis, Loeffler's syndrome, and eosinophilic pneumonia. Allergic granulomatosis can be distinguished by its eosinophilic infiltration on lung biopsy while the latter two diseases lack any renal involvement. Infectious granulomatous diseases include tuberculosis, histoplasmosis, blastomycosis, coccidioidomycosis, syphilis, and lepromatous leprosy. These may be identified with appropriate culture and serologic tests. Pulmonary renal syndromes include Goodpasture's syndrome and streptococcal pneumonia with glomerulonephritis. These two entities are distinguished from Wegener's granulomatosis by renal biopsy. Neoplastic disease, including lymphoma, sarcoma, primary and metastatic lung disease, and Hodgkin's lymphoma will be distinguished by the malignant cells present on biopsy. This lengthy list, although not exhaustive, helps in considering the differential diagnosis in Wegener's granulomatosis.

The pathologic diagnosis of Wegener's granulomatosis, as clarified by Goodman and Churg, involves (1) necrotizing granulomatous lesions of the upper or lower respiratory tracts, (2) focal necrotizing vasculitis of both small arteries and veins with possible widespread dissemination to involve any organ, and (3) glomerulitis with necrosis and thrombosis of the capillary tuft in the kidney.[50] Thus, any organ system may be involved in patients with Wegener's granulomatosis, although the disease predominates in the upper and lower respiratory tracts and kidneys.

The vast majority of patients present with complaints referable to the nose or paranasal sinuses. These initial complaints include rhinorrhea, nasal mucosal crusting, or sinus pain. Lower respiratory tract symptoms or signs include cough, hemoptysis, and pleuritic chest pain. Peripheral manifestations are uncommon initial complaints. Renal impairment is an unusual presenting complaint. Unusual peripheral manifestations such as eye and middle ear problems (Fig. 71–43), arthralgias, skin changes, or constitutional complaints of malaise, fever, and weight loss may bring a patient to the physician.

The nose and paranasal sinuses are the most common upper respiratory tract site of involvement. In more than 90 per cent of the patients, there is involvement of the nose or paranasal sinuses. Increasing nasal obstruction may be the initial symptom. With time, serosanguineous drainage occurs and large mucosal crusts form. Underneath the crust, friable nasal mucosa and septal perforations may be found. Patients who undergo nasal septal operations have postoperative septal perforations as healing fails to occur. Ultimately, mucopurulent rhinorrhea occurs in 75 per cent of patients. Tissue necrosis with the loss of the dorsal septal cartilage results in nasal collapse and saddle-nose deformities in more than half of patients (Fig. 71–44). Scarring and contracture will result in changes in nasal shape in some patients.

Sinus disease develops when the normal sinus ostia are obstructed by inflammatory changes. A pansinusitis is common. The sinuses in order of most to least frequent involvement are maxillary, ethmoid, frontal, and sphenoid. One of the earliest roentgenographic findings is maxillary sinus mucosal thickening. After severe damage to paranasal sinus mucosa has occurred (Fig. 71–45), eradication of secondary bacterial infections becomes problematic because of impaired drainage. The most frequent bacterial agents are *Staphylococcus aureus* and *Pseudomonas aeruginosa*. *Staphylococcus aureus* responds to routine antibiotic therapy. With severe sinus disease, drainage procedures are helpful. The continuation of mild symptoms in patients with sinus involvement may merely indicate chronic sinus problems with or without suprainfection rather than persistent Wegener's disease. Simple mucoperiosteal thickening in these patients requires no therapy.

Nasopharyngeal inflammation is a relatively common occurrence with Wegener's granulomatosis. It is usually

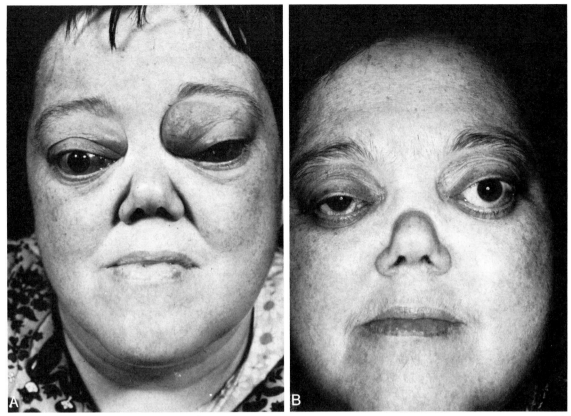

Figure 71–43. (*A*) Wegener's granulomatosis with disease involving the orbits, exophthalmus, and loss of nasal dorsum. (*B*) Same patient 6 months after treatment. Note resolution of orbital masses.

a consequence of suppurative rhinosinusitis. Eustachian tube dysfunction occurs in the majority of these patients from inflammatory changes affecting the tubal orifices. Because many patients continue to experience chronic rhinosinusitis with significant postnasal drip, persistent nasopharyngeal inflammation may make eustachian tube dysfunction a recurrent or protracted problem. When improvement of the rhinosinusitis occurs, eustachian tube dysfunction may improve.

Involvement of the oral cavity or oropharynx is uncommon in Wegener's granulomatosis. When present, it may represent an extension of nasopharyngeal infection.

Laryngitis is a common finding in patients with Wegener's granulomatosis. It usually results from chronic postnasal drip or pharyngeal mucous pooling on the vocal cords. Actual involvement of the larynx by Wegener's granulomatosis is much more unusual. Occurring in 10 to 25 per cent of patients with the disease, the patients will present with hoarseness, odynophagia, dyspnea, or rarely stridor. Laryngeal involvement usually occurs months to years after the presentation in other regions. Edema progresses to congestion and mucosal ulceration, particularly involving the vocal cords and subglottic area. Red, friable, circumferential narrowing of the subglottic region and upper tracheal region may occur, necessitating tracheotomy or alternate therapies including serial dilatations and surgical removal of stenotic material.

In one third or more of these patients there is ear involvement. The pathology is usually persistent or recurrent serous otitis media. Serous otitis media may be the earliest presenting feature of Wegener's granulomatosis and is a presenting complaint in 20 per cent of these patients. Persistent serous otitis media may progress to suppurative otitis media, the predominant organisms being *S. aureus* and *P. aeruginosa*. Biopsy-proven granulomas of the tympanic membrane are unusual but have been documented. Chronic otitis media with tympanic membrane perforation from granulation tissue or from active suppuration may occur. Granulation tissue may involve ossicles with ossicular damage and destruction in rare patients. Fulminant cases with otitis externa and otitis media are difficult to diagnose when the course resembles malignant otitis externa. Mastoidectomy will reveal granulation tissue with minimal amounts of mucous secretion, and biopsy of mastoid granulation tissue rarely yields a pathologic diagnosis. Patients with facial paralysis from nonspecific temporal bone inflammatory changes may undergo mastoidectomy without apparent influence on the facial paralysis. Resolution of facial paralysis, however, may occur with chemotherapy alone.

Although the majority of hearing losses are conductive, sensorineural hearing losses may occur with Wegener's granulomatosis. All patients with sensorineural hearing loss have had additional conductive hearing losses from serous otitis media or tympanic membrane perforations. Improvements in sensorineural hearing loss following chemotherapy have been reported.

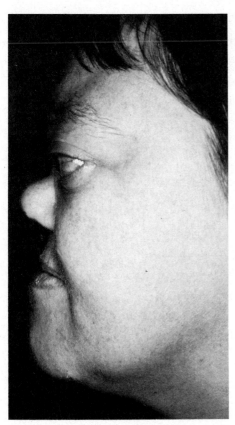

Figure 71–44. Saddle nose deformity from Wegener's granulomatosis.

Surgery with a therapeutic aim is rarely advised until the disease has been controlled. Then, in most patients, hearing may be restored to normal with restoration of middle ear cleft ventilation by tympanostomy tubes. Persistent or recurrent eustachian tube dysfunction in patients with Wegener's granulomatosis mitigates against conservative reconstructive middle ear surgery. Surgery for control of chronic otitis will not control ear disease until the underlying disease is controlled.

Nervous system involvement is an infrequent occurrence. When found, it may be from intracerebral or meningeal granulomas, vasculitis of the vasa nervorum causing neuritis or contiguous spread of granulomas of the paranasal or mastoid sinuses. Vasculitis of the nervous system is the most common cause of neurologic involvement. Between 25 and 50 per cent of cases have some minor neurologic involvement. Facial nerve paralysis has been seen. Although the majority of paralyses resolve with chemotherapy, limited paralysis may persist.

Lower respiratory tract involvement is the most common lesion in patients. Most patients complain of a cough, chest discomfort, hemoptysis, or pleuritic chest pain. Systemic signs of fever, malaise, and weight loss are commonly seen. Secondary bacterial infections are unusual and occur mainly when cavitary lung lesions develop. Roentgenographic changes of single or multiple nodular densities or infiltrates are seen. Unilocular and multilocular cavitations with irregular walls occur (Fig. 71–46). Both lung fields are frequently involved.

Roentgenographic infiltrates may be unrelated to the patient's clinical course. Infiltrates may be transient and may decrease or resolve prior to the institution of chemotherapy.

Although patients with limited Wegener's disease have normal urine, normal renal function, and no glomerulonephritis, 85 per cent of patients with routine Wegener's granulomatosis demonstrate renal disease on percutaneous biopsy. The most common lesion is focal glomerulonephritis. The diagnosis of renal involvement is suspected when proteinuria and red blood cell casts appear in the urinary sediment. Clinically apparent renal disease is rarely part of a patient's early clinical course. Urinary abnormalities may persist for protracted periods. However, once functional renal impairment occurs, with a rising serum creatinine level, the clinical course swiftly deteriorates unless appropriate therapy is instituted. The mean survival after the onset of clinically evident renal disease is 5 months in the absence of therapy. As renal disease progresses, mild proteinuria changes to massive proteinuria with resultant oliguric end-stage renal failure. The diagnosis of limited granulomatosis requires a negative renal biopsy because 10 per cent of patients with Wegener's disease have normal urinalysis and normal urine function but positive biopsies of focal glomerulonephritis. Note that granulomas may be seen in the kidney in limited Wegener's disease, whereas glomerulonephritis will be absent.

Skin involvement with vasculitic changes, with or without granulomas, occurs in one third of patients

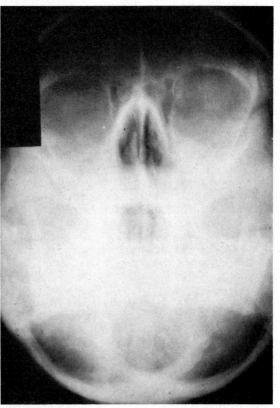

Figure 71–45. Severe sinus changes from Wegener's granulomatosis.

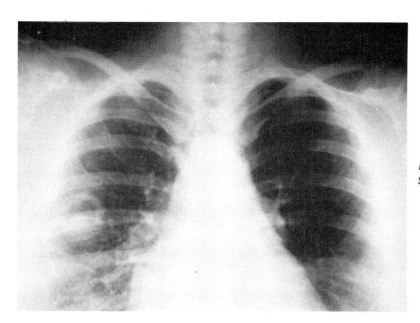

Figure 71–46. Lung cavity in Wegener's granulomatosis.

(Fig. 71–47). Localized necrosis and skin ulceration may occur. Skin lesions tend to occur on the extremities, and biopsy of skin lesions will demonstrate angiitis of dermal vessels with resultant thrombosis and necrosis.

Although arthralgias may occur in 50 per cent of patients, frank arthritis is unusual. Joint symptoms are unrelated to the total disease activity. Patients with severe joint symptoms may have relief with minimal therapy while their renal and pulmonary disease continues unabated. Other patients show improvement of their renal and pulmonary parameters while arthralgias persist.

The diagnosis of Wegener's granulomatosis ultimately depends upon obtaining a characteristic biopsy. The lung is a good source of diagnostic biopsy tissue, revealing necrotizing granulomas and vasculitis. The lung, with an interface between normal and abnormal lung tissue, may offer a better location for biopsy than the nose or paranasal sinuses. Nasal biopsies usually demonstrate positive findings only in tissues with gross inflammatory changes. Superficial biopsies may return the diagnosis of acute and chronic inflammatory changes, overlooking the true nature of the underlying disease. Repeated biopsies may be necessary to obtain the desired combination of necrotizing granuloma with vasculitis. Other common biopsy findings in patients ultimately proved to have Wegener's granulomatosis are acute and chronic inflammation without granulomatous changes or necrotizing granulomas without vasculitis. Because the diagnosis of Wegener's granulomatosis is usually possible following biopsy of the upper and lower respiratory tract, renal biopsy is often unnecessary. One indication for renal biopsy is a clinical suspicion of Wegener's granulomatosis with biopsies from upper and lower respiratory sites supportive of, but nondiagnostic for, Wegener's disease. Here, a renal biopsy of focal glomerulonephritis will confirm the diagnosis.

Although the complete blood cell count, urinalysis, serum creatinine, and blood urea nitrogen are often abnormal, only the erythrocyte sedimentation rate is persistently elevated. Urine specimens for patients with renal involvement usually show hematuria, proteinuria, and red blood cell casts. Normochromic normocytic anemia and leukocytosis are other common findings.

Prior to the 1950s, untreated Wegener's granulomatosis was rapidly fatal with a mean survival of 5 months. Untreated patients died of secondary infection, hemorrhage, and end-stage renal failure. Cytotoxic therapy was first reported to be successful in 1954 by Fahey. Currently, cyclophosphamide is the drug of choice. The use of corticosteroids remains controversial. Occasionally, short courses of steroids are added to relieve symptoms or manifestations of vasculitis or inflammatory changes in skin lesions, ocular lesions, or pericarditis.

Cyclophosphamide is started at a dosage of 1 to 2 mg per kg of body weight, given orally each day. When fulminant renal disease is present, cyclophosphamide is given intravenously for the first week. All patients are given 2 weeks of cyclophosphamide therapy. If renal function based on creatinine clearance is improving, then the same dosage is continued. If renal function is worsening, then the daily dosage of cyclophosphamide is increased weekly by 25 mg each day until either drug toxicity ensues or a favorable clinical response is noted. Major drug toxicity ensues when leukocyte levels drop below 3000 cells per cubic centimeter. When a favorable clinical response is noted, therapy is continued at this dosage schedule. More than 90 per cent of patients treated in this manner have long-term remissions. The remaining 10 per cent of patients will be divided between those having a continued downhill course despite chemotherapy and those who have partial remissions or relapses.

The proper duration of treatment is unknown. When patients have been free of all evidence of disease for 1 year clinically, roentgenographically, and by biopsy examination, then a decrease and eventual discontinuation of cyclophosphamide is entertained. If the disease returns as the therapy is tapered, then dosage levels are raised until the patient again enters remission.

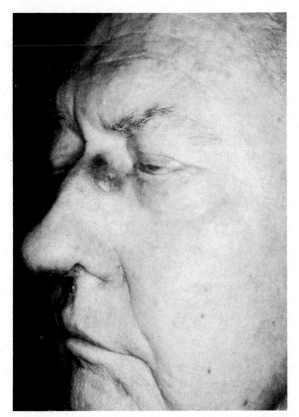

Figure 71–47. Skin lesions of nose from Wegener's granulomatosis.

Persistence of disease requires the adjustment of treatment on an individual basis.

A major complication of cyclophosphamide treatment is leukopenia. This maximal effect occurs 7 to 10 days after starting therapy. Doses of cyclophosphamide must continually be adjusted to prevent the white blood cell count from falling below 3000 cells per cubic centimeter. Hemorrhagic cystitis requiring cessation of cyclophosphamide therapy is rarely seen. Azospermia and ovarian destruction are commonly seen following cyclophosphamide therapy. Combined therapy of cyclophosphamide and glucocorticoids in patients with large mucosal lesions may allow massive secondary infection by microorganisms. Steroid therapy is controversial; some studies recommend starting patients on prednisone at 1 mg per kilogram of body weight per day despite apparent fulminant disease.

Routine nasal care is important in patients either undergoing treatment for Wegener's granulomatosis or in remission. Mucosal crusting is best treated with normal saline irrigations to prevent the development of secondary suprainfection. Secondary suprainfection must be identified and treated appropriately and differentiated from recurrent disease.

Although much has been learned about Wegener's granulomatosis as a disease and about the treatment of this disease since its original description in the 1930s, the precise cause remains elusive. Nonetheless, long-term remission can now be achieved in a majority of patients who receive appropriate therapy. Thus, the otolaryngologist must consider Wegener's granuloma-

tosis in the differential diagnosis of granulomatous disease of the head and neck.

LETHAL MIDLINE GRANULOMA—POLYMORPHIC RETICULOSIS

Lethal midline granuloma is an uncommon entity that has attracted the attention of otolaryngologists since its description by McBride in 1897. In 1933, Stewart reported on 10 cases he called "progressive lethal granulomatous ulceration of the nose." Many other cases have subsequently been described with various names. Lethal midline granuloma has also been called malignant granuloma, granuloma gangrenescens, midline malignant reticulosis, nonhealing granuloma, and polymorphic reticulosis. In 1966, Eichel and associates gave the name of polymorphic reticulosis to this entity, after distinguishing this syndrome from malignant lymphoma of the nose.[60] Polymorphic reticulosis is a preferable term that implies the potentially systemic nature of this disease with angiocentric lymphoproliferation of atypical lymphoid composition. In 1976, McDonald stated that the features of lymphomatoid granulomatosis of the lower respiratory tract with dissemination and the lesions of polymorphic reticulosis of the upper respiratory tract were similar morphologically.[66] Controversy still exists as to whether lethal midline granuloma is a limited form of polymorphic reticulosis that is confined to the upper respiratory tract or whether polymorphic reticulosis and lethal midline granuloma are distinct clinical entities. This author has chosen to follow the pathway of McDonald, believing that these entities are one and the same.

This uncommon disease occurs most frequently in the fourth decade, although patients have been younger than 20 years and older than 70 years. Many different series have demonstrated a male predominance, with a male-to-female ratio ranging from 2:1 to 8:1. This puzzling disease has a long duration, averaging 29 months from the onset of symptoms to diagnosis.

Stewart is credited with describing the three classic phases of this disease:

1. In the first, or *prodromal*, stage nasal stuffiness occurs and may last for years. A watery or serosanguineous discharge is common. No gross nasal lesions are evident. Surgery, such as a submucous resection, performed during this stage will heal with a resultant perforation.

2. In the second, or *active*, stage, a foul-smelling purulent or sanguineous purulent discharge occurs with nasal obstruction. Ulceration leads to septal perforation, and ulceration of the hard palate, usually about its center, may occur. Painless swelling of the face is the result of the continuous spread of disease. Nasal crusting with epistaxis and sequestration of nasal bone and cartilage occur. Epistaxis may be difficult to manage in the presence of a dehiscent nasal floor and septum. Temperature elevations with abscess formation under the cheeks are seen as the disease progresses. During this phase, the relentless, massive destruction of facial tissue is a prominent feature. Granulation tissue advances into normal tissue leaving a path of destroyed tissue behind.

3. In the *terminal* phase, patients remain febrile with

TABLE 71–7. A Comparison of Wegener's Granuloma and Polymorphic Reticulosis

Feature	Wegener's Granulomatosis	Polymorphic Reticulosis (PMR)
Giant cells	Common	Uncommon
Vasculitis	Intense with necrosis of small arteries and veins	Bland necrosis of mature lymphocytes
Sinus involvement	+	+
Focal glomerulonephritis	+	−

repeated episodes of hemorrhage. The sloughing of involved skin and contiguous structures, along with facial swelling, results in a disfiguring facial appearance. Death occurs after a protracted illness, lasting 12 to 18 months after the onset of the active phase. Death is usually the result of meningitis from contiguous erosion, hemorrhage, sepsis, or inanition.

In those forms of polymorphic reticulosis in which the upper airway is not involved, nonspecific symptoms such as fatigue, fever, weight loss, arthritis, and night sweats predominate. Similar symptoms can occur with localized upper airway involvement.

There are no absolute distinctive histopathologic criteria for the diagnosis of polymorphic reticulosis. A nonspecific granulation tissue with widespread necrosis is found. True granulomas with giant cells are uncommon, contrasting with the frequent appearance of giant cells in Wegener's granulomatosis. A bland vascular necrosis, with mature lymphocytes in the intima or beneath the adventitia of small veins and arteries, in polymorphic reticulosis distinguishes this disease from Wegener's granulomatosis, in which an intense arteritis occurs (Table 71–7). In polymorphic reticulosis frequent angiocentric or angioinfiltrative infiltrates result in necrosis from occlusion or secondary thrombosis of small arteries and veins. The polymorphic infiltration of mature and immature lymphocytes with a few atypical reticulum cells sets this process apart from Rappaport's monomorphic lymphoma. Submucosal lymphoid infiltration with necrosis through mucosa, bone, and cartilage characterizes polymorphic reticulosis.

Upper airway involvement, alone or in combination with other sites, occurs in the majority of patients. Lesions most frequently present in the nose. Patients often relate a long history of "sinus trouble." Nasopharyngeal involvement may present without symptoms or with minimal symptoms of headache. Pulmonary involvement is manifested by cough, fever, chest pain, and hemoptysis.

Polymorphic reticulosis of the skin results in maculopapular rashes of the trunk and extremities. In the later stages of the disease, a progression to ulceration may occur. Skin involvement always occurs, together with involvement of other sites. Rare involvement of the gastrointestinal tract, central nervous system, and kidney have been reported.

Repeated biopsies are often necessary in the frustrating attempt to diagnose polymorphic reticulosis. Superficial biopsies of ulcers will often reveal a nondiagnostic acute and chronic inflammation with necrosis. Of major concern is the difficulty of distinguishing polymorphic reticulosis from upper respiratory tract neoplasms with necrosis and inflammation, for superficial biopsies may fail to reveal the underlying malignancy. Culture of biopsy material is necessary to exclude the diagnosis of other entities that may mimic polymorphic reticulosis

of the midface. This includes syphilis, tuberculosis, tularemia, rhinoscleroma, yaws, noma, leprosy, fungal, and protozoal infections. Skin tests for fungi and tuberculosis should be performed. Laboratory tests to exclude collagen vascular diseases, diabetic gangrene, and blood dyscrasias are necessary. Malignant neoplasms, including lymphoma and mycosis fungoides, must be differentiated on pathologic examination. Wegener's granulomatosis has a focal glomerulonephritis that is absent in polymorphic reticulosis.

Routine laboratory tests are of little value in establishing the diagnosis but are necessary to exclude other diagnoses. The single most helpful test is the erythrocyte sedimentation rate. Elevations greater than 60 in the first hour occur in 90 per cent of patients with polymorphic reticulosis.

The necessity of accurate diagnosis has great significance now that proper therapeutic endeavors will both prolong life and result in cure of localized disease. Prior to 1955, no patient treated by antibiotics, extensive surgery, or steroid treatment had prolonged survival. With the appearance of two long-term survivors in 1960, treatment with low-dose irradiation was recommended by Dickson.[59] Further support for the use of radiation therapy in the treatment of localized polymorphic reticulosis of the midface came with the realization that patients originally thought to have lymphoma had greater than 5-year survivals after receiving tumoricidal radiation therapy. It was retrospectively determined that these patients, in fact, were long-term survivors with polymorphic reticulosis.

When polymorphic reticulosis is localized to one region of the upper airway, radiation therapy is the treatment of choice. Supervoltage, wide-field radiation therapy including the nose, palate, and all paranasal sinus areas is used. Combined anterior and lateral radiation portals are often necessary. Daily fractions of 200 rad are given over a period of 4 to 5 weeks for a total dose of 4000 to 5000 rad. Using this therapy, the prognosis of disease localized to the upper respiratory tract has improved dramatically. Greater than 50 per cent of patients are alive a year and a half after the onset of therapy. Some patients are alive and free of disease 19 years after therapy.

Most patients receiving radiation therapy will note skin erythema and mucositis in the treated fields. Some patients will have alopecia. When the orbital cavity is included in the field, loss of vision is a common occurrence. With gross preoperative involvement of the orbital cavity, orbital exenteration may be necessary after radiation therapy.

Supportive therapy for those patients with involvement of the midface includes prevention of secondary paranasal sinus infections. Saline irrigation with débridement of irradiated nonvital tissue on a routine basis is effective. When infections occur, they are usually caused by *Staphylococcus aureus* and respond to appropriate medical management.

The dilemma occurs when multiregional disease exists. Attempts with immunosuppressive agents and steroid therapy have been largely unsuccessful, although temporary improvements in skin lesions occur in patients given large doses of glucocorticoids. The disease invariably continues on a progressive course toward death. Despite various cytotoxic agents used with or without glucocorticoids, the average survival time is approximately 6 months. Patients cured of local nasal disease may die of metachronous multiregional disease.

Polymorphic reticulosis is an unusual non-neoplastic, destructive lesion. When disease is localized to the face, radiation therapy offers a good chance for control. Disseminated polymorphic reticulosis with pulmonary involvement remains fatal regardless of therapy.

MYCOBACTERIAL TUBERCULOSIS

Scrofula (tuberculosis of cervical nodes) was a recognized disease entity during the classical Greek period. The practice of "royal touchings" to cure diseased patients was introduced in France in 481 AD and Louis XVI (1754–1793) reportedly touched 2400 persons with scrofula at the time of his coronation. Late in the 1700s, Laennec proposed that scrofula and pulmonary tuberculosis were different manifestations of the same disease. Then, in the late 1800s, it was recognized that atypical mycobacteria could also cause lymphadenopathy.

The pattern of *Mycobacterium* tuberculosis infections has altered recently. Tuberculosis is no longer a common problem in the United States. Although the incidence of pulmonary disease has decreased, the extrapulmonary manifestations have not. The proportion of tuberculosis presenting as superficial lymphadenopathy has, in fact, increased in the last 20 years. Currently there are approximately 30,000 cases of tuberculosis reported each year in the United States, and 15 per cent of these cases involve extrapulmonary sites. Despite the frequency of the disease, tuberculous lymphadenitis in the head and neck is often clinically confused with the many diseases it mimics. Although laryngeal and otologic involvement are not rare, the otolaryngologist will most commonly encounter cervical lymphadenitis.

The human tubercle bacillus, in contrast to the atypical mycobacteria, is a parasite and will only multiply within warm-blooded animals. After the tubercle bacillus enters a human host, approximately 90 per cent of patients have a positive skin test but have no symptoms, no roentgenographic abnormalities, and no positive bacteriologic studies. The other 10 per cent of patients develop destructive lesions. Untreated infected persons carry the risk of tuberculosis for a lifetime. The vast majority of new cases of tuberculosis in the United States originate from clinically healthy people previously infected by tubercle bacilli in the remote past.

Cervical mycobacterial disease and scrofula are terms often used to refer to the same clinical entity. The occurrence of tuberculous lymphadenopathy is not uncommon. The case rate for tuberculous lymphadenitis is approximately 0.4 per million persons per year, or approximately one tenth the rate of similar disease due to atypical mycobacteria. Cervical lymphadenitis occurs more frequently in Asians and blacks in the United States than in their white counterparts. Almost 75 per cent of the patients are between 40 and 50 years of age. Many series note a large number of immigrants in their patient population. The majority of patients will give a positive history of exposure to tuberculosis.

In most patients the cervical mass itself is the chief complaint, and a minimum of other constitutional symptoms exist. The nodes are often multiple, matted, bilateral, firm, and nontender (Fig. 71–48). The duration from onset is usually 1 to 6 months in 66 per cent of the patients. Some 10 per cent of patients will have moderately tender nodes that may represent secondary bacterial infection. Abscess formation is not uncommon. There are constitutional symptoms of fever, cough, malaise, night sweats, and weight loss present in 10 to 20 per cent of patients, but this will vary with the degree of pulmonary involvement. Most authors note a surprising lack of constitutional symptoms.

In 75 per cent of the patients, lymph node involvement may be confined to the head and neck area. Posterior cervical triangle involvement occurs in a majority of cases. Many of those patients with supraclavicular lymph nodes will have abnormal chest roentgenograms. The more inferior the cervical adenopathy on the patient's neck, the higher the incidence of pulmonary tuberculosis. Thus, the incidence of positive chest roentgenograms in different series will vary with the location of the cervical adenopathy. Although the chest roentgenogram will be abnormal in 50 to 66 per cent of patients, a normal chest roentgenogram cannot be relied upon to exclude the diagnosis of tuberculosis.

Administration of the 5 tuberculin units of PPD-tuberculin is the diagnostic test of choice, as 98 per cent of patients with cervical lymphadenopathy secondary

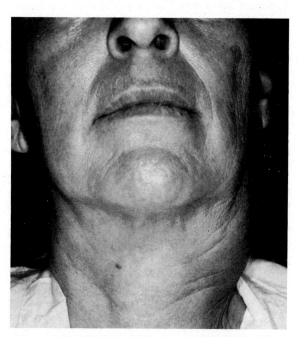

Figure 71–48. Neck node enlargement secondary to tuberculosis (scrofula).

to tuberculosis will have a positive skin test. First-strength skin tests have a lower true positive rate than second-strength skin tests but avoid the occasional skin necrosis sometimes found with reactions to higher doses of antigen. Although a negative tuberculin skin test does not absolutely exclude the diagnosis of tuberculosis, the most common cause of a false negative test is a failure to correctly inject the antigen into the dermal layer. False negative tests may also occur in elderly patients and in the presence of overwhelming infection. False positive tests occur because tuberculosis shares numerous antigens with nontuberculous mycobacterial species. Because the reactivity to tuberculin is dose related, the use of second-strength tuberculin will increase the frequency of these nonspecific reactions.

Once the most common chronic laryngeal disease, laryngeal tuberculosis was present in 37 per cent of autopsy patients with tuberculosis in the 1940s. The introduction of specific chemotherapy has now reduced the incidence of laryngeal involvement to less than 2 per cent. The typical patient with laryngeal tuberculosis is likely to be a male with an average age of 50 years. Unlike tuberculous lymphadenopathy, patients with laryngeal tuberculosis usually have chest roentgenograms that are consistent with findings of tuberculosis.

The first clinical sign of laryngeal involvement is vocal weakness followed by slight hoarseness. With increasing disease hoarseness increases, the cough becomes blood-streaked, and mild dyspnea occurs. The most constant symptom of advanced disease is pain, soreness of the larynx, odynophagia, and referred otalgia. The absence of symptoms is unusual.

Infection of laryngeal tissue by tuberculosis occurs via two routes: bronchogenic spread from infected sputum and miliary hematogenous spread. Bronchogenic spread initially causes invasion of the laryngeal mucous membrane. The lesions are usually ulcerative and may extend deeply to involve perichondrium and cartilage with resulting perichondritis, necrosis, and collapse. Lesions are occasionally verrucous, hyperkeratotic and even dysplastic. Compromise of the laryngeal lumen can occur by edema, cord fixation, cricoarytenoid tuberculous arthritis, cicatricial contraction or by the tuberculous lesion itself.

Hematogenous dissemination more commonly involves the extrinsic larynx, arytenoids and aryepiglottic folds. Pain and dysphagia are more frequent symptoms than hoarseness with hematogenous spread. The onset of acute edematous laryngitis, usually seen with advanced lung disease, is marked by rapid clinical deterioration.

Recent studies note changes in the location of tuberculous laryngitis. The most commonly affected site is the arytenoids, which are involved in 65 per cent of patients, followed by the epiglottis and vocal cords, each with 50 per cent involvement. Some patients, however, have the vocal cord as the sole site of involvement. Papable cervical lymphadenopathy rarely accompanies tuberculous laryngitis.

Although initially difficult to distinguish from carcinoma in some presentations, the clinical differential diagnosis is not difficult once the entity of tuberculous is entertained. Laryngeal biopsy to confirm the diagnosis of tuberculosis is usually unnecessary, for the diagnosis can be made from positive skin tests, positive

sputum examinations, and chest roentgenographic findings. Most physicians prefer a 3- to 4-week period of double- or triple-drug therapy prior to any biopsy. The rapid relief of pain following introduction of antituberculous chemotherapy is striking. Pain is significantly decreased after 7 days of therapy, and gross appearances begin to change after 2 to 3 weeks. If treatment produces rapid improvement, biopsy may be avoided. Indeed, many patients have normal-appearing larynges within 60 days after the onset of antituberculous chemotherapy. Biopsy was previously considered both ill-advised and dangerous because perichondritis developed. With the advent of specific chemotherapy, laryngeal biopsy is no longer hazardous and is recommended when carcinoma is thought to coexist with tuberculosis.

Although it was widely believed that patients with laryngeal tuberculosis were especially contagious, it is now thought that the far-advanced active pulmonary tuberculosis that accompanies laryngeal tuberculosis accounts for the contagiousness of these patients. Infectiousness of patients with pulmonary tuberculosis has best been correlated with the bacteriologic status of their sputum and roentgenographically demonstrated extent of their pulmonary disease. Household contacts have higher tuberculosis prevalence rates when exposed to patients with positive sputum smears and highly advanced disease, as demonstrated on chest roentgenograms, than when exposed to patients with positive sputum and less advanced roentgenographic findings. Those few rare cases of laryngeal tuberculosis in the absence of far-advanced, active pulmonary tuberculosis have not been found to transmit tuberculosis to their household members.

The chest roentgenogram in patients with laryngeal disease usually shows active tuberculosis (Figs. 71–49 and 71–50). The most common radiologic finding is apical cavitary disease (Fig. 71–51) with diffuse, bilateral, small nodular infiltrates typical of extensive endobron-

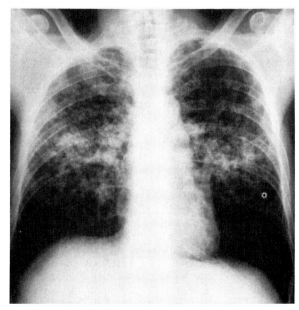

Figure 71–49. Diffuse pulmonary infiltration from TB.

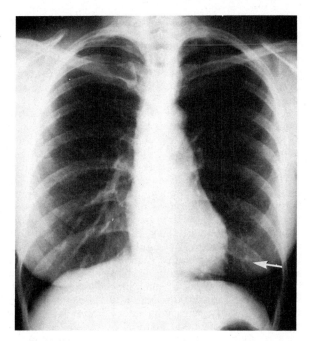

Figure 71–50. Left lower lung infiltrate (arrow) from TB.

chial dissemination. A common error, however, is to diagnose chronic nonspecific laryngitis in a patient in the absence of a chest roentgenogram, for it is the abnormal chest roentgenogram that most often places tuberculosis into the differential diagnosis. Mycotic infections of the larynx may resemble tuberculosis or carcinoma. These have been described with histoplasmosis, blastomycosis, coccidioidomycosis, actinomycosis, and sporotrichosis. Because most fungal laryngeal involvement occurs secondary to fungal pulmonary involvement, chest roentgenograms may resemble those seen with tuberculosis.

Before antituberculosis drugs became available, the presence of an oral lesion indicated a grave prognosis of widespread dissemination. Since the use of effective chemotherapeutic agents, the incidence of secondary oral lesions has shown a greater decrease than that for primary tuberculosis. In general, less than 1 per cent of patients with pulmonary tuberculosis develop oral lesions. Controversy exists regarding the distinction between primary and secondary tuberculous lesions of the oral cavity. Although an occasional convincing report of primary tonsillar tuberculosis in an adult can be found, most cases of upper airway tuberculosis result from the spread of highly infectious sputum of cavitary lung disease.

The typical oral mucous membrane lesion is an irregular nodular ulcer with ragged undermined edges surrounded by a red inflamed peripheral zone with little or no induration. Small tuberculous nodules called "sentinel tubercules" may be seen in the surrounding area in the course of breaking down. The confluence of nodules results in a rapidly enlarging zone. The lesions are quite painful. A lack of induration at the ulcer border and the surrounding tissue may distinguish the lesions from carcinoma, but most lesions are biopsied to exclude the diagnosis of carcinoma. The oral cavity

has certain protective mechanisms against primary tuberculosis, and these mechanisms increase the resistance to infection. These are the cleansing action of saliva with secretory IgA, the presence of saprophytes, and the thickness of the protective epithelial covering. Poor oral hygiene, local trauma, and leukoplakia breach the protective barrier and predispose to invasion. Oral lesions are more prevalent in males, possibly because of increased oral trauma and irritation, the use of chewing and smoking tobacco, and the poorer oral hygiene practiced by many males.

Tuberculous otologic involvement rarely occurs in the United States today. The pathogenesis is mainly hematogenous dissemination from other tuberculous foci. Rarely, aspiration through the eustachian tube occurs. Small caseating granulomas appear as thickened, hyperemic, yellowish spots on the tympanic membrane. Tinnitus or fullness in the ear is noted. When the granulomas coalesce, multiple tympanic membrane perforations occur. A thin, watery discharge follows tympanic membrane perforation. This painless drainage is accompanied by an acute hearing loss that is conductive, neurosensory, or mixed. The middle ear mucosa seen through the tympanic membrane perforation appears as red granulation tissue.

As the disease progresses, the granulation tissue increases and the discharge changes to a thicker cheesey discharge. With blockage of the mastoid antrum, mastoiditis ensues. Subperiosteal abscess and periauricular sinuses also appear. Labyrinthitis and petrositis as well as facial paralysis have been reported. Extradural abscess and tuberculous meningitis may be the presenting signs of temporal bone disease.

Commonly, the disease is treated as chronic otitis media. With mastoidectomy, one finds that slow wound healing, recurring granuloma, persistent otorrhea, and

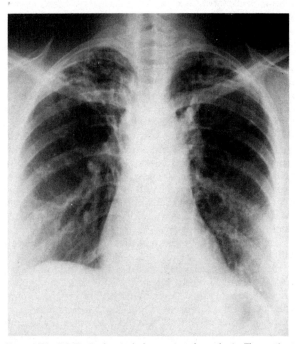

Figure 71–51. Typical apical change in tuberculosis. The patient had laryngeal TB.

sequestration of the bony external ear prompt the suggestion of tuberculosis. The differential diagnosis is extensive and includes disorders such as histoplasmosis, syphilis, Wegener's granulomatosis, histiocytosis X, blastomycosis, nocardiosis, malignant external otitis, lymphoma, polymorphic midline reticulosis, and cholesteatoma. The diagnosis of tuberculosis is confirmed by skin testing, chest roentgenograms, and ear canal culture and smear. Canal cultures are positive for tuberculosis in 5 to 30 per cent of cases, and smears are positive in approximately 20 per cent of cases. Biopsy of mastoid or middle ear mucosa shows miliary changes in superficial infection. Large polyps with superficial bone involvement show granulomatous changes. When bone necrosis and sequestration occur, the pathologic examination demonstrates caseating necrosis.

Mastoid roentgenograms may show only increased soft-tissue density. There is usually no bony destruction. Because the disease process is relatively acute, there is often minimal chronic sclerosis.

If the diagnosis of tuberculosis is confirmed, then treatment with isoniazid, 300 mg given orally each day, and rifampin, 600 mg given orally each day, will cause a cessation of drainage and granulation tissue growth within a few weeks. Surgery is reserved for complications of the disease such as facial paralysis, subperiosteal abscess, labyrinthitis, periauricular fistula persisting after chemotherapy, and central nervous system infection. The indications, techniques, and guidelines are thus the same for the surgical treatment of otologic mycobacterial tuberculosis as for the surgical treatment of chronic bacterial otitis with or without cholesteatoma.

Patients with extensive pulmonary tuberculosis who produce sputum infecting the larynx may also acquire gastrointestinal tuberculosis when such sputum is swallowed. This is responsible for the association of tuberculous laryngitis and tuberculous enteritis. When laryngitis complicates extensive pulmonary tuberculosis, the presence of cramping abdominal pain, tenderness, and changing bowel habits should suggest tuberculous enteritis.

In patients pretreated with appropriate chemotherapy, the culture of tuberculous lymph nodes has a dramatically lower yield despite the presence of acid-fast bacilli demonstrable in histologic sections. Thus, biopsy of lymph nodes should precede the introduction of antituberculous chemotherapy, and all biopsies should be cultured. The normal yield of organisms in lymph node cultures ranges from 25 to 50 per cent. Almost all patients with abscessed lymph nodes, however, have positive cultures. Numerous cases of culture-proved tuberculous involvement of lymph nodes have no acid-fast bacteria on histologic staining. Thus, all nodes should be cultured and stained before the introduction of chemotherapy.

The microscopic differential diagnosis can be divided into three groups:

1. Cases of caseating or noncaseating granuloma with acid-fast bacilli present are included in the first group. The differential diagnosis includes atypical mycobacteria and lepromatous leprosy. Acid-fast bacilli are seen in tissue sections in 20 to 70 per cent of cases. Caseating necrosis is the hallmark of tuberculous lymphadenitis, yet noncaseating necrosis also occurs. Fluorescent staining appears more sensitive than the modified Ziehl-Neelsen staining in demonstrating acid-fast bacilli in tissue sections.

2. Biopsy specimens in this group are associated with a granulomatous reaction, but no acid-fast bacilli are present. The differential diagnosis includes cat scratch disease, lymphogranuloma venereum, syphilis, tularemia, and fungal granuloma.

3. In this group, there is a granulomatous reaction without necrosis. The differential diagnosis here may be sarcoidosis, brucellosis, and all lymphadenopathies of the neck, including systemic disease, multiple infections, and neoplastic diseases.

The mainstay of treatment of tuberculosis of the lungs, larynx, lymph nodes, and oral cavity is chemotherapy. Hospitalization of newly diagnosed cases is not necessary solely to limit transmission of tuberculosis because patient contacts have minimal risk of becoming infected once effective chemotherapy has begun. Since 1975, therapy has changed from an 18-month course of isoniazid and para-aminosalicylic acid to 300 mg of isoniazid and 600 mg of rifampin daily for 9 months. With extensive or life-threatening disease, three drugs are used. Pyridoxine may be added to prevent the side effects of the peripheral neuropathy of isoniazid. Persons receiving isoniazid need monthly evaluation for signs and symptoms of liver dysfunction. Patients at high risk for developing hepatitis may need laboratory evaluation of liver function tests.

Although chemotherapy alone is adequate in most cases of tuberculous lymphadenitis, there are occasional chemotherapeutic failures. The incidence of persistent cervical lymphadenitis is variable. Chemotherapeutic failure often occurs as a result of patient noncompliance. Nonetheless, there are cases in which pulmonary manifestations have cleared but neck disease has worsened. Indications for surgical therapy include lymph node fluctuance and chronic sinus drainage. Resection en bloc of involved lymph nodes is then required. In some cases a modified neck dissection sparing the sternocleidomastoid muscle and spinal accessory nerve is necessary. Surgical excision alone is insufficient therapy, as recurrence rates from 30 to 100 per cent will occur if no chemotherapy is given. When an incisional rather than an excisional biopsy is inadvertently done, persistent wound drainage will occur for at least 1 month despite appropriate antituberculous chemotherapy. In most cases, given sufficient time, the wound will close spontaneously. Some chronic sinus drainage may occasionally need surgical correction. Full-course systemic chemotherapy is the current treatment of choice after surgical removal of affected nodal tissue.

NONTUBERCULOUS MYCOBACTERIAL DISEASE

Microbiologists were aware of nontuberculous mycobacterial disease in the early 1900s. Only after effective chemotherapy for tuberculosis was developed did the medical community appreciate that some cases of apparent resistance of tuberculosis to chemotherapy were caused by infections of nontuberculous mycobacteria. These species of nontuberculous mycobacteria have been known as atypical mycobacteria, or unclassified mycobacteria. Authorities now use the specific name of each organism, referring to the group by the term nontuberculous mycobacteria. The first description of cervical lymphadenitis due to atypical mycobacteria appeared in 1956.

A number of mycobacterial species, other than *Mycobacterium tuberculosis*, are found in a saprophytic state in nature. Although they occasionally colonize the respiratory tract and may even produce invasive disease, they do not require the human as a host. These organisms are common in nature and may exist in medical laboratory water supplies. There are four different categories based on in vitro growth characteristics.

Runyon group 1 contains the species *Mycobacterium kansasii* and *Mycobacterium marinum*. *Mycobacterium kansasii* is an infrequent contaminant commonly associated with pulmonary disease in patients with chronic obstructive pulmonary disease that affects middle-aged men in urban areas and is most often found in the southwestern portion of the United States. In the absence of therapy, most patients show slow progression of their symptoms over a period of years. *Mycobacterium marinum* is commonly found in fresh and salt water. Infections, the result of skin trauma in or around water, cause skin nodules that ulcerate. The infection usually resolves spontaneously.

Runyon group 2 contains the organism *Mycobacterium scrofulaceum*. This organism is isolated from soil, water, raw milk, and other dairy products. The source in human infection remains uncertain. In children, cervical adenitis is the most common manifestation, although pulmonary disease has also been described.

Runyon group 3 contains *Mycobacterium avium* and *M. intracellularis*. Runyon group 4 contains the organisms *Mycobacterium fortuitum* and *Mycobacterium chelonei*.

Runyon group 1 organisms are photochromogens. They require exposure to light to produce yellow pigment. Runyon group 2 organisms are scotochromogens. These organisms produce orange colonies while growing in the dark. Runyon group 3 organisms are nonphotochromogens and do not produce any pigment. Runyon group 4 organisms are rapid growers. They grow colonies in 3 to 5 days rather than the normal 12 to 42 days that are required for Runyon groups 1, 2, and 3.

Lung infections are commonly caused by groups 1 and 3. Atypical mycobacterial lymphadenitis is most commonly caused by *M. scrofulaceum*; it is less commonly caused by *M. avium intracellularis* and least often by *M. kansasii*. *Mycobacterium kansasii* is notable for case reports clustered around Dallas, Texas. Although rare, infections in bone, blood, skin, and meninges can also occur.

Skin tests are available to differentiate all four groups of atypical mycobacteria from one another. Skin tests may, however, be inconclusive, and diagnosis will then depend upon culturing the organism. The FDA removed nontuberculin antigens for skin testings from the market, although supplies do exist at some research centers. These antigens are very useful in children, especially those in whom purified protein derivative (PPD) conversion has not occurred. Positive cutaneous skin testing to atypical mycobacteria occurs in most children with the disease. Indeed, exposure is common, and approximately 10 per cent of children have positive skin tests despite the absence of clinical disease. In this situation over 50 per cent of young patients will have negative

or weakly positive PPDs, thereby giving strong evidence against mycobacterial tuberculosis.

In difficult cases, or in those with extrapulmonary disease, a tissue biopsy demonstrating granulomas supports the diagnosis. Isolation of organisms in sterile areas of the body, such as the cerebrospinal fluid, indicates invasion by definition.

Criteria for diagnosing invasive nontuberculous mycobacteria are (1) isolation of the same organism from the same source on separate occasions, (2) isolation in a single instance from a normally sterile site, (3) clinical evidence of a disease process consistent with nontuberculous mycobacterial infection, and (4) exclusion of other disease processes such as *M. tuberculosis* or fungal infections. The casual isolation of a few colonies from the sputum of a patient without respiratory disease should be ignored, but repeated recovery of large numbers of organisms from the same host raises the likelihood of invasive disease. Many nontuberculous mycobacteria cause disease only in immunocompromised patients, and these organisms can be ignored in the appropriate clinical setting.

Positive identification by culture is the only laboratory test that distinguishes nontuberculous mycobacterial disease from that caused by *M. tuberculosis*. Although some differences exist morphologically on acid-fast stain, the absence of substantial diagnostic differences on history, physical examination, chest roentgenograms, and routine laboratory studies makes accurate identification by culture very important.

Excised lymph node is the most suitable material for culture, as cultures of purulent aspirates are often unsuccessful. Guinea pig inoculation will help distinguish this disorder from tuberculosis, for atypical tuberculosis will not cause a progressive disease, but *M. tuberculosis* will.

The symptoms of nontuberculous mycobacterial infection are usually nonspecific. With pulmonary disease, productive cough, dyspnea, and weight loss are common. In a few patients an acute febrile illness resembling acute tonsillitis may occur. The most common clinical presentation, however, involves cervical lymphadenopathy in children.

Almost all cases of lymphadenitis occur in children 1 to 5 years of age, with extremes of 7 months to 12 years of age reported. Most patients are females. The children present with a neck mass or granulating sinus tract. The lymph nodes are separate and discrete, rather than matted. They arise quickly, stick to the overlying skin, and rapidly progress to sinus or abscess formation. The nodes are usually high in the neck and are in the submandibular, parotid, preauricular, and postauricular areas. No pain or tenderness exists, and there is a lack of constitutional symptoms. The disease is thought to occur as a primary infection at the portal of entry, with subsequent nodal spread. Thus, the oropharynx and conjunctivae drain into the upper area nodes of the neck. The infected nodes are generally unilateral. In contrast, tuberculotic lymph nodes have more random distribution in the neck, suggesting a hematogenous spread from a primary site elsewhere in the body. Furthermore, lymphadenitis of *M. tuberculosis* is often bilateral and progresses more slowly, with abscess formation occurring at a later stage.

Preoperatively, nontuberculous mycobacterial infection is often omitted from the differential diagnosis.

Instead, pediatric lesions such as parotid tumors, branchial cleft cysts, and other pediatric entities more commonly come to mind. Proper treatment of this disease involves surgical excision of all infected tissue. This provides not only the best opportunity for bacteriologic identification of the organism but also provides the best chance for cure. Incision and drainage are contraindicated and result in permanent sinus tracts. A major difficulty in medical therapy of atypical mycobacterial infection is the poor response to most chemotherapeutic agents.

Mycobacterium kansasii is unusual in showing a good in vitro susceptibility to commonly used antituberculosis drugs and an excellent clinical response to therapy. Current recommendations include a combination of rifampin, isoniazid, and ethambutol for 2 years when treating pulmonary disease. Before discontinuing therapy, at least 6 months of negative cultures should be obtained. Relapse following successful therapy may occur, although it is less frequently seen when rifampin is included in the initial therapy. *Mycobacterium scrofulaceum* has been treated with multiple drug regimens of four to five different antituberculous agents; however, results have been disappointing.

No reported cases of transmission from human contacts of atypical mycobacterial disease have been documented. Nonetheless, patients with draining sinuses should not be placed in close proximity to patients with open wounds. The use of the term atypical tuberculosis may result in confusion among patients and their families concerning the transmissibility of this disease. Social or economic embarrassment can be avoided by using the terminology *M. scrofulaceum* lymphadenitis. Nontuberculous mycobacteria will commonly be encountered by the head and neck surgeon. Diagnosis must be based upon lymph node culture, and treatment requires complete excision of infected tissue.

TOXOPLASMOSIS

In 1906 Sam Darling, a pathologist in Panama, described a man in whom a muscle biopsy revealed the presence of an encysted organism, which Darling interpreted with reservation as sarcosporidia. Later pathologists suggest that Darling should receive credit for the first description of toxoplasmosis in the human adult. Adult toxoplasmosis was reported by Pinkerton and Wynman in 1940 in the same issue of the *Journal of the American Medical Association* in which Sapin described acquired toxoplasmosis in juvenile patients. Toxoplasmic lymphadenitis was first recognized in the 1950s by Siim and Gard, and Magnussen.

Toxoplasmosis is a widespread disease. Between 1 in 500 and 1 in 3000 people per year undergo serologic conversion, indicating exposure to toxoplasmosis. There is no difference in prevalence between the sexes. Colder geographic areas demonstrate less human infection than do the warmer geographic areas.

The protozoan *Toxoplasma gondii* is a zoonotic parasite. Cats are the definitive hosts. Toxoplasma exists in three forms: trophozoites, cysts, and oocysts. There is no host specificity, and the only species recovered in nature are *T. gondii*. The oocysts are found only in the cat. Infection in humans occurs after ingestion of cysts or oocysts as a result of the consumption of contaminated water,

uncooked meat, or from direct or indirect contamination with cat feces. The encysted form is resistant to pepsin digestion. The oocysts sporulate in humans, releasing infective toxoplasma trophozoites. Released organisms invade the intestine and spread hematogenously to all organs of the body, where they multiply intracellularly. Cysts form in the brain, heart, and skeletal muscles.

There are three stages of infection, and clinical illness may appear in any, all, or none of these stages. In the acute phase after growth at the portal of entry, parasites spread hematogenously, invade cells, and proliferate. Toxoplasmas require an intracellular habitat to proliferate. Parasites fill the host cells, reproduce, and invade new cells when lysis occurs. The parasitemia lasts 1 to 2 weeks or more. Antibodies appear during the first 3 weeks and coincide with a decrease and then a cessation of parasitemia. Proliferative organisms are eventually found only within the central nervous system. In the brain and eye proliferation continues, owing to failure of sufficient antibody to penetrate the blood-brain barrier or blood-ocular barrier. Cyst formation begins as early as the second week. In the chronic stage cysts are found in the brain, skeletal muscle, and heart. The encysted forms are considered to be dormant and are more resistant to treatment.

In the majority of cases of toxoplasmosis in adults, infection occurs after birth. The clinical manifestations of acquired toxoplasmosis mimic those of more common diseases. Indeed, physicians rarely consider the disease in their differential diagnosis, and many physicians claim to have never diagnosed a case of toxoplasmosis.

Rarely in the normal host does serious disease occur, although chorioretinitis may be the sole manifestation of infection in the normal adult. Symptomatic and asymptomatic lymphadenopathies are present in over 80 per cent. Fever, headache, arthralgias, myalgias, and maculopapular rash are other common manifestations. Rarely, one sees myocarditis, pericarditis, hepatitis, encephalitis, and pneumonitis. In all, some 95 per cent of cases will demonstrate minor symptoms. Congenital toxoplasmosis and toxoplasmosis occurring during pregnancy are entities not of immediate concern to most head and neck surgeons.

Most surgeons do not consider toxoplasmosis in their differential diagnosis of cervical lymphadenopathy. The majority of cases of toxoplasmosis are biopsied in order to exclude a diagnosis of lymphoma. Other considerations of local lymphadenopathy such as localized infections, tuberculosis, lymphoma, leukemia, metastatic disease, sarcoidosis, cat scratch fever, rheumatoid arthritis, and systemic lupus erythematosus must also be considered in the differential diagnosis.

Serologic testing can be the primary method of diagnosis, and early serologic testing may obviate the need for biopsy. A rising serologic titer or a high initial IgM antibody titer indicates acquired acute toxoplasmosis. IgM antibodies detected by the indirect fluorescent antibody technique appear in the first week of infection and peak within a month. A titer greater than 1:80 is high, and that of 1:20 is low. In most cases the titer reverts to negative or less than 1:10 in a matter of months. A negative IgM test indicates that an acute infection of less than 3 weeks' duration has not occurred, but it does not exclude an infection of longer duration.

IgG antibodies are detected by the conventional indirect fluorescent antibody test in most centers. Also available are the Sabin-Feldman dye test, indirect hemagglutination test, and the complement-fixation test. Dye test antibodies appear approximately 11 days after infection. The peak titer of IgG antibodies is reached within 1 to 2 months of onset of infection. Titers may persist at 1:1000 to 1:16,000 levels for months. The titer then falls slowly and remains at low levels for life in some patients. In at least one laboratory-acquired case, antibodies failed to appear until 4 weeks after the onset of symptoms. Complement-fixation antibodies appear much later than those of the dye test. Complement-fixation antibodies are therefore useful to reveal an increase in titer when dye test antibody levels are already high and stable. Hemagglutination test antibodies trail approximately 4 days behind the dye tests antibodies in obtaining their maximum levels. A serial two-tube rise in titer when serum specimens are drawn at 3-week intervals and are tested in parallel is diagnostic of acute infection with any of the antibody tests.

The diagnosis of acute acquired toxoplasmosis is complicated by the high prevalence of antibodies in the normal population, ranging from 10 to 20 per cent among young adults and increasing to 35 to 70 per cent in older adults. With the exception of a single high IgM titer or a serial two-tube rise in titer to high levels in any serologic test, no other serologic test result, by itself, establishes a diagnosis of acute infection. Any other positive test may be seen in chronic asymptomatic infections. An antibody titer as high as 1:4000 may persist for 1 or more years.

A delayed hypersensitivity tuberculin type skin test can be used. In some adults this skin test will not become positive until 1 year after infection. The skin test is a useful procedure to demonstrate that a patient has previously had toxoplasmosis and that a current acute febrile illness is therefore not the result of an acute acquired toxoplasmal infection. During an acute febrile illness of unknown etiology, a positive skin test indicates an old exposure to toxoplasmosis. A negative skin test in a patient with an acute febrile illness would, however, require serologic testing to ascertain whether the illness is due to an acute acquired toxoplasmal infection.

Cervical lymphadenopathy is the most common clinical manifestation of acute acquired toxoplasmosis. Some estimate that 15 per cent of otherwise unexplained lymphadenopathy may be due to toxoplasmosis. Lymphadenopathy may be localized or generalized, superficial or deep. Cervical nodes are the nodes most commonly involved, although mesenteric, retroperitoneal, and mediastinal nodes may also be affected. Of the cervical nodes, 66 per cent will have a single site of adenopathy, but 33 per cent will show adenopathy at several sites. Half of the cervical nodes will be present in the posterior triangle, with 33 per cent in the anterior triangle and the remainder in both. The nodes are often discrete, are of variable firmness, and may or may not be tender. There is no surrounding tissue reaction or suppuration. Malaise and fever may accompany lymphadenopathy and mimic Epstein-Barr virus infectious mononucleosis. The most common groups of nodes involved are the cervical, suboccipital, supraclavicular, axillary, and inguinal nodes. More than 90 per cent of these nodes will be smaller than 3 cm and will be

present for an average of 9 weeks. Resolution occurs in the majority of cases within months. The tonsils can be involved with the acute phase of toxoplasmosis and may also harbor latent infection. Lymph nodes can harbor residual toxoplasmic cysts for months after an apparent cure. Indeed, toxoplasmas have been recovered from lymph nodes 8 months after an acute subclinical infection. Thus, one must be wary of equating the presence of toxoplasmosis with a definitive etiology of current illness unless a temporal relationship exists or unless high or rising serologic titers are present.

Skin rashes are another finding of toxoplasmosis. A maculopapular rash occurs in severe cases. This rash covers the body but spares the scalp, palms, and soles. The rash usually appears in the first week of illness and lasts 1 to 2 weeks. The lesions may appear purpuric secondary to coalescence. In milder cases the rash may be slight or transient.

Both the liver and spleen are invaded early in acute infection, with resultant scattered necrosis occurring. After healing, no histologic damage may be evident. These two organs may become enlarged, with splenomegaly persisting into the chronic stage of infection.

Headache may be the only symptom of brain involvement. In more severe cases, personality changes and psychiatric disorders may result. Focal necrotic lesions with surrounding cellular infiltrates are seen in the acute stages, and cysts without cellular reaction occur in the chronic stages.

Ocular toxoplasmosis usually occurs with chronic rather than acute infection. Both eyes are involved in congenital toxoplasmosis, although ocular involvement may be unilateral with acquired disease. The adult patient may present with loss of central vision from a perimacular lesion, or hazy vision from exudates of peripheral foci. Most patients with adult toxoplasmosis do not have ocular lesions; patients with ocular lesions usually do not have other signs of infection. Nevertheless, the otolaryngologist needs to be aware of this most serious consequence of the disease.

Toxoplasmas may invade and proliferate in skeletal muscle with resultant myalgias and arthralgias as presenting or chronic symptoms. The disease may simulate influenza when fever and chills accompany myalgias and arthralgias. Muscle biopsy may diagnose disease from microscopic identification or cultural isolation of the organism.

Immunocompromised hosts, in addition to having an increased incidence of central nervous system involvement, also are susceptible to myocarditis and pneumonitis. Myocarditis is a common finding in severe infection. The myocardium is invaded early in the acute phase with resultant inflammation; in later stages cysts will form without any surrounding reaction. In the lungs atypical pneumonia can occur anytime during the course of the disease. Lung involvement may be the presenting symptom and the primary cause of death in the immunocompromised patient.

The routine laboratory evaluation is nondiagnostic. The hematologic picture may imitate infectious mononucleosis, with lymphocytosis and atypical lymphocytes appearing. The white blood cell count can show leukopenia and leukemoid reaction and in milder cases may be normal. Eosinophilia occurs in 10 to 20 per cent of patients. The erythrocyte sedimentation rate will be normal in 66 per cent of patients and will be markedly elevated in 10 per cent. Liver function tests may be elevated. The routine serologic testing for syphilis is unchanged. The heterophil antibody test will be absent, thereby excluding the diagnosis of infectious mononucleosis.

Initially, the pathologic diagnosis of toxoplasmic lymphadenopathy based on characteristics described by Piringer-Kuchinka was made with hesitancy in the United States. It now appears that 90 per cent of cases of the lymphadenopathic form of toxoplasmosis may be diagnosed simply by histologic criteria. Visualization of the trophozoite in tissue is diagnostic of acute infection but rarely occurs. Wright-Giemsa stain is required. The isolation of cysts from tissue does not indicate acute infection. Cysts may persist in human tissue such as muscle, heart, and brain for years after an infection. Toxoplasma exists in many tissues in the human body. In the immunocompromised host with previous infections, exacerbation may reflect the release of parasites from cysts.

Encephalitis in the immunocompromised host is an indication for brain biopsy. Electron microscopy and indirect fluorescent methods can demonstrate trophozoites in brain biopsy material. Cysts, however, occur in chronic asymptomatic infections and may be an incidental finding in brain biopsy. Again, the finding of organisms in histologic sections is fortuitous and unnecessary for the pathologic diagnosis of toxoplasmic infection.

In the immunocompetent host, treatment of lymphadenopathic toxoplasmosis is rarely necessary. The infection is almost always self-limited and without sequelae. The only treatment proved efficacious against acute acquired toxoplasmosis is the combination of sulfadiazine (or triple sulfonamides) with pyrimethazine. Pyrimethazine is a variant of an antimalarial drug and acts synergistically with sulfadiazine against toxoplasmosis. Their combined activity is eight times that expected from merely additive effects. The indications for treatment include the presence of severe and persistent constitutional symptoms or evidence of vital organ damage. Treatment of chronically infected individuals does not yield the same radical cure obtained when treating acutely infected patients. The clinical response to treatment has been favorable, although the parasite is not always eliminated by treatment.

The treatment regimen includes a loading dose of pyrimethazine given as 25 mg three times a day for 2 days and a loading dose of 2 to 4 gm of triple sulfonamide. Pyrimethazine is then continued at 25 mg per day for 4 to 6 weeks while triple sulfonamides are continued at 1 gm of triple sulfa a day for 6 weeks. Toxicity has been observed. Pyrimethazine produces a gradual, reversible, dose-related depression of bone marrow. Platelet depression is the gravest consequence, with leukopenia and anemia also being seen. Other side effects include gastrointestinal distress, headache, and dysgeusia. The blood counts return to normal 1 to 2 weeks after cessation of treatment. Of the immunocompromised patients who receive treatment, 80 per cent improve after this therapy.

The immunocompromised patient provides special difficulties. Toxoplasmosis is often fatal in this patient. The immune mechanisms, which keep organisms from previous infections in a dormant state, break down and allow chronic disease to reactivate. Alternatively, initial acute infections in immunocompromised patients may not be contained. The organism will cause encephalitis in 90 per cent of fatal cases. Encephalitis occurs in 50 per cent of all immunocompromised patients with toxoplasmosis and has a fulminant course with death in a matter of days if untreated. Necrotizing myocarditis and pneumonitis also occur. Although the majority of immunocompromised patients with toxoplasmosis have an appropriate antibody response, false negative serologic tests may occur. In summary, less stringent criteria for the diagnosis of acute infection should be utilized to allow immediate institution of therapy while awaiting further diagnostic tests in the immunocompromised host.

Prevention of disease is preferable to treating infection. Because cysts can be killed after heating to 60° C or freezing to −20° C, proper handling of food should be encouraged. In addition, hands should be washed after touching uncooked meats, fruits, or vegetables that may be contaminated with oocysts. Fruit and vegetables should be cleaned before ingestion. Water itself may be a source of infection.

Toxoplasmosis is a common protozoal disease with lymphadenopathy. It can be diagnosed serologically or by lymph node biopsy. Immunocompetent patients have a benign, self-limited course and rarely require therapy. Immunocompromised patients may have a fulminant course despite treatment.

CAT-SCRATCH DISEASE

Cat-scratch disease has a number of synonyms: cat-scratch fever, benign lymphoreticulosis, benign inoculation lymphoreticulosis, regional lymphadenitis, and la maladie des grittes de chat. Generally, the disease is self-limiting, nonfatal, and characterized by malaise, headache, low-grade fever, regional or generalized lymphadenopathy, and development of a papule at the scratch site. Varying degrees of skin involvement have been reported. Cat scratches may be unnoticed or may not even be necessary. Debre, of the University of Paris, first described cat-scratch disease. Hanger recognized similar cases in the United States. He himself had the disease and had an antigen prepared from fluid aspirated from his own lymph nodes. The fluid was aspirated by Rose, hence the name Hanger-Rose skin test antigen.

An estimated 2000 cases of this disease occur annually, 66 per cent of them in children. The true incidence of the disease is unknown, and the number of reported cases varies greatly, depending on the interest of the physician and the availability of skin test antigen. Furthermore, because the natural course of the disease causes minimal symptoms, a large number of cases probably go unrecognized. The disease occurs worldwide in all races and equally in both sexes. In temperate zones, three fourths of the cases occur in the fall and winter. Seasonal variation is minimal in warmer climates.

The transmission of cat-scratch disease has been studied clinically and experimentally. The mode of transmission is presumably by direct contact. Cat contact occurs in 90 per cent of patients, although the disease may also develop from dog bites, other scratches, or following an inoculation with an inanimate object. Although there is no evidence that the disease can be transmitted from human to human, the disease has been transmitted experimentally to humans, monkeys, baboons, and guinea pigs. Regional lymphadenopathy is produced in each of these species following an intradermal injection of material aspirated from suppurative lymph nodes of affected human patients. There are reports of family epidemics, with two to five cases occurring within a few weeks. When a family epidemic occurs, asymptomatic family contacts frequently develop positive skin tests. However, in more than three fourths of cases a patient's siblings and parents do not develop active disease. Patients with the disease require neither isolation nor quarantine, for there is no evidence that the disease can be spread from person to person.

The presumed infectious etiology of cat-scratch disease remains unknown despite extensive analysis. Cultures for bacteria, protozoans, fungi, and viruses have been unsuccessful. Serologic studies have also been unable to elicit an etiologic agent. Attempts to isolate virus from cat saliva or claws have been unsuccessful. The healthy cat, usually a kitten, apparently acts as a mechanical vector for the agent, for skin tests with cat-scratch antigen on the implicated cats have been nonreactive. Studies indicate that the cat will transmit the disease for a time period of approximately 3 weeks. Because the suspect cat is invariably well, the cat should not be disposed of.

The patient usually is not ill despite the impressive appearance of lymphadenopathy. The length of illness is usually 2 to 10 weeks. In some patients relapses occur with repeated glandular tenderness. Clinically persistent disease lasts for 6 to 12 months, but some rare cases have symptoms lasting up to 2 years. Malaise occurs in approximately 50 per cent of these patients, lasting an average of 4 days, and fever is seen in 25 to 50 per cent of patients. In about one third of cases, patients have a fever ranging from 38 to 41° C, lasting an average of 5 to 9 days. Approximately 50 per cent of the patients have no clinical signs other than lymphadenopathy. Splenomegaly occurs in approximately 15 per cent of patients. Exanthems have been reported in 4 per cent of affected patients and usually last 4 to 9 days. The most common skin exanthem is erythema nodosum.

Approximately 90 per cent of patients have a typical clinical course for cat-scratch disease. The remainder have unusual clinical manifestations or complications. These include the oculoglandular syndrome of Parinaud, encephalitis, thrombocytopenic purpura, osteomyelitis, and primary atypical pneumonia. Recovery from thrombocytopenic purpura, osteomyelitis, pneumonitis, and Parinaud's syndrome has been complete.

The following criteria have been recommended to fully establish a diagnosis of cat-scratch disease:

1. The absence of any laboratory evidence supporting another etiologic agent.

2. A lymph node that is histopathologically compatible with the disease.

3. A positive skin test with a reliable antigen.

4. A history of an association with a cat, preferably a cat scratch.

In a typical case, lacking atypical manifestations or complications, three of the four criteria are sufficient for a diagnosis. All four criteria should be met for those cases with atypical symptoms or complications.

Cat-scratch disease is a consideration in all patients with lymphadenopathy persisting for longer than 3 weeks, for it is a very common cause of chronic regional lymphadenitis in children and adolescents. The preoperative diagnosis will strongly suggest cat-scratch disease when an inoculation site is identified. In the absence of an inoculation site, the differential diagnosis commonly includes tumors, lymphoma, infectious mononucleosis, tuberculosis and atypical mycobacterial disease, tularemia, sporotrichosis, syphilis, brucellosis, histoplasmosis, coccidioidomycosis, toxoplasmosis, lymphogranuloma venereum, sarcoidosis, benign tumors, and congenital lesions. Many of these disease states may be excluded preoperatively on the basis of serologic testing or skin testing. Others will be clearly excluded following a lymph node biopsy. A lymph node biopsy must be sent for cultures of the aforementioned organisms as well as pathologic testing.

The physician should search for a healing primary lesion (Fig. 71–52) proximal to the regional adenopathy. From the time of the initial scratch or contact, 3 to 10 days elapse before a primary skin papule or pustule forms. An erythematous papule, 2 to 5 mm in diameter, appears at the inoculation site and may become crusted. The papules are nonpruritic and heal without scarring. Depending on the thoroughness of the examination, an inoculation site will be discovered in approximately 50 per cent or more of patients. Most primary lesions persist for 1 to 3 weeks, but can last 2 to 7 weeks. Approximately 50 per cent of primary inoculations occur in the head and neck region.

Regional lymphadenopathy (Fig. 71–53) without intervening lymphangitis develops approximately 2 weeks following the scratch. Lymphadenopathy occurs in 100 per cent of patients and may be the only clinical finding in up to one third of them. Single lymph nodes are present in 50 per cent, multiple lymph nodes at a single site in 40 per cent, and multiple site involvement occurs in 10 to 20 per cent of cases. The majority of enlarged

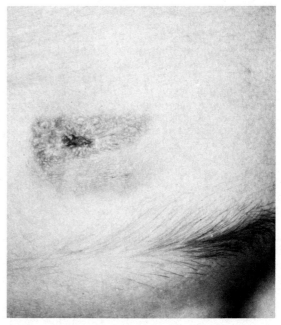

Figure 71–52. Primary skin lesion of cat-scratch disease.

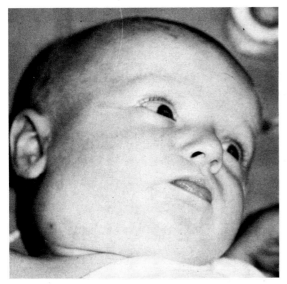

Figure 71–53. Cervical lymphadenopathy secondary to cat-scratch disease.

lymph nodes are tender and are commonly found in the head and neck or axilla. Popliteal, inguinal, femoral, and epitrochlear areas are involved less frequently. Lymph nodes vary from 1 to 5 cm in size in 90 per cent of patients. Ten per cent of patients may have adenopathy greater than 6 cm in size. Gross suppuration occurs in about one tenth to one fourth of patients, and spontaneous drainage may occur. Despite the impressive lymphadenopathy, patients generally do not appear ill.

Histopathologic examination of the lymph nodes is both nonspecific and nonpathognomonic. Early findings show a lymphoproliferative disorder. Microabscesses then form and coalesce into larger abscesses with caseous degeneration. Giant cell infiltration and fibroblastic invasion indicate the start of healing.

The third requirement for the diagnosis of cat-scratch disease is a positive skin test with a reliable antigen giving a delayed hypersensitivity reaction. In patients clinically suspected of having cat-scratch disease with a history of cat scratches or contact, 90 per cent of patients will have a positive skin test. This skin test may remain positive for life. When the duration of illness is less than 3 or 4 weeks, approximately 10 per cent of patients with typical cat-scratch disease will have negative skin tests. One month later, approximately half of those with negative skin tests will have developed a positive skin test. With repeated skin testing at 4-week intervals, with two to three different antigens of known potency, a negative skin test excludes the diagnosis of cat-scratch disease at a high level of confidence. Repeated skin testing will not cause skin test conversion.

A positive reaction consists of a wheal or papule formation with 5 mm or more of induration occurring 48 to 72 hours after intradermal inoculation of 0.1 ml of antigen. Induration may persist for 5 to 6 days following inoculation. Because positive tests may be obtained many years after an initial episode, a positive test does not necessarily indicate current active disease. Positive reactions occur in 30 per cent of veterinarians and approximately 5 per cent of the general healthy popu-

lation. Thus, the limit of confidence for a positive reaction is about 95 per cent.

Cat-scratch antigen is not available commercially. To prepare this antigen, aspirates of purulent material from patients with known cat-scratch disease are mixed in a ratio of one part aspirate to four parts of normal saline and then are heated to 60°C for 72 hours to destroy complement and hepatitis virus. A preservative is not added. This material is then cultured and stored in a frozen state until negative cultures have returned. Each antigen must then be tested on a known priorly positive reactor and on healthy control subjects. Some patients have positive skin tests to one proven antigen but have negative skin tests with other proven antigens. For this reason, some suggest that a mix of two or three different antigens be used. The main difficulty with the use of the skin test antigen, however, involves preparing and validating a skin test antigen, for none is commercially available.

The fourth criterion of association or scratch with a cat will be found in approximately 90 per cent of patients given proper questioning. Studies indicate approximately two thirds of patients will have had cat scratches. Others note dog contact or scratches occurring in approximately 8 per cent.

Laboratory data are nondiagnostic and are used to exclude alternative diagnoses. The most helpful laboratory study is the erythrocyte sedimentation rate. This is usually elevated during the first few weeks of adenopathy, suggesting an inflammatory lymphadenitis. The complete blood count may be normal or may show a mild leukocytosis early in the disease.

The most common unusual manifestation of cat-scratch disease is the oculoglandular syndrome of Parinaud. In the oculoglandular form of cat-scratch disease, the inoculation site presents typically as a granulomatous area on the palpebral conjunctiva. It is often polypoid, measuring 0.5 to 2 cm in diameter, with an irregular border and little surrounding erythema. There is only minimal conjunctival erythema and no purulent exudate. When located beneath ocular conjunctiva, lesions may appear as gray necrotic areas. When the granuloma matures, it enlarges and small, whitish areas of necrosis appear. The site can be identified for several weeks after inoculation and the lesion resolves without scarring. These inoculation sites are only slightly symptomatic. As in typical cat-scratch disease, lymphadenopathy develops in those nodes draining the site of inoculation. Thus, preauricular lymph nodes enlarge in this syndrome. Usually only one node is enlarged, although bilateral enlargement may occur with bilateral inoculation.

Patients with central nervous system involvement develop encephalopathy, meningitis, radiculitis, polyneuritis, and myelitis with paraplegia. The onset of neurologic symptoms is sudden and occurs within 1 to 6 weeks following the onset of lymphadenopathy. The most common neurologic manifestation is encephalitis, accompanied by fever, convulsions, and coma in 66 per cent of patients. Neurologic abnormalities occur in 25 per cent, and lethargy and confusion occur in 15 per cent of patients with neurologic abnormalities. With neurologic involvement of the central nervous system, 50 per cent of patients show cerebrospinal fluid pleocytosis, elevated protein levels, or both. Electroencephalograms are abnormal in most patients. Neurologic manifestations persist for 1 to 2 weeks, with gradual recovery occurring in most patients from 1 to 6 months following the episodes.

Having made the diagnosis of cat-scratch disease with three of the four criteria needed for typical cases and all four needed for atypical cases, the physician must now attempt to treat a disease of unknown etiology. In the vast majority of patients, the disease is self-limited. The best therapy is reassurance that the lymphadenopathy is benign and will subside spontaneously within 2 to 3 months. Management, therefore, consists of reassurance, appropriate periodic re-examination, and analgesics. If suppuration occurs, aspiration will relieve symptoms within 24 to 48 hours unless fluid reaccumulates. Needle aspiration is much preferred to incision and drainage. Aspiration is usually performed on an outpatient basis. After cleansing the skin, a large-gauge needle is inserted at the base of the mass to avoid a chronic sinus tract. Aspiration not only provides material for skin test antigen, but relieves painful lymphadenopathy within 1 to 2 days. If fluid recurs, repeat aspiration is recommended. Antibiotics are of no proved efficacy, and corticosteroids are not recommended.

Because this is a self-limited disease, surgical excision is rarely necessary. Occasionally patients will have persistent sinus tract drainage. Several case reports indicate that following complete excision, pain is relieved and successful primary closure may be accomplished. Excision of infected regional lymph nodes rapidly halts the course of the disease and may be indicated when the disease is severe or life-threatening.

The prognosis of cat-scratch disease is excellent. Lymphadenopathy regresses spontaneously within 2 to 6 months in most patients. The patients are provided with lifelong immunity following one episode of the disease. Complications and sequelae are almost nonexistent. Following the diagnosis of this disease by exclusion of other known etiologies of lymphadenopathy, the best therapy is one of reassurance. Given a disease of unknown etiology, no recommendations to prevent the disease may be reached.

Cat-scratch disease is a common cause of lymphadenopathy. Occurring mainly in children, this self-limited disease has a benign prognosis.

REFERENCES

SINUS HISTIOCYTOSIS

1. Adekeye E, Edwards M, Goubran G: Sinus histiocytosis with massive lymphadenopathy in a Nigerian child. J Laryngol Otol 96:89, 1982.
2. Banacki M, Morris R, Stool S, Paradise J: Sinus histiocytosis with massive lymphadenopathy: Report of its occurrence in two siblings with retropharyngeal involvement in both. Ann Otol Rhinol Laryngol 87:327, 1978.
3. Dearth J, Hunter D, Kelly D, Grist W: Sinus histiocytosis with massive lymphadenopathy. Cancer J Clinicians 30:55, 1980.
4. Foucar E, Rosai J, Dorfman R: Sinus histiocytosis with massive lymphadenopathy. Arch Otolaryngol 104:687, 1978.
5. Foucar E, Rosai J, Dorfman R: The ophthalmologic manifestations of sinus histiocytosis with massive lymphadenopathy. Am J Ophthalmol 87:354, 1979.
6. Kessler E, Srulijes C, Toledo E, Shalit M: Sinus histiocytosis with massive lymphadenopathy and spinal epidural involvement. Cancer 38:1614, 1976.
7. Rosai J, Dorfman R: Sinus histiocytosis with massive lymphadenopathy: A pseudolymphomatous benign disorder. Cancer 30:1174, 1972.
8. Siegel M, Shackelford G, McAlister W: Sinus histiocytosis: Some radiologic observations. Am J Radiol 132:783, 1979.
9. Walker P, Rosai J, Dorfman R: The osseous manifestations of sinus histiocytosis with massive lymphadenopathy. Am J Clin Pathol 75:131, 1981.
10. Weaver D: Atypical lymphadenopathies of the head and neck. CRC Crit Rev Clin Lab Sci 15:1, 1981.

ANGIOIMMUNOBLASTIC LYMPHADENOPATHY

11. Frizzera G, Moran E, Rappaport H: Angio-immunoblastic lymphadenopathy: diagnosis and clinical course. Am J Med 59:803, 1975.
12. Kessler E: Angioimmunoblastic lymphadenopathy: A case study. Cancer 38:1587, 1976.
13. Lukes R, Tindle B: Immunoblastic lymphadenopathy: A hyperimmune entity resembling Hodgkin's disease. N Engl J Med 292:1, 1975.
14. Matloff R, Neiman R: Angioimmunoblastic lymphadenopathy: A generalized lymphoproliferative disorder with cutaneous manifestations. Arch Dermatol 114:92, 1978.
15. Moran E, Rappaport H: Angio-immunoblastic lymphadenopathy. N Engl J Med 292:42, 1975.
16. Myers T, Cole S, Pastuszak W: Angioimmunoblastic lymphadenopathy: Pleural-pulmonary disease. Cancer 40:266, 1978.
17. Nathwani B, Rappaport H, Moran E, et al.: Malignant lymphoma arising in angioimmunoblastic lymphadenopathy. Cancer 41:578, 1978.
18. Neiman R, Dervan P, Haudenschild C, Jaffe R: Angioimmunoblastic lymphadenopathy. An ultrastructural and immunologic study with review of the literature. Cancer 41:507, 1978.
19. Rudders R, DeLellis R: Immunoblastic lymphadenopathy: A mixed proliferation of T and B lymphocytes. Am J Clin Pathol 68:518, 1977.
20. Schultz D, Yunis A: Immunoblastic lymphadenopathy with mixed cryoglobulinemia. N Engl J Med 292:8, 1975.
21. Weisenberger D, Armitage J, Dick F: Immunoblastic lymphadenopathy with pulmonary infiltrates, hypocomplementemia and vasculitis. Am J Med 63:849, 1977.

HISTIOCYTOSIS X

22. Cinberg J: Eosinophilic granuloma in the head and neck: A five year review with report of an instructive case. Laryngoscope 88:1281, 1978.
23. McCaffrey T, McDonald T: Histiocytosis X of the ear and temporal bone: Review of 22 cases. Laryngoscope 89:1735, 1979.
24. Nezelof C, Frileux-Herbet F, Cronier-Sachot J: Disseminated histiocytosis X; analysis of prognostic factors based on a retrospective study of 50 cases. Cancer 44:1824, 1979.
25. Osband M, Lipton J, et al.: Histiocytosis X: Demonstration of abnormal immunity, T-cell histamine H_2 receptor deficiency, and successful treatment with thymic extract. N Engl J Med 304:146, 1981.
26. Schloss A, Klein A, Black B: Histiocytosis X of the head and neck. J Otolaryngol 10:189, 1981.
27. Schuknecht H: Histiocytosis X. Otolaryngol Head Neck Surg 88:544, 1980.
28. Sweet R, Kornblut A, Hyams V: Eosinophilic granuloma in the temporal bone. Laryngoscope 89:1545, 1979.
29. Williams J, Dorfman R: Lymphadenopathy as the initial manifestation of histiocytosis X. Am J Surg Pathol 3:405, 1979.

SARCOIDOSIS

30. Armstrong J, Radke J, Kvale P, et al.: Endoscopic findings in sarcoidosis, characteristics and correlations with radiographic staging and bronchial mucosal biopsy yield. Ann Otol Rhinol Laryngol 90:339, 1981.
31. Block A, Light R: Alternate day steroid therapy in diffuse pulmonary sarcoidosis. Chest 63:495, 1973.
32. Delaney P, Henkin R, Manz H, et al.: Olfactory sarcoidosis. Arch Otolaryngol 103:717, 1977.
33. Huninghake G, Gadek J, Young R Jr, et al.: Maintenance of granuloma formation in pulmonary sarcoidosis by T lymphocytes within the lung. N Engl J Med 302:594, 1980.
34. Hybels R, Rice D: Neuro-otologic manifestations of sarcoidosis. Laryngoscope 86:1873, 1976.
35. Lieberman J: Elevation of serum angiotensin-converting enzyme (ACE) level in sarcoidosis. Am J Med 59:365, 1975.
36. McCaffrey T, McDonald T: Sarcoidosis of the nose and paranasal sinuses. Laryngoscope 93:1281, 1983.
37. Maycock R, Bertrand P, Morrison C, Scott J: Manifestations of sarcoidosis. Am J Med 35:67, 1963.
38. Mitchell D, Scadding J: Sarcoidosis. Am Rev Respir Dis 110:774, 1974.

39. Neel H III, McDonald T: Laryngeal sarcoidosis. Ann Otol Rhinol Laryngol 91:359, 1982.
40. Nessan V, Jacoway J: Biopsy of minor salivary glands in the diagnosis of sarcoidosis. N Engl J Med 301:922, 1979.
41. O'Connor A, McKelvie P: Sarcoid of the larynx and pharynx. ENT J 61:25, 1982.
42. Sharma O: Cutaneous sarcoidosis: Clinical features and management. Chest 61:320, 1972.
43. Sharma O: Diagnosis of sarcoidosis. Arch Intern Med 143:1418, 1983.
44. Solomon D, Horn B, Byrd R, et al.: The diagnosis of sarcoidosis by conjunctival biopsy. Chest 74:271, 1978.
45. Weiss J: Sarcoidosis in otolaryngology—Report of eleven cases: Evaluation of blind biopsy as a diagnostic aid. Laryngoscope 70:1351, 1960.

WEGENER'S GRANULOMATOSIS

46. Carrington C, Liebow A: Limited forms of angiitis and granulomatosis of Wegener's type. Am J Med 41:497, 1966.
47. Cassan S, Coles D, Harrison E Jr: The concept of limited forms of Wegener's granulomatosis. Am J Med 49:366, 1970.
48. DeRemee R, Weiland L, McDonald T: Respiratory vasculitis. Mayo Clin Proc 55:492, 1980.
49. Fauci A, Wolff S: Wegener's granulomatosis: Studies in eighteen patients and a review of the literature. Medicine 52:535, 1973.
50. Godman G, Churg J: Wegener's granulomatosis. Arch Pathol 58:533, 1954.
51. Illum P, Thorling K: Otologic manifestations of Wegener's granulomatosis. Laryngoscope 92:801, 1982.
52. Kornblut A, Wolff S, DeFries H, Fauci A: Wegener's granulomatosis. Laryngoscope 90:1453, 1980.
53. Kornblut A, Wolff S, Fauci A: Ear disease in patients with Wegener's granulomatosis. Laryngoscope 92:713, 1982.
54. McDonald T, DeRemee R: Wegener's granulomatosis. Laryngoscope 93:220, 1983.
55. Novack S, Pearson C: Cyclophosphamide therapy in Wegener's granulomatosis. 284:938, 1971.
56. Wolff S, Fauci A, Horn R, Dale D: Wegener's granulomatosis. Ann Intern Med 81:513, 1974.

LETHAL MIDLINE GRANULOMA

57. Crissman T, Weiss M, Gluckman J: Midline granuloma syndrome. Am J Surg Pathol 6:335, 1982.
58. DeRemee R, Weiland L, McDonald T: Polymorphic reticulosis lymphomatoid granulomatosis: Two diseases or one? Mayo Clin Proc 53:634, 1978.
59. Dickson R, Cantab D: Radiotherapy of lethal midline granuloma. J Chron Dis 12:417, 1960.
60. Eichel B, Harrison E Jr, Devine K, et al.: Primary lymphoma of the nose including a relationship to lethal midline granuloma. Am J Surg 112:597, 1966.
61. Fauci A, Johnson R, Wolff S: Radiation therapy of midline granuloma. Ann Intern Med 84:140, 1976.
62. Fitzgerald R: Irradiation of the nose and paranasal sinuses in idiopathic midline destructive disease. Laryngoscope 92:335, 1982.
63. Friedmann I: The changing pattern of granulomas of the upper respiratory tract. J Laryngol Otol 85:631, 1985.
64. Kassel S, Echevarria R, Guzzo F: Midline malignant reticulosis (so-called lethal midline granuloma). Cancer 23:920, 1969.
65. MacKenzie M, Wolfenden N: Progressive lethal granulomatous ulceration of the nose. J Laryngol Otol 48:657, 1933.
66. McDonald T, DeRemee R, Harrison E Jr, et al.: The protean clinical features of polymorphic reticulosis (lethal midline granuloma). Laryngoscope 86:936, 1976.

MYCOBACTERIAL TUBERCULOSIS

67. Appling D, Miller R: Mycobacterial cervical lymphadenopathy: A 1981 update. Laryngoscope 91:1259, 1981.
68. Brennan T, Vrabec D: Tuberculosis of the oral mucosa. Ann Otol Rhinol Laryngol 79:601, 1970.
69. Brodovsky D: Laryngeal tuberculosis in an age of chemotherapy. Can J Otolaryngol 4:168, 1975.
70. Byrd R, Bopp R, Gracy D, Puritz E: The role of surgery in tuberculous lymphadenitis in adults. Am Rev Respir Dis 103:816, 1971.
71. Cantrell R, Jensen J, Reid D: Diagnosis and management of tuberculous cervical adenitis. Arch Otolaryngol 101:53, 1975.
72. Horowitz G, Kaslow R, Friedland G: Infectiousness of laryngeal tuberculosis. Am Rev Respir Dis 114:241, 1976.

73. Huhti E, Brander E, Paloheimo S, Sutinen S: Tuberculosis of the cervical lymph nodes: A clinical, pathological and bacteriological study. Tubercle 56:27, 1975.
74. Lucente F, Tobias G, Parisier S, Som P: Tuberculous otitis media. Laryngoscope 88:1107, 1978.
75. Rohwedder J: Upper respiratory tract tuberculosis. Ann Intern Med 80:708, 1974.
76. Summers G, McNichol M: Tuberculosis of superficial lymph nodes. Br J Dis Chest 74:369, 1980.
77. Tomblin J, Roberts F: Tuberculous cervical lymphadenitis. CMAJ 121:324, 1979.
78. Travis L, Hybels R, Newman M: Tuberculosis of the larynx. Laryngoscope 86:549, 1976.
79. Wong M, Jafek B: Cervical mycobacterial disease. Trans Am Acad Ophthalmol Otol 78:75, 1974.

NONTUBERCULOUS MYCOBACTERIAL DISEASE

80. Appling D, Miller R: Mycobacterial cervical lymphadenopathy: A 1981 update. Laryngoscope 91:1259, 1981.
81. Bass J Jr, Hawkins E: Treatment of disease caused by nontuberculous mycobacteria. Arch Intern Med 143:1439, 1983.
82. Cantrell R, Jensen J, Reid D: Diagnosis and management of tuberculous cervical adenitis. Arch Otolaryngol 101:53, 1975.
83. Glassroth J, Robins A, Snider D Jr: Tuberculosis in the 1980's. N Engl J Med 302:1441, 1980.
84. Olsen N: Atypical mycobacterial infections of the neck. Laryngoscope 77:1376, 1967.

TOXOPLASMOSIS

85. deLuise V: Toxoplasmosis; an update and overview. Resident Staff Physician 29:62, 1983.
86. Dorfman R, Remington J: Value of lymph node biopsy in the diagnosis of acute acquired toxoplasmosis. N Engl J Med 289:878, 1973.
87. Gray G Jr, Kimball A, Kean B: The posterior cervical lymph node in toxoplasmosis. Am J Pathol 69:349, 1972.
88. Karlan M, Baker D Jr: Cervical lymphadenopathy secondary to toxoplasmosis. Laryngoscope 82:956, 1972.
89. Krick J, Remington J: Toxoplasmosis in the adult—an overview. N Engl J Med 298:550, 1978.
90. Miettinen M, Saxen L, Saxen E: Lymph node toxoplasmosis. Acta Med Scand 208:431, 1980.
91. Rafaty F: Cervical adenopathy secondary to toxoplasmosis. Arch Otolaryngol 103:547, 1977.
92. Remington J: Toxoplasmosis in the adult. Bull NY Acad Med 50:211, 1974.
93. Remington J, Jacobs L, Kaufman H: Toxoplasmosis in the adult. N Engl J Med 262:180, 1960.
94. Remington J, Jacobs L, Kaufman H: Toxoplasmosis in the adult. N Engl J Med 262:237, 1960.
95. Tuetsch S, Juranek D, Sulzer A, et al.: Epidemic toxoplasmosis associated with infected cats. N Engl J Med 300:695, 1979.

CAT-SCRATCH DISEASE

96. Carrithers H: Oculoglandular disease of Parinaud. Am J Dis Child 132:1195, 1978.
97. Carrithers H, Carrithers C, Edwards R Jr: Cat scratch disease. JAMA 207:312, 1969.
98. Daniels W, MacMurray F: Cat scratch disease: Report of one hundred sixty cases. JAMA 154:1247, 1954.
99. Emmons R, Riggs J, Schachter J: Continuing search for the etiology of cat scratch disease. J Clin Microbiol 4:112, 1976.
100. Jorgensen M: Familial cat-scratch disease. Am J Surg 112:124, 1966.
101. Kalter S: Cat scratch disease. Int J Dermatol 8:656, 1978.
102. Margileth A: Cat scratch disease: Nonbacterial regional lymphadenitis. Pediatrics 42:803, 1968.
103. Margileth A: Cat scratch disease in 65 patients, evaluation of cat scratch skin test antigen in 109 subjects. Clin Proc Child Hosp 27:213, 1971.
104. Margileth A: Cat scratch disease. In Beeson PB, et al (eds): Cecil's Textbook of Medicine. Philadelphia, W. B. Saunders Co., 1979, pp 302–305.
105. Small W, Sniffen R: Nonbacterial regional lymphadenitis ("cat-scratch fever") evaluation of surgical treatment. N Engl J Med 255:1029, 1956.
106. Warwick W: The cat-scratch syndrome: Many diseases or one disease? Prog Med Virol 9:256, 1967.

CHAPTER 72

Chemotherapy and Immunotherapy of Head and Neck Tumors

Jay Marion, M.D.

Surgery and radiation therapy have demonstrated curative potential in the treatment of early squamous cell cancer of the head and neck. However, patients who present with extensive local, regional, or metastatic disease are often incompletely palliated with these modalities. Chemotherapy has demonstrated effectiveness in inducing tumor regression, but its role in the management of head and neck cancer patients has been limited by its toxicity and relative ineffectiveness. Even though temporary complete regression of clinically evident disease may occur during chemotherapy, the goal of such treatment has classically been palliation of symptomatically advanced disease. However, a new, and perhaps valuable, role for chemotherapy in the head and neck cancer patient appears to be evolving. The use of chemotherapy, before surgery and radiation in patients at high risk for recurrence, has generally been termed "induction chemotherapy," and its role is now being defined.

Because increasing numbers of patients with head and neck malignancies will be receiving chemotherapy, it is important that the head and neck physician become familiar with the pharmacology, activity, and toxicity of the drugs.

CLINICAL PHARMACOLOGY OF ANTI-NEOPLASTIC DRUGS

The Cell Cycle

Cytotoxic drugs interfere with the growth and reproduction of cells by disrupting some aspect of the cell's growth cycle. A schematic representation of the cell cycle is shown in Figure 72–1. Following mitosis, M phase, cells enter G1—a phase of active RNA and protein synthesis. When this phase is prolonged, as in tissues with a low growth fraction, the cells are said to be in G0, or a resting phase. The G1 phase is followed by the S phase, during which DNA synthesis occurs. The factors that regulate DNA synthesis are poorly understood, but it is felt that a lack of sensitivity to such regulation might account, in part, for the unrestrained growth of neoplastic tissue.[59] Following the S phase, cells enter into the G2 phase, during which the synthesis of proteins essential for mitosis occurs.

Phase Specificity

Drugs that are effective only during a specific phase of the cell cycle are referred to as "phase-specific" agents. For example, an S-phase inhibitor (such as methotrexate) is effective only against cells that are undergoing DNA synthesis. Since only those cells that are in the sensitive phase of growth will be killed by a single exposure to drug, either repeated doses or prolonged continuous infusions of the drug must be used in an attempt to increase the number of cells killed. Examples of phase-specific drugs are shown in Table 72–1.

Drugs that exert their effects independent of cycle phase are referred to as "phase-nonspecific" agents. Since their activity is not dependent upon the cells being in any specific phase of growth, these drugs are oftentimes still effective in tumors with low growth fractions. Examples of phase-nonspecific drugs include cis-platinum, cyclophosphamide, dacarbazine, steroid hormones, and nitrogen mustard.

CLASSIFICATION OF CHEMOTHERAPEUTIC DRUGS COMMONLY USED IN THE TREATMENT OF HEAD AND NECK MALIGNANCIES

Antimetabolites

Antimetabolites are cytotoxic agents that, by virtue of structural similarity with physiologic intermediates, are accepted as fraudulent substrates for vital biochemical reactions, thus interfering with a required cellular process.[22] Examples include 6-mercaptopurine, 6-thioguanine, cytosine arabinoside, 5-fluorouracil (5-FU), and methotrexate.

Methothrexate

Methotrexate exerts its effect by reversibly inhibiting dihydrofolate reductase (DHFR)[22], which is the enzyme responsible for maintaining adequate intracellular levels of reduced folate compounds. The reduced folates are needed for the synthesis of thymidine and purines. By blocking the production of these nucleotides, methotrexate inhibits DNA synthesis. Leucovorin (5-formyl-

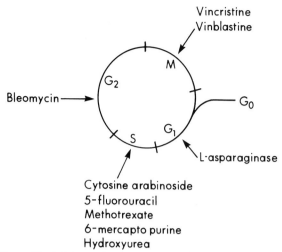

Figure 72–1. Schematic representation of the cell cycle. Phase-specific drugs that affect the cell cycle are shown.

tetrahydrofolate) can "rescue" cells from the effects of methotrexate by providing an alternative source of reduced folate.[50]

Methotrexate can be given orally, intramuscularly, intravenously, or intrathecally. It is excreted almost unchanged in the urine, and dose reduction is required for patients with significant renal dysfunction. Methotrexate accumulates in interstitial fluid spaces, such as pleural and peritoneal effusions. Slow diffusion of the drug back into the systemic circulation then results in prolonged drug exposure, which augments its systemic toxicity.[23] Since it is an S phase–specific inhibitor of cell growth, its toxicity is, in part, dependent upon the duration of exposure to the drug. The longer a cell is exposed to methotrexate, the more likely it is that it will enter the S phase and experience cytotoxicity. Therefore, significant pleural or peritoneal effusions should be completely drained prior to treatment with methotrexate. The inability to drain such effusions is a contraindication to treatment with methotrexate.

Mucositis is a common toxicity associated with methotrexate therapy and may range clinically from mouth soreness to diffuse gastrointestinal ulceration. The myelosuppression that occurs with methotrexate may be severe, but it tends to be of short duration. Hematologic recovery is often evident within 12 to 17 days after treatment. Acute hepatotoxicity is occasionally seen after treatment with high doses of methotrexate. Chronic administration of methotrexate can result in hepatic cirrhosis.[31] Nephrotoxicity may occur after high-dose therapy and may, in part, be due to precipitation of methotrexate in the renal tubules. Since methotrexate precipitates in an acidic environment, such tubular precipitation is favored by an acidic urinary pH. Thus, forced hydration with alkaline fluids is critical to ensure solubility and renal excretion of the drug.[67] Less common toxicities include pneumonitis, vasculitis, and skin rash.

Postulated mechanisms of resistance to methotrexate include alterations in membrane transport mechanisms and increased intracellular levels of dihydrofolate reductase.[68] Conceivably, both mechanisms could be overcome by utilizing higher doses of the drug. Early clinical trials confirmed that high doses of methotrexate could be administered without producing prohibitive toxicity if such therapy was then followed by leucovorin rescue.[49] This form of therapy, however, has the potential for excessive, and even fatal, toxicity and should be administered only under the supervision of physicians experienced in its use.

5-Fluorouracil

A pyrimidine analogue that inhibits DNA synthesis after being converted to an active nucleotide,[15] 5-FU can be given orally, intravenously, or intra-arterially. As a result of its unpredictable absorption and a variable first-pass metabolism in the liver, plasma levels are unpredictable after oral administration.[47] Following intravenous administration, plasma concentrations fall rapidly because of metabolism by the liver and other tissues. Schedules of intravenous dosing have included weekly or daily bolus injections and continuous infusions lasting 1 to 5 days.

The limiting toxic effects of 5-FU are mucositis and myelosuppression. Bolus doses tend to produce more severe myelosuppression, whereas continuous infusion schedules are associated with more severe mucositis.[99] Neurologic dysfunction, characterized by somnolence, cerebellar ataxia, and upper motor neuron signs, has been associated with intracarotid arterial infusions and, less commonly, with intravenous dosing.[22] Conjunctivitis, with lacrimal duct stenosis, and hyperpigmentation are often associated with chronic 5-FU therapy.

Alkylating Agents

Alkylating agents constitute a class of drugs that produce cytotoxicity by alkylation of DNA. This results in cross-linking and strand breakage within the molecule.[26] Examples include cyclophosphamide, nitrogen mustard, the nitrosoureas, and cis-platinum.

The antitumor activity of *cis-platinum* is probably based upon the production of intrastrand and interstrand cross-links in the DNA molecule.[127] Cis-platinum is classically administered by the intravenous route, although intra-arterial therapy is being investigated. Common schedules of administration include single doses of up to 120 mg/m² and lower daily doses (20 mg/m²) for 5 consecutive days. The primary route of drug elimination is urinary excretion.

The most significant toxic effect of cis-platinum is nephrotoxicity,[79] the likelihood of which increases as the kidneys are exposed to high concentrations of the drug for prolonged periods of time. It is thus critical to ensure adequate intravenous hydration in an attempt to maintain a vigorous diuresis. Typically, such a diuresis is initiated 4 to 12 hours prior to cis-platinum administration and continued for 12 to 24 hours after

TABLE 72–1. Cell Cycle Phase-Specific Drugs

S Phase-Specific	M Phase-Specific	G2 Phase-Specific
Cytosine arabinoside	Vincristine	Bleomycin
5-Fluorouracil	Vinblastine	
Methotrexate		
6-Mercaptopurine		
Hydroxyurea		

treatment. All patients should have a creatinine clearance value determined prior to initial therapy with cis-platinum and repeated if there is any significant change in the serum creatinine level. The renal toxicity associated with cis-platinum therapy appears to be augmented by aminoglycoside treatment, and thus concurrent therapy should be avoided.[96]

Cis-platinum can produce severe nausea and vomiting. This toxic effect is often managed effectively with various antiemetic drugs, such as high-dose metoclopramide.[52] Ototoxicity (tinnitus, high-frequency hearing loss) may occur in approximately 20 to 30 per cent of patients treated with cis-platinum.[82] Myelosuppression is moderate, but it can become significant in patients who had previously received cytotoxic chemotherapy. Less common toxicities include distal sensory neuropathy, hypersensitivity reactions, and hypomagnesemia.

Antitumor Antibiotics

Antitumor antibiotics include bleomycin and the anthracyclines—doxorubicin and daunorubicin. *Bleomycin* is thought to act by binding DNA and inducing single- and double-strand breaks in the molecule.[35] The *anthracyclines* damage DNA by intercalation, resulting in the inhibition of DNA, RNA, and protein synthesis.

Bleomycin represents a mixture of at least 13 small-molecular-weight glycopeptides that are produced by the fungus *Streptomyces venticillus*.[113] The drug may be administered subcutaneously, intramuscularly, or intravenously. Since most bleomycin is excreted unchanged in the urine, dose adjustment is needed for patients with significant renal dysfunction.[30]

The toxicities of bleomycin are different from those associated with most other antineoplastic drugs. Bleomycin rarely causes bone marrow supression, but it can lead to lethal pulmonary toxicity in about 1 to 2 per cent of treated patients.[10] Another 2 to 3 per cent of patients will develop nonlethal pulmonary fibrosis.[13] Factors that appear to contribute to the development of pulmonary toxicity include:[51]

1. A prior history of, or concurrent, thoracic radiation therapy.
2. Pre-existing pulmonary disease.
3. High concentrations of inspired oxygen during anesthesia.
4. Age greater than 70 years.
5. Cumulative doses greater than 400 to 450 units.

Other effects include mucositis, fever, chills, hypotension, skin reactions (hyperpigmentation, erythema, sclerosis), and a rare but fulminant, anaphylaxis-like reaction that can be fatal.[76]

Plant Alkaloids

Plant alkaloids include the Vinca alkaloids (vincristine, vinblastine) and the epipodophyllotoxins (VM-26, VP-16). The Vinca alkaloids bind the protein tubulin, resulting in mitotic arrest during metaphase.

Vincristine is administered intravenously and is eliminated primarily by hepatic metabolism. It rarely causes clinically significant myelosuppression. The dose-limiting toxicity of vincristine is a motor and sensory neuropathy. Early signs and symptoms include a decrease in the deep tendon reflexes and paresthesias. Auto-

nomic neuropathy can manifest as constipation, urinary retention, and occasionally paralytic ileus.[121] Although sensory and reflex changes may improve slowly when the drug is stopped, motor deficits often show little improvement. The incidence of neurotoxicity is increased in older patients.

CHEMOTHERAPY OF ADVANCED EPIDERMOID CARCINOMA OF THE HEAD AND NECK

The prognosis for patients with locally recurrent or metastatic epidermoid carcinoma of the head and neck is dismal. Although chemotherapy can produce tumor regression in this setting, treatment is palliative and should be reserved for symptomatic patients or for those in whom tumor growth threatens vital structures. The response to such therapy, however, is not always predictable and appears to be influenced by several factors. Several studies, for example, have documented lower response rates in patients treated after surgery or radiation therapy.[11, 16] This may reflect regional microvascular compromise caused by fibrosis.[94] In addition, malnutrition, poor performance status, and radiation-induced mucositis may limit the patient's tolerance for chemotherapy and thus result in dose reductions and compromised effect.[3] Bertino noted that tumor location affected the response to chemotherapy in that tumors of the oral cavity and oropharynx appeared to respond better to methotrexate than did tumors of the hypopharynx and nasopharynx (response rates 50 to 67 per cent versus 18 to 25 per cent, respectively).[11] Tests of statistical significance were not mentioned in this report, and the response rate for the oral lesions was higher than usually reported with methotrexate. In contrast, the Eastern Cooperative Oncology Group found no significant relationship between the site of disease and the response rate to chemotherapy.[33]

Single-Agent Chemotherapy

Single agents that have demonstrated response rates of at least 10 per cent are listed in Table 72–2. Much of the variation in the reported response rates may reflect differences in the prognostic factors of the patient populations treated. As in other squamous cell malignancies, complete responses are rare with single-agent chemotherapy and the responses obtained are often of brief duration. The combination of low response rate and brief duration of response accounts for the minimal impact of single-agent chemotherapy on the survival of patients with squamous cell carcinomas of the head and neck.

The most active and thoroughly evaluated single agents are methotrexate, cis-platinum, and bleomycin.

Methotrexate was the first drug demonstrated to have activity in epidermoid carcinoma of the head and neck. There has been extensive experience with this drug, and it thus remains the standard to which other single agents and combinations are compared. The most commonly used schedule involves the oral or intravenous administration of 40 to 60 mg/m² weekly. Response rates of 15 to 65 per cent have been reported with a median duration of 2 to 6 months.[33, 34, 58, 70, 74, 117, 125] Methotrexate

TABLE 72–2. Single-Agent Systemic Chemotherapy for Recurrent or Metastatic Disease

Drug*	Number of Patients	Response† (Per Cent)	Range	References
Methotrexate	726	31%	13–68%	33, 58, 70, 117, 125
Bleomycin	362	23%	6–45%	2, 14, 36, 53, 54, 126
Cis-platinum	186	27%	17–31%	27, 62, 85, 91, 95, 124
Doxorubicin	88	18%	0–21%	12, 73
Cyclophosphamide	77	36%	0–39%	21
5-Fluorouracil	59	10%	0–15%	7, 65, 80
Methyl-GAG‡	47	25%	12–41%	85, 111
Vindesine‡	46	11%	8–14%	24, 115
Chlorambucil	35	14%	—	81
Dibromodulcitol‡	25	16%	8–25%	5, 6
Vinblastine	23	17%	—	105

*Data are included only for drugs found to produce a minimum response rate of 10 per cent with *at least* 20 patients treated. Data from intra-arterial therapy are not included. The range is not stated if only one study is performed.
†Response means at least 50 per cent tumor regression.
‡Investigational agents.

has also been administered according to a number of other schedules and over a large range of doses. However, as shown in Table 72–3, prospective randomized trials have not demonstrated the superiority of any schedule or dose over weekly, moderate-dose methotrexate. In particular, high-dose methotrexate with leucovorin rescue is neither more effective nor less toxic. When conventional doses are given, mucositis and myelosuppression are the most frequently encountered toxicities. Nephrotoxicity is more common with high doses than with conventional doses.[33, 125]

Bleomycin has been extensively evaluated in epidermoid carcinoma of the head and neck. Administration of 10 to 20 mg/m² two times weekly produces short responses in approximately 20 per cent of patients with recurrent disease. A variety of other schedules of administration have been used without improvement in the response rate. In particular, continuous intravenous administration does not improve efficacy.[94] Single-agent therapy with bleomycin is limited by mucositis, dermatitis, and pulmonary fibrosis. However, the lack of significant myelosuppression makes this drug ideal for use in combination regimens.

In 1973 Lippman documented the activity of *cis-platinum* in recurrent head and neck cancer.[77] As a single agent, the drug is usually administered in moderate doses, 80 to 120 mg/m², every 3 weeks. Response rates of 17 to 30 per cent have been reported, and as with methotrexate complete responses are rare and the median duration of response is usually short.[27, 62, 83, 91, 95, 124] With vigorous hydration and care to maintain adequate urine output, nephrotoxicity is uncommon. The absence of severe myelosuppression makes cis-platinum an excellent choice for use in combination regimens.

In a randomized, prospective trial, Hong compared single-agent methotrexate at 40 to 60 mg/m²/week to cis-platinum 50 mg/m² on days 1 and 8 repeated at 4-week intervals.[58] A total of 44 patients with recurrent disease were treated. There was no significant difference in response rates—29 per cent for cis-platinum and 23 per cent for methotrexate. Median duration of response was 3 months in each group. Lehane compared results of cis-platinum in the dose and schedule above with methotrexate 15 mg/m² intramuscularly on days 1 to 3 every

3 weeks.[38] Again, there was no significant difference in response rate or duration; however, in both studies, vomiting was more common with cis-platinum and mucositis and myelosuppression were more severe with methotrexate.

Combination Chemotherapy

A number of combination regimens have been used in the treatment of advanced epidermoid carcinoma of the head and neck. These have generally included one or more of the most active single agents—bleomycin, methotrexate, cis-platinum—with or without the other drugs listed in Table 72–2. As with single agents, response rates vary considerably but duration of response has been uniformly short. Studies reporting the highest response rates have often included a substantial proportion of previously untreated or inevaluable patients.[88, 42] Randomized trials comparing single agents with combination therapy are listed in Table 72–4. In each study, such therapy failed to improve response rate or duration, with most combinations producing substantially more toxicity.

The combination of cis-platinum and 4-day continuous infusion 5-FU was initially evaluated at Wayne State University.[71] Of 30 patients with local-regional recurrence or disseminated disease, an overall response rate of 70 per cent was obtained. Complete responses were seen in 27 per cent—a result superior to that documented for any single agent. Although the median survival of the entire group was only 7 months, the median duration of complete remission was 11.3 months. Myelosuppression and mucositis were more severe than would be expected with single-agent cis-platinum. Subsequent trials have confirmed the activity of this combination,[4, 48, 92] but randomized studies will be required to prove its superiority over single-agent cis-platinum.

The use of cis-platinum with optimal schedules of methotrexate has been hampered by severe myelosuppression and mucositis. This is probably the result of decreased renal excretion of methotrexate induced by cis-platinum nephrotoxicity.[29] Dichloromethotrexate is an investigational, dihalogenated methotrexate ana-

TABLE 72–3. Clinical Trials Comparing Various Doses and Schedules of Methotrexate Administration

Study	Regimen	Response Rate* (Per Cent)	Response Duration†	Toxicity
Levitt et al., 1973[75]	*Randomized* a) m 80–230 mg/m² bw b) m 240–1080 mg/m² bw + Lv	44% ⎫NS 60% ⎭	12 weeks 11 weeks	Less heme with b
Vogler et al., 1979[117]	*Randomized* a) m 500 mg/m² po qw + Lv b) m 60 mg/m² po qw c) m 60 mg/m² IV qw	22% ⎫ 27% ⎬NS 15% ⎭	6.3 months ⎫ 5.8 months ⎬NS 5.4 months ⎭	Less heme with b
Kirkwood et al., 1981[70]	*Not randomized* a) m 3.75 gm/m² qw + Lv b) m 40–200 mg/m² biw + Lv	30% ⎫NS 63% ⎭	11 weeks 12 weeks	Less heme with b
Woods et al., 1981[125]	*Randomized* a) m 50 mg/m² qw + Lv b) m 500 mg/m² qw + Lv c) m 5 gm/m² qw + Lv	31% ⎫ 21% ⎬NS 50% ⎭	not given	Less heme and nephro with a
DeConti and Schonfeld, 1981[33]	*Randomized* a) m 40–60 mg/m² qw b) m 240 mg/m² to >4 gm/m² biw + Lv	26% 24%	19 weeks 7 weeks	No difference in toxicity
Taylor et al., 1984[110]	*Randomized* a) m 40 mg/m² ↑ qw b) m 1500 mg/m² ↑ qw + Lv	22% ⎫NS 32% ⎭	5 weeks ⎫P<.05 11 weeks ⎭	Toxicity prevented survival benefit in group b

*Partial plus complete responses.
†Median response duration.
Abbreviations: M = Methotrexate; bw = two times per week; NS = not significant; heme = hematologic toxicity; Lv = leucovorin; qw = weekly; biw = every other week; nephro = nephrotoxicity; ↑ = escalating doses; IV = intravenous; po = by mouth; mg = milligrams; gm = grams; m² = square meters.

TABLE 72–4. Randomized Trials Comparing Single Agents with Combination Chemotherapy in Recurrent or Metastatic Epidermoid Carcinoma of the Head and Neck

Study	Regimen	Response Rate (Per Cent)	Response Duration	Toxicity

Davis and Kessler, 1979[32]	a) DDP 3 mg/kg q 4 wk
	b) DDP 3 mg/kg day 1
	  m 50 mg/m² days 1,15 ⎬ q 4 weeks
	  B 15 mg/m² bw
		13%
		11%
			4.2 months (mn)
			5.2 months
				Combination with greater heme

Baker, 1979[8a]	a) m 40 mg/m² qw
	b) DDP 100 mg/m² day 1
	  O 1 mg days 2,5 ⎬ q 21 days
	  B 30 u days 2,5
		43%
		50%
			Not stated	Overall toxicity similar

DeConti and Schoenfeld, 1981[33]	a) m 240 mg/m² to > 4 biw + Lv b) m as in "a" + Ctx + Ara-C biw	24% 18%	6 weeks (md) 7 weeks	Combination with greater heme

Williams, 1982[123a]	a) m 45–60 mg/m² qw
	b) DDP 60 mg/m² day 1
	  VBL 0.1 mg/kg days 1,15 ⎬ q 28 days
	  B 15 u qw
		16%
		20%
			21 weeks (md)
			16 weeks
				Overall toxicity similar

Jacobs et al., 1983[63]	DDP 80 g/m² qw q 3 weeks DDP as in "a" + m 250 mg/m² qw + Lv	18% ⎫NS 33% ⎭	7 months (md) 4 months	More heme toxicity in combination arm

Abbreviations: mn = Mean; md = median; m = methotrexate; B = bleomycin; O = vincristine; Ctx = cytoxan; DDP = cis-platinum; VBL = vinblastine; Ara-C = cytosine arabinoside; bw = twice a week; NS = not significant; heme = hematologic toxicity; Lv = leucovorin; m² = square meters; mg = milligrams; qw = weekly; biw = every other week; q = for; u = units.

logue that is excreted and metabolized by the liver. Blood levels of this drug are thus not dependent upon renal function. Clinical trials have produced therapeutic results similar to those with methotrexate.[45] A recent study in patients with recurrent head and neck carcinoma combined escalating weekly doses of dichloromethotrexate with cis-platinum 100 mg/m² every 4 weeks.[123] Dichloromethotrexate dose escalation was stopped when mild myelosuppression or mucositis developed. An overall response rate of 43 per cent was obtained, with 20 per cent complete responses. Toxicity was minimal with a single episode of sepsis in a leukopenic patient.

Intra-arterial Chemotherapy

Despite extensive surgery and radiation, most advanced head and neck tumors recur in local-regional sites. This pattern of relapse would seem ideally suited for treatment by regional infusion of chemotherapy. Intra-arterial therapy has the advantage of producing high local concentrations of drug, possibly improving efficacy without increasing systemic toxicity. Prolonged infusion of phase-specific drugs may also improve efficacy by killing tumor cells as they pass through the cell cycle.

For the intra-arterial perfusion of head and neck tumors, the superficial temporal or superior thyroid artery is cannulated and the catheter is advanced into the external carotid artery. Following verification of perfusion by fluorescein or radioisotope injection, branches of the external carotid that do not directly perfuse tumor are ligated. The catheter is then attached to a perfusion pump and the chosen drug is infused for a predetermined period or until toxicity develops.

In 1977, Carter reviewed over 10 years of experience with intra-arterial methotrexate infusions in 340 patients with advanced head and neck tumors.[21] The cumulative response rate of 53 per cent was similar to that obtained in patients with localized tumors receiving systemic methotrexate. In these early studies, life-threatening complications associated with catheter use were common. Hemorrhage, infection, and thromboemboli were associated with a 5 to 15 per cent mortality rate.[18, 118] However, the recent introduction of completely implantable infusion pumps and silicone catheters has significantly reduced the incidence of complications and has allowed for long-term infusions outside the hospital.[9] The clinical value of such therapy is now being investigated.

ADJUVANT CHEMOTHERAPY IN SQUAMOUS CELL CANCERS OF THE HEAD AND NECK

Standard therapies for squamous cell cancers of the head and neck have included surgery and/or radiation therapy. These modalities of treatment are often successful in curing early lesions, but they are rarely curative for more locally advanced lesions. Chemotherapy has demonstrated effectiveness in shrinking locally recurrent and metastatic lesions after failure of primary therapy. However, even though complete regression of all measurable disease may occur during chemotherapy, the goal of such secondary treatment is palliation and the benefits are rarely long-lasting.[25] The tumor ultimately reoccurs, and the patient dies from refractory disease.

This is analogous to the situation faced by many women with breast cancer. Certain subsets of such patients with advanced local-regional disease are unlikely to be cured by primary therapy (surgery and/or radiotherapy). When recurrence becomes evident, disease in these women is very often palliated with systemic chemotherapy, but ultimately relapse occurs and they die of uncontrolled disease. However, when the same "high-risk" subsets of women are treated with adjuvant chemotherapy in the immediate postoperative period, an increased disease-free survival (and possibly cure rate) can be expected.[19] Similar findings have also been noted for some soft-tissue sarcomas and for Wilms' tumors.

Clonal heterogeneity within some tumors has been demonstrated[46, 104, 112] and might explain why drugs that are incapable of curing large tumors can sometimes cure residual microscopic disease following surgical debulking. The failure to cure large lesions with drugs that are known to be effective in a given tumor suggests that microscopic foci of disease remain viable. This may be due to inherent drug resistance by subclones of malignant cells. The larger the primary tumor, the more likely it is that there will be subpopulations of drug-resistant cells. If the tumor can be decreased in size either by surgical debulking or by radiation therapy, it is possible that the number of resistant cells can also be reduced. The advanced head and neck tumor has been estimated to contain 10^{10} cells.[41] If, for example, one of every 10^6 cells is resistant to the chemotherapy being used, there would be 10^4 resistant cells present ($10^{10}/10^6$). If, however, extensive surgical debulking were to remove 99.99 per cent of the malignant cells, the patient's tumor burden would be reduced from 10^{10} to 10^6 cells. Similarly, in this example, the burden of resistant cells would be reduced from 10^4 ($10^{10}/10^6$) to 1 ($10^6/10^6$). Thus, the likelihood of ultimately being cured has been increased, although not guaranteed.

In theory, it should not matter whether the adjuvant chemotherapy is given prior to surgery (and/or radiation therapy) or afterward. In practice, however, the main interest over the past decade has been in the use of chemotherapy before surgery or radiation in high-risk patients. The rationale for this approach (induction chemotherapy) is summarized as follows and has been discussed by Hong and Bromer[57]:

1. Because both surgery and radiation therapy compromise the blood supply of a tumor, it is possible that more efficient drug delivery will occur if the drug is given as the initial therapy.

2. Preoperative cytoreduction may allow for an easier and more efficient resection. Inoperable tumors may thus become operable.

3. There may be better tolerance of the chemotherapy if it is given early to patients with normal nutrition and normal performance statuses.

4. The elimination of subclinical systemic metastases by chemotherapy may result in improved disease-free survival rates.

Induction chemotherapy appears to be tolerated better

TABLE 72—5. Randomized Trials of Chemotherapy Plus Radiation Therapy in Patients with Locally Advanced Squamous Cell Carcinoma of the Head and Neck

Reference	Drug	Number of Patients	Time (Years)	Per Cent Survival Chemotherapy and Radiation Therapy	Radiation Therapy
Knowlton et al., 1975[72]	Methotrexate	96	3	14	17
Lustig et al., 1976[78]	Methotrexate	75	3	20	10
Fazekas, 1980,[43] 1983[44]	Methotrexate	712	3	18–30	12–22
Cachin et al., 1977[20]	Bleomycin	186	3	40	40
Shanta et al., 1977,[101] 1983[102]	Bleomycin	157	5	50	19
Hussey and Abrams, 1975[61]	Hydroxyurea	40	2	30	27
Ansfield et al., 1970[8]	5-Fluorouracil	134	3	45	19

than when the same drugs are administered to patients with more advanced disease,[116] and there does not appear to be an increase in subsequent postoperative complications.[98] Several studies have shown that the response to chemotherapy in previously untreated patients is better than the response observed in patients who had received initial surgery or radiation therapy. For example, Elias and co-workers[39] reported a 73 per cent response rate to combination chemotherapy in previously untreated patients, and a 55 per cent response rate in patients who had received prior surgery or radiation. Price and associates published similar findings.[89] However, the value of induction chemotherapy remains uncertain despite several clinical trials.

Radiation Therapy and Adjuvant Chemotherapy

Multiple reports have described the results of combining chemotherapy with radiotherapy in patients with advanced localized disease. Most of the initial reports involved nonrandomized trials and did not demonstrate a marked benefit over radiation therapy alone. Increased toxicity was suggested.[100] Additionally, several randomized studies have examined the role of combined chemotherapy and radiation therapy (Table 72–5).

The results of the studies with methotrexate, bleomycin, and hydroxyurea have not demonstrated a substantial advantage to the addition of chemotherapy to primary radiation therapy. The Radiation Therapy Oncology Group (RTOG) investigated the role of adjuvant methotrexate in a large study. They randomized 312 patients to receive intravenous methotrexate prior to definitive radiation therapy and 326 patients to radiation therapy only. With no significant survival difference after 4 years of follow-up, the investigators concluded that methotrexate was not effective as an adjuvant to

full-course radiation therapy.[43, 44] A single trial of adjuvant 5-FU did suggest a benefit to combined therapy,[8] but these results have not been duplicated.

In summary, the results of the randomized studies to date have not demonstrated a clear value for the use of adjuvant chemotherapy in patients receiving definitive radiation therapy. Even though increased local tumor regressions have been reported, there does not appear to be an associated improvement in the disease-free interval or overall survival. This form of treatment should thus be considered investigational at the present time. Studies are now ongoing to evaluate the potential role of multidrug adjuvant protocols.

Induction Chemotherapy Prior to Surgery

In 1975, Tarpley and colleagues reported the results of a provocative study in which 30 patients were given two cycles of high-dose methotrexate, (240 mg/m²), and leucovorin rescue as preoperative adjuvant therapy.[109] An impressive objective response rate of 77 per cent was noted, and the combination with surgery did not appear to produce excessive toxicity. Despite this, there did not appear to be an associated survival benefit when compared with matched historical controls. The results of other adjuvant chemotherapy trials are summarized in Table 72–6.

In general, response rates to induction chemotherapy have been excellent in previously untreated patients. However, since the ultimate goal of such therapy is to prolong survival, its value cannot be determined by examining the response rates alone. In the few studies that have provided long-term follow-up, the results have been conflicting. Pennacchio and others[84] reported the follow-up data on 41 patients who were originally part of the trial by Hong.[56] With a median follow-up of

TABLE 72—6. Results of Preoperative Induction Chemotherapy Trials in Previously Untreated Patients with Locally Advanced Squamous Cell Carcinomas of the Head and Neck

Reference	Drug Regimen	Number of Patients	Response Rate (Per Cent)
Tarpley et al., 1975[109]	MTX	30	77%
Weaver et al., 1980[120]	DDP/VCR/B	75	80%
Spaulding et al., 1982[106]	DDP/VCR/B	50	88%
Schuller et al., 1983[98]	DDP/MTX/B/VCR	53	66%
Weaver et al., 1984[119]	DDP/5-FU	88	94%
Jacobs et al., 1984[66]	DDP/5-FU	23	91%

Abbreviations: MTX = Methotrexate; DDP = cis-platinum; VCR = vincristine; B = bleomycin; 5-FU = 5-fluorouracil

TABLE 72–7. Adjuvant Chemotherapy after Surgery and Radiation for Stage III and IV Patients

Group	Patient Number	Recurrence	Death Due to Tumor	Disease-Free Survival/Median (% months)	Overall Survival/Median (% months)
Primary therapy plus adjuvant chemotherapy	20	3 (15%)*	2 (10%)	85%/31 (range 14–76)	70%/31 (range 14–76)
Recurrent retreatment plus adjuvant chemotherapy	11	2 (18%)	2 (18%)	82%/52 (range 19–65) (from recurrence/Rx)	64%/52 (range 27–99) (from Dx)
Primary therapy without adjuvant chemotherapy	24	16 (67%)	13 (54%)	33%/19 (range 5–75)	38%/30 (range 6–77)

*Recurrent disease not documented in one patient, but his progressive symptoms and demise suggested tumor progression.
Source: Huang AT, et al: Ann Surg 200:195, 1984.

20 months, 53 per cent of the patients were alive and 41 per cent were disease-free. A median survival of 29 months was projected. In contrast, the median survival of a historical control group that received only radiation therapy was 4.5 months, and only 5 per cent were disease-free at 24 months. Hill and co-workers reported a similar benefit in patients treated with preoperative vincristine, hydrocortisone, bleomycin, 5-FU, methotrexate, and folinic acid.[55] In their study, chemotherapy responders lived longer than nonresponders and response to chemotherapy thus appeared to be a favorable prognostic sign. The median survival for chemotherapy responders was 34 months in contrast to 14 months for nonresponders (P = 0.006). Furthermore, the degree of response provided prognostic information. Stage IV patients who achieved a complete response (CR) enjoyed a 52.4-month median survival in contrast to 7.8 months for those with overt residual disease (P<0.001). Other studies have also demonstrated encouraging results with induction chemotherapy,[86, 106] but not all studies have demonstrated a beneficial effect on survival. Vogl and associates treated 24 patients with combination chemotherapy prior to planned local treatment with irradiation or surgery.[116] Despite a 77 per cent objective response rate, all but two patients had died within 30 months. The median survival of 10 months was no better than that of historical control. In a large randomized trial, Jacobs and colleagues further evaluated the long-term results of induction chemotherapy.[64] A total of 462 patients were prospectively randomized to one of three treatment groups:

1. Standard therapy of surgery and postoperative radiation.
2. Induction chemotherapy followed by standard therapy.
3. Induction chemotherapy and standard therapy followed by maintenance chemotherapy.

There was no difference in overall or disease-free survival among the three groups. The 2-year disease-free survival for the patients who received standard therapy was 55 per cent and for those who received the initial induction therapy, 57 per cent. Furthermore, no benefit was seen in maintenance chemotherapy.

Prechemotherapy Planning

Pretreatment evaluation of the patient with a locally advanced head and neck cancer should include consul-

tation with a medical oncologist and radiation therapist. If the patient appears to have a resectable lesion, tattooing should be performed prior to the administration of chemotherapy, since precise definition of the original tumor margins may become lost if the patient has a good response to chemotherapy. The initially planned surgical procedure should not be altered as a result of a favorable response to induction chemotherapy.

Postoperative Adjuvant Chemotherapy

Huang and co-workers reported the results of treating high-risk head and neck cancer patients with adjuvant chemotherapy after primary local therapy had been delivered.[60] Twenty consecutive patients with stage III and IV squamous cell carcinomas of the head and neck were treated with adjuvant chemotherapy after undergoing primary resection and radiation therapy. Another group of 11 patients with locally recurrent disease was also treated with adjuvant chemotherapy after undergoing a second resection or radiation. The survival of these 31 patients was then compared with the survival of 24 other patients with stage III and IV disease who were treated similarly but without adjuvant chemotherapy. In this nonrandomized study, patients who received adjuvant chemotherapy enjoyed a better disease-free survival than those who received "standard" therapy alone. The results of their study are shown in Table 72–7.

Based upon the Huang's observations, a randomized study has been initiated to evaluate the role of adjuvant chemotherapy given after surgery and/or radiation for patients with stage III and IV tumors (under joint sponsorship of The National Cancer Institute and Duke University Medical Center).

Thus, postoperative adjuvant chemotherapy may also be shown to play an important role in the management of some patients with locally advanced epidermoid carcinoma of the head and neck. For the present time, however, its role should be considered investigational.

BIOLOGIC RESPONSE MODIFIERS

Immunotherapy remains an area of active interest in the treatment of many malignancies. Data from available trials with head and neck cancers have not demon-

TABLE 72–8. Chemotherapy of Advanced Adenoid Cystic Carcinoma

Study	Regimen	Response Rate*	Response Duration†
Rentschler et al., 1977[93]	Doxo or HMM	3/11 (27%)	3 months (2–3)
Tannock and Sutherland, 1980[108]	5-Fluorouracil	4/12 (33%)	5 months (5–24)
Schramm et al., 1981[97]	Cis-platinum	7/10 (70%)	Not stated
Posner et al., 1982[90]	Cytoxan + Doxo	2/5 (40%)	2+ and 8

*Complete and partial responses/patients entered on study (except Tannock study, in which response was defined as "unequivocal decrease in size of all lesions").
†Median response duration and range of response duration.
Abbreviations: Doxo = Doxorubicin; HMM = hexamethylmelamine.

strated a clear benefit from the use of biologic response modifiers,[1] and thus their use remains investigational.

RECOMMENDATIONS FOR THE USE OF CHEMOTHERAPY IN PATIENTS WITH EPIDERMOID CARCINOMA OF THE HEAD AND NECK

Patients who have primary tumors that can be treated by surgery and/or radiation therapy with curative intent are not appropriate candidates for systemic chemotherapy. However, those who have more locally advanced disease should be offered participation in available adjuvant induction chemotherapy programs.

Patients with inoperable locally recurrent or metastatic disease can be offered single-agent systemic chemotherapy for attempted short-term palliation. Alternately, if available, patients should be offered participation in trials investigating the roles of newer agents and/or multiagent chemotherapy.

CHEMOTHERAPY OF SALIVARY GLAND MALIGNANCIES

Malignant salivary gland tumors represent 5 to 10 per cent of all head and neck cancers.[93] The most common histologic types are adenoid cystic, malignant mixed, adenocarcinoma, mucoepidermoid, and acinic cell carcinoma. Information concerning the chemotherapy of these tumors is limited and difficult to interpret. Most series contain small numbers of patients who were treated over many years with a number of different regimens.

Adenoid cystic carcinomas (cylindromas) comprise 20 to 30 per cent of all salivary gland malignancies.[17] The tendency of these tumors to infiltrate surrounding tissue makes complete resection difficult, resulting in a 65 per cent rate of local-regional recurrence in patients treated by surgery alone.[17, 107] Distant metastases occur in 40 per cent of patients—most commonly involving the lungs.[107, 114] Adenoid cystic tumors usually demonstrate indolent growth patterns and allow for long survival of even the patient with metastatic disease. However, in the series compiled by Spiro, one third of all patients with metastatic disease died within 1 year of diagnosis.[97]

Table 72–8 contains data from the four largest series of patients treated with chemotherapy for recurrent or metastatic adenoid cystic carcinoma. Rentschler's report summarized the experience with salivary tumors over a 25-year period at M.D. Anderson Hospital.[93] During that time, over 25 different chemotherapeutic regimens were used. The series reported by Posner demonstrated activity of doxorubicin in combination with cyclophosphamide.[90] Four other case reports have documented the activity of doxorubicin as a single agent or in combination.[17, 28, 103, 114] The significant activity of cis-platinum reported by Schramm is encouraging, but results await confirmation.[97] As with advanced epidermoid carcinoma, responses are generally short (median < 6 months) and partial.

The value of chemotherapy in the management of other histologic subtypes of salivary gland tumors is also unclear. Doxorubicin, cis-platinum, and cyclophosphamide in combination or as single agents have produced brief responses in 30 to 40 per cent of patients with advanced disease.[2, 28, 37, 90, 93]

The goal of future studies should be the treatment of larger numbers of patients with uniform regimens. In this uncommon group of malignancies, this will best be accomplished by cooperative groups. Combination regimens that include doxorubicin and cis-platinum appear to offer the best chance of a response. Surgical adjuvant trials using a similar regimen in patients with advanced local-regional disease are also indicated.

REFERENCES

1. Alberts DS: Perspectives on adjuvant therapy of head and neck cancer. *In* Salmon S, Jones S (eds): Adjuvant Therapy of Cancer, III. New York, Grune & Stratton, 1981, p. 191.
2. Alberts DS, Manning MR, Coulthard SW, et al: Adriamycin/cis-platinum/cyclophosphamide combination chemotherapy for advanced carcinoma of the parotid gland. Cancer 47:645, 1981.
3. Amer MH, Al-Sarrat M, Vaitkevicius VK: Factors that affect response to chemotherapy and survival of patients with advanced head and neck cancer. Cancer 43:2202, 1979.
4. Amrein P, Weitzman S: 24-hour infusion cisplatin and 5 day infusion 5-fluorouracil in squamous cell carcinoma of the head and neck. Proc of the American Society of Clinical Oncology 4:133, 1985.
5. Andrews NC, Weiss AJ, Ansfield FJ, et al: Phase I study of dibromodulcitol. Cancer Chemother Rep 55:61, 1971.
6. Andrews NC, Weiss AJ, Wilson W, et al: Phase II study of dibromodulcitol. Cancer Chemother Rep 58:653, 1974.
7. Ansfeld FJ, Schroeder JM, Curreri AR: Five years' clinical experience with 5-fluorouracil. JAMA 181:295, 1962.
8. Ansfield FJ, Guillermo R, Davis HL Jr, et al: Treatment of advanced cancer of the head and neck. Cancer 25:78, 1970.
8a. Baker L, Al-Sarraf M: A comparative trial of cisplatinum, oncovin, and bleomycin versus methotrexate in patients with advanced epidermoid carcinoma of the head and neck. Proceedings of the American Association for Cancer Research 20:202, 1979.
9. Baker SR, Wheeler RH, Ensminger WD: Intra-arterial infusion chemotherapy for head and neck cancer using a totally implantable infusion pump. Head Neck Surgery 4:118, 1981.

10. Bennett WM, Pastore L, Houghton DC: Fatal pulmonary bleomycin toxicity in cis-platinum induced renal failure. Cancer Treat Rep 64:921, 1980.
11. Bertino JR, Boston B, Capizzi RL. The role of chemotherapy in the management of cancer of the head and neck: A review. Cancer 36:752, 1975.
12. Blum RH. An overview of studies with adriamycin in the United States. Cancer Chemother Rep 6:247, 1975.
13. Blum RH, Carter SK, Agre K: A clinical review of bleomycin—a new antineoplastic agent. Cancer 31:903, 1973.
14. Bonnadonna G, Tancini G, Bajetta E: Controlled studies with bleomycin in solid tumors and lymphomas. Prog Biochem Pharmacol 11:172, 1976.
15. Bosch L, Harbers E, Heidelberger C: Studies on fluorinated pyrimidines. V. Effects on nucleic acid metabolism in vitro. Cancer Res 18:335, 1958.
16. Brown AW, Blom J, Butler WM, et al: Combination chemotherapy with vinblastine, bleomycin and cis-diammine dichloroplatinum in squamous cell carcinoma of the head and neck. Cancer 45:2830, 1980.
17. Budd GT, Crope CW: Adenoid cystic carcinoma of the salivary gland. Cancer 51:589, 1983.
18. Burn JI, Johnston DA, Davies AJ, et al: Cancer chemotherapy by continuous intra-arterial infusion of methotrexate. Br J Surg 53:329, 1966.
19. Buzdar AU, Smith T, Blumenschein G, et al: Adjuvant chemotherapy with fluorouracil, doxorubicin, and cyclophosphamide (FAC) for stage II or III breast cancer: 5 year results. In Salmon SE, Jones SE (eds): Adjuvant Therapy of Cancer, III. New York, Grune & Stratton, 1981, p. 419–426.
20. Cachin Y, Jortay A, Sancho H, et al: Preliminary results of a randomized E.O.R.T.C. study comparing radiotherapy and concomitant bleomycin, to radiotherapy alone in epidermoid carcinomas of the oropharynx. Eur J Cancer 13:1389, 1977.
21. Carter SK: The chemotherapy of head and neck cancer. Semin Oncol 4:413, 1977.
22. Chabner BA, Myers CE: Clinical pharmacology of cancer chemotherapy. In DeVita VT, Hellman S, Rosemberg SA (ed): Cancer—Principles and Practice of Oncology. Philadelphia, J. B. Lippincott, 1985, pp. 296–298.
23. Chabner BA, Stoller RG, Hande KR, et al: Methotrexate disposition in humans: Case studies in ovarian cancer and following high dose infusion. Drug Metab Rev 8:107, 1978.
24. Cheng E, Young CW, Wittes RE: Phase II trial of vindesine in advanced head and neck cancer. Cancer Treat Rep 64:1141, 1980.
25. Chiuten D, Vogl SE, Kaplan BH, Greenwald E: Effective outpatient combination chemotherapy for advanced cancer of the head and neck. Surg Gynecol Obstet 151:659, 1980.
26. Colvin M, Brundrett RB, Kan MN, et al: Alkylating properties of phosphoramide mustard. Cancer Res 36:1121, 1976.
27. Creagan ET, O'Fallon JR, Woods JE, et al: Cis-diammioedichloroplatinum (II) administered by 24-hour infusion in the treatment of advanced upper aerodigestive cancer. Cancer 51:2020, 1983.
28. Creagan ET, Woods JE, Schutt AJ, O'Fallon JR: Cyclophosphamide, adriamycin and cis-diamminedichloroplatinum (II) in the treatment of advanced nonsquamous cell head and neck cancer. Cancer 52:2007, 1983.
29. Crom WR, Pratt CB, Green AA, et al: The effect of prior cisplatin therapy on the pharmacokinetics of high-dose methotrexate. J Clin Oncol 2:655, 1984.
30. Crooke GT, Comis RL, Einhorn LH, et al: Effects of variation in renal function on the clinical pharmacology of bleomycin administered as an IV bolus. Cancer Treat Rep 61:1631, 1977.
31. Dahl MGC, Gregory MM, Scheuer PJ: Liver damage due to methotrexate in patients with psoriasis. Br Med J 1:625, 1971.
32. Davis S, Kessler W: Randomized comparison of cis-diamminedichloroplatinum versus cis-diamminedichloroplatinum, methotrexate, and bleomycin in recurrent squamous cell carcinoma of the head and neck. Cancer Chemother Pharmacol 3:57, 1979.
33. DeConti RC, Schoenfeld D: A randomized prospective comparison of intermittent methotrexate, methotrexate with leucovorin, and a methotrexate combination in head and neck cancer. Cancer 48:1061, 1981.
34. DePalo GM, Dehena M, Molinari R, et al: Clinical evaluation of high weekly intravenous doses of methotrexate in advanced oropharyngeal carcinoma. Tumori 56:259, 1970.
35. Donehover RC, Myers CE, Chabner BA: Minireview: New developments on the mechanism of action of antineoplastic drugs. Life Sci 25:1, 1979.
36. Durkin WJ, Pugh RP, Jacobs E: Bleomycin therapy of responsive solid tumors. Oncology 33:260, 1976.
37. Eisenberger MA: Supporting evidence for an active treatment program for advanced salivary gland carcinomas. Cancer Treat Rep 69:319, 1985.
38. Eisenberger M, Hoth D, Posada J: New drug development in head and neck oncology. In Wolf GT (ed): Head and Neck Oncology. Boston, Martinus Nijhoff, 1984, pp. 347–373.
39. Elias EG, Chretien PB, Monnard E, et al: Chemotherapy prior to local therapy in advanced squamous cell carcinoma of the head and neck: Preliminary assessment of an intensive drug regimen. Cancer 43:1025, 1979.
40. EORTC (European Organization for Research and Treatment of Cancer) Clinical Screening Group: Study of the clinical efficiency of bleomycin in human cancer. Br Med J 2:643, 1970.
41. Ervin TJ, Karp DD, Weichselbaum RR, et al: Role of chemotherapy in the multidisciplinary approach to advanced head and neck cancer: Potentials and problems. Ann Otol 90:506, 1981.
42. Ervin T, Weishelbaum R, Miller D, et al: Treatment of advanced squamous cell carcinoma of the head and neck with cis-platinum, bleomycin, and methotrexate. Cancer Treat Rep 65:787, 1981.
43. Fazekas JT, Sommer C, Kramer S, et al: Adjuvant intravenous methotrexate or definitive radiotherapy alone for advanced squamous cancers of the oral cavity, oropharynx, supraglottic larynx or hypopharynx. Int J Radiat Oncol Biol Phys 6:533, 1980.
44. Fazekas JT, Sommer C, Kramer S, et al: Tumor regression and other prognosticators in advanced head and neck cancers: A sequel to the RTOG methotrexate study. Int J Radiat Oncol Biol Phys 9:957, 1983.
45. Fernback B, Takahashi I, Ohnuma T, et al: Clinical and laboratory re-evaluation of dichloromethotrexate. Recent Results Cancer Res 74:56, 1979.
46. Fidler IJ, Kripke ML: Metastasis results from preexisting variant cells within a malignant tumor. Science 197:893, 1977.
47. Finche RE, Bending MR, Lant AF: Plasma levels of 5-fluorouracil after oral and intravenous administration in cancer patients. Br J Clin Pharmacol 7:613, 1979.
48. Fosser VP, Paccagnella A, Venturelli E, et al: Cisplatin + 5-fluorouracil 120-hour infusion in patients with recurrent and disseminated head and neck cancer. Proceedings of the American Society of Clinical Oncology 4:150, 1985.
49. Glode LM, Pitman SW, Ensminger WD, et al: A phase I study of high-dose aminopterin administration with leucovorin rescue in patients with advanced metastatic tumor. Cancer Res 39:3707, 1979.
50. Goldin A, Mantel N, Greenhouse SW, et al: Effect of delayed administration of citrovorun factor on antileukemic effectiveness of aminopterin in mice. Cancer Res 14:43, 1954.
51. Goldiner PL, Carlon GC, Critkovic E, et al: Factors influencing postoperative morbidity and mortality in patients treated with bleomycin. Br Med J 1:1164, 1978.
52. Gralla RJ, Itri LM, Pisko SL, et al: Antiemetic efficacy of high dose metoclopramide: Randomized trial with placebo and prochlorperazine patients with chemotherapy-induced nausea and vomiting. N Eng J Med 305:905, 1981.
53. Haas C, Cotman C: Phase II evaluation of bleomycin. Cancer 38:8, 1976.
54. Halman KE, Bleehen NM, Brewin TB, et al: Early experience with bleomycin in the United Kingdom in series of 105 patients. Br Med J 4:635, 1972.
55. Hill BT, Price LA, Busby E, et al: Positive impact of initial 24-hour combination chemotherapy without cis-platinum on 6-year survival figures in advanced squamous cell carcinomas of the head and neck. In Jones SE, Salmon SE (eds): Adjuvant Therapy of Cancer, IV. Orlando, Grune & Stratton, Inc. 1984, pp. 97–106.
56. Hong WK: Induction chemotherapy of advanced previously untreated squamous cell head and neck cancer with cisplatin and bleomycin. In Prestayko AW, Crooke ST, Carter SK (eds): Cisplatin: Current Status and New Developments. New York, Academic Press, Inc, 1980, pp. 431–444.
57. Hong WK, Bromer R: Chemotherapy in head and neck cancer. N Engl J Med 308:75, 1983.
58. Hong WK, Schaefer S, Issell B, et al: A prospective randomized trial of methotrexate versus cisplatin in the treatment of recurrent squamous cell carcinoma of the head and neck. Cancer 52:206, 1983.
59. Houck JC (ed): Chalones. Amsterdam, North-Holland, 1976.
60. Huang AT, Cole TB, Fishburn R, et al: Adjuvant chemotherapy after surgery and radiation for stage III and IV head and neck cancer. Ann Surg 200:195, 1984.
61. Hussey DH, Abrams JP: Combined therapy in advanced head and neck cancer: Hydroxyurea and radiotherapy. Prog Clin Cancer 6:79, 1975.

62. Jacobs C: The role of cisplatin in the treatment of recurrent head and neck cancer. *In* Prestayko AW, Crooke ST, Carter SK (eds): Cisplatin—current status and new developments. New York, Academic Press, 1980, pp. 423–430.

63. Jacobs C, Meyers F, Hendrickson C, et al: A randomized phase III study of cisplatin with or without methotrexate for recurrent squamous cell carcinoma of the head and neck. Cancer 52:1563, 1983.

64. Jacobs C, Wolf GT, Makurch RW, et al: Adjuvant chemotherapy for head and neck squamous carcinomas. Proc Am Soc Clin Oncol 3:182, 1984.

65. Jacobs EM, Luce JK, Wood DA: Treatment of cancer with weekly intravenous 5-fluorouracil. Cancer 22:1233, 1968.

66. Jacobs JR, Kinzie J, Al-Sarraf M, et al: Combination of cis-platinum and 5-fluorouracil infusion before surgery in patients with resectable head and neck cancer. Proc Am Soc Clin Oncol 3:180, 1984.

67. Jacobs SA, Stoller RG, Chabner BA, et al: 7-Hydroxymethotrexate as a urinary metabolite in human subjects and rhesus monkeys receiving high-dose methotrexate. J Clin Invest 57:534, 1976.

68. Kaufman RJ, Brown PC, Schimke RT: Amplified dihydrofolate reductase genes in unstable methotrexate-resistant cells are associated with double minute chromosomes. Proc Natl Acad Sci USA 76:5669, 1979.

69. Kessel D, Hall TC, Roberts D, et al: Uptake as a determinant of methotrexate response in mouse leukemias. Science 150:752, 1965.

70. Kirkwood JM, Canellos GP, Ervin TJ, et al: Increased therapeutic index using moderate-dose methotrexate and leucovorin twice weekly versus weekly high-dose methotrexate—leucovorin in patients with advanced squamous cell carcinoma of the head and neck. Cancer 47:2414, 1981.

71. Kish JA, Weaver A, Jacobs J, et al: Cisplatin and 5-fluorouracil infusion in patients with recurrent and disseminated epidermoid cancer of the head and neck. Cancer 53:1819, 1984.

72. Knowlton AH, Percarpio B, Bobrow S, et al: Methotrexate and radiation therapy in the treatment of advanced head and neck tumors. Radiology 116:709, 1975.

73. Krakoff IH. Adriamycin studies in adult patients. Cancer Chemother Rep 6:253, 1975.

74. Leone LA, Albalba MM, Reye VB: Treatment of carcinoma of the head and neck with intravenous methotrexate. Cancer 21:828, 1968.

75. Levitt M, Mosher MB, DeConti RC, et al: Improved therapeutic index of methotrexate with leucovorin rescue. Cancer Res 33:1729, 1973.

76. Levy RL, Chiarillo S: Hyperpyrexia, allergic type response, and death occurring with low-dose bleomycin administration. Oncology 37:316, 1980.

77. Lippman AJ, Helson C, Helson L, et al: Clinical trials of cis-diamminedichloroplatinum. Cancer Chemother Rep 57:191, 1973.

78. Lustig, RA, DeMare PA, Kramer S: Adjuvant methotrexate in the radiotherapeutic management of advanced tumors of the head and neck. Cancer 37:2703, 1976.

79. Madias NE, Harrington JT: Platinum nephrotoxicity. Am J Med 65:307, 1978.

80. Moore GE, Bross DJ, Ausman R, et al: Effects of 5-fluorouracil in 389 patients with cancer. Cancer Chemother Rep 52:641, 1968.

81. Moore GE, Bross IDJ, Ausman R, et al: Effects of chlorambucil in 374 patients with advanced cancer. Cancer Chemother Rep 52:661, 1968.

82. Nelson L, Okonkwo E, Anton L, et al: Cis-platinum ototoxicity. Clin Toxicol 13:469, 1978.

83. Panettiere F, Lehane D, Gletcher WS, et al: Cis-platinum outpatient treatment for patients with squamous cell carcinomas. Med Pediatr Oncol 8:221, 1980.

84. Pennacchio JL, Hong WK, Shapshay S, et al: Combination of cis-platinum and bleomycin prior to surgery and/or radiotherapy compared with radiotherapy alone for the treatment of advanced squamous cell carcinoma of the head and neck. Cancer 50:2795, 1982.

85. Perry DJ, Carin SM, Weltz MD, et al: Phase II trial of mitoguazone in patients with advanced squamous cell carcinoma of the head and neck. Cancer Treat Rep 67:91, 1983.

86. Price LA, et al: Integration of safe initial combination chemotherapy (without cisplatin) with a high response rate and local therapy for untreated stage III and IV epidermoid cancer of the head and neck: 5-year survival data. Cancer Treat Rep 67:535, 1983.

87. Price LA, Hill BT. Safe and effective combination chemotherapy without cis-platinum for squamous cell carcinomas of the head and neck. Cancer Treat Rep 65:149, 1981.

88. Price LA, Hill BT, Calvert AH, et al: Kinetically based multiple drug treatment for advanced head and neck cancer. Br Med J 3:10, 1975.

89. Price LA, Hill BT, Calvert AH, et al: Improved results in combination chemotherapy of head and neck cancer using a kinetically based approach: A randomized study with and without Adriamycin. Oncology 35:26, 1978.

90. Posner MR, Ervin TJ, Weichselbalm RR, et al: Chemotherapy of advanced salivary gland neoplasms. Cancer 50:2261, 1982.

91. Randolph V, Wittes R: Weekly administration of cis-diamminedichloroplatinum (II) without hydration or osmotic diuresis. Eur J Cancer 14:753, 1978.

92. Raymond MG, Lyman GH: Treatment of unresectable/recurrent epidermoid carcinoma of the head and neck with cisplatin plus 5-fluorouracil infusion. Proceedings of the American Society of Clinical Oncology 4:133, 1985.

93. Rentschler R, Burgess MA, Byers R. Chemotherapy of malignant major salivary gland neoplasms. Cancer 40:619, 1977.

94. Ross WE: General principles for treatment of cancers in the head and neck: Chemotherapy. *In* Million RR, Cassisi N (eds). Management of Head and Neck Cancer. Philadelphia, J. B. Lippincott, 1984, pp. 97–104.

95. Sako K, Razack M, Kalnins I: Chemotherapy for advanced and recurrent squamous cell carcinoma of the head and neck with high- and low-dose cis-diamminedichloroplatinum. Am J Surg 136:529, 1978.

96. Salem PA, et al: Severe nephrotoxicity: A probable complication of cis-dichlorodiammineplatinum (II) and cephalothin-gentamicin therapy. Oncology 39:31, 1982.

97. Schramm VL, Srodes C, Myers EN: Cisplatin therapy for adenoid cystic carcinoma. Arch Otolaryngol 107:739, 1981.

98. Schuller DE, Wilson HE, Smith RE, et al: Preoperative reductive chemotherapy for locally advanced carcinoma of the oral cavity, oropharynx, and hypopharynx. Cancer 51:15, 1983.

99. Seifert P, Baker L, Reed ML, et al: Comparison of continuously infused 5-fluorouracil with bolus injection in treatment of patients with colorectal carcinoma. Cancer 36:123, 1975.

100. Shah PM, Shukla SN, Patel KM, et al: Effect of bleomycin-radiotherapy combination in management of head and neck squamous cell carcinoma. Cancer 48:1106, 1981.

101. Shanta U, Krishnamurthi S: Combined therapy of oral cancer bleomycin and radiation: A clinical trial. Clin Radiol 28:427, 1977.

102. Shanta U, Krishnamurthi S, Sharma M: Irradiation, bleomycin, and hyperbaric oxygen in the treatment of oral carcinoma. Acta Radiol Oncol 22:13, 1983.

103. Skibba JL, Hurley JD, Ravelo HV: Complete response of a metastatic adenoid cystic carcinoma of the parotid gland to chemotherapy. Cancer 47:2543, 1981.

104. Sluyser M, Van Nie R: Estrogen receptor content and hormone-responsive growth of mouse mammary tumors. Cancer Res 34:3253, 1974.

105. Smart CR, Rochlin DB, Nahum AM, et al: Clinical experience with vinblastine sulfate in squamous cell carcinoma and other malignancies. Cancer Chemother Rep 34:31, 1964.

106. Spaulding MB, Kahn A, De Los Santos R, et al: Adjuvant chemotherapy in advanced head and neck cancer: An update. Am J Surg 144:432, 1982.

107. Spiro RH, Huvos AG, Strong EW: Adenoid cystic carcinoma of salivary origin. Am J Surg 128:512, 1974.

108. Tannock IF, Sutherland DJ: Chemotherapy for adenocystic carcinoma. Cancer 46:452, 1980.

109. Tarpley JL, Chretien PB, Alexander JC, et al: High-dose methotrexate as a preoperative adjuvant in the treatment of epidermoid carcinoma of the head and neck: A feasibility study and clinical trial. Am J Surg 130:481, 1975.

110. Taylor SG, McGuire WP, Hauck WW, et al: A randomized comparison of high-dose infusion methotrexate versus standard-dose weekly therapy in head and neck squamous cancer. J Clin Oncol 2:1006, 1984.

111. Thongprasent S, Bosi GJ, Geller NL, et al: Phase II trial of mitoguazone in patients with advanced head and neck cancer. Cancer Treat Rep 68:1301, 1984.

112. Tropé C, Håkansson L, Dencker H: Heterogeneity of human adenocarcinomas of the colon and the stomach as regards sensitivity to cytostatic drugs. Neoplasma 22:423, 1975.

113. Umezawa H, Meada K, Takeuchi T, et al: New antibiotics, bleomycin A and B. J Antibiot 19:200, 1966.

114. Vermeer RJ, Pinedo HM: Partial remission of advanced adenoid cystic carcinoma obtained with adriamycin. Cancer 43:1604, 1979.

115. Vogl SE, Camacho FJ, Kaplan BH, et al: Phase II trial of vindesine in advanced squamous cell cancer of the head and neck. Cancer Treat Rep 68:559, 1984.

116. Vogl SE, Lerner H, Kaplan BH, et al: Failure of effective initial chemotherapy to modify the course of stage IV (M₀) squamous cancer of the head and neck. Cancer 50:840, 1982.

117. Vogler WR, Jacobs J, Moffitt S, et al: Methotrexate therapy with or without citrovorum factor in carcinoma of the head, neck, breast, and colon. Cancer Clin Trials 2:227, 1979.

118. Watkins E, Sullivan RD. Cancer chemotherapy by prolonged arterial infusion. Surg Gynecol Obstet 118:3, 1964.

119. Weaver A, Fleming S, Ensley J, et al: Superior clinical response and survival rates with initial bolus of cisplatin and 120-hour infusion of 5-fluorouracil before definitive therapy for locally advanced head and neck cancer. Am J Surg 148:525, 1984.

120. Weaver A, Loh John JK, Vandenberg H, et al: Combined modality therapy for advanced head and neck cancer. Am J Surg 140:549, 1980.

121. Weiss HD, Walker MD, Wiernik PH: Neurotoxicity of commonly used antineoplastic agents. N Engl J Med 291:127, 1974.

122. Werkheiser WC: The biochemical, cellular and pharmacological action and effects of the folic acid antagonists. Cancer Res 23:1277, 1963.

123. Wheeler RH, Natale RB, Roshon SG, et al: A phase I–II trial of cisplatin and dichloromethotrexate in squamous cell cancer of the head and neck. J Clin Oncol 2:831, 1984.

123a. Williams SD, Einhorn LH, Velez-Garcia E, et al: Chemotherapy of head and neck cancer: Comparison of cisplatin + vinblastine + bleomycin (PVB) versus methotrexate (MTX). Proc Am Soc Clin Oncol 1:202, 1982.

124. Wittes RE, Cvitkovic E, Shah J, et al: cis-Dichlorodiammineplatinum in the treatment of epidermoid carcinoma of the head and neck. Cancer Treat Rep 61:359, 1977.

125. Woods RL, Fox RM, Tattershall MHW: Methotrexate treatment of advanced head and neck cancers: A dose-response evaluation. Cancer Treat Rep 65:155, 1981.

126. Yagoda A, Mukherji B: Bleomycin, an antitumor antibiotic clinical experience in 274 patients. Ann Intern Med 77:861, 1972.

127. Zwelling LA, Kohn KW: Mechanism of action of cis-dichlorodiammineplatinum (II). Cancer Treat Rep 63:1439, 1979.

CHAPTER 73

Head and Neck Surgery in the Aged Patient

Charles F. Koopmann, Jr., M.D., F.A.C.S.

This chapter will be devoted to special considerations involved in head and neck surgery in the elderly. This portion of our population is the most rapidly increasing group in our society. Prior to 1960, elective surgery was avoided in the elderly because the mortality rates were two to five times those of the population as a whole.[4] However, mortality rates for emergency procedures have decreased significantly from 29 per cent in 1960 to 9 per cent in 1972 and to 2.5 per cent for elective procedures.[9] Unfortunately, age alone continues to be used by many referring physicians (as well as many surgeons) in explaining their failure to recommend surgical curative measures to extirpate neoplasms in the head and neck.

Prior to specific details as to the preoperative evaluation, the specific wound healing and metabolic considerations, and brief discussions of site of lesions, it would be advisable to discuss the surgical risks in the elderly in general terms. Risk factors that increase mortality include (1) pre-existing heart disease (mortality rates up to 17 per cent, depending upon type of surgery), (2) diabetes mellitus (mortality rates up to 26 per cent), and (3) dementia (mortality rates to 45 per cent).[19] However, if the American Society of Anesthesiologists Physical Status Scale (Table 73–1) is used to classify the patients, one can more accurately predict the risks of perioperative death. In a study of 500 patients older than 80 years of age, the overall mortality rate within one postoperative month was 6.2 per cent. Less than 1 per cent of class 2 patients died, 4 per cent of class 3 died, and 25 per cent of class 4 died.[5] In the latter high-risk group, Mohr recommends invasive measures (arterial blood

gas measurements and right-sided heart catheterization to evaluate pulmonary wedge pressures and pulmonary resistance) to subcategorize these individuals into those with reversible problems (mortality 8.5 per cent) and those with irreversible parameters (perioperative mortality rate approaching 100 per cent).[17] Such individual risk estimation is much more realistic than using age as the main criterion when making a decision concerning major head and neck surgery.

First, we will explore specific factors that impact upon operative or perioperative mortality in this elderly group. In general, several authors now state that age alone (up to 90 or 95 years) is not a major factor.[5, 16, 18, 26] Most data reveal that any reduction in survival is secondary to intolerance to cardiac or respiratory complications or to inappropriate therapeutic endeavors. Mithoefer and Mithoefer[16] found that although 46 per cent of their 240 patients over 69 years of age had evidence of cardiac disease, only a history of angina pectoris was of significant *preoperative* prognostic importance. Postoperative atelectasis and pneumonia were also of importance in their mortality data. This coincides with the findings of Wilder and Fishbein,[29] who found that respiratory complications accounted for the majority of cases of postoperative morbidity and death.

Steen and associates reviewed the reinfarction rate after anesthesia and surgery in 587 patients at the Mayo Clinic.[25] They found an overall 6.1 per cent reinfarction rate, with the highest incidence (27 per cent) occurring within the first 3 months after initial infarction. The reinfarction rate drops to 11 per cent if surgery occurs between 3 and 6 months after the first episode and stabilizes to 4 to 5 per cent if the interval is 6 months or greater. Risk factors that are associated with an increase in reinfarction rates include preoperative hypertension, intraoperative hypertension, and thoracic (noncardiac) and upper abdominal procedures lasting longer than 3 hours. However, other authors feel that intraoperative time does not correlate with increased incidence of myocardial infarction.[5] In this group, there were no infarctions in 73 patients who underwent procedures lasting longer than 5.5 hours. These patients were monitored with intra-arterial blood pressure and acid-base monitors and titrated with intravenous vasodilators such as nitroglycerin if EKG data suggested myocardial ischemia. Death from pulmonary embolism may be reduced by preoperative low-dose heparin and rapid postoperative mobilization.[5]

TABLE 73–1. American Society of Anesthesiologists Physical Status Scale

Class 1: A normally healthy person

Class 2: A patient with mild systemic disease

Class 3: A patient with severe systemic disease that is not incapacitating

Class 4: A patient with incapacitating systemic disease that is a constant threat to life

Class 5: A moribund patient who is not expected to survive 24 hours with or without operation

ANESTHESIA

The elderly patient requiring head and neck surgery presents specific problems in regard to wound healing, preoperative assessments, intraoperative anesthesia considerations, and aggressive postoperative management. The head and neck surgeon deals with a high percentage of elderly patients. In the last 20 years, the perioperative death rate has declined to less than 6 per cent in patients over 80 years of age. Consequently, although age is no longer a contraindication to general anesthesia, the elderly do present certain problems that must be evaluated prior to major surgery.

The most important aspect of the preoperative evaluation is the history, especially as it relates to exercise tolerance. When obtaining the pertinent details of exercise habits, the surgeon must bear in mind possible limiting factors, such as joint disabilities or visual impairment, that may reduce the individual's exercise capability despite an adequate cardiopulmonary reserve. A history of previous renal or hepatic disease may be of extreme importance, not only in selection of a general anesthetic agent but also in the type and amounts of pain medication, sedation, and antibiotics. Chronic diuretic usage (especially the thiazides) may result in a severe potassium depletion that may take days to correct. Poor sensory input (visual or auditory) may lead to difficulties during the induction or recovery phases unless the patient has been well instructed preoperatively. The status of the mandible, dentition, temporomandibular joint function, and neck flexibility is important for intubation and postoperative airway management. Examination of the chest may reveal expiratory wheezes, which are very suggestive of chronic obstructive pulmonary disease. Such patients should be given bronchodilators preoperatively.

Laboratory studies basically should be individualized. Certainly, the parameters of importance include a complete blood count, urinalysis, serum electrolytes, serum blood urea nitrogen (BUN) and creatinine, and liver function studies as well as an electrocardiogram (EKG) and chest radiograph. Pulmonary evaluation with bedside spirometry is also recommended. Other studies (such as arterial blood gases, creatinine clearance) are obtained on an individual basis.

Certain physiologic parameters are altered in the elderly, thus affecting the anesthetic management. Cardiac alterations may include hypokinesia of the left ventricle due to previous myocardial infarctions, hypertension, and generalized arteriosclerosis. The respiratory changes include a reduction in expiratory flow rate, vital capacity, total lung capacity, forced expiratory volume (FEV), and maximal breathing capacity. The ventilation-perfusion ratio decreases owing to shunting. This leads to a reduction in the PaO_2, resulting in a lower tolerance for hypoxia during induction or recovery. Reduced cough reflexes also lead to an increased risk of atelectasis and pneumonitis.

Renal changes include a reduced glomerular filtration rate due to age-related loss of functioning nephrons. This may markedly alter the metabolism of anesthetic agents, antibiotics, and sedatives. Such effects are compounded by the fact that the central nervous system in the elderly is more sensitive to hypnotic and sedative drugs not only in immediate action but also in the recovery phase. Not only may the drugs trigger a psychotic response but they may also initiate an acute attack of glaucoma. Agents such as the phenothiazines and droperidol (Innovar) should be avoided because of the risk of extrapyramidal side effects.

WOUND HEALING

Wound healing may be significantly affected by the aging process. The rate of cellular multiplication of fibroblasts varies inversely with the age of the donor's plasma, as does the index of cicatrization.[3] Others have observed that reduced healing in the elderly is secondary to increased autocatalysis and an increased inhibitory substance in the wound.[10]

The cellular functional capacity also diminishes with age, as evidenced by a decrease in fibroblasts, collagen, and polysaccharide synthesis. The components of the connective tissue substances change in regard to stability, amount, and relative proportions. Collagenous factors increase in both maturation and polymerization with age. Young subjects form granulation tissue more rapidly. Their wounds heal more quickly with less scarring owing to more rapid collagen turnover with decreasing age.

In evaluating the elderly patient preoperatively, there are many physiologic parameters that should be considered. Unless there are pre-existing disorders, the arterial pH and the blood or plasma volumes per kilogram of body weight do not vary with age. Reductions in plasma volume are associated with disease, and not age alone.

The cardiovascular, renal, metabolic, endocrine, and pulmonary systems do undergo physiologic changes as they age. There is evidence that the capacity of the adrenal cortex to produce adrenocortical hormones is not lessened with age. Instead, there appears to be a decrease in the ratio of 17-ketosteroids to 17-hydroxysteroids (a proportional increase in catabolic steroids in the aged), possibly causing tissue loss. If the adrenal cortex of the average geriatric patient is stimulated *maximally*, it can respond appropriately, but submaximal stimulation will yield a diminished response.[24] Likewise, the thyroid gland's ability to respond to maximal physiologic stimulus is minimally altered with aging (based upon protein-bound iodine, 24-hour ^{131}I uptake, and basal metabolism measurements following a maximal stimulating dose of thyrotropic hormone).[1]

Gregerman and Solomon found that the thyroid function in elderly patients who were subjected to the stress of acute infections responded appropriately in production of thyroxine and tri-iodothyronine. Thus, any decrease in thyroxine in the aged is felt to be due to some change in peripheral function, not in the production of the hormone.[8]

Pulmonary function may change in the geriatric population despite a lack of gross clinical symptoms. In the pulmonary parenchyma, as age increases, there appears to be an increase in the pressure gradient between the alveoli and blood secondary to a disparity in the adjustment of circulatory perfusion to alveolar ventilation. Other factors are decreases in total lung capacity, vital capacity, maximal breathing capacity, thoracic compliance, and muscle strength and increases in residual pulmonary volumes. The combination of these mechanical and physiologic processes can yield significantly reduced pulmonary functional capacity.

Renal function gradually diminishes with age. The ability to concentrate urine (as measured by specific gravity) is impaired during fluid restriction. Conversely, during diuresis, the urea clearance will also decrease, as does renal blood flow (PAH clearance) and the glomerular filtration rate (probably secondary to an increase in renal vasoconstriction).[21] These changes are magnified by anesthesia and surgery but are reversible unless there is a major disruption in the renal blood flow during abdominal or vascular surgery. Finally, there is evidence of a diminution in the excretory and reabsorptive ability of the renal tubules with advancing age. Thus, in a time of crisis, the renal reserve mechanisms may be markedly impaired in the elderly.

The cardiovascular system manifests multiple changes secondary to aging. The cardiac output and cardiac index decline, and the peripheral vascular resistance increases, leading to a reduction in cellular perfusion and oxygen uptake. The hepatic portal, renal, and cerebral blood flow parameters decrease at a range of 1.9 per cent per year for renal blood flow to 0.3 per cent per year for hepatic portal flow.[13]

METABOLISM

Preoperative metabolic assessment and postoperative management of the geriatric patient require very precise clinical expertise. The surgeon should realize that there is a decline (in a linear fashion) of 0.9 to 1.5 per cent per year in the function of organ systems and functions such as basal metabolic rate, cardiac index, vital capacity, and glomerular filtration rate. The red blood cell volume and hematocrit decrease with age and debility, although the total blood volume may remain normal (or may become elevated in congestive heart failure). In hypoproteinemia or severe edema, the oxygen-carrying capacity of the blood may be markedly reduced. This situation should be corrected by diuresis or the administration of colloid or packed red blood cells, as necessary.

Fluid and electrolyte metabolism may be deranged by hypotonic, hypertonic, or isotonic expansion or contraction of fluids. Asymptomatic hypotonic contraction (hyponatremia) occurs in debilitation, chronic pulmonary disease, impaired renal function, or decreased cardiac output and usually becomes clinically evident only when the patient is severely stressed. Symptomatic hyponatremia may occur in the late stages of starvation or from dilutional factors (fluid overloading in surgery) and may lead to hyperkalemia and impaired cardiac contractility as well as a loss of digitalis effect in the patient.[14] Water intoxication should be considered in the postoperative period when the patient shows mental or neurologic aberrations and an increase in weight associated with an unexplained reduction in hematocrit, serum electrolytes, and plasma proteins. Other causes of hypotonic expansion are cirrhosis, congestive heart failure, and inappropriate secretion of antidiuretic hormone. Therapy consists of water restriction or administration of hypertonic saline if cerebral edema becomes evident. Hypertonic expansion occurs in excessive intake of tube feedings (or other hypertonic fluid)

with osmotic diuresis and should be preventable by careful monitoring of urine specific gravity and serum osmolality.

Hypotonic contraction of body fluid may occur in loss of gastrointestinal fluid secondary to nasogastric suctioning, vomiting, diarrhea, or prolonged thiazide diuretic intake. The risk of hypokalemia leading to digitalis intoxication and cardiac arrhythmias is increased in the elderly in the immediate postoperative period. Isotonic fluid contraction is very dangerous because there is reduction of both plasma volume and red blood cells. A patient with impaired cardiac or cerebral circulation is at great risk for catastrophic operative complications (myocardial or cerebral infarction) if the cardiac output cannot sufficiently compensate for the diminished oxygen-carrying ability of the red blood cells. Careful assessment of blood volume and red blood cell mass preoperatively is important in this patient population. Preoperative blood transfusions (given slowly over days to avoid circulatory overload) are occasionally warranted in the chronically depleted patient.

INFECTION

The age of the patient is very important in regard to infection. Senescence not only lowers host resistance but also reduces the ability to successfully conquer infection and sepsis. Host response may be good (only minor diminution in phagocytic, antibody, and complement activity), but the reduction in the vascular supply in the dermis and age-related lymphatic atrophy appear to be of primary importance. Other general factors such as diabetes mellitus, obesity, intraoperative hypotension requiring either transfusions or vasopressors, and increased length of surgical time all contribute to a significant increase in postoperative infections. The interstitial fluid shows a reduction in volume and an increase in certain connective tissue elements.

Each of the preceding factors contributes to a delay in the vascular phase of inflammation with a resultant increase in infection rate in the elderly. The first phase of response to inflammation (vascular phase) allows dilatation and increased permeability of capillaries so that phagocytes and antibodies may reach the affected site to initiate the body's response to an insult. A reduction in blood supply to the affected area (such as the use of epinepherine injected locally or a reduction in blood supply due to hypotension) leads to an increased infection rate.

Bacteriuria in the elderly may be silent and may remain unnoticed until the patient develops septic shock or renal failure during or after the surgical procedure. The most common organisms are *Escherichia coli, Klebsiella, Aerobacter aerogenes, Proteus mirabilis,* and *Pseudomonas aeruginosa.* Thus, the preoperative evaluation of the elderly patient, especially males with a history of prostatic obstruction, should include a clean catch, freshly voided urinalysis to look for leukocytes, erythrocytes, and casts. Appropriate preoperative antimicrobial therapy is recommended when significant bacteriuria is discovered.

The prophylactic administration of antibiotics may significantly reduce infections in head and neck surgery. However, to be effective, the antibiotic must be both effective against the particular organism and present in the host tissue before the infection occurs. Several types of antibiotics are excreted by the kidneys (penicillins, tetracyclines, aminoglycosides). Because the decrease in renal function in the elderly may range from 20 to 50 per cent, the serum creatinine level must be evaluated and drug dosages must be modified accordingly (especially the aminoglycosides gentamicin and kanamycin). These latter drugs are also nephrotoxic and may decrease the glomerular filtration rate. Thus, drugs such as digoxin and chlorpropamide must be given carefully during aminoglycoside therapy because they also are cleared by glomerular filtration. Antibiotics bound by serum albumin (benzylpenicillin, sulfonamides, nalidixic acid) must be given with care because they may affect oral anticoagulant and tolbutamide therapy and can cause bleeding and hypoglycemia (Table 73–2).

SURGICAL CONSIDERATIONS

Dermatologic Aspects

Certain dermatologic entities are of major interest to the head and neck surgeon. Seborrheic dermatitis may occur in up to 20 per cent of the geriatric population,

especially in a chronically debilitated person. Seborrheic dermatitis occurs in the scalp, nasolabial folds, glabellar areas, and postauricular regions. The areas are erythematous and have poor margins. Scalp involvement should be treated with special shampoos (Selsun, Sebulex, Neutrogena). Other areas can be managed with 1 per cent hydrocortisone cream.

Seborrheic keratoses (Fig. 73–1) are characteristically papular, distinct, flat lesions approximately 1 cm in diameter. They vary from a tan to dark brown color. Although these lesions usually require no treatment, they may be removed for cosmetic reasons by a variety of methods (cryosurgery, surgical paring, or chemical peeling with trichloracetic acid or phenol solution).

Actinic keratosis (Fig. 73–2) usually occurs as a scaling, gray or yellow papule that has well-demarcated edges. These lesions must be considered precancerous. Sharply demarcated lesions can be treated by cryotherapy or, if invasion is suspected, by surgical excision. Diffuse areas may be treated chemically with topical 5-fluorouracil.

Keratoacanthomas (Fig. 73–3) are skin lesions that closely resemble nodular squamous cell carcinoma. Keratoacanthomas grow rapidly and have a characteristic central depression that is filled with keratin. It is rec-

TABLE 73–2. Clinically Important Drug Interactions*

Primary Drugs	Interacting Drug(s)	Mechanism	Effect
Augmented drug effects			
1. Warfarin	Phenylbutazone	IM; DA	Hemorrhage
	Metronidazole	IM	
	Aspirin	OM	
2. Antidiabetic sulfonylureas (tolbutamide, chlorpropamide)	Sulfaphenazole	IM	Hypoglycemia
	Chloramphenicol	IM	
	Phenylbutazone	IM; DA; IE	
	Warfarin	IM	
3. Phenytoin	Phenylbutazone	IM	Nystagmus
	Chloramphenicol	IM	Cerebellar ataxia
	Isoniazid	IM	Sedation
4. Azathioprine	Allopurinol	IM	Bone marrow suppression
5. Methotrexate	Sulfisoxazole	DA	Bone marrow suppression
	Aspirin	IE	
6. Digoxin	Diuretics	OM	Digitalis intoxication
	Quinidine	OM	
7. Propranolol	Cimetidine	HBF	Bradycardia
8. Sedative-hypnotics	Ethanol	OM	Excessive sedation
Decreased drug effects			
1. Warfarin	Barbiturates	SM	Loss of anticoagulation control
	Rifampin	SM	
	Glutethimide	SM	
	Disopyramide	SM	
2. Prednisone	Barbiturates	SM	Decreased steroid effects
3. Steroidal orally administered contraceptives	Rifampin	SM	Loss of contraceptive effects
4. Quinidine	Barbiturates	SM	Decreased antiarrhythmic effect
	Rifampin		
5. Lincomycin	Kaolin-pectin	IA	Decreased drug bioavailability
Tetracycline	Antacids-iron	IA	
6. Tolbutamide	Thiazide diuretics	OM	Decreased hypoglycemic effects
Chlorpropamide	Corticosteroids	OM	

*From Bressler R: Otolaryngol Clin North Am 15:459, 1982.
Abbreviations: DA = Displacement from albumin binding; HBF = decreased hepatic blood flow; IA = inhibition of drug absorption; IE = inhibition of renal excretion; IM = inhibition of drug metabolism; OM = other mechanisms (pharmacodynamic effects of drugs on tissue responses); SM = stimulation of drug metabolism.

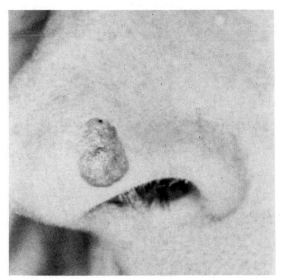

Figure 73–1. Seborrheic keratosis of the nasal ala.

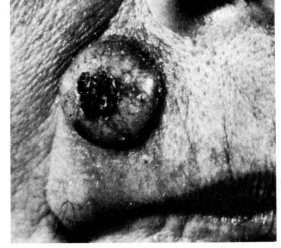

Figure 73–3. Keratoacanthoma of the upper lip.

ommended that these lesions be considered a type of squamous cell carcinoma and thus that they be surgically excised.

Lentigo maligna (Fig. 73–4) lesions are flat and dark brown, with dark sparkling pigment and sharp margins. These lesions should be considered in situ melanoma and should be managed by local excision.

Basal cell carcinoma is primarily a disease associated with the geriatric population. Although this disease will

be covered in great detail elsewhere (Chapter 49), the author feels that one topic of considerable controversy in this age group should be examined here: the management of recurrent basal cell carcinoma, which approximates 5 per cent of all cases; 85 per cent of this group involves the head and neck region, especially the nose (25 per cent), cheek (16 per cent), periorbital area (14 per cent), and ear (11 per cent).[12] It is estimated that there is involvement of margins in 5.5 to 12.5 per cent

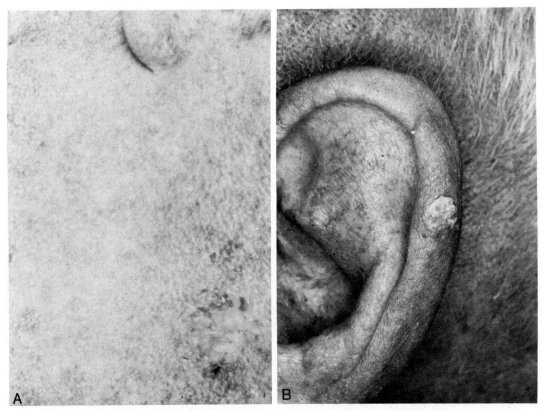

Figure 73–2. (*A*) Actinic keratosis of the face. (*B*) Actinic keratosis of the auricle.

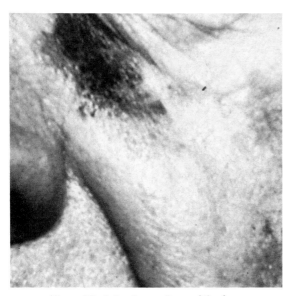

Figure 73–4. Lentigo maligna of the face.

of all cases, with the morphea type having the greatest risk of incomplete excision and the nodular and ulcerated types being most commonly completely excised.[2]

Pascal and co-workers reported a 12 per cent incidence of recurrence if the lesion is within one high-power field (400×) and a 33 per cent recurrence rate if the margin is definitely involved, with a mean recurrence time of 24 months after initial excision. In the evaluation of re-excision data, it appears that the potential for success approaches 100 per cent in several studies.[20, 28] Thus, it would seem appropriate to re-excise lesions after healing of the primary excision site in individuals with positive margins who have a life expectancy of 2 years or greater. However, if the tumor comes to within one high-power field (400×), it is acceptable to carefully observe the site in the elderly person, as the recurrence rate is only 12 per cent.

Thyroid Malignancies

Malignancies of the thyroid gland in the elderly are more likely to be undifferentiated. Even if the lesion is papillary (well differentiated) or follicular, the lesion is likely to be more aggressive in this age group. The geriatric patient may give a history of recent change in the size of a pre-existing goiter (50 per cent in follicular, 50 per cent in anaplastic, 33 per cent in papillary have this history).[22] This is a sign pointing to neoplastic change in this age group.

Diagnosis of a thyroid malignancy in this subset of our population is similar to that in younger individuals. The most common complaint is enlargement of a pre-existing goiter or a low neck mass. Later cervical adenopathy, hoarseness, dysphagia, or dyspnea may be present. Unfortunately, the latter three symptoms are frequently seen in the general geriatric population for a variety of non-neoplastic disorders and are therefore of marginal assistance unless vocal cord paralysis is present. The most useful diagnostic methods to evaluate this problem are cytologic aspiration and radioactive imaging. Suppressive therapy for asymptomatic thyroid

nodules is not recommended in the older person because of the risk of cardiovascular complications. Thus, if a goiter or nodule is enlarging, or if there is adjacent cervical adenopathy, with or without vocal cord paralysis, surgical exploration is warranted.

If the lesion is malignant, surgical resection is the initial treatment of choice.[23] In papillary and follicular carcinomas, one should perform a total or near-total thyroidectomy with modified radical neck dissection if there is clinically positive lymphatic involvement, followed by radioactive iodine ablation and thyroid hormone suppression. Medullary carcinoma should be treated with total or near-total thyroidectomy and resection of regional lymphatics followed by external radiation to the neck and mediastinum plus thyroid hormone replacement therapy. Anaplastic carcinoma should be resected, and postoperative radiation and thyroid hormone replacement therapy, plus possible chemotherapy, should be instituted. Survival for any of these cell types is decreased in the older individual owing to the more aggressive nature of the neoplasm.

Ablative Surgery

Carcinoma of the oral cavity occurs most commonly in the older age group. Johnson and associates[11] reported 27 cases of composite resection in patients over 65 years of age. The surgical complications, both major and minor, were equivalent to or less than those of a paired, younger group. There was an increase in associated medical complications, which included cardiac arrhythmias, pulmonary problems, and a fatality from gastrointestinal hemorrhage. However, the rehabilitation time to oral alimentation and to discharge is essentially the same in both groups.

Age has been used as a relative criterion for withholding conservation laryngeal surgery from persons over 65 years of age because of a fear that there will be an increased mortality rate due to aspiration and other pulmonary complications. In 1977, Tucker[27] reviewed 27 cases of conservation laryngeal surgery in this age group and found that his 11 per cent complication rate with no deaths compared favorably to total laryngectomy or radiation therapy alone. In this population 12 patients had vertical hemilaryngectomies with no fistula, skin breakdown, or delayed discharges. Fifteen persons underwent supraglottic laryngectomy (including one person 92 years of age) with two fistulas, no carotid blowouts, and one delayed discharge. This experience would compare favorably to the complication rate of 5 to 10 per cent in radiation therapy alone.[6] Gall and associates[7] reported no increased incidence in complications in elderly patients undergoing total laryngectomies as well as conservation procedures. McGuirt and associates[15] reported no increased incidence of surgical complications in the above-70 age group, although the medical complications (cerebrovascular accidents, cardiac problems) was 8 per cent greater in the older group.

In summary, it would appear that age alone is not a criterion for withholding curative surgery from a patient. Instead, the postponement of extirpative procedures is unwise. Consequently, the head and neck surgeon should evaluate each patient based upon pre-existing medical problems (are they reversible or controllable or are they irreversible or uncontrollable?), the pre-existing psychological and mental condition, the type of extirpative and reconstructive procedures required, the probable postoperative functional state, and the anesthetic and support facilities in the surgeon's institution. Only after all these factors are weighed should recommendations regarding major head and neck surgery be made.

REFERENCES

1. Baker SP, Gaffney GW, Shock NW, Landowne M: Physiological responses of five middle-aged and elderly men to repeated administration of thyroid stimulating hormone (thyrotropin, TSH). J Gerontol 14:37, 1959.
2. Burg G: Histographic surgery: Accuracy of visual assessment of margins of basal-cell epithelioma. J Dermatol Surg 1:21, 1972.
3. Carrel A, Ebeling AH: Age and multiplication of fibroblasts. J Exp Med 34:599, 1921.
4. Cole WH: Prediction of operative reserve in the elderly patient (editorial). Ann Surg 168:310, 1968.
5. Drokovic JL, Hedley-Whyte J: Prediction of outcome of surgery and anesthesia in patients over 80. JAMA 242:2301, 1979.
6. Ennuyer A, Bataini P: Laryngeal carcinomas. Laryngoscope 85:1467, 1975.
7. Gall AM, Sessions DG, Ogura JH: Complications following surgery for cancer of the larynx and hypopharynx. Cancer 39:624, 1977.
8. Gregerman RI, Solomon N: Acceleration of thyroxine and triiodothyronine turnover during bacterial pulmonary infections and fever: Implications for the functional state of the thyroid during stress and senescence. J Clin Endocrinol 27:93, 1967.
9. Griffiths JMT: Surgical policy in the over-seventies (surgery in the over-seventies). Gerontol Clin (Basel) 14:282, 1972.
10. Howes EL, Harvey SC: Current concepts of wound healing. Clin Plast Surg 4:173, 1977.
11. Johnson JT, Rabuzzi DD, Tucker HM: Composite resection in the elderly: A well-tolerated procedure. Laryngoscope 87:1509, 1977.
12. Koplin L, Zarem HA: Recurrent basal cell carcinoma—a review concerning the incidence, behavior, and management of recurrent basal cell carcinoma with emphasis on the incompletely excised lesion. Plast Reconstr Surg 65:656, 1980.
13. Landownes M, Stanley J: In Shock NW (ed): Aging, Some Social and Biological Aspects. Washington, D.C., American Association for the Advancement of Science, Pub. No. 65, 1961, pp. 177–180.
14. Lown B, Black H, Moore FD: Digitalis, electrolytes, and the surgical patient. Am J Cardiol 6:309, 1960.
15. McGuirt WF, Loevy S, McCabe BF, Krause CJ: The risks of major head and neck surgery in the aged population. Laryngoscope 87:1378, 1977.
16. Mithoefer J, Mithoefer JC: Studies of the aged. Arch Surg 69:58, 1964.
17. Mohr DN: Estimation of surgical risk factors in the elderly: A correlative review. J Am Geriatr Soc 31:99, 1983.
18. Morgan RF, Hirata RM, Jaques DA, Hoopes JE: Head and neck surgery in the aged. Am J Surg 144:449, 1982.
19. Palmberg S, Hirsjarvi E: Mortality in geriatric surgery: With special reference to the type of surgery, anesthesia, complicating diseases, and prophylaxis of thrombosis. Gerontology 25:103, 1979.
20. Pascal R, Hobby L, Lattes R, Crikelair G: Prognosis of "incompletely excised" vs "completely excised" basal cell carcinoma. Plast Reconstr Surg 41:328, 1968.
21. Shock NW: Age changes in renal function. In Lansing AI (ed): Cowdry's Problems of Aging. 3rd ed. Baltimore, Williams & Wilkins Co., 1952, pp. 415–446.
22. Simpson WJ: Anaplastic thyroid carcinoma: A new approach. Can J Surg 23:25, 1980.
23. Simpson WJ: Thyroid malignancy in the elderly. Geriatrics 37:119, 1982.
24. Solomon DH, Shock NW: Studies of adrenal cortical and anterior pituitary function in elderly men. J Gerontol 5:302, 1950.
25. Steen PA, Tinker JH, Tarhan S: Myocardial reinfarction after anesthesia and surgery. JAMA 239:2566, 1978.
26. Trott JA, David DA, Edwards RM: Experience with surgery for head and neck cancer in a geriatric population. Aust NZ J Surg 52:149, 1982.
27. Tucker HM: Conservation laryngeal surgery in the elderly patient. Laryngoscope 87:1995, 1977.
28. Waller G, Weidenbacher M: Recurrent basal cell carcinoma of the facial region—A clinico-pathological challenge. Arch Otorhinolaryngol 215:61, 1977.
29. Wilder RJ, Fishbein RH: Operative experience with patients over 80 years of age. Surg Gynecol Obstet 113:205, 1961.

CHAPTER 74

Statistics of Head and Neck Cancer

William E. Davis, M.D., M.S.P.H.

The significance of experimental data is usually measured by a statistical test. Statistical analysis of oncologic data assumes certain scientific procedures; if these procedures are followed, an organized body of scientific knowledge results that is statistically significant. Opinion concerning cancer therapy is then minimized, and preferably is replaced by scientifically proven principles of treatment. Is this the case?

A controlled clinical trial may be defined as a clinical experiment in which certain scientific procedures are followed. Controlled clinical trials in head and neck cancers are performed infrequently. Retrospective studies using historical control subjects for comparison are the rule. These reviews imply a reduction in validity of conclusions because they are lacking in some aspects of controlled scientific method. "Lack of control" (e.g., absence of randomization, presence of bias, no blinding) means that these studies are more susceptible to procedural error and thus erroneous conclusions. Statistical tests in these series will still show, or fail to show, significance because the statistics can still be generated, but are the conclusions valid?

Physicians have little or no opportunity to be trained in statistical theory, public health, or experimental design. Since these matters are not covered in their basic training programs, physicians are generally left with feelings of inadequacy in these areas. Ability to interpret these data as to validity or methodologic errors is minimal. Therefore, clinical trials designed by them tend to have poor structure, or "beg the question," by looking at only retrospective noncontrolled data. This chapter is written to facilitate understanding of cancer studies by a review of selected concepts in public health, statistics, experimental design, and survival data. Specific references will be made to head and neck cancer, but the chapter is designed to be general, with applications to other areas. Mathematics is minimized, and theory is emphasized.

SELECTED PUBLIC HEALTH CONSIDERATIONS

Cancer is the second leading cause of death in the United States. For the year 1985, it was predicted that 462,000 persons would die of cancer and approximately 15,000 (2.9 per cent) of these would die from head and neck cancer. Of the 910,000 individuals who develop cancer, approximately 50,000 would be afflicted with head and neck cancers. About 5.6 per cent of all new cancer cases are head and neck cancers. Public health issues in head and neck cancer begin with these statistics and then proceed to define the characteristics of the populations involved and the factors that seem to be causal or factors that give clues to causality. From these studies, recommendations on prevention, possible etiology, and needs of the health care system are expounded (Table 74–1).[25, 30]

Epidemiology is the branch of preventive medicine and public health that is concerned with the study of the dynamics and distribution of disease in human populations. Epidemiologists ask questions about disease rates in normal populations and identify populations at risk. Factors implicated as causal in disease states are studied, and if a single cause cannot be found, a "web of causation" is constructed. Clinicians, on the other hand, deal with diseased patients and are not generally concerned with normal populations. Methodologic research and reporting in epidemiology generally complement our clinical understanding of diseases by producing rates, risks, ratios, and similar statistics for a specific illness. The epidemiology of cancer is that of a chronic disease with a (presumed) prolonged latent period between initial causal exposure and onset. A relatively low incidence and high case fatality rate are also characteristic of cancer.

TABLE 74–1. Estimated New Cancer Cases in the United States in 1983, Selected Sites

Site	Number of Cases
Lip	27,100
Tongue	4600
Salivary gland and mouth	9800
Pharynx	7800
Esophagus	9000
Larynx	11,000
Lung	135,000
Brain	12,600
Thyroid	10,200
Leukemia	23,900
Lymphomas	40,300
Skin melanoma	17,400
Breast	114,000

Source: Data extracted from Silverberg E, et al: A review of American Cancer Society estimates of cancer cases and deaths. CA 33, 1983.

Epidemiologic relationships are manifested by ratios and rates such as prevalence, incidence, mortality ratio, and age-adjusted rates. The *incidence rate* is the number of new cases divided by the total number of subjects at risk in the population during a given period of time (usually per year). For example, in 1983 there were 11,000 new cases of carcinoma of the larynx in the United States. The U.S. population is roughly 230 million. The incidence rate per year is then 11,000/230,000,000, or 4.78 cases of larynx cancer per 100,000 persons. An *age-specific rate* can be obtained by taking the number of cases, say, between ages 40 and 50, and dividing this number by the total population in this age group. Incidence rates can thus be defined for a specific age group.

$$\text{Incidence rate} = \frac{\text{Number of new cases}}{\text{Total number at risk}} \text{ per unit of time}$$

In age adjustment or *age-adjusted incidence rates* age is removed as a factor (Table 74–2). By the direct method of age adjustment, the incidence of a particular disease is compared with a standard population and a comparison is made in terms of cases per 100,000 of the standard population. With this statistic, the number of larynx cancers in a typical United States city of 100,000 can be predicted to be approximately 4.5 cases per year.[11]

Table 74–2 gives age-adjusted rates for the incidence of different types of cancer in the United States. These rates are derived by comparing the population at risk to a "standard population," and they indicate the incidence per 100,000 population with age removed as a factor.

Prevalence is defined as the number of cases of a disease in a population at a specified time, divided by the number of persons in the population at that time. It is a "snapshot" at a given instant and includes all cases of the disease both treated and untreated. In cancer studies, this term has limited usefulness because it conceptually cannot handle "cures." Prevalence is frequently confused with incidence.

$$\text{Prevalence} = \frac{\text{Number of persons with a disease}}{\text{Total number in the group}}$$

A *mortality ratio* in epidemiologic terms is the number of persons dying of a particular cause divided by the

TABLE 74–3. Estimated United States Cancer Deaths for Selected Sites, 1983

Site	Deaths
Lip	175
Tongue	2000
Salivary gland	700
Mouth	2000
Esophagus	8500
Larynx	3700
Lung	117,000
Skin	1900
Melanoma	5200
Thyroid	1050
Leukemia	16,100
Lymphoma	20,800
Breast	37,500
Colon and rectum	57,000

Source: Data compiled from Silverberg E, et al: A review of American Cancer Society estimates of cancer cases and deaths. CA 33, 1983.

total number in the normal population group per unit of time (usually per year). This is not, then, the reciprocal of the cure rate. *Case fatality rate* is defined as the number of persons dying from a particular disease divided by the total number with the disease. The number of deaths in the United States for selected cancers is given in Table 74–3.

If a group of patients differ in some characteristic but all have the same disease, the effect attributed to that characteristic may be calculated. This calculated effect is called the *attributable risk*. As an example, let us suppose that a group of larynx cancer patients differ in their cigarette smoking history. Assume for discussion purposes that all other contaminating variables are evenly distributed between the two groups. For the first, say they smoke two packs of cigarettes per day and the incidence rate of larynx cancer is 10.2 cases per 100,000 age-adjusted population. The control group smokes less than five cigarettes per day, and the incidence is 1.2 cases per 100,000 population.* The difference between 10.2 and 1.2 or 9.0 cases per 100,000 is presumptively attributed to the effect of smoking two packs per day. This difference of 9.0 cases per 100,000 is termed the *attributable risk*.

---

*Less than five cigarettes per day for discussion purposes will be considered as equal to the amount consumed by nonsmokers.

TABLE 74–2. Annual Age-Adjusted Incidence Rates of Selected Cancers per 100,000 Population in the United States, 1973–1977

Site	Incidence Rate	Site	Incidence Rate
Lip	1.9/100,000	Major salivary gland	0.9/100,000
Tongue	2.0	Nasal cavity and ear	0.6
Floor of mouth	1.3	Larynx	4.6
Other mouth	1.8	Lung	46.7
Nasopharynx	0.6	Esophagus	3.7
Tonsil	1.1	Melanomas of skin	6.0
Hypopharynx	1.0	Skin cancer	0.6
Oropharynx	0.3	Breast	46.7
Lymphoma	12.0	Colon and rectum	48.5
Leukemia	9.8	Brain tumor	5.3
Thyroid	4.0		

Source: Data abstracted from Young JL, Percy CL, Asire AO (eds): SEER Program: Incidence and Mortality, 1973–77. National Cancer Institute Monograph 57. Washington D.C., U.S. Government Printing Office, 1981.

Attributable risk = Incidence rate of exposure group −
Incidence rate of unexposed group
(usually given in cases per 100,000)

Relative risk, on the other hand, is the ratio of the incidence of those who are exposed to a risk (such as smoking two packs per day) divided by the incidence of the same disease in those who do not possess the characteristics (for example, nonsmokers). In the preceding example, it would be 10.2 divided by 1.2, or 8.5. In other words, the relative risk of larynx cancer would be 8.5 times as great in the exposed group as in the unexposed group.

$$\text{Relative risk} = \frac{\text{Incidence rate of exposed group}}{\text{Incidence rate of unexposed group}}$$

Epidemiologic studies may be prospective, following cohorts over time (a cohort or incidence study), or retrospective, comparing the prevalence of a disease (case-control studies). All types of variables such as sex, socioeconomic status, occupation, smoking history, environmental exposure, and racial factors may be examined. The more factors examined, the greater the chance of finding a significant factor in the web of causation. By increasing the number of variables to a large number, often we do not derive more benefits, but sometimes we introduce the possibility that by chance alone a spurious significant factor may be found. An observed relationship between study variables may indeed appear to exist, when in fact it is spurious and due to unmeasured variables, correlated variables, poor study design, or random error. This spurious relationship is an example of what epidemiologists term the *ecologic fallacy*, that is, the association of variables where no association exists.[11, 21, 22] Ecologic fallacies may not be identifiable per se or preventable even with the best of techniques.

Prospective studies begin with a defined normal population and are used to observe the incidence of disease in this representative population. Numerous factors are catalogued, and at a later time (usually 10 to 20 years) the data are analyzed. The best known *cohort* (prospective) study is the coronary risk factor study from Framingham, Massachusetts.[9] A representative population was followed with numerous variables observed and analyzed in relation to the eventual development of heart disease. Valid estimates of disease incidence referable to the population selected are achieved in this type of study. Prospective epidemiologic studies have the disadvantages of being prolonged and costly, and they are also concerned with diseases of relatively high incidence in order to be cost-effective. Because head and neck cancer is relatively rare, in contrast to conditions such as heart disease, hypertension, and stroke, large samples are needed to determine incidence and risks by this method. In Table 74–4 a typical array of prospective epidemiologic data is shown. These data

TABLE 74–4. Typical Array of Epidemiologic Data

	Exposure*	No Exposure
Disease	A	B
No disease	C	D

*A, B, C, D = Number of patients in each cell.

TABLE 74–5. The Retrospective Case-Control Study

	Cases*	Control Group
Variable present	A	B
Variable absent	C	D

*A, B, C, D = Number of patients in each cell.

Note: Relative odds ratio = $\frac{AD}{BC}$.

may be analyzed by the chi square test or other statistical methods.

Retrospective studies look back over populations and usually compare those who have a disease with a similar or matched (for age, sex, occupation) control group. This is the classic *case-control*, or *prevalence, study*. Retrospective case-control studies are usually only as valid as the selection of the control group. The study must reflect the target population, for a skewed sample will result in inappropriate conclusions. An estimate of incidence and prevalence can be made under certain constraints and assumptions. A measure of relative risk in these studies is also possible and is referred to as the *relative odds ratio*. In Table 74–5, the odds ratio is a cross product of AD/BC, and under certain conditions is a close approximation of relative risk. Attributable risk may also be estimated from this 2 by 2 data array.[23, 29]

STATISTICAL CONSIDERATIONS

Because physicians do not generally have the opportunity to study statistics, they are often "handcuffed" by statistical terminology. This section concentrates on statistical concepts and will explain some of the more common statistical measures.

Statistical consultations should not be sought "after the fact," but rather in the early phases of controlled prospective clinical trials. Infrequent early statistical consultation is problematic and contributes to the small number of planned controlled clinical trials. Late consultation is symptomatic of ignorance of the statistician's function. When called upon after the fact, the statistician looks at retrospective uncontrolled data and offers criticism of the experimental design. Design errors may then be apparent that concede little scientific information. Certainly, this is not the best way to study patients in general and cancer patients in particular. Because the controlled clinical trial is poorly understood, the most common clinical study of head and neck cancer is descriptive, in which only retrospective data are reviewed. Questions are not answered.

Statistics might be defined as the mathematical science dealing with decision making in the face of uncertainty. A *statistic* is a number that represents a set of data. These data may be other numbers, classes (better, worse, unchanged), or ranks (1, 2, 3). Statistically, there is interest in whether an *association* exists between one factor and another; these factors are usually called *variables*. Usually, a question is posed as to whether one group or population is different from another because of some variable. In head and neck cancer, the variable may be a type of treatment, historical characteristics, laboratory values, and so on.

In statistical jargon, if an association between two variables exists, the variables are said to be *dependent*;

that is, in some mathematical way they are related. If there is no association, this indicates variables that are *independent*. If knowing the value of one variable makes no difference in predicting the value of the second variable, the variables are not statistically associated (statistically independent). Statistical association or dependence does not signify a cause-and-effect relationship; it is only a statement of mathematical probability.

p Values

The strength of association between variables is often quantified in relative statistical terms. Such terms as *p-values*, correlation coefficients, and confidence limits give an idea of the degree or certainty of association between variables. The *p* value may be defined as the probability that a statistic is in error. In medical and other scientific literature, by convention, we accept a 5 per cent risk (1 chance in 20 or $p < 0.05$) that a statistic may occur by chance or be in error. That is, we accept a 0.05 error that the value for a statistic would occur by chance less than 1 in 20 times.[17] Any level greater than 0.05 is not considered to be sufficiently rare to be statistically significant.

Figure 74–1 shows the "bell-shaped" curve of the Gaussian distribution. This is the "normal" distribution. The entire population (100 per cent) resides under the curve, and by study of a normal curve, in terms of how far from the center a value is, statements can be made concerning the probability of attaining the specific value. The "Z scale" is used to identify the specific location on the curve. The Z scale pertains to the normal distribution, but is translated into the values of the population or variable under study. This translation will not be discussed.

The *mean* (μ_0) is in the center of the normal distribution. This is the *average* value of the variable (or population) we are examining. A standard deviation represents a fixed distance on the Z scale from the mean. Roughly two standard deviations (SD) to the right of μ_0 is a point on the measurement scale shown as point Z_α ($Z_\alpha = 2.0$ SD). The darkened area (called α to the right

of Z_α represents roughly 2.5 per cent (0.025) of the population we are studying. This is one half of the 5 per cent error we might accept. The area that is two standard deviations to the left of μ_0 represents the other 2.5 per cent (0.025). Thus, 95 per cent of the population resides between -2 and $+2$ SD. At a point $+1.65$ standard deviations to the right of the mean only 5 per cent (0.05) of the population will have a larger value. Conversely at -1.65 SD only 5 per cent of the population has a smaller value.

In a normal distribution with acceptance level at 0.05, we will accept an error of 5 per cent in the experiment to hopefully make the right decision 95 per cent of the time. The decision process may be constructed as we have shown here ("two-tail"), with the *p* value split equally at both ends of the distribution, or we may select only one side ("one-tail"). In this event, we would specify that all 5 per cent of our error would be on the right side or left side of the curve. Suppose, for example, we were interested in an upper (one-tail) significance level; then, only the numbers larger than 1.65 standard deviations to the right of the μ_0 would matter. This area of significance is specified before the statistical test is begun.

An error in decision making might occur when Z_α is exceeded, because in fact the values are in the α region of the same population. These errors are called *type I statistical errors* and occur because of accepting a 5 per cent random error in the expected results.

To be meaningful, a *p* value must be identified by the statistical test used (such as t-test, F Dist, Wilcoxson); otherwise, it is uninterpretable. Statistical tests all have certain assumptions that, if not fulfilled accurately, render the *p* value derived from these tests meaningless.[15, 27]

Beta Values and Power

Beta Values and Statistical Power. The second type of statistical error is the *type II error*. Beta (β) is the probability of a type II error. This error occurs when sample size is insufficient and is manifested in an erroneous conclusion, such as: "There is no difference in treatment A when compared to placebo treatment," when in fact there is a difference. If the question of sufficient sample size is not addressed in planning a clinical trial, this error can be easily introduced. Suppose the normal distributions in which H_0 is the survival distribution of a placebo treated group and H_1 is the survival distribution of an active treatment group (Fig. 74–2).

From our previous discussion, Z_α is the point at which to expect that only one in 20 times ($p < 0.05$) a result will occur that is more extreme. Any value greater than Z_α would be accepted as sufficiently rare as to be considered probably in another distribution (in this case H_1). The shaded area β represents an overlap of the distributions H_0 and H_1. In statistical thought, μ_0 and μ_1 can be considered to be the true population means of H_0 and H_1. On any given trial, however, the mean of these populations will vary. The mean of any given trial of H_0 (the population with mean μ_0) will give a value $\bar{x}_0$. Suppose that $\bar{x}_0$ equals the average survival in months of a sample of untreated patients with mucous membrane melanoma and $\bar{x}_1$ equals the average survival in

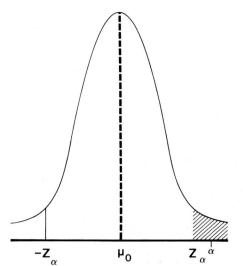

Figure 74–1. "Bell-shaped" (normal) curve of the Gaussian distribution.

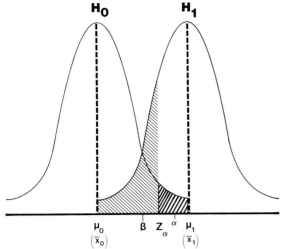

Figure 74–2. Survival distributions in placebo (H_0) and active treatment (H_1) groups.

$(\overline{x}_0)$ & $(\overline{x}_1)$ **are the random values you might get on any trial with a specific sample of population H_0 and H_1**

months of a sample of patients treated with chemotherapy protocol A (the mean of treatment A is $\overline{x}_1$). Let treatment A be population H_1 (with mean μ_1). Because of random variation in numbers, the possibility exists that on any given clinical trial of treatment A, a value to the left of Z_α might occur. This statistic (occurring to the left of Z_α) would lead to acceptance of the statement: "No difference exists between treatment A and placebo." The area under the curve represented by β is the probability of making this type II error.

Type II statistical errors can be eliminated by increasing sample size. It is important to remember that some studies are doomed to failure from the beginning because of this error. If the differences in μ_0 and μ_1 are not great, then the probability of a type II error is enhanced. This is a common problem in cancer studies, and in other clinical studies such as Meniere's.[10, 27] *Statistical power* is defined as the probability of not making a type II error and is mathematically equal to 1 − β. It can be predicted based on an expected difference and given sample size.[20]

In the context of the previous example of placebo versus treatment A, the concept of the null hypothesis and alternative hypothesis was introduced but not explained. A null hypothesis is signified here by H_0, and is the statement we wish to disprove in the preceding example. The alternative hypothesis is represented by the distribution of H_1. We might state that $\mu_0 = \mu_1$. As an alternative, we might hope to find that $\mu_0 < \mu_1$, or that treatment A is superior to placebo. To test the hypotheses, we would decide on our level of significance, say $p < 0.025$ or two standard deviations to the right of μ_0 and apply the statistical test. Any value more extreme than this value would be a cause to reject H_0 (that $\mu_0 = \mu_1$). Our conclusion would be that to equate placebo treatment and treatment A would be in error with a 95 per cent degree of certainty.

Regression Models and Multiple p Values. Another commonly used statistical procedure is the regression model. A dependent variable and an independent variable are identified. Suppose there is interest in two

variables, such as pack-years of cigarettes smoked and age of development of cancer of the larynx. These data could be graphed. The points of this scatter diagram could be summarized by a single regression line derived mathematically (Fig. 74–3). Regression lines summarize data points so that for any value of x you could predict a value of y. Linear regression models convey a measure of confidence for the proximity of points to the line with the "r" value. The "r" value (*correlation coefficient*) is a measure of how close data points conform to a regression line which mathematically best summarizes the data.* An r value of +1 or −1 means all points are on the line, and an r value of 0 means that there is essentially no relationship between the variables and that only random points are on the line. Large correlation coefficients imply a strong statistical relationship and vice versa. The correlation coefficient (r) is derived from sophisticated mathematical equations, but is deceptive in that the important value is really r^2. The *coefficient of determination* (r^2) is the amount of variation explained in one variable by knowing the other variable.

---

*Simple linear regression constructs a straight line that has a y intercept (β_0) and slope (β_1) and compares an independent variable x with a dependent variable y. The resulting equation is $y = \beta_0 + \beta_1 x$.

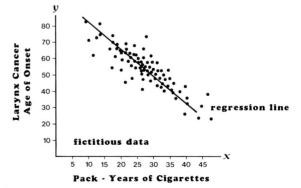

Figure 74–3. Regression model of cigarette smoking and age at development of laryngeal cancer.

They are actually square roots of the amount of variation explained by knowing one or many variables. (Space limits will not allow a discussion of r² and r.) Table 74–6 illustrates how deceptive r values can be in regard to percentage of variation explained.

As a general rule, the r value should be squared and then considered as the amount of variation that is explained by the variables under consideration. Then a decision of how significant the data array is can be made. In public health cancer studies, *multivariable linear regression* models are used to explain the change in one dependent variable while many independent variables that perhaps influence the dependent variable are being examined.[24]

In a multiple linear regression models,* one dependent variable and many independent variables are studied. There will be a *p* value for each variable, and *p* values for variables that are looked at in combination or as interacting. A problem that often occurs when evaluating multiple *p* values is that if 20 *p* values are examined in the study, the probability that at least one of the *p* values becomes positive by random error is magnified. Based on a study of just 20 random independent variables, the chances are actually about 0.6 that more than one *p* value will be significant by random error alone. Logically, we expect only 1 in 20 to be positive, but this is not the case. Because randomness exists in measurement of *each* of these singular variables, the chances of a spurious level of significance being reached from random error grows as the number of variables increases. An application of this principle to our daily practice will lead us to expect at least one positive laboratory test out of 20 (as in multichannel chemistry profiles) and to expect at least one positive test on multiple intradermal allergy skin testing (this may even be higher because of nonindependence of the tests). One final note about regression lines is that projections made outside the actual limits of the data are perilous.

Statistical Data

Statistical data come in different forms. *Parametric data* are data that are normally processed. The parameters of mean standard deviation are well known. These are

---

*Multiple independent variables (x_1, x_2, x_3, etc.) are looked at in relation to one dependent variable. The mathematical model follows the equation $y_i = \beta_0 + \beta_1 + x_1 \beta_2 x_2 + \beta_3 x_3 + \ldots$.

TABLE 74–6. A Comparison of "r" Values

Correlation Coefficient	Coefficient of Determination* (r²)
1.0	1.0
0.9	0.81†
0.5	0.25
0.3	0.09
0.1	0.01

*Amount of variation in dependent variable explained by knowing the value of the independent variable(s). A coefficient of determination of +1 or −1 means that all points are on the regression line and there is perfect prediction of one variable if the other is known.

†This means that 81% of the variation is explained, and on the average the data will be off by 19% if the value of the independent variable(s) is known.

parameters of the normal distribution. Are there other ways to measure variables other than the normal distribution? Data can be measured on three scales, and only one of them is parametric. First is the *nominal scale* in which data are divided into classes (such as male, female, black, white) or results can be measured by gradations such as cured, free of disease, alive with recurrent disease. In chemotherapy, nominal data may be used such as CR (complete response) or PR (partial response). *Nominal scale data* are interpreted by statistical tests that are not based on the normal distribution. They are termed non-normal, or *nonparametric*, distributions or nonparametric statistics. Examples of these tests are the Wilcoxson test, binomical test, and chi square test.[7]

The *ordinal scale* is the second scale on which to measure and analyze data. Ordinal scale data means that the data are based on some ranking system. For example, suppose you study two randomly assigned treatment groups for stage III larynx cancer and assign a No. 1 to the first person who dies, a No. 2 to the second, and so on. After a small number of patients have expired, a test of the hypothesis might be possible as to which treatment is superior based on a nonparametric rank test using the time of death after treatment as the significant event. With nonparametric tests, statistical significance is possible using a much smaller sample size and usually after a shorter interval.

The *interval* or *ratio scale* is the third way data can be measured and analyzed statistically. It assumes a zero point and unit difference. Mean, standard deviation, and variance are the parameters used with this data, and parametric statistical tests are based on the normal (Gaussian) distribution.

Biologic versus Statistical Significance

It is important to reflect upon the concept of "biologic significance" in reference to "statistical significance." Statistical signficance means that the results would occur by chance less than one time in 20 ($p < 0.05$). For a statistically significant event to be "significant" (meaningful), it must be biologically significant. In other words, a difference in treatment groups *should* make a difference in the human beings under study. For example, a 93 per cent cure rate by radiation therapy for carcinoma of the mobile vocal cords, although being statistically better than a 91 per cent cure rate from surgical therapy for the same lesion, is not a biologically significant difference in cure rate. Patient selection and methodologic design could easily account for this variability. There may be a biologically superior result in quality of life in one versus the other, but in terms of cure rate they are equivalent.

Independent Observations and Random Sampling

Sampling error is a major problem in statistics and experimental design. For convenience this concept is included in the statistical section. In order for a sample to be valid in a statistical analysis, it must reflect the target population. For this reason, there may be difficulty in cancer studies if the "random sample" is derived from one group, such as one socioeconomic group or one ethnic group. Results obtained from skewed samples may be applicable only to that group alone and not to the entire target population. The best treatment then may differ from group to group, depending on factors such as age, sex, metabolic status, and socioeconomic status.[1]

Observations must be reliable and independent. A staging system that is not rigid in its placement of patients will lead to data that are "soft." One surgical group cannot stage patients differently than another group and then compare results. Bias must be eliminated from the observers, the patients, and the statistician. Elimination of bias is difficult.

In summary, reaching statistical significance does not guarantee truth; it is only a statement of probability. Invalid assumptions and poor structure can still produce data that, if put to a statistical analysis, will result in a p value. Because of this, the physician's desire to know the truth is often the limiting factor in rejecting some conclusions. Some questions must be asked. Does this study prove anything of biologic significance? Does this study involve a non-issue? Will this conclusion be beneficial? Questions such as these will put the study and the p value in perspective.

SELECTED CONCEPTS IN EXPERIMENTAL DESIGN OF CANCER STUDIES[2, 4–6, 13, 14, 18, 28]

Theoretically, there should be no difference in the construction of clinical trials for cancer and clinical trials for other diseases (for example, rheumatoid arthritis, Meniere's disease). Are there differences? From a pragmatic approach, significant differences appear to exist:

1. Death is the end result of untreated cancer.
2. Control groups should have effective treatment offered to them.
3. Controlled trials in head and neck cancer often involve active agents that make certain aspects of controlling difficult. For example, suppose we wanted to "blind" all our observers in order to eliminate bias. It is very difficult to "blind" observers with regard to type of surgical therapy or surgical therapy versus radiation therapy; however, blinding is easily achieved in chemotherapy trials.
4. Head and neck cancer is relatively rare.
5. Randomization problems exist because of patient and physician feelings and attitudes.

For these and other reasons to be elucidated, the purist should keep in mind that a utopia is not possible. Head and neck cancer patients are not test tubes.

The Diseased Group

In the investigation of any disease, the selection of a group for study involves the assumption that what is said of this sample will be applicable to the total population of those diseased. It is crucial that the group not be skewed to one extreme or the other (e.g., poor, early disease, late disease, ethnic heritage, age), but should be truly representative of the group under study. If the diseased group is skewed, comparison of results with previously studied groups requires clarification. Correct identification of the extent of disease is extremely important. Staging by the JCAH classification (Joint Commission on Accreditation of Hospitals), for example,

cannot be compared to a study staged by the UICC (International Union Against Cancer) because the qualities of the specific stages are not identical.

The Control Group

In randomized controlled clinical trials, enormous energy must be directed toward the control gorup. A purist would insist that a control group should be a nontreated group, that it would be randomly selected from those one is studying, and that a random allocation to treatment or control group would take place. Because of this method of assignment, treatment and control groups would be assumed to have all other contaminating variables equally distributed. The differences in results or responses would then be due to the active treatment agent under study.

Control groups in cancer trials are different. In general, a control group can mean placebo treatment or no treatment. Because the end result in untreated cancer is uniformly death, ethically, a cancer trial control group must be one that is treated by another active or accepted standard agent(s) if such therapy exists. It would be unethical to recommend a treatment thought to be less effective to patients. So, in nearly all clinical cancer trials, the patient must be asked to accept a randomization between the standard treatment and a treatment the physician thinks would (might) be better. Some patients are perhaps being asked to accept a less effective treatment. Randomization as a basic tenet in controlled clinical cancer trials becomes more difficult from both the patient's and physician's perspective. Patients who might be used in these trials decline or may be advised by others to seek treatment elsewhere where a "standard" or "new" therapy is offered exclusively. When a patient declines therapy and selects a different therapy, the process of randomization is stressed and the all-important sample size becomes diminished. Concurrent controls and randomization are the optimum, but this choice may not be pragmatic. The use of literature control groups has been the solution (in theory) of this dilemma.

The use of literature or *historical control groups* has thus found its way into cancer trials as a substitute for randomization into groups. The assumptions that must be valid for a literature control group to be comparable are that the groups (historical control group and current experimental treatment group) are similar in all variables except time, specific physician, institution, and those other variables that will not be important enough to cause an invalid comparison. The use of historical control groups lessens the time needed because fewer patients are needed. Cost is also reduced. Historical control groups allow smaller institutions to proceed with a study they could not do if two groups were randomized.

Historical control data must be well documented. Personal data such as sex, age, socioeconomic class, ethnic grouping, and stage must be clearly equivalent so that cure rates or control rates may be logically compared. With the advent of computer technology the use of historical control data should be more reliable.

Literature control groups are championed by some and criticized by others. The Mayo Clinic series of osteosarcoma clearly points out the difficulty of nonrandomized studies without control groups. Mayo Clinic patients with osteosarcoma were studied for 10 years, and increased survival was noted without significant change in treatment regimen. Even in a single institution, there was increased survival over time without a change in treatment. During that time frame, other institutions were claiming increased survival secondary to adjuvant chemotherapy. This example is a strong argument for the use of concurrent control groups.[26]

Another reason for not randomizing might be to determine dosage. (This routinely occurs in phase 1 chemotherapy protocols or when a new drug is initially being tested for effectiveness [phase 2 chemotherapy protocols].) Also, when a large difference in response between treatments is indicated by preliminary data, it seems unreasonable to randomize.

Sample Size

The concept of adequate sample size was discussed in relation to the beta error in the statistical section. Now, sample size will be discussed in relation to what is to be proved or disproved. Suppose a new treatment for carcinoma of the true vocal cord (stage 1) is to be compared with a historical control group of patients treated with radiation therapy. How many cases are needed in order to show a 5 per cent increase in cure rate if the recognized cure rate of stage I carcinoma of the larynx by radiation therapy is 87 per cent? Suppose the beta error is set at 5 per cent (power 95 per cent) and the alpha error at 1 per cent. To show this difference under these constraints, 7500 patients would be needed.

In order to begin a clinical trial, the number of patients needed to show a significant difference should be predetermined. Larger percentage differences in response require smaller numbers of patients. For example, in the preceding example a 10 per cent improvement would require only 2000 patients. Table 74–7 indicates the number of patients required for a 1 per cent level of significance (α) and a 95 per cent power ($1 - beta$). The number of patients given is the sum of a control and a treatment group. Under the alpha and beta constraints of the preceding, a 50 per cent increase in median improvement would require 110 patients in the control and experimental group or 220 total patients with stage I carcinoma of the larynx. By a decrease of α to 0.05 and β to 0.10, a significant decrease in number of required patients might be achieved without much loss of experimental significance (Table 74–7).

TABLE 74–7. Total Number of Patients Needed

Improvement %	Number of Patients[14, 19]
10	4000
20	1100
50	220
70	128
80	104

$\alpha = 0.01$, $\beta = 0.05$.
The formula to calculate the number of patients required is as follows:

$$n = \frac{(2.58 + 1.65)^2}{[1n(1 + \Delta)]^2}$$

where 2.58 = 9.95 level of significance and 1.65 = 0.95 level of significance.

Elimination of Bias

Bias is defined in mathematical terms as the difference between the estimated value and the true value of a statistic obtained by random sampling. From the definition, it is implicit that an error in measurement of any statistic is to be expected. In fact, the goal of randomized controlled clinical trials is to minimize this error. Bias error involves not only nonprejudicial or expected error but also those errors that might arise from conscious or subconscious patient factors, observer factors, or design factors. To some extent, everyone is biased. There is a way one prefers to do a neck dissection, a way one believes children should be educated, and a definite way one believes the government should be managed. Although a person can be expert in several areas and have logical arguments for decisions in these areas, the fact remains that, using the preceding examples, few are experts in primary education or expert in running the affairs of government. To some extent, then, biased or prejudiced views occur in regard to these issues. So it is that prejudice occurs in clinical trials. A scientist has predetermined expectations of what a study should show. Personal involvement in the study equates to a scientific and economic future written in the results of this study. So it is that there is physician bias, but there is also patient motivation for a significant result in these trials. A significant result for the patient means cure or doing well. Patients would prefer to be doing well, and this colors their interpretation.

Blinding is the process whereby bias is minimized. In head and neck trials this is not always possible. For chemotherapy protocols, it is easier; however, in comparison of surgical treatment or another surgical treatment or radiation treatment, blinding is impaired. The following discussion presents the perfect situation, but pragmatically that is not always attainable. Under ideal conditions, a patient would be selected for a study, would be informed of the selection, and would accept the study (informed consent). Randomization to one of several treatment groups would then occur. Under the best of circumstances, the patient is blinded and does not know his or her grouping (*primary blinding*).

Secondary blinding is the next level of blinding and occurs when the observers who analyze end points are unaware of the group to which the patient is allocated. For hard data analysis such as survival or months until recurrence, observers will not have a difficult problem in entering data. For nonparametric data (quality of life judgments), it is essential to have observer blinding. This will eliminate statements such as: "In my opinion people do better," or "I believe patients feel better on treatment A." Thus instead of "personal" knowledge, actual scientific knowledge will be derived.

Tertiary blinding indicates that the data analyst (statistician) is unaware of the particular treatments and thus looks only at arrays of data.

Follow-up should be specified in terms of how often each parameter is measured and how it is to be measured. Rules should be clear so that a definite schedule will lead to systematic review at designated times. Early termination of clinical trials may be indicated after an early analysis because one treatment is clearly superior or inferior. The natural history of the disease must be considered in a planned termination. Abnormally prolonged or shortened follow-up may be costly to the patient or the study.

SOME SURVIVAL AND RESPONSE CONCEPTS[1, 3, 8, 12, 16]

This section briefly discusses some concepts in survival and response data. Response data and survival data are analogous in that they both are concerned with when an event (death or failure) might occur. In survival data we are interested in death as the event, and in response data the events are the occurrence of a response and its magnitude. Response data do not imply cure, although in certain instances a complete response for 5 years may be a "5-year cure."

Chemotherapy Results

A *complete response* (CR) is defined as the disappearance of all clinical signs and symptoms attributable to the cancer for at least 1 month. As we might imagine, this type of response would be unusual in head and neck cancer because seldom are these solid tumors seen by the oncologist at a small size and the activity of his armamentarium is generally slight. *Partial response* (PR) indicates more than a 50 per cent reduction in the measured tumor mass, without a concomitant increase in size of any other tumor masses. *Progressive disease*, on the other hand, indicates more than a 50 per cent increase in tumor size or the appearance of new lesions after treatment. *Stable disease* after chemotherapy is defined as a decrease in tumor size short of a partial remission. A *relapse* would be defined as new tumor growth or new tumor masses after a complete or a partial response.

Frequently quoted measures of evaluation in chemotherapy protocols are the Karnofsky Performance Status[19] and the Eastern Cooperative Oncologic Group Performance Status. These evaluations are an attempt to quantify whether at the beginning of therapy a person possessed a certain "life-style" and to measure improvement or worsening. Tables 74–8 and 74–9 summarize these rankings.

"T" Year Survival Data

In the surgical world, the most commonly quoted survival parameter is the 5-year cure." Superficially, this

TABLE 74–9. Eastern Cooperative Oncology Group Performance Status

Performance Status	Description
0	Asymptomatic
1	Mild symptoms
2	In bed 50% of the time
3	In bed 50 to 99% of the time
4	In bed all day

concept is simple; however, several qualifications are necessary for the term to convey the appropriate information. Groups must be identified, definitions set forth, and calculations explained. Five-year cure rate is a misnomer. A person passing the magical 5-year mark means only that the person is a 5-year survivor. "Cure" implies a normal life span; cure means there is not one cancer cell remaining, and present knowledge and theory of immune surveillance make this a difficult word to use. Quoting 5-, 10-, or even 15-year statistics for success of therapy should, rather, be stated as *5-, 10-, or 15-year survival rates*, not cure rates.

Group delineation in survival data is extremely important. Criteria for inclusion or exclusion must be clear and concise to avoid misconceptions. A clear profile on the types of patients by age, stage, sex, or socioeconomic status is a basic requirement. In surgical studies, only those diagnosed, treated, and surviving a specific surgical modality or combination therapy would be admitted to the study group. Those who declined treatment or those whose disease was too advanced for treatment are not considered. Intraoperative and postoperative mortality rates would not be reported. After these qualifications are made, attention should be focused on the "survival rates."

Determinate Survival. What are determinate and actuarial survival? Physicians are expected to understand these rates and the methods used in computing them. Yet, the literature is a vacuum should one search for an explanation. Over the past 60 years very few sources can be identified for the nonstatistician to learn of these concepts. For this reason the two survival statistics will be contrasted.

The *determinate survival* method for arriving at 5-year survival is also known as the "direct method" or "ad hoc method." It was first proposed in 1935 by Martin and modified by MacDonald in 1948. Two basic groups are identified:

TABLE 74–8. Karnofsky Performance Status

	Status	Percentage	Description
I.	Able to work and carry on activity	100	Normal
		90	Minor symptoms only
		80	Normal activity with some effort
II.	Unable to work but can care for self at home	70	No assistance needed
		60	Requires occasional assistance
		50	Requires some assistance
III.	Needs institutional support	40	
		30	Disabled, death not imminent
		20	Very sick
		10	Moribund
		0	Dead

Source: abstracted from Karnofsky DA, Burchenal JH: Symposium of Microbiology, New York Academy of Medicine. New York, Columbia University Press, 1949, pp 191–205.

1. The *indeterminate group* includes those lost to follow-up, those dead of intercurrent disease, patients who refused treatment, patients treated by other methods, and patients who accepted treatment elsewhere. This total is then subtracted from the total to arrive at the determinate group.

2. Subjects in the *determinate group* represent the successful results and the treatment failures. Failures are defined as those who are living with recurrence, dead of disease, and lost to follow-up with disease. A 5-year survival rate by the determinate method is derived by the following relationship of the determinate group.

$$\text{Five-year survival rate} \atop \text{(determinate)} = \frac{\text{Number of failures}}{\text{Number in determinate group}}$$

In order to arrive at this figure, an assumption concerning the group lost to follow-up must be made. One must assume the survival rate of the untraced group is equal to that of the traced group. This assumption may or may not be true. As a general statement, if the number of those lost to follow-up is small, the variance is minimal and the assumption need not be questioned. Another problem of the determinate method is that analysis of the data is often delayed far beyond the "T" year period if tumors are encountered infrequently. It may require 10 years to get 100 patients in the determinate group who have been exposed to the risk of dying for 5 years after surgical therapy (assuming 20 new cases per year and none lost to follow-up). The actuarial survival does not suffer from this limitation. Another disadvantage of the determinate method is that it is possible to see increasing survival rates at 10 and 15 years if those with disease are lost to follow-up or the group dying of intercurrent disease becomes relatively larger. At 10 years, for example, only the successes are being followed and the denominator continually becomes smaller from death secondary to intercurrent disease.

Actuarial Survival. *Actuarial survival* was suggested by Berkson and Gage and seems to be more scientific, simpler, and quicker to compute. It will give approximately the same answer in a large series as the determinate method, but in a smaller series or series in which a significant number of cases might be lost to follow-up, the actuarial method is superior. Actuarial survival data also differ in that a survival curve is generated. Because data are analyzed at yearly intervals, the percentage of survival is shown graphically. This graphic representation of survival may be contrasted with the actuarial survival curve of a hypothetical control group using expected fatality rates for a mean age. In this way, the hazard function may be viewed graphically.

In the actuarial survival method, however, the fundamental difference is the use of *censored* patient data. Subject data that have not been exposed to the risk of death for 5 years is used. That is, in year No. 1, for example, we examine all the patients who have been exposed to the risk of failure, not just those in year group No. 1 who have completed 5 years of risk. Again, the analysis at 2 years includes all patients who have completed 2 years, and so on. This utilization of data is done on sound statistical ground that cannot be discussed here because of space limitations. Most cases

can be analyzed and studies completed in much less time than the determinate method might take. Statistically, actuarial survival data are said to be censored data because subjects who are at risk for failure later on in the study or who are lost to follow-up are analyzed early to arrive at statistics contributing to the 5-year survival rates. With the use of standard statistical procedures, standard errors, confidence limits, and probability theory, the results of actuarial survival rates are as good as, and frequently better than, determinate 5-year survival rates.

To better understand the methodologic differences in these two survival rates, suppose that we encounter 125 new stage III (T3, N1, M0) carcinomas of the larynx during the next 5 years and that all 125 patients were treated with preoperative chemotherapy, then by laryngectomy and neck dissection. Suppose that five patients were lost to follow-up and no one died of other causes (intercurrent disease). The data will be displayed by the determinate and actuarial survival methods. The determinate survival is shown in Table 74–10.

The actuarial analysis is shown in Table 74–11, in which column 1 represents the time interval from time of treatment to 1 year after diagnosis. Column 2 indicates the number of patients in the study at its inception, that is, all patients considered together who were exposed to the risk of dying up to 12 months. In this example, the number at risk at inception of our study is 125 patients. Similarly, the number of patients who were exposed to the risk of failure from period 12 months to 24 months is 79, and so on.

Column 3 indicates the deaths during the respective time periods. Column 4 shows when a patient or group of patients were lost to follow-up. In dealing with column 4, we do not accept the fact that all patients lost to follow-up were lost on a given day, say, the first day after the twelfth month or the last day of the twenty-fourth month. An average value is taken, meaning that

TABLE 74–10. Five-Year Determinate Survival of 125 Hypothetical Cases of Carcinoma of the Larynx*

Total number admitted	125
Indeterminate group	
Dead within 5 years of other disease	0
Lost to follow-up within 5 years	5
Treatment elsewhere	0
No treatment	0
Total in indeterminate group	5
Determinate group (125 − 5)	120
Failures	
Dead of disease	40
Alive with disease	10
Dead of other causes—cancer unknown	1
Lost to follow-up with cancer	2
Total number of failures	53
Successes (free of cancer and followed for 5 years) (120 − 53)	67
Net 5-year determinate survival (67 divided by 120)	55.7%

*All cases accepted treatment; no one died intraoperatively or postoperatively (hypothetical data). This study took 10 years to complete because the last group of patients had to be followed for 5 years.

TABLE 74–11. Actuarial Survival Method for the Same 125 Hypothetical Larynx Cancer Cases Followed Five Years

Years after Treatment	Number at Beginning of Interval	Died during Interval	Lost to Follow-up	With-drawn Alive*	Effective Number Exposed to Death	Propor-tion Dying	Propor-tion Surviving Interval	Cumula-tive Survival (%)
0–1	125	20	1	25	112	0.179	0.821	0.821
1–2	79	12	2	20	68	0.176	0.824	0.676
2–3	45	8	2	20	34	0.235	0.764	0.516
3–4	15	—	—	8	11	0.000	1.00	0.516
4–5	7	—	—	7	3.5	—	1.00	0.516†
5–6	7	—	—	—	—	—	—	—

*Those who did not have enough time at risk in the study to advance to the next interval.

†Actuarial 5-year survival is 51.6 per cent. There will be easily calculable standard errors and variances available on these data. This study took less than 6 years to complete.

Number at beginning of interval = number at beginning of previous interval minus those dying in previous interval, those lost to follow-up, and those withdrawn alive: e.g., $79 = 125 - (20 + 1 + 25)$.

Effective number exposed to death = number at beginning of interval minus one half of those lost to follow-up and those withdrawn alive: e.g., $112 = 125 - 1/2 (1 + 25)$.

Proportion dying = the number of deaths in the interval divided by those exposed to death: e.g., $0.178 = 20/112$.

Proportion surviving = $1 -$ proportion dying: e.g., $1 - 0.178 = 0.821$.

Cumulative survival = probability of surviving to point t (time), given survival to point $t - 1$: e.g., probability of 2-year survival is $(0.821) \times (0.824) = 0.676$. Multiply 0.676 by 100 to get 67.6 per cent survival at 2 years.

for computational purposes during the first time period each person is assumed to average one half year of risk, or 0.5 person lost to follow-up in this period. Again, in period two, two patients were lost to follow-up and the average for the 12 month period was one patient.

Column 5 indicates the patients withdrawn from the study during the respective time period. In the first time period, 25 patients were withdrawn alive, meaning that they were removed from consideration because they did not have enough time in the study to be at risk for death in the next time category. These patients would not have over 12 months of risk since treatment. Included at the beginning of the second interval would be the original 125, minus those who died (20), those lost to follow-up (1), and those withdrawn alive (25), or $125 - 20 - 1 - 25 = 79$.

To compute the effective number exposed to the risk of death, we take the total in column 2, minus half the total in those lost to follow-up and half the total of those withdrawn alive. In the first time period, it would be $125 - \frac{1}{2}(1 + 25) = 112$. This figure in column 6 indicates those at risk of death and is admittedly an average figure, but when all time periods are considered, it should be close to the true mean.

The proportion dying will be equal to those dying in the time period divided by those at risk for death. In row 1, the 20/112 equals 0.179, or a 17.9 per cent chance of death in the first year. Conversely, the survival rate is $1 - 0.179 = 0.821$, or a probability of 1-year survival of 82.1 per cent. This is seen in column 9.

Statistically, the probability of surviving the second time period is dependent on surviving the first time period. We first identify those eligible for the group, and again find the risk of dying and the survival rate. Now, survival in period two depends on survival in period one and is given by the product of p^* (survival 2 given survival 1) = p (survival 1) × p (survival 2). In this example, the probability of surviving the second year is (0.821) times (0.824), or 0.676, or 67.6 per cent. As you see, there is another drop in the survival rate at 3 years, but no drop after that period.

---

*Reads as the probability of surviving period two, given survival of period one.

One last word about the example actuarial problem. These data were analyzed in 5 years and gave good information concerning survival. The cost of this study had to be less than the determinate survival study, and the data were available much sooner because censored data were utilized. Often, this type of actuarial survival curve will be presented. This curve starts at 100 per cent of a population and graphs survival data. In the example, the following data array could be graphed as in Figure 74–4. To compare our cancer group survival record with that of the general population, the mean age of our larynx cancer group at year 0 would be used; and by using standard life tables, we would project a curve of a normal population of the same mean age. Let's assume that the 125 patients at 0 years have a mean age of 60 years. With a standard table, 0.01761 of 125 patients (2.21 patients) would die in the next 12 months. This would be graphed as 0.9824 $(1 - 0.1761)$ on the y-axis. A life-table or actuarial curve would thus be established for the control group. Then, graphically, the benefit or lack thereof of a particular treatment could be visualized.

Actuarial survival curves are the complement of the proportion of patients dying. Another important statistic in life tables is the average remaining lifetime, or *life expectancy*. These statistics are shown in Table 74–12 for every year of age. These life tables should sometimes be consulted when we are determining treatment regi-

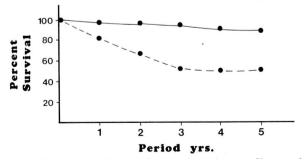

Figure 74–4. Actuarial curves for hypothetical cases of laryngeal cancer.

TABLE 74–12. Abbreviated Life Table for the Total Population of the United States, 1959–1961

Age Interval (Years)	Proportion Dying	Average Life Expectancy	Age Interval (Years)	Proportion Dying	Average Life Expectancy	Age Interval (Years)	Proportion Dying	Average Life Expectancy
0–1	0.02593	69.89	36–37	0.00209	37.58	72–73	0.04530	10.27
1–2	0.00170	70.75	37–38	0.00228	36.66	73–74	0.04915	9.74
2–3	0.00104	69.87	38–39	0.00249	35.74	74–75	0.05342	9.21
3–4	0.00080	68.94	39–40	0.00273	34.83	75–76	0.05799	8.71
4–5	0.00067	67.99	40–41	0.00300	33.92	76–77	0.06296	8.21
5–6	0.00059	67.04	41–42	0.00330	33.02	77–78	0.06867	7.73
6–7	0.00052	66.08	42–43	0.00362	32.13	78–79	0.07535	7.26
7–8	0.00047	65.11	43–44	0.00397	31.25	79–80	0.08302	6.81
8–9	0.00043	64.14	44–45	0.00435	30.37	80–81	0.09208	6.39
9–10	0.00039	63.17	45–46	0.00476	29.50	81–82	0.10219	5.98
10–11	0.00037	62.19	46–47	0.00521	28.64	82–83	0.11244	5.61
11–12	0.00037	61.22	47–48	0.00573	27.79	83–84	0.12195	5.25
12–13	0.00040	60.24	48–49	0.00633	26.94	84–85	0.13067	4.91
13–14	0.00048	59.26	49–50	0.00700	26.11	85–86	0.14380	4.58
14–15	0.00059	58.29	50–51	0.00774	25.29	86–87	0.15816	4.26
15–16	0.00071	57.33	51–52	0.00852	24.49	87–88	0.17355	3.97
16–17	0.00082	56.37	52–53	0.00929	23.69	88–89	0.19032	3.70
17–18	0.00093	55.41	53–54	0.01005	22.91	89–90	0.20835	3.45
18–19	0.00102	54.46	54–55	0.01082	22.14	90–91	0.22709	3.22
19–20	0.00108	53.52	55–56	0.01161	21.37	91–92	0.24598	3.02
20–21	0.00115	52.58	56–57	0.01249	20.62	92–93	0.26477	2.85
21–22	0.00122	51.64	57–58	0.01352	19.87	93–94	0.28284	2.69
22–23	0.00127	50.70	58–59	0.01473	19.14	94–95	0.29952	2.55
23–24	0.00128	49.76	59–60	0.01611	18.42	95–96	0.31416	2.43
24–25	0.00127	48.83	60–61	0.01761	17.71	96–97	0.32915	2.32
25–26	0.00126	47.89	61–62	0.01917	17.02	97–98	0.34450	2.21
26–27	0.00125	46.95	62–63	0.02082	16.34	98–99	0.36018	2.10
27–28	0.00126	46.00	63–64	0.02252	15.68	99–100	0.37616	2.01
28–29	0.00130	45.06	64–65	0.02431	15.03	100–101	0.39242	1.91
29–30	0.00136	44.12	65–66	0.02622	14.39	101–102	0.40891	1.83
30–31	0.00143	43.18	66–67	0.02828	13.76	102–103	0.42562	1.75
31–32	0.00151	42.24	67–68	0.03053	13.15	103–104	0.44250	1.67
32–33	0.00160	41.30	68–69	0.03301	12.55	104–105	0.45951	1.60
33–34	0.00170	40.37	69–70	0.03573	11.96	105–106	0.47662	1.53
34–35	0.00181	39.44	70–71	0.03866	11.38	106–107	0.49378	1.46
35–36	0.00194	38.51	71–72	0.04182	10.82	107–108	0.51095	1.40
						108–109	0.52810	1.35
						109–110	0.54519	1.29

Source: Abstracted from U.S. National Center for Health Statistics, Life Tables, 1959–1961, No. 1, "U.S. Life Tables 1959–1961," Dec. 1964, pp 8–9).

TABLE 74–13. Calculation of Survival Curve from Censored Data on Mucous Membrane Melanoma (Fictitious Data)

Patients at Risk	Survival (Months)	Probability of Failure at Time t	Estimated Probability of No Relapse
12	3	1/12	$p(3) = 0.916$*
11	4	1/11	$p(4) = 0.833$
10	6	1/10	$p(6) = 0.750$
10	6+		
8	8	1/8	$p(8) = 0.656$
7	9	1/7	$p(9) = 0.562$
6	10	1/6	$p(10) = 0.468$
6	10+		
4	12	1/4	$p(12) = 0.351$
4	12+		
2	15+	0/2	$p(15) = 0.351$
1	15+		

*$p(3) = \dfrac{(12-1)}{12} = 0.916 = $ probability of survival at 3 months

$$p(4) = \frac{(12-1)}{12} \times \frac{(11-1)}{11} = 0.833$$

$$p(6) = \frac{(12-1)}{12} \times \frac{(11-1)}{11} \times \frac{(10-1)}{10} = 0.750$$

$$p(8) = \frac{(12-1)}{12} \times \frac{(11-1)}{11} \times \frac{(10-1)}{10} \times \frac{(8-1)}{8} = 0.656$$

$$\dots \dots \text{ to } p(15)$$

$$p(t) = \prod_{j=1}^{i} \frac{(n_j - 1)}{n_j}$$

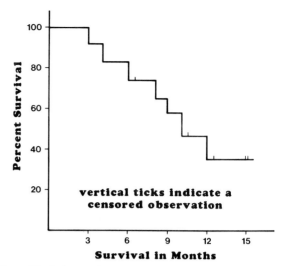

Figure 74–5. A typical Kaplan-Meier actuarial curve for mucous membrane melanoma.

The Gehan extension of the Wilcoxson nonparametric test for the difference of two sample means is often used in small sample cancer studies. A discussion of this test is beyond the scope of this chapter. For those interested, a basic survival textbook is recommended.[3] Other more advanced distributions will be found there also.

GENERAL COMMENTS

This chapter has presented areas the physician or care provider must at least partially understand. Although head and neck cancer may be treated without this knowledge, good decisions sometimes require this knowledge. Just as one cannot judge a book by its cover, one cannot read and accept conclusions from the literature at face value. A critical eye on the data, a question concerning the statistics, a look at the methodology, and finally an analysis of the survival data will perhaps lead the reader to a conclusion different from the author's or will strengthen the credibility.

Deficiency in scientific methodology will eventually lead to inappropriate conclusions, and this can direct patients to unfounded treatments. As a result, useless suffering and loss of time and money might result. Table 74–14 offers a starting point in how to review data.

TABLE 74–14. Areas of Concern in Clinical Studies

What is the goal of this study?
What is the view of the literature?
Is the study goal significant (biologically)?
What is the plan (design)?
Is there a control?
Is there randomness in cases and control subjects?
What is the sample size, and is it adequate?
Is blinding involved?
What about observer bias?
How good is the follow-up?
Is the statistical test appropriate?
Was statistical significance reached?

mens. For example, in prescribing radical surgery for adenoid cystic carcinoma or thyroid carcinoma in an 85-year-old patient, we should take the patient's life expectancy into consideration in relation to treatment methods and circumstances.

Kaplan-Meier Statistic. Other methods of survival analysis need to be mentioned. The Kaplan-Meier Statistic (1958) measures the probability a patient survives beyond point t (time). This method is similar to the actuarial method we have discussed. Data are ordered so that those who survive shorter periods are placed first on the list and those who survive the longest are last on a list. A survival distribution can be found for these ordered data and compared with a group treated by another method. The analogy to the actuarial method is that a survival curve is generated but the control group and treatment groups are not normally distributed, or, rather, the assumption of normality cannot be made. It is a nonparametric test. In addition, the Kaplan-Meier Statistic is one that is valid for small samples, and the time intervals are not fixed at a certain length (such as yearly). In both methods, censored data are observed.

Suppose 12 cases of head and neck mucous membrane melanoma are reviewed and the following survival pattern (in months) is observed: 3, 4, 6, 6+, 8, 9, 10, 10+, 12, 12+, 15+, 15+. Note that the series has been ordered from smallest to largest and that 6+ indicates the patient is a survivor at 6 months, whereas 6 is a fatality or failure at 6 months. If a death and a loss occur at the same time, the death is assumed to have occurred prior to the time period and the loss (censored value) slightly after the time period. Table 74–13 shows the way these data are calculated, and Figure 74–5 is the typical Kaplan-Meier actuarial curve for the data.

REFERENCES

1. Berkson J, Gage RP: Calculation of survival rates for cancer. Proc Staff Meetings Mayo Clin 25:270, 1950.
2. Brown BW: Statistical considerations in clinical trials. *In* Carter SK, Goldstein E, Livingston RB (eds): Principles of Cancer Treatment. New York, McGraw-Hill Book Co, 1982.
3. Brown WB, Hollander M: Statistics, A Biomedical Introduction. New York, John Wiley, 1977.
4. Byar DP, et al: Randomized clinical trials. N Engl J Med 295:74, 1976.
5. Chalmers TC, Block JB, Lee S: Controlled studies in clinical cancer research. N Engl J Med 287:75, 1972.
6. Chalmers TC, et al: A method for assessing the quality of a randomized control trial. Controlled Clin Trials 2:31, 1981.
7. Conover WJ: Practical Nonparametric Statistics. 2nd ed. New York, John Wiley, 1980.
8. Cutler SJ, et al: Maximum utilization of the life table method in analyzing survival. J Chron Dis 8:699, 1958.
9. Dawber TR, et al: An approach to longitudinal studies in a community: The Framingham study. Ann NY Acad Sci, 107:539, 1963.
10. Freiman JA, Chalmers TC, Smith H, Ruebler RR: The importance of Beta, the Type II error and sample size in the design and interpretation of the randomized control plan. N Engl J Med 299:690, 1978.
11. Friedman GD: Primer of Epidemiology. New York, McGraw-Hill Book Co., 1980.
12. Gehan EA: Statistical methods for survival time studies. *In* Staquet MJ (ed): Cancer Therapy: Prognostic Factors and Criteria of Response. New York, Raven Press, 1975.
13. Gehan EA, Freireich EJ: Non-randomized controls in cancer clinical trials. N Engl J Med 290:198, 1974.
14. George SL, Desu MM: Planning the size and duration of a clinical trial studying the time to some critical event. J Chron Dis 27:15, 1974.
15. Glantz SA: Biostatistics: How to detect, correct and prevent errors in the medical literature. Circulation 61:1, 1980.
16. Gross AJ, Clark VA: Survival Distributions: Reliability Applications in the Biomedical Sciences. New York, John Wiley, 1975.
17. Haines SJ: Six statistical suggestions for surgeons. Neurosurgery 9:414, 1981.
18. Haynes SJ: Randomized clinical trials in the evaluation of surgical innovation. J Neurosurg 51:5, 1979.
19. Karnofsky DA, Burchenal JH: Symposium of Microbiology. New York Academy of Medicine, Columbia University Press, 1949.
20. Lachin JM: Introduction to sample size determination and power analysis for clinical trials. Controlled Clin Trials 2:93, 1981.
21. Lillienfeld AM, Lillienfeld DE: Foundations of Epidemiology. New York, Oxford University Press, 1980.
22. Morganstern H: Uses of ecologic analysis in epidemiologic research. Am J Public Health 72:1336, 1982.
23. Murphy JR: The relationship of relative risk and positive predictive value in 2 × 2 tables. Am J Epidemiol 117:86, 1983.
24. Neter J, Wasserman W: Applied Linear Statistical Models. Homewood, Ill. Richard Irwin Publisher, 1974.
25. Silverberg E, Lubera JA: A review of American Cancer Society estimates of cancer cases and deaths. CA, 33:2, 1983.
26. Taylor WF, Irins JC, et al: Trends and variability in survival from osteosarcoma. Mayo Clin Proc 53:695, 1978.
27. Walpole RE: Introduction to Statistics. New York, Macmillan Publishing, 1974.
28. Weinstein MC: Allocation of subjects in medical experiments. N Engl J Med 291:1278, 1974.
29. Whittemore AE: Estimating attributable risk from case control studies. Am J Epidemiol 117:76, 1983.
30. Young JL, Pollack ES: The incidence of cancer in the United States. *In* Schohenfield D, Fraumeni JF (eds): Cancer Epidemiology and Prevention. Philadelphia, W. B. Saunders Co., 1982.

Index